# PRINCIPLES OF CLINICAL PHARMACOLOGY

## Third Edition

# PRINCIPLES OF CLINICAL PHARMACOLOGY

## Third Edition

**Arthur J. Atkinson Jr, MD**
Department of Molecular Pharmacology & Biochemistry,
Feinberg School of Medicine,
Northwestern University,
Chicago, IL 60611

**Shiew-Mei Huang, PhD**
Office of Clinical Pharmacology,
Office of Translational Sciences,
Center for Drug Evaluation and Research,
US Food and Drug Administration,
Silver Spring, MD 20993

**Juan J. L. Lertora, MD, PhD**
Clinical Pharmacology Program,
Clinical Center,
National Institutes of Health,
Bethesda, MD 20892

**Sanford P. Markey, PhD**
Laboratory of Neurotoxicology,
National Institute of Mental Health,
National Institutes of Health,
Bethesda, MD 20892

San Diego • San Francisco • New York
Boston • London • Sydney • Tokyo

Academic Press is an Imprint of Elsevier

Academic Press is an imprint of Elsevier
32 Jamestown Road, London NW1 7BY, UK
225 Wyman Street, Waltham, MA 02451, USA
525 B Street, Suite 1800, San Diego, CA 92101-4495, USA

First edition 2002
Second edition 2007
Third edition 2012

**Notice**
No responsibility is assumed by the publisher for any injury and/or damage to persons or
property as a matter of products liability, negligence or otherwise, or from any use or operation
of any methods, products, instructions or ideas contained in the material herein. Because of
rapid advances in the medical sciences, in particular, independent verification of diagnoses
and drug dosages should be made

**British Library Cataloguing-in-Publication Data**
A catalogue record for this book is available from the British Library

**Library of Congress Cataloging-in-Publication Data**
A catalog record for this book is available from the Library of Congress

ISBN: 978-0-12-385471-1

For information on all Academic Press publications
visit our website at elsevierdirect.com

Typeset by TNQ Books and Journals Pvt Ltd.
www.tnq.co.in

Printed and bound in United States of America
12 13 14 15 16   10 9 8 7 6 5 4 3 2 1

Working together to grow
libraries in developing countries

www.elsevier.com | www.bookaid.org | www.sabre.org

ELSEVIER   BOOK AID International   Sabre Foundation

# Contents

CHAPTER

## 1

## Introduction to Clinical Pharmacology

ARTHUR J. ATKINSON, JR

PART

## I

# PHARMACOKINETICS

CHAPTER

## 2

## Clinical Pharmacokinetics

ARTHUR J. ATKINSON, JR

CHAPTER

## 3

## Compartmental Analysis of Drug Distribution

ARTHUR J. ATKINSON, JR

CHAPTER

8

## Non-Compartmental and Compartmental Approaches to Pharmacokinetic Data Analysis

DAVID M. FOSTER AND PAOLO VICINI

CHAPTER

9

## Distributed Models of Drug Kinetics

PAUL F. MORRISON

CHAPTER

10

## Population Pharmacokinetics

RAYMOND MILLER

PART

# II
# DRUG METABOLISM AND TRANSPORT

CHAPTER

11

## Pathways of Drug Metabolism

SANFORD P. MARKEY

CHAPTER

# 12

## Methods of Analysis of Drugs and Drug Metabolites

SANFORD P. MARKEY

CHAPTER

# 13

## Clinical Pharmacogenetics

DAVID A. FLOCKHART AND SHIEW-MEI HUANG

CHAPTER

# 14

## Mechanisms and Genetics of Drug Transport

JOSEPH A. WARE, LEI ZHANG AND SHIEW-MEI HUANG

CHAPTER

# 15

## Drug Interactions

SARAH ROBERTSON, SCOTT R. PENZAK AND SHIEW-MEI HUANG

CHAPTER

# 16

## Biochemical Mechanisms
## of Drug Toxicity

ARTHUR J. ATKINSON, JR AND SANFORD P. MARKEY

CHAPTER

# 17

## Pharmacogenomic Mechanisms of Drug
## Toxicity

SHIEW-MEI HUANG, LIGONG CHEN, AND
KATHLEEN M. GIACOMINI

PART

# III
# ASSESSMENT OF DRUG
# EFFECTS

CHAPTER

# 18

## Physiological and Laboratory Markers
## of Drug Effect

JANET WOODCOCK, ARTHUR J. ATKINSON, JR
AND PAUL ROLAN

CHAPTER

# 19

## Imaging in Drug Development

RICHARD J. HARGREAVES AND MICHAEL KLIMAS

CHAPTER

# 20

## Dose–Effect and Concentration–Effect Analysis

ELIZABETH S. LOWE AND JUAN J.L. LERTORA

CHAPTER

# 21

## Time Course of Drug Response

NICHOLAS H.G. HOLFORD AND
ARTHUR J. ATKINSON, JR

CHAPTER

# 22

## Disease Progress Models

NICHOLAS H.G. HOLFORD, DIANE R. MOULD AND
CARL C. PECK

PART

# IV
# OPTIMIZING AND EVALUATING PATIENT THERAPY

CHAPTER

## 23

### Pharmacological Differences between Men and Women
AMEETA PAREKH

CHAPTER

## 24

### Drug Therapy in Pregnant and Nursing Women
CATHERINE S. STIKA AND MARILYNN
C. FREDERIKSEN

CHAPTER

## 25

### Pediatric Clinical Pharmacology and Therapeutics
BRIDGETTE L. JONES, JOHN N. VAN DEN
ANKER AND GREGORY L. KEARNS

CHAPTER

# 30

## Drug Discovery

EDWARD A. SAUSVILLE

CHAPTER

# 31

## Non-Clinical Drug Development

CHRIS H. TAKIMOTO AND MICHAEL J. WICK

CHAPTER

# 32

## Preclinical Prediction of Human
## Pharmacokinetics

MALCOLM ROWLAND AND ROBERT L. DEDRICK

CHAPTER

# 33

## Phase I Clinical Studies

JERRY M. COLLINS

# Preface to the First Edition

The rate of introduction of new pharmaceutical products has increased rapidly over the past decade, and details learned about a particular drug become obsolete as it is replaced by newer agents. For this reason, we have chosen to focus this book on the principles that underlie the clinical use and contemporary development of pharmaceuticals. It is assumed that the reader will have had an introductory course in pharmacology and also some understanding of calculus, physiology and clinical medicine.

This book is the outgrowth of an evening course that has been taught for the past three years at the NIH Clinical Center. Wherever possible, individuals who have lectured in the course have contributed chapters corresponding to their lectures. The organizers of this course are the editors of this book and we also have recruited additional experts to assist in the review of specific chapters. We also acknowledge the help of William A. Mapes in preparing much of the artwork. Special thanks are due to Donna Shields, Coordinator for the ClinPRAT training program at NIH, whose attention to myriad details has made possible both the successful conduct of our evening course and the production of this book. Finally, we were encouraged and patiently aided in this undertaking by Robert M. Harington and Aaron Johnson at Academic Press.

# Preface to the Third Edition

In the decade since the first edition of *Principles of Clinical Pharmacology* was published, the discipline of clinical pharmacology has come to play an increasingly important role in drug development and regulatory science, as well as in its continued application to clinical medicine. The third edition remains focused on the principles underlying the development, evaluation, and clinical use of pharmaceuticals. However, recent advances have warranted the inclusion of new chapters on imaging and on the pharmacogenetic basis of adverse drug reactions, as well as a substantial expansion of the scope of the chapters on transporters, pharmacogenetics, and biomarkers.

Since the first edition, the center of gravity of clinical pharmacology as a discipline also has shifted from a primarily academic orientation towards its more practical application by the US Food and Drug Administration (FDA) and the pharmaceutical industry. This is best evidenced by the evolution of the FDA's Division of Biopharmaceutics into the current FDA Office of Clinical Pharmacology, with the concomitant proliferation of Clinical Pharmacology Guidance documents that are now cited in many chapters of this text.

We are indebted to the authors from previous editions who have worked to update their chapters and are delighted to welcome the new authors, several of whom are from the FDA's Office of Clinical Pharmacology, who have stepped in to contribute both new chapters and new versions of other existing chapters. As in previous editions, the authors in many cases continue to be lecturers in the evening course that has been taught for the past 15 years at the National Institutes of Health (NIH) Clinical Center[1]. Many of the illustrations in the text appeared originally in *Clinical Pharmacology and Therapeutics*, and we thank the American Society for Clinical Pharmacology and Therapeutics for allowing us to reproduce these free of charge. Finally, special thanks are due the Elsevier Production Staff who together have provided ongoing support that has been invaluable for the successful production of this book.

[1] Videotapes and slide handouts for the NIH course are available on the Internet at: www.cc.nih.gov/training/training/principles.html.

# Contributors

**Darrell R. Abernethy**
Office of Clinical Pharmacology, Center for Drug Evaluation and Research, US Food and Drug Administration, Silver Spring, MD 20993

**Arthur J. Atkinson, Jr**
Department of Molecular Pharmacology & Biochemistry, Feinberg School of Medicine, Northwestern University, Chicago, IL 60611

**William Budris**
Drug Information Center, Department of Pharmacy, Northwestern Memorial Hospital, Chicago, IL 60611

**Ligong Chen**
Department of Bioengineering and Therapeutic Sciences, University of California, San Francisco, CA 94143

**Jerry M. Collins**
Developmental Therapeutics Program, Division of Cancer Treatment and Diagnosis, National Cancer Institute, National Institutes of Health, Rockville, MD 20852

**Charles E. Daniels**
Skaggs School of Pharmacy and Pharmaceutical Sciences, University of California–San Diego, La Jolla, CA 92093

**Robert L. Dedrick**
National Institute of Biomedical Imaging and Bioengineering, National Institutes of Health, Bethesda, MD 20892

**David A. Flockhart**
Division of Clinical Pharmacology, Indiana University School of Medicine, Indianapolis, IN 46250

**David M. Foster**
Department of Bioengineering, University of Washington, Seattle, WA 98195

**Michael Fotis**
Drug Information Center, Department of Pharmacy, Northwestern Memorial Hospital, Chicago, IL 60611

**Marilynn C. Frederiksen**
Department of Obstetrics and Gynecology, Feinberg School of Medicine, Northwestern University, Chicago, IL 60611

**Pamela D. Garzone**
Clinical Research, Pfizer Inc., South San Francisco, CA 94080

**Kathleen M. Giacomini**
Department of Bioengineering and Therapeutic Sciences, University of California, San Francisco, CA 94143

**Charles T. Gombar**
Project Management, Development & Delivery, Endo Pharmaceuticals, Chadds Ford, PA 19317

**Charles Grudzinskas**
NDA Partners LLC, Annapolis, MD 21401

**Richard J. Hargreaves**
Discovery Neuroscience, Merck Research
Laboratories, West Point, PA 19486

**Nicholas H.G. Holford**
Department of Pharmacology and Clinical
Pharmacology, University of Auckland, Auckland,
New Zealand 1142

**Shiew-Mei Huang**
Office of Clinical Pharmacology, Office of
Translational Sciences, Center for Drug Evaluation
and Research, US Food and Drug Administration,
Silver Spring, MD 20993

**Bridgette L. Jones**
Department of Pediatrics, and Divisions of
Pediatric Clinical Pharmacology and Medical
Toxicology, University of Missouri–Kansas City
School of Medicine, Kansas City, MO 64109;
Department of Medical Research, The Children's
Mercy Hospital, Kansas City, MO 64108

**Gregory L. Kearns**
Department of Pediatrics, and Divisions of
Pediatric Clinical Pharmacology and Medical
Toxicology, University of Missouri–Kansas City
School of Medicine, Kansas City, MO 64109;
Department of Pediatrics, University of Kansas
School of Medicine, Kansas City, KS 66160

**Michael Klimas**
Imaging, Merck Research Laboratories, West Point,
PA 19486

**S.W. Johnny Lau**
Office of Clinical Pharmacology, Center for Drug
Evaluation and Research, US Food and Drug
Administration, Silver Spring, MD 20993

**Juan J.L. Lertora**
Clinical Pharmacology Program, Clinical Center,
National Institutes of Health, Bethesda,
MD 20892

**Lawrence J. Lesko**
Center for Pharmacometrics and Systems
Pharmacology, College of Pharmacy, University of
Florida, Lake Nona in Orlando, Florida 32832

**Elizabeth S. Lowe**
Clinical Development, AstraZeneca
Pharmaceuticals, Wilmington, DE 19803

**Sanford P. Markey**
Laboratory of Neurotoxicology, National Institute
of Mental Health, National Institutes of Health,
Bethesda, MD 20892

**Raymond Miller**
Modeling and Simulation, Daiichi Sankyo Pharma
Development, Edison, NJ 08837

**Paul F. Morrison**
National Institute of Biomedical Imaging and
Bioengineering Intramural Research Program,
National Institute of Biomedical Imaging and
Bioengineering, National Institutes of Health,
Bethesda, MD 20892

**Diane R. Mould**
Projections Research Inc, Phoenixville, PA 19460

**Ameeta Parekh**
Office of Translational Sciences, Center for Drug
Evaluation and Research, US Food and Drug
Administration, Silver Spring, MD 20993

**Carl C. Peck**
Center for Drug Development Science, University
of California at San Francisco, University of
California Washington Center, Washington, DC
20036

**Scott R. Penzak**
Clinical Research Center, Department of Pharmacy,
National Institutes of Health, Bethesda, MD 20892

**Sarah Robertson**
Office of Clinical Pharmacology, Office of
Translational Sciences, Center for Drug Evaluation
and Research, US Food and Drug Administration,
Silver Spring, MD 20993

**Paul Rolan**
Discipline of Pharmacology, School of Medical
Sciences, University of Adelaide, Adelaide,
Australia 5005

**Malcolm Rowland**
Centre for Applied Pharmacokinetic Research,
School of Pharmacy and Pharmaceutical Sciences,
University of Manchester, Manchester M13 9PT,
United Kingdom; Department of Bioengineering
and Therapeutic Sciences, Schools of Pharmacy and
Medicine, University of California, San Francisco,
CA 94117

**Steven W. Ryder**
Astellas Pharma Global Development, Deerfield, IL 60015

**Chandrahas G. Sahajwalla**
Office of Clinical Pharmacology, Office of Translational Sciences, Center for Drug Evaluation and Research, US Food and Drug Administration, Silver Spring, MD 20993

**Edward A. Sausville**
Greenebaum Cancer Center, University of Maryland, Baltimore, MD 21201

**Catherine S. Stika**
Department of Obstetrics and Gynecology, Feinberg School of Medicine, Northwestern University, Chicago, IL 60611

**Gregory M. Susla**
Medical Information, MedImmune, LLC, Gaithersburg, MD 20878

**Chris H. Takimoto**
Translational Medicine Early Development, Janssen Pharmaceutical Companies of Johnson & Johnson, Radnor, PA 19087

**John N. Van Den Anker**
Departments of Pediatrics, Integrative Systems Biology, Pharmacology & Physiology, and Division of Pediatric Clinical Pharmacology, The George Washington University School of Medicine and Health Sciences/Children's National Medical Center, Washington, DC 20010

**Paolo Vicini**
Department of Pharmacokinetics, Dynamics and Metabolism, Pfizer Worldwide Research and Development, San Diego, CA 92121

**Joseph A. Ware**
Clinical Pharmacology, Genentech Research and Early Development, South San Francisco, CA 94080

**Ethan S. Weiner**
Latimer Brook Pharmaceutical Consultants, LLC, East Lyme, CT 06333

**Michael J. Wick**
Preclinical Research, South Texas Accelerated Research Therapeutics, San Antonio, TX 78229

**Janet Woodcock**
Center for Drug Evaluation and Research, US Food and Drug Administration, Silver Spring, MD 20903

**Lei Zhang**
Office of Clinical Pharmacology, Office of Translational Sciences, Center for Drug Evaluation and Research, US Food and Drug Administration, Silver Spring, MD 20993

# Introduction to Clinical Pharmacology

Arthur J. Atkinson, Jr.

*Department of Molecular Pharmacology & Biochemistry, Feinberg School of Medicine, Northwestern University, Chicago, IL 60611*

*Fortunately a surgeon who uses the wrong side of the scalpel cuts his own fingers and not the patient; if the same applied to drugs they would have been investigated very carefully a long time ago.*

Rudolph Bucheim
Beitrage zur Arzneimittellehre, 1849 [1]

## BACKGROUND

*Clinical pharmacology* can be defined as the study of drugs in humans. Clinical pharmacology often is contrasted with basic pharmacology, yet *applied* is a more appropriate antonym for *basic* [2]. In fact, many basic problems in pharmacology can only be studied in humans. This text will focus on the basic principles of clinical pharmacology. Selected applications will be used to illustrate these principles, but no attempt will be made to provide an exhaustive coverage of applied therapeutics. Other useful supplementary sources of information are listed at the end of this chapter.

Leake [3] has pointed out that pharmacology is a subject of ancient interest but is a relatively new science. Reidenberg [4] subsequently restated Leake's listing of the fundamental problems with which the science of pharmacology is concerned:

1. The relationship between dose and biological effect
2. The localization of the site of action of a drug
3. The mechanism(s) of action of a drug
4. The absorption, distribution, metabolism and excretion of a drug
5. The relationship between chemical structure and biological activity.

These authors agree that pharmacology could not evolve as a scientific discipline until modern chemistry provided the chemically pure pharmaceutical products that are needed to establish a quantitative relationship between drug dosage and biological effect.

Clinical pharmacology has been termed a bridging discipline because it combines elements of classical pharmacology with clinical medicine. The special competencies of individuals trained in clinical pharmacology have equipped them for productive careers in academia, the pharmaceutical industry, and governmental agencies, such as the National Institutes of Health (NIH) and the Food and Drug Administration (FDA). Reidenberg [4] has pointed out that clinical pharmacologists are concerned both with the optimal use of existing medications and with the scientific study of drugs in humans. The latter area includes both evaluation of the safety and efficacy of currently available drugs and development of new and improved pharmacotherapy.

### Optimizing Use of Existing Medicines

As the opening quotation indicates, the concern of pharmacologists for the safe and effective use of medicine can be traced back at least to Rudolph Bucheim (1820–1879), who has been credited with establishing pharmacology as a laboratory based

*PRINCIPLES OF CLINICAL PHARMACOLOGY, THIRD EDITION*
DOI: http://dx.doi.org/10.1016/B978-0-12-385471-1.00001-5

discipline [1]. In the United States, Harry Gold and Walter Modell began, in the 1930s, to provide the foundation for the modern discipline of clinical pharmacology [5]. Their accomplishments include the invention of the double-blind design for clinical trials [6], the use of effect kinetics to measure the absolute bioavailability of digoxin and characterize the time course of its chronotropic effects [7], and the founding of *Clinical Pharmacology and Therapeutics*.

Few drugs have focused as much public attention on the problem of adverse drug reactions as thalidomide, which was first linked in 1961 to catastrophic outbreaks of phocomelia by Lenz in Germany and McBride in Australia [8]. Although thalidomide had not been approved at that time for use in the United States, this tragedy prompted passage in 1962 of the Harris-Kefauver Amendments to the Food, Drug, and Cosmetic Act. This act greatly expanded the scope of the FDA's mandate to protect the public health. The thalidomide tragedy also provided the major impetus for developing a number of NIH-funded academic centers of excellence that have shaped contemporary clinical pharmacology in this country. These US centers were founded by a generation of vigorous leaders, including Ken Melmon, Jan Koch-Weser, Lou Lasagna, John Oates, Leon Goldberg, Dan Azarnoff, Tom Gaffney, and Leigh Thompson. Collin Dollery and Folke Sjöqvist established similar programs in Europe. In response to the public mandate generated by the thalidomide catastrophe, these leaders quickly reached consensus on a number of theoretically preventable causes that contribute to the high incidence of adverse drug reactions [5]. These include:

1. Inappropriate polypharmacy
2. Failure of prescribing physicians to establish and adhere to clear therapeutic goals
3. Failure of medical personnel to attribute new symptoms or changes in laboratory test results to drug therapy
4. Lack of priority given to the scientific study of adverse drug reaction mechanisms
5. General ignorance of basic and applied pharmacology and therapeutic principles.

The important observations also were made that, unlike the teratogenic reactions caused by thalidomide, most adverse reactions encountered in clinical practice occurred with drugs that have been in clinical use for a substantial period of time rather than newly introduced drugs, and were dose related rather than idiosyncratic [5, 9, 10].

Recognition of the considerable variation in response of different patients treated with standard drug doses has provided the impetus for the development of what is currently called "personalized medicine" [11]. Despite the recent introduction of this term, it actually describes a continuing story that can be divided into three chapters in which different complementary technologies were developed and are being applied to cope with this variability. In the earliest chapter, laboratory methods were developed to measure drug concentrations in patient blood samples and to guide therapy – an approach now termed "therapeutic drug monitoring" [10]. The routine availability of these measurements then made it possible to apply pharmacokinetic principles in routine patient care to achieve and maintain these drug concentrations within a prespecified therapeutic range. Despite these advances, *serious adverse drug reactions* (defined as those adverse drug reactions that require or prolong hospitalization, are permanently disabling, or result in death) continue to pose a severe problem and recently have been estimated to occur in 6.7% of hospitalized patients [12]. Although this figure has been disputed, the incidence of adverse drug reactions probably is still higher than is generally recognized [13]. In the third chapter, which is still being written, genetic approaches are being developed and applied both to meet this challenge and to improve the efficacy and safety of drug therapy [11]. Thus, pharmacogenetics is being used to identify slow drug-metabolizing patients who might be at increased risk for drug toxicity and rapid metabolizers who might not respond when standard drug doses are prescribed. In a parallel development, pharmacogenomic methods are increasingly used to identify subsets of patients who will either respond satisfactorily or be at increased risk of an adverse reaction to a particular drug.

The fact that most adverse drug reactions occur with commonly used drugs focuses attention on the last of the preventable causes of these reactions: the training that prescribing physicians receive in pharmacology and therapeutics. Bucheim's comparison of surgery and medicine is particularly apt in this regard [5]. Most US medical schools provide their students with only a single course in pharmacology that traditionally is part of the second-year curriculum, when students lack the clinical background that is needed to support detailed instruction in therapeutics. In addition, Sjöqvist [14] has observed that most academic pharmacology departments have lost contact with drug development and pharmacotherapy. As a result, students and residents acquire most of their information about drug therapy in a haphazard manner from colleagues, supervisory house staff and attending physicians, pharmaceutical sales representatives, and whatever independent reading they happen to do on the subject. This unstructured process of learning pharmacotherapeutic technique stands in marked contrast to the rigorously supervised training that is an accepted part of surgical training, in which instantaneous feedback is provided whenever a retractor, let alone a scalpel, is held improperly.

## Evaluation and Development of Medicines

Clinical pharmacologists have made noteworthy contributions to the evaluation of existing medicines and development of new drugs. In 1932, Paul Martini published a monograph entitled *Methodology of Therapeutic Investigation* that summarized his experience in scientific drug evaluation and probably entitles him to be considered the "first clinical pharmacologist" [15]. Martini described the use of placebos, control groups, stratification, rating scales, and the "n of 1" trial design, and emphasized the need to estimate the adequacy of sample size and to establish baseline conditions before beginning a trial. He also introduced the term "clinical pharmacology". Gold [6] and other academic clinical pharmacologists also have made important contributions to the design of clinical trials. More recently, Sheiner [16] outlined a number of improvements that continue to be needed in the use of statistical methods for drug evaluation, and asserted

that clinicians must regain control over clinical trials in order to ensure that the important questions are being addressed.

Contemporary drug development is a complex process that is conventionally divided into preclinical research and development and a number of clinical development phases, as shown in Figure 1.1 for drugs licensed by the United States FDA [17]. After a drug candidate is identified and put through *in vitro* screens and animal testing, an Investigational New Drug application (IND) is submitted to the FDA. When the IND is approved, Phase I clinical development begins with a limited number of studies in healthy volunteers or patients. The goal of these studies is to establish a range of tolerated doses and to characterize the drug candidate's pharmacokinetic properties and initial toxicity profile. If these results warrant further development of the compound, short-term Phase II studies are conducted in a selected group of patients to obtain evidence of therapeutic efficacy and to explore patient therapeutic and toxic responses to several dose regimens. These dose–response relationships are used to design longer Phase III trials to confirm therapeutic efficacy and document safety in a larger patient population. The material obtained during preclinical and clinical development is then incorporated in a New Drug Application (NDA) that is submitted to the FDA for review. The FDA may request clarification of study

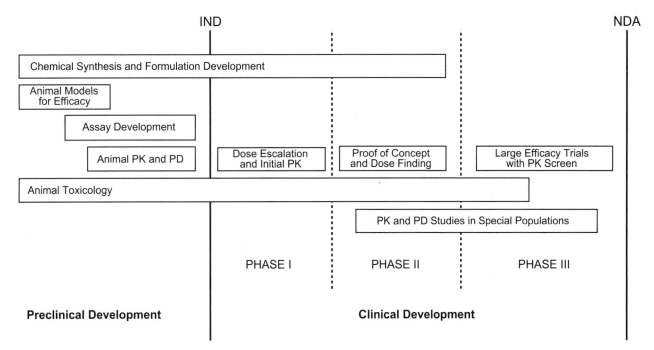

**FIGURE 1.1** The process of new drug development in the United States. PK indicates pharmacokinetic studies; PD indicates studies of drug effect or pharmacodynamics. Further explanation is provided in the text. Modified from Peck CC, Barr WH, Benet LZ *et al.* Clin Pharmacol Ther 1992;51:465–73 [17].

results or further studies before the NDA is approved and the drug can be marketed. Adverse drug reaction monitoring and reporting is mandated after NDA approval. Phase IV studies, conducted after NDA approval, may include studies to support FDA licensing for additional therapeutic indications or "over-the-counter" (OTC) sales directly to consumers.

Although the expertise and resources needed to develop new drugs are primarily concentrated in the pharmaceutical industry, clinical investigators based in academia have played an important catalytic role in championing the development of a number of drugs [18]. For example, dopamine was first synthesized in 1910 but the therapeutic potential of this compound was not recognized until 1963, when Leon Goldberg and his colleagues provided convincing evidence that dopamine mediated vasodilation by binding to a previously undescribed receptor [19]. These investigators subsequently demonstrated the clinical utility of intravenous dopamine infusions in treating patients with hypotension or shock unresponsive to plasma volume expansion. This provided the basis for a small pharmaceutical firm to bring dopamine to market in the early 1970s.

Academically based clinical pharmacologists have a long tradition of interest in drug metabolism. Drug metabolism generally constitutes an important mechanism by which drugs are converted to inactive compounds that usually are more rapidly excreted than the parent drug. However, some drug metabolites have important pharmacologic activity. This was first demonstrated in 1935, when the antibacterial activity of prontosil was found to reside solely in its metabolite, sulfanilamide [20]. Advances in analytical chemistry over the past 30 years have made it possible to measure, on a routine basis, plasma concentrations of drug metabolites as well as parent drugs. Further study of these metabolites has demonstrated that several of them have important pharmacologic activity that must be considered for proper clinical interpretation of plasma concentration measurements [21]. In some cases, clinical pharmacologists have demonstrated that drug metabolites have pharmacologic properties that make them preferable to marketed drugs.

For example, when terfenadine (Seldane™), the prototype of non-sedating antihistamine drugs, was reported to cause *torsades de pointes* and fatality in patients with no previous history of cardiac arrhythmia, Woosley and his colleagues [22] proceeded to investigate the electrophysiologic effects of both terfenadine and its carboxylate metabolite (Figure 1.2). These investigators found that terfenadine, like quinidine, an antiarrhythmic drug with

known propensity to cause *torsades de pointes* in susceptible individuals, blocked the delayed rectifier potassium current. However, terfenadine carboxylate, which actually accounts for most of the observed antihistaminic effects when patients take terfenadine, was found to be devoid of this proarrhythmic property. These findings provided the impetus for commercial development of the carboxylate metabolite as a safer alternative to terfenadine. This metabolite is now marketed as fexofenadine (Allegra™).

The potential impact of pharmacogenetics on drug prescribing and development is illustrated by the example of tamoxifen, a selective estrogen receptor modifier that has been used as therapy and for recurrence prevention in patients with breast cancer. As shown in Figure 1.3, tamoxifen is converted by cytochrome P450 (CYP) enzymes to several metabolites that have more potent anti-estrogenic activity than the parent compound. Although 4-hydroxy-tamoxifen had been thought to be the primary pharmacologically active tamoxifen metabolite, Flockhart and colleagues [23] demonstrated that endoxifen plasma concentrations averaged more than 10 times those of 4–hydroxy-tamoxifen in women treated with tamoxifen, and that both compounds had equal *in vitro* potency in suppressing breast cancer cell proliferation. These investigators subsequently confirmed the clinical relevance of these findings by demonstrating that women who were homozygous for CYP2D6*4, the most common

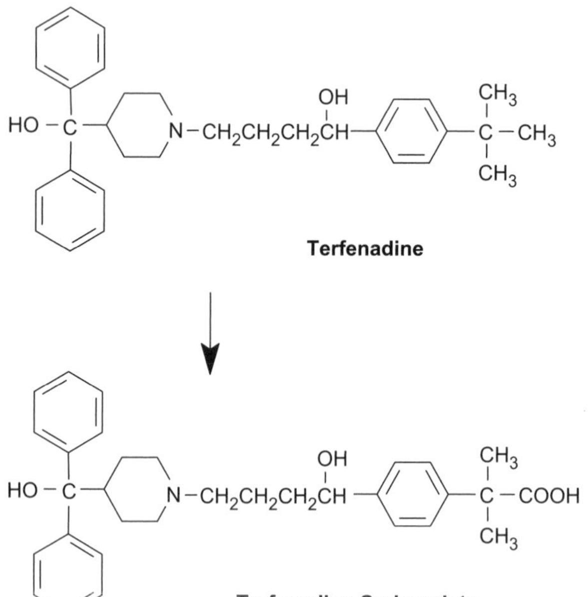

**FIGURE 1.2** Chemical structures of terfenidine and its carboxylate metabolite. The acid metabolite is formed by oxidation of the *t*-butyl side chain of the parent drug.

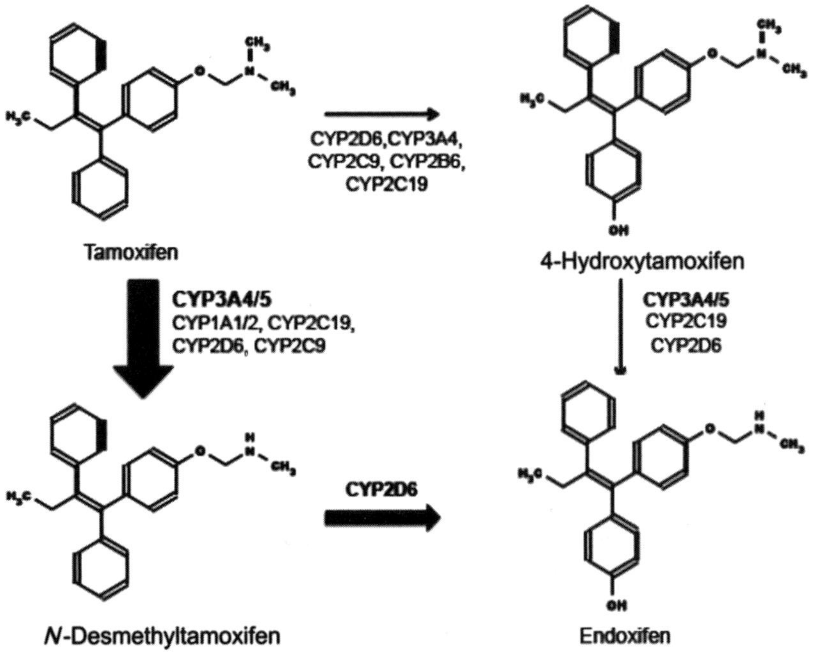

**FIGURE 1.3** Partial metabolic pathway of tamoxifen showing metabolite structures and the CYP enzymes involved. The relative contribution of each metabolic step is indicated by the thickness of the arrows.

allele present in poor CYP2D6 metabolizers, had a shortened duration of relapse-free survival and disease-free survival [24]. These findings support the recommendation for using pharmacogenetic screening to exclude poor CYP2D6 metabolizers as candidates for tamoxifen therapy, and for avoiding co-administration of CYP2D6 inhibitors to patients receiving tamoxifen. In addition, they have provided the rationale for current efforts to develop endoxifen as a replacement for tamoxifen that would not be subject to pharmacogenetic variation or drug interactions affecting CYP2D6 activity [25].

## PHARMACOKINETICS

*Pharmacokinetics* is defined as the quantitative analysis of the processes of drug absorption, distribution, and elimination that determine the time course of drug action. *Pharmacodynamics* deals with the mechanism of drug action. Hence, pharmacokinetics and pharmacodynamics constitute two major subdivisions of pharmacology.

Since as many as 70% to 80% of adverse drug reactions are dose related [9], our success in preventing these reactions is contingent on our grasp of the principles of pharmacokinetics that provide the scientific basis for dose selection. This becomes critically important when we prescribe drugs that have a narrow therapeutic index. Pharmacokinetics is inescapably mathematical. Although 95% of pharmacokinetic calculations required for clinical application are simple algebra, some understanding of calculus is required to fully grasp the principles of pharmacokinetics.

### The Concept of Clearance

Because pharmacokinetics comprises the first few chapters of this book and figures prominently in subsequent chapters, we will pause here to introduce the clinically most important concept in pharmacokinetics: the concept of *clearance*. In 1929, Möller *et al.* [26] observed that, above a urine flow rate of 2 mL/min, the rate of urea excretion by the kidneys is proportional to the amount of urea in a constant volume of blood. They introduced the term "clearance" to describe this constant and defined urea clearance as the volume of blood which 1 minute's excretion serves to clear of urea. Since then, creatinine clearance ($CL_{CR}$) has become most commonly used in clinical practice when renal functional status is directly measured, and is calculated from the following equation:

$$CL_{CR} = UV/P$$

where $U$ is the concentration of creatinine excreted over a certain period of time in a measured volume of urine ($V$) and $P$ is the serum concentration of creatinine. This is really a first-order differential equation since $UV$ is simply the rate at which creatinine is being excreted in urine ($dE/dt$). Hence,

$$dE/dt = CL_{CR} \cdot P$$

If instead of looking at the rate of creatinine excretion in urine we consider the rate of change of creatinine in the body ($dX/dt$), we can write the following equation:

$$dX/dt = I - CL_{CR} \cdot P \qquad (1.1)$$

Here, $I$ is the rate of *synthesis* of creatinine in the body and $CL_{CR} \cdot P$ is the rate of creatinine *elimination*. At steady state, these rates are equal and there is no change in the total body content of creatinine ($dX/dt = 0$), so:

$$P = I / CL_{CR} \qquad (1.2)$$

This equation explains why it is hazardous to estimate the status of renal function solely from serum creatinine results in patients who have a reduced muscle mass and a decline in creatinine synthesis rate. For example, creatinine synthesis rate may be substantially reduced in elderly patients, so it is not unusual for serum creatinine concentrations in these patients to remain within normal limits, even though renal function is markedly impaired.

## Clinical Estimation of Renal Function

In routine clinical practice, it is not practical to collect the urine samples that are needed to measure creatinine clearance directly. However, creatinine clearance in adult patients can be estimated either from a standard nomogram or from equations such as that proposed by Cockcroft and Gault [27]. For men, creatinine clearance can be estimated as follows:

$$CL_{CR} \text{ (mL/min)} = \frac{(140 - \text{age}) \text{ (weight in kg)}}{72 \text{ (serum creatinine in mg/dL)}} \qquad (1.3)$$

For women, this estimate should be reduced by 15%. By comparing Equation 1.2 with Equation 1.3, we see that the term $[(140 - \text{age})(\text{weight in kg})]/72$ simply provides an estimate of the creatinine formation rate in an individual patient.

Since the Cockcroft-Gault equation was introduced there has been substantial improvement in reducing the variability and analytical bias in automated methods for measuring creatinine concentrations, and these measurements are now calibrated to values obtained by isotope dilution mass spectrometry [28]. In addition, the Cockcroft-Gault equation overestimates true glomerular filtration rate (GFR) as measured by inulin clearance because creatinine is secreted by the renal tubule in addition to being filtered at the glomerulus [29]. For these reasons, data from the Modification of Diet in Renal Disease (MDRD) Study have been used by Levey and colleagues [30] to develop a series of equations that more accurately estimate GFR from standardized serum creatinine measurements and other patient characteristics. The most recent of these equations extends the prediction range from patients with chronic kidney disease and GFR less than 60 ml/min/ 1.73 m$^2$ to individuals with higher GFR [31]. This group of investigators [32] has used measured renal clearance of iothalamate to compare drug dosing recommendations based on the Cockcroft-Gault equation with those obtained using the following four-variable version of the MDRD Study equation:

$$\text{GFR} = 175 \times \text{Scr}^{-1.154} \times \text{age}^{-0.203}$$

$$\times 1.212 \text{ (if African American)} \times 0.742 \text{ (if female)}$$

Standardized serum creatinine (SCr) measurements were used in both equations without correcting the Cockcroft-Gault equation for this change in analytical precision. Nonetheless, the concordance rates of dosing recommendations for a panel of 15 medications was 88% for the MDRD Study equation and 85% for the Cockcroft-Gault equation when compared with measured GFR. Consequently, the authors recommended basing drug dosing adjustments in patients with impaired renal function on more recent GFR estimating equations rather than on the Cockcroft-Gault equation.

Patients with low creatinine production due to cirrhosis, cachexia, or age-related skeletal muscle atrophy have not been adequately evaluated, and renal function in these individuals is likely to be overestimated by any estimating equation that is based on serum creatinine measurements. In addition, these estimates are likely to be misleading in patients with anasarca or rapidly changing renal function. In these situations, accurate estimates of creatinine clearance can only be obtained by actually measuring urine creatinine excretion rate in a carefully timed urine specimen or by measuring GFR with another endogenous or administered marker.

Neither the Cockcroft-Gault equation nor the above described GFR estimating equations can be used to estimate creatinine clearance in pediatric patients, because muscle mass has not reached the adult proportion of body weight. Therefore, Schwartz and colleagues [33, 34] developed the following equation to predict creatinine clearance in these patients:

$$CL_{CR} \ (\mathrm{mL/min/1.73 \ m^2})$$
$$= \frac{k \cdot L \ (\mathrm{in \ cm})}{\mathrm{plasma \ creatinine \ in \ mg/dL}}$$

where $L$ is body length and $k$ varies by age and sex. For children 1–13 years of age the value of $k$ had been 0.55, but Schwartz *et al.* [35] revised this to 0.413, to reflect the introduction of SCr measurements. The original Schwartz formula also recommended discrete values of $k$ for neonates and children under 1 year of age (0.45), and for females (0.57) and males (0.70) between the ages of 13 and 20. More recently, Pottel *et al.* [36] have proposed the following modification of the Schwartz formula in which $k$ for children between 1 and 14 years of age is expressed as the following age-dependent continuous variable:

$$k = 0.0414 \times \ln \ (\mathrm{age}) + 0.3018$$

From the standpoint of clinical practice, the utility of using the Cockcroft-Gault equation or more recent methods to estimate GFR stems from the fact that these estimates can alert healthcare workers to the presence of impaired renal function in patients whose creatinine formation rate is reduced. It is in providing appropriate estimates of reduced drug dosage in these patients that pharmacokinetics has perhaps had its greatest impact on patient care.

## Dose-Related Toxicity Often Occurs When Impaired Renal Function is Unrecognized

Failure to appreciate that a patient has impaired renal function is a frequent cause of dose-related adverse drug reactions with digoxin and other drugs that normally rely primarily on the kidneys for elimination. As shown in Table 1.1, an audit of patients with high plasma concentrations of digoxin ($\geq 3.0$ ng/mL)

**TABLE 1.1    Status of Renal Function in 44 Patients with Digoxin Toxicity**

| Serum Creatinine (mg/dL) | $CL_{CR}$ (mL/min) | | % |
| --- | --- | --- | --- |
| | $\geq 50$ | $< 50$ | |
| $\leq 1.7$ | 4 | 19 | 52% |
| $> 1.7$ | 0 | 21 | 48% |

Data from Piergies AA, Worwag EM, Atkinson AJ Jr. Clin Pharmacol Ther 1994;55:353–8 [37].

demonstrated that 19 (or 43%) of 44 patients with digoxin toxicity had serum creatinine concentrations within the range of normal values, yet had estimated creatinine clearances less than 50 mL/min [37]. Hence, assessment of renal function is essential if digoxin and many other drugs are to be used safely and effectively, and is an important prerequisite for the application of clinical pharmacologic principles to patient care.

Decreases in renal function are particularly likely to be unrecognized in older patients whose creatinine clearance declines as a consequence of aging rather than overt kidney disease. It is for this reason that the Joint Commission on Accreditation of Healthcare Organizations has placed the estimation or measurement of creatinine clearance in patients of 65 years of age or older at the top of its list of indicators for monitoring the quality of medication use [38]. Unfortunately healthcare workers have considerable difficulty in using standard equations to estimate creatinine clearance in their patients, and thus this had been done only sporadically until computerized laboratory reporting systems were programmed to report MDRD estimates of GFR – a task that is relatively easy to accomplish because calculations can be performed without access to patient weight. This undoubtedly is an important advance in that it should increase prescriber awareness of a patient's renal functional status.

Although the developers of the MDRD equation advocate its further use in calculating drug dosage [39], this remains controversial and these equations appear to be in a state of continued evolution [40, 41]. Another drawback is that MDRD results are expressed in units of mL/min/1.73 m$^2$, and require further mathematical manipulation before being used to guide drug dosing in an individual patient. In addition, there is a substantial existing body of published dosing guidelines that are based on the Cockcroft-Gault equation. There are also concerns that use of MDRD estimates of renal function could result in excessive drug doses for patients with Stage III renal impairment and subtherapeutic doses for Stage IV and V patients [40], and that the MDRD equation does not predict renal function in elderly patients as well as the Cockcroft-Gault equation [41]. The inclusion of self-identified race in the MDRD equation introduces further complexity that is troublesome in that it excludes some important populations and does not rest on a solid genetic or physiologic basis, whereas the omission of weight in the equation may contribute to its inaccuracy in elderly or other patients whose muscle mass is reduced. In the final analysis it may not matter which equation is used as the basis for adjusting oral doses of many drugs, as the accuracy of either equation in estimating renal function generally exceeds the level of adjustment permitted by available oral formulations, or even the accuracy with which tablets can be split.

# REFERENCES

[1] Holmstedt B, Liljestrand G. Readings in pharmacology. Oxford: Pergamon; 1963.

[2] Reidenberg MM. Attitudes about clinical research. Lancet 1996;347:1188.

[3] Leake CD. The scientific status of pharmacology. Science 1961;134:2069–79.

[4] Reidenberg MM. Clinical pharmacology: The scientific basis of therapeutics. Clin Pharmacol Ther 1999;66:2–8.

[5] Atkinson AJ Jr, Nordstrom K. The challenge of in-hospital medication use: An opportunity for clinical pharmacology. Clin Pharmacol Ther 1996;60:363–7.

[6] Gold H, Kwit NT, Otto H. The xanthines (theobromine and aminophylline) in the treatment of cardiac pain. JAMA 1937;108:2173–9.

[7] Gold H, Catell McK, Greiner T, Hanlon LW, Kwit NT, Modell W, et al. Clinical pharmacology of digoxin. J Pharmacol Exp Ther 1953;109:45–57.

[8] Taussig HB. A study of the German outbreak of phocomelia: The thalidomide syndrome. JAMA 1962;180:1106–14.

[9] Melmon KL. Preventable drug reactions – causes and cures. N Engl J Med 1971;284:1361–8.

[10] Koch-Weser J. Serum drug concentrations as therapeutic guides. N Engl J Med 1972;287:227–31.

[11] Piquette-Miller M, Grant DM. The art and science of personalized medicine. Clin Pharmacol Ther 2007;81:311–5.

[12] Lazarou J, Pomeranz BH, Corey PN. Incidence of adverse drug reactions in hospitalized patients: A meta-analysis of prospective studies. JAMA 1998;279:1200–5.

[13] Bates DW. Drugs and adverse drug reactions. How worried should we be? JAMA 1998;279:1216–7.

[14] Sjöqvist F. The past, present and future of clinical pharmacology. Eur J Clin Pharmacol 1999;55:553–7.

[15] Shelley JH, Baur MP. Paul Martini: The first clinical pharmacologist? Lancet 1999;353:1870–3.

[16] Sheiner LB. The intellectual health of clinical drug evaluation. Clin Pharmacol Ther 1991;50:4–9.

[17] Peck CC, Barr WH, Benet LZ, Collins J, Desjardins RE, Furst DE, et al. Opportunities for integration of pharmacokinetics, pharmacodynamics, and toxicokinetics in rational drug development. Clin Pharmacol Ther 1992;51:465–73.

[18] Flowers CR, Melmon KL. Clinical investigators as critical determinants in pharmaceutical innovation. Nature Med 1997;3:136–43.

[19] Goldberg LI. Cardiovascular and renal actions of dopamine: Potential clinical applications. Pharmacol Rev 1972;24:1–29.

[20] Tréfouël J, Tréfouël Mme J, Nitti F, Bouvet D. Activité du *p*-aminophénylsulfamide sur les infections streptococciques expérimentales de la souris et du lapin. Compt Rend Soc Biol (Paris) 1935;120:756–8.

[21] Atkinson AJ Jr, Strong JM. Effect of active drug metabolites on plasma level–response correlations. J Pharmacokinet Biopharm 1977;5:95–109.

[22] Woosley RL, Chen Y, Freiman JP, Gillis RA. Mechanism of the cardiotoxic actions of terfenadine. JAMA 1993;269:1532–6.

[23] Stearns V, Johnson MD, Rae JM, Morocho A, Novielli A, Bhargava P, et al. Active tamoxifen metabolite plasma concentrations after coadministration of tamoxifen and the selective serotonin reuptake inhibitor paroxetine. J Natl Cancer Inst 2003;95:1758–64.

[24] Goetz MP, Rae JM, Suman VJ, Safgren SL, Ames MM, Visscher DW, et al. Pharmacogenetics of tamoxifen biotransformation is associated with clinical outcomes of efficacy and hot flashes. J Clin Oncol 2005;36:9312–8.

[25] Ahmad A, Shahabuddin S, Sheikh S, Kale P. Krishnappa, M, Rane RC, Ahmad I. Endoxifen, a new cornerstone for breast cancer therapy: Demonstration of safety, tolerability, and systemic bioavailability in healthy human subjects. Clin Pharmacol Ther 2010;88:814–7.

[26] Möller E, McIntosh JF, Van Slyke DD. Studies of urea excretion. II. Relationship between urine volume and the rate of urea excretion in normal adults. J Clin Invest 1929;6:427–65.

[27] Cockroft DW, Gault MH. Prediction of creatinine clearance from serum creatinine. Nephron 1976;16:31–41.

[28] Myers GL, Miller WG, Coresh J, Fleming J, Greenberg N, Greene T, et al. Recommendations for improving serum creatinine measurement: A report from the National Kidney Disease Education Program. Clin Chem 2006;52:5–18.

[29] Bauer JH, Brooks CS, Burch RN. Clinical appraisal of creatinine clearance as a measurement of glomerular filtration rate. Am J Kidney Dis 1982;2:337–46.

[30] Levey AS, Coresh J, Greene T, Stevens LA, Zhang L, Hendriksen S, et al. Using standardized serum creatinine values in the Modification of Diet in Renal Disease Study equation for estimating glomerular filtration rate. Ann Intern Med 2006;145:247–54.

[31] Levey AS, Stevens LA, Schmid CH, Zhang Y, Castro III AF, Feldman HI, et al. A new equation to estimate glomerular filtration rate. Ann Intern Med 2009;150:604–12.

[32] Stevens LA, Nolin TD, Richardson MM, Feldman HI, Lewis JB, Rodby R, et al. Comparison of drug dosing recommendations based on measured GFR and kidney function estimating equations. Am J Kid Dis 2009;54:33–42.

[33] Schwartz GJ, Feld LG, Langford DJ. A simple estimate of glomerular filtration rate in full-term infants during the first year of life. J Pediatr 1984;104:849–54.

[34] Schwartz GJ, Gauthier B. A simple estimate of glomerular filtration rate in adolescent boys. J Pediatr 1985;106:522–6.

[35] Schwartz GJ, Muñoz A, Schneider MF, Mak RH, Kaskel F, Warady BA, et al. New equations to estimate GFR in children with CKD. J Am Soc Nephrol 2009;20:629–37.

[36] Pottel H, Mottaghy FM, Zaman Z, Martens F. On the relationship between glomerular filtration rate and serum creatinine in children. Pediatr Nephrol 2010;25:927–34.

[37] Piergies AA, Worwag EM, Atkinson AJ Jr. A concurrent audit of high digoxin plasma levels. Clin Pharmacol Ther 1994;55:353–8.

[38] Nadzam DM. A systems approach to medication use. In: Cousins DM, editor. Medication use. Oakbrook Terrace, IL: Joint Commission on Accreditation of Healthcare Organizations; 1998. p. 5–17.

[39] Stevens LA, Levey AS. Use of the MDRD Study equation to estimate kidney function for drug dosing. Clin Pharmacol Ther 2009;86:465–7.

[40] Moranville MP, Jennings HR. Implications of using modification of diet in renal disease versus Cockcroft–Gault equations for renal dosing adjustments. Am J Health Syst Pharm 2009;66:154–61.

[41] Spruill WJ, Wade WE, Cobb III HH. Continuing use of the Cockroft–Gault equation for drug dosing in patients with impaired renal function. Clin Pharmacol Ther 2009;86:468–70.

## Additional Sources of Information

### General

Brunton LL, Chabner BA, Knollmann BC, editors. Goodman & Gilman's The pharmacological basis of therapeutics. 12th ed. New York, NY: McGraw-Hill; 2011.

*This is the standard reference textbook of pharmacology. It contains good introductory presentations of the general principles of pharmacokinetics, pharmacodynamics, and therapeutics. Appendix II contains a useful tabulation of the pharmacokinetic properties of many commonly used drugs.*

Waldman SA, Terzic A, editors. Pharmacology and therapeutics: Principles to practice. Philadelphia, PA: Saunders–Elsevier; 2009.

*This is an introductory textbook that is divided into initial chapters that present pharmacologic principles and later chapters that are devoted to therapeutic applications in a wide number of clinical areas.*

Carruthers SG, Hoffman BB, Melmon KL, Nierenberg DW, editors. Melmon and Morrelli's Clinical pharmacology. 4th ed. New York, NY: McGraw-Hill; 2000.

*This is the classic textbook of clinical pharmacology with introductory chapters devoted to general principles and subsequent chapters covering different therapeutic areas. A final section is devoted to core topics in clinical pharmacology.*

## Pharmacokinetics

Gibaldi M, Perrier D. Pharmacokinetics. 2nd ed. New York, NY: Marcel Dekker; 1982.

*This is a standard reference in pharmacokinetics and is the one most often cited in the "methods section" of papers that are published in journals covering this area.*

Rowland M, Tozer TN. Clinical pharmacokinetics and pharamacodynamics: Concepts and applications. 4th ed. Philadelphia, PA: Lippincott Williams & Wilkins; 2010.

*This is a well-written book that is very popular as an introductory text.*

## Drug Metabolism

Pratt WB, Taylor P, editors. Principles of drug action: The basis of pharmacology. 3rd ed. New York, NY: Churchill Livingstone; 1990.

*This book is devoted to basic principles of pharmacology and has good chapters on drug metabolism and pharmacogenetics.*

## Drug Therapy in Special Populations

Evans WE, Schentag JJ, Jusko WJ, editors. Applied pharmacokinetics: Principles of therapeutic drug monitoring. 3rd ed. Vancouver, WA: Applied Therapeutics; 1992.

*This book contains detailed information that is useful for individualizing dose regimens of a number of commonly used drugs.*

## Drug Development

Spilker B. Guide to clinical trials. Philadelphia, PA: Lippincott-Raven; 1996.

*This book contains detailed discussions of many practical topics that are relevant to the process of drug development.*

Yacobi A, Skelly JP, Shah VP, Benet LZ, editors. Integration of pharmacokinetics, pharmacodynamics, and toxicokinetics in rational drug development. New York, NY: Plenum; 1993.

*This book describes how the basic principles of clinical pharmacology currently are being applied in the process of drug development.*

## Journals

Clinical Pharmacology and Therapeutics
British Journal of Clinical Pharmacology
Journal of Pharmaceutical Sciences
Journal of Pharmacokinetics and Biopharmaceutics

## Websites

American Society for Clinical Pharmacology and Therapeutics (ASCPT): http://www.ascpt.org/

The American Board of Clinical Pharmacology (ABCP): http://www.abcp.net/

# PHARMACOKINETICS

# 2

# Clinical Pharmacokinetics

Arthur J. Atkinson, Jr.

*Department of Molecular Pharmacology & Biochemistry, Feinberg School of Medicine, Northwestern University Chicago, IL 60611*

Pharmacokinetics is an important tool that is used in the conduct of both basic and applied research, and is an essential component of the drug development process. In addition, pharmacokinetics is a valuable adjunct for prescribing and evaluating drug therapy. For most clinical applications, pharmacokinetic analyses can be simplified by representing drug distribution within the body by a *single compartment* in which drug concentrations are uniform [1]. Clinical application of pharmacokinetics usually entails relatively simple calculations, carried out in the context of what has been termed *the target concentration strategy*. We shall begin by discussing this strategy.

## THE TARGET CONCENTRATION STRATEGY

The rationale for measuring concentrations of drugs in plasma, serum, or blood is that *concentration–response* relationships are often less variable than are *dose–response* relationships [2]. This is true because individual variation in the processes of drug absorption, distribution, and elimination affects dose–response relationships, but not the relationship between free (non-protein-bound) drug concentration in plasma water and intensity of effect (Figure 2.1). The rationale for therapeutic drug monitoring was first elucidated over 80 years ago when Otto Wuth recommended monitoring bromide levels in patients treated with this drug [3]. However, its more widespread clinical application has been possible only because major advances have been made over the past 40 years in developing analytical methods capable of

routinely measuring drug concentrations in patient serum, plasma, or blood samples, and because of increased understanding of basic pharmacokinetic principles [4].

Because most adverse drug reactions are dose related, therapeutic drug monitoring has been advocated as a means of improving therapeutic efficacy and reducing drug toxicity [5]. Drug concentration monitoring is most useful when combined with pharmacokinetic/pharmacogenetic-based dose selection in an integrated management plan as outlined in Figure 2.2. This approach to drug dosing is termed *the target concentration strategy*. Pharmacokinetics has been most useful in estimating initial drug doses, particularly for loading doses and for maintenance doses of drugs that are primarily eliminated by renal excretion, and in making subsequent dose adjustments based on plasma concentration measurements. Recent advances in pharmacogenetics are finding increasing clinical utility in guiding drug selection and in providing initial dose estimates for drugs that are primarily eliminated by certain metabolic pathways.

### Monitoring Serum Concentrations of Digoxin as an Example

Given the advanced state of modern chemical and immunochemical analytical methods, the greatest current challenge is the establishment of the range of drug concentrations in blood, plasma, or serum that correlate reliably with therapeutic efficacy or toxicity. This challenge is exemplified by the results shown in Figure 2.3, which are taken from the attempt by Smith

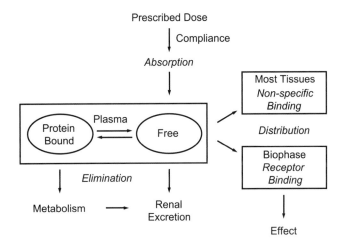

FIGURE 2.1 Diagram of factors that account for variability in observed effects when standard drug doses are prescribed. Some of this variability can be compensated for by using plasma concentration measurements to guide dose adjustments.

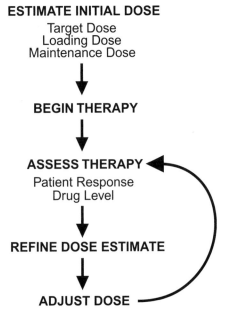

FIGURE 2.2 Target concentration strategy in which pharmacogenetics, pharmacokinetics, and drug concentration measurements are integral parts of a therapeutic approach that extends from initial drug selection and dose estimation to subsequent patient monitoring and dose adjustment.

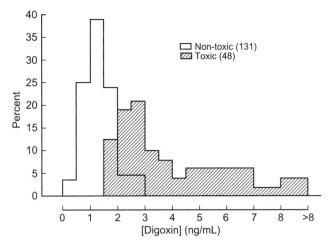

FIGURE 2.3 Superimposed frequency histograms in which serum digoxin concentrations are shown for 131 patients without digoxin toxicity and 48 patients with electrocardiographic evidence of digoxin toxicity. Reproduced with permission from Smith TW, Haber E. J Clin Invest 1970;49:2377–86 [6].

and Haber [6] to correlate serum digoxin levels with clinical manifestations of toxicity. A maintenance dose of 0.25 mg/day is usually prescribed for patients with apparently normal renal function, and this corresponds to a steady-state pre-dose digoxin level of 1.4 ng/mL when measured by the immunoassays that were initially marketed. It can be seen that no patient with digoxin levels below 1.6 ng/mL was toxic, and that all patients with digoxin levels above 3.0 ng/mL had evidence of digoxin intoxication. However, there is a large intermediate range between 1.6 and 3.0 ng/mL in which patients could be either non-toxic or toxic.

Additional clinical information is often necessary to interpret drug concentration measurements that are otherwise equivocal. Thus, Smith and Haber found that all toxic patients with serum digoxin levels less than 2.0 ng/mL had coexisting coronary heart disease – a condition known to predispose the myocardium to the toxic effects of this drug. Conversely, 4 of the 10 non-toxic patients with levels above 2.0 ng/mL were being treated with antiarrhythmic drugs that might have suppressed electrocardiographic evidence of digoxin toxicity. Accordingly, laboratory reports of digoxin concentration have traditionally been accompanied by the following guidelines:

Usual therapeutic range: 0.8–1.6 ng/mL
Possibly toxic levels: 1.6–3.0 ng/mL
Probably toxic levels: > 3.0 ng/mL.

Despite the ambiguity in interpreting digoxin level results, it was demonstrated in a controlled study that routine availability of digoxin concentration measurements markedly reduced the incidence of toxic reactions to this drug [7].

The traditional digoxin serum level recommendations were based largely on studies in which digoxin toxicity or intermediate inotropic endpoints were measured, and the challenge of establishing an appropriate range for optimally effective digoxin serum concentrations is a continuing one [8]. Although control of ventricular rate serves as a useful guide for digoxin dosing in patients with atrial fibrillation, dose recommendations still are evolving for treating congestive heart failure patients who remain in normal sinus rhythm. Recent studies have focused on the long-term clinical outcome of patients with chronic heart failure. The Digitalis Investigation Group trial, in which nearly 1000 patients were enrolled, concluded that, compared to placebo, digoxin therapy decreases the need for hospitalization and reduces the incidence of death from congestive heart failure, but not overall mortality [9]. *Post hoc* analysis of these data indicated that all-cause mortality was only lessened in men whose serum digoxin concentrations ranged from 0.5–0.9 ng/mL [10]. Higher levels were associated with progressively greater mortality and did not confer other clinical benefit. Retrospective analysis of the data from this study suggested that digoxin therapy is associated with increased all-cause mortality in women [11], but inadequate serum concentration data were obtained to identify a dose range that might be beneficial [10]. These findings are consistent with the view that the therapeutic benefits of digoxin relate more to its sympathoinhibitory effects, which are obtained when digoxin serum concentrations reach 0.7 ng/mL, than to its inotropic action, which continues to increase with higher serum levels [8]. As a result of these observations, the proposal has been made that optimally therapeutic digoxin concentrations should lie within the range of 0.5–0.8 ng/mL. Based on the pharmacokinetic properties of digoxin, one would expect levels in this range to be obtained with a daily dose of 0.125 mg. However, a troubling unresolved paradox in the data from the Digoxin Investigation Group trial is that most patients with serum digoxin levels in this range were presumed to be taking a 0.25-mg daily digoxin dose – a dose that in patients with normal renal function generally provides a steady state plasma level of 1.4 ng/mL. In addition, given that digoxin is currently prescribed for less than 30% of these patients and may now be underutilized, it has recently been recommended that its role in treating patients with congestive heart failure be completely re-examined, given their high mortality and rehospitalization rates, and the lack of efficacy shown by newer inotropic agents [12].

## General Indications for Drug Concentration Monitoring

Unfortunately, controlled studies documenting the clinical benefit of drug concentration monitoring are limited. In addition, one could not justify concentration monitoring for all prescribed drugs even if this technical challenge could be met. Thus, drug concentration monitoring is most helpful for drugs that have a low therapeutic index and that have no clinically observable effects that can be easily monitored to guide dose adjustment. Generally accepted indications for measuring drug concentrations are as follows.

1. To evaluate concentration-related toxicity:

   - Unexpectedly slow drug elimination
   - Accidental or purposeful overdose
   - Surreptitious drug taking
   - Dispensing errors

2. To evaluate lack of therapeutic efficacy:

   - Patient non-compliance with prescribed therapy
   - Poor drug absorption
   - Unexpectedly rapid drug elimination.

3. To ensure that the dose regimen is likely to provide effective prophylaxis
4. To use pharmacokinetic principles to guide dose adjustment.

Despite these technical advances, adverse reactions still occur frequently with digoxin, phenytoin, and many other drugs for which drug concentration measurements are routinely available. The persistence in contemporary practice of dose-related toxicity with these drugs most likely reflects inadequate understanding of basic pharmacokinetic principles. This is illustrated by the following case history [4]:

> In October, 1981, a 39-year-old man with mitral stenosis was hospitalized for mitral valve replacement. He had a history of chronic renal failure resulting from interstitial nephritis, and was maintained on hemodialysis. His mitral valve was replaced with a prosthesis and digoxin therapy was initiated postoperatively in a dose of 0.25 mg/day. Two weeks later, he was noted to be unusually restless in the evening. The following day, he died shortly after receiving his morning digoxin dose. Blood was obtained during an unsuccessful resuscitation attempt, and the measured plasma digoxin concentration was 6.9 ng/mL.

Later in this chapter we will demonstrate that the ostensibly surprising delayed onset of this fatal adverse event was pharmacokinetically consistent with this initial therapeutic decision.

## CONCEPTS UNDERLYING CLINICAL PHARMACOKINETICS

Pharmacokinetics provides a scientific basis for dose selection, and the process of dose regimen design can be used to illustrate with a single-compartment model the basic concepts of *apparent distribution volume* ($V_d$), *elimination half-life* ($t_{1/2}$), and *elimination clearance* ($CL_E$). A schematic diagram of this model is shown in Figure 2.4 along with the two primary pharmacokinetic parameters of distribution volume and elimination clearance that characterize it.

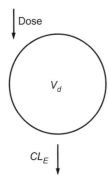

**FIGURE 2.4**   Diagram of a single-compartment model in which the primary kinetic parameters are the apparent distribution volume of the compartment ($V_d$) and the elimination clearance ($CL_E$).

## Initiation of Drug Therapy (Concept of Apparent Distribution Volume)

Sometimes drug treatment is begun with a loading dose to produce a rapid therapeutic response. Thus, a patient with atrial fibrillation might be given a 0.75-mg intravenous loading dose of digoxin as initial therapy to control ventricular rate. The expected plasma concentrations of digoxin are shown in Figure 2.5. Inspection of this figure indicates that the log plasma-concentration vs time curve eventually becomes a straight line. This part of the curve is termed the *elimination phase*. By extrapolating this elimination-phase line back to time zero, we can estimate the plasma concentration ($C_0$) that would have occurred if the loading dose were instantaneously distributed throughout the body. Measured plasma digoxin concentrations lie above the back-extrapolated line for several hours because distribution equilibrium actually is reached only slowly after a digoxin dose is administered. This part of the plasma-level vs time curve is termed the *distribution phase*. This phase reflects the underlying *multi-compartmental* nature of digoxin distribution from the intravascular space to peripheral tissues.

As shown in Figure 2.5, the back-extrapolated estimate of $C_0$ can be used to calculate the apparent volume ($V_{d(extrap)}$) of a hypothetical single compartment into which digoxin distribution occurs:

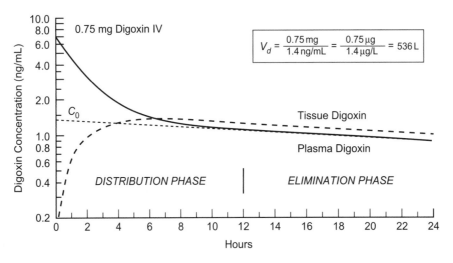

**FIGURE 2.5**   Simulation of plasma (*solid line*) and tissue (*heavy dashed line*) digoxin concentrations after intravenous administration of a 0.75-mg loading dose to a 70-kg patient with normal renal function. $C_0$ is estimated by back extrapolation (*dotted line*) of elimination phase plasma concentrations. $V_d$ is calculated by dividing the administered drug dose by this estimate of $C_0$, as shown. Tissue concentrations are referenced to the apparent distribution volume of a peripheral compartment that represents tissue distribution. Reproduced with permission from Atkinson AJ Jr, Kushner W. Annu Rev Pharmacol Toxicol 1979;19:105–27 [1].

$$V_{d(extrap)} = \text{Loading dose}/C_0 \qquad (2.1)$$

In this case, the apparent distribution volume of 536 L is much larger than anatomically possible. This apparent anomaly occurs because digoxin has a much higher binding affinity for tissues than for plasma, and the apparent distribution volume is the volume of *plasma* that would be required to provide the observed dilution of the loading dose. Despite this apparent anomaly, the concept of distribution volume is clinically useful because it defines the relationship between plasma concentration and the total amount of drug in the body. Further complexity arises from the fact that $V_{d(extrap)}$ is only one of three different distribution volume estimates that we will encounter. Because the distribution process is neglected in calculating this volume, it represents an overestimate of the sum of the volumes of the individual compartments involved in drug distribution.

The time course of the myocardial effects of digoxin parallels its concentration profile in peripheral tissues (Figure 2.5), so there is a delay between the attainment of peak plasma digoxin concentrations and the observation of maximum inotropic and chronotropic effects. The range of therapeutic and toxic digoxin concentrations has been estimated from observations made during the elimination phase, so blood should not be sampled for digoxin assay until distribution equilibrium is nearly complete. In clinical practice, this means waiting for at least 6 hours after a digoxin dose has been administered. In an audit of patients with measured digoxin levels of 3.0 ng/mL or more, it was found that nearly one-third of these levels were not associated with toxicity but reflected procedural error, in that blood was sampled less than 6 hours after digoxin administration [13].

For other drugs, such as thiopental [14] or lidocaine [15], the locus of pharmacologic action (termed the *biophase* in classical pharmacology) is in rapid kinetic equilibrium with the intravascular space. The distribution phase of these drugs represents their somewhat slower distribution from intravascular space to pharmacologically inert tissues, such as skeletal muscle, and serves to shorten the duration of their pharmacologic effects when single doses are administered. Plasma levels of these drugs reflect therapeutic and toxic effects throughout the dosing interval, and blood can be obtained for drug assay without waiting for the elimination phase to be reached.

## Continuation of Drug Therapy (Concepts of Elimination Half-Life and Clearance)

After starting therapy with a loading dose, maintenance of a sustained therapeutic effect often necessitates administering additional drug doses to replace the amount of drug that has been excreted or metabolized. Fortunately, the elimination of most drugs is a *first-order* process in that the rate of drug elimination is directly proportional to the drug concentration in plasma.

### Elimination Half-Life

It is convenient to characterize the elimination of drugs with first-order elimination rates by their *elimination half-life*, the time required for half an administered drug dose to be eliminated. If drug elimination half-life can be estimated for a patient, it is often practical to continue therapy by administering half the loading dose at an interval of 1 elimination half-life. In this way, drug elimination can be balanced by drug administration and a steady state maintained from the onset of therapy. Because digoxin has an elimination half-life of 1.6 days in patients with normal renal function, it is inconvenient to administer digoxin at this interval. When renal function is normal, it is customary to initiate maintenance therapy by administering daily digoxin doses equal to one-third of the required loading dose.

Another consequence of first-order elimination kinetics is that a constant fraction of total body drug stores will be eliminated in a given time interval. Thus, if there is no urgency in establishing a therapeutic effect, the loading dose of digoxin can be omitted and 90% of the eventual steady-state drug concentration will be reached after administering daily doses for a period of time equal to 3.3 elimination half-lives. This is referred to as the *Plateau Principle*. The classical derivation of this principle is provided later in this chapter, but for now brute force will suffice to illustrate this important concept. Suppose that we elect to omit the 0.75 mg digoxin loading dose shown in Figure 2.5 and simply begin therapy with a 0.25-mg/day maintenance dose. If the patient has normal renal function, we can anticipate that one-third of the total amount of digoxin present in the body will be eliminated each day and that two-thirds will remain when the next daily dose is administered. As shown in Scheme 2.1, the patient will have digoxin body stores of 0.66 mg just after the fifth daily dose ($3.3 \times 1.6$-day half-life = 5.3 days), and this is 88% of the total body stores that would have been provided by a 0.75-mg loading dose.

.25 × 2/3 = .17                                              Dose #1
    +.25                                                    Dose #2
.42 × 2/3 = .28
    +.25                                                    Dose #3
.53 × 2/3 = .36
    +.25                                                    Dose #4
.61 × 2/3 = .41
    +.25                                                    Dose #5
.66 × 2/3 = .44
    +.25                                                    Dose #6
.69 × 2/3 = .46
    +.25                                                    Dose #7
    .71

**SCHEME 2.1**

The solid line in Figure 2.6 shows ideal matching of digoxin loading and maintenance doses. When the digoxin loading dose (called the *digitalizing dose* in clinical practice) is omitted, or when the loading dose and maintenance dose are not matched appropriately, steady-state levels are reached only asymptotically. However, the most important concept that this figure demonstrates is that *the eventual steady state level is determined only by the maintenance dose*, regardless of the size of the loading dose. Selection of an inappropriately high digitalizing dose only subjects patients to an interval of added risk without achieving a permanent increase in the extent of digitalization. Conversely, when a high digitalizing dose is required to help control ventricular rate in patients with atrial fibrillation or flutter, a higher than usual maintenance dose also will be required.

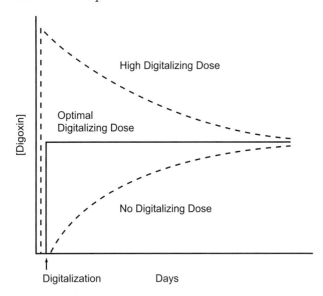

**FIGURE 2.6** Expected digoxin plasma concentrations after administering perfectly matched loading and maintenance doses (*solid line*), no initial loading dose (*bottom dashed line*), or a loading dose that is large in relation to the subsequent maintenance dose (*upper dashed line*).

### Elimination Clearance

Just as creatinine clearance is used to quantitate the renal excretion of creatinine, the removal of drugs eliminated by first-order kinetics can be defined by an *elimination clearance* ($CL_E$). In fact, elimination clearance is the primary pharmacokinetic parameter that characterizes the removal of drugs that are eliminated by first-order kinetics. When drug administration is by intravenous infusion, the eventual steady-state concentration of drug in the body ($C_{ss}$) can be calculated from the following equation, where the drug infusion rate is given by $I$:

$$C_{ss} = I \, / \, CL_E \qquad (2.2)$$

When intermittent oral or parenteral doses are administered at a dosing interval, $\tau$, the corresponding equation is:

$$\overline{C}_{ss} = \frac{\text{Dose}/\tau}{CL_E} \qquad (2.3)$$

where $\overline{C}_{ss}$ is the mean concentration during the dosing interval. Under conditions of intermittent administration, there is a continuing periodicity in maximum ("peak") and minimum ("trough") drug levels so that only a quasi-steady state is reached. However, unless particular attention is directed to these peak and trough levels, no distinction generally is made in clinical pharmacokinetics between the true steady state that is reached when an intravenous infusion is administered continuously and the quasi-steady state that results from intermittent administration.

Because there is a directly proportionate relationship between administered drug dose and steady-state plasma level, Equations 2.2 and 2.3 provide a straightforward guide to dose adjustment for drugs that are eliminated by first-order kinetics. Thus, to double the plasma level, the dose simply should be doubled. Conversely, to halve the plasma level, the dose should be halved. It is for this reason that Equations 2.2 and 2.3 are the most clinically important pharmacokinetic equations. Note that, as is apparent from Figure 2.6, these equations also stipulate that the steady-state level is determined only by the maintenance dose and elimination clearance. The loading dose does not appear in the equations and does not influence the eventual steady-state level.

In contrast to elimination clearance, elimination half-life ($t_{1/2}$) is not a primary pharmacokinetic parameter because it is determined by distribution volume as well as by elimination clearance:

$$t_{1/2} = \frac{0.693 \ V_{d(area)}}{CL_E} \qquad (2.4)$$

The value of $V_d$ in this equation is not $V_{d(extrap)}$, but represents a second estimate of distribution volume, referred to as $V_{d(area)}$ or $V_{d(\beta)}$, that generally is estimated from measured elimination half-life and clearance. The similarity of these two estimates of distribution volume reflects the extent to which drug distribution is accurately described by a single compartment model, and obviously varies from drug to drug [16].

Figure 2.7 illustrates how differences in distribution volume affect elimination half-life and peak and trough plasma concentrations when the same drug dose is given to two patients with the same elimination clearance. If these two hypothetical patients were

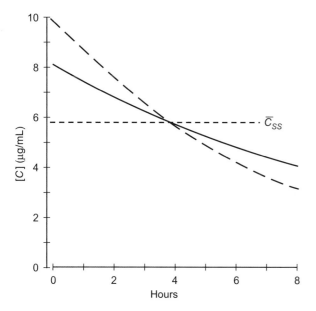

**FIGURE 2.7** Plasma concentrations after repeated administration of the same drug dose to two hypothetical patients whose elimination clearance is the same but whose distribution volumes differ. The patients have the same $\overline{C}_{SS}$, but the larger distribution volume results in lower peak and higher trough plasma levels (*solid line*) than when the distribution volume is smaller (*dashed line*).

given the same nightly dose of a sedative-hypnotic drug for insomnia, $\overline{C}_{ss}$ would be the same for both. However, the patient with the larger distribution volume might not obtain sufficiently high plasma levels to fall asleep in the evening, and might have a plasma level that was high enough to cause drowsiness in the morning.

### Drugs Not Eliminated by First-Order Kinetics

Unfortunately, the elimination of some drugs does not follow first-order kinetics. For example, the primary pathway of phenytoin elimination entails initial metabolism to form 5-(parahydroxyphenyl)-5-phenylhydantoin (*p*-HPPH), followed by glucuronide conjugation (Figure 2.8). The metabolism of this drug is not first order but follows *Michaelis-Menten* kinetics, because the microsomal enzyme system that forms *p*-HPPH is partially saturated at phenytoin concentrations of 10–20 µg/mL that are therapeutically effective. The result is that phenytoin plasma concentrations rise hyperbolically as dosage is increased (Figure 2.9).

For drugs eliminated by first-order kinetics, the relationship between dosing rate and steady-state plasma concentration is given by rearranging Equation 2.3 as follows:

$$\text{Dose}/\tau = CL_E \cdot \overline{C}_{ss} \qquad (2.5)$$

The corresponding equation for phenytoin is:

$$\text{Dose}/\tau = \frac{V_{max}}{K_m + \overline{C}_{ss}} \cdot \overline{C}_{ss} \qquad (2.6)$$

where $V_{max}$ is the maximum rate of drug metabolism and $K_m$ is the apparent Michaelis-Menten constant for the enzymatic metabolism of phenytoin.

Although phenytoin plasma concentrations show substantial interindividual variation when standard doses are administered, they average 10 µg/mL when adults are treated with a 300-mg total daily dose, but rise to an average of 20 µg/mL when the dose is increased to 400 mg [17]. This non-proportional relationship between phenytoin dose and plasma concentration complicates patient management and undoubtedly contributes to the many adverse reactions that are seen in patients treated with this drug. Although several pharmacokinetic approaches have been developed for estimating dose adjustments, it is safest to change phenytoin doses in small increments and to rely on careful monitoring of clinical response and phenytoin plasma levels. The pharmacokinetics of phenytoin were studied in both patients shown in

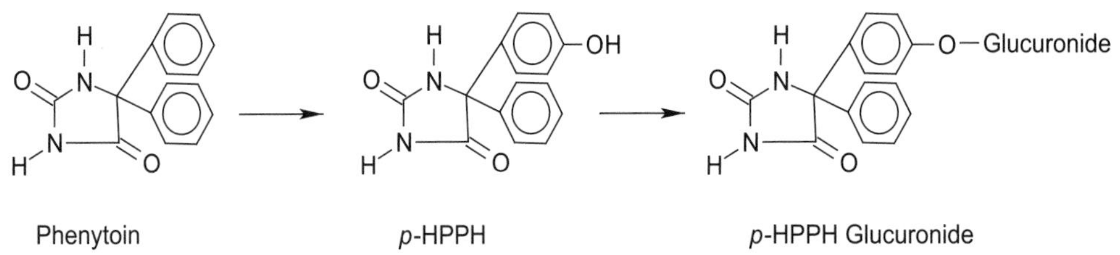

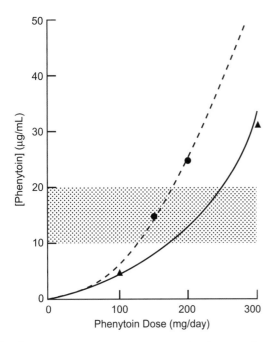

Phenytoin                    *p*-HPPH                    *p*-HPPH Glucuronide

**FIGURE 2.8** Metabolism of phenytoin to form *p*-HPPH and *p*-HPPH glucuronide. The first step in this enzymatic reaction sequence is rate limiting and follows Michaelis-Menten kinetics, showing progressive saturation as plasma concentrations rise within the range that is required for anticonvulsant therapy to be effective.

Hence, for most drugs $\overline{C}_{ss}$ can be ignored in the denominator of Equation 2.6, and this equation reduces to:

$$\text{Dose}/\tau = \frac{V_{max}}{K_m} \cdot \overline{C}_{ss}$$

where the ratio $V_{max}/K_m$ is equivalent to $CL_E$ in Equation 2.5. Thus, even for most metabolized drugs, a change in dose will change steady-state plasma concentrations proportionately – a property that is termed *dose proportionality*.

## MATHEMATICAL BASIS OF CLINICAL PHARMACOKINETICS

In the following sections we will review the mathematical basis of some of the important relationships that are used when pharmacokinetic principles are applied to the care of patients. The reader also is referred to other literature sources that may be helpful [1, 16, 19].

### First-Order Elimination Kinetics

For most drugs, the amount of drug eliminated from the body during any time interval is proportional to the total amount of drug present in the body. In pharmacokinetic terms, this is called *first-order* elimination and is described by the equation:

$$dX/dt = -k\,X \qquad (2.7)$$

where $X$ is the total amount of drug present in the body at any time ($t$) and $k$ is the elimination rate constant for the drug. This equation can be solved by separating variables and direct integration to calculate the amount of drug remaining in the body at any time after an initial dose as follows.

Separating variables:

$$dX/X = -k\,dt$$

**FIGURE 2.9** The lines show the relationship between dose and steady-state plasma phenytoin concentrations predicted for two patients who became toxic after initial treatment with 300 mg/day. Measured steady-state plasma concentrations are shown by the solid circles and triangles. The shaded area shows the usual range of therapeutically effective phenytoin plasma concentrations. Reproduced with permission from Atkinson AJ Jr. Med Clin North Am 1974;58:1037–49 [18].

Figure 2.9 after they became toxic when treated with the 300-mg/day dose that is routinely prescribed as initial therapy for adults [18]. The figure demonstrates that the entire therapeutic range is traversed in these patients by a dose increment of less than 100 mg/day. This presents an obvious therapeutic challenge, because the phenytoin oral formulation that is most commonly prescribed for adults is a 100-mg capsule.

Even though many drugs in common clinical use are eliminated by drug-metabolizing enzymes, relatively few of them have Michaelis-Menten elimination kinetics (e.g., aspirin and ethyl alcohol). The reason for this is that $K_m$ for most drugs is much greater than $\overline{C}_{ss}$.

Integrating from zero time to time $= t$:

$$\int_{X_0}^{X} dX/X = -k \int_0^t dt$$

$$\ln X \Big|_{X_0}^{X} = -kt \Big|_0^t$$

$$\ln \frac{X}{X_0} = -k\,t \qquad (2.8)$$

$$X = X_0\, e^{-kt} \qquad (2.9)$$

Although these equations deal with total amounts of drug in the body, the equation $C = X/V_d$ provides a general relationship between $X$ and drug concentration ($C$) at any time after the drug dose is administered. Therefore, $C$ can be substituted for $X$ in Equations 2.7 and 2.8 as follows:

$$\ln \frac{C}{C_0} = -kt \qquad (2.10)$$

$$C = C_0\, e^{-kt} \qquad (2.11)$$

Equation 2.10 is particularly useful because it can be rearranged in the form of the equation for a straight line ($y = mx + b$) to give:

$$\ln C = -k\,t + \ln C_0 \qquad (2.12)$$

Now when data are obtained after administration of a single drug-dose and $C$ is plotted on base 10 semi-logarithmic graph paper, a straight line is obtained

with 0.434 times the slope equal to $k$ ($\log x/\ln x = 0.434$) and an intercept on the ordinate of $C_0$. In practice $C_0$ is never measured directly because some time is needed for the injected drug to distribute throughout body fluids. However, $C_0$ can be estimated by back-extrapolating the straight line given by Equation 2.12 (Figure 2.5).

### Concept of Elimination Half-Life

If the rate of drug distribution is rapid compared with the rate of drug elimination, the terminal exponential phase of a semilogarithmic plot of drug concentrations vs time can be used to estimate the elimination half-life of a drug, as shown in Figure 2.10. Because Equation 2.10 can be used to estimate $k$ from any two concentrations that are separated by an interval $t$, it can be seen from this equation that when $C_2 = \{1/2\}C_1$:

$$\ln 1/2 = -kt_{1/2}$$

$$\ln 2 = kt_{1/2}$$

so:

$$t_{1/2} = \frac{0.693}{k}, \quad \text{and} \quad k = \frac{0.693}{t_{1/2}} \qquad (2.13)$$

For digoxin, $t_{1/2}$ is usually 1.6 days for patients with normal renal function and $k = 0.43$ day$^{-1}$ ($0.693/1.6 = 0.43$). As a practical point, it is easier to estimate $t_{1/2}$ from a graph such as Figure 2.10 and to then calculate $k$ from Equation 2.13 than it is to estimate $k$ directly from the slope of the elimination-phase line.

### Relationship of $k$ to Elimination Clearance

In Chapter 1, we pointed out that the creatinine clearance equation:

$$CL_{CR} = \frac{U\,V}{P}$$

could be re-written in the form of the following first-order differential equation:

$$dX/dt = -CL_{CR} \cdot P$$

If this equation is generalized by substituting $CL_E$ for $CL_{CR}$, it can be seen from Equation 2.7 that, since $P = X/V_d$:

$$k = \frac{CL_E}{V_d} \qquad (2.14)$$

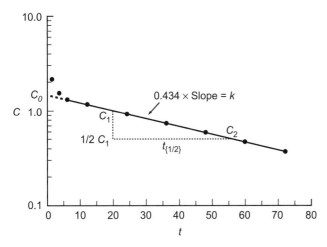

**FIGURE 2.10** Plot of drug concentrations vs time on semi-logarithmic coordinates. Back extrapolation (*dashed line*) of the elimination phase slope (*solid line*) provides an estimate of $C_0$. The elimination half-life ($t_{1/2}$) can be estimated from the time required for concentrations to fall from some point on the elimination-phase line ($C_1$) to $C_2 = 1/2\,C_1$, as shown by the dotted lines. In the case of digoxin, $C$ would be in units of ng/mL and $t$ in hours.

Equation 2.4 is derived by substituting $Cl_E/V_d$ for $k$ in Equation 2.13. Although $V_d$ and $Cl_E$ are the two primary parameters of the single compartment model, confusion arises because $k$ is initially calculated from experimental data. However, $k$ is influenced by changes in distribution volume as well as clearance, and does not reflect just changes in drug elimination.

## Cumulation Factor

In the steady-state condition, the rate of drug administration is exactly balanced by the rate of drug elimination. Gaddum [20] first demonstrated that the maximum and minimum drug levels that are expected at steady state (quasi-steady state) can be calculated for drugs that are eliminated by first-order kinetics. Assume that just maintenance doses of a drug are administered without a loading dose (Figure 2.6, lowest curve). Starting with Equation 2.9:

$$X = X_0 e^{-kt}$$

where $X_0$ is the maintenance dose and $X$ is the amount of drug remaining in the body at time $t$. If $\tau$ is the dosing interval, let:

$$p = e^{-k\tau}$$

Therefore, just before the second dose, $X_{1(min)} = X_0\, p$

Just after the second dose, $X_{2(max)} = X_0 + X_0\, p = X_0 (1+p)$

Similarly, after the third dose, $X_{3(max)} = X_0 + X_0\, p + X_0\, p^2 = X_0(1+p+p^2)$ and after the $n^{th}$ dose, $X_{n(max)} = X_0\,(1 + p + \ldots\ldots + p^{n-1})$, or

$$X_{n(max)} = X_0 \frac{(1 - p^n)}{(1 - p)}$$

Since $p < 1$, as $n \to \infty$, $p^n \to 0$. Therefore,

$$X_{\infty(max)} = X_0/(1-p)$$

or, substituting for $p$:

$$X_{\infty(max)} = \frac{X_0}{(1 - e^{-k\tau})}$$

The value of $X_\infty$ is the maximum *total body content* of the drug that is reached during a dosing interval at steady state. The maximum *concentration* is determined by dividing this value by $V_d$. The *minimum* value is given by multiplying either of these maximum values by $e^{-k\tau}$.

Note that the respective maximum and minimum drug concentrations after the first dose are:

Maximum: $C_0$
Minimum: $C_0\, e^{-k\tau}$.

The expected steady-state counterparts of these initial concentration values can be estimated by multiplying them by the *cumulation factor* (CF):

$$CF = \frac{1}{1 - e^{-kt}} \tag{2.15}$$

## The Plateau Principle

Although the time required to reach steady state cannot be calculated explicitly, the time required to reach *any specified fraction (f) of the eventual steady state* can be estimated. In clinical practice, $f = 0.90$ is usually a reasonable approximation of the eventual steady state. For dosing regimens in which drugs are administered as a constant infusion, the pharmacokinetic counterpart of the Equation 1.1 in which both creatinine synthesis and elimination are considered is:

$$dX/dt = I - k\,X$$

Separation of variables and integration of this equation yields:

$$X = \frac{I}{k}\left(1 - e^{-kt}\right)$$

Because infinite time is required for $X$ to reach its steady state, $X_{SS} = I/k$ and

$$f_{0.90} = X_{0.90}/X_{SS} = \left(1 - e^{-kt_{0.90}}\right)$$

By definition $X_{0.90}/X_{SS} = 0.90$, also $k = \ln 2/t_{1/2}$ (Equation 2.13), so:

$$t_{0.90} = 3.3\; t_{1/2} \tag{2.16}$$

For dosing regimens in which drugs are administered at a constant dosing interval, Gaddum [20] showed that the number of drug doses ($n$) required to reach any fraction of the eventual steady-state amount of drug in the body can be calculated as follows:

$$f = \frac{X_n}{X_\infty} = \frac{X_0 (1 - p^n)}{(1 - p)} \cdot \frac{(1 - p)}{X_0} = 1 - p^n \tag{2.17}$$

Once again, taking $f = 0.90$ as a reasonable approximation of eventual steady state, substituting this value into Equation 2.17, and solving for $n$:

$$0.90 = 1 - e^{-nk\tau}$$

$$e^{-nk\tau} = 0.1$$

$$n = -\frac{\ln 0.1}{k\tau}$$

$$n = \frac{2.3}{k\tau}$$

Again from Equation 2.13, $k = \ln2/t_{[1/2]}$, so the number of doses needed to reach 90% of steady state is:

$$n = 3.3 \frac{t_{1/2}}{\tau} \tag{2.18}$$

and the corresponding time is:

$$n\tau = 3.3 \, t_{1/2} \tag{2.19}$$

Not only are drug accumulations greater and steady-state drug levels higher in patients with a prolonged elimination half-life, but an important consequence of Equation 2.18 is that it also takes these patients longer to reach steady state. For example, the elimination half-life of digoxin in patients with normal renal function is 1.6 days, so that 90% of the expected steady state is reached in 5 days when daily doses of this drug are administered. However, the elimination half-life of digoxin is approximately 4.3 days in functionally anephric patients, such as the one described in the previous case history, and 14 days would be required to reach 90% of the expected steady state. This explains why this patient's adverse reaction occurred 2 weeks after starting digoxin therapy.

### Application of Laplace Transforms to Pharmacokinetics

The Laplace transformation method of solving differential equations falls into the area of *operational calculus* that we will use in deriving several pharmacokinetic equations. Operational calculus was invented by an English engineer, Sir Oliver Heaviside (1850–1925), who had an intuitive grasp of mathematics [21]. Although Laplace provided the theoretical basis for the method, some of Sir Oliver's intuitive contributions remain (e.g., the Heaviside Expansion Theorem utilized in Chapter 3). The idea of operational mathematics and Laplace transforms perhaps is best understood by comparison with the use of logarithms to perform arithmetic operations. This comparison is diagrammed in the flow charts shown in Scheme 2.2.

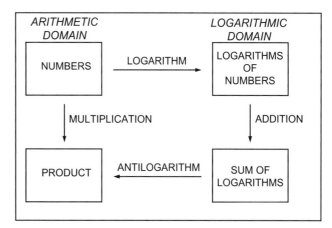

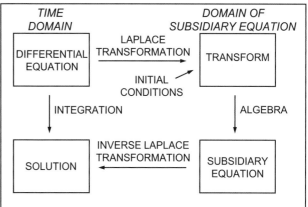

**SCHEME 2.2**

Just as there are tables of logarithms, there are tables to aid the mathematical process of obtaining Laplace transforms ($\mathscr{L}$) and inverse Laplace transforms ($\mathscr{L}^{-1}$). Laplace transforms can also be calculated directly from the integral:

$$\mathscr{L}[F(t)] = f(s) = \int_0^\infty F(t) \, e^{-st} dt$$

We can illustrate the application of Laplace transforms by using them to solve the simple differential equation that we have used to describe the single compartment model (Equation 2.7). Starting with this equation

$$dX/dt = -kX$$

we can use a table of Laplace transform operations (Appendix I) to take Laplace transforms of each side of this equation to create the *subsidiary equation*:

For $X$ on the right side of the equation:

$$\mathscr{L}\, F\,(t) = f\,(s)$$

For $dX/dt$ on the left side of the equation:

$$\mathscr{L}\, F'\,(t) = s\,f\,(s) - F\,(0)$$

Since $F(0)$ represents the *initial condition*, in this case the amount of drug in the model compartment at time zero, $X_0$, the subsidiary equation can be written:

$$s\,f(s) - X_0 = -k\,f(s)$$

This can be rearranged to give: $(s+k)\,f(s) = X_0$ or

$$f(s) = \frac{X_0}{s+k}$$

A table of inverse Laplace transforms indicates

$$\mathscr{L}^{-1}\,\frac{1}{s-a} = e^{at}$$

Therefore, the solution to the differential equation is:

$$X = X_0\,e^{-kt}$$

and this is the same result that we obtained as Equation 2.9.

In other words, the Laplace operation transforms the differential equation from the time domain to another functional domain represented by the subsidiary equation. After algebraic simplification of this subsidiary equation, the inverse transformation is used to return the solved equation to the time domain. We have selected a simple example to illustrate the use of Laplace transform methods. A more advanced application is given in the next chapter, in which equations are derived for a two-compartment model. It will be shown subsequently that Laplace transform methods also are helpful in pharmacokinetics when convolution/deconvolution methods are used to characterize drug absorption processes.

## REFERENCES

1. Atkinson AJ Jr, Kushner W. Clinical pharmacokinetics. Annu Rev Pharmacol Toxicol 1979;19:105–27.
2. Atkinson AJ Jr, Reidenberg MM, Thompson WL. Clinical pharmacology. In: Greenberger N, editor. MKSAP VI Syllabus. Philadelphia, PA: American College of Physicians; 1982. p. 85–96.
3. Wuth O. Rational bromide treatment: New methods for its control. JAMA 1927;88:2013–7.
4. Atkinson AJ Jr, Ambre JJ. Kalman and Clark's drug assay: The strategy of therapeutic drug monitoring. 2nd ed. New York, NY: Masson; 1984.
5. Koch-Weser J. Serum drug concentrations as therapeutic guides. N Engl J Med 1972;287:227–31.
6. Smith TW, Haber E. Digoxin intoxication: the relationship of clinical presentation to serum digoxin concentration. J Clin Invest 1970;49:2377–86.
7. Duhme DW, Greenblatt DJ, Koch-Weser J. Reduction of digoxin toxicity associated with measurement of serum levels. Ann Intern Med 1974;80:516–9.
8. Adams KF Jr, Gheorghiade M, Uretsky BF, Patterson JH, Schwartz TA, Young JB. Clinical benefits of low serum digoxin concentrations in heart failure. J Am Coll Cardiol 2002;39:946–53.
9. The Digitalis Investigation Group. The effect of digoxin on mortality and morbidity in patients with heart failure. N Engl J Med 1997;336:525–33.
10. Rathore SS, Curtis JP, Wang Y, Bristow MR, Krumholz HM. Association of serum digoxin concentration and outcomes in patients with heart failure. JAMA 2003;289:871–8.
11. Rathore SS, Wang W, Krumholz HM. Sex-based differences in the effect of digoxin for the treatment of heart failure. N Engl J Med 2002;347:1403–11.
12. Gheorghiade M, Braunwald E. Reconsidering the role for digoxin in the management of acute heart failure syndromes. JAMA 2009;302:2146–7.
13. Piergies AA, Worwag EW, Atkinson AJ Jr. A concurrent audit of high digoxin plasma levels. Clin Pharmacol Ther 1994;55:353–8.
14. Goldstein A, Aronow L. The durations of action of thiopental and pentobarbital. J Pharmacol Exp Ther 1960;128:1–6.
15. Benowitz N, Forsyth RP, Melmon KL, Rowland M. Lidocaine disposition kinetics in monkey and man. I. Prediction by a perfusion model. Clin Pharmacol Ther 1974;16:87–98.
16. Gibaldi M. Biopharmaceutics and clinical pharmacokinetics. 4th ed. Philadelphia, PA: Lea & Febiger; 1991.
17. Kutt H, McDowell F. Management of epilepsy with diphenylhydantoin sodium. JAMA 1968;203:969–72.
18. Atkinson AJ Jr. Individualization of anticonvulsant therapy. Med Clin North Am 1974;58:1037–49.
19. Rowland M, Tozer TN. Clinical pharmacokinetics and pharmacodynamics: Concepts and applications. 4th ed. Philadelphia, PA: Lippincott Williams & Wilkins; 2010.
20. Gaddum JH. Repeated doses of drugs. Nature 1944;153:494.
21. Van Valkenberg ME. The Laplace transformation. In: Network analysis. Englewood Cliffs, NJ: Prentice-Hall; 1964. p. 159–81.

## STUDY PROBLEMS

Select the *one* lettered answer or statement completion that is BEST. It may be helpful to carry out dimensional analysis by including units in your calculations. Answers are provided in Appendix II.

1. A 35-year-old woman is being treated with gentamicin for a urinary tract infection. The gentamicin plasma level is $4\,\mu g/mL$ shortly after initial intravenous administration of an 80-mg dose of this drug. The distribution volume of gentamicin is:

   A. 5 L
   B. 8 L
   C. 10 L
   D. 16 L
   E. 20 L

2. A 58-year-old man is hospitalized in a cardiac intensive care following an acute myocardial infarction. He has had recurrent episodes of ventricular tachycardia that have not responded to lidocaine and an intravenous infusion of procainamide will now be administered. The patient weighs 80 kg, and expected values for his procainamide distribution volume and elimination half-life are 2.0 L/kg and 3 hours, respectively.

What infusion rate will provide a steady-state plasma procainamide level of 4.0 µg/mL?

A. 2.5 mg/min
B. 5.0 mg/min
C. 7.5 mg/min
D. 10.0 mg/min
E. 12.5 mg/min

3. A patient with peritonitis is treated with gentamicin 80 mg every 8 hours. Plasma gentamicin levels are measured during the first dosing interval. The gentamicin plasma level is 10 µg/mL at its peak after initial intravenous administration of this drug, and is 5 µg/mL when measured 5 hours later.

The cumulation factor can be used to predict an expected steady-state peak level of:

A. 10 µg/mL
B. 12 µg/mL
C. 15 µg/mL
D. 18 µg/mL
E. 20 µg/mL

4. A 20-year-old man is hospitalized after an asthmatic attack precipitated by an upper respiratory infection but fails to respond in the emergency room to two subcutaneously injected doses of epinephrine. The patient has not been taking theophylline-containing medications for the past 6 weeks. He weighs 60 kg, and you estimate that his apparent volume of theophylline distribution is 0.45 L/kg. Bronchodilator therapy includes a 5.6-mg/kg loading dose of aminophylline, infused intravenously over 20 min, followed by a maintenance infusion of 0.63 mg/kg per hour (0.50 mg/kg per hour of theophylline). Forty-eight hours later, the patient's respiratory status has improved. However, he has nausea and tachycardia, and his plasma theophylline level is 24 µg/mL.

For how long do you expect to suspend theophylline administration in order to reach a level of 12 µg/mL before restarting the aminophylline infusion at a rate of 0.31 mg/kg per hour?

A. 5 hours
B. 10 hours
C. 15 hours

C. 20 hours
D. 25 hours

5. Digitoxin has an elimination half-life of approximately 7 days and its elimination is relatively unaffected by decreased renal function. For this latter reason, the decision is made to use this drug to control ventricular rate in a 60-year-old man with atrial fibrillation and a creatinine clearance of 25 mL/min.

If no loading dose is administered and a maintenance dose of 0.1 mg/day is prescribed, how many days would be required for digitoxin levels to reach 90% of their expected steady-state value?

A. 17 days
B. 19 days
C. 21 days
D. 23 days
E. 24 days

6. A 75-year-old man comes to your office with anorexia and nausea. Five years ago he was found to have congestive heart failure that responded to treatment with a thiazide diruetic and an angiotensin-converting enzyme inhibitor. Three years ago digoxin was added to the regimen in a dose of 0.25 mg/day. This morning he omitted his digoxin dose. On hospital admission, electrocardiographic monitoring shows frequent bigeminal extrasystoles and the patient's plasma digoxin level is 3.2 ng/ml. Twenty-four hours later, the digoxin level is 2.7 ng/ml. At that time you decide that it would be appropriate to let the digoxin level fall to 1.6 ng/ml before restarting a daily digoxin dose of 0.125 mg.

For how many more days do you anticipate having to withhold digoxin before your target level of 1.6 ng/ml is reached?

A. 2 days
B. 3 days
C. 4 days
D. 5 days
E. 6 days

7. A 50-year-old man is being treated empirically with gentamicin and a cephalosporin for pneumonia. The therapeutic goal is to provide a maximum gentamicin level of more than 8 µg/mL 1 hour after intravenous infusion and a minimum concentration, just before dose administration, of less than 1 µg/ml. His estimated plasma gentamicin clearance and elimination half-life are 100 mL/min and 2 hours, respectively. Which of the following dosing regimens is appropriate?

A.  35 mg every 2 hours
B.  70 mg every 4 hours
C.  90 mg every 5 hours
D.  110 mg every 6 hours
E.  140 mg every 8 hours

8.  You start a 19-year-old man on phenytoin in a dose of 300 mg/day to control generalized (grand mal) seizures. Ten days later, he is brought to an emergency room following a seizure. His phenytoin level is found to be 5 µg/mL and the phenytoin dose is increased to 600 mg/day. Two weeks later, he returns to your office complaining of drowsiness and ataxia. At that time his phenytoin level is 30 µg/mL.

Assuming patient compliance with previous therapy, which of the following dose regimens should provide a phenytoin plasma level of 15 µg/mL (therapeutic range: 10–20 µg/mL)?

A.  350 mg/day
B.  400 mg/day
C.  450 mg/day
D.  500 mg/day
E.  550 mg/day

# 3

# Compartmental Analysis of Drug Distribution

Arthur J. Atkinson, Jr.

*Department of Molecular Pharmacology & Biochemistry, Feinberg School of Medicine, Northwestern University, Chicago, IL 60611*

*A*ll *models are wrong but some are useful.*

George E. P. Box, 1979 [1]

*Drug distribution* can be defined as the post-absorptive transfer of drug from one location in the body to another. Absorption after various routes of drug administration is not considered part of the distribution process and is dealt with separately. In most cases, the process of drug distribution is symmetrically reversible and requires no input of energy. However, there is increasing awareness that receptor-mediated endocytosis and carrier-mediated active transport also play important roles in either increasing or limiting the extent of drug distribution. The role of these processes in drug distribution will be considered in Chapter 14.

## FIT-FOR-PURPOSE MODELING OF DRUG DISTRIBUTION

In the previous chapter we neglected distribution-phase data and considered drug distribution within the body to be represented by a single homogeneous compartment. Although both anatomically and phys-iologically wrong, this model nonetheless is useful for most clinical applications. In fact, most routine pharmacokinetic studies are performed using *non-compartmental* methods which provide useful estimates of drug elimination clearance and total distribution volume. This approach will be described in greater detail in Chapter 8.

A multicompartmental system was first used to model the kinetics of drug distribution in 1937 by Teorell [2]. The two body distribution compartments of his model consisted of a central compartment corresponding to intravascular space and a peripheral compartment representing non-metabolizing body tissues. Drug elimination was modeled as proceeding from the central compartment. Since then, more complex multicompartmental models have been developed in which different anatomical organs or groups of organs are represented by separate compartments. Price [3] pioneered this approach in 1960, using a four-compartment model to analyze thiopental distribution after intravenous dosing. Distribution was considered to be instantaneous in the central compartment representing intravascular space, and then proceeded at different rates to visceral organ, lean tissue, and fat compartments. The different compartments were characterized by their blood flow rates and thiopental tissue/blood partition coeffi-cients, with brain, heart, splanchnic organs, and kidneys being lumped together into a single visceral compartment because their distribution characteristics were similar. Price used this model to compare measured thiopental concentrations in blood and fat with model-predicted values and to demonstrate that the termination of this drug's central nervous system pharmacologic effect was primarily due to redistri-bution from the brain to skeletal muscle and other lean tissues. Later development of physiologically-based pharmacokinetic models has incorporated increas-ingly detailed information regarding drug physico-chemical properties, information regarding drug absorption and eliminating organ function, and different routes and conditions of drug administration [4–6]. These models can now be implemented using commercially available software and, as described in Chapter 32, are playing an increasingly important role in making *a priori* pharmacokinetic estimates that can then be compared with experimental results [6].

Because physiologically based pharmacokinetic models contain more parameters than can be identified from the analysis of experimental data, compartmental analysis of this data is usually made with systems that model drug distribution with only one, two, or three compartments [7]. Therefore, this chapter will focus on the two- and three-compartment models that are most commonly used for this purpose. In most applications, these models retain Price's assumption that distribution within the intravascular space occurs instantaneously after intravenous administration. However, the onset of pharmacologic action of intravenously administered anesthetic agents occurs within seconds of administration and this necessitates consideration of the kinetics of intravascular mixing [8]. So the appropriate selection of a given modeling approach and model type is very much dependent on the intended purpose of the analysis – what might be termed "fit-for-purpose pharmacokinetics".

Despite their varying complexity, all pharmacokinetic models represent parsimonious simplifications of real-world systems and, in the sense of the opening quotation, are "wrong". However, after reaching that conclusion, Box [1] explained that parsimony is desirable because (i) when essential aspects of the system are simple, simplicity illuminates and complication obscures, (ii) parsimony typically results in increasingly precise model parameter estimates, and (iii) indiscriminate model elaboration is not practical because "the road is endless". Similarly, Cobelli *et al.* [9] pointed out that the validity of a model depends on its adequacy for a well-defined and limited set of objectives, rather than on whether it is a true representation of all facets of an underlying system. Berman [10] made the further distinction between mathematical models in which functions or differential equations are used without regard to the mechanistic aspects of a system, and physical models, which have features that have physiological, biochemical, or physical significance. Dollery [11] has referred to the former as "abstractions derived from curve fitting" that provide minimal mechanistic insight. So this chapter will focus on identifying mechanistic elements of the compartmental models most commonly used for pharmacokinetic data analysis that can be linked to underlying features of human physiology and drug physical chemistry.

## PHYSIOLOGICAL SIGNIFICANCE OF DRUG DISTRIBUTION VOLUMES

Digoxin is typical of most drugs in that its distribution volume, averaging 536 L in 70-kg subjects with normal renal function, is not readily interpreted by reference to physiologically defined fluid spaces. However, some drugs and other compounds appear to have distribution volumes that are physiologically identifiable. Thus, the distribution volumes of inulin, quaternary neuromuscular blocking drugs, and, initially, aminoglycoside antibiotics approximate expected values for extracellular fluid space (ECF). The distribution volumes of urea, antipyrine, ethyl alcohol, and caffeine also can be used to estimate total body water (TBW) [7].

Binding to plasma proteins affects drug distribution volume estimates. Initial attempts to explain the effects of protein binding on drug distribution were based on the assumption that the distribution of these proteins was confined to the intravascular space. However, "plasma" proteins distribute throughout ECF, so the distribution volume of even highly protein-bound drugs exceeds plasma volume and approximates ECF in many cases [7]. For example, thyroxine is 99.97% protein bound, and its distribution volume of 0.15 L/kg [12] approximates recent ECF estimates of $0.16 \pm 0.01$ L/kg made with inulin [13]. Distribution volumes are usually larger than ECF for uncharged drugs that are less tightly protein bound to plasma proteins. Theophylline is a methylxanthine, similar to caffeine, and its non-protein-bound or free fraction distributes in TBW. The fact that theophylline is normally 40% bound to plasma proteins accounts for the finding that its 0.5-L/kg apparent volume of distribution is intermediate between expected values for ECF and TBW (Figure 3.1). The impact on distribution volume ($V_d$) of changes in the extent of theophylline binding to plasma proteins can be estimated from the following equation:

$$V_d = \text{ECF} + f_u(\text{TBW} - \text{ECF}) \qquad (3.1)$$

where $f_u$ is the fraction of unbound theophylline that can be measured in plasma samples [14]. An additional correction has been proposed to account for the fact that interstitial fluid protein concentrations are less than those in plasma [15]. However, this correction does not account for the heterogeneous nature of interstitial fluid composition and entails additional complexity that may not be warranted [7].

Many drugs have distribution volumes that exceed expected values for TBW, or are considerably larger than ECF despite extensive binding to plasma

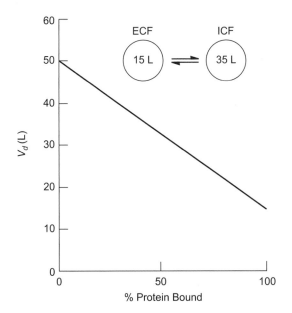

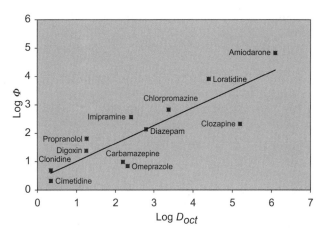

**FIGURE 3.1** Analysis of theophylline $V_d$ in terms of protein binding, ECF, and intracellular fluid (ICF) components of TBW in a hypothetical 70-kg subject. Theophylline is normally 40% bound, so its $V_d$ approximates 35 L, or 0.5 L/kg. Reproduced with permission from Atkinson AJ Jr, Ruo TI, Frederiksen MC. Trends Pharmacol Sci 1991;12:96–101 [7].

**FIGURE 3.2** Relationship between lipophilicity, estimated from $D_{oct}$, and tissue/plasma partition ratio ($\Phi$) for several commonly used drugs.

proteins. The extensive tissue binding of these drugs increases the apparent distribution volume that is calculated by reference to drug concentrations measured in plasma water. By modifying Equation 3.1 as follows,

$$V_d = \text{ECF} + \Phi f_u(\text{TBW} - \text{ECF}) \qquad (3.2)$$

published kinetic data can be used to estimate the tissue-binding affinity ($\Phi$) of these drugs.

For many drugs, the extent of tissue binding is related to their lipophilicity. Although the octanol/water partition coefficient ($P_{oct}$) measured at pH 7.4 is the in vitro parameter traditionally used to characterize lipophilicity and is appropriate for neutral compounds, this coefficient fails to take into account the fact that many acidic and basic drugs are ionized at physiological pH. Because only unionized drug generally partitions into tissues, a distribution coefficient ($D_{oct}$) is thought to provide a better correlation with the extent to which a drug distributes into tissues [16]. Thus, for drugs that are monoprotic bases,

$$\log D_{oct} = \log P_{oct} + [1/(1 + 10^{pK_a - pH})]$$

where $pK_a$ is the dissociation constant of the drug. For monoprotic acids, the exponent in this equation becomes $pH - pK_a$. In Figure 3.2, published experimentally determined values for log $D_{oct}$ are compared

with estimates of log $\Phi$. Equation 3.2 was rearranged to calculate $\Phi$ from literature values for $f_u$ and distribution volume [17, 18], and estimates of ECF (0.16 L/kg) and TBW (0.65 L/kg) that were obtained from a study of inulin and urea distribution kinetics [13].

Since the parameters $f_u$ and $D_{oct}$ can be obtained by in vitro measurements, Lombardo et al. [18] have used the reverse of this type of approach to predict drug distribution volume in humans in order to evaluate its utility in compound optimization and selection during the early stages of drug development. Although this approach would not be expected to provide an accurate prediction of the distribution volume of drugs that bind to specific subcellular components, this is not necessarily the case. For example, digoxin incorporates a steroid molecule (aglycone) but is relatively polar because three glycoside (sugar) groups are attached to it. It is a neutral compound and has an octanol/water partition coefficient of 18, but also binds very tightly to the enzyme Na/K-ATPase that is present in most body tissues. Since digoxin is only 25% bound to plasma proteins ($f_u = 0.75$), Equation 3.2 can be used to estimate that a 536-L distribution volume of this drug corresponds to a $\Phi$ value of 20.4, consistent with the relationship between lipophilicity and tissue partitioning shown in Figure 3.2. However, an important consequence of the specificity of this binding is that digoxin can be displaced from its Na/K-ATPase binding sites by concurrent administration of quinidine, causing a decrease in digoxin distribution volume [19]. As discussed in Chapter 5, Sheiner et al. [20] showed that elevations in serum creatinine concentration, resulting from impaired renal function, also are associated with decreases in digoxin distribution volume. This presumably reflects the same impairment in Na/K-ATPase activity that makes these patients more susceptible to toxicity when digoxin levels are $\geq 3.0\,\mathrm{ng/mL}$ [21].

# PHYSIOLOGICAL BASIS OF MULTICOMPARTMENTAL MODELS OF DRUG DISTRIBUTION

## Formulation of Multicompartmental Models

The construction of multicompartmenal models entails consideration of the *identifiability*, the structural *uniqueness*, and, for physiologically relevant models, the biological *plausibility* of the model. Identifiability of model parameters is problematic when there is a mismatch between the limited data provided by a pharmacokinetic study and the complexity of the proposed model structure [9]. However, a plot of plasma concentration data vs time from a pharmacokinetic experiment can be resolved, in many cases, into a number of discrete exponential phases and characterized by a *sum of exponentials* data equation, such as described later in this chapter. This provides a guide to allowable model complexity in that the minimal number of exponential terms in the data equation corresponds to the number of compartments that can be specified in the model [10]. In addition, the total number of independently identifiable model parameters cannot exceed the number of parameters in the data equation. Thus, drug elimination is usually modeled as proceeding only from the central compartment rather than from several model compartments. Drug transfer between model compartments is best characterized by *intercompartmental clearance*, a term coined by Sapirstein *et al.* [22] to describe the volume-independent parameter that quantifies the rate of analyte transfer between the compartments of a kinetic model. Thus, elimination clearance and intercompartmental clearance are primary pharmacokinetic parameters because they share the property of volume independence and are not affected by changes in compartment volume. However, a number of compartment and parameter configurations are compatible with the data equation in most cases, and additional information about the underlying system may be required to arrive at a unique model structure.

## Basis of Multicompartmental Structure

In contrast to Teorell's model, the central compartment of most two-compartment models often exceeds expected values for intravascular space, and three-compartment models are required to model the kinetics of many other drugs. The situation has been

further complicated by the fact that some drugs have been analyzed with two-compartment models on some occasions and with three-compartment models on others. To some extent, these discrepancies reflect differences in experimental design. Particularly for rapidly distributing drugs, a tri-exponential plasma-level vs time curve is likely to be observed only when the drug is administered by rapid intravenous injection and blood samples are obtained frequently in the immediate post-injection period.

The central compartment of a pharmacokinetic model usually is the only one that is directly accessible to sampling. When attempting to identify this compartment as intravascular space, the erythrocyte/plasma partition ratio must be incorporated in comparisons of central compartment volume with expected blood volume if plasma levels, rather than whole blood levels, are used for pharmacokinetic analysis. Models in which the central compartment corresponds to intravascular space are of particular physiological interest because the process of distribution from the central compartment then can be identified as transcapillary exchange (Figure 3.3). In three-compartment models of this type, it might be tempting to conclude that the two peripheral compartments were connected in series (*catenary* model) and represented interstitial fluid space and intracellular water. Urea is a marker of TBW, and the kinetics of its distribution could be analyzed with a three-compartment catenary model of this type. On the other hand,

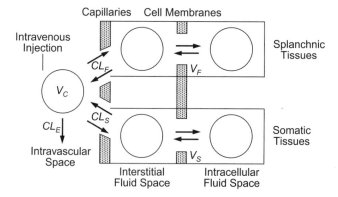

**FIGURE 3.3** Multicompartmental model of the kinetics of inulin and urea distribution and elimination. After injection into a central compartment corresponding to intravascular space ($V_C$), both compounds distribute to rapidly ($V_F$) and slowly ($V_S$) equilibrating peripheral compartments (*rectangles*), at rates of transcapillary exchange that are characterized by intercompartmental clearances $CL_F$ and $CL_S$. These peripheral compartments contain both interstitial and intracellular fluid components, but transfer of urea between them is too rapid to be distinguished kinetically. Inulin is limited in its distribution to the interstitial fluid components of the peripheral compartments. Reproduced with permission from Odeh YK, Wang Z, Ruo TI *et al.* Clin Pharmacol Ther 1993:53:419–25 [13].

a three-compartment model is also required to model distribution of inulin from a central compartment that corresponds to plasma volume. This implies that interstitial fluid is kinetically heterogeneous, and suggests that the *mammillary* system shown in Figure 3.3 is the proper unique configuration for models of both inulin and urea distribution kinetics [7, 13].

The proposed physiological basis for this model is that transfer of relatively small polar compounds, like urea and inulin, occurs rapidly across fenestrated and discontinuous capillaries that are located primarily in the splanchnic vascular bed, but proceeds more slowly through the interendothelial cell junctions of less porous capillaries that have a continuous basement membrane and are located primarily in skeletal muscle and other somatic tissues. Direct evidence to support this proposal has been provided by kinetic studies in which the volume of the rapidly equilibrating compartment was found to be reduced in animals whose spleen and lower intestine had been removed

[23]. Indirect evidence also has been provided by a study of the distribution and pharmacologic effects of *insulin*, a compound with molecular weight and extracellular distribution characteristics similar to *inulin*. As shown in Figure 3.4, insulin distribution kinetics were analyzed together with the rate of glucose utilization needed to stabilize plasma glucose concentrations (glucose clamp) [24]. Since changes in the rate of glucose infusion paralleled the rise and fall of insulin concentrations in the slowly equilibrating peripheral compartment, it was inferred that this compartment is largely composed of skeletal muscle. This *pharmacokinetic–pharmacodynamic* (PK–PD) study is also of interest because it illustrates one of the few examples in which a distribution compartment can be plausibly identified as the site of drug action or *biophase*.

## Mechanisms of Transcapillary Exchange

At this time, the physiological basis for the transfer of drugs and other compounds between compartments can only be inferred for mammillary systems in which the central compartment represents intravascular space and intercompartmental clearance can be equated with transcapillary exchange. In the case of inulin and urea, intercompartmental clearance ($CL_I$) can be analyzed in terms of the rate of blood flow ($Q$) through exchanging capillary beds and the permeability coefficient–surface area product ($P \cdot S$) characterizing diffusion through capillary fenestrae (primarily in splanchnic capillary beds) or small pores (primarily in somatic capillary beds). The following permeability-flow equation,[1] used by Renkin [25] for

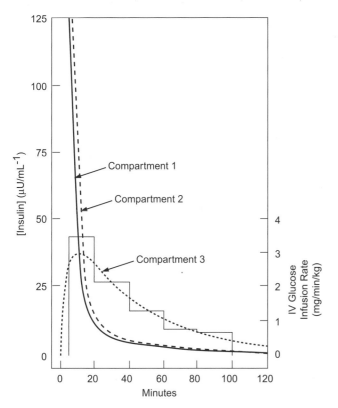

**FIGURE 3.4** Measured plasma concentrations of insulin in compartment 1 (intravascular space) after intravenous injection of a 25-mU/kg dose, and computer-derived estimates of insulin concentration in presumed splanchnic (compartment 2) and somatic (compartment 3) components of interstitial fluid space. The bar graph indicates the glucose infusion rate needed to maintain blood glucose concentrations at the basal level. Reproduced with permission from Sherwin RS, Kramer KJ, Tobin JD *et al.* J Clin Invest 1974;53:1481–92 [24].

---

[1] There is a long history behind attempts to analyze transcapillary exchange in terms of its blood flow and diffusional permeability components. Eugene Renkin appears to be the first to have applied this equation to the transcapillary exchange of non-gaseous solutes. He was guided in this effort by Christian Bohr's derivation of the equation in the context of pulmonary gas exchange (Skand Arch Physiol 1909;22:221–80). Seymour Kety based his derivation of the equation on Bohr's prior work and also applied it to pulmonary gas exchange (Pharmacol Rev 1951;3:1–41). Renkin's derivation was not published along with his original paper [25] but was archived by the American Documentation Institute (document 4648) and serves as the basis for the derivation published in reference [26]. A final independent derivation was published by Christian Crone (Acta Physiol Scand 1963;54:292–305). Renkin concludes that the equation could be eponymously termed the *Bohr/Kety/Renkin/Crone Equation* but prefers to simply refer to it as the *flow-diffusion equation* (Renkin EM. Personal Communication. December 10, 1999).

analyzing transcapillary exchange in an isolated perfused hind limb preparation,

$$CL_I = Q(1 - e^{-P \cdot S/Q}) \qquad (3.3)$$

subsequently was adapted to multicompartmental pharmacokinetic models [26]. Because $CL_I$ is replaced by two terms, $Q$ and $P \cdot S$, it is necessary to study both inulin and urea distribution kinetics simultaneously. In order to estimate all the parameters characterizing the transcapillary exchange of these compounds, it is also necessary to assume that the ratio of their $P \cdot S$ values is the same as the ratio of their free water diffusion coefficients. Calculations based on this assumption yield estimates of the sum of blood flows to the peripheral compartments that are in close agreement with independently measured cardiac output [7, 13].

Although this approach seems valid for small, uncharged molecules, molecular charge appears to slow transcapillary exchange. Large molecular size also retards transcapillary exchange [27]. Molecules considerably larger than inulin are probably transported through small-pore capillaries by convection rather than diffusion (Figure 3.5). Conversely, very lipid-soluble compounds appear to pass directly though capillary walls at rates limited only by blood flow ($P \cdot S >> Q$). Even though theophylline is a relatively polar compound, its transcapillary exchange is also blood-flow limited and presumably occurs by

**TABLE 3.1  Classification of Transcapillary Exchange Mechanisms**

1. Diffusive transfer of small molecules (< 6000 Daltons)
   - Transferred at rates proportional to their free water diffusion coefficients
     Polar, uncharged compounds (e.g., urea, inulin)
   - Transferred more slowly than predicted from free water diffusion coefficients
     Highly charged compounds (e.g., quaternary skeletal muscle relaxants)
     Compounds with intermediate polarity that interact with capillary walls (e.g., procainamide)
   - Transferred more rapidly than predicted from free water diffusion coefficients
     Highly lipid soluble compounds that freely penetrate endo-thelial cells (e.g., anesthetic gases)
     Compounds transferred by carrier-mediated facilitated diffusion (e.g., theophylline)
2. Convective transfer of large molecules (> 50,000 Daltons)

carrier-mediated facilitated diffusion [28]. This leads to the classification shown in Table 3.1.

Although there have been few studies designed to interpret actual drug distribution results in physiological terms, a possible approach is to administer the drug under investigation along with reference compounds such as inulin and urea. This experimental design was used to show that theophylline distributed from intravascular space to two peripheral compartments which had intercompartmental clearances corresponding to the blood flow components of urea and

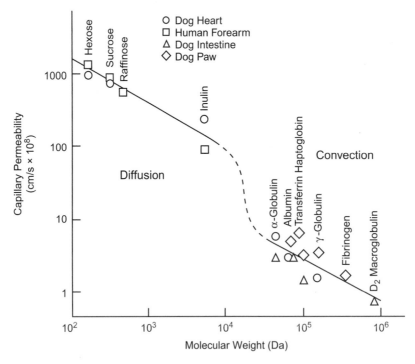

**FIGURE 3.5**  Plot of capillary permeability vs molecular weight. Reproduced with permission from Dedrick RL, Flessner MF. Prog Clin Biol Res 1989;288:429–38 [27].

inulin transcapillary exchange [28]. It also should be emphasized that conventional kinetic studies do not have the resolving power to identify distribution to smaller but pharmacologically important regions such as the brain in which transcapillary exchange is limited by tight junctions or by carrier-mediated active transport (e.g., P-glycoprotein).

## CLINICAL CONSEQUENCES OF DIFFERENT DRUG DISTRIBUTION PATTERNS

The process of drug distribution can account for both the slow onset of pharmacologic effect of some drugs (e.g., digoxin) and the termination of pharmacologic effect after bolus intravenous injection of others (e.g., thiopental and lidocaine). When theophylline was introduced in the 1930s, it was often administered by rapid intravenous injection to asthmatic patients. It was only after several fatalities were reported that the current practice was adopted of initiating therapy in emergency situations with a slow intravenous infusion. Nonetheless, excessively rapid intravenous administration of theophylline still contributes to the frequency of serious adverse reactions to this drug [29]. The rapidity of carrier-mediated theophylline distribution to the brain and heart probably contributes to the infusion-rate dependency of these serious adverse reactions.

The impact of physiological changes on drug distribution kinetics has not been studied extensively. For example, it is known that pregnancy alters the elimination kinetics of many drugs. But physiological changes in body fluid compartment volumes and protein binding also affect drug distribution in pregnant subjects. As discussed in Chapter 24, Equation 3.1 has been used to correlate pregnancy-associated changes in theophylline distribution with this altered physiology [14]. As described in Chapter 6, changes in intercompartmental clearance occur during hemodialysis and have important effects on the extent of drug removal during this procedure.

For most drugs whose plasma-level vs time curve demonstrates more than one exponential phase, the terminal phase primarily, but not entirely, reflects the process of drug elimination, and the initial phase or phases primarily reflect the process of drug distribution. However, the sequence of *distribution* and *elimination phases* is reversed for some drugs, and these drugs are said to exhibit *"flip-flop"* kinetics. For example, Schentag and colleagues [30] have shown that the elimination phase precedes the distribution phase of gentamicin, an aminoglycoside antibiotic, and accounts for the long terminal half-life that is seen

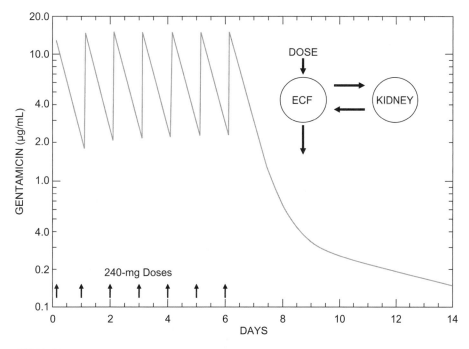

**FIGURE 3.6** Simulated serum gentamicin concentrations in a patient during and after a typical 1-week course of therapy (240 mg infused intravenously every 24 h). The half-life of serum levels observed during repeated dosing is primarily reflective of renal elimination. The terminal half-life seen after therapy was stopped is the actual distribution phase. Data were simulated with the two-compartment model shown in the figure using pharmacokinetic parameters reported by Colburn WA, Schentag JJ, Jusko WJ, Gibaldi M. J Pharmacokinet Biopharm 1978;6:179–86 [35].

after a course of therapy (Figure 3.6). In this case, the reported central compartment of drug distribution probably corresponds to ECF. In one of the few studies in which drug concentrations actually were measured in human tissues, Schentag *et al.* [31] demonstrated that the kidneys account for the largest fraction of drug in the peripheral compartment. Although aminoglycosides are highly charged and do not passively diffuse across mammalian cell membranes, they are taken up by proximal renal tubular cells by a receptor-mediated endocytic mechanism in which megalin serves at the endocytic receptor [32]. Aminoglycosides exhibit *dose-regimen dependency* in that their nephrotoxicity is less with intermittent than with continuous administration of the same total antibiotic dose [33]. This reflects the fact that their uptake by proximal renal tubule cells becomes saturated at the higher glomerular ultrafiltrate concentrations that are achieved with intermittent dosing regimens [34]. The saturability of this uptake is what supports the rationale for administering aminoglycosides in one large daily dose rather than giving one-third of this dose at 8-hour intervals. But even with similar dose regimens, the extent of gentamicin distribution into tissues was found to be much greater in patients who exhibited nephrotoxicity than in those whose renal function was preserved (Figure 3.7) [35].

In technical terms, we can say that the approximation of a single-compartment model represents *misspecification* of what is really a two-compartment system for gentamicin. However, the distribution phase for this drug is not even apparent until therapy is stopped. Nonetheless, the extent to which peak and/or trough levels rise during repetitive dosing can be used to provide an important clue to extensive gentamicin accumulation in the "tissue" compartment. Most clinical pharmacokinetic calculations are made with the initial assumption that gentamicin distributes in a single compartment that roughly corresponds to ECF. If the dose and dose interval are kept constant, steady-state peak and trough levels can be predicted simply by multiplying initial peak and trough levels by the *cumulation factor* (*CF*). As derived in Chapter 2,

$$CF = 1/(1 - e^{-kt}) \qquad (3.4)$$

where $k$ is $\ln 2/t_{1/2}$ and $\tau$ is the dosing interval. If peak and trough levels initially rise more rapidly than predicted from Equation 3.4, this reflects the fact that substantial drug is accumulating in the "tissue" compartment. Of course, deterioration in renal function can also cause gentamicin peak and trough levels to increase, but usually this occurs after 5 or more days of therapy.

An important point about drugs that exhibit flip-flop kinetics is that the terminal exponential phase usually is reached only when plasma drug levels are subtherapeutic. For this reason, the half-life corresponding to this terminal exponential phase (greater than 4 days in the example shown in Figure 3.7) cannot be used in selecting an appropriate dosing interval. If the actual extent of drug accumulation is known from the ratio of steady state/initial plasma levels, the observed cumulation factor (*CF*_obs) during repetitive dosing can be used to estimate an effective elimination rate constant (*k*_eff) by rearranging Equation 3.4 to the form:

$$k_{eff} = \frac{1}{\tau} \ln \left( \frac{CF_{obs}}{CF_{obs} - 1} \right)$$

and the effective half-life (*t*_1/2 eff) can be calculated as:

$$t_{1/2eff} = \ln 2/k_{eff}$$

The effective half-life can then be used to design dose regimens for drugs that have a terminal exponential phase representing the disposition of only a small fraction of the total drug dose [36].

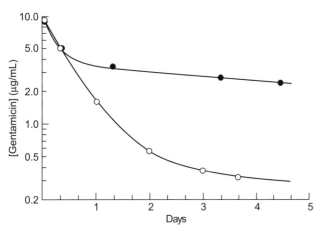

**FIGURE 3.7** Decline in serum gentamicin concentrations after therapy was stopped in a patient with nephrotoxicity (●) and a patient who did not have this adverse reaction (○). Both patients had been treated with gentamicin at an 8-hour dosing interval and had nearly identical elimination-phase half-lives and peak and trough levels. Reproduced with permission from Colburn WA, Schentag JJ, Jusko WJ, Gibaldi M. J Pharmacokinet Biopharm 1978;6:179–86 [35].

## ESTIMATING MODEL PARAMETERS FROM EXPERIMENTAL DATA

### Derivation of Equations for a Two-Compartment Model

After rapid intravenous injection, sequentially measured plasma levels may follow a pattern similar

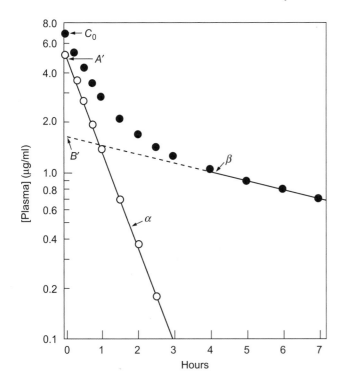

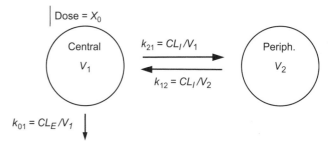

**FIGURE 3.9** Schematic drawing of a two-compartment model with central and peripheral (Periph.) compartments. The number of primary model parameters ($V_1$, $V_2$, $CL_E$, and $CL_I$) that can be identified from the data cannot exceed the total number of coefficients and exponents in the data equation.

**FIGURE 3.8** "Curve-peeling" technique used to estimate the coefficients and exponents of Equation 3.5. Data points (●) are plotted on semilogarithmic coordinates and the points for the $\alpha$-curve (○) are obtained by subtracting back-extrapolated $\beta$-curve values from the experimental data.

to that shown by the solid circles in Figure 3.8. For most drugs, the elimination phase is reached when the data points fall on the line marked $\beta$. The distribution phase occurs prior to that time. In this case, the curve contains two exponential phases and can be described by the following sum of exponentials *data equation*:

$$C = A' \, e^{-\alpha t} + B' \, e^{-\beta t} \qquad (3.5)$$

where $A'$ and $B'$ are the back-extrapolated intercepts, and $\alpha$ and $\beta$ are the slopes shown in the figure. The drug concentration in the central compartment at time zero ($C_0$) equals the sum of $A' + B'$. For convenience in the derivation that follows, we normalize the values of these intercepts:

$$A = A' \, V_1/C_0 \, V_1 = A'/C_0$$

$$B = B' \, V_1/C_0 \, V_1 = B'/C_0$$

Since $A + B = 1$, the administered dose also has a normalized value of 1.

There are two exponential terms in the data equation, so the data are consistent with a two-compartment model and, because the data equation only has a total of four coefficients and exponents, the

model can have only four independently identifiable parameters. In addition, the assumption usually is made that both intravenous administration and subsequent drug elimination proceed via the central compartment. Accordingly, the model is drawn as shown in Figure 3.9. We are interested in obtaining values for the parameters of this model in terms of the parameters of the data equation (Equation 3.5). Whereas the data equation is written in the concentration units of the data, the equations for the model shown in Figure 3.9 usually are developed in terms of the amounts of drug in each compartment ($X_1$ and $X_2$), the micro-rate constants describing drug transfer between or out of compartments ($k$ values), and a single drug dose ($X_0$). The model itself can be described in terms of two first-order linear differential equations (*model equations*):

$$dX_1/dt = -k_{01}X_1 - k_{21}X_1 + k_{12}X_2$$

$$dX_2/dt = k_{21}X_1 - k_{12}X_2$$

Combining terms:

$$dX_1/dt = -(k_{01} + k_{21})X_1 + k_{12}X_2$$

$$dX_2/dt = k_{21}X_1 - k_{12}X_2$$

Laplace transforms can be used to transform this system of linear differential equations in the time domain into a system of linear equations in the Laplace domain. From the table of Laplace operations (Appendix I), we obtain:

$$s \, X_1 - X_1(0) = -(k_{01} + k_{21}) \, X_1 + k_{12} \, X_2$$

$$s \, X_2 - X_2(0) = k_{21} \, X_1 - k_{12} \, X_2$$

If a single drug dose is injected intravenously, the entire administered dose is initially in compartment 1 and, because of normalization, $X_1(0)$ equals 1. The amount of drug in compartment 2 at zero time [$X_2(0)$] is 0. We can now write the following non-homogenous linear equations:

$$(s + k_{01} + k_{21})X_1 - k_{12}X_2 = 1$$

$$- k_{21}X_1 + (s + k_{12})X_2 = 0$$

The method of determinants (Cramer's Rule) can be used to solve the equations for each model compartment. However, we will focus only on the solution for the central compartment, which is the one usually sampled for concentration measurements.

$$X_1 = \frac{\begin{vmatrix} 1 & -k_{12} \\ 0 & s + k_{12} \end{vmatrix}}{\begin{vmatrix} s + k_{01} + k_{21} & -k_{12} \\ -k_{21} & s + k_{12} \end{vmatrix}}$$

$$X_1 = \frac{s + k_{12}}{s^2 + (k_{01} + k_{21} + k_{12})s + k_{01}k_{12}} \quad (3.6)$$

This solution is in the form of a quotient of two polynomials, $P(s) / Q(s)$. $Q(s)$ can be expressed in terms of its factors as follows:

$$X_1 = \frac{s + k_{12}}{(s + \alpha)(s + \beta)}$$

where the roots of the polynomial $Q(s)$ are $R_1 = -\alpha$ and $R_2 = -\beta$. The Heaviside Expansion Theorem states:

$$X_i = \sum_{i=1}^{n} \frac{P(R_i)}{Q'(R_i)} e^{R_i t}$$

Since:

$$Q(s) = s^2 + (\alpha + \beta)s + \alpha\beta \quad (3.7)$$

$$Q'(s) = 2s + \alpha + \beta$$

Therefore,

$$X_1 = \frac{k_{12} - \alpha}{-2\alpha + \alpha + \beta} e^{-\alpha t} + \frac{k_{12} - \beta}{-2\beta + \alpha + \beta} e^{-\beta t}$$

$$X_1 = \frac{k_{12} - \alpha}{\beta - \alpha} e^{-\alpha t} + \frac{k_{12} - \beta}{\alpha - \beta} e^{-\beta t} \quad (3.8)$$

In order to estimate the model parameters from the data equation, we also need to specify the rate of drug elimination from the central compartment ($V_1$). The rate of elimination from this compartment, $dE/dt$, is given by the equation:

$$dE/dt = k_{01} X_1$$

so total elimination is:

$$E = k_{01} \int_0^\infty X_1 \, dt$$

Since $E$ equals the administered dose, which has been normalized to 1,

$$k_{01} = \frac{1}{\int_0^\infty X_1 \, dt} \quad (3.9)$$

If $X_1$ is written in the form of the data equation (Equation 3.5):

$$X_1 = A e^{-\alpha t} + B e^{-\beta t} \quad (3.10)$$

we obtain

$$\int_0^\infty X_1 \, dt = -(A/\alpha)e^{-\alpha t} - (B/\beta)e^{-\beta t} \Big|_0^\infty$$

$$= A/\alpha + B/\beta$$

Substituting this result into Equation 3.9:

$$\boxed{k_{01} = \frac{1}{A/\alpha + B/\beta}} \quad (3.11)$$

By comparing Equations 3.6 and 3.7, it is apparent that:

$$Q(s) = s^2 + (k_{01} + k_{21} + k_{12})s + k_{01}k_{12}$$

So, from Equation 3.7,

$$\alpha + \beta = k_{01} + k_{21} + k_{12} \quad (3.12)$$

$$\alpha\beta = k_{01} k_{12} \quad (3.13)$$

Rearranging Equation 3.13:

$$k_{12} = \frac{\alpha\beta}{k_{01}}$$

Substituting for $k_{01}$ as defined by Equation 3.11:

$$\boxed{k_{12} = \beta A + \alpha B} \quad (3.14)$$

Equation 3.12 can be rearranged to give:

$$k_{21} = \alpha + \beta - k_{01} - k_{12}$$

$$= \alpha + \beta - \frac{\alpha\beta}{k_{12}} - k_{12}$$

$$= -\frac{k_{12}^2 - (\alpha + \beta)k_{12} + \alpha\beta}{k_{12}}$$

$$= -\frac{(k_{12} - \alpha)(k_{12} - \beta)}{k_{12}}$$

By comparing Equations 3.8 and 3.10,

$$A = \frac{k_{12} - \alpha}{\beta - \alpha}$$

so

$$k_{12} - \alpha = -A(\alpha - \beta)$$

and

$$B = \frac{k_{12} - \beta}{\alpha - \beta}$$

so

$$k_{12} - \beta = B(\alpha - \beta)$$

Therefore:

$$k_{21} = \frac{AB(\alpha - \beta)^2}{k_{12}} \qquad (3.15)$$

These techniques also can be applied to develop equations for three-compartment and other commonly used pharmacokinetic models.

## Calculation of Rate Constants and Compartment Volumes from Data

Values for the data equation parameters can be obtained by the technique of "curve peeling", which is illustrated in Figure 3.8. After plotting the data, the first step is to identify the terminal exponential phase of the curve, in this case termed the $\beta$-phase, and then back-extrapolate this line to obtain the ordinate intercept ($B'$). It is easiest to calculate the value of $\beta$ by first calculating the half-life of this phase. The value for $\beta$ then can be estimated from the relationship: $\beta = \ln 2/t_{1/2\beta}$. The next step is to subtract the corresponding value on the back-extrapolated $\beta$-phase line from each of the data point values obtained during the previous exponential phase. This generates the $\alpha$-line

from which the $\alpha$-slope and $A'$ intercept can be estimated.

After calculating the normalized intercept values $A$ and $B$, the rate constants for the model can be obtained from Equations 3.11, 3.14 and 3.15. The volume of the central compartment is calculated from the ratio of the administered dose to the back-extrapolated value for $C_0$ (which equals $A' + B'$) as follows:

$$V_1 = \frac{Dose}{C_0}$$

Since $k_{21} = CL_I/V_1$ and $k_{12} = CL_I/V_2$,

$$k_{21} V_1 = k_{12} V_2$$

and

$$V_2 = V_1(k_{21}/k_{12})$$

The sum of $V_1$ and $V_2$ is termed the apparent volume of distribution at steady state ($V_{d(ss)}$) and is the third distribution volume that we have described. Note also that $CL_I = k_{21}V_1 = k_{12}V_2$.

Even though computer programs now are used routinely for pharmacokinetic analysis, most require initial estimates of the model parameters. As a result of the least-squares fitting procedures employed, these computer programs generally yield the most satisfactory results when the technique of curve peeling is used to make reasonably accurate initial estimates of parameter values.

## Different Estimates of Apparent Volume of Distribution

The three estimates of distribution volume that we have encountered have slightly different properties [37]. Of the three, $V_{d(ss)}$ has the strongest physiologic rationale for multicompartment systems of drug distribution. It is independent of the rate of both drug distribution and elimination, and is the volume that is referred to in Equations 3.1 and 3.2. On the other hand, estimates of $V_{d(area)}$ are most useful in clinical pharmacokinetics, since it is this volume that links elimination clearance to elimination half-life in the equation:

$$t_{1/2} = \frac{0.693 V_{d(area)}}{CL_E}$$

Because the single-compartment model implied by this equation makes no provision for the contribution of intercompartmental clearance to elimination half-life, estimates of $V_{d(area)}$ are larger than $V_{d(ss)}$.

Estimates of $V_{d(extrap)}$ are also based on a single-compartment model in which drug distribution is assumed to be infinitely fast. However, slowing of intercompartmental clearance reduces estimates of $B'$, the back-extrapolated $\beta$-curve intercept in Figure 3.8, to a greater extent than it prolongs elimination half-life. As a result, $V_{d(extrap)}$ calculated from the equation

$$V_{d(extrap)} = Initial\ Dose/\ B'$$

is even larger than $V_{d(area)}$. Thus, when the plasma-level vs time curve includes more than a single exponential component, the relationship of the three distribution volume estimates to each other is:

$$V_{d(extrap)} > V_{d(area)} > V_{d(ss)}$$

# REFERENCES

[1] Box GEP. Robustness in the strategy of scientific model building. In: Launer RL, Wilkinson GN, editors. Robustness in statistics. New York, NY: Academic Press; 1979. p. 231–6.

[2] Teorell T. Kinetics of distribution of substances administered to the body: I. The extravascular modes of administration. Arch Intern Pharmacodyn 1937;57:205–25.

[3] Price HL, Kovnat PJ, Safer JN, Conner EH, Price ML. The uptake of thiopental by body tissues and its relation to the duration of narcosis. Clin Pharmacol Ther 1960;1:16–22.

[4] Bischoff KB, Dedrick RL. Thiopental kinetics. J Pharm Sci 1968;57:1346–51.

[5] Oliver RE, Jones AF, Rowland M. A whole-body physiologically based pharmacokinetic model incorporating dispersion concepts: Short and long time characteristics. J Pharmacokinet Pharmacodyn 2001;28:27–55.

[6] Jamei M, Dickinson GL, Rostami-Hodjegan A. A framework for assessing inter-individual variability in pharmacokinetics using virtual human populations and integrating general knowledge of physical chemistry, biology, anatomy, physiology and genetics: A tale of "bottom-up" vs "top down" recognition of covariates. Drug Metab Pharmacokinet 2009;24:53–75.

[7] Atkinson AJ Jr, Ruo TI, Frederiksen MC. Physiological basis of multicompartmental models of drug distribution. Trends Pharmacol Sci 1991;12:96–101.

[8] Henthorn TK, Krejcie TC, Avram MJ. Early drug distribution: A generally neglected aspect of pharmacokinetics of particular relevance to intravenously administered anesthetic agents. Clin Pharmacol Ther 2008;84:18–22.

[9] Cobelli C, Carson ER, Finkelstein L, Leaning MS. Validation of simple and complex models in physiology and medicine. Am J Physiol 1984;246:R259–66.

[10] Berman M. The formulation and testing of models. Ann NY Acad Sci 1963;108:182–94.

[11] Dollery CT. The challenge of complexity. Clin Pharmacol Ther 2010;88:13–5.

[12] Larsen PR, Atkinson AJ Jr, Wellman HN, Goldsmith RE. The effect of diphenylhydantoin on thyroxine metabolism in man. J Clin Invest 1970;49:1266–79.

[13] Odeh YK, Wang Z, Ruo TI, Wang T, Frederiksen MC, Pospisil PA, Atkinson AJ Jr. Simultaneous analysis of inulin and $^{15}N_2$-urea kinetics in humans. Clin Pharmacol Ther 1993;53:419–25.

[14] Frederiksen MC, Ruo TI, Chow MJ, Atkinson AJ Jr. Theophylline pharmacokinetics in pregnancy. Clin Pharmacol Ther 1986;40:321–8.

[15] Øie S, Tozer TN. Effect of altered plasma protein binding on apparent volume of distribution. J Pharm Sci 1979;68:1203–5.

[16] Lombardo F, Shalaeva MY, Tupper KA, Gao F. ElogD$_{oct}$: A tool for lipophilicity determination in drug discovery. 2. Basic and neutral compounds. J Med Chem 2001;44:2490–7.

[17] Thummel KE, Shen DD, Isoherranen N, Smith HE. Design and optimization of dosage regimens: Pharmacokinetic data. In: Bruton LL, Lazo JS, Parker KL, editors. Goodman & Gilman's The pharmacological basis of therapeutics. 11th edn. New York, NY: McGraw-Hill; 2006. p. 1787–8.

[18] Lombardo F, Obach RS, Shalaeva MY, Gao F. Prediction of human volume of distribution values for neutal and basic drugs. 2. Extended data set and leave-class-out statistics. J Med Chem 2004;47:1242–50.

[19] Hager WD, Fenster P, Mayersohn M, Perrier D, Graves P, Marcus FI, Goldman S. Digoxin–quinidine interaction: Pharmacokinetic evaluation. N Engl J Med 1979;300:1238–41.

[20] Sheiner LB, Rosenberg B, Marathe VV. Estimation of population characteristics of pharmacokinetic parameters from routine clinical data. J Pharmacokinet Biopharm 1977;5:445–79.

[21] Piergies AA, Worwag EW, Atkinson AJ Jr. A concurrent audit of high digoxin plasma levels. Clin Pharmacol Ther 1994;55:353–8.

[22] Sapirstein LA, Vidt DG, Mandel MJ, Hanusek G. Volumes of distribution and clearances of intravenously injected creatinine in the dog. Am J Physiol 1955;181:330–6.

[23] Sedek GS, Ruo TI, Frederiksen MC, Frederiksen JW, Shih S-R, Atkinson AJ Jr. Splanchnic tissues are a major part of the rapid distribution spaces of inulin, urea and theophylline. J Pharmacol Exp Ther 1989;251:963–9.

[24] Sherwin RS, Kramer KJ, Tobin JD, Insel PA, Liljenquist JE, Berman M, Andres R. A model of the kinetics of insulin in man. J Clin Invest 1974;53:1481–92.

[25] Renkin EM. Effects of blood flow on diffusion kinetics in isolated perfused hindlegs of cats: A double circulation hypothesis. Am J Physiol 1953;183:125–36.

[26] Stec GP, Atkinson AJ Jr. Analysis of the contributions of permeability and flow to intercompartmental clearance. J Pharmacokinet Biopharm 1981;9:167–80.

[27] Dedrick RL, Flessner MF. Pharmacokinetic considerations on monoclonal antibodies. Prog Clin Biol Res 1989;288:429–38.

[28] Belknap SM, Nelson JE, Ruo TI, Frederiksen MC, Worwag EM, Shin S-G, Atkinson AJ Jr. Theophylline distribution kinetics analyzed by reference to simultaneously injected urea and inulin. J Pharmacol Exp Ther 1987;243:963–9.

[29] Camarta SJ, Weil MH, Hanashiro PK, Shubin H. Cardiac arrest in the critically ill. I. A study of predisposing causes in 132 patients. Circulation 1971;44:688–95.

[30] Schentag JJ, Jusko WJ, Plaut ME, Cumbo TJ, Vance JW, Abrutyn E. Tissue persistence of gentamicin in man. JAMA 1977;238:327–9.

[31] Schentag JJ, Jusko WJ, Vance JW, Cumbo TJ, Abrutyn E, DeLattre M, Gerbracht LM. Gentamicin disposition and tissue accumulation on multiple dosing. J Pharmacokinet Biopharm 1977;5:559–77.

[32] Nagai J, Takano M. Molecular aspects of renal handling of aminoglycosides and strategies for preventing the nephrotoxicity. Drug Metab Pharmacokinet 2004;19:159–79.

[33] Reiner NE, Bloxham DD, Thompson WL. Nephrotoxicity of gentamicin and tobramycin given once daily or continuously in dogs. J Antimicrob Chemother 1978;4(Suppl. A):85–101.

[34] Verpooten GA, Giuliano RA, Verbist L, Eestermans G, De Broe ME. Once-daily dosing decreases renal accumulation of gentamicin and netilmicin. Clin Pharmacol Ther 1989;45:22–7.

[35] Colburn WA, Schentag JJ, Jusko WJ, Gibaldi M. A model for the prospective identification of the prenephrotoxic state during gentamicin therapy. J Pharmacokinet Biopharm 1978;6:179–86.

[36] Boxenbaum H, Battle M. Effective half-life in clinical pharmacology. J Clin Pharmacol 1995;35:763–6.

[37] Gibaldi M, Perrier D. Pharmacokinetics. 2nd edn. New York, NY: Marcel Dekker; 1982.

## STUDY PROBLEMS

1. Single dose and steady-state multiple dose plasma-concentration vs time profiles of tolrestat, an aldose reductase inhibitor, were compared. The terminal exponential-phase half-life was 31.6 hours at the conclusion of multiple dose therapy administered at a 12-hour dosing interval. However, there was little apparent increase in plasma concentrations with repetitive dosing and the cumulation factor, based on measurements of the area under the plasma-level vs time curve ($AUC$), was only 1.29. Calculate the effective half-life for this drug. (*Reference*: Boxenbaum H, Battle M. Effective half-life in clinical pharmacology. J Clin Pharmacol 1995;35:763–6 [36].)

2. The following data were obtained in a Phase I dose-escalation tolerance study after administering a 100-mg bolus of a new drug to a healthy volunteer:

### Plasma Concentration Data

| Time (h) | (µg/mL) |
| --- | --- |
| 0.10 | 6.3 |
| 0.25 | 5.4 |
| 0.5 | 4.3 |
| 0.75 | 3.5 |
| 1.0 | 2.9 |
| 1.5 | 2.1 |
| 2.0 | 1.7 |
| 2.5 | 1.4 |
| 3.0 | 1.3 |
| 4.0 | 1.1 |
| 5.0 | 0.9 |
| 6.0 | 0.8 |
| 7.0 | 0.7 |

a. Use two-cycle, semilogarithmic graph paper to estimate $\alpha$, $\beta$, $A$, and $B$ by the technique of curve peeling.

b. Draw a two-compartment model with elimination proceeding from the central compartment ($V_1$). Use Equations 3.11, 3.14 and 3.15 to calculate the rate constants for this model.

c. Calculate the central compartment volume and the elimination and intercompartmental clearances for this model.

d. Calculate the volume for the peripheral compartment for the model. Sum the central and peripheral compartment volumes to obtain $V_{d(ss)}$ and compare your result with the volume estimates, $V_{d(extrap)}$ and $V_{d(area)}$, that are based on the assumption that the $\beta$-slope represents elimination from a one-compartment model. Comment on your comparison.

## COMPUTER-BASED TUTORIALS

Pharmacokinetic data usually are analyzed using computers, and several software programs are available that incorporate curve-fitting algorithms for estimating the parameters of a selected model. Interested readers can find tutorials and data files available free of charge at the following website (http://www.saam.com/case_studies_pharmacokinetic.htm).

Of particular relevance to this chapter are the pharmacokinetic case studies on inulin kinetics and gentamicin kinetics. The latter is a heuristic simulation exercise that provides insight on the features of flip-flop kinetics and the basis for this drug's dose-regimen dependency.

# 4

# Drug Absorption and Bioavailability

Arthur J. Atkinson, Jr.

*Department of Molecular Pharmacology & Biochemistry, Feinberg School of Medicine, Northwestern University, Chicago, IL 60611*

## DRUG ABSORPTION

The study of drug absorption is of critical importance in developing new drugs and in establishing the therapeutic equivalence of new formulations or generic versions of existing drugs. A large number of factors can affect the rate and extent of absorption of an oral drug dose. These are summarized in Figure 4.1.

Biopharmaceutic factors include drug solubility and formulation characteristics that impact the rate of drug disintegration and dissolution. From the physiologic standpoint, passive non-ionic diffusion is the mechanism by which most drugs are absorbed once they are in solution. However, attention also has been focused on the role that specialized small intestine transport systems play in the absorption of some drugs [1]. Thus, levodopa, α–methyldopa, and baclofen are amino acid analogs that are absorbed from the small intestine by the large neutral amino acid (LNAA) transporter. Similarly, some amino-β-lactam antibiotics, captopril, and other angiotensin-converting enzyme inhibitors are absorbed via an oligopeptide transporter (PEPT-1), and salicylic acid and pravastatin by a monocarboxylic acid transporter.

Absorption by passive diffusion is largely governed by the molecular size and shape, degree of ionization, and lipid solubility of a drug. Classical explanations of the rate and extent of drug absorption have been based on the pH-partition hypothesis. According to this hypothesis, weakly acidic drugs are largely unionized and lipid soluble in acid medium, and hence should be absorbed best by the stomach. Conversely, weakly basic drugs should be absorbed primarily from the more alkaline contents of the small intestine. Absorption would not be predicted for drugs that are permanently ionized, such as quaternary ammonium compounds. In reality, the stomach does not appear to be a major site for the absorption of even acidic drugs. The surface area of the intestinal mucosa is so much greater than that of the stomach that this more than compensates for the decreased absorption rate per unit area. Table 4.1 shows results that were obtained when the stomach and small bowel of rats were perfused with solutions of aspirin at two different pH values [2]. Even at a pH of 3.5, gastric absorption of aspirin makes only a small contribution to the observed serum level, and the rate of gastric absorption of aspirin is less than the rate of intestinal absorption even when normalized to organ protein content. Furthermore, it is a common misconception that the pH of resting gastric contents is always 1–2 [3]. Values exceeding pH 7 may occur after meals, and achlorhydria is common in the elderly.

Since absorption from the stomach is poor, the rate of gastric emptying becomes a prime determinant of the rate of drug absorption. Two patterns of gastric motor activity have been identified that reflect whether the subject is fed or fasting [4, 5]. Fasting motor activity has a cyclical pattern. Each cycle lasts 90–120 minutes and consists of the following four phases:

Phase 1: A period of quiescence lasting approximately 60 minutes.
Phase 2: A 40-minute period of persistent but irregular contractions that increase in intensity as the phase progresses.

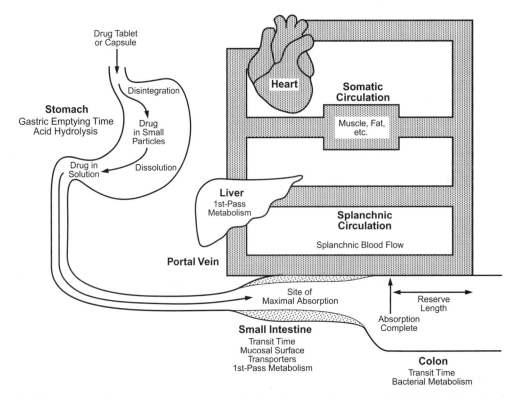

**FIGURE 4.1**   Summary of biopharmaceutic and physiologic processes that affect the rate and extent of absorption of an orally administered drug dose. Further explanation is provided in the text.

Phase 3: A short burst of intense contractions that are propagated distally from the stomach to the terminal ileum. These have been termed migrating motor complexes (MMC) or "housekeeper waves".
Phase 4: A short period of transition with diminished contractile activity.

After feeding, the MMCs are inhibited and there is uncoupling of proximal and distal gastric motility such that the resting tone of the antrum is decreased. However, solid food stimulates intense and sustained antral contractions that reduce the particle size of gastric contents. The pylorus is partially constricted

**TABLE 4.1   Aspirin (ASA) Absorption from Simultaneously Perfused Stomach and Small Intestine**

| pH | ASA Absorption (μmol/100 mg protein/h) | | ASA Serum level (mg/100 ml) |
| | Stomach | Small bowel | |
|---|---|---|---|
| 3.5 | 346 | 469 | 20.6 |
| 6.5 | 0 | 424 | 19.7 |

Data from Hollander D, Dadugalza VD, Fairchild PA. J Lab Clin Med 1981;98:591–8 [2].

and, although liquids and particles less than 1 mm in diameter can pass through to the small bowel, larger particles are retained in the stomach. Studies employing γ-scintigraphy have confirmed that, as a result of these patterns of motor activity, a tablet taken in the fasting state will generally leave the stomach in less than 2 hours but may be retained in the stomach for more than 10 hours if taken following a heavy meal [6].

Slow gastric emptying may not only retard drug absorption but, in some cases, lead to less complete drug absorption as well. Thus, penicillin is degraded under acid conditions and levodopa is decarboxylated by enzymes in the gastric mucosa. Accordingly, patients should be advised to take these medications before meals. On the other hand, the prolonged gastric residence time that follows feeding may be needed to optimize the bioavailability of saquinavir and other drugs that are either poorly soluble or are prepared in formulations that have a slow rate of disintegration [7]. Concurrent administration of drugs that modify gastric motility may also affect drug absorption. Hence, metaclopramide stimulates gastric emptying and has been shown to increase the rate of acetaminophen absorption, whereas propantheline delays gastric emptying and retards acetaminophen absorption [8].

Transit through the small intestine is more rapid than generally has been appreciated. Small intestinal transit time averages $3 \pm 1$ hours ($\pm$ SE), is similar for large and small particles, and is not appreciably affected by fasting or fed state [6]. Rapid transit through the small intestine may reduce the bioavailability of compounds that either are relatively insoluble or are administered as extended-release formulations that have an absorption window with little reserve length. *Reserve length* is defined as the anatomical length over which absorption of a particular drug can occur, less the length at which absorption is complete (Figure 4.1) [9]. Digoxin is an important example of a compound that has marginal reserve length. Consequently, the extent of absorption of one formulation of this drug is influenced by small bowel motility, being decreased when co-administered with metoclopramide and increased when an atropinic was given shortly before the digoxin dose [10].

Administered drug also may be lost in transit through the intestine due to metabolism by intestinal bacteria. Most enteric bacteria reside in the large intestine, so this is seldom a problem for drugs that are rapidly and completely absorbed in the small bowel. However, at least 30 drugs have been identified as substrates for intestinal bacteria, and this is most likely to have important consequences for drugs that have minimal reserve length [11]. Thus, digoxin is metabolized to inactive dihydro compounds by *Eubacterium lentum*, a constituent of normal bacterial flora in some individuals (see Chapter 11, Scheme 11.12) [12]. Intestinal metabolism of sorivudine, an oral antiviral drug introduced in Japan to treat patients with herpes zoster, had particularly serious consequences and resulted in the death of 18 patients who were treated concurrently with the anticancer drug 5-fluorouracil (5-FU). Okuda *et al.* [13] found that sorivudine undergoes intestinal metabolism by *Bacteroides* species to (E)-5-(2-bromovinyl)-uracil (BVU) which, when absorbed and further converted in the liver to dihydro-BVU, binds covalently to and inactivates dihydropyrimidine dehydrogenase (*suicide inhibition*). Because this enzyme is primarily responsible for metabolizing 5-FU, plasma 5-FU concentrations reached toxic levels in the patients who died while being treated with these two drugs; thus it was decided to withdraw sorivudine from the market. On the other hand, intestinal metabolism has been beneficially exploited to target topical therapy for patients with inflammatory bowel disease. This was accomplished first with sulfasalazine, a prodrug in which 5–aminosalicylic acid (5-ASA) is linked by an azo bond to sulfapyridine [14]. This drug was particularly effective in treating patients with ulcerative colitis because azoreductase in enteric bacteria liberates 5-ASA

in the colon, thus maximizing delivery of its topical anti-inflammatory effects to the affected mucosa. However, the sulfopyridine moiety limits the tolerability of sulfasalazine, so delayed-release formulations of 5-ASA, now referred to as mesalamine, currently are used to target colonic delivery of this compound.

In addition to their effects on gastrointestinal motility, drug–drug and food–drug interactions can have a direct effect on drug absorption [15]. These interactions are discussed in Chapter 15. Mucosal integrity of the small intestine also may affect the bioavailability of drugs that have little reserve length. Thus, the extent of digoxin absorption was found to be less than one-third of normal in patients with D-xylose malabsorption due to sprue, surgical resection of the small intestine, or intestinal hypermotility [16]. Drug efflux transporters located on the apical membrane of intestinal epithelial cells can also reduce the extent of drug absorption. P-Glycoprotein (P-gp) is the transporter that has been studied most extensively, but multidrug resistance-associated protein 2 (MRP2) and breast cancer related protein (BCRP) are other ATP-dependent efflux transporters that have been shown to limit the extent to which some drugs are absorbed [17]. In this case of sulfasalazine, this lipophilic drug would be expected to cross the small intestinal mucosa rapidly but it reaches the colon without significant prior absorption because it is a substrate for both MRP2 and BCRP efflux transport in the small intestine [18].

Drugs also can be metabolized before reaching the systemic circulation, either in their first pass through intestinal mucosal cells or after delivery by the portal circulation to the liver. Cytochrome P450 (CYP) 3A4 plays the major role in the intestinal metabolism of drugs and other xenobiotics, and is strategically placed at the apex of intestinal villi [19]. Studies in anhepatic patients have demonstrated that intestinal CYP3A4 may account for as much as half of the first-pass metabolism of cyclosporine that normally is observed [20]. P-gp shares considerable substrate specificity with CYP3A4 and may act in concert with intestinal CYP3A4 to reduce the net absorption of a variety of lipophilic drugs, although some drugs (e.g., digoxin) are substrates for P-gp but not CYP3A4 and others (e.g., midazolam) are substrates for CYP3A4 but not P-gp [17]. Marzolini *et al.* [21] compiled a list of drugs that are P–gp substrates, and some of these are listed in Table 4.2 along with the extent to which they are absorbed after oral administration [22]. The underlined names indicate drugs that also are known to be CYP3A4 substrates. As expected, many of these drugs are poorly absorbed. However, what is surprising is that the absorption of some P-gp substrate drugs exceeds 70%. In part, this can be explained by the fact

**TABLE 4.2   Extent of Absorption (*F*) of some P-glycoprotein Substrates[a]**

| > 70% Absorption | | 30%—70% Absorption | | < 30% Absorption | |
|---|---|---|---|---|---|
| Drug | F % | Drug | F % | Drug | F % |
| Phenobarbital | 100 | Digoxin | 70 | Cyclosporine | 28 |
| Levofloxacin | 99 | Indinavir | 65 | Tacrolimus | 25 |
| Methadone | 92 | Ondanseton | 62 | Morphine | 24 |
| Phenytoin | 90 | Cimetidine | 60 | Verapamil | 22 |
| Methylprednisolone | 82 | Clarithromycin | 55 | Nicardipine | 18 |
| Tetracycline | 77 | Itraconazole | 55 | Sirolimus | 15 |
| | | Etoposide | 52 | Saquinavir | 13 |
| | | Amitriptyline | 48 | Atorvastatin | 12 |
| | | Amiodarone | 46 | Paclitaxel | 10 |
| | | Diltiazem | 38 | Doxorubicin | 5 |
| | | Losartan | 36 | | |
| | | Erythromycin | 35 | | |
| | | Chlorpromazine | 32 | | |

[a]Underlined drugs are also substrates for CYP3A4.

that some drugs reach millimolar concentrations in the intestinal lumen that exceed the Michaelis-Menten constant of P-gp, thus saturating this transport mechanism [23]. This is particularly likely to occur with drugs such as indinavir that are administered in greater than 100-mg doses. In addition P-gp transport is non-destructive, so, provided there is adequate reserve length, some of the drug that is extruded by P-gp in the proximal small intestine may be reabsorbed distally, as shown in Figure 4.2. On the other hand, repeated exposure to metabolism in the intestinal mucosa would further reduce the absorption of drugs that also are CYP3A4 substrates [23, 24]. The rate and extent of drug absorption across the intestinal mucosa can also be affected by splanchnic blood flow rate [25], but only a few clinical studies have attempted to demonstrate its

significance [26]. The liver represents a final barrier that orally administered drugs must traverse before reaching the systemic circulation, and hepatic first-pass metabolism of a number of drugs, in many cases reflecting the activity of cytochrome P450 enzymes, has been well documented [27].

Morphine, organic nitrates, propranolol, lidocaine, and cyclosporine are some commonly used drugs that have extensive first-pass metabolism or intestinal P-gp transport. As a result, effective oral doses of these drugs are substantially higher than intravenously administered doses. Despite the therapeutic challenge posed by presystemic elimination of orally administered drugs, first-pass metabolism provides important protection from some potentially noxious dietary xenobiotics. Thus, hepatocytes contain monamine oxidase that inactivates tyramine present in Chianti wine, and in Cheddar and other aged cheeses. Patients treated with monamine oxidase inhibitors lack this protective barrier and tyramine in foods and beverages can reach the systemic circulation, causing norepinephrine release from sympathetic ganglia and potentially fatal hypertensive crises [28]. On the other hand, first-pass sulfation of swallowed isoproterenol minimizes the systemic side effects experienced by patients using isoproterenol nebulizers.

## BIOAVAILABILITY

Bioavailability is the term most often used to characterize drug absorption. This term has been defined as

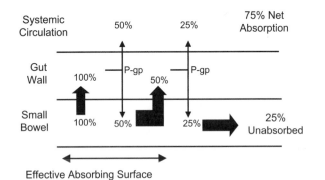

**FIGURE 4.2**   Possible explanation for > 70% absorption of some P-glycoprotein (P-gp) substrates that have a reserve length that permits repeated absorption opportunities.

the relative amount of a drug administered in a pharmaceutical product that enters the systemic circulation in an unchanged form, and the rate at which this occurs [29]. Implicit in this definition is the concept that a comparison is being made. If the comparison is made between an oral and an intravenous formulation of a drug, which by definition has 100% bioavailability, the *absolute bioavailability* of the drug is measured. If the comparison is made between two different oral formulations, then the *relative bioavailability* of these formulations is determined. As shown in Figure 4.3, three indices of drug bioavailability usually are estimated: the maximum drug concentration in plasma ($C_{max}$), the time needed to reach this maximum ($t_{max}$), and the area under the plasma- or serum-concentration vs time curve ($AUC$). Generally there is also an initial lag period ($t_{lag}$) that occurs before drug concentrations are measurable in plasma.

The $AUC$ measured after administration of a drug dose is related to the extent of drug absorption in the following way. Generalizing from the analysis of creatinine clearance that we presented in Chapter 1, the first-order differential equation describing rate of drug elimination from a single-compartment model is:

$$dE/dt = CL \cdot C$$

where $dE/dt$ is the rate of drug elimination, $CL$ is the elimination clearance, and $C$ is the concentration of drug in the compartment. Separating variables and integrating yields the result:

$$E = CL \int_0^\infty C \, dt \qquad (4.1)$$

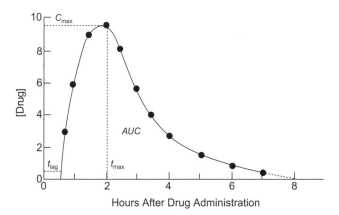

**FIGURE 4.3** Hypothetical plasma-concentration vs time curve after a single oral drug dose. Calculation of the area under the plasma-level vs time curve ($AUC$) requires extrapolation of the elimination phase curve beyond the last measurable plasma concentration, as shown by the dotted line.

where $E$ is the total amount of drug eliminated in infinite time. By mass balance, $E$ must equal the amount of the drug dose that is absorbed. The integral is simply the $AUC$. Thus, for an oral drug dose ($D_{oral}$):

$$D_{oral} \cdot F = CL \cdot AUC_{oral} \qquad (4.2)$$

where $F$ is the fraction of the dose that is absorbed and $AUC_{oral}$ is the $AUC$ resulting from the administered oral dose.

## Absolute Bioavailability

In practice, absolute bioavailability most often is measured by sequentially administering single intravenous and oral doses ($D_{IV}$ and $D_{oral}$) of a drug and comparing their respective $AUCs$. Extent of absorption of the oral dose can be calculated by modifying Equation 4.2 as follows:

$$\%\text{Absorption} = \frac{CL \cdot D_{IV} \cdot AUC_{oral}}{CL \cdot D_{oral} \cdot AUC_{IV}} \times 100$$

$$= \frac{D_{IV} \cdot AUC_{oral}}{D_{oral} \cdot AUC_{IV}} \times 100$$

A two-formulation, two-period, two-sequence crossover design is usually used to control for administration sequence effects. $AUCs$ frequently are estimated using the linear trapezoidal method, the log trapezoidal method or a combination of the two [30]. Alternatively, bioavailability can be assessed by comparing the amounts of unmetabolized drug recovered in the urine after giving the drug by the intravenous and oral routes. This follows directly from Equation 4.1, since urinary excretion accounts for a constant fraction of total drug elimination when drugs are eliminated by first-order kinetics.

In either case, the assumption usually is made that the elimination clearance of a drug remains the same in the interval between drug doses. This problem can be circumvented by administering an intravenous formulation of the stable-isotope-labeled drug intravenously at the same time that the test formulation of unlabeled drug is given orally. Although the feasibility of this technique was first demonstrated in normal subjects [31], the method entails only a single study and set of blood samples and is ideally suited for the evaluation of drug absorption in patients, as shown in Figure 4.4 [26]. More recently, accelerator mass spectrometry has been used to extend this approach to microdosing studies with radiolabeled drugs [32].

In a study of $N$–acetylprocainamide (NAPA) pharmacokinetics in patients [26], a computer program employing a least-squares fitting algorithm was used to

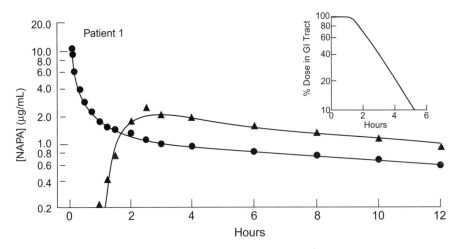

**FIGURE 4.4** Kinetic analysis of plasma concentrations resulting from the intravenous injection of NAPA-¹³C (*circles*) and the simultaneous oral administration of a NAPA tablet (*triangles*). The solid lines are a least-squares fit of the measured concentrations shown by the data points. The calculated percentage of the oral dose remaining in the gastrointestinal (GI) tract is plotted in the insert. Reproduced with permission from Atkinson AJ Jr, Ruo TI, Piergies AA *et al.* Clin Pharmacol Ther 1989;46:182–9 [26].

analyze those data in terms of the pharmacokinetic model shown in Figure 4.5. The extent of NAPA absorption was calculated from model parameters representing the absorption rate ($k_a$) and nonabsorptive loss ($k_0$) from the gastrointestinal tract, as follows:

$$\%\text{Absorption} = \frac{k_a}{k_a + k_0} \times 100$$

The extent of absorption also was assessed by comparing the 12-hour urine recovery of NAPA and NAPA-¹³C. A correction was made to the duration of NAPA recovery to compensate for the lag in NAPA absorption that was observed after the oral dose was administered. The results of these two methods of assessing extent of absorption are compared in Table 4.3. The discrepancy was less than 2% for all but one of the subjects.

Slow and incomplete absorption of procainamide has been reported in patients with acute myocardial infarction, and has been attributed to decreased splanchnic blood flow [33]. Decreased splanchnic blood flow also may reduce the bioavailability of NAPA, the acetylated metabolite of procainamide. Although an explicit relationship between $CL_F$ and $k_a$ is not shown in Figure 4.5, splanchnic blood flow is proposed as a major determinant of $CL_F$, and it is noteworthy that the extent of NAPA absorption in patients was well correlated with $CL_F$ estimates ($r = 0.89$, $P = 0.045$). This illustrates how a model-based approach can provide important insights into patient factors affecting drug absorption.

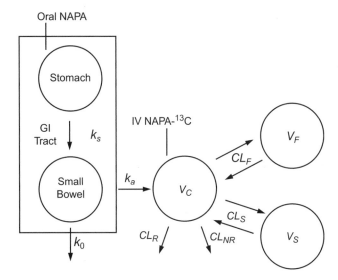

**FIGURE 4.5** Multicompartment system used to model the kinetics of NAPA absorption, distribution, and elimination. NAPA labeled with ¹³C was injected intravenously (IV) to define the kinetics of NAPA disposition. NAPA distribution from intravascular space ($V_C$) to fast ($V_F$) and slow ($V_S$) equilibrating peripheral compartments is characterized by the intercompartmental clearances $CL_F$ and $CL_S$. NAPA is cleared from the body by both renal ($CL_R$) and non-renal ($CL_{NR}$) mechanisms. A NAPA tablet was administered orally with the intravenous dose to analyze the kinetics of NAPA absorption from the gastrointestinal (GI) tract. After an initial delay that consisted of a time lag (not shown) and presumed delivery of NAPA to the small bowel ($k_s$), the rate and extent of NAPA absorption were determined by $k_a$ and $k_o$, as described in the text. Reproduced with permission from Atkinson AJ Jr, Ruo TI, Piergies AA *et al.* Clin Pharmacol Ther 1989;46:182–9 [26].

**TABLE 4.3   Comparison of Bioavailability Estimates**

| Patient number | Kinetic analysis (%) | NAPA Recovery in urine[a] (%) |
|---|---|---|
| 1 | 66.1 | 65.9 |
| 2 | 92.1 | 92.1 |
| 3 | 68.1 | 69.9 |
| 4 | 88.2 | 73.1 |
| 5 | 75.7 | 75.6 |

[a]Corrected for absorption lag time.

## Relative Bioavailability

If the bioavailability comparison is made between two oral formulations of a drug, then their relative bioavailability is measured. Two formulations generally are regarded as being *bioequivalent* if the 90% confidence interval of the ratios of the population average estimates of *AUC* and $C_{max}$ for the test and reference formulations lie within a pre-established bioequivalence limit, usually 80% to 125% [34]. Bioequivalence studies are needed during clinical investigation of a new drug product in order to ensure that different clinical trial batches and formulations have similar performance characteristics. They are also required when significant manufacturing changes occur after drug approval. Following termination of marketing exclusivity, generic drugs that are introduced are expected to be bioequivalent to the innovator's product. Population average metrics of the test and reference formulations have traditionally been compared to calculate an *average bioequivalence*. However, more sophisticated statistical approaches have been advocated to compare full population distributions or estimate intraindividual differences in bioequivalence [34].

Although *therapeutic equivalence* is assured if two formulations are bioequivalent, the therapeutic equivalence of two bioinequivalent formulations can be judged only within a specific clinical context [29]. Thus, if we ordinarily treat streptococcal throat infections with a 10-fold excess of penicillin, a formulation having half the bioavailability of the usual formulation would be therapeutically equivalent since it still would provide a 5-fold excess of antibiotic. On the other hand, bioinequivalence of cyclosporine formulations, and of other drugs that have a narrow therapeutic index, could have serious therapeutic consequences.

## *In Vitro* Prediction of Bioavailability

The introduction of combinatorial chemistry and high-throughput biological screens has placed increasing stress on the technology that traditionally has been used to assess bioavailability. Insufficient time and resources are available to conduct formal *in vivo* kinetic studies for each candidate compound that is screened. Consequently, there is a clear need to develop *in vitro* methods that can be integrated into biological screening processes as reliable predictors of bioavailability. For reformulation of some immediate-release compounds it is even possible that *in vitro* data will suffice and that the regulatory requirement for repeated *in vivo* studies can be waived [35]. Waivers for immediate-release formulations, granted initially only for scale-up and post-approval changes, have since been extended to the approval of new generic products [36].

An important part of this development effort has been the establishment of a theoretical basis for drug classification that focuses on three critical biopharmaceutical properties: drug solubility relative to drug dose ($D_0$), dissolution rate of the drug formulation, and the intestinal permeability of the drug [37]. A $D_0$ value $\leq 1$ indicates high solubility and can be measured *in vitro* as the number of 250-mL glasses of water required to completely dissolve the maximum-strength drug dose over a pH range of 1–7.5 at 37° C [36, 37]. *In vitro* dissolution tests have been standardized and are widely used for manufacturing quality control and in the evaluation of new formulations and generic products. However, proper selection of the apparatus and dissolution medium for these tests needs to be based on the physical chemistry of the drug and on the dosage form being evaluated [38]. For immediate-release products, a dissolution specification of at least 85% dissolved within 30 minutes is considered sufficient to exclude dissolution-rate limitations to bioavailability [35]. Based on these considerations, the following biopharmaceutic drug classification system (BCS) has been established [35, 37].

**Class 1: High solubility–high permeability drugs.** Drugs in this class are well absorbed but their bioavailability may be limited either by first-pass metabolism or by P-gp-mediated efflux from the intestinal mucosa. *In vitro–in vivo* correlations of dissolution rate with the rate of drug absorption are expected if dissociation is slower than gastric emptying rate. If dissociation is sufficiently rapid, gastric emptying will limit absorption rate.

**Class 2: Low solubility–high permeability drugs.** Poor solubility may limit the extent of absorption of high drug doses. The rate of absorption is limited by dissolution rate and generally is slower than for drugs in Class 1. *In vitro–in vivo* correlations are tenuous in view of the many formulation and physiological variables that can affect the dissolution profile.

**Class 3: High solubility–low permeability drugs.**
Intestinal permeability limits both the rate and
extent of absorption for this class of drugs and
intestinal reserve length is marginal. Bioavailability
is expected to be variable but, if dissolution is
at least 85% complete within 30 minutes, this
variability will reflect differences in physiological
variables such as intestinal permeability and intestinal transit time.

**Class 4: Low solubility–low permeability drugs.**
Effective oral delivery of this class of drugs presents
the most difficulties, and reliable *in vitro–in vivo*
correlations are not expected.

The rapid evaluation of the intestinal membrane
permeability of drugs represents a continuing challenge. Human intubation studies have been used to
measure jejunal effective permeability of a number of
drugs, and these measurements have been compared
with the extent of drug absorption. It can be seen from
Figure 4.6 that the expected fraction absorbed exceeds
95% for drugs with a jejunal permeability of more
than $2.4 \times 10^{-4}$ cm/s [29]. Currently, compounds are
considered to be highly permeable if they achieve at
least 90% absorption in humans [35].

Although human intubation studies are even more
laborious than formal assessment of absolute
bioavailability, they have played an important role in
validating *in vitro* methods that have been developed.
The most commonly used *in vitro* method is based on

measurement of drug transfer across a monolayer of
cultured Caco-2 cells derived from a human colorectal
carcinoma. Artursson and Karlsson [39] found that the
apparent permeability of 20 drugs measured with
the Caco-2 cell model was well correlated with the
extent of drug absorption in human subjects, and
that drugs with permeability coefficients exceeding
$1 \times 10^{-6}$ cm/s were completely absorbed (Figure 4.7).
However, Caco-2 cells, being derived from colonic
epithelium, have less paracellular permeability than
jejunal mucosa, and the activity of drug-metabolizing
enzymes, transporters, and efflux mechanisms in these
cells does not always reflect what is encountered *in
vivo*. In addition, the Caco-2 cell model provides no
assessment of the extent of hepatic first-pass metabolism. Despite these shortcomings, this *in vitro* model
has been useful in accelerating biological screening
programs, and further methodological improvements
can be expected [40].

Several alternative methods have been proposed
to characterize drug permeability. Thus, Wu and
Benet [41] observed that Class 1 and 2 drugs are
mainly eliminated by metabolism, whereas Class 3
and 4 drugs are mainly eliminated by biliary or renal
excretion of unchanged drug. On this basis they
proposed an alternate biopharmaceutics drug disposition classification system (BDDCS) in which permeability is replaced by predominant route of
elimination, initially defined as $\geq$ 50% but later 70% or
90% of an oral dose in humans [36]. Wu and Benet [41]
went on to predict that transporter effects would be
minimal for BDDCS Class 1 drugs but would
predominate for Class 2 drugs, that absorptive

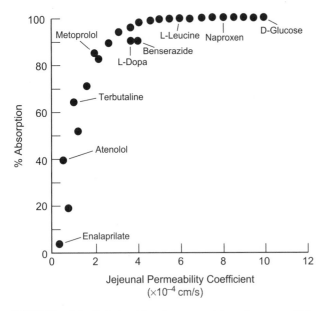

**FIGURE 4.6** Relationship between jejunal permeability
measured by intestinal intubation and extent of absorption of
a series of compounds. Reproduced with permission from Amidon
GL, Lennerås H, Shah VP, Crison JR. Pharm Res 1995;12:413–20 [37].

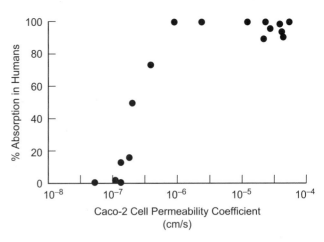

**FIGURE 4.7** Relationship for a series of 20 compounds between
apparent permeability coefficients in a Caco-2 cell model and the
extent of absorption after oral administration to humans. Reproduced with permission from Artursson P, Karlsson J. Biochem Biophys Res Commun 1991;175:880–5 [39].

transporters would be necessary for Class 3 drugs, and that no Class 4 compounds would become effective drugs. Additional predictions also were made regarding the effects of food on the bioavailability of these different drug classes. Although somewhat promising, the BDDCS fails correctly to classify drugs like amoxicillin, trimethoprim, and chloroquine that are highly absorbed even though they are excreted unchanged into urine and bile [36].

The ability of combinatorial chemistry to synthesize large numbers of compounds has stimulated interest in developing *in silico* methods that can predict bioavailability as part of the drug discovery process. In a study of drugs comprising the WHO Essential Medicines List and other widely prescribed drugs, Dahan *et al.* [36] used readily available *in silico* estimates of both log P and ClogP drug *n*-octanol/water partition coefficients as surrogates for permeability. Metoprolol (log P = 1.72) was taken as the cut-off for low- vs high-permeability drugs. Despite the shortcoming that this approach does not account for the effects of transporters on drug absorption, the authors found that it gave results that were sufficiently similar to the established BCS classification to be a useful screen in the preclinical setting of drug discovery. Currently, the most sophisticated method for predicting drug bioavailability utilizes an extremely detailed physiologically-based pharmacokinetic model in which the gastrointestinal tract is divided into nine separate compartments [42]. Drug physicochemical properties and *in vitro* measurements of drug dissolution and metabolism can then be used as inputs to simulate drug absorption in a hypothetical patient population under varying physiological and pathological conditions.

## KINETICS OF DRUG ABSORPTION AFTER ORAL ADMINISTRATION

After drug administration by the oral route, some time passes before any drug appears in the systemic circulation. This lag time ($t_{lag}$) reflects the time required for disintegration and dissolution of the drug product, and the time for the drug to reach the absorbing surface of the small intestine. After this delay, the plasma drug concentration vs time curve shown in Figure 4.3 reflects the combined operation of the processes of drug absorption and of drug distribution and elimination. The peak concentration, $C_{max}$, is reached when drug entry into the systemic circulation no longer exceeds drug removal by distribution to tissues, metabolism, and excretion. Thus, drug absorption is not completed when $C_{max}$ is reached.

In Chapters 2 and 3 we analyzed the kinetic response to a bolus injection of a drug, an input that can be represented by a single impulse. Similarly, the input resulting from administration of an oral or intramuscular drug dose, or a constant intravenous infusion, can be regarded as a series of individual impulses, $G(\theta)d\theta$, where $G(\theta)$ describes the rate of absorption over a time increment between $\theta$ and $\theta + d\theta$. If the system is linear and the parameters are time invariant [43], we can think of the plasma response [$X(t)$] observed at time $t$ as resulting from the sum or integral over each absorption increment occurring at prior time $\theta[G(\theta)d\theta$ where $0 \le \theta \le t$] reduced by the fractional drug disposition that occurs between $\theta$ and $tH(t - \theta)$], that is:

$$X(t) = \int_0^t G(\theta) \cdot H(t - \theta)d\theta$$

The function $H(t)$ describes drug disposition after intravenous bolus administration of a unit dose at time $t$. The interplay of these functions and associated physiological processes is represented schematically in Figure 4.8. This expression for $X(t)$ is termed the *convolution* of $G(t)$ and $H(t)$ and can be represented as:

$$X(t) = G(t) * H(t)$$

where the operation of convolution is denoted by the symbol $*$. The operation of convolution in the time domain corresponds to multiplication in the domain of the subsidiary algebraic equation given by Laplace transformation. Thus, in Laplace transform notation:

$$x(s) = g(s) \cdot h(s)$$

In the disposition model shown in Figure 4.9, the kinetics of drug distribution and elimination are represented by a single compartment with first-order elimination as described by the equation:

$$dH/dt = -kH$$

Since

$$\mathscr{L}F(t) = f(s)$$

and

$$\mathscr{L}F'(t) = sf(s) - F_0$$

$$s\,h(s) - H_0 = -k\,h(s)$$

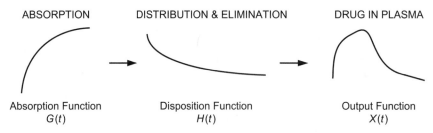

**FIGURE 4.8** The processes of drug absorption and disposition (distribution and elimination) interact to generate the observed time course of drug in the body. Similarly, the output function can be represented as an interaction between absorption and disposition functions.

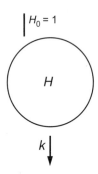

**FIGURE 4.9** Disposition model representing the elimination of a unit impulse drug dose ($H_0 = 1$) from a single body compartment. Drug in this compartment ($H$) is removed as specified by the first-order elimination rate constant $k$.

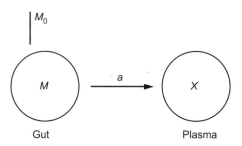

**FIGURE 4.10** Model representing the absorption of a drug dose ($M_0$) from a gut compartment to a plasma compartment. The first-order absorption constant $a$ determines the rate at which drug remaining in the gut ($M$) is transferred to plasma ($X$).

$H_0$ is a unit impulse function, so $h(s)$ is given by:

$$h(s) = \frac{1}{s+k} \qquad (4.3)$$

Although the absorption process is quite complex, it often follows simple first-order kinetics. To obtain the appropriate absorption function, consider absorption under circumstances where there is no elimination [44]. This can be diagrammed as shown in Figure 4.10. In this absorption model, drug disappearance from the gut is described by the equation:

$$\frac{dM}{dt} = -a\,M$$

so

$$M = M_0\,e^{-at}$$

But the rate of drug appearance in plasma is

$$\frac{dX}{dt} = a\,M$$

The absorption function is defined as this rate, so $G(t)$ is:

$$G(t) = a\,M_0 e^{-at}$$

By definition

$$g(s) = \int_0^\infty G(t)e^{-st}\,dt$$

so

$$g(s) = a\,M_0 \int_0^\infty e^{-at}e^{-st}\,dt$$

$$g(s) = -\left.\frac{a\,M_0}{s+a}e^{-(s+a)t}\right|_0^\infty$$

Therefore:

$$g(s) = \frac{a\,M_0}{s+a} \qquad (4.4)$$

Multiplication of Equations 4.3 and 4.4 gives:

$$x(s) = g(s) \cdot h(s) = \frac{a\,M_0}{s+a} \cdot \frac{1}{s+k}$$

and

$$X(t) = \mathscr{L}^{-1}\frac{a\,M_0}{(s+a)(s+k)}$$

The table of inverse Laplace transforms shows that there are two solutions for this equation. Usually, $a \neq k$ and:

$$X(t) = \frac{a\,M_0}{k-a}\left(e^{-at} - e^{-kt}\right) \tag{4.5}$$

In the special case, where $a = k$:

$$X(t) = a\,M_0\,t\,e^{-kt} \tag{4.6}$$

## Time to Peak Level

The time needed to reach the peak level ($t_{max}$) can be determined by differentiating $X(t)$. For $a \neq k$:

$$X'(t) = \left[\frac{a\,M_0}{k-a}\right]\left(-a\,e^{-at} + k\,e^{-kt}\right)$$

At the peak level, $X'(t) = 0$. Therefore:

$$k\,e^{-kt_{max}} = a\,e^{-at_{max}} \tag{4.7}$$

$$a/k = e^{(a-k)t_{max}}$$

and

$$t_{max} = \frac{1}{a-k}\ln(a/k) \tag{4.8}$$

The absorption half-life is another kinetic parameter that can be calculated as $\dfrac{\ln 2}{a}$.

## Value of Peak Level

The value of the peak level ($C_{max}$) can be estimated by substituting the value for $t_{max}$ back into the equation for $X(t)$. For $a \neq k$, we can use Equation 4.7 to obtain:

$$e^{-at_{max}} = \frac{k}{a}\,e^{-kt_{max}}$$

Substituting this result into Equation 4.5:

$$X_{max} = \frac{a\,M_0}{k-a}\left(\frac{k}{a} - 1\right)e^{-kt_{max}}$$

Hence:

$$X_{max} = M_0\,e^{-kt_{max}}$$

But from Equation 4.8:

$$-k\,t_{max} = \frac{k}{k-a}\ln(a/k)$$

so

$$e^{-kt_{max}} = (a/k)^{k/(k-a)}$$

Therefore:

$$X_{max} = M_0(a/k)^{k/(k-a)} \tag{4.9}$$

The maximum plasma concentration would then be given by $C_{max} = X_{max}/V_d$, where $V_d$ is the distribution volume. It can be seen from Equations 4.8 and 4.9 that $C_{max}$ and $t_{max}$ are complex functions of both the absorption rate, $a$, and the elimination rate, $k$, of a drug.

## Use of Convolution/Deconvolution to Assess in Vitro–in Vivo Correlations

Particularly for extended-release formulations, the simple characterization of drug absorption in terms of $AUC$, $C_{max}$ and $t_{max}$ is inadequate and a more comprehensive comparison of in vitro test results with in vivo drug absorption is needed [45]. Both $X(t)$, the output function after oral absorption, and $H(t)$, the disposition function, can be obtained from experimental data, and the absorption function, $G(t)$, estimated by the process of deconvolution. This process is the inverse of convolution and, in the Laplace domain, $g(s)$ can be obtained by dividing the transform of the output function, $x(s)$, by the transform of the disposition function, $h(s)$:

$$g(s) = \frac{x(s)}{h(s)}$$

Since this approach requires that $X(t)$ and $H(t)$ be defined by explicit functions, deconvolution is usually performed using numerical methods [46]. Alternatively, the absorption function can be obtained from a pharmacokinetic model, as shown by the insert in Figure 4.4 [26]. Even when this approach is taken, numerical deconvolution methods may be helpful in developing the appropriate absorption model [31]. As a second step in the analysis, linear regression commonly is used to compare the time course of drug absorption with dissolution test results at common time points, as shown in Figure 4.11 [47]. The linear relationship in this figure, with a slope and a coefficient of determination ($R^2$) of nearly 1, would be expected primarily for Class 1 drugs. The non-zero intercept presumably reflects the time lag in gastric emptying.

Another approach is to convolute a function representing in vitro dissolution with the disposition function in order to predict the plasma-level vs time curve following oral drug administration. Obviously, correlations will be poor if there is substantial

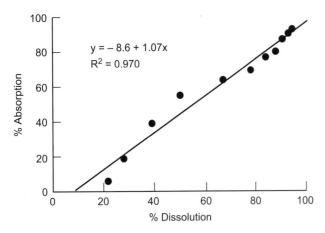

$y = -8.6 + 1.07x$
$R^2 = 0.970$

**FIGURE 4.11** Linear regression comparing the extent of drug dissolution and oral absorption at common time points. Reproduced with permission from Rackley RJ. Examples of *in vitro–in vivo* relationships with a diverse range of quality. In: Young D, Devane JG, Butler J, editors. *In vitro–in vivo* correlations. New York, NY: Plenum Press; 1997. pp. 1–15 [47].

first-pass metabolism of the drug or if *in vivo* conditions, such as rapid intestinal transit that results in inadequate reserve length, are not reflected in the dissolution test system.

## REFERENCES

[1] Tsuji A, Tamai I. Carrier-mediated intestinal transport of drugs. Pharm Res 1996;13:963–77.

[2] Hollander D, Dadugalza VD, Fairchild PA. Intestinal absorption of aspirin: Influence of pH, taurocholate, ascorbate, and ethanol. J Lab Clin Med 1981;98:591–8.

[3] Meldrum SJ, Watson BW, Riddle HC, Sladen GE. pH profile of gut as measured by radiotelemetry capsule. Br Med J 1972;2:104–6.

[4] Wilding IR, Coupe AJ, Davis SS. The role of γ-scintigraphy in oral drug delivery. Adv Drug Del Rev 1991;7:87–117.

[5] Rees WDW, Brown CM. Physiology of the stomach and duodenum. In: Haubrich WS, Schaffner F, Berk JE, editors. Bockus gastroenterology. Philadelphia, PA: WB Saunders; 1995. p. 582–614.

[6] Davis SS, Hardy JG, Fara JW. Transit of pharmaceutical dosage forms through the small intestine. Gut 1986;27:886–92.

[7] Kenyon CJ, Brown F, McClelland, Wilding IR. The use of pharmacoscintigraphy to elucidate food effects observed with a novel protease inhibitor (saquinavir). Pharm Res 1998;15:417–22.

[8] Nimmo I, Heading RC, Tothill P, Prescott LF. Pharmacological modification of gastric emptying: Effects of propantheline and metcolopromide on paracetamol absorption. Br Med J 1973;1:587–9.

[9] Higuchi WI, Ho NFH, Park JY, Komiya I. Rate-limiting steps in drug absorption. In: Prescott LF, Nimmo WS, editors. Drug absorption. Sydney: ADIS Press; 1981. p. 35–60.

[10] Manninen V, Melin J, Apajalahti A, Karesoja M. Altered absorption of digoxin in patients given propantheline and metoclopramide. Lancet 1973;1:398–9.

[11] Dobkin JF, Saha JR, Butler VP Jr, Neu HC, Lindenbaum J. Digoxin-inactivating bacteria: Identification in human gut flora. Science 1983;220:325–7.

[12] Sousa T, Paterson R, Moore V, Carlsson A, Abrahamsson B, Basit AW. The gastrointestinal microbiota as a site for the biotransformation of drugs. Intl J Pharm 2008;363:1–25.

[13] Okuda H, Ogura K, Kato A, Takubo H, Watabe T. A possible mechanism of eighteen patient deaths caused by interactions of sorivudine, a new antiviral drug, with oral 5-fluorouracil prodrugs. J Pharmacol Exp Ther 1998;287:791–9.

[14] Kao A, Kwak K, Das KM. Introducing and maintaining remission in ulcerative colitis: Role of high-dose, extended-release mesalamine. J Clin Gastroenterol 2010;44:531–5.

[15] Welling PG. Interactions affecting drug absorption. Clin Pharmacokinet 1984;9:404–34.

[16] Heizer WD, Smith TW, Goldfinger SE. Absorption of digoxin in patients with malabsorption syndromes. N Engl J Med 1971;285:257–9.

[17] Takano M, Yumoto R, Murakami T. Expression and function of efflux drug transporters in the intestine. Pharmacol Ther 2006;109:137–61.

[18] Dahan A, Amidon GL. Small intestinal efflux mediated by MRP2 and BCRP shifts sulfasalazine intestinal permeability from high to low, enabling its colonic targeting. Am J Physiol Gastrointest Liver Physiol 2009;297:G371–7.

[19] Doherty MM, Charman WN. The mucosa of the small intestine. How clinically relevant as an organ of drug metabolism? Clin Pharmacokinet 2002;41:235–53.

[20] Kolars JC, Merion RM, Awni WM, Watkins PB. First-pass metabolism of cyclosporine by the gut. Lancet 1991;338:1488–90.

[21] Marzolini C, Paus E, Buclin T, Kim R. Polymorphisms in human MDR1 (P-glycoprotein): Recent advances and clinical relevance. Clin Pharmacol Ther 2004;75:13–33.

[22] Thummel KE, Shen DD, Isoherranen N, Smith HE. Design and optimization of dosage regimens: Pharmacokinetic data. In: Bruton LL, Lazo JS, Parker KL, editors. Goodman & Gilman's The pharmacological basis of therapeutics. 11th ed. New York, NY: McGraw-Hill; 2006. p. 1787–8.

[23] Lin JH. Drug–drug interaction mediated by inhibition and induction of P-glycoprotein. Adv Drug Deliv Rev 2003;55:53–81.

[24] Benet LZ. The drug transporter–metabolism alliance: Uncovering and defining the interplay. Mol Pharm 2009:1631–43.

[25] Winne D. Influence of blood flow on intestinal absorption of xenobiotics. Pharmacology 1980;21:1–15.

[26] Atkinson AJ Jr, Ruo TI, Piergies AA, Breiter HC, Connelly TJ, Sedek GS, et al. Pharmacokinetics of N-acetylprocainamide in patients profiled with a stable isotope method. Clin Pharmacol Ther 1989;46:182–9.

[27] Watkins PB. Drug metabolism by cytochromes P450 in the liver and small bowel. Gastroenterol Clin N Amer 1992;21:511–26.

[28] Lippman SB, Nash K. Monamine oxidase inhibitor update. Potential adverse food and drug interactions. Drug Saf 1990;5:195–204.

[29] Koch-Weser J. Bioavailability of drugs. N Engl J Med 1974;291:233–7.

[30] Yeh KC, Kwan KC. A comparison of numerical integrating algorithms by trapezoidal, Lagrange, and spline approximation. J Pharmacokinet Biopharm 1978;6:79–98.

[31] Strong JM, Dutcher JS, Lee W-K, Atkinson AJ Jr. Absolute bioavailability in man of N–acetylprocainamide determined by a novel stable isotope method. Clin Pharmacol Ther 1975;18:613–22.

[32] Lappin G, Rowland M, Garner RC. The use of isotopes in the determination of absolute bioavailability of drugs in humans. Expert Opin Drug Metab Toxicol 2006;2:419–27.

[33] Koch-Weser J. Pharmacokinetics of procainamide in man. Ann NY Acad Sci 1971;179:370–82.

[34] Patnaik RN, Lesko LJ, Chen ML, Williams RL, the FDA Individual Bioequivalence Working Group. Individual bioequivalence: New concepts in the statistical assessment of bioequivalence metrics. Clin Pharmacokinet 1997;33:1–6.

[35] Biopharmaceutic Classification Working Group. Biopharmaceutics Coordinating Committee, CDER. Waiver of *in vivo* bioavailability and bioequivalence studies for immediate-release solid oral dosage forms based on a biopharmaceutics classification system. Guidance for Industry, Rockville: FDA (Internet at, www.fda.gov/downloads/Drugs/Guidance ComplianceRegulatoryInformation/Guidances/UCM070246. pdf; 2000).

[36] Dahan A, Miller JM, Amidon GL. Prediction of solubility and permeability class membership: Provisional BCS classification of the world's top oral drugs. AAPS J 2009;11:740–6.

[37] Amidon GL, Lennerås H, Shah VP, Crison JR. A theoretical basis for a biopharmaceutic drug classification: The correlation of *in vitro* drug product dissolution and *in vivo* bioavailability. Pharm Res 1995;12:413–20.

[38] Rohrs BR, Skoug JW, Halstead GW. Dissolution assay development for *in vitro–in vivo* correlations: Theory and case studies. In: Young D, Devane JG, Butler J, editors. *In vitro–in vivo* correlations. New York, NY: Plenum Press; 1997. p. 17–30.

[39] Artursson P, Karlsson J. Correlation between oral drug absorption in humans and apparent drug permeability coefficients in human intestinal epithelial (Caco-2) cells. Biochem Biophys Res Commun 1991;175:880–5.

[40] Artursson P, Borchardt RT. Intestinal drug absorption and metabolism in cell cultures: Caco–2 and beyond. Pharm Res 1997;14:1655–8.

[41] Wu C-Y, Benet LZ. Predicting drug disposition via application of BCS: Transport/absorption/elimination interplay and the development of a biopharmaceutics drug discposition classification system. Pharm Res 2005;22:11–23.

[42] Jamei M, Turner D, Yang J, Neuhoff S, Polak S, Rostami-Hodjegan A, et al. Population-based mechanistic prediction of oral drug absorption. AAPS J 2009;11:225–37.

[43] Sokolnikoff IS, Redheffer RM. Mathematics of physics and modern engineering. 2nd ed. New York, NY: McGraw-Hill; 1966.

[44] Atkinson AJ Jr, Kushner W. Clinical pharmacokinetics. Ann Rev Pharmacol Toxicol 1979;19:105–27.

[45] Langenbucher F, Mysicka J. *In vitro* and *in vivo* deconvolution assessment of drug release kinetics from oxprenolol Oros preparations. Br J Clin Pharmacol 1985;19:151S–62S.

[46] Vaughan DP, Dennis M. Mathematical basis of point-area deconvolution method for determining *in vivo* input functions. J Pharm Sci 1978;67:663–5.

[47] Rackley RJ. Examples of *in vitro–in vivo* relationships with a diverse range of quality. In: Young D, Devane JG, Butler J, editors. *In vitro–in vivo* correlations. New York, NY: Plenum Press; 1997. p. 1–15.

## STUDY PROBLEMS

1. An approach that has been used during drug development to measure the absolute bioavailability of a drug is to administer an initial dose intravenously in order to estimate the area under the plasma-level vs time curve from zero to infinite time (*AUC*). Subjects then are begun on oral therapy. When steady state is reached, the *AUC* during a dosing interval ($AUC_{0\rightarrow\tau}$) is measured. The extent of absorption of the oral formulation is calculated from the following equation:

$$\% \ Absorption = \frac{D_{IV} \cdot AUC_{0\rightarrow\tau(oral)}}{D_{oral} \cdot AUC_{IV}} \times 100$$

This approach requires AUC to equal $AUC_{0\rightarrow\tau}$ if the same doses are administered intravenously and orally and the extent of absorption is 100%. Derive the proof for this equality.

2. When a drug is administered by constant intravenous administration, this zero-order input can be represented by a "step function". Derive the appropriate absorption function and convolute it with the disposition function to obtain the output function. (*Clue:* Remember that the absorption function is the *rate* of drug administration.)

3. A 70-kg patient is treated with an intravenous infusion of lidocaine at a rate of 2 mg/min. Assume a single-compartment distribution volume of 1.9 L/kg and an elimination half-life of 90 minutes.

   a. Use the output function derived in Problem 2 to predict the expected steady-state plasma lidocaine concentration.

   b. Use this function to estimate the time required to reach 90% of this steady-state level.

   c. Express this 90% equilibration time in terms of number of elimination half-lives.

## COMPUTER-BASED TUTORIALS

Interested readers might find it helpful to access the tutorials and data files that are available free of charge at the following: (http://www.saam.com/case_studies_pharmacokinetic.htm).

Of particular relevance to this chapter are the pharmacokinetic case studies on theophylline kinetics after oral administration and *N*-acetylprocainamide (NAPA) kinetics. The former study illustrates the use of *a priori* identifiability to obtain the appropriate model configuration when more than one mathematical solution exists and provides another example of "flip-flop" kinetics in which the terminal exponential phase of the plasma-level vs time curve in this case reflects slow absorption of theophylline from an extended-release formulation. Data for the latter exercise was taken from the study described in reference [26] in which an oral formulation of NAPA was administered simultaneously with an intravenous dose of NAPA-C[13].

# 5

# Effect of Renal Disease on Pharmacokinetics

**Arthur J. Atkinson, Jr.**[1] **and Juan J.L. Lertora**[2]

[1]*Department of Molecular Pharmacology & Biochemistry, Feinberg School of Medicine, Northwestern University, Chicago, IL 60611*
[2]*Pharmacology Program, Clinical Center, National Institutes of Health, Bethesda, MD 20892*

A 67-year-old man had been functionally anephric, requiring outpatient hemodialysis for several years. He was hospitalized for revision of his arteriovenous shunt and postoperatively complained of symptoms of gastroesophageal reflux. This complaint prompted institution of cimetidine therapy. In view of the patient's impaired renal function, the usually prescribed dose was reduced by half. Three days later, the patient was noted to be confused. An initial diagnosis of dialysis dementia was made and the family was informed that dialysis would be discontinued. On teaching rounds, the suggestion was made that cimetidine be discontinued. Two days later the patient was alert and was discharged from the hospital to resume outpatient hemodialysis therapy.

Although drugs are developed to treat patients who have diseases, relatively little attention has been given to the fact that these diseases themselves exert important effects that affect patient response to drug therapy. Accordingly, the case presented above is an example from the past that illustrates a therapeutic problem that persists today. In the idealized scheme of contemporary drug development shown in Figure 1.1 (Chapter 1), the pertinent information would be generated in pharmacokinetic/pharmacodynamic (PK/PD) studies in special populations that are carried out concurrently with Phase II and Phase III clinical trials [1]. Additional useful information can be obtained by using population pharmacokinetic methods to analyze data obtained in the large-scale Phase III trials themselves [2]. However, a review of labeling in the *Physicians' Desk Reference* indicates that there often is scant information available to guide dose selection for individual patients [3].

Illness, aging, sex, and other patient factors may have important effects on *pharmacodynamic* aspects of patient response to drugs. For example, patients with advanced pulmonary insufficiency are particularly sensitive to the respiratory depressant effects of narcotic and sedative drugs. In addition, these patient factors may affect the *pharmacokinetic* aspects of drug elimination, distribution, and absorption. In this regard, renal impairment has been estimated to account for one-third of the prescribing errors resulting from inattention to patient pathophysiology [4]. Even when the necessary pharmacokinetic and pharmacodynamic information is available, appropriate dose adjustments often were not made for patients with impaired renal function because assessment of this function usually was based solely on serum creatinine measurements without concomitant estimation of creatinine clearance [5]. Fortunately, prescriber awareness of patients with impaired renal function is likely to improve as routine reporting of estimated glomerular filtration rate (GFR) becomes standard clinical laboratory practice [6].

Because there is a large population of functionally anephric patients who are maintained in relatively stable condition by hemodialysis, a substantial number of pharmacokinetic studies have been carried out in these individuals. Patients with intermediate levels of impaired renal function have not been studied to the same extent, but studies in these patients are recommended in current FDA guidelines [7].

## DRUG DOSING IN PATIENTS WITH IMPAIRED RENAL FUNCTION

The effects of decreased renal function on drug elimination have been examined extensively. This is appropriate since only elimination clearance ($CL_E$) and drug dose determine the steady state concentration of drug in the body ($C_{ss}$). This is true whether the drug is given by constant intravenous infusion ($I$), in which case

$$C_{ss} = I/CL_E \qquad (5.1)$$

or by intermittent oral or parenteral doses, in which case the corresponding equation is:

$$\overline{C}_{ss} = \frac{\text{Absorbed Dose}/\tau}{CL_E} \qquad (5.2)$$

where $\overline{C}_{ss}$ is the mean concentration during the dosing interval $\tau$.

For many drugs, $CL_E$ consists of additive renal ($CL_R$) and non-renal ($CL_{NR}$) components, as indicated by the following equation:

$$CL_E = CL_R + CL_{NR} \qquad (5.3)$$

Non-renal clearance is usually equated with drug metabolism and/or transport by the liver, but also could include hemodialysis and other methods of drug removal. In fact, even the metabolic clearance of a drug frequently consists of additive contributions from several parallel metabolic pathways. The characterization of drug metabolism by a clearance term usually is appropriate, since the metabolism of most drugs can be described by first-order kinetics within the range of therapeutic drug concentrations.

Dettli [8] proposed that the additive property of *elimination rate constants* representing parallel elimination pathways provides a way of either using Equation 5.3 or constructing nomograms to estimate the dose reductions that are appropriate for patients with impaired renal function. This approach also can be used to estimate *elimination clearance*, as illustrated for cimetidine in Figure 5.1 [9]. In implementing this approach, creatinine clearance ($CL_{CR}$) has been estimated in adults from the Cockcroft and Gault equation (Equation 1.3) [10], and in pediatric patients from other simple equations (see Chapter 1). Although a more accurate prediction method has been proposed for estimating creatinine clearance in adults [11], as discussed in Chapter 1, its routine adoption for estimating drug dosage remains controversial. Calculations or nomograms for many drugs can be made after consulting tables in Appendix II of Goodman and Gilman [12] or other reference sources to obtain values

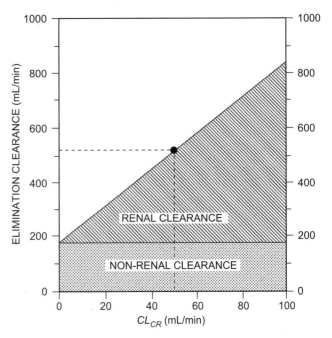

**FIGURE 5.1** Nomogram for estimating cimetidine elimination clearance ($CL_E$) for a 70-kg patient with impaired renal function. The right-hand ordinate indicates cimetidine $CL_E$ measured in young adults with normal renal function, and the left-hand ordinate indicates expected cimetidine $CL_E$ in a functionally anephric patient, based on the fact that 23% of an administered dose is eliminated by non-renal routes in healthy subjects. The *heavy line* connecting these points can be used to estimate cimetidine $CL_E$ from creatinine clearance ($CL_{CR}$). For example, a 70-kg patient with $CL_{CR}$ of 50 mL/min (*large dot*) would be expected to have a cimetidine $CL_E$ of 517 mL/min, and to respond satisfactorily to doses that are 60% of those recommended for patients with normal renal function. Reproduced with permission from Atkinson AJ Jr, Craig RM. Therapy of peptic ulcer disease. In: Molinoff PB, editor. Peptic ulcer disease. Mechanisms and management. Rutherford, NJ: Healthpress Publishing Group, Inc.; 1990. pp. 83–112 [9].

of $CL_E$ and the fractional dose eliminated by renal excretion (percentage urinary excretion) in subjects with normal renal function.

Schentag *et al.* [13] obtained slightly lower estimates of cimetidine percentage urinary excretion in healthy subjects and of $CL_E$ in patients with duodenal ulcer and in older healthy subjects than shown in Figure 5.1, which is based on reports by previous investigators who studied only young adults [14]. Nonetheless, there is apparent internal discrepancy in the labeling for cimetidine [15]. Under "Dosage Adjustment for Patients with Impaired Renal Function", the label states that "Patients with creatinine clearance less than 30 cc/min who are being treated for prevention of upper gastrointestinal bleeding should receive half the recommended dose". However, under "Pharmacokinetics" it indicates that "following I.V. or I.M. administration, approximately

75% of the drug is recovered from the urine after 24 hours as the parent compound". Since only one-fourth of the dose is eliminated by non-renal mechanisms, it can be expected that functionally anephric patients who receive half the usual cimetidine dose, such as the man whose case is described at the beginning of this chapter, will have potentially toxic blood levels that are twice those recommended for patients with normal renal function.

When dose adjustments are needed for patients with impaired renal function, they can be made by reducing the drug dose or by lengthening the dosing interval. Either approach, or a combination of both, may be employed in practice. For example, once the expected value for $CL_E$ has been estimated, the daily drug dose can be reduced in proportion to the quotient of the expected clearance divided by the normal clearance. This will maintain the average drug concentration at the usual level, regardless of whether the drug is administered by intermittent doses or by continuous infusion. On the other hand, it is often convenient to administer doses of drugs that have a short elimination half-life at some multiple of their elimination half-life. The multiple that is used is determined by the therapeutic index of the drug. The expected half-life can be calculated from the following equation:

$$t_{1/2} = \frac{0.693 \ V_{d(area)}}{CL_E} \qquad (5.4)$$

and the usual dose can be administered at an interval equal to the same multiple of the increased half-life. Dose-interval adjustment is usually necessary when safety and efficacy concerns specify a target range for both peak and trough plasma levels, or when selection of drug doses is limited.

The reliability of the Dettli method of predicting drug clearance depends on two critical assumptions:

1. The non-renal clearance of the drug remains constant when renal function is impaired.
2. $CL_E$ declines in a linear fashion with $CL_{CR}$.

There are important exceptions to the first assumption that will be considered when we discuss the effects of impaired renal function on drug metabolism. Nonetheless, this approach is widely used for individualizing drug dosage for patients with impaired renal function. In addition, Equations 5.3 and 5.4 provide a useful tool for hypothesis generation during drug development when pharmacokinetic studies are planned for subjects with impaired renal function.

# EFFECTS OF RENAL DISEASE ON RENAL DRUG EXCRETION MECHANISMS

The important mechanisms involved in the renal excretion and reabsorption of drugs that are summarized in Table 5.1 were extensively reviewed by Reidenberg [16] over 40 years ago, and more recently by Masereeuw and Russel [17].

## Excretion Mechanisms

Glomerular filtration affects all drugs of small molecular size and is *restrictive* in the sense that it is limited by drug binding to plasma proteins. On the other hand, renal tubular secretion is *non-restrictive* since both protein-bound and free drug concentrations in plasma are available for elimination. In fact, the proximal renal tubular secretion of *p*–aminohippurate is rapid enough that its elimination clearance is used to estimate renal blood flow. There are many proteins in renal tubular cells that actively transport compounds against a concentration gradient. These include P-glycoprotein (P-gp), six multiple drug resistance proteins, five cation and nine organic anion transporters, along with a number of genetic variants [18, 19]. The transporters

**TABLE 5.1  Important Mechanisms of Renal Elimination of Drugs**

I.  Glomerular filtration
- Affects all drugs and metabolites of appropriate molecular size
- Influenced by protein binding ($f_u$ = free fraction)
  Drug filtration rate = GFR $\times f_u \times$ [drug]

II.  Renal tubular secretion
- Not influenced by protein binding
- May be affected by competition with other drugs, etc.

   *Examples:*
   Active drugs:       Acids – penicillin
                              Bases – procainamide
   Metabolites:       Glucuronides, hippurates, etc.

III.  Reabsorption by non-ionic diffusion
- Affects weak acids and weak bases
- Only important if excretion of free drug is major elimination path

   *Examples:*
   Weak acids:    Phenobarbital
   Weak bases:    Quinidine

IV.  Active reabsorption
- Affects ions, not proved for other drugs
   *Examples:*
   Halides:          Fluoride, bromide
   Alkaline metals:    Lithium

involved in drug secretion are located at both the baso-lateral membrane of renal tubule cells, where they transport drugs from blood into these cells, and the brush border membrane, where they transport drugs into proximal tubular urine. Despite the progress that has been made in cloning these transporters and in establishing their binding affinities for various model substrates, more work needs to be done to identify which transporters are actually responsible for the renal secretion of most drugs.

Competition by drugs for renal tubular secretion is an important cause of drug–drug interactions. Inhibitors of P-gp slow excretion by this pathway. Anionic drugs compete with other anionic drugs for these active transport pathways, as do cationic drugs for their pathways. When two drugs secreted by the same pathway are given together, the renal clearance of each will be less than when either drug is given alone. For example, methotrexate is actively secreted by renal tubular cells, but its renal clearance is halved when salicylate is co-administered with it [20].

## Reabsorption Mechanisms

Net drug elimination also may be affected by drug reabsorption in the distal nephron, primarily by non-ionic passive diffusion. Because only the non-ionized form of a drug can diffuse across renal tubule cells, the degree of reabsorption of a given drug depends on its degree of ionization at a given urinary pH. For this reason, sodium bicarbonate is administered to patients with salicylate or phenobarbital overdose in order to raise urine pH, thereby increasing the ionization and minimizing the reabsorption of these acidic drugs. This therapeutic intervention also reduces reabsorption by increasing urine flow. Lithium and bromide are examples of drugs that are extensively reabsorbed by active transport mechanisms. Present evidence suggests that lithium is reabsorbed at the level of the proximal tubule by a $Na^+/H^+$ exchanger (NHE-3) at the brush border and extruded into the blood by sodium–potassium ATPase and the sodium bicarbonate cotransporter located at the basolateral membrane [21].

Proximal tubular endocytosis, mediated by the apical cell membrane receptors megalin and cipolin, plays an important role in removing proteins and peptides that pass through glomerular filtration pores [22]. This accounts for the absence of protein in normal urine and for the essential conservation of protein-carrier-bound vitamins and trace elements which are returned to the systemic circulation. However, the absorbed peptides and proteins are degraded by lysosomal proteases within the renal tubular cells. Aminoglycosides are freely filtered at the glomerulus and are nephrotoxic because of their subsequent active uptake by this endocytic receptor complex [23]. The fact that this uptake is saturable accounts for the fact that aminoglycosides are less nephrotoxic when administered as single daily doses rather than when one-third of that dose is given every 8 hours, a phenomenon referred to as *dose-regimen dependency* [24, 25].

## Renal Metabolism

The kidney plays a major role in the clearance of insulin from the systemic circulation, removing approximately 50% of endogenous insulin and a greater proportion of insulin administered to diabetic patients [26]. Insulin is filtered at the glomerulus, reabsorbed by the proximal tubule cell endocytotic mechanism described above, and then degraded by lysosomal proteolytic enzymes. Consequently, insulin requirements are markedly reduced in diabetic patients with impaired renal function. Imipenem and other peptides and peptidomimetics are also filtered at the glomerulus, absorbed by endocytosis, then metabolized by proximal renal tubule cell proteases [27]. Cilastatin, an inhibitor of proximal tubular dipeptidases, is co-administered with imipenem to enhance the clinical effectiveness of this antibiotic. Other examples of renal drug metabolism are provided in the review by Lohr and colleagues [28].

## Analysis and Interpretation of Renal Excretion Data

Renal tubular mechanisms of excretion and reabsorption can be analyzed by stop-flow and other standard methods used in renal physiology, but detailed studies are seldom performed. For most drugs, all that has been done is to correlate renal drug clearance with the reciprocal of serum creatinine or with creatinine clearance. Even though creatinine clearance primarily reflects GFR, it serves as a rough guide to the renal clearance of drugs that have extensive renal tubular secretion or reabsorption. This is a consequence of the glomerulo-tubular balance that is maintained in damaged nephrons by intrinsic tubule and peritubular capillary adaptations that parallel reductions in single nephron GFR [29]. For this reason, $CL_R$ usually declines fairly linearly with reductions in $CL_{CR}$. However, some discrepancies can be expected. For example, Reidenberg *et al.* [30] have shown that with aging, renal secretion of some basic drugs declines more rapidly than GFR. Also studies with N-1-methylnicotinamide, an endogenous marker of renal tubular secretion, have demonstrated some degree of glomerulo-tubular imbalance in patients with impaired renal function [31].

Despite the paucity of detailed studies, it is possible to draw two general mechanistic conclusions from renal clearance values:

1. If renal clearance *exceeds* drug filtration rate (Table 5.1), there is net renal tubular secretion of the drug.
2. If renal clearance *is less than* drug filtration rate, there is net renal tubular reabsorption of the drug.

## EFFECTS OF IMPAIRED RENAL FUNCTION ON NON-RENAL METABOLISM

Most drugs are not excreted unchanged by the kidneys but first are biotransformed to metabolites that then are excreted. Renal failure may not only retard the excretion of these metabolites, which in some cases have important pharmacologic activity, but in some cases alters the non-renal as well as the renal clearance of drugs [32, 33]. Hepatic drug clearance ($CL_H$) is mediated by transporter uptake and excretion mechanisms, as well as by metabolic processes within hepatocytes. In some cases hepatocyte uptake is the rate limiting step in drug elimination, and the expression and uptake function of hepatic organic anion transport polypeptides (OATPs) has been shown to be depressed in an animal model of chronic renal failure whereas P-gp expression appeared to be increased [34]. Subsequently, Sun *et al.* [35] found that $CL_H$ of intravenously administered erythromycin, a drug in which enzyme metabolism accounts for $< 15\%$ of $CL_H$, was markedly reduced in patients with end-stage renal disease and suggested that this might have been the result of depressed OATP function.

Impaired renal function impacts the hepatic clearance of drugs that are metabolized by a number of enzymatic pathways, as indicated in Table 5.2. Both Phase I biotransformations (cytochrome P450 (CYP) and non-CYP enzymes) and Phase II biotransformations (e.g., acetylation by NAT-2, glucuronidation by UGT2B) may be impaired to varying degrees, which are particularly pronounced in patients with end-stage renal disease (ESRD).

Recent attention has been focused primarily on the effects of impaired renal function on the hepatic elimination of drugs that are substrates for CYP enzymes [32, 33]. Rowland Yeo *et al.* [36] have estimated the

**TABLE 5.2  Effect of Renal Disease on Drug Metabolism**

| I. Oxidations | Variably slowed[a] |
|---|---|
| | *Example:* CYP substrates |
| II. Reductions | Slowed |
| | *Example:* Hydrocortisone |
| III. Hydrolyses | |
| • Plasma esterase | Slowed |
| | *Example:* Procaine |
| • Plasma peptidase | Normal |
| | *Example:* Angiotensin |
| • Tissue peptidase | Slowed |
| | *Example:* Insulin |
| IV. Syntheses | |
| • Glucuronide formation | Normal |
| | *Example:* Hydrocortisone |
| • Acetylation | Slowed |
| | *Example:* Procainamide |
| • Glycine conjugation | Slowed |
| | *Example:* Para-aminosalicylic acid |
| • O-Methylation | Normal |
| | *Example:* Methyldopa |
| • Sulfate conjugation | Normal |
| | *Example:* Acetaminophen |

[a]See Figure 5.2.

effect on metabolism of moderate and severe renal impairment for several of these enzymes by back-calculating clinical estimates of $CL_H$ to account for protein and erythrocyte binding for the following drug–CYP enzyme pairs: midazolam–CYP3A4, bufuralol–CYP2D6, bosentan–CYP2C9, theophylline–CYP1A2, omeprazole–CYP2C19, and rosiglitazone–CYP2C8. It can be seen from Figure 5.2 that these enzymes vary in their sensitivity to the adverse effects of impaired renal function, but that the extent of their impairment increases as renal function deteriorates. Relatively little information is available about the effects of impaired renal function on Phase II metabolic pathways. In an early study, Gibson *et al.* [37] found that NAT2-mediated procainamide acetylation in hemodialysis-dependent patients was reduced by 61% in phenotypic slow acetylators and by 69% in rapid acetylators. Subsequently, Kim *et al.* [38] reported that isoniazid acetylation by NAT2 was decreased by 63% in ESRD slow acetylators but by only 23% in rapid acetylators. Osborne *et al.* [39] have shown that Phase II metabolism of morphine to form glucuronide conjugates is reduced by 48% in functionally anephric patients. More importantly, these patients accumulated much higher concentrations of the morphine-6-glucuronide metabolite that is a much more potent narcotic than

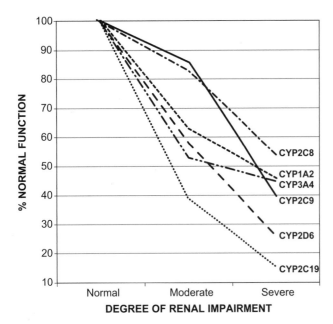

**FIGURE 5.2** Effect of increasing degrees of renal impairment on hepatic clearance mediated by different CYP enzymes. Moderate impairment = $CL_{CR}$ 30–59 mL/min, Severe impairment = $CL_{CR} < 30$ mL/min, – – – – CYP3A4, – – CYP2D6, — CYP2C9, – – – – CYP1A2, ···· CYP2C19, – – – – CYP2C8. Figure based on data from Rowland Yeo K, Aarabi M, Jamei M, Rostami-Hodjegan A. Expert Rev Clin Pharmacol 2011;4:261–74 [36].

morphine. Both of these factors account for the serious adverse events that have been reported in some patients with severely impaired renal function who have been treated with morphine [40].

The effects of impaired renal function on hepatic drug elimination have been attributed to the accumulation of 3–carboxy-4-methyl-5-propyl-2-furan propanoic acid (CMPF), indoxyl sulfate, parathyroid hormone (PTH), cytokines, and perhaps other toxins that inhibit drug metabolism and transport [34, 41, 42]. On the basis of experiments in rodent and *in vitro* models of chronic renal failure it has been shown that impairment occurs in some cases at the level of gene transcription, as indicated by decreased levels of the mRNA that encodes OATP2 [34], a number of CYP enzymes [41], and NAT2 [42]. In attempting to identify the toxin responsible for these effects, Sun *et al.* [35] documented that CMPF and indoxyl sulfate were increased in ESRD patients but found that plasma levels of these uremic toxins were not correlated with the extent to which erythromycin $CL_H$ was decreased. On the other hand, Michaud *et al.* [43] showed that PTH antibodies could prevent the downregulation of CYP mRNA that was observed when rat hepatocytes were incubated with serum from ESRD patients. In subsequent studies, these investigators used this *in vitro* model to further demonstrate that this

downregulation results from PTH stimulation of nuclear factor-κB (NF-κB), since it was prevented by adding andrographolide, an NF-κB inhibitor, to the incubation mixture [44]. This downregulation also was shown to be reversible by hemodialysis, since it did not occur when the hepatocytes were incubated with post-dialysis patient serum. In this regard, it had previously been shown by Nolin *et al.* [45] that hemodialysis increased CYP3A4 activity acutely and by De Martin *et al.* [46] that the elimination clearance of lidocaine, a substrate for CYP1A2 and 3A4, was impaired in ESRD patients not undergoing regular hemodialysis but was normal in dialyzed ESRD patients. However, the fact that the hepatic elimination of many drugs is not normalized by hemodialysis suggests the existence of other important inhibitory mechanisms, and there is a clear need for further study of the effects of impaired renal function on drug metabolism [47].

## EFFECTS OF RENAL DISEASE ON DRUG DISTRIBUTION

Impaired renal function is associated with important changes in the binding of some drugs to *plasma proteins*. In some cases, the *tissue binding* of drugs is also affected.

### Plasma Protein Binding of Acidic Drugs

Reidenberg and Drayer [48] have stated that protein binding in serum from uremic patients is decreased for every acidic drug that has been studied. Most acidic drugs bind to the bilirubin binding site on albumin, but there are also different binding sites that play a role. The reduced binding that occurs when renal function is impaired has been variously attributed to reductions in serum albumin concentration, structural changes in the binding sites, or displacement of drugs from albumin binding sites by organic molecules that accumulate in uremia. As described in Chapter 3, reductions in the protein binding of acidic drugs result in increases in their distribution volume. In addition, the elimination clearance of *restrictively eliminated* drugs is increased. However, protein-binding changes do not affect distribution volume or clearance estimates when they are referenced to unbound drug concentrations. For restrictively eliminated drugs, the term *intrinsic clearance* is used to describe the clearance that would be observed in the absence of any protein-binding restrictions. As discussed in Chapter 7, $CL_H$ for restrictively eliminated drugs, when referenced to total drug concentrations, simply equals the product of the unbound fraction of drug ($f_u$) and this intrinsic clearance ($CL_{int}$):

$$CL_H = f_u \cdot CL_{int} \qquad (5.5)$$

Phenytoin is an acidic, restrictively eliminated drug that can be used to illustrate some of the changes in drug distribution and elimination that occur in patients with impaired renal function. In patients with normal renal function, 92% of the phenytoin in plasma is protein bound. However, the percentage that is unbound or "free" rises from 8% in these individuals to 16% (or more) in hemodialysis-dependent patients. In a study comparing phenytoin pharmacokinetics in normal subjects and uremic patients, Odar-Cederlöf and Borgå [49] administered a single low dose of this drug so that first-order kinetics were approximated. The results shown in Table 5.3 can be inferred from their study.

The uremic patients had an increase in distribution volume that was consistent with the observed decrease in phenytoin binding to plasma proteins. The three-fold increase in hepatic clearance that was observed in these patients also was primarily the result of decreased phenytoin protein binding. Although $CL_{int}$ for this CYP2C9, CYP2C19, and P–gp substrate also appeared to be increased in the uremic patients, the difference did not reach statistical significance at the $P = 0.05$ level.

A major problem arises in clinical practice when only total (protein-bound + free) phenytoin concentrations are measured and used to guide therapy of patients with severely impaired renal function. The decreases in phenytoin binding that occur in these patients result in commensurate decreases in total plasma levels (Figure 5.3). Even though therapeutic and toxic pharmacologic effects are correlated with unbound rather than total phenytoin concentrations in plasma, the decrease in total concentrations can mislead physicians into increasing phenytoin doses inappropriately. Fortunately, rapid ultrafiltration procedures are available that make it possible to

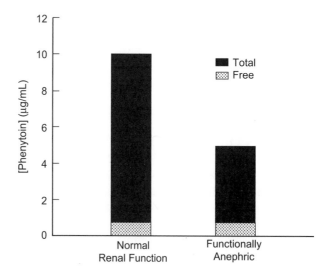

**FIGURE 5.3** Comparison of free and total plasma phenytoin levels in a patient with normal renal function and a functionally anephric patient who are both treated with a 300-mg daily phenytoin dose and have identical $CL_{int}$. Although free phenytoin levels are 0.8 μg/mL in both patients, phenytoin is only 84% bound (16% free) in the functionally anephric patient, compared to 92% bound (8% free) in the patient with normal renal function. For that reason total phenytoin levels in the functionally anephric patient are only 5 μg/mL, whereas they are 10 μg/mL in the patient with normal renal function.

measure free phenytoin concentrations in these patients on a routine basis.

## Plasma Protein Binding of Basic and Neutral Drugs

The protein binding of basic drugs tends to be normal or only slightly reduced [48]. In some cases, this may reflect the facts that these drugs bind to $\alpha_1$-acid glycoprotein and that concentrations of this glycoprotein are higher in hemodialysis-dependent patients than in patients with normal renal function.

## Tissue Binding of Drugs

The distribution volume of some drugs also can be altered when renal function is impaired. As described in Chapter 3, Sheiner *et al.* [50] have shown that impaired renal function is associated with a decrease in digoxin distribution volume that is described by the following equation:

$$V_d \text{ (in L)} = 3.84 \text{ weight (in kg)}$$
$$+ 3.12 \, CL_{CR} \text{ (in mL/min)}$$

This presumably reflects a reduction in tissue levels of Na/K-ATPase, an enzyme that represents a major tissue-binding site for digoxin [51]. In other cases

**TABLE 5.3   Effect of Impaired Renal Function on Phenytoin Kinetics**

|  | Healthy subjects ($n = 4$) | Uremic patients ($n = 4$) |
|---|---|---|
| Percent unbound ($f_u$) | 12% | 26% |
| Distribution volume ($V_{d(area)}$) | 0.64 L/kg | 1.40 L/kg |
| Hepatic clearance ($CL_H$) | 2.46 L/h | 7.63 L/h |
| Intrinsic clearance ($CL_{int}$) | 20.3 L/h | 29.9 L/h |

in which distribution volume is decreased in patients with impaired renal function, the relationship between the degree of renal insufficiency and reduction in distribution volume has not been characterized and neither have plausible mechanisms been proposed.

## EFFECTS OF RENAL DISEASE ON DRUG ABSORPTION

The bioavailability of most drugs that have been studied has not been found to be altered in patients with impaired renal function. However, the absorption of D-xylose, a marker compound used to evaluate small intestinal absorptive function, was slowed (absorption rate constant: $0.555\ h^{-1}$ vs $1.03\ h^{-1}$) and less complete (% dose absorbed: 48.6% vs 69.4%) in patients with chronic renal failure than in healthy subjects [52]. Although these results were statistically significant, there was considerable interindividual variation in both patients and healthy subjects. This primary absorptive defect may explain the fact that patients with impaired renal function have *reduced* bioavailability of furosemide [53] and pindolol [54]. However, it also is possible that impaired renal function will result in *increased* bioavailability of drugs exhibiting first-pass metabolism when the function of drug-metabolizing enzymes is compromised. In this regard, Sun *et al.* [35] observed a 36% increase in erythromycin bioavailability in ESRD patients that was attributed to decreased hepatic extraction rather than any change in gut availability. However, Wood *et al.* [55] found no difference in propranolol absolute bioavailability between healthy subjects and either hemodialyzed or non-dialyzed ESRD patients.

The paucity of reliable bioavailability data in patients with impaired renal function underscores the cumbersome nature of most absolute bioavailability studies in which oral and intravenous drug doses are administered on two separate occasions. The validity of this approach rests on the assumption that the kinetics of drug distribution and elimination remain unchanged in the interval between the two studies – an assumption that obviously is more tenuous for patients than for healthy subjects. As discussed in Chapter 4, these shortcomings can be overcome by conducting a single study in which an intravenous formulation of an isotope-labeled drug is administered simultaneously with the oral drug dose. Radioisotopically labeled propranolol was used by Wood and colleagues [55], but intravenous administration of a stable isotope-labeled drug would currently be preferred for absolute bioavailability studies in patients [56].

## REFERENCES

[1] Yacobi A, Batra VK, Desjardins RE, Faulkner RD, Nicolau G, Pool WR, et al. Implementation of an effective pharmacokinetics research program in industry. In: Yacobi A, Skelly JP, Shah VP, Benet LZ, editors. Integration of pharmacokinetics, pharmacodynamics, and toxicokinetics in rational drug development. New York, NY: Plenum; 1993. p. 125–35.

[2] Peck CC. Rationale for the effective use of pharmacokinetics and pharmacodynamics in early drug development. In: Yacobi A, Skelly JP, Shah VP, Benet LZ, editors. Integration of pharmacokinetics, pharmacodynamics, and toxicokinetics in rational drug development. New York, NY: Plenum; 1993. p. 1–5.

[3] Spyker DA, Harvey ED, Harvey BE, Harvey AM, Rumack BH, Peck CC, et al. Assessment and reporting of clinical pharmacology information in drug labeling. Clin Pharmacol Ther 2000;67:196–200.

[4] Lesar TS, Briceland L, Stein DS. Factors related to errors in medication prescribing. JAMA 1997;277:312–7.

[5] Piergies AA, Worwag EM, Atkinson AJ Jr. A concurrent audit of high digoxin plasma levels. Clin Pharmacol Ther 1994;55:353–8.

[6] Accetta NA, Gladstone EH, DiSogra C, Wright EC, Briggs M, Narva AS. Prevalence of estimated GFR reporting among US clinical laboratories. Am J Kidney Dis 2008;52:778–87.

[7] CDER, CBER. Pharmacokinetics in patients with impaired renal function – study design, data analysis, and impact on dosing and labeling. Draft Guidance for Industry. Rockville: FDA (Internet at, http://www.fda.gov/downloads/Drugs/GuidanceComplianceRegulatoryInformation/Guidances/UCM204959.pdf; 2010).

[8] Dettli L. Individualization of drug dosage in patients with renal disease. Med Clin North Am 1974;58:977–85.

[9] Atkinson AJ Jr, Craig RM. Therapy of peptic ulcer disease. In: Molinoff PB, editor. Peptic ulcer disease. Mechanisms and management. Rutherford, NJ: Healthpress Publishing Group, Inc.; 1990. p. 83–112.

[10] Cockroft DW, Gault MH. Prediction of creatinine clearance from serum creatinine. Nephron 1976;16:31–41.

[11] Stevens LA, Padala S, Levey AS. Advances in glomerular filtration rate-estimating equations. Curr Opin Nephrol Hypertens 2010;19:298–307.

[12] Thummel KE, Shen DD, Isoherranen N. Design and Optimization of Dosage Regimens: Pharmacokinetic Data. In: Brunton LL, Chabner BA, Knollmann BC, editors. Goodman & Gilman's The pharmacological basis of therapeutics. 12th ed. New York, NY: McGraw-Hill; 2011.

[13] Schentag JJ, Cerra FB, Calleri GM, Leising ME, French MA, Bernhard H. Age, disease, and cimetidine disposition in healthy subjects and chronically ill patients. Clin Pharmacol Ther 1981;29:737–43.

[14] Grahnén A, von Bahr C, Lindström B, Rosén A. Bioavailability and pharmacokinetics of cimetidine. Eur J Clin Pharmacol 1979;16:335–40.

[15] Physician's Desk Reference. 59th ed. Montvale, NJ: Medical Economics; 2005.

[16] Reidenberg MM. Renal function and drug actions. Philadelphia, PA: Saunders; 1971.

[17] Masereeuw R, Russel FG. Mechanisms and clinical implications of renal drug excretion. Drug Metab Rev 2001;33:299–351.

[18] International Transporter Consortium Giacomini KM, Huang SM, Tweedie DJ, Benet LZ, Brouwer KL, Chu X, et al. Membrane transporters in drug development. Nat Rev Drug Discov 2010;9:215–36.

[19] Yee SW, Chen L, Giacomini KM. Pharmacogenomics of membrane transporters: Past, present and future. Pharmacogenomics 2010;11:475–9.

[20] Liegler DG, Henderson ES, Hahn MA, Oliverio VT. The effect of organic acids on renal clearance of methotrexate in man. Clin Pharmacol Ther 1969;10:849–57.

[21] Ng LL, Quinn PA, Baker F, Carr SJ. Red cell $Na^+/Li^+$ counter-transport and $Na^+/H^+$ exchanger isoforms in human proximal tubules. Kidney Intl 2000;58:229–35.

[22] Christensen EI, Verroust PJ, Nielsen R. Receptor-mediated endocytosis in renal proximal tubule. Pflugers Arch 2009;458:1039–48.

[23] Quiros Y, Vincente-Vincente L, Morales AI, López-Novoa JM, López-Hernández FJ. An integrative overview on the mechanisms underlying the renal tubular cytotoxicity of gentamicin. Toxicol Sci 2011;119:245–56.

[24] Lui EC-C, Bendayan R. Gentamicin uptake by $LLCPK_1$ cells: Effect of intracellular and extracellular pH changes. Can J Physiol Pharmacol 1998;76:155–60.

[25] Freeman CD, Nicolau DP, Belliveau PP, Nightingale CH. Once-daily dosing of aminoglycosides: Review and recommendations for clinical practice. J Antimicrob Chemother 1997;39:677–86.

[26] Duckworth WC, Bennett RG, Hamel FG. Insulin degradation: Progress and potential. Endocr Rev 1998;19:608–24.

[27] Brater DC. Measurement of renal function during drug development. Br J Clin Pharmacol 2002;54:87–95.

[28] Lohr JW, Willsky GR, Acara MA. Renal drug metabolism. Pharmacol Rev 1998;50:107–41.

[29] Brenner BM. Nephron adaptation to renal injury or ablation. Am J Physiol 1985;249:F324–37.

[30] Reidenberg MM, Camacho M, Kluger J, Drayer DE. Aging and renal clearance of procainamide and acetylprocainamide. Clin Pharmacol Ther 1980;28:732–5.

[31] Maiza A, Waldek S, Ballardie FW, Daley-Yates PT. Estimation of renal tubular secretion in man, in health and disease, using endogenous $N$-1-methylnicotinamide. Nephron 1992;60:12–6.

[32] Nolin TD, Naud J, Leblond FA, Pichette V. Emerging evidence of the impact of kidney disease on drug metabolism and transport. Clin Pharmacol Ther 2008;83:898–903.

[33] Dreisbach AW. The influence of chronic renal failure on drug metabolism and transport. Clin Pharmacol Ther 2009;86:553–6.

[34] Naud J, Michaud J, Leblond FA, Lefrançois S, Bonnardeaux A, Pichette V. Effects of chronic renal failure on liver drug transporters. Drug Metab Disp 2008;36:124–8.

[35] Sun H, Frassetto LA, Huang Y, Benet LZ. Hepatic clearance, but not gut availability, of erythromycin is altered in patients with end-stage renal disease. Clin Pharmacol Ther 2010;87:465–72.

[36] Rowland Yeo K, Aarabi M, Jamei M, Rostami-Hodjegan R. Modeling and predicting drug pharmacokinetics in patients with renal impairment. Expert Rev Clin Pharmacol 2011;4:261–74.

[37] Gibson TP, Atkinson AJ Jr, Matusik E, Nelson LD, Briggs WA. Kinetics of procainamide and $N$-acetylprocainamide in renal failure. Kidney Intl 1977;12:422–9.

[38] Kim Y-G, Shin J-G, Shin S-G, Jang I-J, Kim S, Lee J-S, et al. Decreased acetylation of isoniazid in chronic renal failure. Clin Pharmacol Ther 1993;54:612–20.

[39] Osborne R, Joel S, Grebenik K, Trew D, Slevin M. The pharmacokinetics of morphine and morphine glucuronides in kidney failure. Clin Pharmacol Ther 1993;54:158–67.

[40] Lagas JS, Wagenaar JFP, Huitema ADR, Hillebrand MJX, Koks CHW, Gerdes VEA, et al. Lethal morphine intoxication in a patient with a sickle cell crisis and renal impairment: Case report and a review of the literature. Hum Exp Toxicol 2011;30:1399–403.

[41] Dani M, Boisvert C, Michaud J, Naud J, Lefrançois S, Leblond FA, et al. Down-regulation of liver drug-metabolizing enzymes in a murine model of chronic renal failure. Drug Metab Dispos 2010;38:357–60.

[42] Simard E, Naud J, Michaud J, Leblond FA, Bonnardeaux Guillemette C, Sim E, et al. Downregulation of hepatic acetylation of drugs in chronic renal failure. J Am Soc Nephrol 2008;19:1352–9.

[43] Michaud J, Naud J, Chouinard J, Désy F, Leblodn FA, Desbiens K, et al. Role of parathyroid hormone in the downregulation of liver cytochrome P450 in chronic renal failure. J Am Soc Nephrol 2006;17:3041–8.

[44] Michaud J, Nolin TD, Naud J, Dani M, Lafrance J-P, Leblond FA, et al. Effect of hemodialysis on hepatic cytochrome P450 functional expression. J Pharmacol Sci 2008;108:157–63.

[45] Nolin TD, Appiah K, Kendrick SA, Le P, McMonagle E, Himmelfarb J. Hemodialysis acutely improves hepatic CYP3A4 metabolic activity. J Am Soc Nephrol 2006;17:2363–7.

[46] De Martin S, Orlando R, Bertoli M, Pegoraro P, Palatini P. Differential effect of chronic renal failure on the pharmacokinetics of lidocaine in patients receiving and not receiving hemodialysis. Clin Pharmacol Ther 2006;80:597–606.

[47] Zhang Y, Zhang L, Abraham S, Apparaju S, Wu T-C, Strong JM, et al. Assessment of the impact of renal impairment on systemic exposure of new molecular entities: Evaluation of recent new drug applications. Clin Pharmacol Ther 2009;85:305–11.

[48] Reidenberg MM, Drayer DE. Alteration of drug–protein binding in renal disease. Clin Pharmacokinet 1984;9(Suppl. 1):18–26.

[49] Odar-Cederlöf I, Borgå O. Kinetics of diphenylhydantoin in uremic patients: Consequences of decreased plasma protein binding. Eur J Clin Pharmacol 1974;7:31–7.

[50] Sheiner LB, Rosenberg B, Marathe VV. Estimation of population characteristics of pharmacokinetic parameters from routine clinical data. J Pharmacokinet Biopharm 1977;5:445–79.

[51] Aronson JK, Grahame-Smith DG. Altered distribution of digoxin in renal failure – a cause of digoxin toxicity? Br J Clin Pharmacol 1976;3:1045–51.

[52] Craig RM, Murphy P, Gibson TP, Quintanilla A, Chao GC, Cochrane C, et al. Kinetic analysis of D-xylose absorption in normal subjects and in patients with chronic renal failure. J Lab Clin Med 1983;101:496–506.

[53] Huang CM, Atkinson AJ Jr, Levin M, Levin NW, Quintanilla A. Pharmacokinetics of furosemide in advanced renal failure. Clin Pharmacol Ther 1974;16:659–66.

[54] Chau NP, Weiss YA, Safar ME, Lavene DE, Georges DR, Milliez P. Pindolol availability in hypertensive patients with normal and impaired renal function. Clin Pharmacol Ther 1977;22:505–10.

[55] Wood AJJ, Vestal RE, Spannuth CL, Stone WJ, Wilkinson GR, Shand DG. Propranolol disposition in renal failure. Br J Clin Pharmacol 1980;10:561–6.

[56] Atkinson AJ Jr, Ruo TI, Piergies AA, Breiter HC, Connely TJ, Sedek GS, et al. Pharmacokinetics of $N$-acetylprocainamide in patients profiled with a stable isotope method. Clin Pharmacol Ther 1989;46:182–9.

## STUDY PROBLEM

The following pharmacokinetic data for $N$-acetyl-procainamide (NAPA) were obtained in a Phase I study[1] in which procainamide and NAPA kinetics were compared in volunteers with normal renal function:

Elimination half-life: 6.2 hours
Elimination clearance: 233 mL/min
% Renal excretion: 85.5%

a. Use these results to predict the elimination half-life of NAPA in functionally anephric patients,

---

[1] Dutcher JS, Strong JM, Lucas SV, Lee W-K, Atkinson AJ Jr. Procainamide and $N$–acetylprocainamide kinetics investigated simultaneously with stable isotope methodology. Clin Pharmacol Ther 1977;22:447–57.

assuming that non-renal clearance is unchanged in these individuals.

b. Create a nomogram similar to that shown in Figure 5.1 to estimate the elimination clearance of NAPA that would be expected for a patient with a creatinine clearance of 50 mL/min. Assume that a creatinine clearance of 100 mL/min is the value for individuals with normal renal function.

c. If the usual starting dose of NAPA is 1 g every 8 hours in patients with normal renal function, what would be the equivalent dosing regimen for a patient with an estimated creatinine clearance of 50 mL/min if the dose is decreased but the 8-hour dosing interval is maintained?

d. If the usual starting dose of NAPA is 1 g every 8 hours in patients with normal renal function, what would be the equivalent dosing regimen for a patient with an estimated creatinine clearance of 50 mL/min if the 1-g dose is maintained but the dosing interval is increased?

# Pharmacokinetics in Patients Requiring Renal Replacement Therapy

Arthur J. Atkinson, Jr.[1] and Gregory M. Susla[2]

[1]*Department of Molecular Pharmacology & Biochemistry, Feinberg School of Medicine, Northwestern University, Chicago, IL 60611*
[2]*Medical Information, MedImmune, LLC, Gaithersburg, MD 20878*

Although measurements of drug recovery in the urine enable reasonable characterization of the renal clearance of most drugs, analysis of drug elimination by the liver is hampered by the types of measurements that can be made in routine clinical studies. Hemodialysis and hemofiltration are considered at this point in the text because they provide an unparalleled opportunity to measure blood flow to the eliminating organ, drug concentrations in blood entering and leaving the eliminating organ, and recovery of eliminated drug in the dialysate or ultrafiltrate. The measurements that can be made in analyzing drug elimination by different routes are compared in Table 6.1. Unfortunately, few pharmacokinetic studies in patients undergoing intermittent hemodialysis or continuous renal replacement therapy have incorporated all of the measurements that are shown in the table. However, the US Food and Drug Administration [1] recently has issued draft

guidance that specifies the essential measurements that should be made in these studies, and this approach will be emphasized in this chapter.

Hemodialysis is an area of long-standing interest to pharmacologists. The pioneer American pharmacologist, John Jacob Abel, can be credited with designing the first artificial kidney [2]. He conducted extensive studies in dogs to demonstrate the efficacy of hemodialysis in removing poisons and drugs. European scientists were the first to apply this technique to humans, and Kolff sent a rotating-drum artificial kidney to the United States when the Second World War ended [3, 4]. Repetitive use of hemodialysis for treating patients with chronic renal failure finally was made possible by the development of techniques for establishing long-lasting vascular access in the 1960s. By the late 1970s, continuous peritoneal dialysis had become a therapeutic alternative for these patients and offered the advantages of simpler, non-machine-dependent home therapy and less hemodynamic stress [5]. In 1977, continuous arteriovenous hemofiltration (CAVH) was introduced as a method for removing fluid from diuretic-resistant patients, whose hemodynamic instability made them unable to tolerate conventional intermittent hemodialysis [6]. Since then, this and related techniques have become the preferred treatment modality for critically ill patients with acute renal failure.

Several variations of continuous renal replacement techniques have been developed that use hemodialysis and/or hemofiltration to remove both solutes and fluid, and some of these are listed in Table 6.2 [7]. Also

**TABLE 6.1 Measurements Made in Assessing Drug Elimination by Different Routes**

| Measurements | Renal elimination | Hepatic elimination | Hemodialysis |
|---|---|---|---|
| Blood flow | +[a] | +[a] | + |
| Afferent blood concentration | + | + | + |
| Efferent blood concentration | 0 | 0 | + |
| Recovery of eliminated drug | + | 0 | + |

[a]Not actually measured in routine pharmacokinetic studies

**TABLE 6.2   Summary of Selected Renal Replacement Therapies**

| Procedure | Abbreviation | Diffusion | Convection | Vascular access | Replacement Fluid |
|---|---|---|---|---|---|
| Intermittent hemodialysis | HD | ++++ | + | Fistula or vein—vein | No |
| Intermittent high-flux dialysis | HFD | +++ | ++ | Fistula or vein—vein | No |
| Short-duration daily hemodialysis | SDHD | ++++ | + | Fistula or vein—vein | No |
| Nightly hemodialysis | NHD | ++++ | + | Fistula or vein—vein | No |
| Sustained low-efficiency dialysis | SLED | ++++ | + | Fistula or vein—vein | No |
| Continuous ambulatory peritoneal dialysis | CAPD | ++++ | + | None | No |
| Continuous arteriovenous hemofiltration | CAVH | 0 | ++++ | Artery—vein | Yes |
| Continuous venovenous hemofiltration | CVVH | 0 | ++++ | Vein—vein | Yes |
| Continuous arteriovenous hemodialysis | CAVHD | ++++ | + | Artery—vein | Yes |
| Continuous venovenous hemodialysis | CVVHD | ++++ | + | Vein—vein | Yes |
| Continuous arteriovenous hemodiafiltration | CAVHDF | +++ | +++ | Artery—vein | Yes |
| Continuous venovenous hemodiafiltration | CVVHDF | +++ | +++ | Vein—vein | Yes |

listed are three recently popularized hemodialysis modalities that differ from conventional hemodialysis in that they are administered daily in order to minimize the extent of intradialytic weight gain and changes in body fluid composition. Short-duration daily hemodialysis (SDHD) utilizes only the most productive initial 2 hours during which most low molecular weight solutes are removed during conventional hemodialysis, whereas the 6- to 8-hour duration of nightly hemodialysis (NHD) results in increased phosphate and middle molecule clearance [8]. Sustained low-efficiency dialysis (SLED) provides an alternative to continuous renal replacement therapy for treating patients with acute renal failure and has advantages in that it utilizes conventional dialysis machines and routine dialysate fluids, and affords some patient mobility since it lasts for only 6–12 hours [9]. All of these methods can affect pharmacokinetics, but we will focus on conventional intermittent hemodialysis and selected aspects of continuous renal replacement therapy in this chapter.

## KINETICS OF INTERMITTENT HEMODIALYSIS

### Solute Transfer across Dialyzing Membranes

In Abel's artificial kidney, blood flowed through a hollow cylinder of dialyzing membrane that was immersed in a bath of dialysis fluid. However, in modern hollow-fiber dialysis cartridges, there is a continuous countercurrent flow of dialysate along the outside of the dialyzing membrane that maximizes the concentration gradient between blood and dialysate. Mass transfer across the dialyzing membrane occurs by diffusion and ultrafiltration. The rate of transfer has been analyzed with varying sophistication by a number of investigators [10]. A simple approach is that taken by Eugene Renkin, who likened this transfer process to mass transfer across capillary walls (see Chapter 3) [11]. Renkin expressed dialysis clearance ($CL_D$) as:

$$CL_D = Q\left(1 - e^{-P \cdot S/Q}\right) \qquad (6.1)$$

where $Q$ is blood flow through the dialyzer and $P \cdot S$ is the permeability coefficient—surface area product of the dialyzing membrane, defined by Fick's First Law of Diffusion as:

$$P \cdot S = DA/\lambda$$

In this equation, $A$ is the surface area, $\lambda$ is the thickness of the dialyzing membrane, and $D$ is the diffusivity of a given solute in the dialyzing membrane. Solute diffusivity is primarily determined by molecular weight. Non-spherical molecular shape also may affect the diffusivity of larger molecules. This approach also neglects the effects of ultrafiltration,

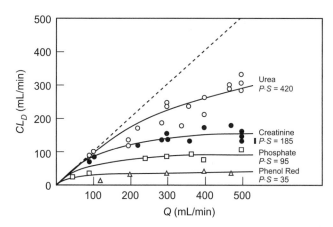

**FIGURE 6.1** Plot of dialysis clearance ($CL_D$) vs dialyzer blood flow ($Q$). The theoretical curves were fit to experimental data points to obtain estimates of the permeability coefficient–surface area product ($P \cdot S$) for each solute. Flow-limited clearance is indicated by the dashed line. The data were generated with a Kolff-Brigham type hemodialysis apparatus. Reproduced with permission from Renkin EM. Tr Am Soc Artific Organs 1956;2:102–5 [11].

**TABLE 6.3** Dialyzer Permeability Coefficient–Surface Area Products for PA and NAPA

| Column | $CL_{PA}$ mL/min | $CL_{NAPA}$ mL/min | $P \cdot S_{PA}$ mL/min | $P \cdot S_{NAPA}$ mL/min | Ratio $P \cdot S_{PA}/P \cdot S_{NAPA}$ |
|---|---|---|---|---|---|
| Dow 4 | 79.9 | 55.3 | 102.0 | 64.7 | 1.58 |
| Dow 5 | 114.6 | 89.9 | 170.2 | 119.4 | 1.43 |
| Gambro 17 | 50.8 | 33.3 | 58.6 | 36.4 | 1.61 |
| ULTRA-FLOW II | 78.5 | 63.8 | 99.7 | 76.8 | 1.30 |
| ULTRA-FLOW 145 | 63.4 | 50.4 | 76.3 | 58.1 | 1.31 |
| VIVACELL | 37.1 | 27.8 | 41.0 | 29.9 | 1.37 |
| Ex 23 | 50.4 | 50.4 | 58.1 | 58.1 | 1.00 |
| Ex 25 | 71.6 | 62.6 | 88.6 | 75.1 | 1.18 |
| Ex 29 | 81.4 | 78.0 | 104.5 | 98.9 | 1.06 |
| Ex 55 | 51.8 | 53.9 | 60.0 | 62.8 | 0.93 |
| **MEAN ± SD** | | | | | 1.28 ± 0.23 |

Clearance data obtained by Gibson *et al.* [12] with dialyzer blood flow set at 200 mL/min and single-pass dialysate flow at 400 mL/min.

non-membrane diffusive resistance, and drug binding to dialysis membranes.

Renkin used Equation 6.1 to estimate $P \cdot S$ values for several solutes from flow and clearance measurements made on the Kolff-Brigham artificial kidney (Figure 6.1). This theoretical analysis seems reasonably consistent with the experimental results. In the figure, the dashed line indicates a flow limitation to transport because clearance can never exceed dialyzer blood flow – a result that is obvious from inspection of Equation 6.1 (i.e., $e^{-P \cdot S/Q}$ is never less than 0).

An analysis of relative dialysis clearance and dialyzer $P \cdot S$ values for the closely related compounds procainamide (PA) and *N*-acetylprocainamide (NAPA) is summarized in Table 6.3. Dialyzer clearance measurements of PA ($CL_{PA}$) and NAPA ($CL_{NAPA}$) made by Gibson *et al.* [12] were used together with Equation 6.1 to calculate $P \cdot S$ values for PA ($P \cdot S_{PA}$) and NAPA ($P \cdot S_{NAPA}$). The ratio of these $P \cdot S$ values is also shown, since this ratio indicates the relative diffusivity of PA and NAPA. The utility of Renkin's approach is confirmed by the fact that the mean $P \cdot S$ ratio of 1.28 ± 0.23 (± SD) is in close agreement with the diffusion coefficient ratio of 1.23 that was obtained for PA and NAPA by the porous plate method of McBain and Liu [13].

## Calculation of Dialysis Clearance

Currently, the efficiency of hemodialysis is expressed in terms of *dialysis clearance*. Dialysis clearance ($Cl_D$) is usually estimated from the Fick equation as follows:

$$CL_D = Q \left[ \frac{A - V}{A} \right] \qquad (6.2)$$

where $A$ is the solute concentration entering (arterial) and $V$ the solute concentration leaving (venous) the dialyzer. This approach to calculating $CL_D$ has been referred to as the $A - V$ *difference* method [14]. The terms in brackets collectively describe what is termed the *extraction ratio* ($E$). As a general principle, clearance from an eliminating organ can be thought of as the product of organ blood flow and extraction ratio.

Single-pass dialyzers are now standard for patient care, and clearance calculations suffice for characterizing their performance. However, recirculating dialyzers were used in the early days of hemodialysis. Dialysis bath solute concentration (*Bath*) had to be considered in describing the performance of recirculating dialyzers and was included in the equation for calculating *dialysance* ($D$), as shown in the following equation [10]:

$$D = Q \left[ \frac{A - V}{A - Bath} \right]$$

Considerable confusion surrounds the proper use of Equation 6.2 to calculate dialysis clearance. There is general agreement that *blood clearance* is calculated when $Q$ is set equal to blood flow and $A$ and $V$ are expressed as blood concentrations. Unfortunately, *plasma clearance* often is obtained by setting $Q$ equal to plasma flow and expressing $A$ and $V$ as plasma concentrations. In fact, this estimate of plasma clearance usually results in erroneous clearance estimates that are not comparable to plasma clearance calculated by standard pharmacokinetic techniques for other eliminating organs [15]. This error occurs because, when $Q$ is set equal to plasma flow through the dialyzer, this approach yields valid clearance estimates only for those few solutes that are totally excluded from red blood cells.

This dilemma is best avoided by calculating dialysis clearance using an equation that is analogous to the equation used to determine renal clearance:

$$CL_P = \frac{C_D \cdot Vol_D}{P \cdot t} \qquad (6.3)$$

where the amount of drug recovered by dialysis is calculated as the product of the drug concentration in dialysate ($C_D$) and total volume of dialysate ($Vol_D$) collected during the dialysis time ($t$), and $P$ is the average concentration of drug in plasma entering the dialyzer. The term *recovery clearance* has been coined for this clearance estimate, and it is regarded as the "gold standard" of dialysis clearance estimates [16].

Equation 6.3 provides an estimate of dialysis plasma clearance ($CL_P$) that is *pharmacokinetically consistent* with estimates of elimination and inter-compartmental clearance that are based on plasma concentration measurements. On the other hand, if the average drug concentration in blood entering the dialyzer ($B$) is substituted for $P$, a valid estimate of blood clearance ($CL_B$) is obtained:

$$CL_B = \frac{C_D \cdot Vol_D}{B \cdot t} \qquad (6.4)$$

We can use these recovery clearances to examine the *effective* flow of plasma ($Q_{EFF}$) that is needed if Equation 6.2 is to yield an estimate of dialysis clearance that is consistent with the corresponding recovery clearance value. Since $CL_B = Q_B E$, it follows from Equation 6.4 that:

$$\frac{C_D \cdot Vol_D}{B \cdot t} = Q_B E$$

Rearranging,

$$\frac{C_D \cdot Vol_D}{E \cdot t} = Q_B B$$

But from Equation 6.3,

$$\frac{C_D \cdot Vol_D}{t} = CL_P P$$

Therefore,

$$CL_P/E = Q_B \cdot B/P$$

However, $CL_P = Q_{EFF} \cdot E$. So,

$$Q_{EFF} = Q_B \cdot B/P$$

For drugs like NAPA that partition preferentially into red blood cells and are fully accessible to the dialyzer from both plasma and erythrocytes, the effective plasma flow will not be less than but will *exceed* measured blood flow [15].

Some authorities argue that it is improper to combine organ *blood* flow and *plasma* concentrations in Equation 6.2 [10, 16]. However, in many cases the ratio of red cell/plasma drug concentrations remains constant over a wide concentration range, so the same estimate of extraction ratio is obtained regardless of whether plasma concentrations or blood concentrations are measured.

As shown in Figure 6.2, pharmacokinetic models can be constructed that incorporate all the measurements made during hemodialysis [17]. For this purpose, it is convenient to rearrange Equation 6.2 to the form:

$$V = [(Q_{PK} - CL_D)/Q_{PK}] \cdot A \qquad (6.5)$$

where $Q_{PK}$ is the pharmacokinetically calculated flow of blood or plasma through the dialysis machine. Since $CL_D$ is calculated from the recovery of drug in dialysis

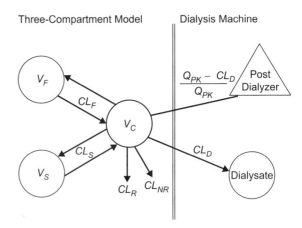

**FIGURE 6.2** Multicompartmental system for modeling pharmacokinetics during hemodialysis. Drug is delivered to the dialysis machine from the central compartment ($V_C$) and represents $A$ in the Fick Equation. The dialysis machine is modeled by a compartment representing drug recovery in dialysis bath fluid and a proportionality (*triangle*) representing the drug concentration in blood returning to the patient.

bath fluid, an estimate of $Q_{PK}$ can be obtained from the observed ratio of $V/A$ (Equation 6.5 and Figure 6.2).

In a study of NAPA hemodialysis kinetics, blood flow measured through the dialyzer averaged 195 mL/min [17]. When evaluated by paired $t$ test this was significantly less than $Q_{PK}$, which averaged 223 mL/min. However, $Q_{PK}$ was similar to estimates of $Q_{EFF}$, which averaged 217 mL/min. In this case NAPA concentrations in erythrocytes were 1.5 times as high as in plasma, and this preferential distribution of drug into red blood cells enhanced drug removal by hemodialysis. Unfortunately, most hemodialysis studies have not incorporated the full range of readily available measurements in an integrated pharmacokinetic analysis.

## Patient Factors Affecting Hemodialysis of Drugs

Because elimination clearances are additive, total solute clearance during hemodialysis ($CL_T$) can be expressed as the sum of dialysis clearance ($CL_D$), and the patient's renal clearance ($CL_R$) and non-renal clearance ($CL_{NR}$):

$$CL_T = CL_D + CL_R + CL_{NR} \qquad (6.6)$$

When $CL_D$ is small relative to the sum of $CL_R$ and $CL_{NR}$, hemodialysis can be expected to have little impact on the overall rate of drug removal. The extent of drug binding to plasma proteins is the most important patient factor affecting dialysis clearance of most drugs, and in that sense dialysis clearance is restrictive. However, partitioning into erythrocytes has been shown to enhance rather than retard the clearance of at least some drugs. A large distribution volume also reduces the fraction of total body stores of a drug that can be removed by hemodialysis, and limits the effect of hemodialysis on shortening drug elimination half-life since:

$$t_{1/2} = \frac{0.693 \ V_d}{CL_T}$$

An assumption made in the analysis of most hemodialysis studies is that drug distribution and elimination kinetics remain unchanged during this procedure. However, Nolin *et al.* [18] used the erythromycin breath test to show that hepatic CYP3A4 activity increases by 27% as early as 2 hours after hemodialysis, presumably reflecting the dialytic removal of low molecular weight uremic toxins that inhibit cytochrome P450 activity. Finally, there are significant hemodynamic changes during hemodialysis that not only may affect the extent of drug removal by this procedure but also may have an important impact on patient response.

### Hemodynamic Changes during Dialysis

Few studies of pharmacokinetics during hemodialysis have utilized the recovery method of calculating dialysis clearance that is necessary to evaluate the impact of hemodynamic changes that may affect the efficiency of this procedure. The fall in both $A$ and $V$ drug concentrations that occurs during hemodialysis is generally followed by a post-dialysis rebound, as shown for NAPA in Figure 6.3. However, if no change in drug distribution is assumed, two discrepancies are likely to be encountered when the recovery method is incorporated in an integrated analysis of hemodialysis kinetics:

1. The total amount of drug recovered from the dialysis fluid is less than would be expected from the drop in plasma concentrations during hemodialysis.
2. The extent of the rebound in plasma levels is less than would be anticipated.

The only single parameter change that can resolve these discrepancies is a reduction in the intercompartmental clearance for the slowly equilibrating compartment ($CL_S$). This is illustrated in the bottom panel of Figure 6.3, and in this study the extent of reduction in $CL_S$ was found to average 77% during hemodialysis [17]. This figure also shows that a reduction in $CL_S$ persisted for some time after hemodialysis was completed.

The hemodynamic basis for these changes in $CL_S$ was investigated subsequently in a dog model [19]. Urea and inulin were used as probes, and were injected simultaneously 2 hours before dialysis. The pharmacokinetic model shown in Figure 6.2 was used for data analysis, and representative results are shown in Figure 6.4. During hemodialysis, $CL_S$ for urea and inulin fell on average to 19% and 63% of their respective predialysis values, and it was estimated that the efficiency of urea removal was reduced by 10%. In the 2 hours after dialysis, urea $CL_S$ averaged only 37% of predialysis values but returned to its predialysis level for inulin. Compartmental blood flow and permeability coefficient–surface area products of the calculated intercompartmental clearances were calculated as described in Chapter 3 from the permeability-flow equation derived by Renkin [20]. During and after dialysis, blood flow to the slow equilibrating compartment ($Q_S$) on average was reduced to 10% and 20%, respectively, of predialysis values. The permeability coefficient–surface area product did not change significantly. There were no changes in either fast compartment blood flow or permeability coefficient–surface

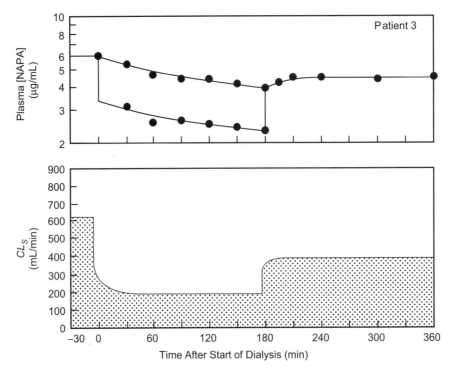

**FIGURE 6.3** Computer-fitted curves from pharmacokinetic analysis of NAPA plasma concentrations (●) measured before, during and after hemodialysis. NAPA plasma concentrations entering (*A*) and leaving (*V*) the artificial kidney are shown during dialysis. The bottom panel shows changes occurring in slow compartment intercompartmental clearance ($CL_S$) during and after dialysis. Reproduced with permission from Stec GP, Atkinson AJ Jr, Nevin MJ *et al.* Clin Pharmacol Ther 1979;26:618–28 [17].

area product. Measurements of plasma renin activity in these dogs with intact kidneys (lower panel of Figure 6.4) suggest that these hemodynamic changes, both during and after hemodialysis, were mediated at least in part by the renin–angiotensin system.

Since the slow equilibrating compartment is largely composed of skeletal muscle, it is not surprising that the hemodynamic changes associated with hemodialysis result in the skeletal muscle cramps that have been estimated to complicate more than 20% of hemodialysis sessions [21]. Plasma volume contraction appears to be the initiating event which triggers blood pressure homeostatic responses. Those patients who are particularly prone to cramps appear to have a sympathetic nervous system response to this volume stress that is not modulated by activation of a normal renin–angiotensin system [22].

## KINETICS OF CONTINUOUS AND SUSTAINED RENAL REPLACEMENT THERAPY

Hemofiltration is a prominent feature of many continuous renal replacement therapies (Table 6.2).

However, continuous hemodialysis can also be employed to accelerate solute removal [23]. The contribution of both processes to extracorporeal drug clearance will be considered separately in the context of continuous renal replacement therapy.

### Clearance by Continuous Hemofiltration

Hemofiltration removes solutes by convective mass transfer down a hydrostatic pressure gradient [24, 25]. As plasma water passes through the hemofilter membrane, solute is carried along by solvent drag. Convective mass transfer thus mimics the process of glomerular filtration. The pores of hemofilter membranes are larger than those of dialysis membranes, and permit passage of solutes having a molecular weight of up to 50 kDa. Accordingly, a wider range of compounds will be removed by hemofiltration than by hemodialysis. Since large volumes of fluid are removed, fluid replacement solutions need to be administered at rates exceeding 10 L/day [26]. This fluid can be administered either before (predilution mode) or after (postdilution mode) the hemofilter. In contemporary practice, roller pumps are used to generate the hydrostatic driving force for

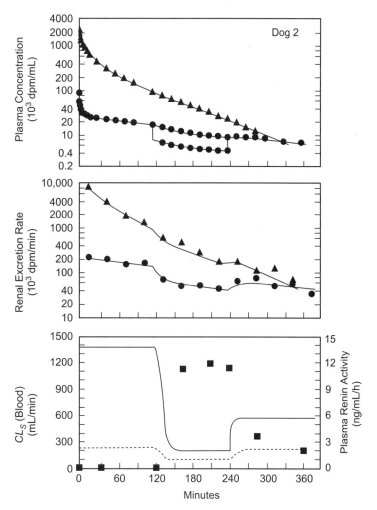

**FIGURE 6.4**  Kinetic analysis of urea $^{14}$C (●) and inulin $^{3}$H (▲) plasma concentrations (*upper panel*) and renal excretion rates (*middle panel*) before, during, and after dialysis of a dog with intact kidneys. Inulin was not dialyzable but urea concentrations entering and leaving the dialyzer are both shown. The *lower panel* shows $CL_S$ estimates for urea (——) and inulin (– – –), and measured plasma renin activity (■). Reproduced with permission from Bowsher DJ, Krejcie TC, Avram MJ *et al.* J Lab Clin Med 1985;105:489–97 [19].

ultrafiltration, and the need for arterial catheterization has been obviated by the placement of double-lumen catheters into a large vein [23].

Albumin and other drug-binding proteins do not pass through the filtration membrane, so only unbound drug in plasma water is removed by ultrafiltration. In addition, albumin and other negatively charged plasma proteins exert a Gibbs-Donnan effect that retards the transmembrane convection of some polycationic drugs, such as gentamicin [27, 28]. The situation with regard to erythrocyte drug binding is less clear. Although predilution reduces the efficiency of solute removal because solute concentrations in the hemofilter are less than in plasma water [29], it has been reported that net urea

removal is enhanced when replacement fluid is administered in the predilution mode, because it can diffuse down its concentration gradient from red blood cells into the diluted plasma water before reaching the hemofilter [26].

The extent to which a solute is carried in the ultrafiltrate across a membrane is characterized by its *sieving coefficient*. An approximate equation for calculating sieving coefficients (*SC*) is:

$$SC = \frac{UF}{A} \qquad (6.7)$$

where *UF* is the solute concentration in the ultrafiltrate and *A* is the solute concentration in plasma water entering the hemofilter [30]. The convective clearance of solute across an ultrafilter ($CL_{UF}$) is given by the product of $SC$ and the rate at which fluid crosses the ultrafilter ($UFR$):

$$CL_{UF} = SC \cdot UFR \qquad (6.8)$$

Since $UFR$ cannot exceed blood flow through the hemofilter, that establishes the theoretical upper limit for $CL_{UF}$. The major determinants of $SC$ are molecular size and the unbound fraction of a compound in plasma water. Values of $SC$ may range from 0 for macromolecules that do not pass through the pores of the hemofilter membrane, to 1 for small molecule drugs that are not protein bound. Although less information has been accumulated about the ultrafiltration clearance of drugs than about their dialysis clearance, in many cases the unbound fraction of drug in plasma water can be used to approximate $SC$.

Measured values of $SC$ and fraction of unbound drug in plasma ($f_u$) are compared for several drugs in Figure 6.5. Values of $f_u$ and $SC$ were taken from data published by Golper and Marx [28], with the following exceptions. For both theophylline and phenytoin, measurements of $f_u$ are much higher in serum from uremic patients than in serum from normal subjects, and agree more closely with experimental values of $SC$. Accordingly, uremic patient $f_u$ values for theophylline [31] and phenytoin [32] were chosen for the figure, as well as values of $SC$ that were obtained in clinical studies of ceftazidime [33], ceftriaxone [34],

ciprofloxacin [35], cyclosporine [36], and phenytoin [32]. The fact that $SC$ values for gentamicin and vancomycin are less than expected on the basis of their protein binding reflects the retarding Gibbs-Donnan effect referred to previously [27, 28]. On the other hand, $SC$ values for cyclosporine and ceftazidime are considerably greater than expected from $f_u$ measurements. Hence, factors other than plasma protein binding may affect the sieving of some drugs during hemofiltration [37].

## Clearance by Continuous Hemodialysis and SLED

Some of the renal replacement therapies listed in Table 6.2 incorporate continuous hemodialysis, or a combination of continuous hemofiltration and hemodialysis. Continuous hemodialysis differs importantly from conventional intermittent hemodialysis and SLED in that the flow rate of dialysate is much lower than countercurrent blood flow through the dialyzer. As a result, concentrations of many solutes in dialysate leaving the dialyzer ($C_D$) will have nearly equilibrated with their plasma concentrations in blood entering the dialyzer ($C_P$) [23, 38]. The extent to which this equilibration is complete is referred to as the *dialysate saturation* ($S_D$), and is calculated as the following ratio:

$$S_D = \frac{C_D}{C_P}$$

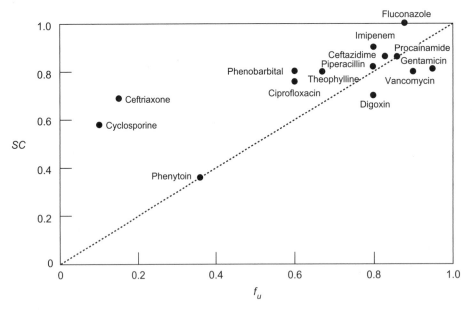

**FIGURE 6.5** Relationship between free fraction ($f_u$) and hemofiltration sieving coefficient ($SC$) for selected drugs. The line of identity (*dashed line*) indicates what would be expected if $SC$ were equal to $f_u$. (See text for further details).

Under conditions of minimal ultrafiltration, diffusive drug clearance ($CL_D$) is calculated from the equation:

$$CL_D = Q_D \cdot S_D \qquad (6.9)$$

Because $Q_D = V_D / t$, Equation 6.9 can be re-written as follows:

$$CL_D = \frac{C_D \cdot V_D}{C_P \cdot t} \qquad (6.10)$$

which is identical to Equation 6.3. Both Equations 6.10 and 6.3 are non-mechanistic descriptions of clearance that do not incorporate the factors of molecular size or protein binding that account for incomplete equilibration of plasma and dialysate solute concentrations. However, in contrast with intermittent hemodialysis, in which dialyzer blood flow is rate limiting, diffusive drug clearance during continuous renal replacement therapy is limited by dialysate flow ($Q_D$), which typically is only 25 mL/min. Another important characteristic of dialysate saturation is that it becomes progressively less complete as dialysate flow approaches blood flow [23]. Few studies have been conducted in which SLED is compared with other modalities, but the *SC* of linezolid during SLED is similar to CVVH, although higher than with intermittent hemodialysis [39].

## Extracorporeal Clearance during Continuous Renal Replacement Therapy

Extracorporeal clearance during continuous renal replacement therapy ($CL_{EC}$) can be regarded as the sum of convective and hemodialytic clearance [23, 38]:

$$CL_{EC} = SC \cdot UFR + Q_D \cdot S_D \qquad (6.11)$$

Because solute diffusivity decreases with increasing molecular weight, diffusion becomes relatively inefficient even with large-pore hemofilter membranes, and convection becomes the primary mechanism involved in the extracorporeal clearance of vancomycin (MW: 1448 Da) and other high molecular weight drugs [29]. Unfortunately, ultrafiltration rate (*UFR*) tends to decrease with time, falling rather rapidly during the first 6 hours of therapy and reaching about half of its original value in approximately 20 hours [23]. Conversely, drug adsorption to the dialyzer membrane may decrease during therapy, resulting in an increase in the sieving coefficient (*SC*) [40]. For these reasons, estimates of extracorporeal drug clearance during continuous renal replacement therapy are

**TABLE 6.4  Factors Affecting the Extent of Drug Removal by Renal Replacement Therapy**

**Characteristics of hemodialysis or hemofiltration**
- Extracorporeal clearance ($CL_{EC} = CL_D + CL_{UF}$)
- Duration of hemodialysis or hemofiltration

**Patient characteristics**
- Distribution volume of drug
- Drug binding to plasma proteins
- Drug partitioning into erythrocytes
- Reduction in intercompartmental clearance

most reliable when made from measurements of drug recovery in dialysate, as discussed for conventional hemodialysis. Under conditions of combined dialysis and ultrafiltration, extracorporeal clearance still can be calculated using the recovery method. Thus,

$$CL_{EC} = \frac{C_D \cdot V_{UF}}{C_P \cdot t} \qquad (6.12)$$

By analogy with Equation 6.6, the contribution of $CL_{EC}$ to total solute clearance during continuous renal replacement therapy is given by:

$$CL_T = CL_{EC} + CL_R + CL_{NR} \qquad (6.13)$$

## CLINICAL CONSIDERATIONS

From the clinical standpoint, the two main pharmacokinetic considerations regarding renal replacement therapy deal with the use of these therapeutic modalities to treat drug toxicity and, more frequently, the need to administer supplemental drug doses to patients whose impaired renal function necessitates intervention. The factors that determine the extent of drug removal by renal replacement therapy are summarized in Table 6.4. As yet, there has been no attempt to analyze the interaction of all these factors with sufficient rigor to provide precise guidelines for clinical practice. However, extensive protein binding and large distribution volume are the most important factors limiting the extent to which most drugs are removed by hemodialysis or hemofiltration. Accordingly, neither conventional intermittent hemodialysis nor continuous renal replacement therapy will significantly enhance the removal of drugs such as phenytoin, which is extensively bound to plasma proteins, or digoxin, which has a large distribution volume.

Reduction in intercompartmental clearance during hemodialysis may result in a greater than expected decrease in drug concentrations in plasma and rapidly-equilibrating tissues, since hemodynamic changes during hemodialysis may effectively sequester a substantial amount of drug in skeletal muscle. This tourniquet-like effect, and its persistence in the post-dialysis period, may be useful in treating patients with central nervous system or cardiovascular toxic reactions to drugs [41]. Although inter-compartmental clearance has not been studied during continuous renal replacement therapy or SLED, these modalities produce less hemodynamic instability and would be expected to provoke a smaller cardiovascular homeostatic response.

## Drug Dosing Guidelines for Patients Requiring Renal Replacement Therapy

Drug doses need to be increased or supplemented for patients requiring renal replacement therapy only if $CL_{EC}$, representing extracorporeal clearance from either intermittent hemodialysis or continuous renal replacement therapy, is substantial when compared to $CL_R + CL_{NR}$ (Equations 6.6 and 6.13). Levy [42] has proposed that supplementation is needed only when $CL_{EC}$ is greater than 30% of $CL_R + CL_{NR}$. Several approaches will be considered that can be used to make appropriate drug dose adjustments for patients requiring renal replacement therapy.

Perhaps the simplest approach is to guide dosage using standard reference tables, such as those published by Aronoff and colleagues [43]. These tables are based on published literature and suggest drug dose reductions for adult and pediatric patients with various levels of renal impairment, as well as for patients requiring conventional hemodialysis, chronic ambulatory peritoneal dialysis, and continuous renal replacement therapy. Unfortunately, there is considerable variation in dialyzer membrane characteristics and surface area, so estimates of $CL_D$ obtained with any one dialyzer usually do not reflect the performance of other dialyzers. In particular, data obtained before the development of high-efficiency and high-flux membranes may no longer be clinically useful. It has been proposed that a suitable standard compound could be selected for *in vitro* studies, such as that described by Gibson *et al.* [12], so that Equation 6.1 could be used to facilitate the extrapolation of results to different dialyzers [15].

Although fewer data are available for patients treated with continuous renal replacement therapy than with conventional intermittent hemodialysis, *UFR* generally ranges from 10 to 16 mL/min during hemofiltration without extracorporeal blood pumping and from 20 to 30 mL/min when blood pumps are used

[28]. Accordingly, for many drugs, the dose recommendation for patients treated with continuous renal replacement therapy is considered simply to be that which is appropriate for patients with a glomerular filtration rate of 10–50 mL/min. For patients undergoing SLED for 6–12 hours per day, doses of renally eliminated drugs such as antibiotics should be adjusted for a creatinine clearance of 10–50 mL/min [44].

A second approach is to calculate supplemental doses to replace drug lost during hemodialysis or continuous renal replacement therapy by directly measuring drug loss by extracorporeal removal or by estimating this loss from drug levels measured in plasma [28, 30]. It is relatively easy to make repeated plasma level measurements of some drugs, and to use these to refine supplemental dose estimates. In this case, the supplemental dose ($D_{sup}$) can be estimated from a plasma level measured at the conclusion of dialysis, or at a convenient interval during continuous renal replacement therapy ($C_{measured}$):

$$D_{sup} = (C_{target} - C_{measured})V_d \qquad (6.14)$$

Gentamicin, theophylline, and vancomycin are several drugs for which plasma concentration measurements are routinely available and can be used to provide a more accurate assessment of dosing requirements when these drugs are used to treat patients requiring renal replacement therapy.

In the setting of conventional intermittent hemodialysis, caution is warranted when using this method to estimate doses of drugs that have a narrow therapeutic index because drug redistribution to the intravascular space from the periphery is slowed by the marked hemodynamic changes that occur during and for some time after hemodialysis, so Equation 6.14 is likely to overestimate the supplemental dose that is needed [17]. For example, Pollard *et al.* [45] reported that the postdialysis rebound in serum vancomycin concentrations following high-flux hemodialysis ranged from 19% to 60% of the intradialytic concentration drop and did not peak for an average of 6 hours (range: 1–12 h). On the other hand, Equation 6.14 provides a reasonably reliable guide to drug dosing during continuous renal replacement therapy and SLED because hemodynamic changes are minimized and the rate of drug removal by these modalities is usually less than the rate of drug redistribution from the periphery. For example, postdialysis rebound in patients on SLED has been reported to be < 4% for gentamicin [46] and < 10% for vancomycin [47]. Thus, serum trough levels should be measured immediately after SLED to determine if post-SLED supplemental doses are needed [44]. For medications that are significantly removed during dialysis, specifically antimicrobials administered every 24 hours, the daily dose or a supplemental dose should be administered immediately after SLED. For dialyzable agents that require administration every 12 hours, supplemental doses should be administered after SLED and 12 hours later [44].

An exception to this approach is that *postdialysis* dosing is suboptimal for therapy with gentamicin and other drugs that exhibit concentration-dependent antibiotic efficacy, a prolonged post-antibiotic effect, and increased toxicity when trough levels are elevated [48, 49]. Doses of these drugs should be administered 2–6 hours *before* intermittent hemodialysis in order to achieve optimally effective peak levels. Subsequent dialysis then acts to minimize trough antibiotic concentrations.

A third approach is to use the principles discussed above to calculate a maintenance dose multiplication factor (*MDMF*) that can be used to augment the dose that would be appropriate in the absence of renal replacement therapy [40]. For continuous renal replacement therapy, *MDMF* is given simply by the following ratio of clearances:

$$MDMF = \frac{CL_{EC} + CL_R + CL_{NR}}{CL_R + CL_{NR}} \quad (6.15)$$

The relative time on ($t_{ON}$) and off ($t_{OFF}$) extracorporeal therapy during a dosing interval also must be taken into account for conventional hemodialysis and other intermittent interventions such as SLED. In this situation:

$$MDMF$$

$$= \frac{(CL_{EC} + CL_R + CL_{NR})t_{ON} + (CL_R + CL_{NR})t_{OFF}}{(CL_R + CL_{NR})(t_{ON} + t_{OFF})}$$

$$MDMF = \left(\frac{CL_{EC}}{CL_R + CL_{NR}}\right)\left(\frac{t_{ON}}{t_{ON} + t_{OFF}}\right) + 1 \quad (6.16)$$

Estimates of *MDMF* for several drugs are listed in Table 6.5. With the exception of vancomycin, baseline drug clearance values for functionally anephric patients ($CL_{aneph.}$) are taken from either the intermittent hemodialysis or the continuous renal replacement references that are cited. In the first 2 weeks after the onset of acute renal failure, vancomycin $CL_{aneph.}$ falls from approximately 40 mL/min to the value of 6.0 mL/min that is found in patients with chronic renal failure [50]. This latter value is included in Table 6.5 (the abbreviations used for treatment modality are defined in Table 6.2). In the studies of intermittent hemodialysis, $CL_{EC}$ was calculated by the recovery method except for the studies of ceftazidime [51], ceftriaxone [52], and ciprofloxacin [53], in which this clearance was estimated from the reduction in elimination half-life during dialysis. Equation 6.15 was used to estimate *MDMF* for a dialysis time of 4 hours during a single 24-hour period. In the studies of continuous renal replacement therapy, $CL_{EC}$ was calculated from

**TABLE 6.5  Estimated Drug Dosing Requirements for Patients Requiring Renal Replacement Therapy**

| Drug | $CL_{(aneph.)}$ (mL/min) | Intermittent hemodialysis | | | | Continuous renal replacement therapy | | | | | | | |
| | | Mode | $CL_D$ (mL/min) | MDMF | Ref. | Mode | SC | UFR (mL/min) | $CL_{UF}$ (mL/min) | $CL_{HD}$ (mL/min) | $CL_{EC}$ (mL/min) | MDMF | Ref. |
|---|---|---|---|---|---|---|---|---|---|---|---|---|---|
| Ceftazidime | 11.2 | HD | 43.6 | 1.6 | [51] | CAVHD | 0.86 | 7.5 | 6.5 | 6.6 | 13.1 | 2.2 | [33] |
| Ceftriazone | 7.0 | HD | 11.8 | 1.0 | [52] | CVVH | 0.69 | 24.1 | 16.6 | | 16.6 | 3.4 | [34] |
| Ciprofloxacin | 188[a] | HD | 40.0 | 1.0 | [53] | CAVHD/ CVVHD | 0.76 | 7.2 | 4.8 | 7.3 | 12.1 | 2.4 | [35] |
| Cyclosporine | 463 | HD | 0.31 | 1.0 | [54] | CAVH | 0.58 | 4.4 | 2.6 | | 2.6 | 1.0 | [36] |
| Gentamicin | 15.3 | HFD | 116 | 2.0 | [55] | CAVHD | | | | | 5.2 | 1.3 | [60] |
| Phenytoin | 83[b] | HD | 12.0 | 1.0 | [56] | CAVH | 0.36 | 2.8 | 1.0 | | 1.0 | 1.0 | [32] |
| Theophylline | 57.4 | HD | 77.9 | 1.1 | [57] | CAVHD | | | 23.3 | | 23.3 | 1.4 | [61] |
| Vancomycin | 6 | HFD | 106 | 3.9 | [58] | CVVH | 0.89 | 26.2 | 23.3 | | 23.3 | 4.9 | [62] |
| Levofloxacin | 37 | SLED | 49 | 1.4 | [59] | CVVH | 0.96 | 21.7 | 21 | | 21 | 1.6 | [63] |
| Linezolid | 76 | SLED | 33 | 1.2 | [39] | CVVH | 0.69 | 40 | 31 | | 31 | 1.4 | [64] |
| Meropenem | 21 | SLED | 38 | 1.6 | [47] | CVVH | 0.63 | 28 | 17 | | 17 | 1.8 | [65] |
| Vancomycin | 6 | SLED | 35 | 2.9 | [47] | CVVH | 0.88 | 25 | 23 | | 23 | 4.8 | [66] |

[a]Calculated from $CL/F$ with $F$ assumed to be 60% as in normals.
[b]Elimination of this drug follows Michaelis–Menten kinetics. Apparent clearance will be lower when plasma levels are higher than those obtained in this study.

drug recovery in ultrafiltrate/dialysate in all but the case report of theophylline removal by CAVHD [61]. In this study, $CL_{EC}$ was estimated from the change in theophylline clearance before and during extracorporeal therapy. Dialysate flow also was not specified in this report. However, the $CL_{EC}$ values for ceftazidime [33], ciprofloxacin [35], and gentamicin [60] all were obtained with a dialysate flow rate of 1 L/h. Estimates of MDMF were made from Equation 6.14. Equation 6.16 can be used to calculate the MDMF for linezolid [39], levofloxacin [59], meropenem [47], and vancomycin [47] for patients on SLED for a typical 8-hour dialysis session. Values of $CL_{EC}$ for these agents were calculated using the recovery method with blood flow and dialysis flow rates ranging from 100–300 mL/min and are compared to $CL_{EC}$ obtained during CVVH in Table 6.5.

It is apparent from Table 6.5 that drug dose adjustments generally are required more frequently for patients receiving continuous renal replacement therapy than for those requiring intermittent hemodialysis. In addition, it is evident that drug dosing need not be altered with any modality for phenytoin, cyclosporine, and other drugs that are extensively bound to plasma proteins. As in treating other patients with impaired renal function, maintenance drug doses for patients receiving renal replacement therapy can be adjusted by increasing the dosing interval as well as by reducing the drug dose. An estimate of the increased dosing interval ($\tau'$) can be made by dividing the maintenance dosing interval ($\tau$) by MDMF [40].

## Extracorporeal Therapy of Patients with Drug Toxicity

Intensive supportive therapy is all that is required for most patients suffering from dose-related drug toxicity, and drug removal by extracorporeal methods generally is indicated only for those patients whose condition deteriorates despite institution of these more conservative measures [67]. However, a decision to intervene with extracorporeal therapy may be prompted by other clinical and pharmacologic considerations that are listed in Table 6.6. For example, most intoxications with phenobarbital can be managed by a combination of supportive care and minimization of renal tubular reabsorption of this drug by forced diuresis and urine alkalinization. However, extracorporeal therapy is indicated for patients who are severely hypotensive or exhibit respiratory depression or deep and prolonged coma [68].

Conventional intermittent hemodialysis remains the mainstay for extracorporeal treatment of drug toxicity, and newer high-flux membranes have extended its applicability to higher molecular weight compounds [68]. Continuous renal replacement therapy also has been utilized and may have advantages for patients who are hemodynamically unstable or have intoxications with large molecular weight compounds such as heparin. However, hemodialysis provides higher clearance rates for most drugs and is generally regarded as preferable [69, 70]. Because SLED is a novel hybrid technique that combines features of both conventional hemodialysis and continuous renal replacement therapy, it may find increasing future application in treating patients with life-threatening drug toxicity, and case reports already have been published in which variants of SLED have been used successfully to treat patients with valproate [71] and metformin [72] intoxication.

Although hemodialysis and continuous renal replacement therapy effectively remove low molecular weight compounds that have a relatively small distribution volume and are not extensively protein bound, the technique of hemoperfusion has greater

**TABLE 6.6  Considerations for Extracorporeal Treatment of Drug Intoxications**

**General clinical considerations**
- Clinical deterioration despite intensive supportive therapy
- Severe intoxication indicated by depression of midbrain function or measured plasma or serum level
- Condition complicated by pneumonia, sepsis or other coexisting illness

**Pharmacologic considerations**
- Extracorporeal intervention can increase drug elimination significantly
- Drug clearance is slow due to pharmacologic properties of intoxicant or patient's impaired renal or hepatic function
- Intoxicant has a toxic metabolite or has toxic effects that are delayed

**TABLE 6.7  Comparison of Hemodialysis and Hemoperfusion Efficiency[a]**

| Intoxicant | Hemodialysis | Charcoal hemoperfusion | Resin hemoperfusion |
|---|---|---|---|
| Acetaminophen | ++[b] | ++ | +++ |
| Acetylsalicylic acid | ++ | ++ | |
| Amobarbital | ++ | ++ | +++ |
| Phenobarbital | ++ | ++ | +++ |
| Theophylline | ++ | +++ | +++ |
| Tricyclic antidepressants | ++ | ++ | +++ |

[a]Calculated for blood flow of 200 mL/min (based on data from Winchester [67]).
[b]++ = extraction ratio 0.2–0.5, +++ = extraction ratio > 0.5.

efficiency in treating patients with toxicity resulting from higher molecular weight drugs or those that are highly bound to plasma proteins [67, 68]. Hemoperfusion relies on the physical process of adsorption, and entails passage of blood in an extracorporeal circuit through a sorbent column of activated charcoal or resin. Several common intoxicants are listed in Table 6.7, along with the relative efficiency with which they can be removed by hemodialysis and hemoperfusion. Complications of hemoperfusion include platelet and leukocyte depletion, hypocalcemia, and a mild reduction in body temperature [67]. In many cases, these complications are outweighed by the fact that intoxicants are removed more rapidly by hemoperfusion than by hemodialysis. However, an additional consideration is that hemoperfusion clearance tends to decline during therapy as column efficiency declines, presumably reflecting saturation of adsorbent sites [73]. In addition, intercompartmental clearance from skeletal muscle and other slowly equilibrating tissues can limit the extent of drug removal by hemoperfusion and result in a rebound of blood levels and possible toxicity at the conclusion of this procedure [74]. Despite its efficacy, the utilization of hemoperfusion has declined in the past 10 years and it is not routinely available in many hospitals [68, 75].

In some instances, alternative approaches for treating intoxications have been developed that are even more efficient than hemodialysis or hemoperfusion. For example, methanol and ethylene glycol are low molecular weight compounds that are converted to toxic metabolites. Methanol is metabolized by hepatic alcohol dehydrogenase (ADH) to formaldehyde and formic acid, which causes metabolic acidosis and, after a 12- to 18-hour latent period, retinal injury and blindness [76]. Ethylene glycol is also metabolized by ADH to glycoaldehyde and further oxidized to glycolic and oxalic acid. Formation of glycolic acid causes metabolic acidosis, whereas calcium oxalate precipitation results in severe kidney damage. Ethyl alcohol has traditionally been used to treat both of these intoxications because it competitively inhibits ADH. However, ethyl alcohol exhibits Michaelis-Menten elimination kinetics that make appropriate drug dosing difficult, must be infused continuously in large fluid volumes that may be deleterious, and depresses the central nervous system, thus complicating patient evaluation. Fomepizole (4–methylpyrazole) is a more effective inhibitor of ADH that can be administered at a convenient interval and does not depress the central nervous system [72]. Accordingly, it has replaced ethyl alcohol as the standard of care in managing patients who have ingested either methanol or ethylene glycol. However, current guidelines recommend hemodialysis as adjunctive therapy when serum methanol or ethylene glycol concentrations reach or exceed 50 mg/dL [77, 78]. Although some patients with higher concentrations have been treated successfully with fomepizole alone, hemodialysis effectively reduces exposure risk from both these alcohols and their toxic metabolites. Therefore, hemodialysis remains an important adjunctive therapy, particularly for patients in whom treatment is only begun several hours after ingestion.

The development of drug-specific antibody fragments (Fab) represents a possible strategy for rapidly treating drug intoxications for which hemodialysis and hemoperfusion are suboptimal. For example, digoxin-specific Fab now are available for treating severe intoxication with either digoxin or digitoxin [79]. In most patients, initial improvement is observed within 1 hour of Fab administration and toxicity is resolved completely within 4 hours. Tricyclic antidepressant Fab also are being developed and appear to have potential in minimizing manifestations of tricyclic antidepressant cardiotoxicity [80].

## REFERENCES

[1] CDER, CBER. Pharmacokinetics in patients with impaired renal function – study design, data analysis, and impact on dosing and labeling. Draft guidance for industry. Rockville, MD: FDA (Internet at, www.fda.gov/downloads/Drugs/GuidanceComplianceRegulatoryInformation/Guidances/UCM204959.pdf; 2010).

[2] Abel JJ, Rowntree LG, Turner BB. On the removal of diffusible substances from the circulating blood of living animals by dialysis. J Pharmacol Exp Ther 1914;5:275–317.

[3] Kolff WJ. First clinical experience with the artificial kidney. Ann Intern Med 1965;62:608–19.

[4] Uribarri J. Past, present and future of end-stage renal disease therapy in the United States. Mt Sinai J Med 1999;66:14–9.

[5] Baillie GR, Eisele G. Continuous ambulatory peritoneal dialysis: A review of its mechanics, advantages, complications, and areas of controversy. Ann Pharmacother 1992;26:1409–20.

[6] Kramer P, Wigger W, Rieger J, Matthaei D, Scheler F. Arteriovenous haemofiltration: A new and simple method for the treatment of overhydrated patients resistant to diuretics. Klin Wochenschr 1977;55:1121–2.

[7] Ronco C, Bellomo R. Continuous renal replacement therapies: The need for a standard nomenclature. Contrib Nephrol 1995;116:28–33.

[8] Blagg CR, Ing TS, Berry D, Kjellstrand CM. The history and rationale of daily and nightly hemodialysis. Contrib Nephrol 2004;145:1–9.

[9] Tolwani AJ, Wheeler TS, Wille KM. Sustained low-efficiency dialysis. Contrib Nephrol 2007;156:320–4.

[10] Henderson LW. Hemodialysis: Rationale and physical principles. In: Brenner BM, Rector Jr FC, editors. The kidney. Philadelphia, PA: WB Saunders; 1976. p. 1643–71.

[11] Renkin EM. The relation between dialysance, membrane area, permeability and blood flow in the artificial kidney. Tr Am Soc Artific Organs 1956;2:102–5.

[12] Gibson TP, Matusik E, Nelson LD, Briggs WA. Artificial kidneys and clearance calculations. Clin Pharmacol Ther 1976;20:720–6.

[13] McBain JW, Liu TH. Diffusion of electrolytes, non-electrolytes and colloidal electrolytes. J Am Chem Soc 1931;53:59–74.

[14] Lee CS, Marbury TC. Drug therapy in patients undergoing haemodialysis. Clin Pharmacokinet 1984;9:42–66.

[15] Atkinson AJ Jr, Umans JG. Pharmacokinetic studies in hemodialysis patients. Clin Pharmacol Ther 2009;86:548–52.

[16] Gibson TP. Problems in designing hemodialysis drug studies. Pharmacotherapy 1985;5:23–9.

[17] Stec GP, Atkinson AJ Jr, Nevin MJ, Thenot J-P, Ruo TI, Gibson TP, et al. N-Acetylprocainamide pharmacokinetics in functionally anephric patients before and after perturbation by hemodialysis. Clin Pharmacol Ther 1979;26:618–28.

[18] Nolin TD, Appiah K, Kendrick SA, Le P, McMonagle E, Himmelfarb J. Hemodialysis acutely improves hepatic CYP3A4 metabolic activity. J Am Soc Nephrol 2006;17: 2363–7.

[19] Bowsher DJ, Krejcie TC, Avram MJ, Chow MJ, del Greco F, Atkinson AJ Jr. Reduction in slow intercompartmental clearance of urea during dialysis. J Lab Clin Med 1985;105:489–97.

[20] Renkin EM. Effects of blood flow on diffusion kinetics in isolated perfused hindlegs of cats: A double circulation hypothesis. Am J Physiol 1953;183:125–36.

[21] Bregman H, Daugirdas JT, Ing TS. Complications during hemodialysis. In: Daugirdas JT, Ing TS, editors. Handbook of dialysis. Boston, MA: Little, Brown; 1988. p. 106–20.

[22] Sidhom OA, Odeh YK, Krumlovsky FA, Budris WA, Wang Z, Pospisil PA, et al. Low dose prazosin in patients with muscle cramps during hemodialysis. Clin Pharmacol Ther 1994;56:445–51.

[23] Sigler MH, Teehan BP, Van Valceknburgh D. Solute transport in continuous hemodialysis: A new treatment for acute renal failure. Kidney Intl 1987;32:562–71.

[24] Bressolle F, Kinowski J-M, de la Coussaye JE, Wynn N, Eledjam J-J, Galtier M. Clinical pharmacokinetics during continuous haemofiltration. Clin Pharmacokinet 1994;26:457–71.

[25] Meyer MM. Renal replacement therapies. Critical Care Clin 2000;16:29–58.

[26] Golper TA. Continuous arteriovenous hemofiltration in acute renal failure. Am J Kidney Dis 1985;6:373–86.

[27] Golper TA, Saad A-MA. Gentamicin and phenytoin in vitro sieving characteristics through polysulfone hemofilters: Effect of flow rate, drug concentration and solvent systems. Kidney Intl 1986;30:937–43.

[28] Golper TA, Marx MA. Drug dosing adjustments during continuous renal replacement therapies. Kidney Intl 1998;53(Suppl. 66):S165–8.

[29] Clark WR, Ronco C. CRRT efficiency and efficacy in relation to solute size. Kidney Intl 1999;56(Suppl. 72):S3–7.

[30] Golper TA, Wedel SK, Kaplan AA, Saad A-M, Donta ST, Paganini EP. Drug removal during continuous arteriovenous hemofiltration: Theory and clinical observations. Intl J Artif Organs 1985;8:307–12.

[31] Vanholder R, Van Landschoot N, De Smet R, Schoots A, Ringoir S. Drug protein binding in chronic renal failure: Evaluation of nine drugs. Kidney Intl 1988;33:996–1004.

[32] Lau AH, Kronfol NO. Effect of continuous hemofiltration on phenytoin elimination. Ther Drug Monitor 1994;16:53–7.

[33] Davies SP, Lacey LF, Kox WJ, Brown EA. Pharmacokinetics of cefuroxime and ceftazidime in patients with acute renal failure treated by continuous arteriovenous haemodialysis. Nephrol Dial Transplant 1991;6:971–6.

[34] Kroh UF, Lennartz H, Edwards DJ, Stoeckel K. Pharmacokinetics of ceftriaxone in patients undergoing continuous venovenous hemofiltration. J Clin Pharmacol 1996;36:1114–9.

[35] Davies SP, Azadian BS, Kox WJ, Brown EA. Pharmacokinetics of ciprofloxacin and vancomycin in patients with acute renal failure treated by continuous haemodialysis. Nephrol Dial Transplant 1992;7:848–54.

[36] Cleary JD, Davis G, Raju S. Cyclosporine pharmacokinetics in a lung transplant patient undergoing hemofiltration. Transplantation 1989;48:710–2.

[37] Lau AH, Pyle K, Kronfol NO, Libertin CR. Removal of cephalosporins by continuous arteriovenous ultrafiltration (CAVU) and hemofiltration (CAVH). Intl J Artif Organs 1989;12:379–83.

[38] Schetz M, Ferdinande P, Van den Berghe G, Verwaest C, Lauwers P. Pharmacokinetics of continuous renal replacement therapy. Intensive Care Med 1995;21:612–20.

[39] Fiaccadori E, Maggiore H, Rotelli C, Giacosa R, Parenti E, Picetti E, et al. Removal of linezolid by conventional intermittent hemodialysis, sustained low-efficiency dialysis, or continuous venovenous hemofiltration in patients with acute renal failure. Crit Care Med 2004;32:2437–42.

[40] Reetze-Bonorden P, Böhler J, Keller E. Drug dosage in patients during continuous renal replacement therapy: Pharmacokinetic and therapeutic considerations. Clin Pharmacokinet 1993;24:362–79.

[41] Atkinson AJ Jr, Krumlovsky FA, Huang CM, del Greco F. Hemodialysis for severe procainamide toxicity. Clinical and pharmacokinetic observations. Clin Pharmacol Ther 1976;20: 585–92.

[42] Levy G. Pharmacokinetics in renal disease. Am J Med 1977;62: 461–5.

[43] Aronoff GR, Bennett WM, Berns JS, Brier ME, Kasbekar N, Mueller BA, et al. Drug prescribing in renal failure: Dosing guidelines for adults and children. 5th ed. Philadelphia, PA: American College of Physicians; 2007.

[44] Mushatt DM, Mihm LB, Dreisbach AW, Simon EE. Antibiotic dosing in slow extended daily dialysis. Clin Infect Dis 2009;49:433–7.

[45] Pollard TA, Lampasona V, Akkerman S, Tom K, Hooks MA, Mullins RE, et al. Vancomycin redistribution: Dosing recommendations following high-flux hemodialysis. Kidney Intl 1994;45:232–7.

[46] Manley HJ, Bailie GR, McClaran ML, Bender WL. Gentamicin pharmacokinetics during slow daily home hemodialysis. Kidney Intl 2003;63:1072–8.

[47] Kielstein JT, Czock D, Schöpke T, Hafer C, Bode-Böger SM, Kuse E, et al. Pharmacokinetics and total elimination of meropenem and vancomycin in intensive care unit patients undergoing extended daily dialysis. Crit Care Med 2006;34:51–6.

[48] Decker BS, Mueller BA, Sowinski KM. Drug dosing considerations in alternative hemodialysis. Adv Chronic Kidney Dis 2007;14:17–25.

[49] O'Shea S, Duffull S, Johnson DW. Aminoglycosides in hemodialysis patients: Is the current practice of post dialysis dosing appropriate? Semin Dial 2009;22:225–30.

[50] Macias WL, Mueller BA, Scarim KS. Vancomycin pharmacokinetics in acute renal failure: Preservation of nonrenal clearance. Clin Pharmacol Ther 1991;50:688–94.

[51] Ohkawa M, Nakashima T, Shoda R, Ikeda A, Orito M, Sawaki M, et al. Pharmacokinetics of ceftazidime in patients with renal insufficiency and in those undergoing hemodialysis. Chemotherapy 1985;31:410–6.

[52] Ti T-Y, Fortin L, Kreeft JH, East DS, Ogilvie RI, Somerville PJ. Kinetic disposition of intravenous ceftriaxone in normal subjects and patients with renal failure on hemodialysis or peritoneal dialysis. Antimicrob Agents Chemother 1984;25:83–7.

[53] Singlas E, Taburet AM, Landru I, Albin H, Ryckelinck JP. Pharmacokinetics of ciprofloxacin tablets in renal failure: Influence of haemodialysis. Eur J Clin Pharmacol 1987;31:589–93.

[54] Venkataramanan R, Ptachcinski RJ, Burckart GJ, Yang SL, Starzl TE, van Theil DH. The clearance of cyclosporine by hemodialysis. J Clin Pharmacol 1984;24:528–31.

[55] Amin NB, Padhi ID, Touchette MA, Patel RV, Dunfee TP, Anandan JV. Characterization of gentamicin pharmacokinetics in patients hemodialyzed with high-flux polysulfone membranes. Am J Kidney Dis 1999;34:222–7.

[56] Martin E, Gambertoglio JG, Adler DS, Tozer TN, Roman LA, Grausz H. Removal of phenytoin by hemodialysis in uremic patients. JAMA 1977;238:1750–3.

[57] Kradjan WA, Martin TR, Delaney CJ, Blair AD, Cutler RE. Effect of hemodialysis on the pharmacokinetics of theophylline in chronic renal failure. Nephron 1982;32:40–4.

[58] Touchette MA, Patel RV, Anandan JV, Dumler F, Zarowitz BJ. Vancomycin removal by high-flux polysulfone hemodialysis membranes in critically ill patients with end-stage renal disease. Am J Kidney Dis 1995;26:469–74.

[59] Czock D, Husig-Linde C, Langhoff A, Schopke T, Hafer C, de Groot K, et al. Pharmacokinetics of moxifloxacin and levofloxacin in intensive care unit patients who have acute renal failure and undergo extended daily dialysis. Clin J Am Soc Nephrol 2006;1:1263–8.

[60] Ernest D, Cutler DJ. Gentamicin clearance during continuous arteriovenous hemodiafiltration. Crit Care Med 1992; 20:586–9.

[61] Urquhart R, Edwards C. Increased theophylline clearance during hemofiltration. Ann Pharmacother 1995;29:787–8.

[62] Boereboom FTJ, Ververs FFT, Blankestijn PJ, Savelkoul THE, van Dijk A. Vancomycin clearance during continuous venovenous haemofiltration in critically ill patients. Intensive Care Med 1999;25:1100–4.

[63] Hansen E, Bucher M, Jakob W, Lemberger P, Kees F. Pharmacokinetics of levofloxacin during continuous veno-venous hemofiltration. Intensive Care Med 2001;27:371–5.

[64] Meyer B, Kornek GV, Nikfardjam M, Delle Karth G, Heinz G, Locker GJ, et al. Multiple-dose pharmacokinetics of linezolid during continuous venovenous haemofiltration. J Antimicrob Chemother 2005;56:172–9.

[65] Ververs TFT, van Dijk A, Vinks SATMM, Blankestijn PJ, Savelkoul JF, Meulenbelt J, et al. Pharmacokinetics and dosing regimen of meropenem in critically ill patients receiving continuous venovenous hemofiltration. Crit Care Med 2000;28:3412–6.

[66] Boereboom ETJ, Verves FFT, Blankestijn PJ, Savelkoul TJF, van Dijk A. Vancomycin clearance during continuous venovenous hemofiltration in critically ill patients. Intensive Care Med 1999;25:1100–4.

[67] Winchester JF. Active methods for detoxification. In: Haddad LM, Shannon MW, Winchester JF, editors. Clinical management of poisoning and drug overdose. 3rd ed. Philadelphia, PA: WB Saunders; 1998. p. 175–88.

[68] de Pont A- C. Extracorporeal treatment of intoxications. Curr Opin Crit Care 2007;13. 688–73.

[69] Goodman JW, Goldfarb DS. The role of continuous renal replacement therapy in the treatment of poisoning. Semin Dial 2006;19:402–7.

[70] Kim Z, Goldfarb DS. Continuous renal replacement therapy does not have a clear role in the treatment of poisoning. Nephron Clin Pract 2010;115:c1–6.

[71] Kahn E, Huggan P, Celi L, Macginley R, Schollum J, Walker R. Sustained low-efficiency dialysis with filtration (SLEDD-f) in the management of acute sodium valproate intoxication. Hemodial Intl 2008;12:211–4.

[72] Tukcuer I, Erdur B, San I, Yuksel A, Tura P, Yuksel S. Severe metformin intoxication treated with prolonged haemodialyses and plasma exchange. Eur J Emerg Med 2009;16:11–3.

[73] Shah G, Nelson HA, Atkinson AJ Jr, Okita GT, Ivanovich P, Gibson TP. Effect of hemoperfusion on the pharmacokinetics of digitoxin in dogs. J Lab Clin Med 1979;93:370–80.

[74] Gibson TP, Atkinson AJ Jr. Effect of changes in intercompartment rate constants on drug removal during hemoperfusion. J Pharm Sci 1978;67:1178–9.

[75] Shalkham AS, Kirrane BM, Hoffman RS, Goldfarb DS, Nelson LS. The availability and use of charcoal hemoperfusion in the treatment of poisoned patients. Am J Kidney Dis 2006;48:239–41.

[76] Brent J. Fomepizole for ethylene glycol and methanol poisoning. N Engl J Med 2009;360:2216–23.

[77] Barceloux DG, Krenzelok EP, Olson K, Watson W. American Academy of Clinical Toxicology practice guidelines on the treatment of ethylene glycol poisoning. J Toxicol Clin Toxicol 1999;37:537–60.

[78] Barceloux DG, Bond GR, Krenzelok EP, Cooper H, Vale JA. ACCT Ad Hoc Committee on the Treatment Guidelines for Methanol Poisoning. American Academy of Clinical Toxicology practice guidelines on the treatment of methanol poisoning. J Toxicol Clin Toxicol 2002;40:415–46.

[79] Antman E, Wenger TL, Butler VP Jr, Haber E, Smith TW. Treatment of 150 cases of life-threatening digitalis intoxication with digoxin-specific Fab antibody fragments: Final report of a multicenter study. Circulation 1990;81:1744–52.

[80] Heard K, Dart RC, Gogdan G, O'Malley GF, Burkhart KK, Donovan JW, et al. A preliminary study of tricyclic antidepressant (TCA) ovine FAB for TCA toxicity. Clin Toxicol 2006;44:275–81.

## COMPUTER-BASED TUTORIAL

Readers interested in hands-on analysis of hemodialysis kinetic data can access the tutorials and data files that are available free of charge at the following website: (http://www.saam.com/case_studies_pharmacokinetic. htm)

Of relevance to this chapter is the pharmacokinetic case study on *N*–Acetylprocainamide (NAPA) Kinetics in a Hemodialysis Patient. Data for this exercise were taken from the study described in reference [17].

# Effect of Liver Disease on Pharmacokinetics

**Gregory M. Susla[1] and Juan J.L. Lertora[2]**
[1]*Medical Information, MedImmune, LLC, Gaithersburg, MD 20878*
[2]*Clinical Pharmacology Program, Clinical Center, National Institutes of Health, Bethesda, MD 20892*

## HEPATIC ELIMINATION OF DRUGS

Hepatic clearance ($CL_H$) may be defined as the volume of blood perfusing the liver that is cleared of drug per unit time. Usually, hepatic clearance is equated with non-renal clearance and is calculated as total body clearance ($CL_E$) minus renal clearance ($CL_R$).

$$CL_H = CL_E - CL_R \qquad (7.1)$$

Accordingly, these estimates may include a component of extrahepatic nonrenal clearance.

The factors that affect hepatic clearance include blood flow to the liver ($Q$), the fraction of drug not bound to plasma proteins ($f_u$), and intrinsic clearance ($CL_{int}$)[1, 2]. Intrinsic clearance is simply the hepatic clearance that would be observed in the absence of blood flow and protein binding restrictions. As discussed in Chapter 2, hepatic clearance usually can be considered to be a first-order process. In those cases, intrinsic clearance represents the ratio of $V_{max}/K_m$, and this relationship has been used as the basis for correlating *in vitro* studies of drug metabolism with *in vivo* results [3]. However, for phenytoin and several other drugs the Michaelis-Menten equation is needed to characterize intrinsic clearance.

The well-stirred model, shown in Figure 7.1, is the model of hepatic clearance that is used most commonly in pharmacokinetics. If we apply the Fick Equation (see Chapter 6) to this model, hepatic clearance can be defined as follows [2]:

$$CL_H = Q \left[ \frac{C_a - C_v}{C_a} \right] \qquad (7.2)$$

The ratio of concentrations defined by the terms within the brackets is termed the *extraction ratio* (ER). An expression for the extraction ratio also can be obtained by applying the following mass balance equation to the model shown in Figure 7.1:

$$V \frac{dC_a}{dt} = Q\,C_a - Q\,C_v - f_u\,CL_{int}\,C_v$$

At steady state,

$$Q(C_a - C_v) = f_u\,CL_{int}\,C_v \qquad (7.3)$$

Also,

$$Q\,C_a = (Q + f_u\,CL_{int})C_v \qquad (7.4)$$

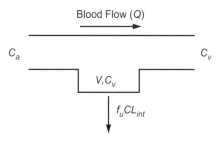

**FIGURE 7.1** The well-stirred model of hepatic clearance, in which the liver is viewed as a single compartment having a volume ($V$) and blood flow ($Q$). Drug concentrations reaching the liver via the hepatic artery and portal vein are designated by $C_a$, and those in emergent hepatic venous blood by $C_v$. Drug concentrations within the liver are considered to be in equilibrium with those in emergent venous blood. Intrinsic clearance ($CL_{int}$) acts to eliminate the fraction of drug not bound to plasma proteins ($f_u$).

since

$$ER = \frac{C_a - C_v}{C_a}$$

Equation 7.3 can be divided by Equation 7.4 to define extraction ratio in terms of $Q$, $f_u$, and $CL_{int}$:

$$ER = \frac{f_u\ CL_{int}}{Q + f_u\ CL_{int}} \qquad (7.5)$$

By substituting this expression for extraction ratio into Equation 7.2, hepatic clearance can be expressed as:

$$CL_H = Q\left[\frac{f_u\ CL_{int}}{Q + f_u\ CL_{int}}\right] \qquad (7.6)$$

Two limiting cases arise when $f_u\ CL_{int} << Q$ and when $f_u\ CL_{int} >> Q$ [2]. In the former instance Equation 7.5 can be simplified to

$$CL_H = f_u\ CL_{int} \qquad (7.7)$$

Hepatic clearance is termed *restrictive* in this case, since it is limited by protein binding. This situation is analogous to the elimination of drugs by glomerular filtration. Drugs that are restrictively eliminated have extraction ratios $< 0.3$.

When $f_u\ CL_{int} >> Q$, Equation 7.5 can be reduced to:

$$CL_H = Q \qquad (7.8)$$

In this case hepatic clearance is *flow limited*, similar to the renal tubular excretion of $p$–aminohippurate. Because protein binding does not affect their clearance, drugs whose hepatic clearance is flow limited are said to be *non-restrictively* eliminated and have extraction ratios $> 0.7$.

Yang *et al.* [4] point out that the well-stirred model equates whole blood clearance, rather than plasma clearance, to liver blood flow because the liver is capable of extracting drug from both plasma and red blood cells. This situation is similar to that encountered for drugs removed by hemodialysis (see Chapter 6). So if plasma drug clearance is to be estimated from plasma concentration measurements, then Equation 7.6 must be modified as follows by including the total blood to plasma drug concentration ratio (B/P):

$$CL_H = Q\left[\frac{f_u\ CL_{int}}{Q + f_u\ CL_{int}/(B/P)}\right] \qquad (7.9)$$

In addition to this modification of the well-stirred model, several other kinetic models of hepatic clearance have been developed [5]. However, the following discussion will be based on the relationships defined by Equation 7.6, and the limiting cases represented by Equations 7.7 and 7.8.

## Restrictively Metabolized Drugs (*ER* < 0.3)

The product of $f_u$ and $CL_{int}$ is small relative to liver blood flow (usually about 1500 mL/min) for drugs that are restrictively metabolized. Although the extraction ratio of these drugs is less than 0.3, hepatic metabolism often constitutes their principle pathway of elimination and they frequently have long elimination-phase half-lives (e.g., diazepam: $t_{1/2} = 43$ h). The hepatic clearance of these drugs is affected by changes in their binding to plasma proteins, by induction or inhibition of hepatic drug-metabolizing enzymes, and by age, nutrition, and pathological factors. However, as indicated by Equation 7.7, their hepatic clearance is not affected significantly by changes in hepatic blood flow.

### Effect of Changes in Protein Binding on Hepatic Clearance

It usually is assumed that the free drug concentration in blood is equal to the drug concentration to which hepatic drug-metabolizing enzymes are exposed. Although protein binding would not be anticipated to change hepatic clearance significantly for restrictively metabolized drugs that have $f_u > 80\%$, displacement of highly bound ($f_u < 20\%$) drugs from their plasma protein binding sites will result in a significant increase in their hepatic clearance. However, steady-state concentrations of unbound drug will be unchanged as long as there is no change in $CL_{int}$. This occurs in some drug interactions, as diagrammed in Figure 7.2 [6]. This situation also is encountered in pathological conditions in which plasma proteins or plasma protein binding are decreased, as described in Chapter 5 for phenytoin kinetics in patients with impaired renal function. Since pharmacological effects are related to concentrations of unbound drug, pure displacement-type drug interactions put patients at risk for only a brief period of time. Similarly, dose adjustments are not needed for patients whose protein binding is impaired. In fact, as pointed out in Chapter 5, measurement of total rather than unbound drug levels in these patients actually may lead to inappropriate dose increases.

### Effect of Changes in Intrinsic Clearance on Hepatic Drug Clearance

Both hepatic disease and drug interactions can alter the intrinsic clearance of restrictively eliminated drugs. Drug interactions will be considered in more detail in Chapter 15. The effects of liver disease on

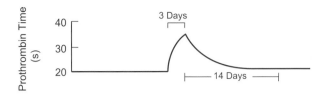

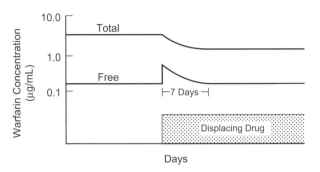

**FIGURE 7.2** Time course of an interaction in which warfarin, a restrictively metabolized drug, is displaced from its plasma protein binding sites. Although free warfarin concentrations rise initially as a result of the interaction, they subsequently return to pre-interaction levels. As a result, the increase in prothrombin time is only transient. Because $f_u$ is increased, total (bound plus free) warfarin levels remain depressed as long as treatment with the displacing drug is continued. Reproduced with permission from Atkinson AJ Jr, Reidenberg MM, Thompson WL. Clinical Pharmacology. In: Greenberger N, editor. MKSAP VI Syllabus. Philadelphia, PA: American College of Physicians; 1982. pp. 85–96 [6].

drug elimination will be discussed in the following sections. Although a number of probe drugs have been used to characterize hepatic clearance, analysis of the factors influencing the intrinsic clearance of drugs is hampered by the fact that, in contrast to the use of creatinine clearance to assess renal function, there are no simple measures that can be applied on a routine clinical basis to assess hepatic clearance.

## Drugs with an Intermediate Extraction Ratio (0.3 < *ER* < 0.7)

Few drugs exhibit an intermediate extraction ratio. Evaluation of the hepatic clearance of these drugs requires consideration of all of the parameters included in Equation 7.6. Disease-associated or drug-induced alterations in protein binding, hepatic blood flow, or intrinsic clearance may alter hepatic clearance significantly.

## Non-Restrictively Metabolized Drugs (*ER* > 0.70)

The product of $f_u$ and $CL_{int}$ is large relative to liver blood flow for drugs that are non-restrictively

metabolized. These drugs characteristically have short elimination-phase half-lives (e.g., propranolol: $t_{1/2} = 3.9$ h), and changes in hepatic blood flow have a major effect on their hepatic clearance (Equation 7.8). Accordingly, hemodynamic changes, such as congestive heart failure, that reduce liver blood flow will reduce the hepatic clearance of these drugs and may necessitate appropriate adjustments in intravenous dosage. Changes in hepatic blood flow will also affect the first-pass metabolism of oral doses of non-restrictively metabolized drugs, but the effects of this on patient exposure are not intuitively obvious.

### First-Pass Metabolism

Because non-restrictively metabolized drugs have an extraction ratio that exceeds 0.7, they undergo extensive first-pass metabolism which reduces their bioavailability after oral administration (Chapter 4). If there is no loss of drug due to degradation or metabolism within the gastrointestinal tract or to incomplete absorption, the relationship between bioavailability (*F*) and extraction ratio is given by the following equation:

$$F = 1 - ER \qquad (7.10)$$

Because Equation 7.8 implies that $ER = 1$ for non-restrictively metabolized drugs, yet the oral route of administration can be used for many drugs in this category (e.g., $F > 0$ for morphine and propranolol), it is apparent that Equation 7.10 represents only a rough approximation. By using Equation 7.5 to substitute for *ER* in Equation 7.10, we obtain a more precise estimate of the impact of first-pass metabolism on bioavailability:

$$F = \frac{Q}{Q + f_u \, CL_{int}} \qquad (7.11)$$

Considering the case in which a drug is eliminated only by hepatic metabolism, Equation 4.2 from Chapter 4 can be re-written as follows:

$$D_{oral} \cdot F = CL_H \cdot AUC_{oral}$$

Using Equations 7.6 and 7.11 to substitute respectively for $CL_H$ and *F*, yields the result that

$$D_{oral} = f_u \, CL_{int} \cdot AUC_{oral} \qquad (7.12)$$

It can be seen from Equation 7.12 that oral doses of non-restrictively metabolized drugs should not need to be adjusted in response to changes in hepatic blood flow. Equation 7.12 also forms the basis for using

*AUC_oral* measurements to calculate so-called "oral clearance" as an estimate of $f_u CL_{int}$. However, if renal excretion contributes to drug elimination, it will reduce *AUC_oral* and lead to overestimation of $f_u CL_{int}$ unless the contribution of renal clearance is accounted for [2].

## Biliary Excretion of Drugs

Relatively few drugs are taken up by the liver and without further metabolism excreted into bile which, as an aqueous solution, generally favors excretion of more water soluble-compounds [7]. On the other hand, many polar drug metabolites, such as glucuronide conjugates, undergo biliary excretion. In order for compounds to be excreted in bile they must first pass the fenestrated endothelium that lines the hepatic sinusoids, then cross both the luminal and canalicular membrane surfaces of hepatocytes. Passage across these two hepatocyte membrane surfaces often is facilitated by active transport systems that will be discussed in Chapter 14. Consequently, chemical structure, polarity, and molecular weight are important determinants of the extent to which compounds are excreted in bile. In general, polar compounds with a molecular weight range of 500–600 Da are excreted in bile, whereas those with a lower molecular weight tend to be eliminated preferentially by renal excretion. However, 5-fluorouracil has a molecular weight of only 130 Da, yet is excreted in bile with a bile/plasma concentration ratio of 2.0 [8]. Nonetheless, biliary excretion of parent drug and metabolites accounts for only 2–3% of the elimination of an administered 5–fluorouracil dose in patients with normal renal function [9].

Compounds that enhance bile production stimulate biliary excretion of drugs normally eliminated by this route, whereas biliary excretion of drugs will be decreased by compounds that decrease bile flow or pathophysiologic conditions that cause cholestasis [10]. Route of administration may also influence the extent of drug excretion into bile. Oral administration may cause a drug to be extracted by the liver and excreted into bile to a greater degree than if the intravenous route were used.

### Enterohepatic Circulation

Drugs excreted into bile traverse the biliary tract to reach the small intestine where they may be reabsorbed [7]. Drug metabolites that reach the intestine also may be converted back to the parent drug and be reabsorbed. This is particularly true for some glucuronide conjugates that are hydrolyzed by β–glucuronidase present in intestinal bacteria. The term *enterohepatic circulation* refers to this cycle in which a drug or metabolite is excreted in bile and then reabsorbed from the intestine

either as the metabolite or after conversion back to the parent drug. Thus, enterohepatic cycling of a drug increases its bioavailability, as assessed from the area under the plasma-level vs time curve, and prolongs its elimination-phase half-life.

Studies in animals have demonstrated that biliary clearance actually may exceed plasma clearance for some drugs and species with extensive enterohepatic circulation [11]. Interruption of enterohepatic circulation reduces both the area under the plasma-level vs time curve and the elimination-phase half-life. Enterohepatic circulation also increases the total exposure of the intestinal mucosa to potentially toxic drugs. Thus, the intestinal toxicity of indomethacin is most marked in those species that have a high ratio of biliary to renal drug excretion [11].

Enterohepatic circulation may result in a second peak in the plasma-level vs time curve, as shown in Figure 7.3A. The occurrence of this second peak in plasma drug concentrations appears to reflect intermittent gallbladder contraction and pulsatile delivery of drug-containing bile to the intestine, because this double peak phenomenon is not encountered in animal species that lack a gallbladder [12]. Realistic pharmacokinetic modeling of this process entails incorporation of a variable lag-time interval that can reflect intermittent gallbladder emptying, as in Figure 7.3B. Cimetidine is typical of many drugs that undergo enterohepatic circulation, in that secondary plasma concentration peaks occur after oral but not intravenous administration [12]. These secondary peaks were seen after meals in individuals who were given cimetidine while fasting but were allowed subsequent food intake that presumably triggered gallbladder contraction and the discharge of drug-containing bile into the small intestine. Secondary peaks were not seen when cimetidine was administered intravenously or co-administered orally with food. On the other hand, ranitidine differs from cimetidine and is unusual in that secondary peaks occur after both intravenous and oral administration to fasting patients who subsequently were fed, as shown in Figure 7.3A [13]. This difference reflects the fact that cimetidine reaches the bile from the liver primarily during first-pass transit via the portal circulation ($k_1$ in Figure 7.3B), whereas there is substantial hepatic uptake of ranitidine from the systemic circulation ($k_2$ in Figure 7.3B).

## EFFECTS OF LIVER DISEASE ON PHARMACOKINETICS

Liver disease in humans encompasses a wide range of pathological disturbances that can lead to

**(A)**

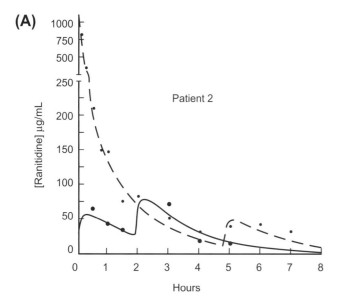

**(B)**

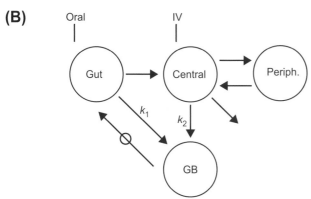

**FIGURE 7.3** (A) Pharmacokinetic analysis of secondary plasma concentration peaks following the oral and intravenous administration of single 20-mg doses of ranitidine to a healthy subject. The lines are based on the pharmacokinetic model shown in (B) and represent a least-squares fit of the plasma concentrations measured after the intravenous (*dashed line*) and oral (*solid line*) doses. (B) Pharmacokinetic model used for the analysis of the enterohepatic cycling of cimetidine and ranitidine. Drug enters the gallbladder via the liver, for which a separate compartment is not required, either during first-pass transit from the gut via the portal circulation ($k_1$) or directly from the systemic circulation ($k_2$). The irregular discharge of drug-containing bile from the gallbladder is indicated by the arrow going from gallbladder (GB) to gut. Drug distribution within the body is modeled as a two-compartment system. Reproduced with permission from Miller R. J Pharm Sci 1984;73:1376–9 [13].

a reduction in liver blood flow, extrahepatic or intrahepatic shunting of blood, hepatocyte dysfunction, quantitative and qualitative changes in serum proteins, and changes in bile flow. Different forms of hepatic disease may produce different alterations in drug absorption, disposition, and pharmacologic effect. The pharmacokinetic or pharmacodynamic consequences of a specific hepatic disease may differ between individuals or even within a single individual over time. Each of the major determinants of hepatic clearance, $CL_{int}$, $f_u$, $Q$, and vascular architecture may be independently altered.

Although there are numerous causes of hepatic injury, it appears that the hepatic response to injury is a limited one and that the functional consequences are determined more by the extent of the injury than by the cause. At this time there is no generally available test that can be used to correlate changes in drug absorption and disposition with the degree of hepatic impairment.

## Acute Hepatitis

Acute hepatitis is an inflammatory condition of the liver that is caused by viruses or hepatotoxins. In acute viral hepatitis inflammatory changes in the hepatocyte are generally mild and transient, although they can be chronic (chronic active hepatitis) and severe, resulting in cirrhosis or death. Blaschke and Williams and their colleagues [14–17] have conducted informative studies of the effects of acute viral hepatitis on drug disposition. These investigators used a longitudinal study design in which each of a small number of patients was studied initially during the time that they had acute viral hepatitis and subsequently after recovery (Table 7.1). The drugs that were administered included phenytoin [14], tolbutamide [15], warfarin [16], and lidocaine [17]. The most consistent significant finding was that the plasma protein binding of both phenytoin and tolbutamide was reduced during acute hepatitis. For both drugs, this was partly attributed to drug displacement from protein-binding sites by elevated bilirubin levels. As a result of these changes, the distribution volume of phenytoin increased slightly during hepatitis (see Chapter 3). Although no significant change was noted in the average values of either phenytoin $CL_H$ or $CL_{int}$, $CL_{int}$ was reduced by approximately 50% in the two patients with the greatest evidence of hepatocellular damage. On the other hand, the reduction in tolbutamide binding to plasma proteins had no observable effect on distribution volume or $CL_{int}$ but did result in an increase in $CL_H$. No consistent changes were observed in warfarin kinetics during acute viral hepatitis. However, prothrombin time was prolonged to a greater extent than expected in two of the five patients, reflecting impaired synthesis of Factor VII. Lidocaine kinetics also was not altered consistently during acute viral hepatitis, although clearance decreased in four of the six patients that were studied.

In general, drug elimination during acute viral hepatitis is either normal or only moderately impaired.

**TABLE 7.1    Pharmacokinetics of Some Drugs During and After Acute Viral Hepatitis**

| | $f_u$ | | $V_d$ | | $CL_H$ | | $CL_{int}$ | | |
|---|---|---|---|---|---|---|---|---|---|
| | During | After | During (L/kg) | After (L/kg) | During (mL/h/kg) | After (mL/h/kg) | During (mL/h/kg) | After (mL/h/kg) | Ref. |
| Phenytoin[a] | 0.126[b] | 0.099 | 0.68[b] | 0.63 | 0.0430 | 0.0373 | 0.352 | 0.385 | [14] |
| Tolbutamide | 0.087[b] | 0.068 | 0.15 | 0.15 | 26[b] | 18 | 300 | 260 | [15] |
| Warfarin | 0.012 | 0.012 | 0.09 | 0.21 | 6.1 | 6.1 | 519 | 514 | [16] |
| Lidocaine | 0.56 | 0.49 | 3.1 | 2.0 | 13.0 | 20.0 | 23.2[c] | 40.8[c] | [17] |

[a]A low dose of phenytoin was administered so that first-order kinetics would be approximated.
[b]Difference in studies during and after recovery from acute viral hepatitis was significant at $P < 0.05$ by paired t-test.
[c]Protein binding results for individual patients were not given so $CL_{int}$ was estimated from average values.

Observed changes tend to be variable and related to the extent of hepatocellular damage incurred. If the acute hepatitis resolves, drug disposition returns to normal. Drug elimination is likely to be impaired most significantly in patients who develop chronic hepatitis B virus-related liver disease, but even then only late in the evolution of this disease [18]. This stands in marked contrast to the severity of acute hepatitis that can be caused by hepatotoxins. For example, Prescott and Wright [19] found that liver damage can occur within 2–3 hours after ingestion of an acetaminophen overdose. The elimination-phase half-life of acetaminophen averaged only 2.7 hours in patients without liver damage, but ranged from 4.3 to 7.7 hours (mean = 5.8 h) in four patients with liver damage and from 4.3 to 13.9 hours (mean = 7.7 h) in three patients with both liver and kidney damage resulting from acetaminophen toxicity. These authors observed that a fatal outcome was likely in patients whose acetaminophen elimination half-life exceeded 10–12 hours.

## Chronic Liver Disease and Cirrhosis

Chronic liver disease is usually secondary to chronic alcohol abuse or chronic viral hepatitis. Alcoholic liver disease is most common and begins with the accumulation of fat vacuoles within hepatocytes and hepatic enlargement. There is a decrease in cytochrome P450 content per weight of tissue, but this is compensated for by the increase in liver size so that drug metabolism is not impaired [20]. Alcoholic fatty liver may be accompanied or followed by alcoholic hepatitis, in which hepatocyte degeneration and necrosis become evident. In neither of these conditions is there significant diversion of blood flow past functioning hepatocytes by functional or anatomic shunts.

Cirrhosis occurs most frequently in the setting of alcoholic liver disease, and represents the final common pathway of a number of chronic liver diseases. The development of cirrhosis is characterized by the appearance of fibroblasts and collagen deposition. This is accompanied by a reduction in liver size and the formation of nodules of regenerated hepatocytes. As a result, total liver content of cytochrome P450 is reduced in these patients. Initially, fibroblasts deposit collagen fibrils in the sinusoidal space, including the space of Disse [20]. Collagen deposition not only produces characteristic bands of connective scar tissue but also forms a basement membrane devoid of microvilli along the sinusoidal surface of the hepatocyte. This process thickens and defenestrates the endothelial barrier between the sinusoid and the hepatocytes, a process referred to as *capillarization* [21]. This process, in conjunction with alterations in the sinusoidal membrane of the hepatocyte, results in functional shunting of blood past the remaining hepatocyte mass. These changes can interfere significantly with the function of hepatic transporters and the hepatic uptake of oxygen, nutrients, and plasma constituents, including drugs and metabolites.

The deposition of fibrous bands also disrupts the normal hepatic vascular architecture and increases vascular resistance and portal venous pressure. This reduces portal venous flow that normally accounts for 70% of total liver blood flow [22]. However, the decrease in portal venous flow is compensated for by an increase in hepatic artery flow, so that total blood flow reaching the liver is maintained at the normal value of 18 mL/min·kg in patients with either chronic viral hepatitis or cirrhosis [23]. The increase in portal venous pressure also leads to the formation of extrahepatic and intrahepatic shunts. Extrahepatic shunting occurs through the extensive collateral network that connects the portal and systemic circulations [22]. Important examples include collaterals at the gastroesophageal junction, which can dilate to form varices, and the umbilical vein. In a study of cirrhotic patients with bleeding esophageal varices, an average of 70% of mesenteric and 95% of splenic blood flow was found to be diverted through extrahepatic shunts [24]. Intrahepatic shunting results both from intrahepatic vascular anastamoses that bypass hepatic sinusoids and from the functional sinusoidal barrier caused by collagen deposition. Iwasa *et al.* [22] found that the combination of anatomic and functional intrahepatic shunting averaged 25% of total liver blood flow in normal subjects, but was increased to 33% in patients with chronic viral hepatitis and to 52% in cirrhotic patients.

## Pharmacokinetic Consequences of Liver Cirrhosis

The net result of chronic hepatic disease that leads to cirrhosis is that pathophysiologic alterations may result in both decreased hepatocyte function, with as much as a 50% decrease in cytochrome P450 content, and/or shunting of blood away from optimally functioning hepatocytes. Accordingly, cirrhosis affects drug metabolism more than any other form of liver disease does. In fact, cirrhosis may decrease the clearance of drugs that are non-restrictively eliminated in subjects with normal liver function to the extent that it no longer approximates hepatic blood flow but is influenced to a greater extent by hepatic intrinsic clearance [25]. By reducing first-pass hepatic metabolism, cirrhosis also may cause a clinically significant increase in the extent to which non-restrictively eliminated drugs are absorbed.

### Influence of Portosystemic Shunting

When portosystemic shunting is present, total hepatic blood flow ($Q$) equals the sum of perfusion flow ($Q_p$) and shunt flow ($Q_s$). Portocaval shunting will impair the efficiency of hepatic extraction and reduce the extraction ratio, as indicated by the following modification of Equation 7.5 [26]:

$$ER = \frac{f_u\, CL_{int}}{Q + f_u\, CL_{int}} \cdot \frac{Q_p}{Q} \qquad (7.13)$$

The corresponding impact on hepatic clearance is given by the following equation:

$$CL_H = Q_p \left[ \frac{f_u\, CL_{int}}{Q + f_u\, CL_{int}} \right] \qquad (7.14)$$

Because $Q$ and $Q_p$ are both reduced in patients with severe cirrhosis, in whom portocaval shunting is most pronounced, hepatic clearance will be reduced more for non-restrictively than for restrictively metabolized drugs.

Similarly, restrictively metabolized drugs exhibit little first-pass metabolism even in subjects with normal liver function, so portocaval shunting will have little impact on drug bioavailability. On the other hand, portocaval shunting will decrease the extraction ratio and increase the bioavailability of non-restrictively metabolized drugs as follows:

$$F = 1 - \frac{f_u\, CL_{int}}{Q + f_u\, CL_{int}} \cdot \frac{Q_p}{Q} \qquad (7.15)$$

For example, if the extraction ratio of a completely absorbed but non-restrictively metabolized drug falls from 0.95 to 0.90, the bioavailability will double from 0.05 to 0.10. Because this increase in absorption is accompanied by a decrease in elimination clearance, total exposure following oral administration of non-restrictively eliminated drugs will increase to an even greater extent than will the increase in bioavailability, as shown in Table 7.2 for meperidine [27], pentazocine [27], and propranolol [28]. Cirrhosis also is associated with a reduction in propranolol binding to plasma proteins, so this also contributes to increased exposure following either intravenous or oral doses of this drug (see the following section). Accordingly, the relative exposure estimates for propranolol in Table 7.2 are based on comparisons of area under the plasma-level vs time curve of non-protein-bound plasma concentrations. The increase in drug exposure resulting from these changes may cause unexpected increases in

**TABLE 7.2 Impact of Cirrhosis on Bioavailability and Relative Exposure to Doses of Non-restrictively Eliminated Drugs**

|  | Absolute bioavailability | | Relative exposure (cirrhotics/controls) | | |
|---|---|---|---|---|---|
|  | Controls (%) | Cirrhotics (%) | IV | Oral | Reference |
| Meperidine | 48 | 87 | 1.6 | 3.1 | [27] |
| Pentazocine | 18 | 68 | 2.0 | 8.3 | [27] |
| Propranolol | 38 | 54 | 1.5[a] | 2.0[a] | [28] |

[a]These estimates also incorporate the 55% increase in propranolol free fraction that was observed in cirrhotic patients.

intensity of pharmacologic response or in toxicity when the usual doses of these drugs are prescribed for patients with liver disease.

### Consequences of Decreased Protein Binding

Hypoalbuminemia frequently accompanies chronic liver disease, and may reduce drug binding to plasma proteins [29]. In addition, endogenous substances such as bilirubin and bile acids accumulate and may displace drugs from protein-binding sites. Reductions in protein binding will tend to increase the hepatic clearance of restrictively metabolized drugs. For drugs that have low intrinsic clearance and tight binding to plasma proteins, it is possible that liver disease results in a decrease in $CL_{int}$ but also an increase in $f_u$. The resultant change in hepatic clearance will depend on changes in both these parameters. Thus, hepatic disease generally produces no change in warfarin clearance, a decrease in diazepam clearance, and an increase in tolbutamide clearance. However, as discussed in Chapter 5, unbound drug concentrations will not be affected by decreases in the protein binding of restrictively metabolized drugs. Therefore, no dosage alterations are required for these drugs when protein binding is the only parameter that is changed.

Although reduced protein binding will not affect the clearance or total (bound plus free) plasma concentration of non-restrictively eliminated drugs, it will increase the plasma concentration of free drug. This may increase the intensity of pharmacological effect that is observed at a given total drug concentration [29]. Therefore, even in the absence of changes in other pharmacokinetic parameters, a reduction in the plasma protein binding of non-restrictively eliminated drugs will necessitate a corresponding reduction in drug dosage.

As previously discussed in the context of renal disease (Chapter 5), reduced protein binding will increase the distribution volume referenced to total drug concentrations and this will tend to increase elimination-phase half-life [29].

### Consequences of Hepatocellular Changes

Intrinsic clearance depends on the activity of sinusoidal and canalicular transporters and hepatocyte metabolic enzymes [30, 31]. The liver content of cytochrome P450 enzymes is decreased in patients with cirrhosis. In these patients, intrinsic clearance is the main determinant of the systemic clearance of lidocaine and indocyanine green, two drugs that have non-restrictive metabolism in subjects with normal liver function. In general, enzyme activities and drug

**TABLE 7.3   Differential Alterations of Cytochrome P450 Enzyme Content in Cirrhosis**

| Enzyme | Representative substrate | % Change in cirrhosis | |
| | | Guengerich and Turvy [33] | George [34] |
| --- | --- | --- | --- |
| CYP1A2 | Theophylline | ↓ 53%[a] | ↓ 71%[b] |
| CYP2C19 | Omeprazole | ↑ 95% | ↓ 43% |
| CYP2E1 | Acetaminophen | ↓ 59%[a] | ↓ 19% |
| CYP3A | Midazolam | ↓ 47% | ↓ 75%[c] |

[a]$P < 0.05$, [b]$P < 0.005$, [c]$P < 0.0005$.

binding protein concentrations are progressively reduced as disease severity increases. However, cirrhosis does not reduce the function of different drug metabolizing enzymes uniformly [31, 32]. As can be seen from the results of the two *in vitro* studies summarized in Table 7.3, CYP1A2 content is consistently reduced in cirrhosis [33, 34]. Significant reductions in CYP2E1 and CYP3A also have been found by some investigators. Although CYP2C19 appears to be somewhat more resilient in these *in vitro* studies, content of this enzyme was markedly reduced in patients with cholestatic types of cirrhosis [34]. More recent studies in patients with liver disease, in whom the presence or absence of cholestasis was not noted, have indicated that clearance of S-mephenytoin, a CYP2C19 probe, was decreased by 63% in cirrhotic patients with mild cirrhosis and by 96% in patients with moderate cirrhosis [35]. On the other hand, administration of debrisoquine to these patients indicated normal function of CYP2D6. In contrast, in patients with non-alcoholic fatty liver disease (NAFLD), the expression and activity of CYP1A2, CYP2C19, CYP2D6, and CYP3A4 tend to decrease with increasing severity of NAFLD, while the activity of CYP2A6 and CYP2C9 tend to increase with progressive disease [36]. Glucuronide conjugation of morphine and other drugs is relatively well preserved in patients with mild and moderate cirrhosis [32], but morphine clearance was 59% reduced in patients whose cirrhosis was severe enough to have caused previous hepatic encephalopathy [37]. Although glucuronidation may be spared in patients with mild to moderate liver disease, it has been shown to be reduced in patients with severe liver disease [38].

## USE OF THERAPEUTIC DRUGS IN PATIENTS WITH LIVER DISEASE

A number of clinical classification schemes and laboratory measures have been proposed as a means

**TABLE 7.4   Pugh Modification of Child's Classification of Liver Disease Severity**

| Assessment parameters | Assigned score | | |
| --- | --- | --- | --- |
| | 1 Point | 2 Points | 3 Points |
| Encephalopathy Grade | 0 | 1 or 2 | 3 or 4 |
| Ascites | Absent | Slight | Moderate |
| Bilirubin (mg/dL) | 1–2 | 2–3 | >3 |
| Albumin (g/dL) | >3.5 | 2.8–3.5 | <2.8 |
| Prothrombin time (seconds > control) | 1–4 | 4–10 | >10 |
| **Classification of clinical severity** | | | |
| Clinical Severity | Mild | Moderate | Severe |
| Total Points | 5–6 | 7–9 | >9 |
| **Encephalopathy grade** | | | |
| Grade 0 | Normal consciousness, personality, neurological examination, EEG | | |
| Grade 1 | Restless, sleep disturbed, irritable/agitated, tremor, impaired hand writing, 5 cps waves on EEG | | |
| Grade 2 | Lethargic, time-disoriented, inappropriate, asterixis, ataxia, slow triphasic waves on EEG | | |
| Grade 3 | Somnolent, stuporous, place-disoriented, hyperactive reflexes, rigidity, slower waves on EEG | | |
| Grade 4 | Unrousable coma, no personality/behavior, decerebrate, slow 2- to 3-cps delta waves on EEG | | |

Adapted from Pugh RNH, Murray-Lyon IM, Dawson JL *et al.* Br J Surg 1973;60:646–9 [39], and CDER, CBER. Guidance for Industry, Rockville, FDA, 2003. (Internet at, www.fda.gov/downloads/Drugs/GuidanceComplianceRegulatoryInformation/Guidances/ucm072123.pdf [40].)

of guiding dose adjustments in patients with liver disease, much as creatinine clearance has been used to guide dose adjustments in patients with impaired renal function. The Pugh modification of Child's classification of liver disease severity (Table 7.4) is the classification scheme that is used most commonly in studies designed to formulate drug dosing recommendations for patients with liver disease [39, 40]. Another classification scheme, the model for end-stage liver disease (MELD), is based on serum bilirubin, serum creatinine, the international normalized prothrombin time ratio (INR), and the underlying cause of liver disease [41]. Unfortunately, these classification schemes are unable to precisely quantify the effect that liver disease has on the drug-metabolizing capability of individual patients. Because only patients with mild or moderately severe liver disease usually are enrolled in these studies, there are relatively few data from patients with severe liver disease, in whom both pharmacokinetic changes and altered pharmacologic response are expected to be most pronounced. The administration of narcotic, sedative, and psychoactive drugs to patients with severe liver disease is particularly hazardous because these drugs have the potential to precipitate life-threatening hepatic encephalopathy.

Prediction of pharmacokinetic alterations resulting from varying degrees of hepatic dysfunction remains a challenge, given the multiple factors that may impact on the hepatic clearance of drugs. Whole-body *physiologically based* pharmacokinetic modeling has been proposed by Edginton and Willman [42] and, more recently, by Johnson *et al.* [43]. These approaches are based on the "well-stirred" model of hepatic drug clearance and incorporate *in vitro–in vivo* extrapolation of intrinsic metabolic clearance for each enzymatic pathway, with corrections for estimated abundance of individual specific enzyme and liver weight, and utilize the Monte Carlo method to generate *virtual populations* of individuals with varying physiological and pathophysiologic characteristics [43]. Reasonable predictions were generated for orally administered midazolam, oral caffeine, oral and intravenous theophylline, oral and intravenous metoprolol, oral nifedipine, oral quinidine, oral diclofenac, oral sildenafil, and oral omeprazole, but not for intravenous omeprazole [43]. The clinical applicability of these predictive modeling approaches remains to be determined.

## Effects of Liver Disease on the Hepatic Elimination of Drugs

Equation 7.14 emphasizes the central point that changes in perfusion and protein binding, as well as intrinsic clearance, will affect the hepatic clearance of a number of drugs. The intact hepatocyte theory has been proposed as a means of simplifying this complexity [44]. This theory is analogous to the intact nephron theory (see Chapter 5) in that it assumes that the increase in portocaval shunting parallels the loss of functional cell mass, and that the reduced mass of normally functioning liver cells is perfused normally. Other theories have been proposed to account for the effects of chronic liver disease on hepatic drug clearance and it currently is not clear which, if any, of these theories is most appropriate [45]. However, what is apparent from studies in patients with significantly impaired liver function is that the intrinsic clearance of some drugs that normally are non-restrictively metabolized is reduced to the extent that $f_{u}CL_{int}$ now becomes rate limiting and clearance is no longer approximated by hepatic perfusion rate [25]. It also is apparent from Equation 7.14 that the presence of portosystemic shunting and hepatocellular damage will significantly increase the bioavailability of drugs that normally have extensive first-pass hepatic metabolism.

### Correlation of Laboratory Tests with Drug Metabolic Clearance

Bergquist *et al.* [46] presented examples in which several laboratory tests that are commonly used to assess liver function provide a more reliable indication of impaired drug metabolic clearance than the Child-Pugh clinical classification scheme (Table 7.5). Serum albumin concentrations were of greatest predictive value for two of the drugs shown in the table. However, this marker was not correlated with the hepatic clearance of lansoprazole, and a combination of all three laboratory tests was better correlated with hepatic clearance of atorvastatin than serum albumin alone. Serum concentrations of aspartate aminotransferase (AST) or alanine aminotransferase (ALT) were not correlated with hepatic drug clearance, as might be expected from the fact that these enzymes reflect hepatocellular damage rather than hepatocellular function.

TABLE 7.5   Correlation of Laboratory Test Results with Impaired Hepatic Clearance

|  |  | Laboratory test | | |
| --- | --- | --- | --- | --- |
| Drug | Enzyme(s) | Albumin | PT[a] | Bilirubin |
| "A" | CYP2C9 | X | | |
| "B" | Not given | X | | |
| Atorvastatin | CYP3A4 | X | X | X |
| Lansoprazole | CYP3A4 + CYP2C19 | | X | |

[a]Prothrombin time.
Data from Bergquist C, Lindergård J, Salmonson T. Clin Pharmacol Ther 1999;66:201–4 [46].

### Use of Probe Drugs to Characterize Hepatic Drug Clearance

A number of probe drugs have been administered to normal subjects and to patients to evaluate hepatic clearance. Quantitative liver function tests using probe drugs can be categorized either as specific for a given metabolic pathway or as more generally reflective of hepatic metabolism, perfusion, or biliary function. An example of the latter category is the *aminopyrine breath test*, which is a broad measure of hepatic microsomal drug metabolism, since aminopyrine is metabolized by at least six cytochrome P450 enzymes [47]. Other tests in this category are the *galactose elimination test*, to measure cytosolic drug metabolism; *sorbitol clearance*, to measure liver parenchymal perfusion; and *indocyanine green clearance*, reflecting both parenchymal perfusion and biliary secretory capacity. Figure 7.4 illustrates the relationship between the degree of impairment in these tests and Child-Pugh class of liver disease severity in patients with chronic hepatitis B and C [48]. These results indicate that hepatic metabolic capacity is impaired before portosystemic shunting becomes prominent in the pathophysiology of chronic viral hepatitis. However, these non-specific tests are, by their nature, of limited value in predicting the clearance of a specific drug in an individual patient.

The monoethylglycinexylidide (MEGX) test is an example of a test that specifically evaluates the function of a single metabolic pathway. In this test, a 1-mg/kg dose of lidocaine is administered intravenously and plasma concentrations of its N–dealkylated metabolite, MEGX, are measured either 15 or 30 minutes later. Testa *et al.* [49] found that a 30-minute post-dose MEGX concentration of 50 ng/ml provided the best discrimination between chronic hepatitis and cirrhosis (sensitivity, 93.5%; specificity, 76.9%). These authors concluded that both hepatic blood flow and the enzymatic conversion of lidocaine to MEGX, initially thought to be mediated by CYP3A4 but subsequently shown to be due primarily to CYP1A2 [50], were well preserved in patients with mild and moderate chronic hepatitis. However, MEGX levels fell significantly in patients with cirrhosis and were well correlated with the clinical stage of cirrhosis, as shown in Figure 7.5. Muñoz *et al.* [51] subsequently reported that serum lidocaine levels measured 120–180 minutes after administering a 5-mg/kg oral lidocaine dose had greater sensitivity (100%) than serum bilirubin (57%), serum albumin (62%), prothrombin concentrations (43%), or MEGX serum concentrations (57%) in differentiating cirrhotic patients from healthy controls, and suggested that this

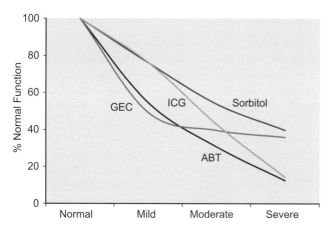

**FIGURE 7.4** Relationship between Child-Pugh stages of liver disease severity and extent of impairment in antipyrine breath test (ABT), galactose elimination capacity (GEC), sorbitol clearance, and indocyanine green clearance (ICG). Adapted from data published by Herold C, Heinz R, Niedobitek G *et al.* Liver 2001;21:260–5 [48].

approach would be better than either standard liver function tests or the MEGX test for evaluating liver function in cirrhotic patients.

Morphine, S-mephenytoin, debrisoquin, and erythromycin also have been used as selective probes to evaluate, respectively, glucuronidation and the CYP2C19, CYP2D6, and CYP3A4 metabolic pathways in patients with different Child-Pugh classes of liver disease severity, and these results are included in Figure 7.5 [35, 37, 52]. To increase the efficiency of evaluating specific drug metabolic pathways, the

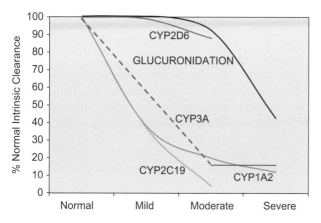

**FIGURE 7.5** Schematic diagram showing the relationship between Child-Pugh stages of liver disease severity and the intrinsic clearance of drugs mediated by specific cytochrome P450 metabolic pathways. Estimates for glucuronidation [36], CYP2D6 [35], CYP1A2 [46], CYP3A4 [47], and CYP2C19 [35] pathways are based on the literature sources indicated in parentheses. The erythromycin breath test was used to assess hepatic CYP3A in a study in which no patients with mild liver disease were included and results in patients with moderate and severe liver disease were combined.

strategy has been developed of simultaneously administering a combination of probes [53]. As many as five probe drugs have been administered in this fashion to provide a profile of CYP1A2, CYP2E1, CYP3A, CYP2D6, CYP2C19, and N–acetyltransferase activity [54]. The method was evaluated to exclude the possibility of a significant metabolic interaction between the individual probes. Although a number of different versions of the cocktail approach have been described, these all are too cumbersome for routine clinical use [55]. In addition, even when the metabolic pathway for a given drug is known, prediction of hepatic drug clearance in individual patients is complicated by the effects of pharmacogenetic variation and drug interactions.

## Effects of Liver Disease on the Renal Elimination of Drugs

Drug therapy in patients with advanced cirrhosis is further complicated by the fact that renal blood flow and glomerular filtration rate are frequently depressed in these patients in the absence of other known causes of renal failure. Renal hemodynamics are compromised long before cirrhosis is categorized as severe because even moderate portal hypertension triggers increased production of nitric oxide and other factors that cause arterial vasodilation in the splanchnic circulation [56]. Initially, cardiac output can increase to compensate for the decrease in systemic vascular resistance. However, in advanced cirrhosis, the sympathetic nervous system, the renin–angiotensin system, and the non-osmotic release of arginine vasopressin must be activated to maintain arterial pressure. Activation of these additional compensatory mechanisms causes intrarenal vasoconstriction and hypoperfusion that adversely affect renal sodium excretion and solute-free water retention, leading to the formation of ascites and edema, and ultimately results in renal failure. This etiology of renal failure has been termed the *hepatorenal syndrome* (HRS) and has been subdivided into Type I HRS, which presents as acute renal failure characterized by a doubling of a previously measured serum creatinine, or a 50% reduction in creatinine clearance, within 2 weeks; and Type II HRS, in which refractory ascites is prominent and progression to serum creatinine concentrations of 1.5–2.5 mg/dL occurs more gradually over a period of weeks to months [57]. However, a number of factors, including administration of certain drugs or spontaneous bacterial peritonitis resulting from the bacterial translocation from the intestine to the peritoneum, can precipitate acute renal failure in patients with Type II HRS.

Ginès *et al.* [58] monitored 234 patients with cirrhosis, ascites and a glomerular filtration rate (GFR) of more than 50 mL/min. These authors found that HRS developed within 1 year in 18%, and within 5 years in 39%, of these patients. Although the Pugh score was of no prognostic value, high plasma renin activity, low serum sodium concentrations, small liver size, and baseline estimates of renal function were independent predictors of the onset of this syndrome. However, conventional assessment of renal function in patients with advanced liver disease is complicated by the fact that GFR is overestimated when it is based on serum creatinine concentration measurements. Thus many patients with cirrhosis and ascites have a normal serum creatinine concentration with a GFR < 60 mL/min and serum creatinine concentrations may remain within the normal range even when inulin clearance falls as low as 10 mL/min [59]. This occurs because creatinine production is reduced, due to the reduced skeletal muscle mass that occurs in patients with advanced liver disease, and renal tubular secretion of creatinine increases as glomerular filtration rate is reduced. Consequently, both the Cockcroft and Gault and MDRD equations [60], and even the actual measurement of creatinine clearance based on timed urine collections, provide an inaccurate guide to the status of renal function in these patients [61]. But until a better approach is developed for evaluating renal function in liver disease patients, the current version of the MDRD equation is recommended as most suitable for routine clinical use [57].

The need for caution in estimating drug dosage for patients with hepatorenal syndrome is exemplified by carbenicillin, an antipseudomonal, semisynthetic penicillin that is excreted primarily by the kidneys, with biliary excretion normally accounting for less than 20% of total elimination. The decline in renal function that is associated with severe liver disease prolongs the elimination half-life of this drug from 1 hour in subjects with normal renal and liver function to approximately 24 hours [62]. Although studies in patients with hepatorenal syndrome were not reported, similar half-life prolongations have been described in patients with combined renal and hepatic functional impairment who were treated with the newer but pharmacokinetically similar antipseudomonal penicillins piperacillin [63] and mezlocillin [64]. Consequently, it is advisable to consider reducing doses even for drugs that are eliminated to a significant extent by renal excretion when treating patients with cirrhosis that is severe enough to be accompanied by ascites.

## Effects of Liver Disease on Patient Response

The relationship between drug concentration and response also can be altered in patients with advanced liver disease. Of greatest concern is the fact that customary doses of sedatives may precipitate the confusion, disorientation, and eventual coma that are characteristic of portal-systemic or hepatic encephalopathy that frequently occurs in the terminal phase of advanced liver disease [65]. Hepatic encephalopathy is primarily caused by the synergistic effects of excess ammonia production and inflammation that together result in astrocyte swelling and brain edema. Specific measures to treat patients with hepatic encephalopathy include oral administration of lactulose and the poorly absorbed antibiotic rifaximin to reduce ammonia formation by intestinal bacteria. However, experimental hepatic encephalopathy also is associated with increased γ–aminobutyric acid-mediated inhibitory neurotransmission, and there has been some success in using the benzodiazepine antagonist flumazenil to reverse this syndrome [66]. This provides the rationale for using flumazenil to treat patients who fail to respond to ammonia-reduction therapy, as well as those whose hepatic encephalopathy is triggered by exogenous benzodiazepines [67], and provides a theoretical basis for the finding that brain hypersensitivity, together with impaired drug elimination, is responsible for the exaggerated sedative response to diazepam that is exhibited by some patients with chronic liver disease [68]. Changes in the cerebrospinal fluid/serum concentration ratio of cimetidine have been reported in patients with liver disease, suggesting an increase in blood–brain barrier permeability that also could make these patients more sensitive to the adverse central nervous system effects of a number of other drugs [69].

Although cirrhotic patients frequently are treated with diuretic drugs to reduce ascites, they exhibit a reduced responsiveness to loop diuretics that cannot be overcome by administering larger doses. This presumably is related to the pathophysiology of increased sodium retention that contributes to the development of ascites [70]. In addition, decreases in renal function, which is often unrecognized in these patients [59], may lead to decreased delivery of loop diuretics to their renal tubular site of action. Because hyperaldosteronism is prevalent in these patients and spironolactone is not dependent on glomerular filtration for efficacy, it should be the mainstay of diuretic therapy in this clinical setting [71].

When diuretic therapy does result in effective fluid removal in cirrhotic patients, it is associated with a very high incidence of adverse reactions. In

TABLE 7.6   Some Drugs Requiring a Dose Reduction in Patients with Moderate Cirrhosis

| | F (%) | Parameter values or changes in cirrhosis | | | |
| | | F (%) | Clearance | $f_u$ | Ref(s) |
| --- | --- | --- | --- | --- | --- |
| *Analgesic drugs:* | | | | | |
| Morphine | 47 | 100 | ↓ 59% | | [36] |
| Meperidine | 47 | 91 | ↓ 46% | | [27] |
| Pentazocine | 17 | 71 | ↓ 50% | | [27] |
| *Cardiovascular drugs:* | | | | | |
| Propafenone | 21 | 75 | ↓ 24% | ↑ 213% | [75] |
| Verapamil | 22 | 52 | ↓ 51% | No change | [76] |
| Nifedipine | 51 | 91 | ↓ 60% | ↑ 93% | [77] |
| Nitrendipine | 40 | 54 | ↓ 34% | ↑ 43% | [78] |
| Nisoldipine | 4 | 15 | ↓ 42% | | [79] |
| Losartan | 33 | 66 | ↓ 50% | | [80–85] |
| *Other:* | | | | | |
| Omeprazole | 56 | 98 | ↓ 89% | | [82, 86] |
| Tacrolimus | 27 | 36 | ↓ 72% | | [83, 84, 87, 88] |

one study of diuretic therapy in cirrhosis, furosemide therapy precipitated HRS in 12.8%, and hepatic coma in 11.6%, of the patients [72]. Although daily doses of this drug did not differ, patients who had adverse drug reactions received total furosemide doses that averaged 1384 mg, whereas patients without adverse reactions received lower total doses that averaged 743 mg. Accordingly, when spironolactone therapy does not provide an adequate diuresis, only small frequent doses of loop diuretics should be added to the spironolactone regimen [71]. Cirrhotic patients also appear to be at an increased risk of developing acute renal failure after being treated with angiotensin-converting enzyme inhibitors and non-steroidal anti-inflammatory drugs [73].

## Modification of Drug Therapy in Patients with Liver Disease

It is advisable to avoid using certain drugs in patients with advanced liver disease. For example, angiotensin-converting enzyme inhibitors and non-steroidal anti-inflammatory drugs should be avoided because of their potential to cause acute renal failure. Paradoxically, administration of captopril to cirrhotic patients with ascites actually impairs rather than promotes sodium excretion [74]. Since coagulation disorders are common in patients with advanced cirrhosis, alternatives should be sought for therapy with β-lactam antibiotics that contain the *N*-methyl-thiotetrazole side chain (e.g., cefotetan) that inhibits γ-carboxylation of vitamin K-dependent clotting factors [73].

It also is prudent to reduce the dosage of a number of other drugs that frequently are used to treat patients with liver disease [30, 75–77]. Delcò and colleagues [76] recommend that although drug conjugation pathways also may be impaired in patients with liver failure, drugs that are mainly metabolized by these pathways are preferred because only one metabolic pathway usually is involved. Particular attention has been focused on drugs whose clearance is significantly impaired in patients with moderate hepatic impairment, as assessed using the Child-Pugh classification scheme shown in Table 7.4. Even greater caution should be exercised in using these drugs to treat patients with severely impaired liver function. Table 7.6 lists several drugs whose dose should be reduced in treating patients with moderate hepatic impairment. Most of the drugs in this table have first-pass metabolism that is greater than 50% in normal subjects but is substantially reduced when liver function is impaired [27, 36, 75–88].

Although initial and maintenance oral drug doses may need to be reduced in patients with moderate to severe liver disease, the extent of reduction cannot be accurately predicted since neither the extent of portosystemic shunting nor the actual hepatic blood flow usually are known in a given patient [76]. Given this uncertainty, maintenance doses need to be adjusted empirically to achieve the desired pharmacologic effect while avoiding toxicity. When medications are administered intravenously, a normal initial or loading dose may be administered, but the maintenance dose should be lowered to reflect the reduction in hepatic clearance [76]. Although not routinely evaluated in most studies of patients with liver disease, drug binding to plasma proteins also may be reduced in

**TABLE 7.7  Dosage Adjustments in Patients with Liver Disease**[a]

| Clinical setting | Recommendation |
| --- | --- |
| Drugs with a relatively high extraction ratio ($> 70\%$) | The dose should be reduced because the oral bioavailability can be significantly increased |
| Drugs with a low hepatic extraction ratio ($< 30\%$) and high plasma protein binding ($> 90\%$) | Pharmacokinetic evaluations should be based on the unbound blood/plasma concentrations because the unbound fraction of drug may be significantly increased. Dosage adjustments may be necessary even though total blood/plasma concentrations are within the normal range |
| Drugs with a low hepatic extraction ratio ($< 30\%$) and low plasma protein binding ($< 90\%$) | Dosage adjustment may be necessary and should be targeted at maintaining normal total (bound plus unbound) plasma concentrations |
| The elimination of drugs partly excreted unchanged by the kidneys will be impaired in patients with hepatorenal syndrome | Consider that creatinine clearance significantly over estimates glomerular filtration rate in these patients |
| The distribution volume of hydrophilic drugs may be increased in patients with edema or ascites | The loading dose may have to be increased if a rapid and complete response to the drug is required. Many of these drugs are eliminated by the kidneys so renal function should be taken into consideration |
| Drug selection and dosing in patients with severe liver disease (Child-Pugh classification) | Use caution when administering drugs with narrow therapeutic indices to patients with liver disease and any drug to patients with severe liver disease |

[a]Recommendations from Verbeeck RK. Eur J Clin Pharmacol 2008;64:1147–61 [30].

these patients and may contribute to exaggerated responses to non-restrictively metabolized drugs. Formation of pharmacologically active metabolites is another complicating factor that deserves consideration. For example, losartan has an active metabolite, EXP3174, which is primarily responsible for the extent and duration of pharmacological effect in patients treated with this drug [83]. Although standard doses produce plasma concentrations of losartan that are four to five times higher in patients with cirrhosis than those observed in normal subjects, plasma levels of EXP3174 are only increased by a factor of 1.5–2.0 [85]. This provided the rationale for reducing the usual losartan dose by only half in a trial in which this drug was used to reduce portal pressure in patients with cirrhosis and esophageal varices [89].

When no drug-specific recommendations are available, Delcò et al. [76] recommend using the Child-Pugh classification as a guide to reduce normal maintenance drug doses by 50% in patients with mild, and by 75% in patients with moderate, liver disease. In patients with severe liver disease, they recommend using drugs whose safety is known, or whose pharmacokinetics is not affected by liver disease, or for which therapeutic drug monitoring is available. Verbeeck [30] has provided the more detailed guidelines, listed in Table 7.7, for adjusting drug dosage in patients with liver failure. None of these guidelines obviates the need to monitor patient response closely and to make the further dose adjustments that may be required to both achieve the desired therapeutic response and avoid toxicity.

# REFERENCES

[1] Rowland M, Benet LZ, Graham GG. Clearance concepts in pharmacokinetics. J Pharmacokinet Biopharm 1973;1:123–36.
[2] Wilkinson GR, Shand DG. A physiological approach to hepatic drug clearance. Clin Pharmacol Ther 1975;18:377–90.
[3] Rane A, Wilkinson GR, Shand DG. Prediction of hepatic extraction ratio from in vitro measurement of intrinsic clearance. J Pharmacol Exp Ther 1977;200:420–4.
[4] Yang J, Jamei M, Yeo KR, Rostami-Hodjegan A, Tucker GT. Misuse of the well-stirred model of hepatic drug clearance. Drug Metab Dispos 2007;35:501–2.
[5] Roberts MS, Donaldson JD, Rowland M. Models of hepatic elimination: Comparison of stochastic models to describe residence time distributions and to predict the influence of drug distribution, enzyme heterogeneity, and systemic recycling on hepatic elimination. J Pharmacokinet Biopharm 1988;16:41–83.
[6] Atkinson AJ Jr, Reidenberg MM, Thompson WL. Clinical Pharmacology. In: Greenberger N, editor. MKSAP VI Syllabus. Philadelphia, PA: American College of Physicians; 1982. p. 85–96.
[7] Roberts MS, Magnusson BM, Burczynski FJ, Weiss M. Enterohepatic circulation: Physiological, pharmacokinetic and clinical implications. Clin Pharmacokinet 2002;41:751–90.
[8] Rollins DE, Klaassen CD. Biliary excretion of drugs in man. Clin Pharmacokinet 1979;4:368–79.
[9] Heggie GD, Sommadossi J-P, Cross DS, Huster WJ, Diasio RB. Clinical pharmacokinetics of 5-fluorouracil and its metabolites in plasma, urine, and bile. Cancer Res 1987;47:2203–6.
[10] Siegers C-P, Bumann D. Clinical significance of the biliary excretion of drugs. Prog Pharmacol Clin Pharmacol 1991;8:537–49.
[11] Duggan DE, Hooke KF, Noll RM, Kwan KC. Enterohepatic circulation of indomethacin and its role in intestinal irritation. Biochem Pharmacol 1975;24:1749–54.

[12] Veng Pedersen P, Miller R. Pharmacokinetics and bioavailability of cimetidine in humans. J Pharm Sci 1980;69:394–8.

[13] Miller R. Pharmacokinetics and bioavailability of ranitidine in humans. J Pharm Sci 1984;73:1376–9.

[14] Blaschke TF, Meffin PJ, Melmon KL, Rowland M. Influence of acute viral hepatitis on phenytoin kinetics and protein binding. Clin Pharmacol Ther 1975;17:685–91.

[15] Williams RL, Blaschke TF, Meffin PJ, Melmon KL, Rowland M. Influence of acute viral hepatitis on disposition and plasma binding of tolbutamide. Clin Pharmacol Ther 1977;21:301–9.

[16] Williams RL, Schary WL, Blaschke TF, Meffin PJ, Melmon KL, Rowland M. Influence of acute viral hepatitis on disposition and pharmacologic effect of warfarin. Clin Pharmacol Ther 1976;20:90–7.

[17] Williams RL, Blaschke TF, Meffin PJ, Melmon KL, Rowland M. Influence of viral hepatitis on the disposition of two compounds with high hepatic clearance: Lidocaine and indocyanine green. Clin Pharmacol Ther 1976;20:290–9.

[18] Villeneuve JP, Thibeault MJ, Ampelas M, Fortunet-Fouin H, LaMarre L, Côtè J, et al. Drug disposition in patients with HB$_s$Ag-positive chronic liver disease. Dig Dis Sci 1987;32:710–4.

[19] Prescott LF, Wright N. The effects of hepatic and renal damage on paracetamol metabolism and excretion following overdosage. A pharmacokinetic study. Br J Pharmacol 1973;49:602–13.

[20] Sotaniemi EA, Niemelä O, Risteli L, Stenbäck F, Pelkonen RO, Lahtela JT, et al. Fibrotic process and drug metabolism in alcoholic liver disease. Clin Pharmacol Ther 1986;40:46–55.

[21] Le Couteur DG, Fraser R, Hilmer S, Rivory LP, McLean AJ. The hepatic sinusoid in aging and cirrhosis. Clin Pharmacokinet 2005;44:187–200.

[22] Boyer TD, Henderson JM. Portal hypertension and bleeding esophageal varices. In: Zakim D, Boyer TD, editors. Hepatology: A textbook of liver disease. 4th ed. Philadelphia, PA: Saunders; 2003. p. 581–629.

[23] Iwasa M, Nakamura K, Nakagawa T, Watanabe S, Katoh H, Kinosada Y, et al. Single photon emission computed tomography to determine effective hepatic blood flow and intrahepatic shunting. Hepatology 1995;21:359–65.

[24] Lebrec D, Kotelanski B, Cohn JN. Splanchnic hemodynamics in cirrhotic patients with esophageal varices and gastrointestinal bleeding. Gastroenterology 1976;70:1108–11.

[25] Huet P-M, Villeneuve J-P. Determinants of drug disposition in patients with cirrhosis. Hepatology 1983;3:913–8.

[26] McLean A, du Souich P, Gibaldi M. Noninvasive kinetic approach to the estimation of total hepatic blood flow and shunting in chronic liver disease – a hypothesis. Clin Pharmacol Ther 1979;25:161–6.

[27] Neal EA, Meffin PJ, Gregory PB, Blaschke TF. Enhanced bioavailability and decreased clearance of analgesics in patients with cirrhosis. Gastroenterology 1979;77:96–102.

[28] Wood AJJ, Kornhauser DM, Wilkinson GR, Shand DG, Branch RA. The influence of cirrhosis on steady-state blood concentrations of unbound propranolol after oral administration. Clin Pharmacokinet 1978;3:478–87.

[29] Blaschke TF. Protein binding and kinetics of drugs in liver diseases. Clin Pharmacokinet 1977;2:32–44.

[30] Verbeeck RK. Pharmacokinetics and dosage adjustment in patients with hepatic dysfunction. Eur J Clin Pharmacol 2008;64:1147–61.

[31] Kusuhara H, Sugiyama Y. In vitro–in vivo extrapolation of transporter-mediated clearance in the liver and kidney. Drug Metab Pharmacokinet 2009;24:37–52.

[32] Elbekai RH, Korashy HM, El-Kadi AOS. The effect of liver cirrhosis on the regulation and expression of drug metabolizing enzymes. Curr Drug Metab 2004;5:157–67.

[33] Guengerich FP, Turvy CG. Comparison of levels of several human microsomal cytochrome P-450 enzymes and epoxide hydrolase in normal and disease states using immunochemical analysis of surgical liver samples. J Pharmacol Exp Ther 1991;256:1189–94.

[34] George J, Murray M, Byth K, Farrell GC. Differential alterations of cytochrome P450 proteins in livers from patients with severe chronic liver disease. Hepatology 1995;21:120–8.

[35] Adedoyin A, Arns PA, Richards WO, Wilkinson GR, Branch RA. Selective effect of liver disease on the activities of specific metabolizing enzymes: Investigation of cytochromes P450 2C19 and 2D6. Clin Pharmacol Ther 1998;64:8–17.

[36] Fisher CD, Lickteig AJ, Augustine LM, Ranger-Moore J, Jackson JP, Ferguson SS, et al. Hepatic cytochrome p450 alterations in humans with progressive stages of nonalcoholic fatty liver disease. Drug Metab Dispos 2009;37:2087–94.

[37] Hasselström J, Eriksson S, Persson A, Rane A, Svensson O, Säwe J. The metabolism and bioavailability of morphine in patients with severe liver cirrhosis. Br J Clin Pharmacol 1990;29:289–97.

[38] Hoyumpa AM, Schenker S. Is glucuronidation truly preserved in patients with liver disease? Hepatology 1991;13:786–95.

[39] Pugh RNH, Murray-Lyon IM, Dawson JL, Pietroni MC, Williams R. Transection of the oesophagus for bleeding oesophageal varices. Br J Surg 1973;60:646–9.

[40] CDER, CBER. Pharmacokinetics in patients with impaired hepatic function: Study design, data analysis, and impact on dosing and labeling. Guidance for Industry. Rockville, MD: FDA (Internet at www.fda.gov/downloads/Drugs/GuidanceComplianceRegulatoryInformation/Guidances/ucm072123.pdf; 2003).

[41] Wieisner R, Edwards E, Freeman R, Harper A, Kim R, Kamath P, et al. United Network for Organ Sharing Liver Disease Severity Score Committe. Model for end-stage liver disease (MELD) and allocation of donor livers. Gastroenterology 2003;124:91–6.

[42] Edginton AN, Willman S. Physiology-based simulations of a pathological condition. Prediction of pharmacokinetics in patients with liver cirrhosis. Clin Pharmacokinet 2008;47:743–52.

[43] Johnson TN, Boussery K, Rowland-Yao K, Tucker GT, Rostami-Hodjegan A. A semi-mechanistic model to predict the effects of liver cirrhosis on drug clearance. Clin Pharmacokinet 2010;49:189–206.

[44] Wood AJJ, Villeneuve JP, Branch RA, Rogers LW, Shand DG. Intact hepatocyte theory of impaired drug metabolism in experimental cirrhosis in the rat. Gastroenterology 1979;76:1358–62.

[45] Tucker GT. Alteration of drug disposition in liver impairment. Br J Clin Pharmacol 1998;46:355.

[46] Bergquist C, Lindergård J, Salmonson T. Dosing recommendations in liver disease. Clin Pharmacol Ther 1999;66:201–4.

[47] Engel G, Hofmann U, Heidemann H, Cosme J, Eichelbaum M. Antipyrine as a probe for human oxidative drug metabolism: Identification of the cytochrome P450 enzymes catalyzing 4-hydroxyantipyrine, 3-hydroxymethylantipyrine, and norantipyrine formation. Clin Pharmacol Ther 1996;59:613–23.

[48] Herold C, Heinz R, Niedobitek G, Schneider T, Hahn EG, Schuppan D. Quantitative testing of liver function in relation to fibrosis in patients with chronic hepatitis B and C. Liver 2001;21:260–5.

[49] Testa R, Caglieris S, Risso D, Arzani L, Campo N, Alvarez S, et al. Monoethylglycinexylidide formation measurement as a hepatic function test to assess severity of chronic liver disease. Am J Gastroenterol 1997;92:2268–73.

[50] Orlando R, Piccoli P, De Martin S, Padrini R, Floreani M, Palatini P. Cytochrome P50 1A2 is a major determinant of lidocaine metabolism in vivo: Effects of liver function. Clin Pharmacol Ther 2004;75:80–8.

[51] Muñoz AE, Miguez C, Rubio M, Bartellini M, Levi D, Podesta A, et al. Lidocaine and monoethylglycinexylidide serum determinations to analyze liver function of cirrhotic patients after oral administration. Dig Dis Sci 1999;44:789–95.

[52] Lown K, Kolars J, Turgeon K, Merion R, Wrighton SA, Watkins PB. The erythromycin breath test selectively measures P450IIIA in patients with severe liver disease. Clin Pharmacol Ther 1992;51:229–38.

[53] Breimer DD, Schellens JHM. A "cocktail" strategy to assess *in vivo* oxidative drug metabolism in humans. Trends Pharmacol Sci 1990;11:223–5.

[54] Frye RF, Matzke GR, Adedoyin A, Porter JA, Branch RA. Validation of the five-drug "Pittsburgh cocktail" approach for assessment of selective regulation of drug-metabolizing enzymes. Clin Pharmacol Ther 1997;62:365–76.

[55] Tanaka E, Kurata N, Yasuhara H. How useful is the "cocktail approach" for evaluating human hepatic drug metabolizing capacity using cytochrome P450 phenotyping probes *in vivo*? J Clin Pharm Ther 2003;28:157–65.

[56] Ginès P, Schrier RW. Renal failure in cirrhosis. N Engl J Med 2009;361:1279–90.

[57] Wong F, Nadim MK, Kellum JA, Salerno F, Bellomo R, Gerbes A, et al. Working Party proposal for a revised classification system of renal dysfunction in patients with cirrhosis. Gut 2011;60:702–9.

[58] Ginès A, Escorsell A, Ginès P, Saló J, Jiménez W, Inglada L, et al. Incidence, predictive factors, and prognosis of the hepatorenal syndrome in cirrhosis with ascites. Gastroenterology 1993;105:229–36.

[59] Papadakis MA, Arieff AI. Unpredictability of clinical evaluation of renal function in cirrhosis: Prospective study. Am J Med 1987;82:945–52.

[60] MacAulay J, Thompson K, Kiberd BA, Barnes DC, Peltekian KM. Serum creatinine in patients with advanced liver disease is of limited value for identification of moderate renal dysfunction: Are the equations for estimating renal function better? Can J Gastroenterol 2006;20:521–6.

[61] Proulx NL, Akbari A, Garg AX, Rostom A, Jaffey J, Clark HD. Measured creatinine clearance from timed urine collections substantially overestimates glomerular filtration rate in patients with liver cirrhosis: A systematic review and individual patient meta-analysis. Nephrol Dial Transplant 2005;20:1617–22.

[62] Hoffman TA, Cestero R, Bullock WE. Pharmacodynamics of carbenicillin in hepatic and renal failure. Ann Intern Med 1970;73:173–8.

[63] Green L, Dick JD, Goldberger SP, Anelopulos CM. Prolonged elimination of piperacillin in a patient with renal and liver failure. Drug Intell Clin Pharm 1985;19:427–9.

[64] Cooper BE, Nester TJ, Armstrong DK, Dasta JF. High serum concentrations of mezlocillin in a critically ill patient with renal and hepatic dysfunction. Clin Pharm 1986;5:764–6.

[65] Prakash R, Mullen KD. Mechanisms, diagnosis and management of hepatic encephalopathy. Nat Rev Gastroenterol Hepatol 2010;7:515–25.

[66] Ferenci P, Grimm G, Meryn S, Gangl A. Successful long-term treatment of portal-systemic encephalopathy by the benzodiazepine antagonist flumazenil. Gastroenterology 1989;96:240–3.

[67] Romero-Gómez M. Pharmacotherapy of hepatic encephalopathy in cirrhosis. Expert Opin Pharmacother 2010;11:1317–27.

[68] Branch RA, Morgan MH, James J, Read AE. Intravenous administration of diazepam in patients with chronic liver disease. Gut 1976;17:975–83.

[69] Schentag JJ, Cerra FB, Calleri GM, Leising ME, French MA, Bernhard H. Age, disease, and cimetidine disposition in healthy subjects and chronically ill patients. Clin Pharmacol Ther 1981;29:737–43.

[70] Brater DC. Resistance to loop diuretics: Why it happens and what to do about it. Drugs 1985;30:427–43.

[71] Brater DC. Use of diuretics in cirrhosis and nephrotic syndrome. Semin Nephrol 1999;19:575–80.

[72] Naranjo CA, Pontigo E, Valdenegro C, González G, Ruiz I, Busto U. Furosemide-induced adverse reactions in cirrhosis of the liver. Clin Pharmacol Ther 1979;25:154–60.

[73] Westphal J-F, Brogard J- M. Drug administration in chronic liver disease. Drug Saf 1997;17:47–73.

[74] Daskalopoulos G, Pinzani M, Murray N, Hirschberg R, Zipser RD. Effects of captopril on renal function in patients with cirrhosis and ascites. J Hepatol 1987;4:330–6.

[75] Rodighiero V. Effects of liver disease on pharmacokinetics: An update. Clin Pharmacokinet 1999;37:399–431.

[76] Delcò F, Tchambaz L, Schlienger R, Drewe J, Krähenbühl S. Dose adjustment in patients with liver disease. Drug Saf 2005;28:529–45.

[77] Nguyen HM, Cutie AJ, Pham DQ. How to manage medications in the setting of liver disease with the application of six questions. Intl J Clin Pract 2010;64:858–67.

[78] Lee JT, Yee Y-G, Dorian P, Kates RE. Influence of hepatic dysfunction on the pharmacokinetics of propafenone. J Clin Pharmacol 1987;27:384–9.

[79] Somogyi A, Albrecht M, Kliems G, Schäfer K, Eichelbaum M. Pharmacokinetics, bioavailability and ECG response of verapamil in patients with liver cirrhosis. Br J Clin Pharmacol 1981;12:51–60.

[80] Kleinbloesem CH, van Harten J, Wilson JPH, Danhof M, van Brummelen P, Breimer DD. Nifedipine: Kinetics and hemodynamic effects in patients with liver cirrhosis after intravenous and oral administration. Clin Pharmacol Ther 1986;40:21–8.

[81] Dylewicz P, Kirch W, Santos SR, Hutt HJ, Mönig H, Ohnhaus EE. Bioavailability and elimination of nitrendipine in liver disease. Eur J Clin Pharmacol 1987;32:563–8.

[82] van Harten J, van Brummelen P, Wilson JHP, Lodewijks MTM, Breimer DD. Nisoldipine: Kinetics and effects on blood pressure in patients with liver cirrhosis after intravenous and oral administration. Eur J Clin Pharmacol 1988;34:387–94.

[83] Lo M-W, Goldberg MR, McCrea JB, Lu H, Furtek CI, Bjornsson TD. Pharmacokinetics of losartan, an angiotensin II receptor antagonist, and its active metabolite EXP3174 in humans. Clin Pharmacol Ther 1995;58:641–9.

[84] Goa KL, Wagstaff AJ. Losartan potassium. A review of its pharmacology, clinical efficacy and tolerability in the management of hypertension. Drugs 1996;51:820–45.

[85] McIntyre M, Caffe SE, Michalak RA, Reid JL. Losartan, an orally active angiotensin ($AT_1$) receptor antagonist: A review of its efficacy and safety in essential hypertension. Pharmacol Ther 1997;74:181–94.

[86] Andersson T, Olsson R, Regårdh C-G, Skänberg I. Pharmacokinetics of [$^{14}$C]omeprazole in patients with liver cirrhosis. Clin Pharmacokinet 1993;24:71–8.

[87] Venkataramanan R, Jain A, Cadoff E, Warty V, Iwasaki K, Nagase K, et al. Pharmacokinetics of FK 506: Preclinical and clinical studies. Transplant Proc 1990;22(Suppl. 1):52–6.

[88] Jain AB, Venkataramanan R, Cadoff E, Fung JJ, Todo S, Krajack A, et al. Effect of hepatic dysfunction and T tube clamping on FK 506 pharmacokinetics and trough concentrations. Transplant Proc 1990;22(Suppl. 1):57–9.

[89] Schneider AW, Kalk JF, Klein CP. Effect of losartan, and angiotensin II receptor antagonist, on portal pressure in cirrhosis. Hepatology 1999;29:334–9.

# Non-Compartmental and Compartmental Approaches to Pharmacokinetic Data Analysis

David M. Foster[1] and Paolo Vicini[2]

[1]*Department of Bioengineering, University of Washington, Seattle, WA 98195*
[2]*Pfizer Worldwide Research and Development, San Diego, CA 92121*

## INTRODUCTION

From previous chapters, it is clear that the evaluation of pharmacokinetic parameters is an essential part of understanding how drugs function in the body. To estimate these parameters, studies are undertaken in which time-dependent measurements are collected. These studies can be conducted in animals at the preclinical level, through all stages of clinical trials, and can be data rich or sparse. No matter what the situation, there must be some common means by which to communicate the experimental results and summarize key features of a drug's properties. Pharmacokinetic parameters serve this purpose. Thus, in the field of pharmacokinetics, the definitions and formulas for the parameters must be agreed upon, and the methods used to calculate them understood. This understanding includes assumptions and domains of validity, for the utility of the parameter values depends upon them. This chapter examines the assumptions and domains of validity for the two commonly used methods of pharmacokinetic modeling analysis – non-compartmental and compartmental. Compartmental models have been presented in earlier chapters. This chapter will expand upon this, and compare the two methods.

Pharmacokinetic parameters fall basically into two categories. One category is qualitative or descriptive, in that the parameters are observational and require no formula for calculation. Examples would include the maximal observed concentration of a drug or the amount of drug excreted in the urine during a given time period. The other category is quantitative. Quantitative parameters require a mathematical formalism for calculation. Examples here would include mean residence times, clearance rates, and volumes of distribution. Estimation of terminal slopes would also fall into this category.

The quantitative parameters require not only a mathematical formalism but also data from which to estimate them. As noted, the two most common methods used for pharmacokinetic estimation are non-compartmental and compartmental analysis. Gillespie [1] has compared the two methods as applied to pharmacokinetics. Comparisons regarding the two methodologies as applied to metabolic studies have been provided by DiStefano [2] and Cobelli and Toffolo [3]. Covell *et al.* [4] have made an extensive theoretical comparison of the two methods. It is worth noting that in the literature the term "non-compartmental" has been used in two different contexts: not only to indicate methods based on the statistical analysis (i.e., averaging or integration) of time-dependent drug concentration profiles, but also to describe modeling formalisms (i.e., distributed systems [5] or recirculatory models [6]) that essentially relax the assumption of "lumping" (i.e., combining processes with similar space–time characteristics) that is inherent in the compartmental models used both in pharmacokinetics and tracer kinetics. We will not be concerned with these latter classes of models but will focus on the commonly used moment-based method of non-compartmental pharmacokinetic data analysis.

The use of compartment-based and moment-based methods for determining pharmacokinetic parameters has been the subject of intense discussion in the literature, and various clarifications have been proposed to deal with some of the issues we will cover here [7, 8]. Despite this, questions still remain regarding the circumstances under which these two methods can be used to estimate the pharmacokinetic parameters of interest. To begin to formulate an answer, one must start with a definition of kinetics, since it is through this definition that one can rigorously introduce the mathematical and statistical analyses needed to study the dynamic characteristics of a system and proceed to define specific parameters of interest that can be estimated from the experimental data. From the definition of kinetics, the types of equations that can be used to provide a mathematical description of the system can be given. The assumptions underlying non-compartmental analysis and estimation techniques for the different parameters for different experimental input–output configurations can then be discussed. One then moves to compartmental analysis with the understanding that models set in full generality are very difficult to practically solve. With appropriate assumptions that are commonly made in pharmacokinetic studies, a simpler set of compartmental models will evolve. These models are easy to solve, and it will be seen that all parameters estimated using non-compartmental analysis can be recovered from these compartmental models. Under conditions when the two methods should, in theory, yield the same estimates, differences can be attributed to the numerical techniques used (e.g., sums of exponentials vs trapezoidal integration). With this knowledge, the circumstances under which the two methods will provide the same or different estimates of the pharmacokinetic parameters can be discussed. Thus, it is not the point of this chapter to favor one method over another; rather, the intent is to describe the assumptions and consequences of using either method.

An interesting facet of our discussion is that estimating parameters from data provides a vehicle for communicating information about a drug (e.g., summarizing the pharmacokinetics of a drug by way of its residence time, half-life, or apparent volume of distribution) to what may be a diverse audience. Non-compartmental parameters are usually easy to grasp in their implication and fit this role very well. Our purpose here is to discuss the implications

of different parameter estimation methods, all the while describing a reliance on conceptual models that has stimulated much debate in both the pharmacokinetic [9] and integrative physiology [2] literature.

Most of the theoretical details of the material covered in this chapter can be found in Covell *et al.* [4], Jacquez and Simon [10], and Jacquez [11]. Of particular importance to this chapter is the material covered in Covell *et al.* [4] in which the relationship between the calculation of kinetic parameters from statistical moments and the same parameters calculated from the rate constants of a linear, constant coefficient compartmental model are derived. Jacquez and Simon [10] discuss in detail the mathematical properties of systems that depend upon local mass balance; this forms the basis for understanding compartmental models and the simplifications that result from certain assumptions about a system under study. Berman [12] gives examples using metabolic turnover data, while the pharmacokinetic examples provided in Gibaldi and Perrier [13] and Rowland and Tozer [14] are more familiar to clinical pharmacologists.

## KINETICS, PHARMACOKINETICS AND PHARMACOKINETIC PARAMETERS

### Kinetics and the Link to Mathematics

Substances being processed in a biological system are constantly undergoing change. These changes can include transport (e.g., transport via the circulation or transport into or out from a cell) or transformation (e.g., biochemically changing from one substance to another). These changes and the concomitant outcomes form the basis for the system in which the substance interacts. How can one formalize these changes, and once formalized, how can one describe their quantitative nature? Dealing with these questions involves an understanding and utilization of concepts related to kinetics.

The *kinetics* of a substance in a biological system is its spatial and temporal distribution in that system. Kinetics is the result of several complex events including entry into the system, subsequent distribution (which may entail circulatory dynamics and transport into and from cells), and elimination (which usually requires biochemical transformations). Together these events characterize both the transformations undergone by the substance and the system in which it resides.

In this chapter, the substance will be assumed to be a drug that is not normally present in the system, but in other contexts it could be an element such as calcium or zinc, or a compound such as amino acids, proteins, or sugars that exist normally in the body. Thus, in this chapter, *pharmacokinetics* is defined as the spatial and temporal distribution of a drug in a system. Unlike endogenous substances which are normally present, input of drugs into the system normally occurs from exogenous sources. In addition, unless otherwise noted, the system under consideration will be the whole body. When the therapeutic drug is an endogenous substance (e.g., recombinant endogenous proteins or hormones such as insulin), then more general considerations apply. It should be noted that this definition of pharmacokinetics differs somewhat from the more conventional definition given in Chapter 1. The reason for this is seen in the following section.

Our definition of pharmacokinetics contains a spatial component, so location of the substance in the biological system is important. From the temporal component of the definition, it follows that the amount of substance at a specific location is changing with time. Mathematically, the combination of these temporal and spatial components leads to partial derivatives,

$$\frac{\partial}{\partial t}, \frac{\partial}{\partial x}, \frac{\partial}{\partial y}, \frac{\partial}{\partial z} \tag{8.1}$$

which, mathematically, reflect change in time and space. Here $t$ is time, and a three-dimensional location in the system is represented by the spatial coordinates $(x, y, z)$.

If one chooses to use partial derivatives to describe drug kinetics in the body, then expressions for each of $\partial/\partial t$, $\partial/\partial x$, $\partial/\partial y$, and $\partial/\partial z$ must be written. That is, a system of partial differential equations must be specified. Writing these equations involves knowledge of physical chemistry, irreversible thermodynamics, and circulatory dynamics. Such equations will incorporate parameters that can be either deterministic (known) or stochastic (contain statistical uncertainties). Although such equations can sometimes be written for specific systems, defining and then estimating the unknown parameters is in most cases impossible because of the difficulty in obtaining sufficient measurements to resolve the spatial components of the system. In pharmacokinetic applications, partial differential equations are sometimes used to describe distributed systems models, such as those described in Chapter 9.

How does one resolve the difficulty associated with partial differential equations? The most common way is to reduce the system into a finite number of components. This can be accomplished by lumping together processes based upon time, location, or a combination of the two. One thus moves from partial derivatives to ordinary derivatives, where space is not taken directly into account. This reduction in complexity results in the compartmental models discussed later in this chapter. The same lumping process also forms the basis for the non-compartmental models discussed in the next section, although the resulting models are much simpler than compartmental models in that they have a less explicitly defined structure.

One can now appreciate why conventional definitions of pharmacokinetics are a little different from the definition given here. The conventional definitions make references to events other than temporal and spatial distribution. These events are, in fact, consequences of a drug's own kinetics, and thus the two should be conceptually separated. The processes of drug absorption, distribution, metabolism, and elimination relate to quantitative parameters that can only be estimated from a mathematical model describing the kinetics of the drug. The point is that, to understand the mathematical basis of pharmacokinetic parameter estimation, it is necessary to keep in mind the separation between the general concepts of kinetics *per se* and the use of data to estimate pharmacokinetic parameters of practical interest.

Using the general definition of pharmacokinetics given in terms of spatial and temporal distribution and transformation processes, one can easily progress to a description of the underlying assumptions and mathematics of non-compartmental and compartmental analysis, and, from there, proceed to the processes involved in estimating the pharmacokinetic parameters. This will permit a better understanding of the domain of validity of non-compartmental vs compartmental parameter estimation.

## The Pharmacokinetic Parameters

What is desired from the pharmacokinetic parameters is a quantitative measure of how a drug behaves in the system. To estimate these parameters, one must design an experiment to collect transient data that can then be used, in combination with an appropriate mathematical formalism, to estimate the parameters of interest. These fundamental concepts have been reviewed in the past from a variety of viewpoints [15].

To design such an experiment, the system must contain at least one *accessible pool*; that is, the system must contain a "site" that is available for drug input and data collection. As we will see, this site must have certain properties. If the system contains an accessible pool, this implies that other parts of the system are not accessible for test input and/or data collection. This divides the system into accessible and non-accessible pools. A drug (or drug metabolite) in each pool interacts with other components of the system. The only difference between non-compartmental and compartmental models is the way in which the non-accessible portion of the system is described.

The pharmacokinetic parameters defined in the following section can be used to characterize both the accessible pool and the system (i.e., the totality of accessible and non-accessible pools), although accessible pool and system parameters are usually distinct. This situation is illustrated by the two models shown in Figure 8.1. For example, Figure 8.1A could describe the situation where plasma is the accessible pool and is used for both drug input and sampling. Figure 8.1B accommodates extravascular input (e.g., oral dosing or intramuscular injection) followed by the collection of serial blood samples, but it can also accommodate the situation where the input is intravascular and only urine samples are collected. Thus, the schematic in Figure 8.1 describes the experimental situation for most pharmacokinetic studies. The case with a single accessible pool is of most frequent interest, while the case with two accessible pools has been studied in the context of substances involved in intermediary metabolism and studied with multiple-input, multiple-output experiments.

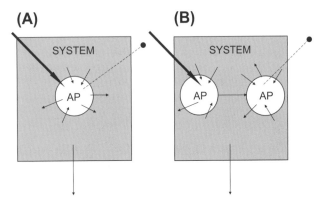

**FIGURE 8.1** (A) A system in which an accessible pool (AP) is available for test input (*bold arrow*) and sampling (*dashed line with bullet*). Loss of material from the system is indicated by the arrow leaving the system box. Material exchanging between the accessible pool and the rest of the system is indicated by the small arrows leaving and entering the accessible pool. The pharmacokinetic parameters estimated from kinetic data characterize the accessible pool and the system in which the accessible pool is embedded. (B) A system in which there are two accessible pools, one of which is available for test input (*bold arrow*) and a second which is available for sampling (*dashed line with bullet*); the test input is transported to the second accessible pool as indicated by the transfer arrow. Other transfer arrows are as explained in (A).

### Accessible Pool Parameters

The pharmacokinetic parameters descriptive of the accessible pool are given as follows (these definitions apply both to non-compartmental and compartmental models; how they relate to the situation where there are two accessible pools will be discussed for the individual cases):

*Volume of distribution*: $V_a$ (units: volume). The volume of the accessible pool is the volume in which the drug, upon introduction into the system, intermixes uniformly (kinetically homogeneous) and instantaneously.

*Clearance rate*: $CL_a$ (units: volume/time). This is the rate at which the accessible pool is irreversibly cleared of drug per unit time. The fundamental concept of clearance rate is perhaps one of the most important in pharmacokinetics, and has been recently reviewed in the context of the original considerations that brought about its definition [16].

*Elimination rate constant*: $k_e$ (units: 1/time). This is the fraction of drug that is irreversibly cleared from the accessible pool per unit time. (In some literature, this is referred to as the fractional clearance or fractional catabolic rate.)

*Mean residence time*: $MRT_a$ (units: time). This is the average time a drug spends in the accessible pool during all passages through the system before being irreversibly cleared. A useful commentary on mean residence time determination has been provided by Landaw and Katz [17].

### System Parameters

The pharmacokinetic parameters descriptive of the system are as follows (although these definitions apply both to the non-compartmental and compartmental models, some modification will be needed for two accessible pool models as well as compartmental models):

*Total equivalent volume of distribution*: $V_{tot}$ (units: volume). This is the total volume of the system seen from the accessible pool; it is the volume in which the total amount of drug would be distributed, assuming the concentration of material throughout the system is uniform and equal to the concentration in the accessible pool. As in Chapter 3, this is also often referred to as the apparent volume of distribution at steady state, $V_{d(ss)}$.

*System mean residence time*: $MRT_s$ (units: time). This is the average time the drug spends in the system before leaving the system for the last time.

*Mean residence time outside the accessible pool*: $MRT_o$ (units: time). This is the average time the drug spends outside the accessible pool before leaving the system for the last time.

*Extent of absorption*: $F$ (units: dimensionless, or percent). This is the fraction of drug that appears in a second accessible (to measurement, but not test input) pool following administration in a first accessible (to test input, but not to measurement) pool.

*Absorption rate constant*: $k_a$ (units: 1/time). This is the fraction of drug that appears per unit time in a second accessible (to measurement, but not test input) pool following administration in a first accessible (to test input, but not to measurement) pool. As discussed in Chapter 4, both $F$ and $k_a$ are components of *bioavailability*.

## Moments

Moments are the weighted integrals of a function and play an essential role in estimating specific pharmacokinetic parameters. The modern use of moments in the analysis of pharmacokinetic data and the notions of non-compartmental or integral equation analysis can be traced to Yamaoka *et al.* [18], although these authors correctly point out that the formulas were known since the pioneering effort of Torsten Teorell [19] in the late 1930s. Beal [7] places the method of moments as early as the work of Karl Pearson [20] in 1902. In other areas of kinetics, specifically tracer (indicator) kinetics, seminal references on the theory of moments are provided by Zierler [21] and Perl [22], with considerations that extend to non-steady state conditions [23].

The moments of a function are defined as follows; how they are used will be described later. Suppose $C(t)$ is a real-valued function defined on the interval $[0, \infty]$, where $C(t)$ is used to denote a functional description of a set of pharmacokinetic measurement data. The zeroth and first order moment of $C(t)$, denoted $S_0$ and $S_1$, are defined as:

$$S_0 = \int_0^\infty C(t)dt = AUC \qquad (8.2)$$

$$S_1 = \int_0^\infty t \cdot C(t)dt = AUMC \qquad (8.3)$$

In these equations, $S_0$ and $S_1$ are also defined, respectively, as $AUC$, "area under the curve", and $AUMC$, "area under the first moment curve". $AUC$ was introduced in the discussion of bioavailability in Chapter 4, and it and $AUMC$ are the more common expressions in pharmacokinetics and will be used in

the following discussions. Higher order moments are rarely used in our context of interest.

The following discussion will describe how $AUC$ and $AUMC$ are estimated, how they are used to estimate specific pharmacokinetic parameters (including related assumptions), and what their relationship is to specific pharmacokinetic parameters estimated from compartmental models. Both moments, however, are used for other purposes that relate to model building. For example, $AUC$ acts as a surrogate for drug exposure, and values of $AUC$ from different dose levels of a drug are used to justify assumptions of pharmacokinetic linearity. Error analyses of moment-based non-compartmental analysis have been described, with reference both to pharmacokinetics [24] and to more general biological systems [25], and also against other formalisms such as those incorporated in circulatory models [26].

## NON-COMPARTMENTAL ANALYSIS

### Non-Compartmental Model

The non-compartmental model provides a framework to introduce and use statistical moment analysis to estimate pharmacokinetic parameters. There are basically two forms of the non-compartmental model: the single accessible pool model and the two accessible pool model. These are schematized in Figure 8.2.

What is the relationship between the situation described in Figure 8.1 and the two models shown in Figure 8.2? Consider first the single accessible pool model shown in Figure 8.2A. The accessible pool here, denoted by the circle into which drug is input (*bold arrow*) and from which samples are taken (*dotted line with bullet*), is the same as that shown in Figure 8.1A. The entire interaction of the accessible pool with the rest of the system is indicated by the arrow leaving and returning to the accessible pool. This is called the

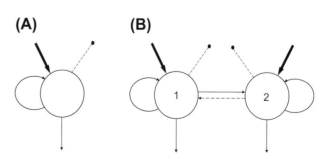

**FIGURE 8.2** The single (A) and two (B) accessible pool models. See text for explanation.

*recirculation-exchange* arrow, and encompasses all interactions the drug undergoes in the system outside of the accessible pool. Notice that a drug introduced into this pool has two routes by which it can leave the accessible pool. One is via recirculation-exchange, and the other is via irreversible loss, denoted by the arrow leaving the accessible pool. As indicated in Figure 8.2A, drug can only enter and leave the system via the accessible pool. Drug can neither enter nor leave the system along the recirculation-exchange arrow. This is called the equivalent sink and source constraint, and is fundamental in understanding the domain of validity of the pharmacokinetic parameters estimated from this model (2). The single accessible pool model is used primarily when the accessible pool is plasma, and the drug is administered directly into plasma.

In the case of more involved experimental designs, including extraplasma administration and measurements, the two accessible pool model depicted in Figure 8.2B may apply. This model is derived from the model shown in Figure 8.1B in a fashion that is similar to that used to derive the single accessible pool model. The difference between the single and two accessible pool models is as follows: While both pools have recirculation-exchange arrows, material can flow from pool 1 to pool 2. Thus, this model is suitable for describing oral or other extravascular drug input, or the situation in which either plasma concentrations of a drug and its metabolite are measured or both plasma and urine data are collected.

Note that there is a dashed arrow from pool 2 to pool 1 in Figure 8.2B. This indicates that exchange can occur in this direction also. Although analysis of this exchange is frequently incorporated in metabolic kinetic studies, there are relatively few examples in pharmacokinetics in which this has been studied. It is essential to note that this arrow is not equivalent to an arrow in a multicompartmental model! This arrow represents transfer of material from pool 2 to pool 1 by whatever routes exist, and can be a composite of many activities including delays.

The two accessible pool model accommodates even more complex experimental formats. For example, one could have inputs into both pools, and samples from both as well. However, in most pharmacokinetic studies with the two accessible pool model, pool 2 is plasma and input is only into pool 1, as with oral dosing. In this situation, the pharmacokinetic parameters depend on bioavailability and can only be estimated up to a proportionality constant, as is the case with so-called *oral clearance* (*CL/F*), referred to as *relative clearance* in this chapter

and elsewhere sometimes referred to as *apparent clearance*.

## Kinetic Parameters of the Non-Compartmental Model

The kinetic parameters of the non-compartmental model are those defined above for the accessible pool and system. However, the formulas depend upon the experimental protocol, especially on the mode of drug administration. In this chapter, only the canonical inputs will be considered, such as an intravenous bolus (or multiple boluses) or constant infusion (or multiple constant infusions). References will be given for those interested in more complex protocols.

The relationships among the accessible pool parameters in the non-compartmental model are given in the following equations:

$$k_e = \frac{CL_a}{V_a} \qquad (8.4)$$

$$MRT_a = \frac{1}{k_e} = \frac{V_a}{CL_a} \qquad (8.5)$$

Note that

$$V_a = \frac{d}{C(0)}$$

where $C(0)$ is the concentration of drug in the system at time zero and $d$ is the amount of drug injected, for a pulse input in the accessible pool. Equation 8.5 can be rearranged to yield

$$k_e \cdot V_a = CL_a \qquad (8.6)$$

In addition, Equations 8.5 and 8.6 can be combined to yield the more familiar

$$V_a = MRT_a \cdot CL_a \qquad (8.7)$$

The relationships among the system parameters for the non-compartmental model are:

$$V_{tot} = MRT_s \cdot CL_a \qquad (8.8)$$

$$MRT_o = MRT_s - MRT_a \qquad (8.9)$$

Other commonly used non-compartmental parameters include $T_{\max}$ (the time at which the concentration in the accessible pool reaches its observed maximum) and $C_{\max}$ (the observed maximum of the concentration in the accessible pool). These parameters are often reported based on inspection of the measured pharmacokinetic data.

## The Single Accessible Pool Model

Assume either a single bolus injection of drug whose amount is denoted by $d$ or a constant infusion of drug whose infusion rate is $u$ over the time interval $[0, t]$. Then, the pharmacokinetic parameters of interest can be calculated from features of the measurements and the test input as:

| Bolus | Infusion | |
|---|---|---|
| $V_a = \dfrac{d}{C(0)}$ | $V_a = \dfrac{u}{\dot{C}(0)}$ | (8.10) |
| $CL_a = \dfrac{d}{AUC}$ | $CL_a = \dfrac{u}{\overline{C}}$ | (8.11) |
| $MRT_s = \dfrac{AUMC}{AUC}$ | $MRT_s = \dfrac{\int_0^\infty [\overline{C} - C(t)]dt}{\overline{C}}$ | (8.12) |

In these formulas, $C(0)$ is the concentration of drug in the system at time zero, $\dot{C}(0)$ is the first derivative of $C(t)$ evaluated at time zero, and $\overline{C}$ is the steady-state value for the concentration of drug in the accessible pool following a constant infusion into that pool. The remaining single accessible pool parameters, $k_e$, $V_{tot}$, and $MRT_0$ can be calculated for either test input format using Equations 8.4, 8.8, and 8.9. For example, the mean residence time outside the accessible pool is calculated as

$$MRT_0 = MRT_s - MRT_a = \frac{AUMC}{AUC} - \frac{V_a}{CL_a}$$
$$= \frac{AUMC}{AUC} - \frac{AUC}{C(0)}.$$

Although these formulas are for a single-input format, formulas also exist for generic inputs including multiple boluses or infusions. If $u(t)$ is a generic input function, the formulas for $V_a$, $CL_a$ and $MRT_s$ are:

$$V_a = \frac{u(0)}{\dot{C}(0)} \tag{8.13}$$

$$CL_a = \frac{\int_0^\infty u(t)dt}{AUC} \tag{8.14}$$

$$MRT_s = \frac{\int_0^\infty t \cdot C(t)dt}{AUC} - \frac{\int_0^\infty t \cdot u(t)dt}{\int_0^\infty u(t)dt} \tag{8.15}$$

What is the origin of these formulas? That is, how are Equations 8.10–8.12 and 8.13–8.15 obtained? The answer is not obvious, although the definitions of mean residence time can be intuitively interpreted as

"weighted averages" (with respect to concentration values) of times. In an excellent description of mean residence times, Weiss [27] points out that, besides an accessible pool that must be available for test input and measurement, the system must be linear and time-invariant for the equations to be valid. Veng-Pedersen [28] has reviewed the concept of linearity with reference to non-compartmental and compartmental formalisms, and we will discuss the notions of linearity and time invariance later. For a formal derivation of these equations, the reader is referred to Weiss [27], Cobelli *et al.* [29], the already cited Covell *et al.* [4] or Gibaldi and Perrier [13]. In practice, *AUC* and *AUMC* are calculated from concentration measurements in the accessible pool. However, an understanding of the derivation of these equations is essential to understanding the domain of validity of the pharmacokinetic parameters obtained by non-compartmental methods, no matter what method of evaluating the integrals or extrapolations is employed.

## The Two Accessible Pool Model

The two accessible pool model presents problems in estimating the pharmacokinetic parameters characterizing this situation. This is largely because the desired parameters such as clearance, volumes, and residence times cannot be estimated from a single-input–single-output experiment with input into the first pool and samples from the second pool. To deal with this situation, recall first the notion of absolute bioavailability discussed in Chapter 4. Let $D_{oral}$ be the total dose of drug input into the first accessible pool, and let $D_{iv}$ be the dose into the second accessible pool, assumed to be intravascular space. Let $AUC[2]$ be the area under the concentration–time curve in the second accessible pool following the dose $D_{oral}$ (this is $AUC_{oral}$ in the notation of Chapter 4), and let $AUC_{iv}$ be the area under the concentration–time curve in the second accessible pool following the bolus dose $D_{iv}$ (in a separate experiment). Since the amounts of $D_{oral}$ and $D_{iv}$ are usually different, the absolute bioavailability is defined as

$$F = \frac{AUC[2]}{AUC_{iv}} \cdot \frac{D_{iv}}{D_{oral}} \tag{8.16}$$

The following parameters can be calculated from data following a bolus injection into the first accessible pool. Let $CL[2]$ and $V[2]$, respectively be the clearance from and volume of the second accessible pool, and let $CL[2,rel]$ and $V[2,rel]$ be the relative clearance (oral clearance) from and volume of the second accessible pool. Then

$$MRT[2, 1] = \frac{\int_0^\infty tC[2](t)dt}{\int_0^\infty C[2](t)dt} \qquad (8.17)$$

$$CL[2, rel] = \frac{CL[2]}{F} = \frac{D_{oral}}{AUC[2]} \qquad (8.18)$$

$$V[2, rel] = \frac{V[2]}{F} = CL[2, rel] \cdot MRT[2, 1] \qquad (8.19)$$

$MRT[2,1]$ is the mean residence time of drug in the second accessible pool following introduction of drug into the first accessible pool.

Clearly this situation is not as rich in information as the single accessible pool situation. Of course the parameters $CL[2]$ and $V[2]$ can be calculated in the event that $F$ is known or when a separate intravenous dose is administered. Information on other input formats or the situation when there is a two-input–four-output experiment can be found in Cobelli *et al.* [29].

## Estimating the Kinetic Parameters of the Non-Compartmental Model

For the canonical input of drug, what information is needed? For the bolus input, an estimate of the drug concentration at time zero, $C(0)$, is needed in order to estimate $V_a$. For a constant infusion of drug, an estimate of $\dot{C}(0)$ is needed to estimate $V_a$, and an estimate of the plateau concentration, $\overline{C}$, is needed to estimate clearance and the system mean residence time.

The most important estimates, however, involve AUC and AUMC. These integrals are supposed to be calculated from time zero to time infinity, whereas an experiment has only a finite time domain $[0, t_n]$, where $t_n$ is the time of the last measurement. In addition, it is rarely the case that the first measurement is obtained at time zero. Consequently, accurate calculation of the integrals requires extrapolation both to time zero and to infinite time. Hence, assuming that the time of the first measurement is $t_1$, one must partition the integral as follows to numerically estimate AUC and AUMC:

$$AUC = \int_0^\infty C(t)dt$$
$$= \int_0^{t_1} C(t)dt + \int_{t_1}^{t_n} C(t)dt + \int_{t_n}^\infty C(t)dt \qquad (8.20)$$

$$AUMC = \int_0^\infty t \cdot C(t)dt$$
$$= \int_0^{t_1} t \cdot C(t)dt + \int_{t_1}^{t_n} t \cdot C(t)dt + \int_{t_n}^\infty t \cdot C(t)dt$$
$$(8.21)$$

The first and third integrals in either equation require extrapolation beyond the experimental start and end times, while the middle integral only requires interpolation of existing data. One approach to solve these issues is to fit the available data to suitable functions of time that can automatically provide the needed extrapolations. Clearly, the use of such functional descriptors also implies that non-compartmental analysis is not truly "model-independent", as has been sometimes claimed [9]. This characteristic is in addition to the other limitations that arise from incomplete knowledge of elimination routes.

### Estimating AUC and AUMC Using Sums of Exponentials

For the single accessible pool model, following a bolus injection of amount $D$ into the pool, the pharmacokinetic data can be described by a sum of exponentials equation of the general form shown in Equation 8.22.

$$C(t) = A_1 e^{-\lambda_1 t} + \dots + A_n e^{-\lambda_n t} \qquad (8.22)$$

In this, and subsequent equations, the $A_i$ are called *coefficients* and the $\lambda_i$ are *exponentials* (in mathematical parlance, they are called *eigenvalues*). Following a constant infusion into the accessible pool, Equation 8.22 changes to Equation 8.23 with the restriction that the sum of the coefficients equals zero, reflecting the fact that no drug is present in the system at time zero.

$$C(t) = A_0 + A_1 e^{-\lambda_1 t} + \dots + A_n e^{-\lambda_n t} \qquad (8.23)$$
$$A_0 + A_1 + \dots + A_n = 0$$

What is the advantage of using sums of exponentials to describe pharmacokinetic data in the situation of the single accessible pool model following a bolus injection or constant infusion? The reason is that the integrals required to estimate the pharmacokinetic parameters are very easy to calculate!

Assuming the data can be fit (for example, by using non-linear regression techniques) to exponential functions, the coefficients and the exponentials can be used to calculate *AUC* and *AUMC* and, hence, the pharmacokinetic parameters. For the bolus injection, from Equation 8.22,

$$AUC = \int_0^\infty C(t)dt = \frac{A_1}{\lambda_1} + \ldots + \frac{A_n}{\lambda_n} \qquad (8.24)$$

$$AUMC = \int_0^\infty t \cdot C(t)dt = \frac{A_1}{\lambda_1^2} + \ldots + \frac{A_n}{\lambda_n^2} \qquad (8.25)$$

In addition, for the bolus injection,

$$C(0) = A_1 + \ldots + A_n \qquad (8.26)$$

provides an estimate for $C(0)$. Thus, with knowledge of the amount of drug in the bolus dose, $D$, all pharmacokinetic parameters can be estimated.

For a constant infusion, the steady state concentration, $\overline{C}$, can be seen from Equation 8.23 to equal $A_0$. An estimate for $\dot{C}(0)$ can be obtained

$$\dot{C}(0) = -A_1\lambda_1 - \ldots - A_n\lambda_n \qquad (8.27)$$

and since the estimate for $\overline{C}$ is $A_0$,

$$\int_0^\infty [\overline{C} - C(t)]dt = \frac{A_1}{\lambda_1} + \ldots + \frac{A_n}{\lambda n} \qquad (8.28)$$

Thus, all the pharmacokinetic parameters for the constant infusion case can be estimated in a straightforward manner from the coefficients and the exponentials.

An advantage of using sums of exponentials is that error estimates (precisions) for all the pharmacokinetic parameters can also be obtained as part of the fitting process. As discussed in the following section, this is not the case for most of the so-called "numerical" techniques for calculating *AUC* and *AUMC*, for which calculation of precision is not straightforward. In addition, for multiple inputs (i.e., multiple boluses or infusions) sums of exponentials can be used over each experimental time period for a specific bolus or infusion, recognizing that the exponentials $\lambda_i$ remain the same (i.e., assuming the system is linear and time invariant) across dosing intervals. The reason is that the exponentials are system parameters, and do not depend on a particular mode of introducing drug into the system [30].

### Estimating **AUC** *and* **AUMC** *Using Other Functions*

While sums of exponentials may seem the logical function to use to describe $C(t)$ and hence estimate *AUC* and *AUMC*, the literature is full of other

recommendations for estimating AUC and AUMC (see, for example, Yeh and Kwan [31] or Purves [32]). These include the trapezoidal rule, the log-trapezoidal rule, combinations of the two, splines, and Lagrangians, among others. All result in formulas for calculations over the available time domain of the data, and are left with the problem of estimating the integrals $\int_{t_n}^\infty C(t)dt$ and $\int_{t_n}^\infty t \cdot C(t)dt$. The problem of estimating $\int_0^{t_1} C(t)dt$ and $\int_0^{t_1} t \cdot C(t)dt$, and estimating a value for $C(0)$, $\dot{C}(0)$, or $\overline{C}$, is rarely discussed in the context of these methods.

There are two problems with this approach. First, estimating *AUMC* is very difficult. While one hopes that the experiment has been designed so that $\int_{t_n}^\infty C(t)dt$ contributes 5% or less to the overall *AUC*, $\int_{t_n}^\infty t \cdot C(t)dt$ can contribute as much as 50% or more to *AUMC* if the drug is cleared relatively slowly. Hence estimates of *AUMC* can be subject to large errors. The second problem is that it can be difficult to obtain error estimates for *AUC* and *AUMC* that will translate into error estimates for the pharmacokinetic parameters derived from them. For example, there are interesting statistical considerations to be made when circumstances dictate that only a single time point can be obtained in each experimental subject, thus making it difficult to separate measurement noise and biological variability between subjects [33]. As a result, it is normal practice in individual studies to ignore error estimates for these parameters, and hence the pharmacokinetic parameters that rely upon them. One attempt to circumvent this statistical problem entails conducting studies in a number of subjects and basing statistical analysis on averages and standard errors of the mean, although this approach includes biological variation among subjects. This distinction is particularly important in population pharmacokinetic studies, such as those described in Chapter 10.

### *Estimating* $\int_{t_1}^{t_n} C(t)dt$ *and* $\int_{t_1}^{t_n} t \cdot C(t)dt$

In what follows, some comments will be made on the commonly used functional approaches to estimating $\int_{t_1}^{t_n} C(t)dt$ and $\int_{t_1}^{t_n} t \cdot C(t)dt$ (i.e., the trapezoidal rule, or a combination of the trapezoidal and log-trapezoidal rule) [15, 16]. Other methods such as splines and Lagrangians will not be discussed. The interested reader is referred to Yeh and Kwan [31] or Purves [32].

Suppose $[(y_{obs}(t_i), t_i)]_{i=1}^n$ is a set of pharmacokinetic data. For example, this can be $n$ plasma samples starting with the first measurable sample obtained at time $t_1$ and the last measurable sample at time $t_n$.

If $[t_{i-1}, t_i]$ is the $i^{th}$ interval, then the AUC and AUMC for this interval calculated using the trapezoidal rule are

$$AUC_{i-1}^i = \frac{1}{2}(y_{obs}(t_i) + y_{obs}(t_{i-1}))(t_i - t_{i-1}) \quad (8.29)$$

$$AUMC_{i-1}^i = \frac{1}{2}(t_i \cdot y_{obs}(t_i) + t_{i-1} \cdot y_{obs}(t_{i-1}))(t_i - t_{i-1}) \quad (8.30)$$

For the log-trapezoidal rule, the formulas are

$$AUC_{i-1}^i = \frac{1}{\ln\left(\frac{y_{obs}(t_i)}{y_{obs}(t_{i-1})}\right)}(y_{obs}(t_i) + y_{obs}(t_{i-1}))(t_i - t_{i-1}) \quad (8.31)$$

$$AUMC_{i-1}^i = \frac{1}{\ln\left(\frac{y_{obs}(t_i)}{y_{obs}(t_{i-1})}\right)}$$

$$(t_i \cdot y_{obs}(t_i) + t_{i-1} \cdot y_{obs}(t_{i-1}))(t_i - t_{i-1}) \quad (8.32)$$

One method by which AUC and AUMC can be estimated from $t_1$ to $t_n$ is to use the trapezoidal rule and add up the individual terms $AUC_{i-1}^i$ and $AUMC_{i-1}^i$. If one chooses this approach, then it is possible to obtain an error estimate for AUC and AUMC using the quadrature method proposed by Katz and D'Argenio [34]. Some software systems use a combination of the trapezoidal and log-trapezoidal formulas to estimate AUC and AUMC, and the formulas resulting from them. The idea here is that the trapezoidal approximation is a good approximation when $y_{obs}(t_i) \geq y_{obs}(t_{i-1})$ (i.e., when the data are rising), and the log-trapezoidal rule is a better approximation when $y_{obs}(t_i) < y_{obs}(t_{i-1})$ (i.e., the data are falling). The rationale is that the log-trapezoidal formula takes into account some of the curvature in the falling portion of the curve. However, the method of Katz and D'Argenio cannot be used with this combination of formulas to obtain an error estimate for AUC and AUMC from $t_1$ to $t_n$.

### Extrapolating from $t_n$ to Infinity

One now has to deal with estimating $\int_{t_n}^{\infty} C(t)dt$ and $\int_{t_n}^{\infty} t \cdot C(t)dt$. The most common way to estimate these integrals is to assume that the data decay mono-exponentially beyond the last measurement at time $t_n$. Such a function can be written

$$y(t) = A_z e^{-\lambda_z t} \quad (8.33)$$

Here the exponent $\lambda_z$ characterizes the terminal decay and is used to calculate the half-life of the terminal decay

$$t_{z,1/2} = \frac{\ln(2)}{\lambda_z} \quad (8.34)$$

Assuming the single exponential decay is applicable from the last observation onwards, estimates for $\int_{t_n}^{\infty} C(t)dt$ and $\int_{t_n}^{\infty} t \cdot C(t)dt$ can be based on the last available measurement:

$$AUC_{extrap-dat} = \int_{t_n}^{\infty} C(t)dt = \frac{y_{obs}(t_n)}{\lambda_z} \quad (8.35)$$

$$AUMC_{extrap-dat} = \int_{t_n}^{\infty} t \cdot C(t)dt$$

$$= \frac{t_n \cdot y_{obs}(t_n)}{\lambda_z} + \frac{y_{obs}(t_n)}{\lambda_z^2} \quad (8.36)$$

or from the model-predicted value at the last measurement time;

$$AUC_{extrap-calc} = \int_{t_n}^{\infty} C(t)dt = \frac{A_z e^{-\lambda_z t_n}}{\lambda_z} \quad (8.37)$$

$$AUMC_{extrap-calc} = \int_{t_n}^{\infty} t \cdot C(t)dt$$

$$= \frac{t_n \cdot A_z e^{-\lambda_z t_n}}{\lambda_z} + \frac{A_z e^{-\lambda_z t_n}}{\lambda_z^2} \quad (8.38)$$

There are a variety of ways that one can use to estimate $\lambda_z$. Most rely on the fact that the last two or three data often appear to decrease mono-exponentially, and thus Equation 8.33 can be fitted to these data. Various options for including or excluding other data have been proposed (e.g., Gabrielsson and Weiner [35], Marino et al. [36]) but will not be discussed here. What is certain is that all parameters and area estimates will have statistical (precision) information, since they are obtained by fitting Equation 8.33 to the data.

It is of interest to note that an estimate for $\lambda_z$ could differ from $\lambda_n$, the terminal slope of a multiexponential function describing the pharmacokinetic data. The reason is that all data are considered in estimating $\lambda_n$ as opposed to a finite (terminal) subset used to estimate $\lambda_z$. Thus, a researcher checking both methods should not be surprised if there are slight differences.

### Estimating AUC and AUMC from 0 to Infinity

Estimating AUC and AUMC from zero to infinity is now simply a matter of adding the two components (i.e., the *AUC* and *AUMC*) over the time domain of the data and the extrapolation from the last measurement to infinity. The zero-time value is handled in a number of ways. For the bolus injection, it can be estimated using a modification of the methodology used to estimate $\lambda_z$ , where extrapolation is from the first measurements back to time zero. In this way, statistical information on $C(0)$ would be available. Otherwise, if an arbitrary value is assigned, no such information is available.

Error estimates for the pharmacokinetic parameters will be available only if error estimates for *AUC* and *AUMC* are calculated. In general, this will not be the case when numerical formulas are used over the time domain of the data. As mentioned previously, the error estimates we are referring to here pertain to a single subject and are not the same as those that are obtained from studies on several individuals. Unfortunately, sums of exponentials are not used as the function of choice as often as they could be, especially since the canonical inputs, boluses and infusions, are the most common ways to introduce a drug into the system. Possible reasons for this include the sensitivity of exponential estimates to noise in the data, which often allows quantifying reliably only a relatively small number of exponential functions. However, this potential limitation has to be considered on a case by case basis that should explicitly take into account experimental design considerations [37].

## COMPARTMENTAL ANALYSIS

### Definitions and Assumptions

As noted earlier in this chapter, it is very difficult to use partial differential equations to describe the kinetics of a drug. A convenient way to deal with this situation is to lump portions of the system into discrete entities and then discuss movement of material among these entities. These lumped portions of the system essentially contain subsets of the material whose kinetics share a similar time frame. Thus, the act of lumping portions of a system together for the purpose of kinetic analysis is based on a combination of known system physiology and biochemistry on the one hand, and the time frame of a particular experiment on the other. Lumping based on *a priori* known organ physiology, as opposed to empirical temporal and spatial kinetic characteristics, forms the basis of physiologically-based pharmacokinetic models. These models are described in Chapter 32 and have been reviewed elsewhere [38, 39].

Compartmental models are the mathematical result of such lumping. Whereas compartments were referenced to *physiological spaces* in Chapter 3, in this chapter we will define a *compartment* as an amount of *material* that is kinetically homogeneous. *Kinetic homogeneity* means that material introduced into a compartment mixes instantaneously, and that each particle in the compartment has the same probability as all other particles in the compartment of leaving the compartment along the various exit pathways from the compartment. A *compartmental model* consists of a finite number of compartments with specified interconnections, inputs, and losses. In addition, a compartmental model specifies the interactions occurring among accessible and inaccessible portions of the system in more (mechanistic) detail than the non-compartmental formalism.

Let $X_i(t)$ be the mass of a drug in the $i^{th}$ compartment. The notation for input, loss, and transfers is summarized in Figure 8.3. In Figure 8.3, the rate constants describe mathematically the mass transfer of material among compartments interacting with the $i^{th}$ compartment ($F_{ji}$ is transfer of material from compartment i to compartment j, $F_{ij}$ is the transfer of material from compartment $j$ to compartment $i$), the new input $F_{i0}$ (this corresponds to $X_0$ in Chapter 4) and loss to the environment $F_{0i}$ from compartment *i*. We are using (engineering) matrix notation here as opposed to the more common pharmacokinetic notation, where $F_{ij}$ would be the transfer of material from compartment *i* to compartment *j*. The notation in this chapter, the same as that used in Chapter 3, describes the compartment in full generality, making it easier to transition to linear compartmental models

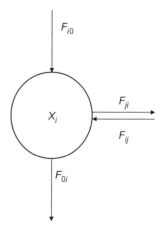

**FIGURE 8.3** The $i^{th}$ compartment of an *n*-compartment model. See text for explanation.

and to write some of the equations that we will discuss. The mathematical expression describing the rate of change for $X_i(t)$ is derived from the mass balance equation:

$$\frac{dX_i(t)}{dt} = \frac{dX_i}{dt} = \sum_{\substack{j=0 \\ j \neq i}}^{n} F_{ij} - \sum_{\substack{j=0 \\ j \neq i}}^{n} F_{ji} \qquad (8.39)$$

There are several important features to understand about the $F_{ij}$ that derive from the fact that the compartmental model is being used to describe a biological system, and hence conservation of mass must be obeyed. First, the $F_{ij}$ must be non-negative for all times $t$ (assumed to be between time zero and infinity). In fact, the $F_{ij}$ can be either stochastic (have uncertainly associated with them) or deterministic (known exactly). In this chapter, the $F_{ij}$ will be assumed to be deterministic but can be functions of the $X_i$ and/or time $t$. (Readers interested in stochastic compartmental models can find references to numerous articles in Covell *et al.* [4], and Macheras *et al.* [40]). Second, as pointed out by Jacquez and Simon [10], if $X_i = 0$, then $F_{ji} = 0$ for all $j \neq i$ and hence $dX_i/t \geq 0$. An important consequence of this, as shown by these authors, is that the $F_{ji}$, with the exception of $F_{i0}$, which remains unchanged, can be written:

$$F_{ji}(\overrightarrow{X}, \overrightarrow{p}, t) = k_{ji}(\overrightarrow{X}, \overrightarrow{p}, t) \cdot X_i(t) \qquad (8.40)$$

The function $F_{i0}$ is either a constant or a function of $t$ alone. The $k_{ji}$ written in this format are called the *fractional transfer functions*. $\overrightarrow{X} = (X_1, ..., X_n)$ is a notation for compartmental masses (mathematically called a vector), $\overrightarrow{p}$ is a descriptor of other elements (parameters) such as blood flow, pH, and temperature that control the system, and $t$ is time. We are using vector notation here (as in $\overrightarrow{X}$) to signify that, in general, the fluxes can be functions of any $X_i(t)$ (the vector $\overrightarrow{X}$ contains all of them) and especially a set of (most often unknown) parameters $\overrightarrow{p}$.

Equation 8.40 is a subtle but important step in moving from the general compartment model to the linear, constant coefficient model because it shows explicitly that the fractional transfers can be functions of time and other system entities, not necessarily constants, and that, as functions, the mass terms can be split out from the fractional transfer term. Written in this format, Equation 8.39 becomes

$$\frac{dX_i}{dt} = -\left( \sum_{\substack{j=0 \\ j \neq i}}^{n} k_{ji}(\overrightarrow{X}, \overrightarrow{p}, t) \right) X_i(t)$$

$$+ \sum_{\substack{j=1 \\ j \neq i}}^{n} k_{ij}(\overrightarrow{X}, \overrightarrow{p}, t) X_j(t) + F_{i0} \qquad (8.41)$$

Define

$$k_{ii}(\overrightarrow{X}, \overrightarrow{p}, t) = -\left( \sum_{\substack{j=0 \\ j \neq i}}^{n} k_{ji}(\overrightarrow{X}, \overrightarrow{p}, t) \right) \qquad (8.42)$$

and write

$$K(\overrightarrow{X}, \overrightarrow{p}, t) = \begin{bmatrix} k_{11} & k_{12} & \cdots & k_{1n} \\ k_{21} & k_{22} & \cdots & k_{2n} \\ \vdots & \vdots & \ddots & \vdots \\ k_{n1} & k_{n2} & \cdots & k_{nn} \end{bmatrix} \qquad (8.43)$$

where in Equation 8.43 the individual terms of the matrix, for convenience, do not contain the $(\overrightarrow{X}, \overrightarrow{p}, t)$. The matrix $K(\overrightarrow{X}, \overrightarrow{p}, t)$ is called the *compartmental matrix*. This matrix is key to deriving many kinetic parameters, and in making the conceptual link between compartmental and non-compartmental analysis.

There are several reasons for starting at this level of mathematical generality for the $n$-compartment model.

- First, this approach clearly points out that the theories underlying non-compartmental and compartmental models are very different. While the theory underlying non-compartmental models relies more on statistical theory and data-based approaches, especially in developing residence time concepts (see, for example, Weiss [27], the theory underlying compartmental models is really the theory of ordinary, first-order differential equations, with some special features due to the nature of the biological applications. These are reviewed in detail in Jacquez and Simon [10] and in many other texts and research articles written on the subject.

- Second, these ideas demonstrate the complexity involved in postulating the structure of a compartmental model to describe the kinetics of a particular drug. As illustrated by the presentation in Chapter

3, it is very difficult to postulate a model structure in which the model compartments have physiological relevance as opposed to simply being a mathematical construct, especially when one is dealing with a single-input–single-output experiment and the limited amount of information it provides. Although the most general compartmental model must be appreciated in its potential application to the interpretation of kinetic data, the fact is that such complex models are not often used. Thus, the most common models are the linear, constant coefficient compartmental models described in the next section. In this discussion, it also will be assumed that all systems are open (i.e., drug introduced into the system will eventually irreversibly leave the system). This means that some special situations discussed by Jacquez and Simon [10] do not have to be considered (i.e., compartmental models with submodels – called traps – from which material cannot escape).

## Linear, Constant Coefficient Compartmental Models

Suppose the compartmental matrix is a constant matrix (i.e., all $k_{ij}$ are constants). In this situation, one can write $K$ instead of $K(\overrightarrow{X}, \overrightarrow{p}, t)$ to indicate that the elements of the matrix no longer depend on $(\overrightarrow{X}, \overrightarrow{p}, t)$. As will be seen, there are several important features of the $K$ matrix that will be used in recovering pharmacokinetic parameters of interest. In addition, as described many times in the kinetic analysis literature, the solution to the compartmental equations, which in this case are a system of linear, constant coefficient equations, involves sums of exponentials.

What is needed for the compartmental matrix to be constant? Recall that the individual elements of the matrix $k_{ij}(\overrightarrow{X}, \overrightarrow{p}, t)$ are functions of several variables. For the $k_{ij}(\overrightarrow{X}, \overrightarrow{p}, t)$ to be constant, $\overrightarrow{X}$ and $\overrightarrow{p}$ must be constant (actually this assumption can be relaxed, but for purposes of this discussion constancy will be assumed), and the $k_{ij}(\overrightarrow{X}, \overrightarrow{p}, t)$ cannot depend explicitly on time (i.e., the $k_{ij}(\overrightarrow{X}, \overrightarrow{p}, t)$ are time invariant). Notice with this concept that the time-invariant $k_{ij}(\overrightarrow{X}, \overrightarrow{p}, t)$ can assume different values depending upon the constant values for $\overrightarrow{X}$ and $\overrightarrow{p}$. This leads naturally to the steady state concepts that have been historically so useful in tracer kinetics.

Under what circumstances are compartmental models linear, constant coefficient? This normally depends upon a particular experimental design and should be consistently tested and verified in practice. The reason is that most biological systems, including those in which drugs are analyzed, are inherently non-

linear. However, the assumption of linearity holds reasonably well over the dose range studied for most drugs, and pharmacokinetic studies often are carried out under stable conditions of minimal physiological perturbation.

## Parameters Estimated from Compartmental Models

### Experimenting on Compartmental Models: Input and Measurements

In postulating a compartmental model such as that shown in Figure 8.4A, one is actually making a statement concerning how the system is believed to behave. To know if a particular model structure can predict the behavior of a drug in the body, one must be able to obtain kinetic data from which the parameters characterizing the system of differential equations can be estimated; the model predictions can then be compared against the data. Experiments are designed to generate the data, so the experimental design must then be reproduced on the model. This is done by specifying inputs and samples, as shown in Figure 8.4B, which reflect the actual conduct of the experiment. More specifically, the input specifies the $F_{i0}$ terms in the differential equations, and the samples provide the measurement equations that link the model's predictions, which are normally in units of drug mass, with the samples, that are usually measured in concentration units.

To emphasize this point, once a model structure is postulated, the compartmental matrix can be estimated in principle, since it depends only upon the defined arrangement of compartments and their transfers and losses. The input, the $F_{i0}$, represents the experimental perturbation and thus is determined by the investigator. In addition, the units of the differential equation (i.e., the units of the $X_i$) are determined by the units of the input. In practical terms, if the data

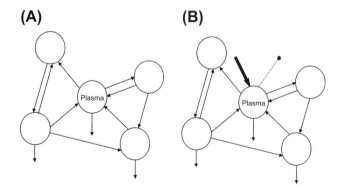

**FIGURE 8.4** (A) A compartmental model of drug behavior in the body. (B) An experimental protocol on (A) showing drug administration (*bold arrow*) and plasma sampling (*dashed line with bullet*).

obtained from a particular experimental design permit the parameters of the postulated compartmental model to be estimated, then the specific form of the input is not important, as long as it is informative on the model structure and parameters (concepts and applications of *a priori* identifiability have been extensively reviewed by Cobelli and DiStefano [41]). In theory, data arising from a bolus injection or constant infusion should be equally rich from an information point of view, although extracting this information would require different practical experimental designs involving sampling frequency.

The final point to make in dealing with experiments on the model relates to the measurement variable(s). The units of the $X_i$ are determined by the experimental input units, and are usually in units of mass (e.g., grams, or moles). The units of the data are normally concentration. No matter what the units of the data, there must be an appropriately dimensioned measurement equation linking the $X_i$ with the data. For example, if the measurement was taken from compartment 1 and the units of the data are concentration, one would need to write the measurement equation

$$C_1(t) = \frac{X_1(t)}{V_1} \quad (8.44)$$

Here $V_1$ is the volume of compartment 1, and is a parameter to be estimated from the data.

Clearly, once a compartmental structure is postulated, there are many experimental protocols and measurement variables that can be accommodated. One just needs to be sure that the parameters characterizing the compartmental matrix, $K$, and the parameters characterizing the measurement variables can be reliably estimated from the data generated by the experiment.

### Non-Linearities in Compartmental Models

Some fractional transfer functions of compartmental models may actually be functions of compartmental masses or concentrations (i.e., the model may actually be non-linear). The most common example is when a transfer or loss is saturable. Here, a Michaelis-Menten type of transfer function can be defined, as was shown in Chapter 2 for the elimination of phenytoin. In this case, loss from compartment 1 is concentration dependent and saturable, and one can write

$$CL_1 = k_{01} \cdot V_1 = \frac{V_{max}}{K_m + C_1} \cdot V_1 \quad (8.45)$$

where $V_{max}$ (in units of concentration per unit time) and $K_m$ (having units of concentration) are parameters

that can be estimated from the pharmacokinetic data. The concentration in the accessible compartment is still defined as in Equation 8.44,

$$C_1(t) = \frac{X_1(t)}{V_1}$$

The corresponding differential equation $dX_1/dt$ can then be written:

$$\frac{dX_1(t)}{dt} = -k_{01} \cdot X_1(t) = -\frac{V_{max}}{K_m + C_1(t)} \cdot X_1(t) \quad (8.46)$$

Another example of a function-dependent transfer function is given in Chapter 6, in which hemodynamic changes during and after hemodialysis reduce inter-compartmental clearance between the intravascular space and a peripheral compartment, as shown in Figure 6.3.

If one has pharmacokinetic data and knows that the situation calls for non-linear kinetics, then compartmental models, no matter how difficult to postulate, are really required. Non-compartmental models cannot deal with the time-varying situation, and estimates derived from them will be prone to varying degrees of error. However, non-compartmental analysis can be useful to investigate the presence or absence of non-linearities, for example by calculating *AUC* at various doses and checking that linearity holds.

### Calculating Pharmacokinetic Parameters from a Compartmental Model

Realizing the full generality of the compartmental model, consider now only the limited situation of linear, constant coefficient models. What parameters can be calculated from a model? The answer to this question can be addressed in the context of Figure 8.5.

### Model Parameters

Once a specific multicompartmental structure has been developed to explain the pharmacokinetics of a particular drug, the parameters characterizing this model are the components of the compartmental matrix, $K$, and the distribution space (volume) parameters associated with the individual measurements. The components of the compartmental matrix are the rate constants $k_{ij}$. Together, these comprise the primary *mathematical* parameters of the model. The parameters of clearance and distribution volume, which are of primary physiological relevance, are secondary from a mathematical standpoint. For this

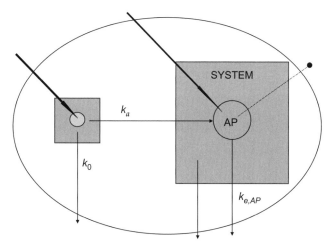

**FIGURE 8.5** The system model shown on the right contains an accessible pool (AP) embedded in an arbitrary multicompartmental model indicated by the shaded box. The drug can be introduced directly into this pool, as indicated by the bold arrow. The drug can also be introduced into a second compartment, indicated by the circle in the small, shaded box on the left. Drug can move from this compartment, as denoted by the arrow passing through the shaded small box and large box, into the accessible pool at a rate denoted by $k_a$. Material also can be lost from the second compartment; this is denoted $k_0$. Finally, material has two ways by which it can leave the system. One is directly from the accessible pool, $k_{e,AP}$, and the other is from non-accessible pools, denoted by the arrow leaving the large box. That both small and large boxes exist in the context of a larger system is denoted by the ellipse surrounding the individual components of the system. See text for additional explanation.

reason, the mathematical parameters of compartmental models often have to be reparameterized in order to recover the physiological parameters of interest (e.g., see Figure 3.8). Although this works relatively well for simple models, it can be a difficult exercise once one moves to more complex models.

The next question is whether the parameters characterizing a model can be estimated from a set of pharmacokinetic data. The answer to the question has two parts. The first is called *a priori identifiability*. This answers the question, "given a particular model structure and experimental design, if the data are 'perfect' can the model parameters be estimated?" The second is *a posteriori identifiability*. This answers the question, "given a particular model structure and experimental design and a set of pharmacokinetic data, can the model parameters be estimated with a reasonable degree of statistical precision?"

*A priori* identifiability is a critical part of model development. While the answer to the question for many of the simpler models used in pharmacokinetics is well known, the general answer, even for linear, constant coefficient models, is more difficult. Figure 8.6 illustrates the situation with some specific model structures (A–F); the interested reader is

referred to Cobelli *et al.* [29] for precise details. Model A is a standard two-compartment model with input and sampling from a "plasma" compartment. There are three $k_{ij}$ and a volume term to be estimated. This model can be shown to be *a priori* identifiable. Model B has four $k_{ij}$ and a volume term to be estimated. The parameters for this model cannot be estimated from a single set of pharmacokinetic data, no matter how information rich they are. In fact, there are an infinite number of values for the $k_{ij}$ and volume term that will fit the data equally well. If one insists on using this model structure (e.g., for reasons of biological plausibility), then some independent constraint will have to be placed on the parameters, such as fixing the volume or defining a relationship among the $k_{ij}$. Model C, while *a priori* identifiable, will have a different compartmental matrix from that of Model A, and hence some of the pharmacokinetic parameters will be different between the two models.

Two commonly used three-compartment models are shown in Figures 8.6D and E. Of the two peripheral compartments, one exchanges rapidly and one slowly with the central compartment. Model D is *a priori* identifiable while Model E is not, since it will have two different compartmental matrices that will produce the same fit of the data. The reason is that the loss in Model E is from a peripheral compartment. Finally, Model F, a model very commonly used to describe the pharmacokinetics of drug absorption, is not *a priori* identifiable. Again, there are two values for the compartmental $K$ matrix that will produce the same fit to the data, one resulting in slow elimination and fast absorption, and the other reversing the two.

*A posteriori* identifiability is linked to the theory of optimization in mathematics and statistics because one normally uses a software package that has an optimization (data-fitting) capability in order to estimate parameter values for a multicompartmental model from a set of pharmacokinetic data. Typically, one obtains an estimate for the parameter values, an estimate for their errors, and a value for the correlation (or covariance) matrix of the estimates. The details of optimization and how to deal with the output from an optimization routine are beyond the scope of this chapter, but they have been discussed extensively with reference to compartmental models. The point to be made here is that the output from these routines is crucial in assessing the goodness-of-fit – that is, how well the model performs when compared to the data – since inferences about a drug's pharmacokinetics will be made from these parameter values. Most often, inference about model selection – i.e., the desired level of model complexity – can also be made on the basis of the performance of such fitting routines.

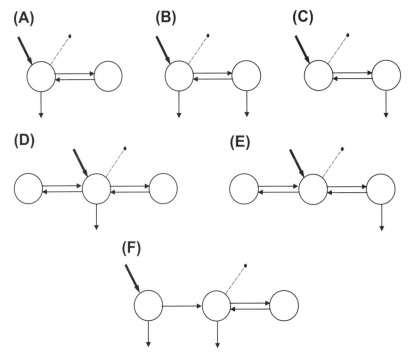

**FIGURE 8.6**  Examples of multicompartmental models. See text for explanation.

### Residence Time Calculations

As we have discussed in the context of non-compartmental analysis, the notion of residence times can be very important in assessing the pharmacokinetics of a drug, the information about residence times available from a linear, constant coefficient compartmental model also is very rich, and will be reviewed in the following comments.

Residence time calculations are a direct result of manipulating the compartmental matrix $K$. Let $\Theta = -K^{-1}$ be the negative inverse of the compartmental matrix, and let $\vartheta_{ij}$ be the $ij^{th}$ element of $\Theta$. The matrix $\Theta$ is called the mean residence time matrix and has units of time (since the rates in $K$ have units of inverse time). The following information given concerning the interpretation of this matrix comes from the original reference of Covell *et al.* [4] and Cobelli *et al.* [29]. Further detail is beyond the scope of this chapter; and the interested reader is directed to these two references.

The elements of the mean residence time matrix have important probabilistic interpretations for linear, constant coefficient models. First, the generic element $\vartheta_{ij}$ represents the average time a drug particle entering the system in compartment $j$ spends in compartment $i$ before irreversibly leaving the system by any route. Second, the ratio $\vartheta_{ij} / \vartheta_{ii}$, $i \neq j$, equals the probability that a drug particle in compartment $j$ will eventually reach compartment $i$. Finally, if a compartmental model

has loss from a single compartment only, say compartment 1, then it can be shown that $k_{01} = 1/\vartheta_{11}$. Clearly if one is analyzing pharmacokinetic data using compartmental models in which the $K$ matrix is constant, this information can be critical in assessing the behavior of a particular drug in various non-accessible pools.

However, more can be said about the $\vartheta_{ij}$ that is important in comparing compartmental and non-compartmental models. Suppose there is a generic input into compartment 1 only, $F_{10}$ (remember in this situation $F_{10}$ can be a function). Then it can be shown that the area under $X_i(t)$, the drug mass in the $i^{th}$ compartment, equals:

$$\int_0^\infty X_i(t)dt = \vartheta_{i1} \int_0^\infty F_{10}\, dt \qquad (8.47)$$

whence

$$\vartheta_{i1} = \frac{\int_0^\infty X_i(t)dt}{\int_0^\infty F_{10}\, dt} \qquad (8.48)$$

More generally, suppose $F_{j0}$ is an arbitrary input into compartment $j$, and $X_i^j(t)$ is the amount of drug in compartment $i$ following an initial administration in compartment $j$. Then:

$$\vartheta_{ij} = \frac{\int_0^\infty X_i^j(t)dt}{\int_0^\infty F_{j0}\, dt} \qquad (8.49)$$

This equation shows that $\vartheta_{ij}$ equals the area under the model predicted drug mass curve in compartment $i$ resulting from an input compartment $j$, normalized to the dose. An example of the application of these concepts is provided by a study of monoclonal immunoglobulin kinetics in mice [42].

The use of the mean residence time matrix can be a powerful tool in pharmacokinetic analysis with a compartmental model, especially if one is dealing with a model of the system in which physiological and/or anatomical correlates are being assigned to specific compartments [2]. Information about the mean residence time matrix is usually available from the compartmental matrix, which can be obtained from many commonly used modeling software tools.

## NON-COMPARTMENTAL VS COMPARTMENTAL MODELS

In comparing non-compartmental with compartmental models, it should now be clear that this is not a question of declaring one method better than the other. It is a question of considering: (1) what information about the system is desired from the data, and (2) what is the most appropriate method to obtain this information. It is hoped that the reader of this chapter will be enabled to make an informed decision on this issue, and especially to grasp the limitations and implications of each method.

This discussion will rely heavily on the following sources. First, the publications of DiStefano and Landaw [37, 43] deal with issues related to compartmental vs single accessible pool non-compartmental models. Second, Cobelli and Toffolo [3] discuss the two accessible pool non-compartmental model. Finally, Covell *et al.* [4] provide the theory to demonstrate the link between non-compartmental and compartmental models in estimating the pharmacokinetic parameters.

### Models of Data vs Models of System

Suppose one has a set of pharmacokinetic data. The question is how to obtain information from the data related to the disposition of the drug in question. DiStefano and Landaw [43] deal with this question by making the distinction between models of data and models of system. Understanding this distinction is useful in understanding the differences between compartmental and non-compartmental models.

As discussed, the non-compartmental model divides the system into two components: an accessible

pool and non-accessible pools. The kinetics of the non-accessible pools are lumped into the recirculation-exchange process. From this, as has been discussed, we can estimate pharmacokinetic parameters describing the accessible pool and system.

What happens in the compartmental model framework? A very common way to deal with pharmacokinetic data is by fitting a sum of exponential functions to them, taking advantage of the fact that in a linear, constant coefficient system, the number of exponential phases in the plasma-level vs time curve equals the number of compartments in the model.

Consider the situation in which plasma data are obtained following a bolus injection of the drug. Suppose that the data can be described by:

$$C(t) = A_1 e^{-\lambda_1 t} + A_2 e^{-\lambda_2 t} \tag{8.50}$$

While the presence of two exponential functions in this equation supports the presence of two distinct compartments, the data could be modeled equally well by the model in Figure 8.7A. In this case, both the exponential equation and the compartmental model serve only to describe the data and to allow extrapolation of the pharmacokinetic time course beyond the experimental boundaries. That is, no comment is being made about a physiological, biochemical and/or anatomical significance to the extravascular compartment 2. This is what DiStefano and Landaw [43] would call a *model of data* because little to nothing is being said about the system into which the drug is administered. Incidentally, if the model in Figure 8.7A were physiologically the most appropriate for the drug, the non-compartmental formulas would be valid.

Suppose, on the other hand, additional information is known about the disposition of the drug. For example, suppose it is known that a major tissue in the body is where virtually all of the drug is taken up extravascularly, and that it is known from

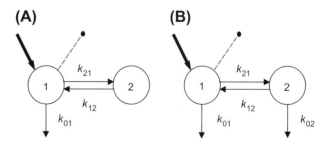

**FIGURE 8.7** Two two-compartment models in which drug is administered intravenously into compartment 1; samples are taken from this compartment. See text for explanation.

independent experiments approximately what fraction of the drug is metabolized in that compartment. Now, given that the plasma data can be fitted by a sum of two exponentials, one can start to develop a *model of system* for the drug, and the mechanistically most appropriate model seems to be the one in Figure 8.7B. While this model is not *a priori* identifiable, one can write an equation in which the loss rate constants $k_{01}$ and $k_{02}$ are related through knowledge of how much of the drug is metabolized in the tissue; compartment 2 can thus be conceptually associated with the tissue.

Such modeling techniques have been the subject of intense debate. First, one has used the fact that the data support a two-compartment model, and the fact that a relationship between the irreversible loss rate constants can be written based upon *a priori* knowledge. A physiological significance can thus be associated with the compartments and the $k_{ij}$ that goes beyond the descriptive model of data just discussed. A criticism of such a statement is that the model does not contain all elements of the system in which the drug is known to interact. If this critique is justified, then one has to design a new experiment to uncover information on these parts of the system. One may have to change the sampling schedule to resolve more components in the data, or to design a different series of input–output experiments. One even may have to conduct a study in which marker compounds for known physiological spaces are co-administered with the study drug [44].

This is not a shortcoming of the modeling approach, but illustrates how knowledge of compartmental modeling can be a powerful tool for understanding the pharmacokinetics of a drug. Such an understanding is not often available from non-compartmental models or when compartmental models are used only as models of data, except that these can be used as preliminary data analysis approaches to uncover more detailed information. Thus, predicting detailed events in non-accessible portions of the system model is the underlying rationale for developing models of systems – remembering, of course, that such predictions are only as good as the assumptions in the model.

## The Equivalent Sink and Source Constraints

When are the parameter estimates from the non-compartmental model equal to those from a linear, constant coefficient compartmental model? As DiStefano and Landaw [43] explain, they are equal when the equivalent sink and source constraints are valid. The equivalent source constraint means that all drug enters the same accessible pools; this is almost universally the case in pharmacokinetic studies. The equivalent sink constraint means that irreversible loss of drug can occur only from the accessible pools. If any irreversible loss occurs from the non-accessible part of the system, this constraint is not valid. For the single accessible pool model, for example, the system mean residence time and the total equivalent volume of distribution will be underestimated [2].

The equivalent sink constraint is illustrated in Figure 8.8. In Figure 8.8A, the constraint holds and hence the parameters estimated either from the non-compartmental model (*left*) or multicompartmental model (*right*) will be equal. If the multicompartmental model is a model of the system, then, of course, the information about the drug's disposition will be much richer, since many more specific parameters can be estimated to describe each compartment.

In Figure 8.8B, the constraint is not satisfied, and the non-compartmental model is not appropriate. As previously described, if used, it will underestimate certain parameters. On the other hand, the multi-compartmental model shown on the right can account for sites of loss from non-accessible compartments, providing a richer source of information about the drug's disposition.

## Linearity and Time-Invariance

If the system cannot be adequately described by a linear, constant coefficient model, then linearity and time invariance cannot be assumed. In this case, non-compartmental parameters do not provide an adequate description of the pharmacokinetics and can be at times misleading. Studying the pharmacokinetics over an adequate dose range usually uncovers these situations and other areas where non-compartmental hypotheses may not apply, and provides insight for the definition of non-linear models of the system from which parameters of interest can be determined [45]. Such models, when mechanistically appropriate, can be a generalization of the compartmental framework that, for example, can account for extraplasma drug removal or for non-linear disposition of both drug and drug target. These issues have been studied in detail to describe the disposition of antibody drugs [46].

## Recovering Pharmacokinetic Parameters from Compartmental Models

We will now use a simple example to demonstrate how non-compartmental and compartmental approaches can be studied together. Assume a linear,

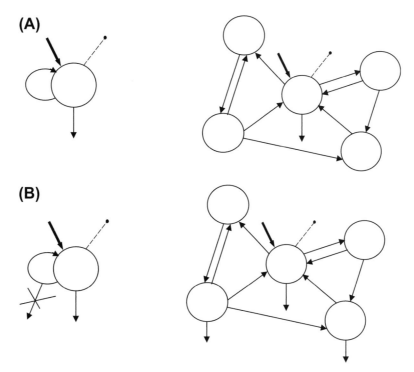

**FIGURE 8.8** (A) A single accessible pool model (*left*) and a multicompartmental model showing a structure for the recirculation-exchange arrow (*right*). (B) A single accessible pool model with an irreversible loss from the recirculation-exchange arrow (*left*) and a multicompartmental model showing a structure for the recirculation-exchange arrow that includes loss from peripheral compartments (*right*). See text for additional explanation.

constant coefficient compartmental model in which compartment 1 is the accessible compartment into which the drug is administered and from which samples are taken. Following a bolus injection of the drug, the volume $V_1$ will be estimated as a parameter of the model. $V_1$ thus will correspond to $V_a$ for the non-compartmental model. The clearance rate from compartment 1, $CL_1$, is equal to the product of $V_1$ and $k_{01}$:

$$CL_1 = V_1 \cdot k_{01} \qquad (8.51)$$

If the only loss is from compartment 1, then $k_{01}$ equals $k_e$, and one has

$$CL_a = CL_1 = V_1 \cdot k_{01} = V_a \cdot k_e \qquad (8.52)$$

showing the equivalence of the two methods. From the residence time matrix,

$$\vartheta_{11} = \frac{\int_0^\infty X_1(t)dt}{d} = \frac{1}{k_{01}} \qquad (8.53)$$

hence, the mean residence time in compartment 1, $MRT_1$, equals the reciprocal of $k_{01}$. Again if the only

loss from the system is via compartment 1, then $MRT_1$ equals $MRT_a$.

Similar results hold for the constant infusion or generic input. In other words, the parameters can be shown to be equal if the equivalent sink and source constraints are valid. Again, the interested reader is referred to the bibliography for details and for consideration of the situation in which the equivalent source and sink constraints are not valid.

## CONCLUSION

In conclusion, non-compartmental models and linear, constant coefficient models have different domains of validity. When the domains are identical, then the pharmacokinetic parameters estimated by either method should, in theory, be equal. If they are not, then differences are due to the methods used to estimate them. When linearity and time invariance cannot be assumed, then more complex system models are required for pharmacokinetic analysis.

Information provided in this chapter should make it easier for a researcher to choose a particular method and to have greater confidence in evaluating reported results of pharmacokinetic analyses.

# REFERENCES

[1] Gillespie WR. Noncompartmental versus compartmental modelling in clinical pharmacokinetics. Clin Pharmacokinet 1991;20:253–62.

[2] DiStefano JJ III. Noncompartmental vs compartmental analysis: Some bases for choice. Am J Physiol 1982;243:R1–6.

[3] Cobelli C, Toffolo G. Compartmental vs noncompartmental modeling for two accessible pools. Am J Physiol 1984;247:R488–96.

[4] Covell DG, Berman M, Delisi C. Mean residence time – theoretical development, experimental determination, and practical use in tracer analysis. Math Biosci 1984;72:213–44.

[5] Norwich K. Noncompartmental models of whole-body clearance of tracers: A review. Ann Biomed Eng 1997;25:421–39.

[6] Weiss M, Förster W. Pharmacokinetic model based on circulatory transport. Eur J Clin Pharmacol 1979;16:287–93.

[7] Beal SL. Some clarifications regarding moments of residence times with pharmacokinetic models. J Pharmacokinet Biopharm 1987;15:75–92.

[8] Mordenti J, Rescigno A. Estimation of permanence time, exit time, dilution factor, and steady-state volume of distribution. Pharm Res 1992;9:17–25.

[9] Wagner JG. Linear pharmacokinetic equations allowing direct calculation of many needed pharmacokinetic parameters from the coefficients and exponents of polyexponential equations which have been fitted to the data. J Pharmacokinet Biopharm 1976;4:443–67.

[10] Jacquez JA, Simon CP. Qualitative theory of compartmental systems. SIAM Rev 1993;35:43–79.

[11] Jacquez JA. Compartmental analysis in biology and medicine. 3rd ed. Ann Arbor, MI: BioMedware; 1996.

[12] Berman M. Kinetic analysis of turnover data. Prog Biochem Pharmacol 1979;15:67–108.

[13] Gibaldi M, Perrier D. Pharmacokinetics. 2nd ed. New York, NY: Marcel Dekker; 1982.

[14] Rowland M, Tozer TN. Clinical pharmacokinetics: Concepts and applications. 3rd ed. Baltimore, MD: Williams & Wilkins; 1995.

[15] Rescigno A. Fundamental concepts in pharmacokinetics. Pharmacol Res 1997;35:363–90.

[16] Benet L. Clearance (née Rowland) concepts: A downdate and an update. J Pharmacokinet Pharmacodyn 2010;37:529–39.

[17] Landaw EM, Katz D. Comments on mean residence time determination. J Pharmacokinet Biopharm 1985;13:543–7.

[18] Yamaoka K, Nakagawa T, Uno T. Statistical moments in pharmacokinetics. J Pharmacokinet Biopharm 1978;6:547–58.

[19] Teorell T. Kinetics of distribution of substances administered to the body. Arch Intern Pharmacodyn Ther 1937;57:205–25.

[20] Pearson K. On the systematic fitting of curves to observations and measurements. Biometrika 1902;1:265–303.

[21] Zierler KL. Theory of use of indicators to measure blood flow and extracellular volume and calculation of transcapillary movement of tracers. Circ Res 1963;12:464–71.

[22] Perl W, Effros RM, Chinard FP. Indicator equivalence theorem for input rates and regional masses in multi-inlet steady-state systems with partially labeled input. J Theor Biol 1969;25:297–316.

[23] Zierler KL. Theory of the use of arteriovenous concentration differences for measuring metabolism in steady and nonsteady states. J Clin Invest 1961;40:2111–25.

[24] Rescigno A. The rise and fall of compartmental analysis. Pharm Res 2001;44:337–42.

[25] DiStefano III JJ. Concepts, properties, measurement, and computation of clearance rates of hormones and other substances in biological systems. Ann Biomed Eng 1976;4:302–19.

[26] Mari A. Circulatory models of intact-body kinetics and their relationship with compartmental and non-compartmental analysis. J Theor Biol 1993;160:509–31.

[27] Weiss M. The relevance of residence time theory to pharmacokinetics. Eur J Clin Pharmacol 1992;43:571–9.

[28] Veng-Pedersen P. Noncompartmentally-based pharmacokinetic modeling. Adv Drug Deliv Rev 2001;48:265–300.

[29] Cobelli C, Foster D, Toffolo G. Tracer kinetics in biomedical research: From data to model. New York, NY: Kluwer Academic/Plenum Publishers; 2000.

[30] Berman M, Schoenfeld R. Invariants in experimental data on linear kinetics and the formulation of models. J Appl Phys 1956;27:1361–70.

[31] Yeh KC, Kwan KC. A comparison of numerical integrating algorithms by trapezoidal, Lagrange, and spline approximation. J Pharmacokinet Biopharm 1978;6:79–98.

[32] Purves RD. Optimum numerical integration methods for estimation of area-under-the-curve (AUC) and area-under-the-moment-curve (AUMC). J Pharmacokinet Biopharm 1992;20:211–26.

[33] Bailer AJ. Testing for the equality of area under the curves when using destructive measurement techniques. J Pharmacokinet Biopharm 1988;16:303–9.

[34] Katz D, D'Argenio DZ. Experimental design for estimating integrals by numerical quadrature, with applications to pharmacokinetic studies. Biometrics 1983;39:621–8.

[35] Gabrielsson J, Weiner D. Pharmacokinetic/pharmacodynamic data analysis: Concepts and applications. 2nd ed. Stockholm: Swedish Pharmaceutical Press; 1997.

[36] Marino AT, DiStefano III JJ, Landaw EM. DIMSUM: An expert system for multiexponential model discrimination. Am J Physiol 1992;262:E546–56.

[37] Landaw EM, DiStefano III JJ. Multiexponential, multicompartmental, and noncompartmental modeling. II. Data analysis and statistical considerations. Am J Physiol 1984;246: R665–77.

[38] Pang KS, Weiss M, Macheras P. Advanced pharmacokinetic models based on organ clearance, circulatory, and fractal concepts. AAPS J 2007;9:E268–83.

[39] Nestorov I. Whole body pharmacokinetic models. Clin Pharmacokinet 2003;42:883–908.

[40] Macheras P, Iliadis A. Stochastic compartmental models. In: Modeling in biopharmaceutics, pharmacokinetics, and pharmacodynamics. New York, NY: Springer; 2006. p. 205–87.

[41] Cobelli C, DiStefano III JJ. Parameter and structural identifiability concepts and ambiguities: A critical review and analysis. Am J Physiol 1980;239:R7–24.

[42] Covell DG, Barbet J, Holton OD, Black CD, Parker RJ, Weinstein JN. Pharmacokinetics of monoclonal immunoglobulin G1, F(ab')2, and Fab' in mice. Cancer Res 1986;46: 3969–78.

[43] DiStefano JJ III, Landaw EW. Multiexponential, multicompartmental, and noncompartmental modeling. I. Methodological limitations and physiological interpretations. Am J Physiol 1984;246:R651–64.

[44] Belknap SM, Nelson JE, Ruo TI, Frederiksen MC, Worwag EM, Shin S-G, et al. Theophylline distribution kinetics analyzed by reference to simultaneously injected urea and inulin. J Pharmacol Exp Ther 1987;287:963–9.

[45] Mager DE. Target-mediated drug disposition and dynamics. Biochem Pharmacol 2006;72:1–10.

[46] Lobo ED, Hansen RJ, Balthasar JP. Antibody pharmacokinetics and pharmacodynamics. J Pharm Sci 2004;93:2645–68.

CHAPTER

# 9

# Distributed Models of Drug Kinetics

Paul F. Morrison

*National Institute of Biomedical Imaging and Bioengineering Intramural Research Program, National Institute of Biomedical Imaging and Bioengineering, National Institutes of Health, Bethesda, MD 20892*

## INTRODUCTION

The hallmark of distributed models of drug kinetics is their ability to describe not only the time dependence of drug distribution in tissue but also its detailed spatial dependence. Previous discussion has mostly revolved around methods meant to characterize the time history of a drug in one or more spatially homogeneous compartments. In these earlier approaches, the end results of pharmacokinetic modeling were time-dependent concentrations, $C(t)$, of the drug or metabolite of interest for each body compartment containing one or more organs or tissue types. In these situations, the agent is also delivered homogeneously and reaches a target organ, either via blood capillaries whose distribution is assumed to be homogeneous throughout the organ, or via infusion directly into that organ, followed by instantaneous mixing with the extravascular space. In contrast, distributed pharmacokinetic models require that neither the tissue architecture nor the delivery source be uniform throughout the organ. The end results of this type of modeling are organ concentration functions (for each drug or metabolite) that depend on two independent variables, one describing spatial dependence and the other time dependence – that is, $C(\vec{r}, t)$ where $\vec{r}$ is a spatial vector to a given location in an organ. As might be expected, the pharmacokinetic analysis and equations needed to incorporate spatial dependence in this function require a more complicated formalism than used previously with compartment models.

It is the goal of this chapter to describe the general principles behind distributed models and to provide an introduction to the formalisms employed with them. Emphasis will be placed on the major physiological, metabolic, and physical factors involved. Following this, we will present several examples where distributed kinetic models are necessary. These will include descriptions of drug delivery to the tissues forming the boundaries of the peritoneal cavity following intraperitoneal infusion, to the brain tissues comprising the ventricular walls following intraventricular infusion, and to the parenchymal tissue of the brain following direct interstitial infusion. The chapter will end by identifying still other applications where distributed kinetic models are required.

## CENTRAL ISSUES

The central issue with distributed models is to answer the question, "What is the situation that leads to a spatially dependent distribution of drug in a tissue and how is this distribution described quantitatively?"

The situation leading to spatial dependence involves the delivery of an agent to a tissue from a geometrically non-uniform source followed by movement of the agent away from the source along a path on which local clearance or binding mechanisms deplete it, thus causing its concentration to vary with location. Several modes of drug delivery lead to this situation. The most common is the delivery of an agent from a spatially restricted source to a homogeneous tissue. One such example is the slow infusion of drugs directly into the interstitial space of tissues via implanted needles or catheters. The infused drug concentration decreases

*PRINCIPLES OF CLINICAL PHARMACOLOGY, THIRD EDITION*
DOI: http://dx.doi.org/10.1016/B978-0-12-385471-1.00009-X

**117**

due to local clearances as the drug moves out radially from the catheter tip. Another example is the delivery of drugs from solutions bathing the surface of a target organ, in which the drug concentration decreases with increasing penetration depth and residence time in the tissue. Modes of drug delivery in which either the source or target tissue are non-uniform are also encountered. One such example is the intravenous delivery of drugs to tumor tissue. In this case, especially in larger tumors, the distribution of capillaries is often highly heterogeneous and microvasculature is completely absent in the necrotic core. Certain tumors are also characterized by cystic inclusions and channeling through the interstitial space, all of which lead to drug concentrations that are spatially dependent throughout the target tissue. Still another example is the intravenous delivery of very tight binding proteins (e.g., high-affinity antibody conjugates) to a homogeneous tissue. In this case, the concentration of protein between adjacent capillaries often exhibits a spatially-dependent profile, even though the capillary bed itself is homogeneously distributed. Such profiles arise because the tight binding causes the concentration fronts, spreading out from capillaries into the space between them, to be extremely steep; if intravascular concentrations are sufficiently low relative to binding capacity, these fronts may move slowly, thus producing time-dependent spatial concentration profiles [1].

## DRUG MODALITY I: DELIVERY ACROSS A PLANAR-TISSUE INTERFACE

### General Principles

The formalisms required to describe these time- and spatially-dependent concentration profiles, as introduced in Chapter 8, are essentially microscopic mass balances expressed as partial differential equations. As previously noted, the ordinary differential equations used to describe well-mixed compartments are no longer sufficient, since they only account for the time-dependence of concentration. To see how these equations are formulated, and to visualize the underlying physiology and metabolism, consider the specific example of drug delivery from a solution across a planar-tissue interface (e.g., as might occur during continuous intraperitoneal infusion of an agent).

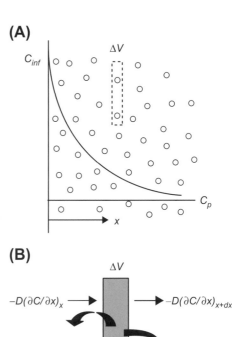

**FIGURE 9.1** (A) Representative concentration profile that develops in tissue when delivering a drug across a fluid–tissue interface. Differential volume element $\Delta V$ is indicated by the rectangle and circles denote capillaries. $C_{inf}$ is the concentration of infusate solution in contact with the tissue surface and $C_p$ is the plasma concentration. (B) Elements contributing to the mass balance over $\Delta V$. On the left, $-D(\partial C/\partial x)_x$ is the diffusive (Fickian) flux entering the volume element at $x$. On the right, $-D(\partial C/\partial x)_{x+dx}$ is the outgoing flux at $x + dx$. Other terms denote the metabolic rate constant ($k_m$) and microvascular permeability coefficient–surface area product ($P{\cdot}s$).

Figure 9.1A shows a typical concentration profile that might develop across an interface. The region to the left of the $y$-axis corresponds to the region containing the peritoneal infusate at drug concentration $C_{inf}$, while the region at the right corresponds to the tissue in contact with the infusate. Small circles depict capillaries, and they are assumed to be homogeneously distributed. In this figure, $x$ is the distance from the fluid–tissue interface. The rectangular box represents a typical differential volume element in the tissue. The transport of drug from the infusate into the tissue in this example is taken to be purely diffusional – that is, no convection (pressure-driven flow) is present. The mathematical model leading to an expression for the concentration profile is a differential mass balance over the volume element $\Delta V$:

$$\underset{\substack{\text{rate of conc} \\ \text{change in } \Delta V}}{\frac{\partial C}{\partial t}} = \underset{\substack{\text{net diffusion} \\ \text{in } \Delta V}}{D\frac{\partial^2 C}{\partial x^2}} - \underset{\substack{\text{metabolism} \\ \text{in } \Delta V}}{\frac{k_m}{R}C} - \underset{\substack{\text{net transport} \\ \text{across microvasculature}}}{P{\cdot}s\left(\frac{C}{R} - C_p\right)}$$

(9.1)

This equation says that the change in total drug concentration within $\Delta V$ over a small increment of time (left-hand term; see Figure 9.1B) is equal to the sum of all the mass fluxes generating this change, namely the net change in mass due to diffusion into and out of $\Delta V$ (first right-hand term) less mass loss due to metabolism within $\Delta V$ (second right-hand term) less net mass loss across the microvasculature within $\Delta V$ (third right-hand term). In this equation, $C = C(x, t)$ is the tissue concentration of bound plus free drug, $R$ is a constant of proportionality that relates $C$ to the free extracellular concentration of drug $C_e$, that is:

$$C = R\,C_e, \qquad (9.2)$$

$k_m/R$ is the metabolic rate constant[1], $P{\cdot}s$ is the product of permeability coefficient and surface area per volume of tissue accounting for passive movement across the microvasculature, and $C_p$ is the free plasma concentration of drug. The parameter $s$ is analogous to $S$ in Chapter 3 that refers to the surface area of an entire capillary bed. In Equation 9.1, $D$ is the apparent tissue diffusion constant and is equal to $\varphi_e D_e/R$, where $\varphi_e$ is the extracellular volume fraction of the tissue and $D_e$ is the diffusion constant within just the extracellular space. For non-binding substances distributed solely in the extracellular space of a tissue, $R = \varphi_e$ and $D = D_e$. For non-binding substances that partition equally into the intracellular and extracellular spaces, $R = 1$ and $D = \varphi_e D_e$.

Formulation of the model is completed by the specification of initial and boundary conditions. The initial condition, the state of the system just before exposing the interface to drug (the beginning of the intraperitoneal infusion in our example), is that the tissue concentration is everywhere zero, that is, $C(x, 0) = 0$. At all times at the fluid–tissue interface, the extracellular concentration equals the infusate concentration, that is:

---

[1] When drug exchanges rapidly between the intracellular (ICS) and extracellular (ECS) spaces, and also equilibrates rapidly between bound and free forms, it can be shown [2] that $R = \varphi_e(1 + K_e B_e) + (1 - \varphi_e)(1 + K_i B_i)K_\pi$. Here $\varphi_e$ is the extracellular volume fraction, $K_e$ and $K_i$ are affinity constants for binding, and $B_e$ and $B_i$ are binding capacities in the ECS and ICS respectively. $K_\pi$ is the equilibrium ratio of the free intracellular concentration to the free extra-cellular concentration ($K_\pi = 0$ for substances confined solely to the ECS). Similarly, $k_m = \varphi_e k_e + (1 - \varphi_e)k_i\,K_\pi$, where $k_e$ and $k_i$ are fundamental rate constants describing the rates of metabolism in the individual ECS and ICS regions.

$$C_e(0, t) = C(0, t)/R = C_{inf}$$

where $C_{inf}$ is the constant peritoneal infusate concentration. Far from the interface, the concentration of drug [$C(\infty, t)$] is determined by the tissue's transport balance with the plasma. If the plasma concentration is zero, then [$C(\infty, t)$] $= 0$.

With these initial and boundary conditions, the solution to Equation 9.1 is [3]:

$$\frac{C(x,t)}{R\,C_{inf}} = \frac{1}{2}exp\left[-x\,\sqrt{k/D}\right]\;erfc\left[\frac{x}{\sqrt{4D\,t}} - \sqrt{k\,t}\right]$$
$$+ \frac{1}{2}exp\left[x\,\sqrt{k/D}\right]erfc\left[\frac{x}{\sqrt{4D\,t}} + \sqrt{k\,t}\right] \quad (9.3)$$

where $k = (k_m + P{\cdot}s)/R$ and $erfc$ is the complementary error function (available in standard spreadsheet programs). If no reaction or microvascular loss is present, then this solution simplifies to:

$$\frac{C(x,t)}{R\,C_{inf}} = erfc\left[\frac{x}{\sqrt{4Dt}}\right] \qquad (9.4)$$

When reaction or microvascular loss is present, the steady state limit of Equation 9.3 is just

$$\frac{C(x)}{R\,C_{inf}} = exp\left[-x\,\sqrt{k/D}\right] \qquad (9.5)$$

In the special steady-state case where the plasma concentration is constant *but not zero* (e.g., as may happen when a large intraperitoneal infusion delivers sufficient mass to increase the plasma concentration to a level consistent with a mass balance between intra-peritoneal delivery and whole-body clearance), a generalized form of Equation 9.5 applies – that is,

$$\frac{\dfrac{C(x)}{R} - \dfrac{P{\cdot}s}{P{\cdot}s + k_m}C_p}{C_{inf} - \dfrac{P{\cdot}s}{P{\cdot}s + k_m}C_p} = exp\left[-x\,\sqrt{k/D}\right] \qquad (9.5')$$

where $C_p$ is now the constant plasma concentration.

Equation 9.4 provides a relationship between time and the distance at which a particular concentration is achieved. When clearance rates are small relative to diffusion rates, it states that the distance from the surface (penetration depth) at which a particular concentration $C$ is achieved advances as the square root of time. In other words, to double the penetration of a compound, the exposure time must quadruple. Equation 9.5 states that, given sufficient time and negligible plasma concentration, most compounds will develop a semilogarithmic concentration profile whose slope is determined by the ratio of the clearance rate to the diffusion constant. Note also that the distance over which the concentration decreases to one-half its surface value, defined as its penetration distance $\Gamma$, is derivable from Equation 9.5 as

$$\Gamma = (\ln 2)/\sqrt{k/D} \qquad (9.6)$$

while the approximate time to penetrate this distance by diffusion is

$$t_\Gamma = \Gamma^2/D \qquad (9.6')$$

The results of Equations 9.5 and 9.6 are very useful and we will refer to them repeatedly. One implication of these results is that drug can be delivered to a tissue layer near the exposed surface of an organ, but its penetration depth depends strongly on the rate of metabolism of the agent. Another is that the delivery of non- or slowly-metabolized substances across surfaces for purposes of systemic drug administration is dominated by distributed microvascular uptake in the tissue layer underlying the surface. In the particular case of intraperitoneal administration, the barrier to uptake of drug into the circulation is thus the resistance to transfer across distributed capillary walls and not, as assumed in the early literature, the resistance to transfer across the thin peritoneal membrane that is relatively permeable.

Distributed pharmacokinetics is characterized not only by spatially dependent concentration profiles but also by dose–response relationships that become spatially dependent. For example, biological responses such as cell kill are often quantified as functions of area under the concentration vs time curve ($AUC$). In compartment models, response is frequently correlated with the area under the plasma-concentration vs time curve, where

$$AUC = \int_0^\infty C_p(t)dt \qquad (9.7)$$

or, alternatively, with the $AUC$ formed by integration over the tissue concentration $C(t)$. With distributed pharmacokinetics, however, the response within each local region of the tissue will vary according to its local exposure to drug. The appropriate correlate of response in this case is thus a spatially dependent $AUC$ formed over the local tissue concentration – that is

$$AUC(x) = \int_0^\infty C(x,t)\,dt \qquad (9.8)$$

In distributed pharmacokinetics, threshold models, in which a biological response is associated with the rise of concentration above a threshold value, are likewise dependent on spatial location.

The use of distributed pharmacokinetic models to estimate expected concentration profiles associated with different modes of drug delivery requires that various input parameters be available. The most commonly required parameters, as seen in Equation 9.1, are diffusion coefficients, reaction rate constants, and capillary permeabilities. As will be encountered later, hydraulic conductivities are also needed when pressure-driven rather than diffusion-driven flows are involved. Diffusion coefficients (i.e., the $D_e$ parameter described previously) can be measured experimentally or can be estimated by extrapolation from known values for reference substances. Diffusion constants in tissue are known to be proportional to their aqueous value, which in turn is approximately proportional to a power of the molecular weight. Hence,

$$D_e = \lambda^2\,\alpha\,D_{aqueous}^{37\,^\circ C} \propto \lambda^2\alpha(MW)^{-0.50} \qquad (9.9)$$

in which $\lambda$ accounts for the tortuosity of the diffusion path in tissue, $\alpha$ accounts for any additional diffusional drag of the interstitial matrix over that of pure water, and $MW$ is the molecular weight of the diffusing species. The 0.50 exponent applies to most small molecular weight species. The diffusion constant for a substance of arbitrary molecular weight can be obtained from the ratio of Equation 9.9 for the desired substance to that for a reference substance – that is, from

$$\left(\frac{D_e}{D_{e,\,ref}}\right) = \left(\frac{MW_{ref}}{MW}\right)^{0.50} \qquad (9.10)$$

Reference values are available for many substances but the one available for a wide variety of tissues is sucrose [4]. In the macromolecular range ($>3$ kDa), albumin values are available in the literature and the exponent is similar.

Capillary permeability coefficient–surface area product values ($P{\cdot}s$) are also available from molecular weight scaling of reference values [5, 6]. In the small molecular weight range shown in Figure 3.4, a relationship very similar to Equation 9.10 is valid – that is:

$$\left(\frac{P{\cdot}s}{P{\cdot}s_{\,ref}}\right) = \left(\frac{MW_{ref}}{MW}\right)^{0.63} \qquad (9.11)$$

The similarity of the diffusion and permeability scaling relationships leads to the prediction that, for slowly metabolized substances, the *steady-state* concentration profiles that develop in a tissue following diffusion across an interface (as in Figure 9.1) are nearly independent of molecular weight. This follows from Equation 9.5, since nearly identical molecular weight scaling factors for $k$ (proportional to $P \cdot s$ in this case) and $D$ appear in both the numerator and denominator of the $k/D$ argument. Hence, one would predict that the penetration depths of inulin (MW 5000 Da) and urea (MW 60 Da) would be similar within the interstitial fluid space.

Reaction rate parameters required for the distributed pharmacokinetic model generally come from independent experimental data. One source is the analysis of rates of metabolism of cells grown in culture. However, the parameters from this source are potentially subject to considerable artifact, since cofactors and cellular interactions may be absent *in vitro* that are present *in vivo*. Published enzyme activities are a second source, but these are even more subject to artifact. A third source is previous compartmental analysis of a tissue dosed uniformly by intravenous infusion. If a compartment in such a study can be closely identified with the organ or tissue later considered in distributed pharmacokinetic analysis, then its compartmental clearance constant can often be used to derive the required metabolic rate constant.

### Case Study 1: Intraperitoneal Administration of Chemotherapeutic Agents for Treatment of Ovarian Cancer

Some aspects of this mode of delivery have already been introduced as part of our discussion of the general principles for transfer across a planar interface, but now the focus will narrow to two specific chemical agents and the use of one of them in the treatment of ovarian cancer.

The goal of ovarian cancer chemotherapy is to achieve sufficient penetration of the surfaces of tumor nodules to allow effective treatment. These nodules lie on the serosal surfaces of the peritoneum, are not invasive, and are not associated with high probabilities of metastasis. When the cancer is diagnosed early, or the larger nodules are removed surgically in more advanced disease, the residual nodules in 73% of the cases have maximum diameters of $< 5\,mm$ [7]. Collectively, these characteristics suggest that, if complete irrigation of the serosal surfaces can be achieved, ovarian tumors may be good candidates for treatment by peritoneal infusion.

The present drug of choice for this purpose is cisplatin (*cis*-diamminedichloroplatinum II) or its analog, carboplatin. Early compartmental models predicted a substantial pharmacokinetic advantage of intraperitoneal over intravenous delivery [8]. A later

Phase III trial [7] confirmed that a comparative survival advantage could be achieved with intraperitoneal administration of cisplatin.

The effectiveness of cisplatin depends on its ability to penetrate target tissue. Therefore, we need to estimate its penetration depth from a distributed model such as that represented by Equation 9.1. However, this is difficult to do with ovarian tumor because the permeabilities and reaction rates are not available. Hence, a first estimate is made for penetration of normal peritoneal cavity tissues by ethylenediaminetetraacetic acid (EDTA), a molecule of similar molecular weight to cisplatin. The steady-state concentration profiles of EDTA should resemble those of cisplatin in normal peritoneal tissues because both compounds are cleared primarily by permeation through the fenestrated capillaries in these tissues, and the small molecular weight-related differences in $P \cdot s$ and $D$ should cancel out in Equations 9.5 and 9.5'. By first focusing on EDTA, experimental data also become available for assessing the ability of the distributed model to account for the observed concentration profiles.

EDTA concentration profiles were determined experimentally from data such as those shown in Figure 9.2 [9]. In these experiments, a $^{14}$C-EDTA solution was infused into the peritoneal cavity of a rat. After 1 hour of exposure (sufficient time to establish steady-state profiles in the tissues), the animal was sacrificed, frozen, and sectioned for autoradiography. The upper panel of Figure 9.2 shows a transverse section across the rat in which a cross-section of the large intestine is identified. This cross-section is magnified in the lower panel and a grid is shown from which the concentration profile was estimated by quantitative autoradiography. Concentration profiles for most of the peritoneal viscera were obtained in this manner, and the aggregated profiles for the stomach, small intestine, and large intestine are plotted (circles) in Figure 9.3. The concentrations in this figure are all expressed relative to the infusate concentration. Because the mass of EDTA that was infused was sufficiently large to distribute throughout the entire body of the rat, the plasma concentration at the end of the experiment could not be neglected. It is shown as the single data point labeled "Plasma", and is expressed as the ratio of the actual plasma concentration to the infusate concentration. Because EDTA distributes only in the extracellular space, the deep tissue concentration only approaches the "Plasma" concentration reduced by the extracellular volume fraction $\varphi_e$.

The steady state formalism of Equation 9.5', which includes the effects of a constant plasma concentration,

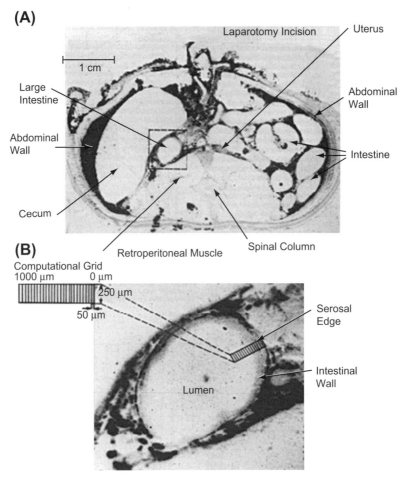

**FIGURE 9.2** (A) Autoradiogram of a cross-section of peritoneal cavity from a study of transport from the peritoneal cavity to plasma. (B) Close-up of dashed area (box) in (A). Reproduced from Flessner MF, Fenstermacher JD, Dedrick RL, Blasberg RG. Am J Physiol 1985;248:F425–35 [9].

should describe these data. Noting from EDTA's distribution into the extracellular space that $R = \varphi_e$, and from its negligible metabolism that $P{\cdot}s/(P{\cdot}s + k_m) \to 1$, Equation 9.5′ can be simplified to:

$$\frac{C(x) - \phi_e\, C_p}{\phi_e\, C_{inf} - \phi_e\, C_p} = exp\left[-x\,\sqrt{k/D}\,\right] \qquad (9.12)$$

When this equation is fit to the data of Figure 9.3 using $\varphi_e$ and $\sqrt{k/D}$ as fitting parameters, the solid line results. The value of $\varphi_e$ so obtained is reasonable (an extracellular volume fraction of 0.27), and the permeability derived from the $\sqrt{k/D}$ term $\left(= \sqrt{P{\cdot}s/(\varphi_e D_e)}\right)$ agrees with that expected from molecular weight correlations. The theory largely accounts for the data, although it tends to overestimate the concentrations at the deepest penetration, perhaps because vascularity increases as one passes toward the luminal side of the organs.

However, the fit is sufficiently good to conclude that the theory has captured most of the relevant physiology and that it can be used to account for or, given availability of parameters, to predict the observed results.

As a predictor of the concentration of cisplatin in normal peritoneal tissues, these data indicate a steady state penetration depth (distance to half the surface layer concentration) of about 0.1 mm (100 μm). If this distance is applied to tumor tissue, penetration even to three or four times this depth would make it difficult to effectively dose tumor nodules of 1–2 mm diameter. Fortunately, crude data are available from proton-induced X-ray emission studies of cisplatin transport into intraperitoneal rat tumors, indicating that the penetration into tumor is deeper and in the range of 1 to 1.5 mm [10]. Such distances are obtained from Equations 9.5 or 9.5′ only if $k$ is much smaller than in normal peritoneal tissues – that is, theory suggests that

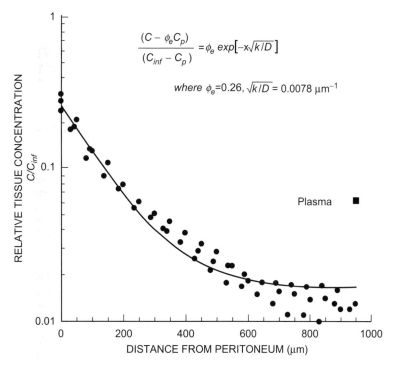

**FIGURE 9.3**  Profile of $^{14}$C-EDTA concentrations (expressed relative to $C_{inf}$) in gastrointestinal tissues following intraperitoneal infusion. The equation shown in the graph was used to fit the experimental tissue (●) and plasma (■) concentration data, resulting in the solid-line curve.

low permeability coefficient–surface area products in tumor (e.g., due to a developing microvasculature and a lower capillary density) may be responsible for the deeper tumor penetration.

### Case Study 2: Intraventricular Administration of Cytosine Arabinoside for the Treatment of JC Virus Infection in Patients with Progressive Multifocal Leukoencephalopathy

Another example of a situation in which distributed pharmacokinetics plays an important role is in the infusion of drug solutions into the lateral ventricles or cisternal space of the brain. Drugs that have been delivered this way include chemotherapeutic agents for the treatment of tumors, antibacterial, antifungal, and antiviral agents for the treatment of infection, and neurotrophic factors for the treatment of neurodegenerative disease.

The principle reason for using this route of administration is to deliver drugs behind the blood–brain barrier (BBB) by taking advantage of the fact that no equivalent barrier exists at the interface between the ventricular fluid space and the interstitial space of the brain parenchyma. That the BBB is often a major problem to be overcome is suggested by the image of

Figure 9.4. This autoradiograph shows a longitudinal cross-section of a rat that was sacrificed 5 minutes after an intravenous injection of $^{14}$C-histamine [11]. The compound has distributed throughout most organs of the body, but the brain and spinal cord remain white in this image, indicating no significant delivery of histamine to the central nervous system. With intraventricular delivery of agents, high brain interstitial fluid levels can be achieved since the BBB now tends to block microvascular efflux of the drug and trap it in the interstitial space, only allowing the drug to be slowly cleared to the plasma and systemic tissues via bulk flow of cerebrospinal fluid through the arachnoid villi.

This approach has been explored in attempts to treat progressive multifocal leukoencephalopathy, a rapidly fatal disease caused by the JC virus and characterized by regions of central nervous system demyelination and markedly altered neuroglia. The virus is known to be sensitive *in vitro* to the action of cytosine arabinoside (ARA-C) concentrations of 40 μM (10 μg/mL) or more [12]. Because the agent crosses the BBB slowly, Hall *et al.* [13] designed a study to test whether intraventricular/intrathecal administration of ARA-C could successfully treat JC virus in humans. ARA-C was administered as a bolus into the

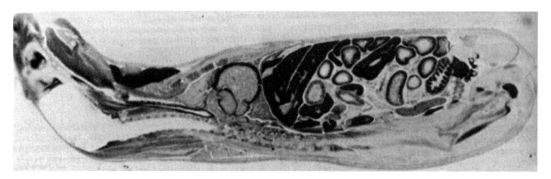

**FIGURE 9.4**   Autoradiogram showing a sagittal cross section of a rat 5 minutes after an intravenous injection of [14]C-histamine. Reproduced with permission from Pardridge WM, Oldendorf WH, Cancilla P, Frank HJ. Ann Intern Med 1986;105:82–95 [11].

cerebrospinal fluid (CSF) space at the initial rate of 50 mg every 7 days. Although this ARA-C regimen was found to be ineffective, Zimm *et al.* [14] had previously shown that, after a 30-mg bolus intraventricular injection of ARA-C, CSF concentrations of this drug have a terminal elimination half-life of 3.4 h and fall below 40 µM in less than 15 hours. Thus, for much of the 7-day dosing period, even the surface concentrations of this drug would not have been expected to exceed the lowest ARA-C concentration found to have antiviral activity *in vitro*. Therefore, choice of the delivery regimen used in the clinical trial probably provided an inadequate test of the potential efficacy of this therapeutic approach.

Groothuis *et al.* [15] used sucrose, an unmetabolized marker compound that has very low capillary permeability, to initially evaluate the therapeutic feasibility of administering chemotherapy by the intraventricular route. Sucrose was infused by osmotic minipump into the lateral ventricle of a rat for 7 days, yielding the concentration profile exhibited in Figure 9.5A, a profile well-fit by theoretical Equation 9.5 using published diffusion and permeation constants for sucrose [16]. In this experiment, the penetration distances to half and one-tenth the surface concentration were 0.9 mm and 3 mm respectively. In a subsequent study, Groothuis *et al.* [17] continuously infused ARA-C into the ventricles of rat brain over 7 days. They found that even with continuous administration of ARA-C, tissue concentrations dropped to one-half the surface concentration at a penetration distance of 0.4 mm and to about one-tenth the surface concentration at a penetration distance of 1.0 mm (Figure 9.5B). These distances are of the same order of magnitude but are somewhat less than those achieved with intraventricular delivery of sucrose.

This indicates (see Equation 9.5) that ARA-C is cleared more rapidly than sucrose, consistent with the known presence of nucleoside transporters in the microvascular walls of the brain as well as metabolic deamination of ARA-C to uracil arabinoside [14]. However, the clearance rate is not so rapid as to prevent the achievement of millimeter penetration depths in accessible time frames. Indeed, evaluation of Equation 9.6′ (assuming equal partitioning of drug between intracellular and extracellular spaces so that $D = \phi_e D_e$) indicates that 1-mm penetration depths can be achieved in roughly 3 hours. This suggests that a 40-µM effective concentration could have been maintained at this depth throughout the multiple-week exposures of the study conducted by Hall *et al.*, provided the surface concentration was constantly maintained near 400 µM (see Figure 9.5B). In turn, if this concentration were to exist throughout the 140-ml CSF volume (so that total mass in the CSF = 13.6 mg), the 3.4-h half-time for clearance of the CSF implies that the concentration could only be maintained if the cleared mass were constantly resupplied by infusion at the rate of (13.6/2 mg/3.4 h) = 2 mg/h or, equivalently, 336 mg/week. This continuous infusion rate is nearly seven-fold the 50-mg/week bolus rate employed in the Hall *et al.* study. Thus, our example suggests that further trials employing more optimized drug delivery may be indicated before ARA-C can be ruled out definitively as a potential therapeutic agent for patients with progressive multifocal leukoencephalopathy.

## Differences between the Delivery of Small Molecules and Macromolecules across a Planar Interface

Previous discussion has indicated that unmetabolized small molecular weight, hydrophilic molecules (MW < 500 Da) typically penetrate tissues to (half-surface-concentration) depths that range at steady state from 0.1 to 1 mm. The depth is on the order of 0.1 mm for most tissues of the body, as we have seen in

**(A)**

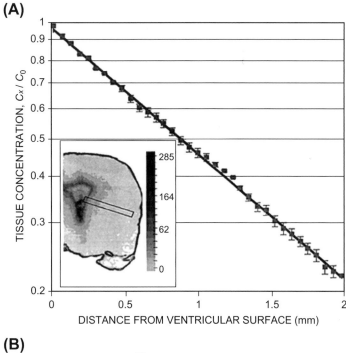

**(B)**

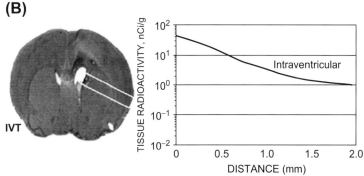

**FIGURE 9.5** (A) Concentration profile of $^{14}$C-sucrose in rat caudate following intraventricular infusion to steady state (expressed relative to average tissue concentration at tissue surface $C_0$). The inset shows the auto-radiogram of a coronal brain section and the rectangular area used to generate the concentration profile. (B) The concentration profile in brain tissue following 7-day intraventricular (IVT) delivery of labeled cytosine arabinoside to rat brain. The tissue radioactivity data were collected from the rectangular area shown at left. (A) Reproduced with permission from Groothuis DR, Ward S, Itskovich AC *et al.* J Neurosurg 1999;90:321–31 [15]; (B) modified from Groothuis DR, Benalcazar H, Allen CV *et al.* Brain Res 2000;856:281–90 [17].

the case of EDTA's penetration of normal peritoneal tissues. The depth increases 10-fold, to 1 mm, for tissues characterized by a tight microvascular endothelium (e.g., brain or spinal cord) because the capillary permeability of those endothelial barriers is nearly 100-fold lower. The times for unmetabolized and unbound small molecular weight species to achieve steady-state concentration profiles in tissues are relatively short and tend not to exceed the 4-hour value of sucrose in brain. When metabolism is present and binding remains negligible, the time to steady state will shorten inversely with an increase in the rate of metabolism, and the penetration depth will fall well below the millimeter value. If linear binding is present, it has no effect on the penetration depth at steady state but proportionally increases the time to attain this steady state. The depth and times can be calculated from Equations 9.6 and 9.6′.

What sort of penetration depth is expected for macromolecules? As with small molecules the depth is again determined by Equation 9.6, but some differences emerge [6]. Were both $k$ and $D$ for non-metabolized macromolecules (for which $k = (P \cdot s)/R$) given as mere extensions of the molecular weight functions for smaller compounds, the penetration depth would remain relatively independent of molecular weight. However, unmetabolized macromolecules (MW > 10 kDa) have been observed to penetrate more deeply at steady state than their non-metabolized small molecular weight counterparts such as sucrose (of the order of two- to three-fold deeper in visceral or muscle tissues). The primary reason is that capillary $P \cdot s$ values for macromolecules are relatively smaller and are related to molecular weight by a power formula of the form

$$P \cdot s = A(MW)^{0.6} \qquad (9.13)$$

where the exponent is similar to that for small molecules, but $A$ is nearly 10-fold lower [6]. Since the penetration depth $\Gamma$ is inversely proportional to the square root of this coefficient, the depth for unmetabolized macromolecules will be about three-fold larger than for small unmetabolized compounds. As with small molecules, steady-state penetration depths are of the order of a few millimeters at best.

One other important difference exists between small and macromolecular weight molecules: the time required to achieve steady-state concentration profiles across an interface. Maximum penetration is obtained by unmetabolized molecules and the time to steady state is largely controlled by the rate of diffusion through the tissue. For sucrose in brain, this time is approximately 4 hours. However, for a macromolecule of 67 kDa, the diffusion constant decreases 19-fold [4, 18], leading to a corresponding 19-fold increase in the time required to achieve the steady state profile (*cf.* Equation 9.4). The 4 hours required for sucrose thus increases to 3 days or more. For both small molecules and macromolecules, these times will greatly decrease as metabolism begins to play a greater role, but only at the cost of a much reduced penetration depth.

Examples of the effects of binding and rapid reaction with macromolecules are demonstrated in Figures 9.6 and 9.7. Figure 9.6 shows the distribution of $^{125}$I-labeled brain-derived neurotrophic factor (BDNF; MW ~17 kDa) following 20 hours of intraventricular infusion into the brain of a rat [19]. The penetration depth is very shallow (~0.2 mm), far less than the few-millimeter distance theoretically obtainable from an unmetabolized and unbound molecule of this size. Part of the reason for the shallow penetration is that the infusion time is, at most, a third of the time required for unmetabolized and unbound molecules to reach this theoretical distance. An even more important factor is that BDNF receptors, whose

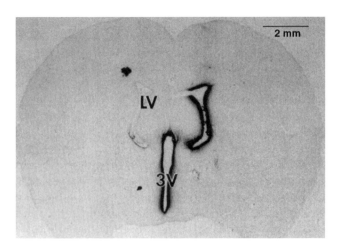

**FIGURE 9.6** Autoradiogram and unstained photograph showing the distribution of $^{125}$I-labeled BDNF in the vicinity of the intraventricular foramen in rat brain following a 20-hour intraventricular infusion. Reproduced with permission from Yan Q, Matheson C, Sun J *et al.* Exp Neurol 1994;27:23–36 [19].

mRNA (trkB) is known from *in situ* hybridization analyses to be present on neurons and glia, bind BDNF and further retard progress to steady state [19]. Figure 9.7 shows the distribution of $^{125}$I-labeled nerve growth factor (NGF; MW ~14 kDa) 48 hours after the implantation of a poly(ethylene-covinyl acetate) disk

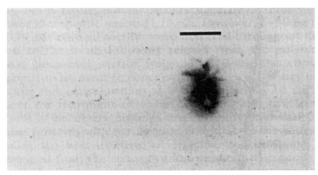

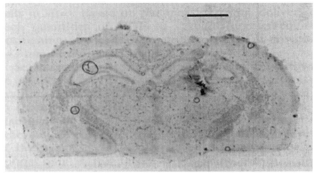

**FIGURE 9.7** Autoradiogram (*top*) and unstained photograph (*bottom*) obtained from a coronal section of rat brain 48 hours after implantation of an $^{125}$I-labeled NGF-loaded polymer. Bars = 2.5 mm. Reproduced with permission from Krewson CE, Klarman ML, Saltzman WM. Brain Res 1995;680:196–206 [20].

(2-mm diameter × 0.8-mm thickness) containing this neurotrophic factor [20]. The upper panel shows the location of radioactivity in a coronal brain section, including the 0.8-mm wide contribution from the disk in this view. In this image, the maximum observable extent of diffusion out from the disk is about 0.4 mm on either side of the disk, corresponding to a penetration depth of 0.25 mm [20]. This is a steady-state penetration depth since the same distribution shown in Figure 9.7 is also observed after 7 days of infusion. Therefore, the shallow penetration of this protein is due neither to slow diffusion nor to the presence of NGF receptors, since none are present in this region [20], but rather is attributable to degradative metabolic processes that result in an NGF half-life of approximately 30 minutes.

# DRUG MODALITY II: DELIVERY FROM A POINT SOURCE, DIRECT INTERSTITIAL INFUSION

## General Principles

As has been seen with the examples of intraperitoneal and intraventricular infusion, tissue penetration

depths of only a few millimeters are generally achievable by diffusive transport across an interface. If the goal of therapy is to dose entire tissue masses such as glioblastomas or structures of the basal ganglia, millimeter penetrations are insufficient and another mode of drug delivery is required. A mode capable of achieving multicentimeter instead of multimillimeter depths is direct interstitial infusion [21, 22]. It is the description of the distributed pharmacokinetics of this modality that is next examined.

In direct interstitial infusion, a narrow-gauge cannula is inserted into tissue and infusate is pumped through it directly into the interstitial space of a target tissue. Figure 9.8, for example, shows a 32-gauge cannula placed stereotactically into the center of the caudate nucleus of a rat. This type of drug delivery uses volumetric flow rates ranging from 0.01 μL/min to 4.0 μL/min. The lower end of this range corresponds to flows provided by osmotic minipumps while the upper end corresponds to flows provided by

microinjection (syringe) pumps. For small molecular weight compounds, the lowest flow rates allow all transport to occur by diffusion, even near the tip of the cannula. At higher flow rates, sufficiently high fluid velocities are generated so that pressure-driven bulk flow processes (convection) dominate most transport for both small molecules and macromolecules. Delivery of mass to a tissue thus involves the outward radial flow of infused drug solution from the cannula tip, and the concentration of drug changes along that radial path as the drug is progressively exposed to clearance processes. A distributed model is required to quantitatively describe this spatially dependent concentration profile.

## Low-Flow Microinfusion Case

The simplest model describing this mode of drug delivery applies to the low volumetric flow range for small molecules – for example, cisplatin delivered at 0.9 μL/hour [23]. The model is a differential mass balance for a typical shell volume surrounding the cannula tip. Deriving it in the same fashion as Equation 9.1, except taking the spherical geometry of the distribution into account, it is:

$$
\underbrace{\frac{\partial C}{\partial t}}_{\substack{\text{rate of conc} \\ \text{change in } \Delta V}} = \underbrace{D\frac{1}{r^2}\frac{\partial}{\partial r}r^2\frac{\partial C}{\partial r}}_{\substack{\text{net diffusion} \\ \text{in } \Delta V}} - \underbrace{\frac{k_m}{R}C}_{\substack{\text{metabolism} \\ \text{in } \Delta V}} - \underbrace{P\cdot s\left(\frac{C}{R}-C_p\right)}_{\substack{\text{net transport} \\ \text{across microvasculature}}}
\tag{9.14}
$$

All parameters have the same definitions as used previously. The initial condition is that drug concentration in the tissue is everywhere zero. The boundary conditions are, first, that the drug concentration remains zero at all times far from the cannula tip, and, second, that the mass outflow from the cannula be equal to the diffusive flux through the tissue at the cannula tip – that is, that

$$
C(\infty, t) = 0 \quad \text{and} \quad q\,C_{inf} = -4\,\pi\,r_o^2 D\frac{\partial C}{\partial r}\bigg|_{r_o}
\tag{9.15}
$$

where $q$ is the volumetric flow rate, $C_{inf}$ is the infusate concentration, and $r_o$ is the radius of the cannula. The steady-state solution to this model is:

$$
C(r) = \frac{q\,C_{inf}}{4\pi D\,r}\exp\left(-r\sqrt{k/D}\right)
\tag{9.16}
$$

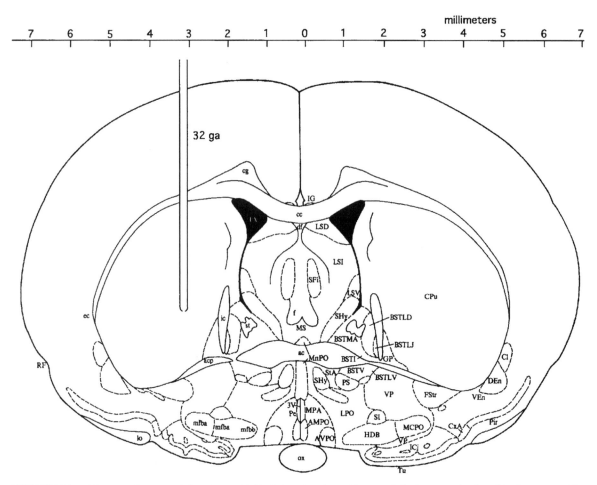

**FIGURE 9.8**  Schematic drawing of direct interstitial infusion showing a 32-gauge infusion cannula placed in the center of the rat caudate nucleus-putamen.

where, again, $k = (k_m + P \cdot s)/R$ and $D = \varphi_e D_e/R$. For cisplatin, $R = 1$. Equation 9.16 is the radial concentration profile of drug about a cannula tip in homogeneous tissue. It is similar in form to Equation 9.5, including the same parameter dependence of the argument of the exponential, but differs by an extra $r$ factor in the denominator that causes the concentration to drop off faster with distance. For cisplatin, the time to achieve this steady-state profile 4 mm distant from the cannula tip is about 3 hours. Figure 9.9 shows the measured steady-state concentration profile of cisplatin in normal rat brain achieved after 160 hours of infusion at 0.9 μL/h. The solid line is the theoretical fit to the data showing that the $r$-damped exponential of Equation 9.16 accounts well for the data. The penetration depth is of the order of 0.6 mm, several-fold deeper than observed with EDTA penetration across the peritoneal interface because of the much lower brain capillary permeability, but generally of the same order of magnitude.

## High-Flow Microinfusion Case

The submillimeter penetration distances found to hold for transport across tissue interfaces or for low-flow microinfusion are insufficiently large to provide effective dosing for many targets. For example, some brain structures such as the human putamen or cortex have centimeter-scale dimensions. Likewise, highly invasive glioblastoma multiforma tumors of the brain are characterized by protrusions of tumor that extend for centimeter distances along vascular and fiber pathways. This mismatch of low-flow microinfusion penetration distance with target dimension provides a rationale for raising the volumetric infusion rate with the intent of increasing the velocity with which materials move through the interstitium. This retards their exposure to capillary or metabolic clearance mechanisms and increases their penetration depth. In the next few paragraphs, simple estimators of the concentration profiles and distribution volumes that result from high-flow microinfusion will be

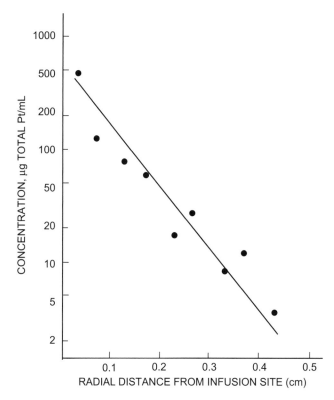

**FIGURE 9.9** Concentration profile of cisplatin in rat brain following slow infusion at 0.9 μL/h for 160 hours. *Solid line* is fit of Equation 9.16 to data ( ● ). Reproduced from Morrison PF, Dedrick RL. J Pharm Sci 1986;75:120–9 [23].

developed for brain from an appropriate distributed drug model [21].

At its core, the distributed model for high-flow microinfusion is once again a differential mass balance on the drug solute in the infusate. However, because the pumps used in this method generate relatively high fluid velocities, transport of molecules through tissue is not just diffusive but also convective (i.e., pressure driven). This necessitates additional model equations so that these velocities may be computed. Once again, partial differential equations are required because of the spatial and time dependence involved. If the tissue is recognized as a porous medium, then these velocities may be

computed from Darcy's Law, which states that the fluid velocity is proportional to the local pressure gradient – that is,

$$v = -\kappa \frac{\partial p}{\partial r} \tag{9.17}$$

where $\kappa$ is defined as the hydraulic conductivity, $v$ is the average fluid velocity in the tissue at position $r$, and $p$ is the hydrostatic pressure. This equation can be combined with another describing the differential mass balance of water in the brain – that is, the continuity equation,

$$\frac{\partial \rho}{\partial t} = -\frac{1}{r^2}\frac{\partial}{\partial r}r^2 \rho v + \Sigma$$

in which $\rho$ is the density of water (infusate) and $\Sigma$ is the sum of any source and sink terms. If the brain is considered an incompressible fluid medium and water losses across the microvascular are negligible [21], then the water density is invariant with time and $\Sigma$ is negligible so that the continuity equation reduces to just

$$0 = \frac{1}{r^2}\frac{\partial}{\partial r}r^2 v \tag{9.18}$$

Equations 9.17 and 9.18 can then be combined to generate a single differential equation in pressure; combined with the pressure boundary conditions that (1) pressure is zero at the brain boundary and that (2) the volumetric flow of infusate $q$ equals the flow across the tissue interface at the cannula tip (i.e., $q = 4\pi r_0^2 v = -4\pi r_0^2[\kappa(\partial p/\partial r)]$ at $r = r_0$), this pressure equation yields the simple result that

$$v = \frac{q}{4\pi r^2} \tag{9.19}$$

The distributed model is completed by forming a differential mass balance for the drug solute in a manner completely analogous to that shown previously in deriving Equation 9.14, except for the inclusion of an additional term describing convective flow:

$$\underset{\substack{\text{rate of conc}\\ \text{change in } \Delta V}}{\frac{\partial C}{\partial t}} = \underset{\substack{\text{net diffusion}\\ \text{in } \Delta V}}{D\frac{1}{r^2}\frac{\partial}{\partial r}r^2\frac{\partial C}{\partial r}} - \underset{\substack{\text{net convective}\\ \text{flow in } \Delta V}}{\frac{1}{R}\frac{1}{r^2}\frac{\partial}{\partial r}r^2 v\,C} - \underset{\substack{\text{metabolism}\\ \text{in } \Delta V}}{\frac{k_m}{R}C} - \underset{\substack{\text{net transport across}\\ \text{microvasculature}}}{P\!\cdot\! s\!\left(\frac{C}{R} - C_p\right)} \tag{9.20}$$

As with low-flow microinfusion, the initial condition is that drug concentration in the tissue is everywhere zero, and the outer boundary condition is that the drug concentration remains zero at all times far from the cannula tip. The boundary condition at the cannula tip (at $r_o$) differs in that the mass outflow from the cannula is equal to the convective (not diffusive) flux at the cannula tip – that is,

$$q \ C_{inf} = 4 \ \pi \ r_o^2 (v \ C) \mid_{r=r_o} \tag{9.21}$$

where $q$ is the volumetric flow rate, $C_{inf}$ is the infusate concentration, and $r_o$ is the radius of the cannula.

In general, the mathematical solution to Equation 9.20 is numerical. However, in the special case of non-endogenous macromolecules (MW > 50 kDa) and high flow (e.g., 3 μL/min), Equation 9.20 can be greatly simplified because diffusive contributions to transport are negligibly small. Hence it becomes just:

$$\frac{\partial \ C}{\partial \ t} = -\frac{1}{R \ r^2}\frac{\partial}{\partial \ r}r^2 v \ C - k \ C \tag{9.22}$$

where, as previously in Equation 9.3, $k = (k_m + P{\cdot}s)/R$. This equation has a very simple and useful solution for the concentration profile at steady state:

$$\frac{C(r)}{C_{inf}} = R \ exp\left[ -\frac{4 \ \pi \ ( \ k_m + P{\cdot}s)}{3 \ q}(r^3 - r_o^3) \right] \tag{9.23}$$

For non-binding macromolecules confined principally to the extracellular space, $R = \varphi_e$ (~0.2 in brain) and the interstitial concentration $C_e$ equals $C/R$ (cf. Equation 9.2).

Very simple estimators of the penetration depths that can be achieved by high-flow infusion of macromolecules can be derived from Equation 9.23. The penetration depth at steady state $(r_p)$ and the time required to reach this steady state $(t_p)$ are

$$r_p = \sqrt[3]{2 \ q/[4\pi \ (k_m + P{\cdot}s)]} \ and$$
$$t_p = 2R \ /[3 \ ( \ k_m + P{\cdot}s)] \tag{9.24}$$

When the characteristic time for degradation of a macromolecule is 33 hours (i.e., $k = \ln2/33$ h) and the flow rate $q$ is 3 μL/min, Equation 9.24 predicts that the penetration depth will be 1.8 cm. This is far in excess of the penetration depth that can be achieved by simple diffusive transport, and is the theoretical result that indicates that high-flow microinfusion can provide brain tissue penetrations that intraventricular infusion

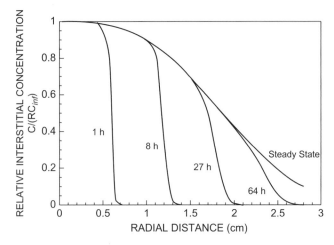

**FIGURE 9.10** Simulated interstitial concentration profiles of a 180-kDa macromolecule in non-binding brain tissue at various times during high-flow microinfusion at 3 μL/min. Model parameters were taken from Table 9.1.

cannot. Equation 9.24 also predicts that the time required to achieve this depth is 1.2 days, so that long-term infusion into the brain parenchyma is necessary.

Simulated concentration profiles for non-binding macromolecules in brain tissue (e.g., albumin or non-binding antibodies) are presented in Figure 9.10 for $k = \ln2/33$ h and $q = 3$ μL/min. Other parameters representative of 180-kDa proteins are given in Table 9.1 [4, 18, 21, 24, 25]. The curve in Figure 9.10 labeled "steady state" and forming an envelope over the other curves from top left to lower right corner is the relative concentration profile, $C_e/C_{inf} = C/(RC_{inf}) = C/(\varphi_e C_{inf})$, given by Equation 9.23. The curves at 1, 8, 27, and 64 hours are numerical results showing the kinetics of approach to the steady state. Note the characteristic shape of these curves. Up to well beyond 8 hours of infusion, the initial portion of the curve (nearest the cannula tip) follows the steady-state profile and then drops off dramatically, approximating a step function. This concentration front moves radially outward over time with a small degree of diffusion superimposed on the advancing front, giving rise to the small curvatures observable in Figure 9.10 at the top and bottom of the leading edge. Hence, over much of the infused tissue volume, the interstitial concentration remains relatively close to the infusate concentration and provides for relatively uniform tissue dosing.

The steep concentration profiles and large penetration distances predicted for non-binding macromolecules have been confirmed by experiment. Figure 9.11 presents an autoradiogram obtained from rat brain following a 4-μL infusion of $^{14}$C-albumin at 0.5 μL/min into the gray matter of the caudate through a 32-gauge cannula [26].

**TABLE 9.1    Representative Macromolecular Parameters[a]**

| Parameter | Symbol | Value | Source |
|---|---|---|---|
| Tissue hydraulic conductivity ($cm^4/dyne/s$) | $\kappa$ | $0.34 \times 10^{-8}$ | Morrison *et al.* [21] |
| Capillary permeability (cm/s) | P | $1.1 \times 10^{-9}$ | Blasberg *et al.* [24] |
| Capillary area/tissue volume ($cm^2/cm^3$) | $s$ | 100 | Bradbury [25] |
| Extracellular fraction | $\varphi_e$ | 0.2 | Patlak *et al.* [4] |
| Radius of 32 gauge catheter (cm) | $r_o$ | 0.0114 | |
| Diffusion coefficient ($cm^2/s$) | $D_e$ | $0.7 \times 10^{-7}$ | Tao and Nicholson [18] [b] |
| Volumetric infusion rate ($cm^3/s$) | $q$ | $5.0 \times 10^{-5}$ | Typical high-flow infusion rate (3 µL/min) |
| Metabolic rate constant ($sec^{-1}$) | $k_m$ | $1.15 \times 10^{-6}$ | Arbitrary value[c] |

[a]Typical of a 180-kDa protein.
[b]The value of $D_e$ value for gray matter obtained by these authors was scaled to 180-kDa molecular weight.
[c]This corresponds to a half-life of 33 hours and is roughly five times the average turnover rate of brain protein.

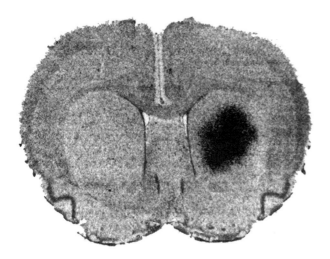

**FIGURE 9.11**  Autoradiogram of the distribution of [14]C-albumin in rat caudate following a 4-µL infusion at 0.5 µL/min. Reproduced from Chen MY, Lonser RR, Morrison PF *et al.* J Neurosurg 1999;90:315–20 [26].

The image shows a relatively uniform concentration (density) over an approximately spherical infusion volume, the symmetry resulting from the isotropic structure of the gray matter on the spatial scale of these observations. Figure 9.12 is an autoradiogram obtained after infusing 75 µL of [111]In-labeled transferrin (MW 80 kDa) at 1.1 µL/min into the white matter tracts of the corona radiata of the cat [22]. Two findings are immediately apparent. First, with this much larger volume of infusion, delivery distances of at least a centimeter have been achieved in accordance with theoretical prediction. Second, the anisotropy of the white matter tracts is evident, indicating that the models of Equations 9.17 and 9.20 must be modified to account for such anisotropy before they are predictive of any details of white matter spread. Figure 9.13 presents both an autoradiogram and a single photon emission computed tomographic (SPECT) image of [111]In-labeled

diethylenetriaminepentaacetic acid (DTPA-transferrin; MW 81 kDa) following a 10-mL continuous infusion at 1.9 µL/min into the centrum semiovale (white matter) of a primate [27]. In this case, the infused protein filled over one-third of the infused hemisphere before finding avenues of exit (10 mL exceeds the capacity of the primate hemisphere). The concentration was relatively uniform across the white matter, dropping off to only about 28% of the infusate concentration at a point over a centimeter from the cannula tip. The larger numbers reflect the presence of edema as well as tissue damage and fluid pockets in the vicinity of the cannula tip near the bottom of the section. The spread as determined from SPECT measurements was similar in the anterior–posterior, medial–lateral, and dorsal–ventral directions, ranging from 2 to 3 cm in each direction.

The high-flow distributed model of Equations 9.17, 9.20, and 9.23 describes the concentration profile that is generated in isotropic tissue at the very end of infusion. However, if these profiles are ultimately to be used to predict tissue response to a drug, these are not sufficient since they do not describe the entire history of tissue exposure to the drug. Once the pumps are turned off, there is *a post-infusion phase* during which further transport through the tissue occurs by diffusion, before clearance mechanisms finally reduce the agent's concentration to a negligible value. This phase is critical in dose–response estimation since it may last a long time relative to the duration of the infusion and may broaden the sharp concentration fronts often present at the termination of infusion. Hence, the distributed model is now extended to include a description of this phase and used in its entirety to assess likely treatment volumes as a function of degradation rate.

For isotropic tissue, the spherical distribution about the cannula tip at the end of infusion may be imagined as composed of a collection of concentric concentration shells. The post-infusion phase can then be described as

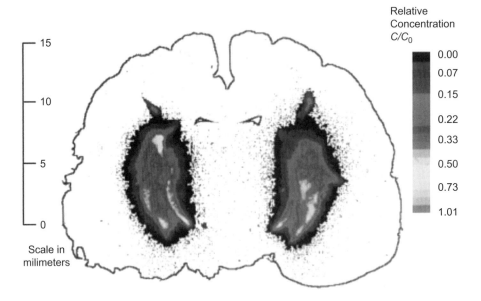

**FIGURE 9.12** Autoradiogram of the distribution of [111]In-labeled transferrin in cat brain following a 75-µL infusion at 1.15 µL/min into the corona radiata.

the superimposed diffusion of the material from each one of these shells acting independently. Mathematically, at the start of the post-infusion period, the concentration of each shell at distance $r$ from the cannula tip is the value of $C(r,t_{inf})$ obtained from Equation 9.20

(or 9.23, if applicable). Each of these shell concentrations can be multiplied by a function that accounts for its diffusional broadening in the post-infusion phase [28], and integration over all such shells leads to the formula for the post-infusion concentration profile, $C(r,\hat{t})$:

$$C(r,\hat{t}) = \frac{e^{-k\hat{t}}}{2\,r\,(\pi D\,\hat{t})^{1/2}} \int_{\infty}^{0} C(r',t_{inf}) \left[ e^{-(r-r')^2/(4D\hat{t})} - e^{-(r+r')^2/(4D\hat{t})} \right] r'\,dr' \tag{9.25}$$

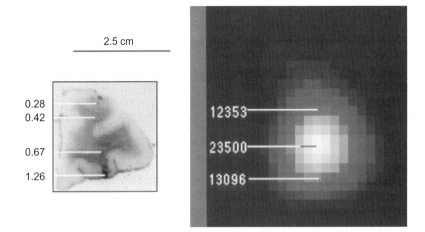

**FIGURE 9.13** *Left:* Autoradiogram of a coronal section of the frontal lobe of a rhesus monkey 13h after completing a 10-mL infusion of [111]In-labeled DTPA-transferrin into the centrum semiovale at 1.9 µL/min. Numerical values represent local tissue concentrations relative to the infusate concentration. *Right:* SPECT image corresponding to the autoradiogram. Numerical values are pixel counts used to assess spread in the dorsal–ventral and medial–lateral directions. Reproduced from Laske DW, Morrison PF, Lieberman DM *et al.* J Neurosurg 1997;87:586–94 [27].

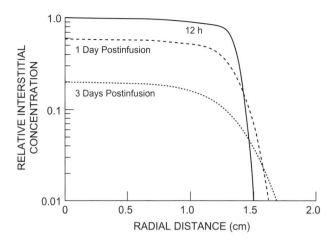

**FIGURE 9.14** Simulated interstitial concentration profiles of a 180-kDa macromolecule in non-binding brain tissue at the end of a 12-hour high-flow infusion at 3 μL/min and at 1 and 3 days post-infusion. Model parameters were taken from Table 9.1. Reproduced from Morrison PF, Laske DW, Bobo RH *et al.* Am J Physiol 1994;266:R292–305 [21].

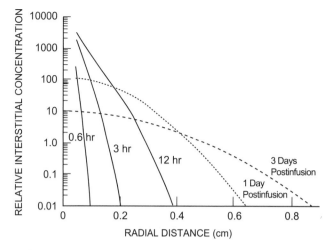

**FIGURE 9.15** Simulated interstitial concentration profiles of a 180-kDa macromolecule in non-binding brain tissue at various times during a 12-hour low-flow infusion at 0.05 μL/h and at 1 and 3 days post-infusion. Model parameters were taken from Table 9.1. Reproduced from Morrison PF, Laske DW, Bobo RH *et al.* Am J Physiol 1994;266:R292–305 [21].

for $\hat{t} > 0$ where $\hat{t} = t - t_{inf}$ is the time after the end of infusion [21]. When this formula is applied to our macromolecule which has a 33-hour degradation time in brain (the example in Figure 9.10), the concentration profiles of Figure 9.14 are generated. The solid line represents the concentration profile (the $C(r', t_{inf})$ in Equation 9.25) at 12 hours ($= t_{inf}$) after the initiation of a 3-μL/min infusion. The dotted lines show the profile at 1 and 3 days post-infusion. In the interior of the infused volume, the profile drops in value as the degradative processes exert their effect. However, beyond the initial 12-hour line, concentrations increase to appreciable values (after 1 day, to around 10% of the infusate concentration at 1.5 cm) and then decrease as degradation continues. Although not immediately apparent in this figure, this outward shift could easily account for a 20% increase in dosage volume if the drug remained biologically active at 1% of its infusate concentration.

For comparison with low-flow infusion (pure diffusion) behavior, the same type of plot as Figure 9.14 is shown in Figure 9.15. In this case, computations based on Equation 9.14 were performed in which the same mass of macromolecule is infused over 12 hours but at a much lower flow rate of 0.05 μL/h (0.00083 μL/min) to assure pure diffusive transport. Because the same infusion time is employed in both the low- and high-flow simulations, the constraint of identical delivered mass at low flow requires that the infusate concentration be raised by several logs. Hence the upper end of the concentration scale in Figure 9.15 is greatly expanded relative to that of Figure 9.14. The more highly sloped lines show the movement of the concentration profile into the tissue by diffusion, with

the 12-hour line being the profile at the end of the infusion. At this time, all regions interior to 0.3 cm are exposed to concentrations that are one to several thousand-fold of that seen in the high-flow profile of Figure 9.14, and the penetration depth at 0.01 relative concentration is only 0.4 cm for low infusion vs 1.5 cm for high infusion. However, it is apparent in Figure 9.15 that the steep concentration profiles at the end of 12 hours of low-flow infusion lead to considerable additional penetration in the post-infusion phase, and the penetration depth at 0.01 relative concentration increases to nearly 0.9 cm by 3 days post-infusion. This raises the question of how much dose–response difference actually exists between the two delivery modes when total exposure time is considered.

Figure 9.16 answers this question for one particular dose–response metric. As discussed previously, the response of a tissue to a drug is often correlated with an *AUC* value in which the integrated concentration is the tissue concentration. In our example of non-binding macromolecular infusion, the tissue concentration is a strong function of the distance from the cannula tip. Hence, the relevant *AUC* is distance dependent and must be computed from an integral of the form presented in Equation 9.8 (with $r$ replacing the $x$ variable). Figure 9.16 shows this $AUC(r)$ function computed for both the low- and high-flow modes of infusion and plotted, not against $r$, but against the corresponding spherical volume $(4/3)\pi r^3$. All cells contained within this volume will have a response equal to or greater than the response at the surface of the volume corresponding to $AUC(r)$. From independent biological information, a particular response in

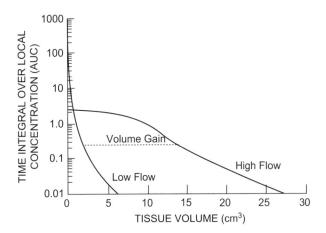

**FIGURE 9.16** Simulated area-under-the-curve [$AUC(r)$] as a function of the tissue volume [$(4/3)\pi r^3$] corresponding to radial position ($r$). Curves correspond to the high- and low-flow infusion rates of Figures 9.14 and 9.15. The dotted line denotes a particular value of $AUC$ corresponding to a particular response level ($AUC_o$). Reproduced from Morrison PF, Laske DW, Bobo RH *et al.* Am J Physiol 1994;266:R292–305 [21].

the target (e.g., a certain percentage of cell kill) is assumed to be identifiable with a particular $AUC$ value, $AUC_o$, shown as the dotted line in Figure 9.16. The infusate concentration would be selected so that the $AUC_o$ would lie sufficiently far below the uppermost value of the high-flow line to just assure response at a maximum desired target distance from the tip of the cannula. The difference in spherical volumes between the intersection of the $AUC_o$ line with the low- and high-flow lines may be interpreted as the gain in treatment volume of high-flow over low-flow infusion. This gain is 12 cm$^3$ for the $AUC_o$ shown, and ranges only between 9 and 20 cm$^3$ for $AUC_o$ selections over the two logs from 1 to 0.01. The conclusion from this analysis is that the post-infusional spreading seen with low-flow infusion is not sufficient to compensate for the large delivery volume advantage gained during the infusion phase of high-flow microinfusion.

Tissue treatment volumes of the substance being infused are a strong function of the tissue elimination half-life, which reflects the sum of both metabolic and microvascular tissue clearances. Table 9.2 summarizes how this treatment volume and associated penetration distance varies with the characteristic tissue

elimination half-life of the infused species. Various elimination half-lives were used for these simulations and an infusion rate of 3 μL/min into brain for 12 hours was assumed. For the extreme case of a macromolecule undergoing no metabolism, the treatment volume is 27 cm$^3$ with a penetration distance of 1.9 cm. For a more realistic tissue elimination half-life, as might be encountered with weakly binding monoclonal antibodies or stabilized analogs of somatostatin or enkephalin peptides, this volume and distance decline only to 14 cm$^3$ and 1.5 cm. When the elimination half-life drops to 1 hour, as is characteristic of the rates encountered with nerve growth factor or stabilized analogs of substance P peptide or glucocerebrosidase enzyme, the treatment volume drops to 2.7 cm$^3$, with a penetration distance of 0.9 cm. In a rapid metabolism situation, when the elimination half-life drops to just 10 minutes, as expected for substances such as native somatostatin, enkephalin, and substance P, the treatment volume diminishes to only 0.5 cm$^3$. However, the penetration distance is still 0.5 cm and still in excess of the penetration distances encountered with modes of delivery that depend on diffusional transport across tissue interfaces. Finally, it should be noted that these penetration distances, computed here for a volumetric infusion rate of 3 μL/min, will drop with decreases in the flow rate only as the cube root of the reduction factor (*cf.* Equation 9.24). For example, there will be only a 30% decrease in penetration distance for a three-fold drop in flow rate to 1 μL/min.

### Case Study 3: Chemopallidectomy in Patients with Parkinson's Disease Using Direct Interstitial Infusion

Direct interstitial infusion has been applied to the treatment of patients with advanced Parkinson's disease, and the design of the protocol is instructive [29]. Motor control is severely compromised in these patients because degradation of the substantia nigra ultimately results in massive over-inhibition of the motor cortex by the globus pallidus interna (Gpi). One therapeutic approach is to thermally ablate a portion of the Gpi to reduce this inhibition and restore freedom of movement. However, thermal ablation also risks destroying the optic nerve that forms the floor of the Gpi structure. Hence, a chemical means of destroying the Gpi has been evaluated as a potentially more selective alternative.

Controlled chemical destruction of the Gpi is possible using direct interstitial infusion of the excitotoxin quinolinic acid (pyridine dicarboxylate, MW 167 Da). The property of quinolinic acid that makes it attractive for this purpose is its ability to selectively

**TABLE 9.2    Tissue Treatment Volume as a Function of Tissue Elimination Half-life**

| Tissue elimination half-life[a] | Infinity | 33.5 h | 1.0 h | 0.17 h |
|---|---|---|---|---|
| Treatment volume (cm$^3$) | 27 | 14 | 2.7 | 0.49 |
| Penetration distance (cm) | 1.9 | 1.5 | 0.9 | 0.49 |

[a]Equal to $(\ln 2)/k$.

bind to and kill neurons that express the *N*-methyl-D-aspartate (NMDA) receptor but not the myelinated receptor-free fibers forming the optic nerve. Use of this compound does, however, pose a potential toxic risk to other basal ganglia surrounding the Gpi since these other structures are populated with NMDA-expressing cells. Thus, the goal is to devise a quinolinic acid delivery procedure that targets just the Gpi while sparing its nearest neighbor, the globus pallidus externa (GPe), and other nearby ganglia.

Development of an administration protocol began with identifying the toxic threshold concentration for quinolinic acid as 1.8 mM. This was based on literature data describing neuronal cell kill in the hippocampus [30] and the assumption that an excitotoxin's toxic response is more determined by whether its concentration exceeds a threshold concentration than by an *AUC* measure. The target volume was taken as the largest inscribed sphere that would fit inside the Gpi. A conservative inflow rate of 0.1 µl/min was chosen to avoid any possibility of infusate leak back along the infusion cannula. A 50-minute infusion time was chosen, partly on the basis of its being the longest time easily maintained in surgery and partly because the associated delivery volume of 5 µL would suffice to initially fill the interstitial fluid volume of the inscribed sphere. The infusate concentration was then determined from theory using published transport parameters [29, 31]. The complete diffusion–convection model of Equation 9.20 was solved numerically for various infusion times. This theoretical analysis was necessary to account for both convection and the substantial diffusion that results from the small molecular weight of this agent and the relatively low infusion rate. The results are expressed as the solid lines in Figure 9.17, which show tissue concentration relative to the infusate concentration. Post-infusional changes were computed using Equation 9.25, and these results are shown in the figure as the dashed lines. In this example, it is apparent that diffusion occurring after termination of infusion has little effect on extending the volume of distribution, principally because so much diffusive transport is involved even during the infusion. The horizontal line at 0.036 is the relative concentration that at the end of the 50-minute infusion is just met at the radius of the inscribed sphere ($r = 1.5$ mm), and is equivalent to the relative toxic threshold concentration – that is, $0.036 = C_{threshold}/C_{inf}$. Using the $C_{threshold}$ of 1.8 mM, the infusate concentration $C_{inf}$ is found to be 50 mM.

Figure 9.18 shows that the 5-µL infusion volume indeed provided localized dosing of the Gpi alone when biotinylated albumin was infused. The results of a 5-µL infusion of 50-mM quinolinic acid on the Gpi of

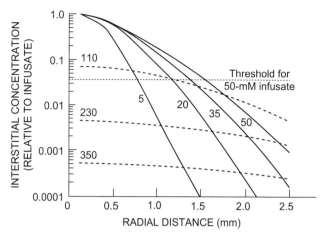

**FIGURE 9.17** Relative interstitial concentration of quinolinic acid computed for a 5-µL infusion at 0.1 µL/min of an isotonic 50-mM solution in CSF into the globus pallidus interna of a primate (50-minute infusion time). The horizontal dotted line represents the threshold concentration in relative units. Solid curved lines denote profiles generated at the indicated times (minutes) during the infusion; dashed curved lines denote the profiles during the post-infusion period, where the numbers are minutes after the initiation of infusion. Reproduced from Lonser RR, Corthesy ME, Morrison PF *et al.* J Neurosurg 1999;91:294–302 [29].

hemi-parkinsonized primates are shown in Figure 9.19. The top panel shows the histology of the Gpi tissue on the infused side of the brain, and the bottom panel B shows the histology of the non-infused, control side. It is apparent that the large neuronal nuclei seen in the

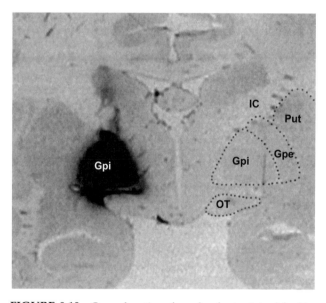

**FIGURE 9.18** Coronal section of monkey brain stained for biotinylated albumin immediately after infusion of 5 µL at 0.1 µL/min. Gpi = globus pallidus interna, Gpe = globus pallidus externa, OT = optic tract, Put = putamen, IC = internal capsule. Reproduced from Lonser RR, Corthesy ME, Morrison PF *et al.* J Neurosurg 1999;91:294–302 [29].

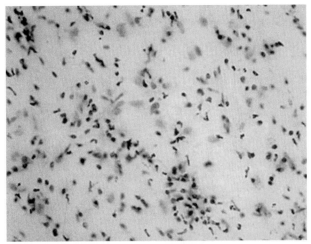

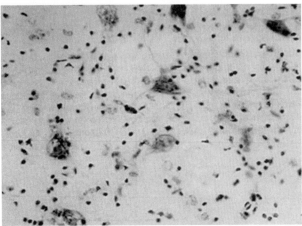

**FIGURE 9.19** Photomicrographs of tissue obtained from the globus pallidus interna (Gpi) of a parkinsonian primate. There is complete neuronal ablation and minimal gliosis in the infused Gpi (Panel A) relative to the unlesioned control side (Panel B). Reproduced from Lonser RR, Corthesy ME, Morrison PF *et al.* J Neurosurg 1999;91:294–302 [29].

control section are virtually absent in the section from the infused side. The selectivity of Gpi targeting was confirmed by quantifying the number of nuclei in nearby gray-matter structures. It was found that 87% of the neurons within the Gpi were destroyed, while less than 10% in the Gpe, 4% in the thalamus, 1% in the subthalamus, and 0% in the hippocampus were destroyed. In addition, no toxic changes were observed in the optic tract. Clinically, the treatment resulted in a stable and pronounced improvement in the principal measures of parkinsonism, including rigidity, tremor, bradykinesia, and gross motor skills.

## SUMMARY

The general principles underlying distributed kinetic models of drug delivery by transfer across tissue interfaces (intraperitoneal and intraventricular delivery) and by direct interstitial infusion (low- and high-flow microinfusion) have been presented and exemplified for both small and large molecular weight substances. Formulas have been provided to assess the concentration profiles that are likely to be obtained in tissue with these delivery methods, including rough estimators of penetration depth and time to achieve steady-state penetration. Rules for obtaining needed parameters by scaling from reference values also have been provided.

Many other applications of distributed drug kinetics exist, including the spatial and time dependence of drug delivery by microdialysis [2, 31–34], by the two-step delivery of targeting toxic moieties to tumors [35, 36], by the percolation of tightly binding antibodies into the intervascular spaces of tissue [1, 37, 38], and by direct interstitial infusion into the spinal cord [39, 40] and peripheral nerves [41]. Recently developed direct interstitial infusion models go beyond simple geometric and homogeneous assumptions and include three-dimensional effects within the central nervous system. These new models account for realistic anatomical boundaries, differences in drug transport and kinetic properties between tissue regions, structural tissue effects such as transport in preferred directions (anisotropy), and the effects of alternative cannula tip configurations. These approaches entail the development of three-dimensional models of the brain and spinal cord from magnetic resonance imaging data and the solution of their corresponding mass transport equations by finite element or computational fluid dynamic methods. As an example of an integrated finite element formalism, Sarntinoranont *et al.* [42–44] developed a mathematical model that optimizes the spinal cord delivery of substance P-associated protein toxins for the treatment of chronic pain by accounting for simple fiber-associated anisotropic transport, realistic gray-white anatomical boundaries, receptor binding and uptake, metabolism, and dose response. Other computational studies have incorporated the fibrous structure of the brain by using diffusion tensor imaging (DTI), an MRI technique that provides a highly detailed way to track axonal alignment in white matter by measuring the restricted diffusion of water in tissue [43, 45, 46]. These DTI-infusion models can account for directions of diffusion and fluid flow which vary from point to point within complex brain structures such as the hippocampus [45]. Other studies have investigated distributions from non-spherical cannula tips and multiple cannula configurations [47].

In addition, there are mechanical distribution issues during direct interstitial infusion that are associated with local tissue swelling and backflow along the cannula tract. Locally high pressures may result in expansion of the interstitial fluid space in the vicinity of the needle tip. Fluid–solid interaction (e.g., poroelastic) models have been combined with mass transport models to quantify local tissue expansion as well as the extent of the diversion of infusate backwards along the cannula surface [48–51]. The formulations of the biological and physical phenomena involved in these cases are necessarily somewhat different from those presented in our earlier examples. Nonetheless, the general concepts of drug delivery presented in this chapter still apply and serve as a starting point for analysis of these more complex systems.

## REFERENCES

[1] Fujimori K, Covell DG, Fletcher JE, Weinstein JN. A modeling analysis of monoclonal antibody percolation through tumors; A binding site barrier. J Nucl Med 1990;31:1191–8.

[2] Morrison PF, Bungay PM, Hsiao JK, Mefford IN, Dykstra KH, Dedrick RL. Quantitative microdialysis. In: Robinson TE, Justice Jr JB, editors. Microdialysis in the neurosciences. Amsterdam: Elsevier; 1991. p. 47–80.

[3] Crank J. The mathematics of diffusion. 2nd ed. Oxford: Oxford University Press; 1975.

[4] Patlak CS, Fenstermacher JD. Measurements of dog blood–brain transfer constants by ventriculocisternal perfusion. Am J Physiol 1975;229:877–84.

[5] Rapoport SI, Ohno K, Pettigrew KD. Drug entry into the brain. Brain Res 1979;172:354–9.

[6] Dedrick RL, Flessner MF. Pharmacokinetic considerations on monoclonal antibodies. Prog Clin Biol Res 1989;288:429–38.

[7] Alberts DS, Liu PY, Hannigan EV, O'Toole R, Williams SD, Young JA, et al. Intraperitoneal cisplatin plus intravenous cyclophosphamide versus intravenous cisplatin plus intravenous cyclophosphamide for stage III ovarian cancer. N Engl J Med 1996;335:1950–5.

[8] Dedrick RL, Myers CE, Bungay PM, DeVita VT. Pharmacokinetic rationale for peritoneal drug administration in the treatment of ovarian cancer. Cancer Treat Rep 1978;62:1–11.

[9] Flessner MF, Fenstermacher JD, Dedrick RL, Blasberg RG. A distributed model of peritoneal-plasma transport: Tissue concentration gradients. Am J Physiol 1985;248:F425–35.

[10] Los G, Mutsaers PHA, van der Vijgh WJF, Baldew GS, de Graaf PW, McVie JG. Direct diffusion of cis-diamminedichloroplatinum(II) in intraperitoneal rat tumors after intraperitoneal chemotherapy: A comparison with systemic chemotherapy. Cancer Res 1989;49:3380–4.

[11] Pardridge WM, Oldendorf WH, Cancilla P, Frank HJ. Blood–brain barrier: Interface between internal medicine and the brain. Ann Intern Med 1986;105:82–95.

[12] Hou J, Major EO. The efficacy of nucleoside analogs against JC virus multiplication in a persistently infected human fetal brain cell line. J Neurovirol 1998;4:451–6.

[13] Hall CD, Dafni U, Simpson D, Clifford D, Wetherill PE, Cohen B, et al. Failure of cytarabine in progressive multifocal leukoencephalopathy associated with human immunodeficiency virus infection. N Engl J Med 1998;338:1345–51.

[14] Zimm S, Collins JM, Miser J, Chatterji D, Poplack DG. Cytosine arabinoside cereberospinal fluid kinetics. Clin Pharmacol Ther 1984;35:826–30.

[15] Groothuis DR, Ward S, Itskovich AC, Dobrescu C, Allen CV, Dills C, et al. Comparison of $^{14}$C-sucrose delivery to the brain by intravenous, intraventricular, and convection-enhanced intracerebral infusion. J Neurosurg 1999;90:321–31.

[16] Fenstermacher JD. Pharmacology of the blood–brain barrier. In: Neuwelt EA, editor. Implications of the blood–brain barrier and its manipulation, vol 1. New York, NY: Plenum Press; 1989. p. 137–55.

[17] Groothuis DR, Benalcazar H, Allen CV, Wise RM, Dills C, Dobrescu C, et al. Comparison of cytosine arabinoside delivery to rat brain by intravenous, intrathecal, intraventricular and intraparenchymal routes of administration. Brain Res 2000;856:281–90.

[18] Tao L, Nicholson C. Diffusion of albumins in rat cortical slices and relevance to volume transmission. Neuroscience 1996;75:839–47.

[19] Yan Q, Matheson C, Sun J, Radeke MJ, Feinstein SC, Miller JA. Distribution of intracerebral ventricularly administered neurotrophins in rat brain and its correlation with trk receptor expression. Exp Neurol 1994;27:23–36.

[20] Krewson CE, Klarman ML, Saltzman WM. Distribution of nerve growth factor following direct delivery to brain interstitium. Brain Res 1995;680:196–206.

[21] Morrison PF, Laske DW, Bobo RH, Oldfield EH, Dedrick RL. High-flow microinfusion: Tissue penetration and pharmacodynamics. Am J Physiol 1994;266:R292–305.

[22] Bobo RH, Laske DW, Akbasak A, Morrison PF, Dedrick RL, Oldfield EH. Convection-enhanced delivery of macromolecules in the brain. Proc Natl Acad Sci USA 1994;91:2076–80.

[23] Morrison PF, Dedrick RL. Transport of cisplatin in rat brain following microinfusion: An analysis. J Pharm Sci 1986;75:120–9.

[24] Blasberg RG, Nakagawa H, Bourdon MA, Groothuis DR, Patlak CS, Bigner DD. Regional localization of a glioma-associated antigen defined by monoclonal antibody 81C6 in vivo: Kinetics and implications for diagnosis and therapy. Cancer Res 1987;47:4432–43.

[25] Bradbury M. The concept of a blood–brain barrier. New York, NY: John Wiley; 1979.

[26] Chen MY, Lonser RR, Morrison PF, Governale LS, Oldfield EH. Variables affecting convection-enhanced delivery to the striatum: A systematic examination of rate of infusion, cannula size, infusate concentration, and tissue-cannula sealing time. J Neurosurg 1999;90:315–20.

[27] Laske DW, Morrison PF, Lieberman DM, Corthesy ME, Reynolds JC, Stewart-Henney PA, et al. Chronic interstitial infusion of protein to primate brain: Determination of drug distribution and clearance with SPECT imaging. J Neurosurg 1997;87:586–94.

[28] Carslaw HS, Jaeger JC. Conduction of heat in solids. 2nd ed. Oxford: Oxford University Press; 1959.

[29] Lonser RR, Corthesy ME, Morrison PF, Gogate N, Oldfield EH. Convective-enhanced selective excitotoxic ablation of the neurons of the globus pallidus interna for treatment of primate parkinsonism. J Neurosurg 1999;91:294–302.

[30] Vezzani A, Forloni GL, Serafini R, Rizzi M, Samanin R. Neurodegenerative effects induced by chronic infusion of quinolinic acid in rat striatum and hippocampus. Eur J. Neurosci 1991;3:40–6.

[31] Beagles KE, Morrison PF, Heyes MP. Quinolinic acid in vivo synthesis rates, extracellular concentrations, and intercompartmental distributions in normal and immune activated brain as determined by multiple isotope microdialysis. J Neurochem 1998;70:281–91.

[32] Bungay PM, Morrison PF, Dedrick RL. Steady-state theory for quantitative microdialysis of solutes and water in vivo and in vitro. Life Sci 1990;46:105–19.

[33] Morrison PF, Bungay PM, Hsiao JK, Ball BA, Mefford IN, Dedrick RL. Quantitative microdialysis: Analysis of transients and application to pharmacokinetics in brain. J Neurochem 1991;57:103–19.

[34] Morrison PF, Morishige GM, Beagles KE, Heyes MP. Quinolinic acid is extruded from the brain by a probenecid-sensitive carrier system. J Neurochem 1999;72:2135–44.

[35] van Osdol WW, Sung CS, Dedrick RL, Weinstein JN. A distributed pharmacokinetic model of two-step imaging and treatment protocols: Application to streptavidin conjugated monoclonal antibodies and radiolabeled biotin. J Nucl Med 1993;34:1552–64.

[36] Sung CS, van Osdol WW, Saga T, Neumann RD, Dedrick RL, Weinstein JN. Streptavidin distribution in metastatic tumors pretargeted with a biotinylated monoclonal antibody: Theoretical and experimental pharmacokinetics. Cancer Res 1994;54:2166–75.

[37] Juweid M, Neumann R, Paik C, Perez-Bacete J, Sato J, van Osdol WW, et al. Micropharmacology of monoclonal antibodies in solid tumors: Direct experimental evidence for a binding site barrier. Cancer Res 1992;54:5144–53.

[38] Baxter LT, Yuan F, Jain RK. Pharmacokinetic analysis of the perivascular distribution of bifunctional antibodies and haptens: Comparison with experimental data. Cancer Res 1992;52:5838–44.

[39] Lonser RR, Gogate N, Wood JD, Morrison PF, Oldfield EH. Direct convective delivery of macromolecules to the spinal cord. J Neurosurg 1998;9:616–22.

[40] Wood JD, Lonser RR, Gogate N, Morrison PF, Oldfield EH. Convective delivery of macromolecules in to the naïve and traumatized spinal cords of rats. J Neurosurg 1999;90:115–20.

[41] Lonser RR, Weil RJ, Morrison PF, Governale LS, Oldfield EH. Direct convective delivery of macromolecules to peripheral nerves. J Neurosurg 1998;89:610–5.

[42] Sarntinoranont M, Banerjee RK, Lonser RR, Morrison PF. A computational model of direct interstitial infusion of macromolecules into the spinal cord. Ann Biomed Eng 2003;31:448–61.

[43] Sarntinoranont M, Chen XM, Zhao JB, Mareci TH. Computational model of interstitial transport in the spinal cord using diffusion tensor imaging. Ann Biomed Eng 2006;34:1304–21.

[44] Sarntinoranont M, Iadarola MJ, Lonser RR, Morrison PF. Direct interstitial infusion of NK1 targeted neurotoxin into the spinal cord: A computational model. Am J Physiol 2003;285:R243–54.

[45] Kim JH, Astary GW, Chen XM, Mareci TH, Sarntinoranont M. Voxelized model of interstitial transport in the rat spinal cord following direct infusion into white matter. J Biomech Eng 2009;131. 071007.

[46] Linninger AA, Somayaji MR, Erickson T, Guo XD, Penn RD. Computational methods for predicting drug transport in anisotropic and heterogeneous brain tissue. J Biomech Eng 2008;41:2176–87.

[47] Motion JPM, Huynh GH, Szoka FC, Siegel RA. Convection and retro-convection enhanced delivery: Some theoretical considerations related to drug targeting. Pharm Res 2011;28:472–9.

[48] Chen XM, Sarntinoranont M. Biphasic finite element model of solute transport for direct infusion into nervous tissue. Ann Biomed Eng 2007;35:2145–58.

[49] Morrison PF, Chen MY, Chadwick RS, Lonser RR, Oldfield EH. Focal delivery during direct infusion to brain: Role of flow rate, catheter diameter, and tissue mechanics. Am J Physiol 1999;277:R1218–29 (Corrigendum 2002;282:U4.).

[50] Raghavan R, Mikaelian S, Brady M, Chen ZJ. Fluid infusions from catheters into elastic tissue: I. Azimuthally symmetric backflow in homogeneous media. Phys Med Biol 2010;55:281–304.

[51] Smith JH, Garcia JJ. A nonlinear biphasic model of flow-controlled infusions in brain: Mass transport analyses. J Biomech 2011;44:524–31.

# 10

# Population Pharmacokinetics

**Raymond Miller**

*Modeling and Simulation, Daiichi Sankyo Pharma Development, Edison, NJ 08837*

## INTRODUCTION

The aim of pharmacokinetic modeling is to define mathematical models to describe and quantify drug behavior in individuals. The development of a successful pharmacokinetic model allows one to summarize large amounts of data into a few values that describe the whole data set. The general procedure used to develop a pharmacokinetic model is outlined in Table 10.1. Certain aspects of this procedure have also been described in Chapters 3 and 8. For example, the technique of "curve peeling" frequently is used to indicate the number of compartments that are included in a compartmental model. In any event, the eventual outcome should be a model that can be used to interpolate or extrapolate to other conditions. Pharmacokinetic studies in patients have led to the appreciation of the large degree of variability in pharmacokinetic

parameter estimates that exists across patients. Many studies have quantified the effects of factors such as age, gender, disease states, and concomitant drug therapy on the pharmacokinetics of drugs, with the purpose of accounting for the interindividual variability. Finding a population model that adequately describes the data may have important clinical benefits in that the dose regimen for a specific patient may need to be individualized based on relevant physiological information. This is particularly important for drugs with a narrow therapeutic range.

Population pharmacokinetic analysis can be thought of as an extension of the modeling procedures described in previous chapters, and can be defined as the study of the variability in plasma drug concentrations between individuals when a standard dosage regimen is administered. The purpose of population pharmacokinetic analysis is summarized in Table 10.2. This definition in fact describes the procedure that has been in place for many years; however, the term has more recently been associated with the population pharmacokinetic analysis of sparse data obtained in late-stage clinical trials. The reason for this is that it has become clear that the pharmacokinetics of a drug needs to be defined in those individuals who are likely

### TABLE 10.1 Steps in Developing a Pharmacokinetic Model

| Step | Activity |
|------|----------|
| 1. | Design an experiment |
| 2. | Collect the data |
| 3. | Develop a model based on the observed characteristics of the data |
| 4. | Express the model mathematically |
| 5. | Analyze the data in terms of the model |
| 6. | Evaluate the fit of the data to the model |
| 7. | If necessary, revise the model in Step 3 to eliminate inconsistencies in the data fit and repeat the process until the model provides a satisfactory description of the data |

### TABLE 10.2 The Purpose of Population Pharmacokinetic Analysis

Estimate the population mean of parameters of interest

Identify and investigate sources of variability that influence drug pharmacokinetics

Estimate the magnitude of intersubject variability

Estimate the random residual variability

*PRINCIPLES OF CLINICAL PHARMACOLOGY, THIRD EDITION*
DOI: http://dx.doi.org/10.1016/B978-0-12-385471-1.00010-6

**139**

to receive the drug. Therefore, the traditional procedure, which involves the determination of each individual's pharmacokinetic parameters, is not feasible under these clinical trial conditions. Although the term "population pharmacokinetics" has come to be associated with the analysis of pharmacokinetic studies involving sparse data, this approach can be applied equally well to conventional pharmacokinetic studies.

## ANALYSIS OF PHARMACOKINETIC DATA

### Structure of Pharmacokinetic Models

As discussed in Chapters 3 and 8, it is often found that the relationship between drug concentrations and time may be described by a sum of exponential terms. This lends itself to compartmental pharmacokinetic analysis in which the pharmacokinetics of a drug is characterized by representing the body as a system of well-stirred compartments with the rates of transfer between compartments following first-order kinetics. The required number of compartments is equal to the number of exponents in the sum of exponentials equation that best fits the data. In the case of a drug that seems to be distributed homogeneously in the body a one-compartment model is appropriate, and this relationship can be described in a single individual by the following monoexponential equation:

$$A = \text{Dose} \cdot e^{-kt} \qquad (10.1)$$

This equation describes the typical time course of amount of drug in the body ($A$) as a function of initial dose, time ($t$), and the first-order elimination rate constant ($k$). As described in Equation 2.14, this rate constant equals the ratio of the elimination clearance ($CL_E$) relative to the distribution volume of the drug ($V_d$), so that Equation 10.1 can then be expressed in terms of concentration in plasma ($C_p$).

$$C_p = \frac{\text{Dose}}{V_d} \cdot e^{-\frac{CL_E}{V_d} \cdot t} \qquad (10.2)$$

Therefore, if one has an estimate of clearance and volume of distribution, the plasma concentration can be predicted at different times after administration of any selected dose. The quantities that are known because they are either measured or controlled, such as dose and time, are called "fixed effects", in contrast to effects that are not known and are regarded as random. The parameters $CL_E$ and $V_d$ are called fixed-effect parameters because they quantify the influence of the fixed effects on the dependent variable, $C_p$.

### Fitting Individual Data

Assuming that we have measured a series of concentrations over time, we can define a model structure and obtain initial estimates of the model parameters. The objective is to determine an estimate of the parameters ($Cl_E$, $V_d$) such that the differences between the observed and predicted concentrations are comparatively small. Three of the most commonly used criteria for obtaining a best fit of the model to the data are ordinary least squares (OLS), weighted least squares (WLS), and extended least squares (ELS), which is a maximum likelihood procedure. These criteria are achieved by minimizing the following quantities, which are often called the objective function ($O$).

Ordinary least squares (OLS) (where $\hat{C}_i$ denotes the predicted value of $C_i$ based on the model):

$$O_{OLS} = \sum_{i=1}^{n} (C_i - \hat{C}_i)^2 \qquad (10.3)$$

Weighted least squares (WLS) (where $W$ is typically 1/ the observed concentration):

$$O_{WLS} = \sum_{i=1}^{n} W_i (C_i - \hat{C}_i)^2 \qquad (10.4)$$

Extended least squares (ELS):

$$O_{ELS} = \sum_{i=1}^{n} [W_i (C_i - \hat{C}_i)^2 + \ln \text{ var}(\hat{C}_i)] \qquad (10.5)$$

The correct criterion for best fit depends upon the assumption underlying the functional form of the variances (var) of the dependent variable $C$. The model that fits the data from an individual minimizes the differences between the observed and the model predicted concentrations (Figure 10.1). What one observes is a measured value which differs from the model-predicted value by some amount called a residual error (also called intrasubject error or within-subject error). There are many reasons why the actual observation may not correspond to the predicted value. The structural model may only be approximate, or the plasma concentrations may have been measured with error. It is too difficult to model all the sources of error separately, so the simplifying assumption is made that each difference between an observation and its prediction is random. When the data are from an

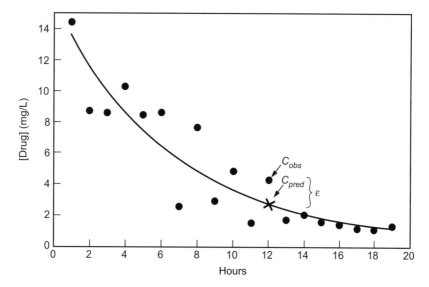

**FIGURE 10.1**   Fit obtained using a one-compartment model (see Equation 10.6) to fit plasma concentration vs time data observed following intravenous bolus administration of a drug: $C_{obs}$ designates the actual measured concentrations and $C_{pred}$ represents the concentrations predicted by the pharmacokinetic model. Adapted from Grasela TH Jr, Sheiner LB. J Pharmacokinet Biopharm 1991;19(Suppl):25S–36S [5].

individual, and the error model is the additive error model, the error is denoted by ε.

$$C = \frac{\text{Dose}}{V_d} \cdot e^{-\frac{CL_E}{V_d} \cdot t} + \varepsilon \qquad (10.6)$$

## POPULATION PHARMACOKINETICS

Population pharmacokinetic parameters quantify population mean kinetics, between-subject variability (intersubject variability), and residual variability. Residual variability includes within-subject variability, model misspecification, and measurement error. This information is necessary to design a dosage regimen for a drug. If all patients were identical, the same dose would be appropriate for all. However, since patients vary, it may be necessary to individualize a dose depending on how large the between-subject variation is. For example, to choose an initial dose one needs to know the relationship between the administered dose and the concentration achieved, and thus the pharmacological response anticipated in a patient. This is the same as knowing the typical pharmacokinetics of individuals of similar sex, age, weight, and function of elimination organs. This information is available if one knows the fixed-effect pharmacokinetic parameters governing the relationship of the pharmacokinetics to sex, age, weight, renal function, liver function, and so on. Large, unexplained

variability in pharmacokinetics in an apparently homogeneous population can lead to an investigation as to the reason for the discrepancy, which in turn may lead to an increased understanding of fundamental principles.

### Population Analysis Methods

Assume an experiment in which a group of subjects selected to represent a spectrum of severity of some condition (e.g., renal insufficiency) is given a dose of drug and drug concentrations are measured in blood samples collected at intervals after dosing. The structural kinetic models used when performing a population analysis do not differ at all from those used for analysis of data from an individual patient. One still needs a model for the relationship of concentration to dose and time, and this relationship does not depend on whether the fixed-effect parameter changes from individual to individual or with time within an individual. The population pharmacokinetic parameters can be determined in a number of ways of which only a few are described in the following sections.

### *The Naïve Pooled Data Method*

If interest focuses entirely on the estimation of population parameters, then the simplest approach is to combine all the data as if they came from a single individual [1]. The doses may need to be normalized so that the data are comparable. Equation 10.6 would be applicable if an intravenous bolus dose were administered. The minimization procedure is similar to that described in Figure 10.1.

The advantages of this method are its simplicity and familiarity, and the fact that it can be used with sparse data and differing numbers of data points per individual. The disadvantages are that it is not possible to determine the fixed effect sources of interindividual variability, such as creatinine clearance ($CL_{CR}$). It also cannot distinguish between variability within and between individuals, and an imbalance between individuals results in biased parameter estimates.

Although pooling has the risk of masking individual behavior, it might still serve as a general guide to the mean pharmacokinetic parameters. If this method is used, it is recommended that a spaghetti plot be made to visually determine if any individual or group of individuals deviates from the central tendency with respect to absorption, distribution, or elimination.

### The Two-Stage Method

The two-stage method is so called because it proceeds in two steps [1]. The first step is to use OLS to estimate each individual patient's parameters, assuming a model such as Equation 10.6. The minimization procedure described in Figure 10.1 is repeated for each individual independently (Figure 10.2).

The next step is to estimate the population parameters across the subjects by calculating the mean of each parameter, its variance, and its covariance. The relationship between fixed-effect parameters and covariates of interest can be investigated by regression techniques. To investigate the relationship between drug clearance ($CL$) and creatinine clearance ($CL_{CR}$), one could try a variety of models depending on the shape of the relationship. As described in Chapter 5, a linear relationship often is applicable, such as that given by Equation 10.7 (Figure 10.3):

$$CL = INT + SLOPE \cdot CL_{CR} \qquad (10.7)$$

The intercept in this equation provides an estimate of non-renal clearance.

The advantages of this method are that it is easy and most investigators are familiar with it. Because parameters are estimated for each individual, these estimates have little or no bias. Pharmacokinetic–pharmacodynamic models can be applied since individual differences can be considered. Covariates can be included in the model. Disadvantages of the method are that variance–covariance of parameters across subjects is biased and contains elements of interindividual variability, intraindividual variability, assay error, time error, model misspecification, and variability from the individual parameter estimation process. In addition, the same

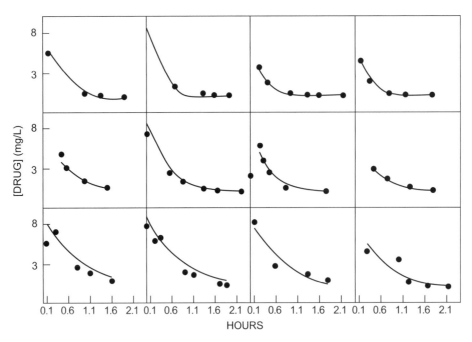

**FIGURE 10.2**  Fit obtained using a one-compartment model to fit plasma concentration vs time data observed following intravenous bolus administration of a drug. Each panel represents an individual subject.

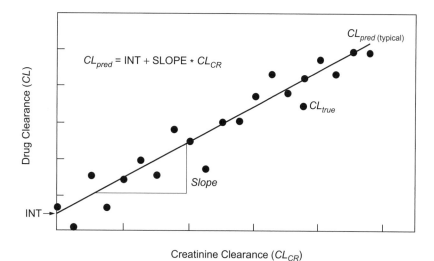

**FIGURE 10.3** Linear regression analysis of drug clearance ($CL$) vs creatinine clearance ($CL_{CR}$). Typical values of drug clearance are generated for an individual or group of individuals with a given creatinine clearance. The discrepancy between the true value for drug clearance ($CL_{true}$) and the typical value ($CL_{pred}$) necessitates the use of a statistical model for interindividual variability. INT denotes the intercept of the regression line. Adapted from Grasela TH Jr, Sheiner LB. J Pharmacokinet Biopharm 1991;19(Suppl):25S–36S [5].

structural model is required for all subjects, and numerous blood samples must be obtained at appropriate times to obtain accurate estimates for each individual subject.

### Non-Linear Mixed Effects Modeling Method

The non-linear mixed-effects method is depicted in Figure 10.4 and is described using the conventions of the NONMEM software [2, 3] and the description by Vozeh *et al.* [3]. It is based on the principle that the individual pharmacokinetic parameters of a patient population arise from a distribution that can be described by the population mean and the interindividual variance. Each individual pharmacokinetic parameter can be expressed as a population mean and a deviation, typical for that individual. The deviation is the difference between the population mean and the individual parameter and is assumed to be a random variable with an expected mean of zero and variance $\omega^2$. This variance describes the biological variability of the population. The clearance and volume of distribution for subject $j$ using the structural pharmacokinetic model described in Equation 10.6 are represented by the following equations:

$$C_{ij} = \frac{\text{Dose}}{V_{dj}} \cdot e^{\frac{CL_j}{V_{dj}} \cdot t_{ij}} + \varepsilon_{ij}$$

where

$$CL_j = \overline{CL} + \eta_j^{CL}$$

and

$$V_{dj} = \overline{V_d} + \eta_j^{V_d}$$

where $\overline{CL}$ and $\overline{V_d}$ are the population mean of the elimination clearance and volume of distribution, respectively, and $\eta^{CL}$ and $\eta_j^{V_d}$ are the differences between the population mean and the clearance ($CL_j$) and volume of distribution ($V_{dj}$) of subject $j$. These equations can be applied to subject $k$ by substituting a $k$ for $j$ in the equations, and so on for each subject. There are, however, two levels of random effects. The first level, described previously, is needed in the parameter model to help model unexplained interindividual differences in the parameters. The second level represents a random error ($\varepsilon_{ij}$), familiar from classical pharmacokinetic analysis, which expresses the deviation of the expected plasma concentration in subject $j$ from the measured value. Each $\varepsilon$ variable is assumed to have a mean zero and a variance denoted by $\sigma^2$. Each pair of elements in $\eta$ has a covariance which can be estimated. A covariance between two elements of $\eta$ is a measure of statistical association between these two random variables.

NONMEM is a one-stage analysis that simultaneously estimates mean parameters, fixed-effect parameters, interindividual variability, and residual

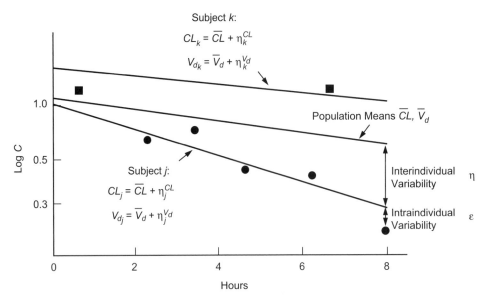

**FIGURE 10.4**   Graphical illustration of the statistical model used in NONMEM for the special case of a one-compartment model following intravenous bolus administration of a drug. ●, Subject j; ■, Subject k. Adapted from Vozeh S, Katz G, Steiner V, Follath F. Eur J Clin Pharmacol 1982;23:445–51 [3].

random effects. The fitting routine makes use of the ELS method. A global measure of goodness of fit is provided by the objective function value based on the final parameter estimates, which, in the case of NONMEM, is minus twice the log likelihood of the data [1]. Any improvement in the model would be reflected by a decrease in the objective function. The purpose of adding independent variables to the model, such as $CL_{CR}$ in Equation 10.7, is usually to explain kinetic differences between individuals. This means that such differences were not explained by the model prior to adding the variable and were part of random interindividual variability. Therefore, inclusion of additional variables in the model is warranted only if it is accompanied by a decrease in the estimates of the intersubject variance, and under certain circumstances intrasubject variance.

The advantages of the one-stage analysis are that interindividual variability of the parameters can be estimated, random residual error can be estimated, covariates can be included in the model, parameters for individuals can be estimated, and pharmacokinetic–pharmacodynamic models can be used. Since allowance can be made for individual differences, this method can be used with routine data, sparse data, and unbalanced number of data points per patient [4, 5]. The models are also much more flexible than when the other methods are used. For example, a number of studies can be pooled into one analysis while accounting for differences between study sites, and all fixed-effect covariate relationships and any

interindividual or residual error structure can be investigated.

Disadvantages arise mainly from the complexity of the statistical algorithms and the fact that fitting models to data is time consuming. The first-order method (FO) used in NONMEM also results in biased estimates of parameters, especially when the distribution of interindividual variability is specified incorrectly. The first-order conditional estimation procedure (FOCE) is more accurate, but is even more time consuming. The objective function and adequacy of the model are based in part on the residuals, which for NONMEM are determined from the predicted concentrations for the mean pharmacokinetic parameters rather than the predicted concentrations for each subject. Therefore, the residuals are confounded by intraindividual, interindividual, and linearization errors.

## MODEL APPLICATIONS

### Mixture Models

The first example is a study to evaluate the efficacy of drug treatment or placebo as add-on treatment in patients with partial seizures, and how this information can assist in formulating dosing guidelines. A mixed-effects model was used to characterize the relationship between monthly seizure frequency over 3 months and pregabalin daily dose (0, 50, 150, 300 and 600 mg) as add-on treatment in three double-blind, parallel group studies in patients with refractory partial seizures ($n = 1042$) [6]. A subject-specific random-effects model was used to characterize the relationship between seizure frequency and pregabalin dose in individual patients, taking into account placebo effect. Maximum likelihood estimates were obtained with use of the Laplacian estimation method implemented in the NONMEM program (version V 1.1) [2]. The response was modeled as a Poisson process with mean $\lambda$. The probability that the number of seizures per 28 days ($Y$) equals $x$ is given by the equation:

$$P(Y = x) = e^{-\lambda}\frac{\lambda^x}{x!}$$

The mean number of seizures per 28 days ($\lambda$) was modeled as a function of drug effect, placebo effect, and subject-specific random effects, based on the following relationship.

$$\lambda = \text{Base} \cdot (1 + f_d + f_p) \cdot e^{\eta}$$

where "Base" is the estimated number of seizures per 28 days reported in the baseline period before treatment. The functions $f_d$ and $f_p$ describe the drug effect and placebo effect, and $\eta$ is the subject-specific random effect.

The structural model that best described the response was an asymptotic decrease in seizure frequency from baseline, including a placebo effect (PLAC) in addition to the drug effect:

$$\lambda = \text{BASE} \cdot \left(1 - \frac{E_{\max} \cdot D}{ED_{50} + D} - \text{PLAC}\right) \cdot e^{\eta_1}$$

In this equation, $E_{\max}$ is the maximal fractional reduction in seizure frequency and $ED_{50}$ is the dose that produces a 50% decrease in seizure frequency from maximum. PLAC is the fractional change in seizure frequency from baseline after placebo treatment. Drug treatment was modeled as an $E_{\max}$ model (see Chapter 20) and placebo treatment was modeled as a constant. This model describes a dose-related reduction in seizure frequency with a maximum decrease in seizure frequency of 38%. Half that reduction ($ED_{50}$) was achieved with a dose of 48.7 mg/day. However, the $ED_{50}$ was not well estimated, since the symmetrical 95% confidence interval included zero. After placebo treatment the average increase in seizure frequency was 10% of baseline.

This analysis suggested that pregabalin reduces seizure frequency in a dose-dependent fashion. However, the results are questionable because of the variability in the prediction of $ED_{50}$. This may be due to the fact that some patients with partial seizures are refractory to any particular drug and would be non-responders at any dose. It would be sensible, then, to explore the dose–response relationship for this drug separately in those patients that are not refractory to pregabalin. Actually, it is only this information that is useful in adjusting dose (and setting therapeutic expectations) for those patients who will benefit from treatment. As is often the case, the clinical trials to evaluate this drug were not designed to first identify patients tractable to pregabalin treatment and then to study dose–response in only the subset of tractable patients. Thus, to obtain the dose–response relationship for this subset we would need to use the available trial data to first classify each patient (as either refractory or responsive), and then assess the degree of pregabalin anticonvulsant effect as a function of dose in the responders.

In order to justify this approach, it was necessary to evaluate if the patients in these studies represented a random sample from a population comprised of at least two subpopulations, one with one set of typical values for response and a second with another set of typical values for response. A mixture model describing such a population can be represented by the following equations.

Subpopulation A (proportion $= p$):

$$\lambda_1 = \text{BASE} \cdot \left(1 - \frac{E_{\max A} \cdot D}{ED_{50} + D} - \text{PLAC}\right) \cdot e^{\eta_1}$$

Subpopulation B (proportion $= 1 - p$):

$$\lambda_2 = \text{BASE} \cdot \left(1 - \frac{E_{\max B} \cdot D}{ED_{50} + D} - \text{PLAC}\right) \cdot e^{\eta_2}$$

Where:
BASE = baseline seizure frequency over 28 days
$E_{\max A}$ = maximal fractional change in baseline seizures due to drug treatment for subpopulation A
$E_{\max B}$ = maximal fractional change in baseline seizures due to drug treatment for subpopulation B
$ED_{50}$ = Daily dose that produces a 50% reduction in seizure frequency from maximum (mg/day)
PLAC = fractional change in seizure frequency from baseline due to placebo treatment
$p$ = proportion of subjects in subpopulation A (by default, $1 - p$ is the proportion in subpopulation B).
$\eta_1$ = intersubject random effect for Population A
$\eta_2$ = intersubject random effect for Population B
$\text{Var}(\eta_1) = \text{Var}(\eta_2) = \omega$

A mixture model implicitly assumes that some fraction ($p$) of the population has one set of typical values of response, and that the remaining fraction ($1 - p$) has another set of typical values. In this model, the only difference initially allowed in the typical values between the two groups was the maximal fractional reduction in seizure frequency after treatment with pregabalin, i.e. $E_{\max A}$ and $E_{\max B}$. Values for these two parameters and the mixing fraction $p$ were estimated. Random interindividual variability effects $\eta_1$ and $\eta_2$ were assumed to be normally distributed with zero means and common variance $\omega$. The estimation method assigns each individual to both subpopulations repeatedly and computes different likelihoods, depending on variables assigned to the subpopulations. This process is carried out for each individual patient record repeatedly as parameter values are varied. The fitting algorithm assigns individuals to the two categories, so that the final fit gives the most probable distribution of patients into the two subpopulations. Introducing the mixture model resulted in a significant improvement in the model fit.

In this case, the maximal response in the one subgroup (subpopulation B) tended towards zero, so the inclusion of an $ED_{50}$ estimate in this population appeared unwarranted. In the final model, the $ED_{50}$ parameter was dropped in this subpopulation so that treatment response in this subgroup defaulted to a constant with random variability that was independent of drug dose. Consequently, the calculated $ED_{50}$ value is representative of only those patients who fall into the subpopulation of pregabalin-responsive patients (subpopulation A), and a dose of approximately 186 mg daily is expected to decrease their seizure frequency by about 50% of baseline. Monte Carlo simulation was used together with the pharmacodynamic parameters and variance for subpopulation A to generate the relationship between expected reduction in seizure frequency and increasing pregabalin dose that is shown in Figure 10.5. Seizure frequency values were simulated for 11,000 individuals (50% female) at doses from 50 to 700 mg pregabalin daily. Exclusion of patients with a baseline value less than six seizures per 28 days to emulate the inclusion criteria for these studies resulted in a total of 8852 individuals of which 51% were female. The percent reduction from baseline seizure frequency was calculated for each individual simulated. Percentiles were determined for percent reduction in seizure frequency at each dose, and are presented in Figure 10.5. In patients who are likely to respond to pregabalin treatment, daily pregabalin doses of 150 mg, 300 mg, and 600 mg are expected to produce at least a 71%, 82%, and 90% reduction in seizure frequency, respectively, in 10% of this population. Similarly, with these doses, 50% of this population is

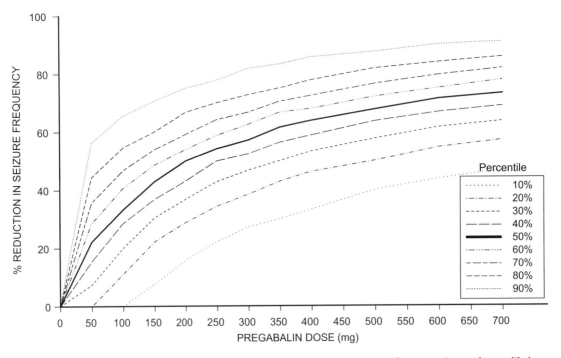

**FIGURE 10.5** Expected percent reduction in seizure frequency with increasing dose in patients who are likely to respond, expressed as percentiles. Adapted with permission from Miller R, Frame B, Corrigan B. Clin Pharmacol Ther 2003;73:491–505 [6].

expected to show a 43%, 57%, and 71% reduction in seizure frequency, respectively. These expectations serve as a useful dosing guide for a clinician when treating a patient.

## Exposure–Response Models

The second example involves the impact of population modeling of exposure–response data on the approval of an application to market a new drug by the US Food and Drug Administration (FDA). Usually, evidence of efficacy from two or more adequate and well-controlled clinical trials, along with safety information, is required for the regulatory approval of a new indication for a drug. The idea is that replication of the results of a single trial is needed to rule out the possibility that a finding of efficacy in a single trial is due to chance. This example describes the application of exposure–response analysis to establish an FDA-approvable claim of drug efficacy based on a dose–reponse relationship that was obtained from two pivotal clinical trials that used different final treatment doses.

Response data for two studies were submitted to the FDA for approval for the treatment of post-herpetic neuralgia (PHN). Both studies were randomized, double-blind, placebo-controlled multicenter studies that evaluated the safety and efficacy of gabapentin administered orally three times a day, compared with placebo. In both studies the patients were titrated to their final treatment dose by the end of either week 3 or 4, and then maintained on these doses for 4 weeks.

However, in one study the final treatment dose was 3600 mg/day, and in the other study, the patients were randomized to the final treatment doses of either 1800 mg/day or 2400 mg/day. The primary efficacy parameter was the daily pain score, as measured by the patient in a daily diary on an 11-point Likert scale with 0 equaling no pain and 10 equaling the worst possible pain. Each morning, the patient self-evaluated pain for the previous day. The dataset consisted of 27,678 observations collected from 554 patients, of which 226 received placebo and 328 received treatment approximately evenly distributed over the three doses. Daily pain scores were collected as integral, ordinal values, and the change from baseline pain score was treated as a continuous variable. The mean of the most recent available pain scores observed during the baseline study phase was used for each patient's baseline score. The individual daily pain score was modeled as change from baseline minus effect of drug and placebo:

Daily Change From Baseline Pain Score

$$= -(\text{Placebo} + \eta) - (\text{Gabapentin Effect} + \eta) + \varepsilon$$

where $\varepsilon$ is the residual variability and $\eta$ is the inter-individual variability.

The placebo effect was described using a model made up of two components, an immediate-effect component and an asymptotic time-dependent component, as described in Chapter 22. The gabapentin effect was described by an $E_{max}$ model using the daily dose corrected for estimated bioavailability. Observed and predicted mean population responses

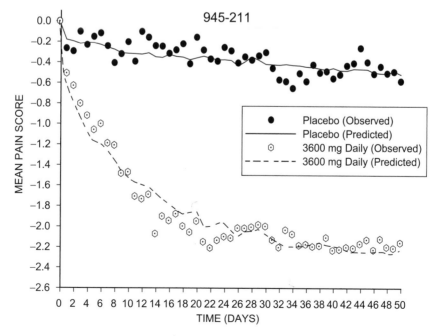

**FIGURE 10.6**   Change in pain score from baseline over time for Study 945-211.

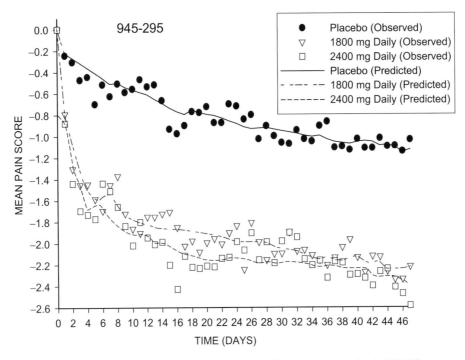

**FIGURE 10.7**   Change in pain score from baseline over time for Study 945-295.

are described in Figures 10.6 and 10.7. The advantage of the population approach is that all the data were included in the analysis, allowing valuable information to be captured, such as time of onset of drug response relative to placebo response, as well as intraindividual dose response. The exposure–response model served as a useful tool for integrating information about the characteristics of the drug over the time course of the study.

This analysis also provided the FDA with a clear understanding of the underlying nature of the gabapentin dose–response relationship to help with their decision-making. Because patients in Study 1 were randomized to a final dose of 3600 mg/day and patients in Study 2 were randomized to either 1800 mg/day or 2400 mg/day, replicate data confirming the efficacy of gabapentin at these doses were not available. This presented a challenging regulatory obstacle to approving gabapentin for the PHN treatment indication. However, to further explore the underlying dose–response relationship, the FDA did their own analysis of the data: an initial summary statistical analysis to compare the observed clinical pain score at various levels or days after starting therapy, followed by a modeling and simulation analysis to check the concordance across the different studies. The use of this pharmacokinetic–pharmacodynamic information confirmed evidence of efficacy across the three studied doses to the satisfaction of the FDA review staff, and the clinical trials section of the package insert

for gabapentin describes Studies 1 and 2 and further states "Pharmacokinetic–pharmacodynamic modeling provided confirmatory evidence of efficacy across all doses" to explain the basis for establishing the effectiveness of this drug for the PHN indication [7].

## CONCLUSIONS

Population pharmacokinetics describes the typical relationships between physiology and pharmacokinetics, the interindividual variability in these relationships, and their residual intraindividual variability. Knowledge of population kinetics can help one choose initial drug dosage, modify dosage appropriately in response to observed drug levels, make rational decisions regarding certain aspects of drug regulation, and elucidate certain research questions in pharmacokinetics. Patients with the disease for which the drug is intended are probably a better source of pharmacokinetic data than are healthy subjects. However, this type of data is contaminated by varying quality, accuracy, and precision, as well as by the fact that generally only sparse data are collected from each patient.

Although population pharmacokinetic parameters have been estimated either by fitting all individuals' data together as if there were no kinetic differences, or by fitting each individual's data separately and then combining the individual parameter estimates, these methods have certain theoretical problems which can only be aggravated when the deficiencies of typical clinical data are present. The non-linear mixed-effect analysis avoids many of these deficiencies and provides a flexible means of estimating population pharmacokinetic parameters.

# REFERENCES

[1] Sheiner LB. The population approach to pharmacokinetic data analysis: Rationale and standard data analysis methods. Drug Met Rev 1984;15:153–71.

[2] Beal SL, Sheiner LB. NONMEM user's guides, NONMEM Project Group. San Francisco, CA: University of California; 1989.

[3] Vozeh S, Katz G, Steiner V, Follath F. Population pharmacokinetic parameters in patients treated with oral mexiletine. Eur J Clin Pharmacol 1982;23:445–51.

[4] Sheiner LB, Rosenberg B, Marathe VV. Estimation of population characteristics of pharmacokinetics parameters from routine clinical data. J Pharmacokinet Biopharm 1997;5:445–79.

[5] Grasela TH Jr, Sheiner LB. Pharmacostatistical modeling for observational data. J Pharmacokin Biopharm 1991;19(Suppl):25S–36S.

[6] Miller R, Frame B, Corrigan B, Burger P, Bockbrader H, Garofalo E, et al. Exposure–response analysis of pregabalin add-on treatment of patients with refractory partial seizures. Clin Pharmacol Ther 2003;73:491–505.

[7] Physician's Desk Reference. 59th ed. Montvale, NJ: Medical Economics; 2005.

## Suggested Additional Reading

Beal SL, Sheiner LB. Estimating population kinetics. CRC Crit Rev Biomed Eng 1982;8:195–222.

Ludden TM. Population pharmacokinetics. J Clin Pharmacol 1988;28:1059–63.

Samara E, Grannenman R. Role of population pharmacokinetics in drug development. Clin Pharmacokinet 1997;32:294–312.

Sheiner LB, Ludden TM. Population pharmacokinetics/dynamics. Annu Rev Pharmacol Toxicol 1992;32:185–209.

Whiting B, Kelman AW, Grevel J. Population pharmacokinetics: Theory and clinical application. Clin Pharmacokinet 1986;11:387–401.

Yuh L, Beal SL, Davidian M, Harrison F, Hester A, Kowalski K, et al. Population pharmacokinetic/pharmacodynamic methodology and applications. A bibliography. Biometrics 1994;50:566–75.

# DRUG METABOLISM AND TRANSPORT

# 11

# Pathways of Drug Metabolism

**Sanford P. Markey**

*Laboratory of Neurotoxicology, National Institute of Mental Health, National Institutes of Health, Bethesda, MD 20892*

## INTRODUCTION

Most drugs are chemically modified or metabolized in the body. The biochemical processes governing drug metabolism largely determine the duration of a drug's action, elimination, and toxicity. The degree to which these processes can be controlled to produce beneficial medical results relies on multiple variables that have been the subject of considerable study, best illustrated by examining several representative drugs. Drug metabolism may render an administered active compound inactive, or activate an inactive precursor, or produce a toxic by-product.

Phenobarbital typifies drugs that are active when administered and then converted to inactive and more polar metabolites in the liver, as shown in Scheme 11.1A. When phenobarbital is hydroxylated, it becomes more water soluble and less lipid-membrane soluble. *p*-Hydroxyphenobarbital is pharmacologically inactive and is either excreted directly, or glucuronidated and then excreted.

Phenobarbital metabolism exemplifies the principles propounded by Richard Tecwyn Williams, a pioneering British pharmacologist active in the mid-twentieth century [1]. Williams introduced the concepts of Phase I and Phase II drug metabolism. He described *Phase I* biotransformations as primary covalent chemical modifications to the administered drug (oxidation, reduction, hydrolysis, etc.), such as the hydroxylation of phenobarbital. On the other hand, *Phase II* reactions involved synthesis or conjugation of an endogenous polar species to either the parent drug or the Phase I modified drug, as exemplified by the glucuronidation of *p*-hydroxyphenobarbital in Scheme 11.1A. These concepts have been useful to catalog and categorize newly described chemical biotransformations, especially as the field of drug metabolism developed.

Pyrimidine nucleotides exemplify a class of pharmaceuticals designed to be biotransformed in the body from inactive to active cancer chemotherapeutic agents. In order to effectively interfere with thymidine synthetase, 5-fluorouracil (5-FU) must be biotransformed to 5-fluorouracil monophosphate (5-FUMP), as shown in Scheme 11.1B. The base 5-FU is not well absorbed as a drug and consequently is administered parenterally. The polar monophosphate is formed within the targeted, more rapidly dividing cancer cells, enhancing the specificity of its action.

Sometimes an active pharmaceutical produces another active agent after biotransformation. An example of a previously commercially popular antihistamine drug with an active metabolite is terfenadine (Seldane™), as shown in Scheme 11.1C. As discussed in Chapter 1, the terfenadine oxidative metabolite fexofenadine (Allegra™) is now marketed as a safer alternative that avoids potentially fatal cardiac terfenadine side effects.

An example of a popular pharmaceutical with a hepatotoxic metabolite is acetaminophen [2, 3]. A portion of the acetaminophen metabolized in the liver is converted to a reactive intermediate, *N*-acetyl-*p*-benzoquinoneimine (NAPQI), which is an excellent substrate for nucleophilic attack by free sulfhydryl groups in proteins or glutathione, as shown in Scheme 11.2. However, the predominant

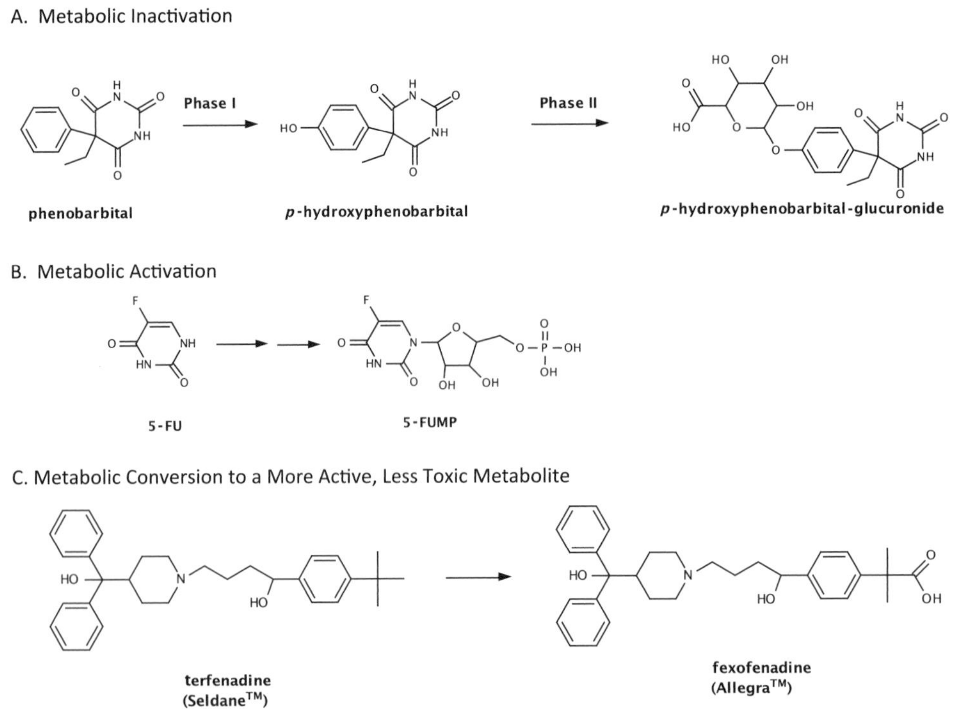

A. Metabolic Inactivation

phenobarbital          p-hydroxyphenobarbital          p-hydroxyphenobarbital-glucuronide

B. Metabolic Activation

5-FU          5-FUMP

C. Metabolic Conversion to a More Active, Less Toxic Metabolite

terfenadine
(Seldane™)

fexofenadine
(Allegra™)

SCHEME 11.1   Metabolism of phenobarbital results in inactive, more polar metabolites; metabolism of 5-fluorouracil produces the active phosphorylated drug within a cell; and the antihistamine terfenadine is oxidized to fexofenadine, another active antihistamine lacking the cardiac side-effects of terfenadine.

pathways for acetaminophen metabolism produce non-toxic polar glucuronide and sulfate conjugates and other minor metabolites that are excreted in urine. By substituting a high concentration of an alternative thiol for the –SH group in cysteine in liver proteins and removing the reactive NAPQI from contact with liver proteins, N-acetylcysteine (NAcCys) is an effective antidote for acetaminophen overdose [4]. The N-acetylcysteine adduct is inactive and is excreted in urine.

Scheme 11.2 demonstrates the complexity of metabolism that can be documented even for a relatively simple drug like acetaminophen when thoroughly analyzed by liquid chromatography-mass spectrometry, a technique described in Chapter 12 [5].

Knowledge of basic principles of drug metabolism may lead to rational development of more effective pharmaceuticals, as illustrated in Scheme 11.3 by the historical progression from procaine to procainamide and then N-acetylprocainamide (NAPA). Procaine was observed in 1936 to elevate the threshold of ventricular muscle to electrical stimulation, making it a promising antiarrhythmic agent [6]. However, it was too rapidly hydrolyzed by esterases to be used in vivo, and its amide analog procainamide was evaluated [7]. Procainamide had similar effects to

procaine and is used clinically as an antiarrhythmic drug. It is relatively resistant to hydrolysis; about 60–70% of the dose is excreted as unchanged drug and 20% acetylated to NAPA, which also has antiarrhythmic activity. NAPA has been investigated as a candidate to replace procainamide because it has a longer elimination half-life than does procainamide (2.5 times in patients with normal renal function) and fewer toxic side effects, representing a third generation of procaine development [8].

These examples indicate the relevance of understanding drug metabolism in the context of patient care and drug development. Presenting an overview of drug metabolism in a single chapter is challenging because the field has developed markedly in the past century, with many important scientific contributions. Recent books summarize advances in understanding fundamental mechanisms of metabolic processes [9] and the encyclopedic information available regarding the metabolism of specific drugs [10]. The broad concepts outlined by R. T. Williams of Phase I and Phase II metabolism are still a convenient framework for introducing the reader to metabolic processes, but these designations do not apply readily to all biotransformations. For

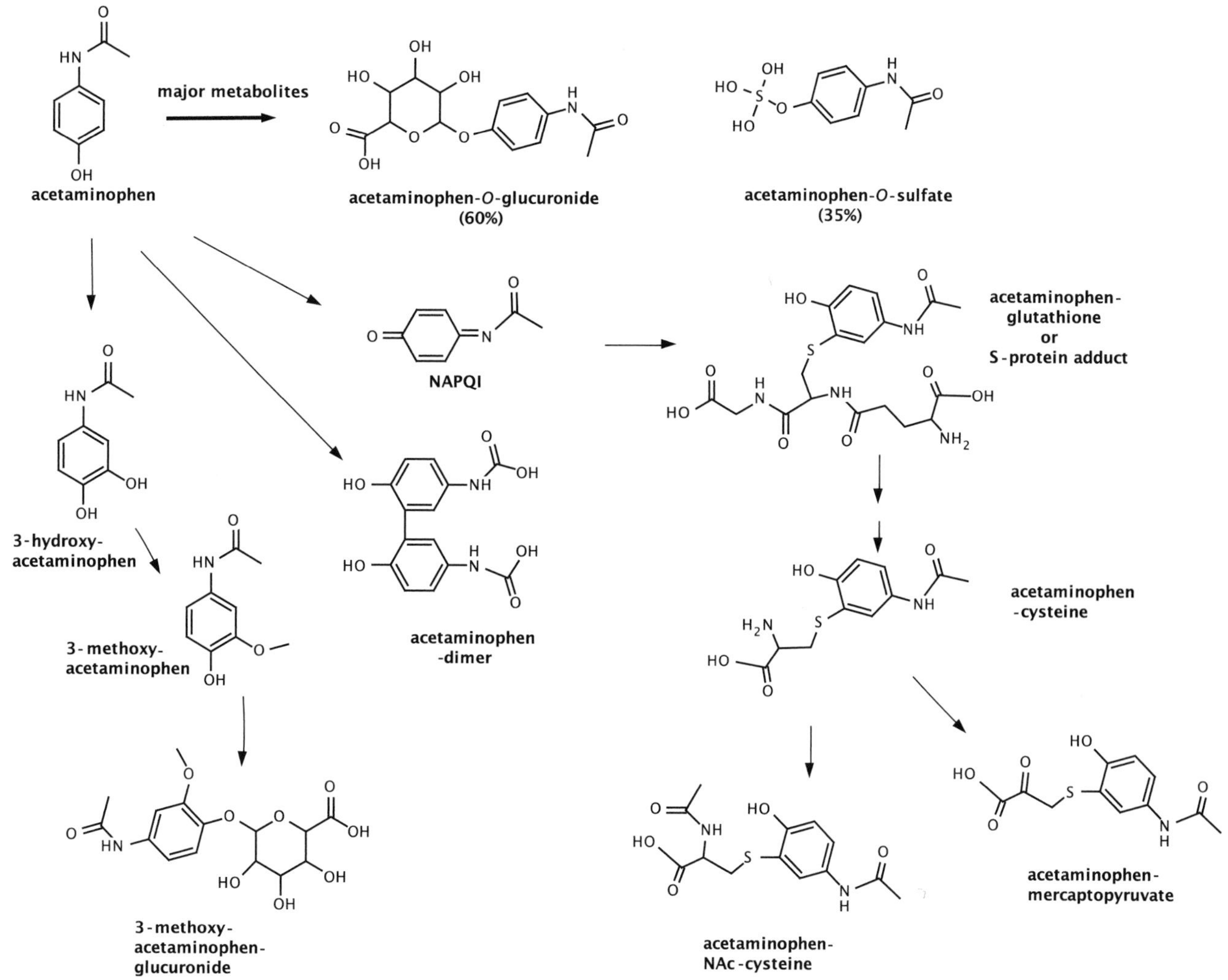

**SCHEME 11.2** Acetaminophen is metabolized mainly to phenolic *O*-glucuronide and *O*-sulfate conjugates. However, acetaminophen is a significant contributor to liver failure, so its metabolism has been extensively studied leading to elucidation of the metabolic pathways depicted in this scheme. NAPQI is a toxic intermediate formed principally by CYP2E1 and CYP3A11, and it can be detoxified by conjugation with glutathione of *N*-acetylcysteine.

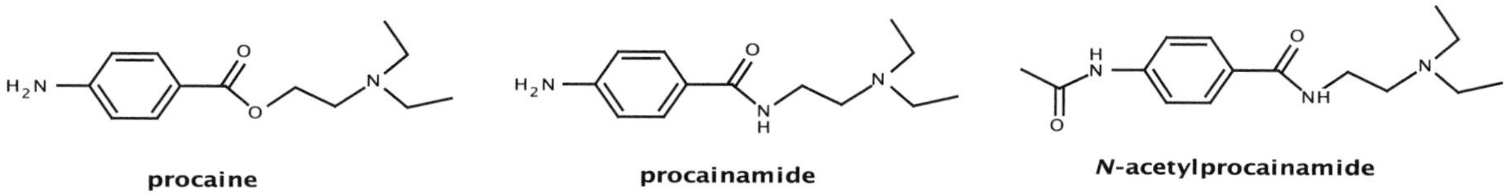

**SCHEME 11.3** The structures of procaine, procainamide, and *N*-acetylprocainamide exemplify development of more effective therapeutic agents based upon understanding the principles of drug metabolism.

example, the metabolic activation of 5-FU and the complexity of the metabolic transformations and toxic protein binding of acetaminophen (Scheme 11.2) are more usefully described with regard to the specific type of chemical transformation, the enzymes involved, and the tissue site of transformation. Because the liver is a major site of drug metabolism, this chapter introduces first the hepatic Phase I enzymes and the biotransformations they effect.

## PHASE I BIOTRANSFORMATIONS

### Liver Microsomal Cytochrome P450 Monooxygenases

Among the major enzyme systems effecting drug metabolism, cytochrome P450 monooxygenases[1] are dominant. In humans, there are 12 gene families of functionally related proteins comprising this group of enzymes. The cytochrome P450 enzymes, abbreviated CYPs (for cytochrome Ps) catalyze drug and endogenous compound oxidations in the liver, and also in the kidneys, gastrointestinal tract, skin, and lungs. Chemically, the processes of oxidation can be written as follows:

$$Drug + NADPH + H^+ + O_2 \rightarrow$$

$$Oxidized\ Drug + NADP^+ + H_2O$$

The requirement for NADPH as an energy and electron source necessitates the close association, within the endoplasmic reticulum of the cell, of CYPs with NADPH-cytochrome P reductase. To reconstitute the enzyme activity *in vitro*, it is necessary to include the CYP heme protein; the reductase, NADPH; molecular oxygen; and phosphatidylcholine, a lipid

---

[1] In an historical review, R. Snyder detailed the history of discovery of cytochrome P450 (Toxicol Sci 2000;58:3–4 [82]). Briefly, David Keilin (1887–1963) of Cambridge University coined the name "cytochromes" for light-absorbing pigments that he isolated from dipterous flies. He named the oxygen activating enzyme "cytochrome oxidase". Otto Warburg (1883–1970), in Berlin, studied cytochrome oxidase and measured its inhibition by carbon monoxide. He reported that the inhibitory effects of carbon monoxide were reversed by light and that the degree of reversal was wavelength dependent. Otto Rosenthal learned these spectroscopic techniques in Warburg's lab and brought them to the University of Pennsylvania when he fled Germany in the 1930s. There, with David Cooper and Ronald Estabrook, the mechanism of steroid hydroxylation was investigated. Using the Yang-Chance spectrophotometer, they determined the characteristic spectroscopic signature of the cytochrome P450–CO complex and recognized in 1963 that it was the same as that of pig and rat liver microsomal pigments reported in 1958 independently by both M. Klingenberg and D. Garfield. These spectroscopic characteristics were used in 1964 by T. Omura and R. Sato to identify cytochrome P450 as a heme protein. Rosenthal, Cooper, and Estabrook studied the metabolism of codeine and acetanilide, and demonstrated in 1965 that cytochrome P450 is the oxygen-activating enzyme in xenobiotic metabolism as well as in steroid hydroxylation.

surfactant. The electron flow in the CYP microsomal drug oxidizing system is illustrated in Figure 11.1.

The name cytochrome P450 derives from the spectroscopic observation that when drug is bound to the reduced heme enzyme ($Fe^{+2}$), carbon monoxide can bind to the complex and absorb light at a characteristic and distinctive 450 nm. The carbon monoxide complex can be dissociated with light, and can then absorb oxygen. The spectroscopic properties of the CYP enzyme complex were of significant utility to investigators who characterized this family of enzymes with respect to their substrate specificity, kinetics, induction, and inhibition.

Of the 12 CYP gene families, most of the drug-metabolizing enzymes are in the CYP 1, 2, and 3 families. All have molecular weights of 45–60 kDa. Their naming and classification relate to their degree of amino acid sequence homology. Subfamilies have been assigned to isoenzymes with significant sequence homology to the family (e.g., CYP1A). An additional numerical identifier is added when more than one subfamily has been identified (e.g., CYP1A2). Frequently, two or more enzymes can catalyze the same type of oxidation, indicating redundant and broad substrate specificity. Thus, early efforts by different investigators to categorize CYPs on the basis of the catalyzed biochemical transformations led to confusion that has now been

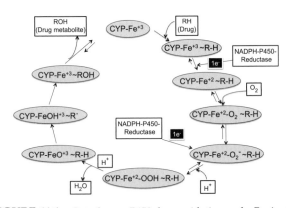

**FIGURE 11.1** Cytochrome P450 drug oxidation cycle. Beginning with CYP heme iron in the ferric (+3) state, the substrate drug is bound to the CYP near the heme center. One electron is transferred from NADPH-dependent P450 reductase. The resulting ferrous (+2) CYP binds molecular oxygen, and a second electron is supplied by P450 reductase, either directly or through cytochrome b5 intermediacy. A proton is added, and the O–O bond cleaves with the addition of a second proton and the release of water. The resulting high-energy ferric complex is used to rationalize most of the resulting reactions. The electron-deficient complex abstracts a hydrogen atom and the intermediate collapses in a step referred to as "oxygen rebound". The oxidized product dissociates from the CYP complex, and the cycle repeats with the CYP heme returned to the ferric state.

resolved with gene sequences. Some of the principle drug-metabolizing CYPs are listed in Table 11.1 [11, 12]. Three of the CYP families, 1A2, 2C, and 3A4, are shown in boldface in the table because they account for >50% of the metabolism of most drugs. Their levels can vary considerably, requiring further clinical evaluation when patient responses suggest that either too much or too little of a prescribed drug is present.

It is instructive to examine which drugs are substrates for various isoforms of CYP enzymes. Table 11.2 lists some of the substrates for different CYP isoforms [11, 12]. There are several examples of a single compound that is metabolized by multiple CYP enzymes (acetaminophen, diazepam, caffeine, halothane, warfarin, testosterone, zidovudine), and CYP enzymes that metabolize bioactive endogenous molecules (prostaglandins, steroids) as well as drugs.

The activity of various CYP enzymes may be influenced by a variety of factors. For example, genetic polymorphisms are most significant in CYP1A, 2A6, 2C9, 2C19, 2D6, and 2E1 families. Factors that either induce or inhibit CYP enzyme activity include nutrition effects that have been documented in CYP1A1, 1A2, 1B1, 2A6, 2B6, 2C8, 2C9, 2C19, 2D6, and 3A4 families [11, 12]; smoking influences the CYP1A1, 1A2, and 2E1 families [13]; alcohol, the CYP2E1 family [14]; drugs, the CYP1A1, 1A2, 2A6, 2B6; 2C, 2D6, 3A3, 3A4,5 families; and environmental xenobiotics such as polycyclic aromatic hydrocarbons, dioxins, organic solvents and organophosphate insecticides the CYP1A1, 1A2, 2A6, 1B, 2E1, 3A4 families [11].

**TABLE 11.1 Human CYP Enzymes Important in Liver Metabolism of Drugs**

| CYP enzyme[a] | Level (% total) | Extent of variability |
|---|---|---|
| 21A2 | ~ 13 | ~ 40-fold |
| 1B1 | < 1 | |
| 2A6 | ~ 4 | ~ 30- to 100-fold |
| 2B6 | < 1 | ~50-fold |
| **2C** | **~ 18** | **25- to 100-fold** |
| 2D6 | Up to 2.5 | > 1000-fold |
| 2E1 | Up to 7 | ~20-fold |
| 2F1 | | |
| 2J2 | | |
| **3A4** | **Up to 28** | **~20-fold** |
| 4A, 4B | | |

[a]Boldface: enzymes that account for >50% of the metabolism of most drugs.

Data from Rendic S, Di Carlo FJ. Drug Metab Rev 1997;29: 413–580 [12].

**TABLE 11.2 Participation of the CYP Enzymes in Metabolism of Some Clinically Important Drugs**

| CYP enzyme | Participation in drug metabolism (%) | Examples of substrates |
|---|---|---|
| 1A1 | 3 | Caffeine, testosterone, (R)-warfarin |
| 1A2 | 10 | Acetaminophen, caffeine, phenacetin, (R)-warfarin |
| 1B1 | 1 | 17β-Estradiol, testosterone |
| 2A6 | 3 | Acetaminophen, halothane, zidovudine |
| 2B6 | 4 | Cyclophosphamide, erythromycin, testosterone |
| 2C-family | 25 | Acetaminophen (2C9), hexobarbital (2C9,19) Phenytoin (2C8,9,19) Testosterone (2C8,9,19), tolbutamide (2C9) (R)-Warfarin (2C8,8,18,19), (S)-Warfarin (2C9,19) Zidovudine (2C8,9,19), |
| 2E1 | 4 | Acetaminophen, caffeine, chlorzoxazone, halothane |
| 2D6 | 18.8 | Acetaminophen, codeine debrisoquine |
| 3A4 | 34.1 | Acetaminophen, caffeine, carbamazepine, codeine, cortisol, erythromycin, cyclophosphamide, (S)- and (R)-Warfarin, phenytoin, testosterone, halothane, zidovudine |

Data from Rendic S. Drug Metab Rev 2002;34:83–448 [11].

Rendic and Guengerich [15, 16] have published a comprehensive review of the effects of environmental factors and diseases on CYPs and transporters.

The diverse nature of these effects is illustrated by recounting the experience of clinical pharmacologists who studied the pharmacokinetics of felodipine, a dihydropyridine calcium channel antagonist [17]. They designed a study to test the effects of ethanol on felodipine metabolism. To mask the flavor of ethanol from the subjects, they tested a variety of fruit juices, selecting double-strength grapefruit juice prepared from frozen concentrate as most effective. The resulting plasma felodipine concentrations did not differ between the ethanol/felodipine and felodipine groups,

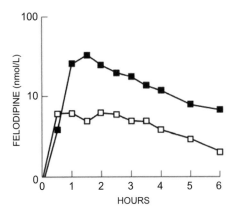

**FIGURE 11.2**  Plasma felodipine concentrations after oral administration of a 5-mg dose to an individual with (■) and without (□) grapefruit juice. Reproduced with permission from Bailey DG, Malcolm J, Arnold O, Spence JD. Br J Clin Pharmacol 1998:46;101–10 [17].

but the plasma concentrations in both groups were considerably higher than those seen in any previous study. The effects of repeated grapefruit juice doses are cumulative and, as shown in Figure 11.2, may increase felodipine concentrations as much as five-fold.

Upon further investigation, it was determined that grapefruit juice administration for 6 consecutive days causes a 62% reduction in small bowel enterocyte CYP3A4 protein, thereby inhibiting the first-pass metabolism of felodipine to oxidized felodipine shown in Scheme 11.4 [18]. The effects of grapefruit juice are highly variable among individuals depending on their basal levels of small bowel CYP3A4, but grapefruit juice does not affect the pharmacokinetics of intravenously administered felodipine because the active constituents of the juice are not absorbed and do not affect liver CYPs. Subsequent studies have shown that the degradation half-life of CYP3A4 normally is 8 hours, and that at least 3 days are required to regain normal CYP3A4 function after exposure to grapefruit juice [19].

The effect of grapefruit juice on felodipine kinetics illustrates several of the difficulties and pitfalls that not only confound clinical studies of new drug products, but are also a source of concern in clinical medicine. There are likely to be other food and diet

supplements with similar constituents and pharmacological activity. For example, Seville orange juice contains some of the same fucocoumarins as grapefruit juice and exhibits the same effect with respect to felodipine pharmacokinetics [20]. The differing composition of fucocoumarin mixtures in fruit juices produces variability in responses to drugs transported and metabolized by multiple mechanisms. Grapefruit juice constituents also inhibit the multidrug transporter P-glycoprotein, MDR-1, and the multidrug resistance protein 2 (MRP2), resulting in pharmacokinetic effects on cyclosporin metabolism [21]. Seville orange juice does not interact with cyclosporin concentrations – evidence for the fact that the orange juice does not contain those components that interfere with MDR-1 and MRP2 [20]. Thus, pharmacologically active CYP inducers or inhibitors may derive from dietary or environmental origin (e.g., insecticides or perfumes) and can only be recognized when appropriate *in vitro* or *in vivo* kinetic studies have been performed. However, particular attention has focused on the topic of drug–drug interactions, which is discussed in greater detail in Chapter 15. At this point, it can be appreciated that elderly patients are particularly at risk because they are likely to use multiple drugs as well as dietary and food supplements [22].

The example of felodipine also demonstrates that CYPs outside of the liver may have significant effects on drug concentrations. In addition to the dominant CYP3A family, the GI tract contains CYPs 2D6, 2C, 2B6, and 1A1. Similarly, CYPs are found in lung (CYPs 1A1, 2A6, 2B6, 2C, 2E, 2F and 4B1), kidney (CYPs 1A1, 1B1, 3A, 4A11), skin, placenta, prostate, and other tissues where their inhibition or activation may be of clinical relevance to the efficacy or toxicity of a therapeutic agent.

## CYP-Mediated Chemical Transformations

Most drugs are relatively small organic compounds with molecular weights below 500 Da. The action of various CYP isoforms is predictable in that there are

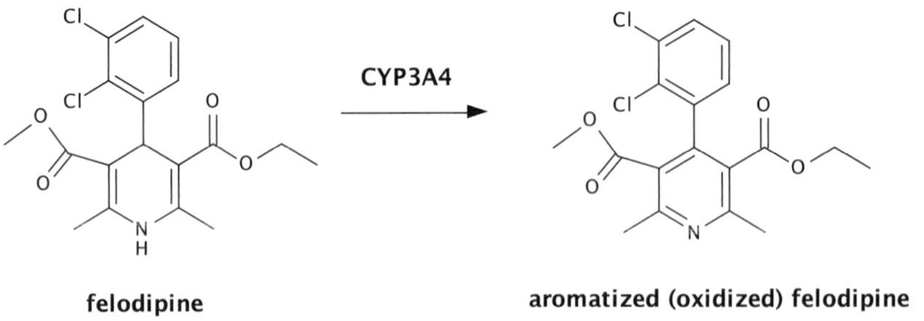

**felodipine**                    **aromatized (oxidized) felodipine**

**SCHEME 11.4**  Oxidation of felodipine by intestinal CYP3A4 limits its bioavailability.

several organic structural elements that are principal targets for metabolic transformations. However, the metabolism of any specific drug is not entirely predictable in that a specific site of metabolism may be favored for one compound and a different site for another, but structurally related, compound. Nevertheless, there are some unifying concepts governing the mechanisms of CYP-mediated reactions that are helpful for classification of potential transformations. Guengerich [23, 24] described four common major reaction types: (1) carbon hydroxylation; (2) heteroatom (N, S, O, P, halogen) release; (3) heteroatom oxygenation; and (4) epoxidation, group migration, and olefinic suicide inactivation, illustrated in Scheme 11.5.

The major reaction types share in common an $FeO^{3+}$ intermediate and odd electron abstraction/oxygen rebound steps that are useful to describe many drug biotransformations. The heme $FeO^{3+}$ is a highly reactive oxidant, responsible for the CYPs' promiscuous attacks on very different substrates. There are, in addition to these four common reaction types, multiple other types of biotransformations (reduction, including dehalogenation, desaturation,

ester cleavage, ring expansion, ring formation, etc.) that require alternative mechanisms [24]. The following examples are chosen to illustrate the four most common characteristic metabolic CYP-mediated oxidative pathways for drugs, as well as the reductive dehalogenation pathway.

### Carbon Hydroxylation

Hydroxylation occurs at *aliphatic* carbon atoms, frequently at secondary or tertiary sites in preference to primary carbon atoms. Hydrogen atom abstraction is followed by oxygen rebound in a stepwise mechanism [23]. Ibuprofen is an example of aliphatic hydroxylation, as shown in Scheme 11.6 [25]. Hydroxylation occurs at primary and secondary carbon atoms, but the major hydroxylated metabolite is at the tertiary site (metabolite 1). Hydroxylation at a primary carbon atom (metabolite 2) is followed by two subsequent carbon hydroxylations to produce the carboxylic acid metabolite 3. The parent ibuprofen and its metabolites are conjugated to varying degrees with glucuronic acid as esters prior to urinary excretion [26].

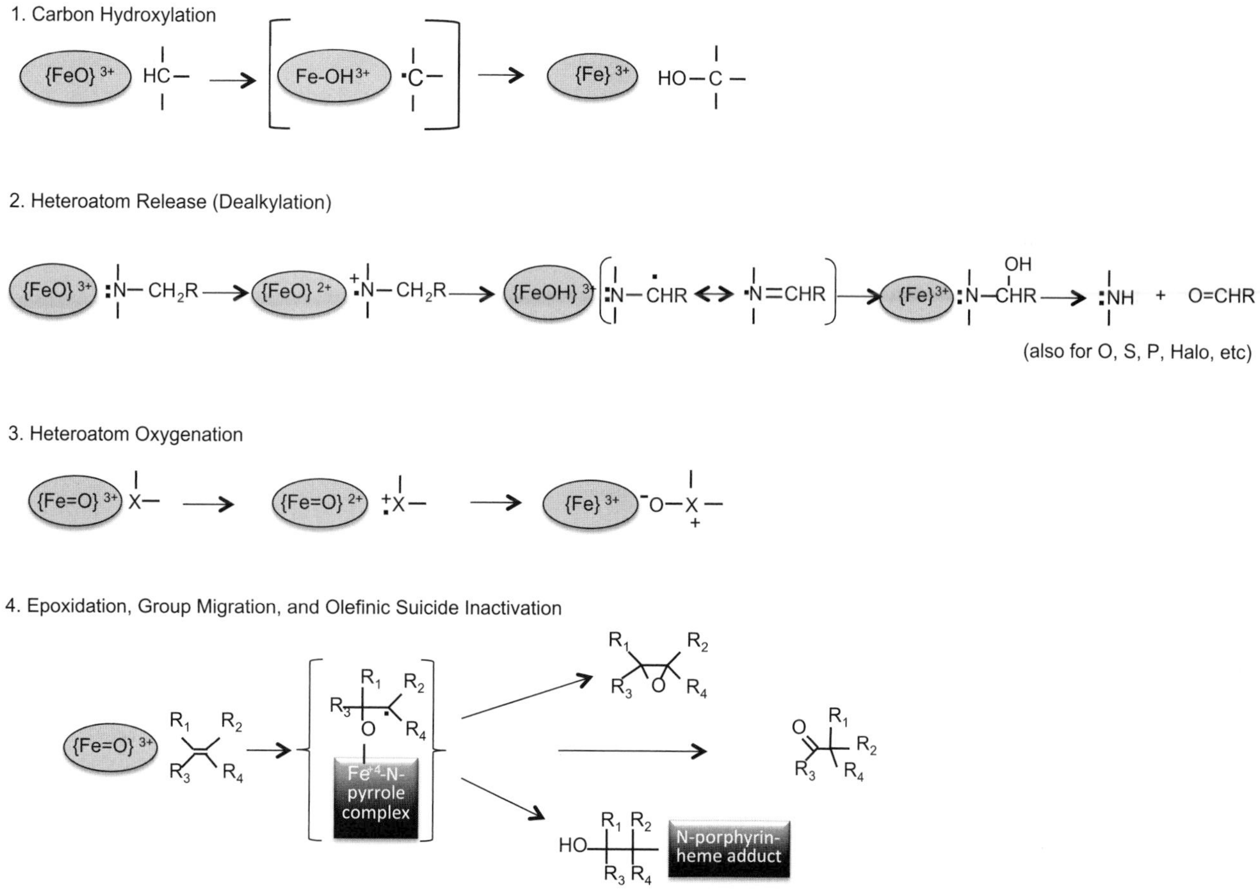

1. Carbon Hydroxylation

2. Heteroatom Release (Dealkylation)

(also for O, S, P, Halo, etc)

3. Heteroatom Oxygenation

4. Epoxidation, Group Migration, and Olefinic Suicide Inactivation

**SCHEME 11.5**  Four common CYP-mediated drug transformation mechanisms according to Guengerich [23, 24].

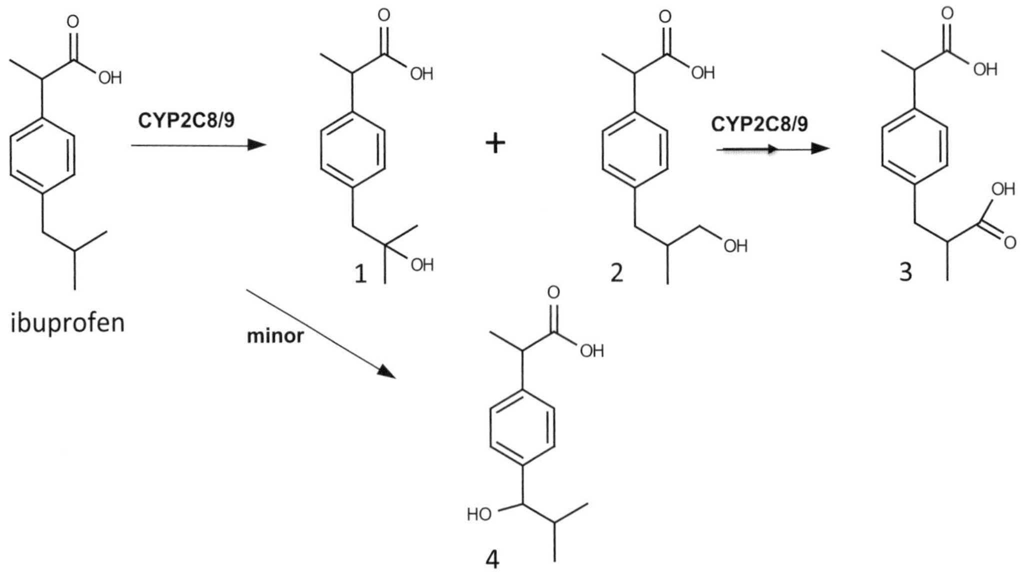

**SCHEME 11.6** Aliphatic carbon hydroxylation of ibuprofen in humans results primarily in metabolite 1. Metabolite 2 undergoes two additional oxidation–hydroxylation steps to form the carboxylic acid 3. Metabolite 4 is barely detectable in urine. All of the ibuprofen acid metabolites are excreted also as ester glucuronide conjugates.

Hydroxylation at *aromatic* carbon atoms proceeds through stepwise oxygen transfer, as shown in Scheme 11.5. More recent studies on selectively deuterated mono-substituted benzenes as well as various epoxides provided strong evidence for a stepwise mechanism rather than the initially proposed pathways that proceeded entirely through symmetrical arene oxide intermediates [27]. As shown for phenytoin in Scheme 11.7, there is an initial attack of $FeO^{3+}$ on the aromatic system to form a tetrahedral carbon intermediate, followed by oxygen rebound with electron transfer and release of metabolites. The resulting products may include mono-hydroxylated aromatics, as well as arene oxides formed from the same tetrahedral intermediate. For example, the major metabolite of phenytoin formed by CYP2C9 is 4-hydroxyphenytoin, which is then excreted in urine after glucuronide conjugation [28]. The 4-hydroxy- and 3-hydroxyphenytoins are further metabolized by CYPs to 3,4 dihydroxyphenytoin, a catechol [29]. The phenytoin catechol also may be oxidized by peroxidases in skin to a reactive quinone, possibly a causative agent for phenytoin idiosyncratic drug reactions [30, 31].

### Heteroatom Release: N-Dealkylation (O-Dealkylation, S-Dealkylation)

N-Demethylation is a frequent route of metabolism of drugs containing alkylamine functionalities. For example, the predominant metabolism of amodiaquine is through CYP2C8 N-de-ethylation (Scheme 11.8) [32, 33]. The stepwise one-electron transfer mechanism

for dealkylation with $[FeO^{2+}]$ as an intermediate base to remove a proton is based on extensive kinetic studies [34]. Formally, O- and S-dealkylation are related to N-dealkylation, although the details of their mechanisms may differ.

### Epoxidation

CYP stepwise metabolism may produce short-lived and highly reactive arene oxide intermediates, not directly characterized, but, as in the example of phenytoin, their formation is inferred from the resulting dihydrodiol metabolites (Scheme 11.7). As described in Chapter 16, the phenytoin arene oxide has been associated with teratogenic effects in children born to women who were treated with phenytoin during pregnancy, and may produce a constellation of congenital abnormalities, including cleft palate [35]. Microsomal epoxide hydrolase (HYL1) is widely distributed in tissues and serves a protective role in converting arene oxide intermediates to diols [36]. The teratogenic effects of phenytoin are associated with phenytoin oxide reactivity with cellular DNA in tissues lacking the protective effects of HYL1 [35, 37]. Gaedigk *et al.* [38] demonstrated that there is tissue-specific expression of microsomal HYL1, and not a single HYL1 transcript and promoter region. Liang *et al.* [39] identified several potential *cis*-regulatory elements, and found that GATA-4 is probably the principal factor regulating liver-specific expression.

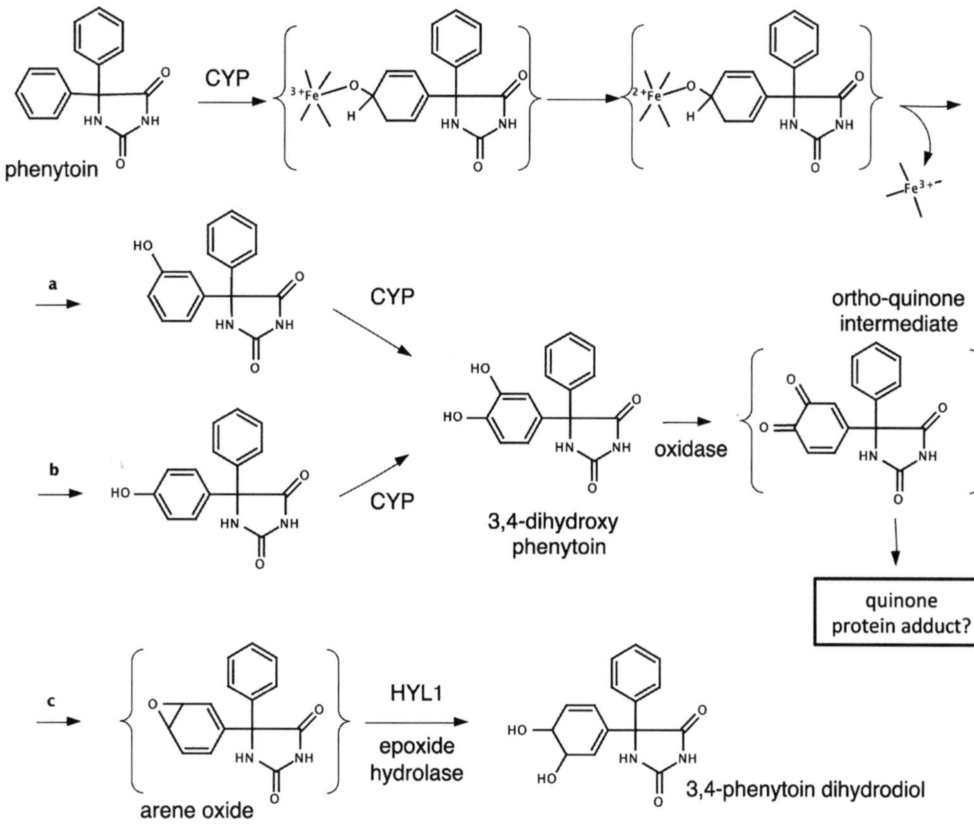

**SCHEME 11.7** Metabolism of phenytoin proceeds through step-wise carbon hydroxylation to yield predominantly 4-hydroxyphenytoin (Pathway b) that can be further metabolized to the 3,4-dihydroxy catechol metabolite. The catechol is a substrate for mixed function oxidases that may yield reactive ortho-quinone intermediates responsible for phenytoin idiosyncratic toxicity. The presence of the 3,4-dihydrodiol metabolite in urine suggests that it is formed from an arene oxide intermediate (Pathway c).

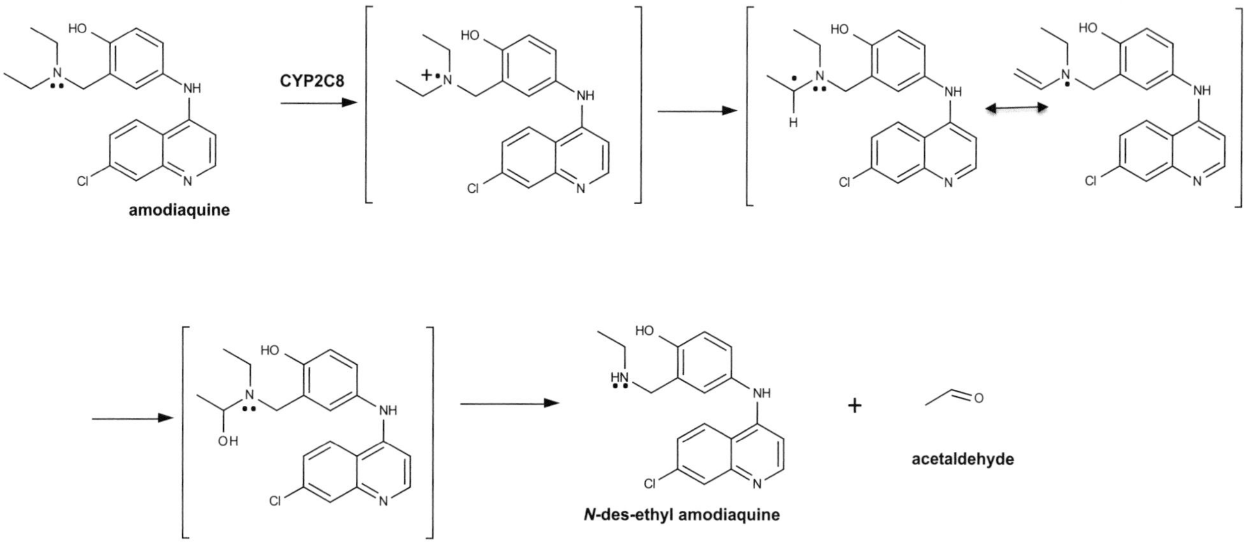

**SCHEME 11.8** The predominant metabolism of amodiaquine is through CYP2C8 N-dealkylation (de-ethylation) in a step-wise mechanism, beginning with one electron loss from nitrogen, followed by proton abstraction from an alpha carbon; oxygen collapse forms an unstable carbinolamine intermediate leading to the des-ethyl amodiaquine and acetaldehyde.

## Heteroatom oxygenation

CYPs add oxygen directly to the heteroatoms nitrogen, sulfur, phosphorous, and iodine through two single electron transfers (Scheme 11.5) or a one-electron transfer/recombination mechanism [23]. Aliphatic amines are converted to hydroxylamines that are less basic than their parents. Aromatic amines are oxidized to products that are more toxic than their parent amines, frequently producing hypersensitivity or carcinogenicity. As shown in Scheme 11.9, dapsone is oxidized by CYP2C8/9 at concentrations used clinically [40]. Methemoglobinemia, a major side effect of dapsone, is linked to its N-oxidation to dapsone hydroxylamine [41]. Additionally, dapsone therapy is associated with decreased erythrocyte lifetime, apparently through direct binding of its hydroxylamine metabolite to membrane proteins. However, the aromatic amine N-hydroxylation products formed by CYP2C8/9 are identical to those produced by flavin monooxygenases (FMOs), so enzymatic studies are required to identify which enzyme system is responsible for dapsone metabolism *in vivo*.

Sulfur is readily oxidized, by CYPs as well as by FMOs. As shown in Scheme 11.10, chlorpromazine metabolism provides an example of preferential S- vs N-oxidation by CYP1A2 [42]. CYP1A2 is the active isoform responsible for the major N-dealkylation and S-oxidation metabolic pathways in humans. There are significant implications for drug interactions when a single CYP isoform is active, because other drug substrates for CYP1A2 (e.g., caffeine, phenacetin, imipramine, propranolol, clozapine) may slow chlorpromazine metabolism and result in undesirable side-effects.

## Dehalogenation

As discussed in Chapter 16, reductive dehalogenation by liver CYP enzymes of a number of inhalation anesthetics (halothane, methoxyflurane) and halogenated solvents yields chemically reactive free radicals that play an important role in the hepatotoxicity of these compounds. CYP ferrous one-electron reductive dehalogenation produces a free radical intermediate that may be detected by its interaction with cellular lipids. Dehalogenation of carbon tetrachloride generates chloroform and free radicals by this pathway [23].

## Non-CYP Biotransformations

### Hydrolysis

Hydrolyses of esters or amides are common reactions catalyzed by ubiquitous esterases, amidases, and proteases found in every tissue and physiological fluid. These enzymes exhibit widely differing substrate specificities. The hydrolytic reactions are the reverse of Phase II conjugation reactions, especially for the acetylation reaction discussed later in this chapter.

Aspirin (acetylsalicylic acid) is an example of a compound that is hydrolyzed readily in plasma to salicylic acid (Scheme 11.11). Hydrolyzed salicylate is further metabolized by conjugation, accounting for the metabolism of 90% of the administered dose in humans [43]. Aspirin has a half-life of 15 minutes in plasma. Salicylic acid, the active anti-inflammatory metabolite of aspirin, has a much longer half-life of 12 hours. However, salicylic acid irritates the gastric mucosa, necessitating the use of acetylsalicylic acid or sodium salicylate in clinical practice.

### Reduction

Although most drugs are metabolized by oxidative processes, reduction may be a clinically important pathway of drug metabolism, as noted for reductive dehalogenation by CYPs. In some cases, these metabolic transformations are carried out by reductase

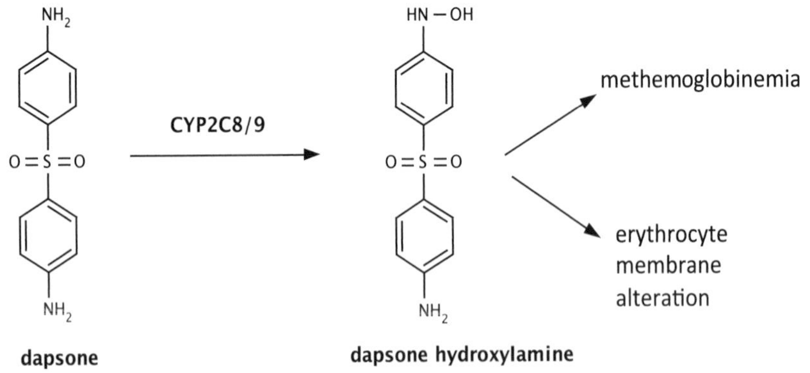

**SCHEME 11.9**   Dapsone is a substrate for N-oxidation, and the resulting hydroxylamine has been demonstrated to cause methemoglobinemia and impair erythrocyte longevity.

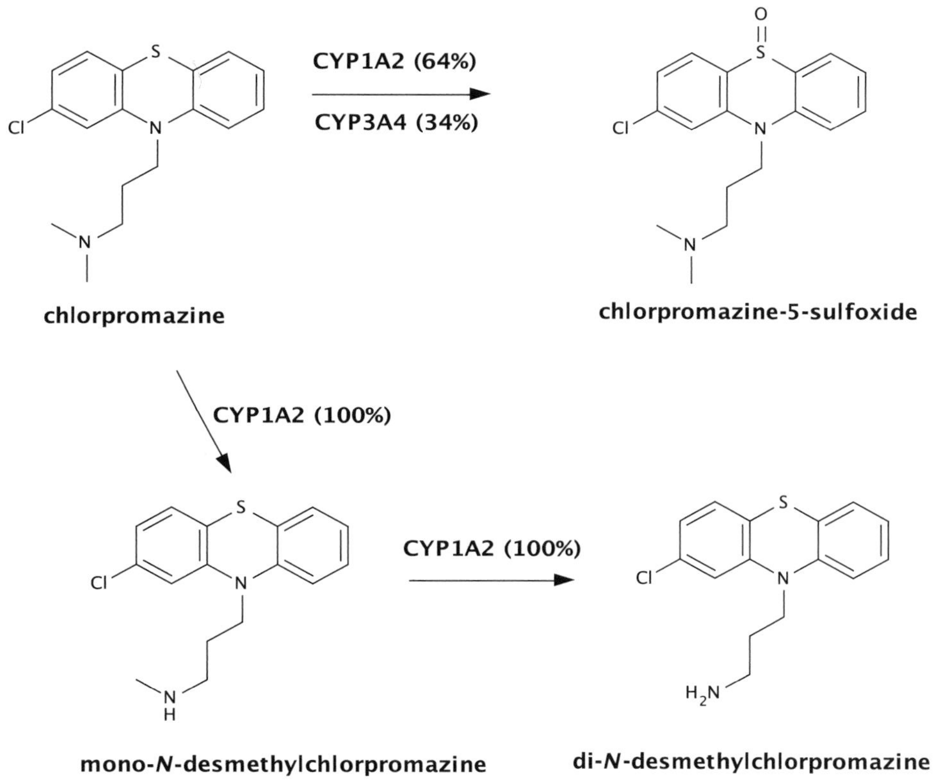

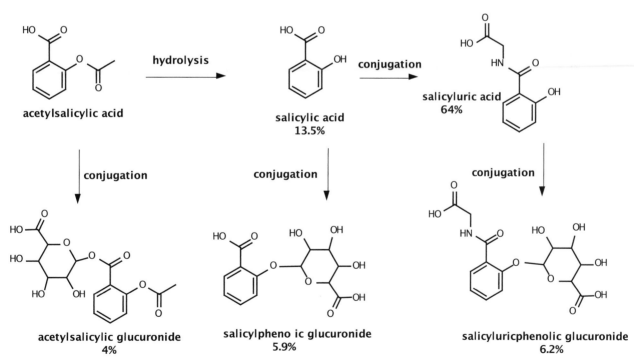

**SCHEME 11.10**  Chlorpromazine at therapeutic doses is metabolized mostly by CYP1A2, either to the 5-sulfoxide or to the des-*N*-methyl metabolites.

**SCHEME 11.11**  Aspirin (acetylsalicylic acid) administered to humans is excreted predominantly (90%) as either its hydrolysis product, salicylic acid, or a conjugate of salicylic acid.

enzymes in intestinal anaerobic bacteria. In the case of prontosil (Scheme 11.12) an aromatic azo-function ($Ar_1$–N=N–$Ar_2$) is reduced, forming two aniline moieties ($Ar_1$–$NH_2$, $Ar_2$–$NH_2$). One of the reduced metabolites is sulfanilamide, the active antibacterial agent that was first recognized in 1935 by an Institute Pasteur team to account for the antibacterial activity of prontosil that was observed *in vivo*, but not in *vitro* [44]. Since biotransformation is required for antibacterial activity, prontosil is referred to as a *prodrug*.

The second example shown in Scheme 11.12 is the metabolic inactivation of digoxin by *Eubacterium lentum* in the intestine [45]. Approximately 10% of patients taking digoxin excrete large quantities of the inactive reduction product dihydrodigoxin [46]. As discussed in Chapter 4, the enteric metabolism of digoxin reduces digoxin bioavailability significantly in some patients. Conversely, when such patients require antibiotic therapy, the resulting blood levels of digoxin may reach toxic levels because the antibiotic halts the previously robust inactivation by *E. lentum* and digoxin bioavailability is thereby increased.

## Oxidations

### Flavine Monooxygenases

Flavine monooxygenases (FMOs) are microsomal enzymes that catalyze the oxygenation of nucleophilic heteroatom-containing (nitrogen, sulfur, phosphorus, selenium) compounds, producing structurally similar metabolites to those produced by CYPs. Unlike CYPs, the FMOs do not require tight substrate binding to the enzyme, but only a single point contact with the very reactive hydroperoxyflavin monooxygenating agent. FMOs are also unlike CYPs in that FMOs do not contain metal and are very heat labile. Experimentally, heat lability may be used as an initial indication of FMO vs CYP intermediacy. The quantitative role of FMOs vs CYPs in the metabolism of any specific drug cannot be predicted from an examination of the drug structure; in fact, many compounds are substrates of both enzymes. Five different human FMO gene subfamilies have been identified, and polyclonal antibodies have permitted identification of FMO isoforms from liver and lung from different

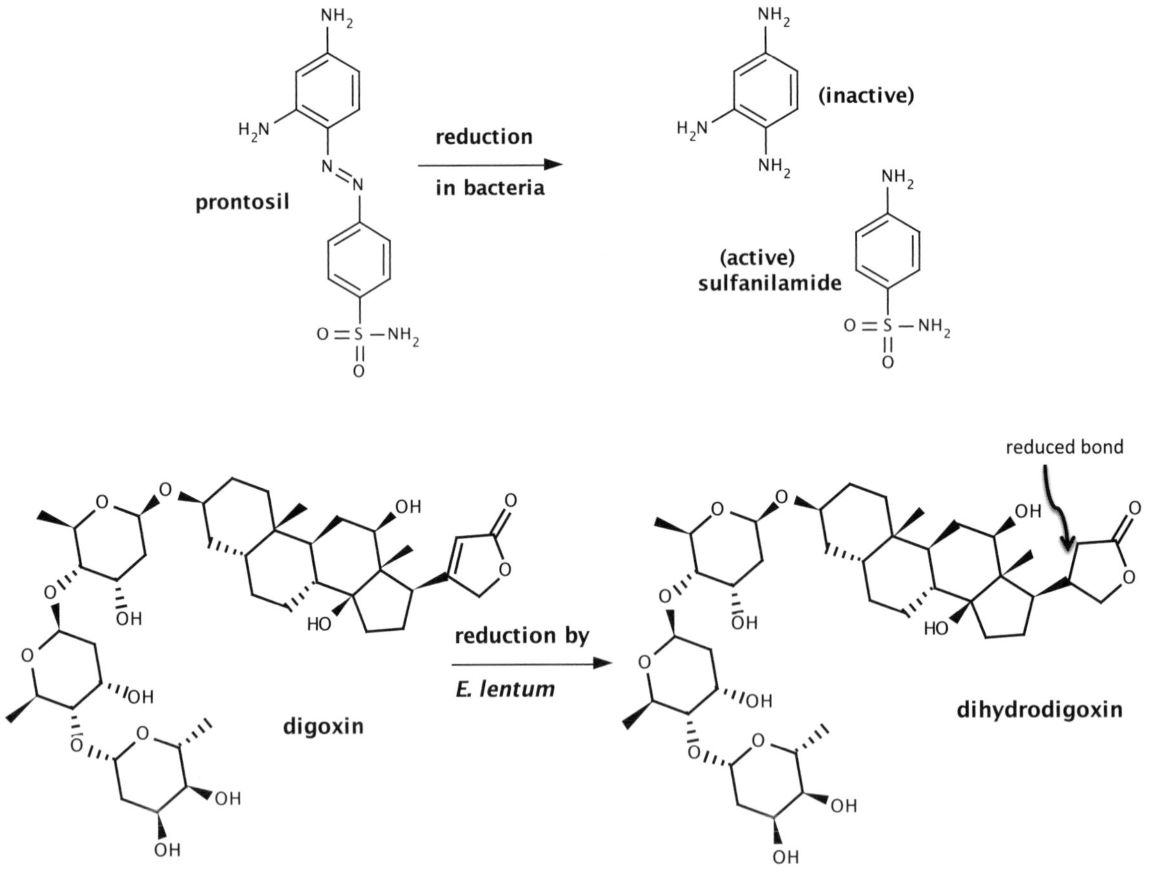

SCHEME 11.12   Examples of bacterial reduction to produce drug activation (prontosil to sulfanilamide) and inactivation (digoxin to dihydrodigoxin).

species (humans, pigs, rabbits) [47, 48]. FMOs exhibit a very broad ability to oxidize structurally different substrates, suggesting that they contribute significantly to the metabolism of a number of drugs. FMOs require molecular oxygen, NADPH, and flavin adenosine dinucleotide. Factors affecting FMOs (diet, drugs, sex) have not been as highly studied as they have for CYPs, but it is clear that FMOs are prominent metabolizing enzymes for common drugs such as nicotine, cimetidine [47], and tamoxifen [49].

Nicotine is an example of a compound that undergoes FMO3 catalyzed N-oxidation, as shown in Scheme 11.13. About 3–7% of nicotine is stereoselectively metabolized to trans-(S)-(−)-nicotine N-1′ oxide in humans by FMO3, whereas more than 80% of an administered dose appears as cotinine or cotinine metabolites, the result of a CYP2A6 oxidation [50]. Other examples of FMO N-oxidation include trimethylamine, amphetamine and the phenothiazines [47, 51].

### Monoamine Oxidases

Monoamine oxidases (MAO-A and MAO-B) are mitochondrial FAD-dependent enzymes that oxidatively deaminate endogenous biogenic amine neurotransmitters such as dopamine, serotonin, norepinephrine, and epinephrine [52]. MAOs are like FMOs in that they may catalyze the oxidation of drugs to produce drug metabolites that are identical in chemical structure to those formed by CYPs. Because the resulting structures are identical, oxidative deamination by MAO can only be distinguished from CYP oxidative deamination by drug and enzyme characterization, not by metabolite structure. MAOs are found in liver, kidney, intestine, and brain. Some drugs (tranylcypromine, selegiline) have been designed as irreversible "suicide" substrates to inhibit MAO in order to alter the balance of CNS neurotransmitters. Both the response to these inhibitors and the study of *in vitro* enzyme preparations are used to distinguish this enzymatic process.

Similarly, diamine oxidases and non-FAD containing amine oxidases catalyze oxidative deamination of endogenous amines such as histamine and the polyamines putrescine and cadaverine, and can contribute to the oxidative deamination of drugs [53]. Diamine oxidase is found in high levels in liver, intestine, and placenta, and converts amines to aldehydes in the presence of oxygen, similar to the action of CYPs.

### Alcohol and Aldehyde Dehydrogenases

Alcohols and aldehydes are metabolized by liver dehydrogenases that are nonmicrosomal and by nonspecific liver enzymes that are important in the catabolism of endogenous compounds. Ethanol is a special example of a compound whose metabolism is clinically relevant in that ethanol may interact with

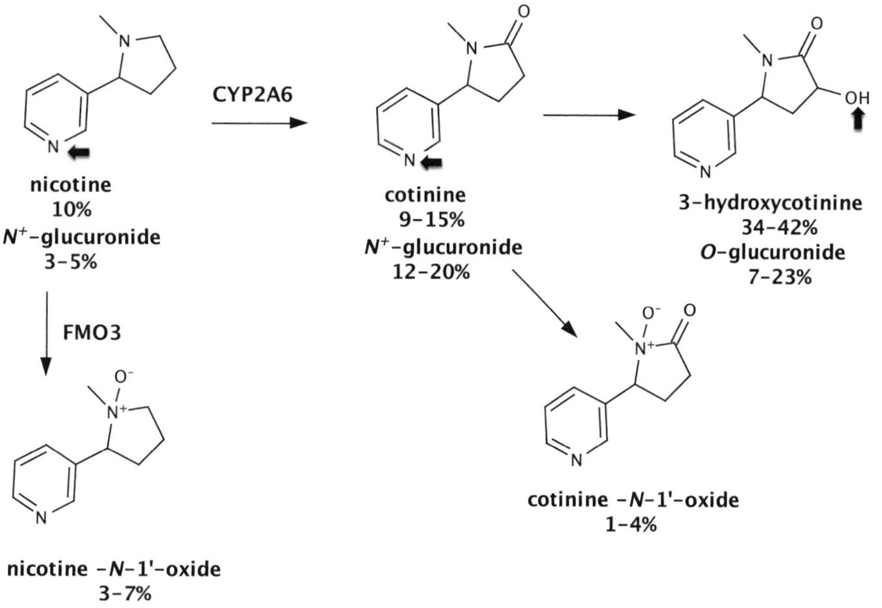

**SCHEME 11.13** Nicotine is metabolized by human smokers to urinary metabolites as summarized above. A relatively small percentage is stereospecifically metabolized by FMO3 to nicotine-N-oxide, and the majority is oxidized by CYP2A6 to cotinine and its metabolites. Arrows point to the sites of glucuronidation.

prescribed pharmaceuticals either metabolically or pharmacodynamically. Ethanol is metabolized first to acetaldehyde by alcohol dehydrogenase and then to acetic acid by aldehyde dehydrogenase. These enzymes also play an important role in the metabolism of other drugs containing alcohol functional groups. There are also CYP-dependent microsomal ethanol oxidizing enzymes that provide metabolic redundancy, but alcohol and aldehyde dehydrogenases are the major enzymes involved in ethanol metabolism under normal physiological conditions.

## PHASE II BIOTRANSFORMATIONS (CONJUGATIONS)

Drugs are frequently metabolized by covalent addition of an endogenous species such as a sugar or an amino acid. This addition, or conjugation, usually converts a lipophilic drug into a more polar product, as noted in the example of phenobarbital metabolism to hydroxyphenobarbital-glucuronide (Scheme 11.1A). There are multiple conjugation reactions – glucuronidation, sulfonation, acetylation, methylation, and amino acid conjugation (glycine, taurine, glutathione). Taken together, these Phase II biotransformations are analogous and comparable. However, their catalytic enzyme systems differ greatly from each other, as do the properties of resulting metabolites. Not all of these metabolites are pharmacologically inactive; some have therapeutic activity whereas others are chemically reactive and toxic intermediates. As a consequence, it is more useful to separately present and discuss each of the three major conjugation reactions. In humans, glucuronidation is a high-capacity pathway, sulfonation is a low-capacity pathway, and acetylation exhibits high interindividual variability.

### Glucuronidation

The glucuronidation pathway often accounts for a major portion of drug metabolites that are found excreted in urine. Glucuronides are formed by a family of soluble liver microsomal enzymes, the uridine diphosphate(UDP)-glucuronosyltransferases (UGTs). The substrate functional groups for UGTs are hydroxyl and carboxylic acid groups (forming O-glucuronides), primary, secondary, and tertiary amines (forming N-glucuronides), and thiols and sulfoxides (forming S-glucuronides). Although glucuronide formation occurs predominantly in the liver, it also takes place in the kidneys and brain. There are two subfamilies comprising multiple (at least 20) isoforms with very

different primary amino acid structures [54, 55]. The UGT1 subfamily glucuronidates phenols and bilirubin; the substrates for UGT2 include steroids and bile acids. The subfamilies that have been cloned and expressed exhibit limited substrate specificity. The high capacity of human liver for glucuronidation may be due to the broad substrate redundancy in this family. UGTs catalyze the transfer of glucuronic acid from UDP-glucuronic acid to an oxygen, nitrogen, or sulfur atom in a drug substrate, as shown in Scheme 11.14. There is considerable variation allowed in the substrates for glucuronidation, and phenols (metabolites of phenobarbital, Scheme 11.1A; acetaminophen, Scheme 11.2; acetylsalicylic acid, Scheme 11.11), alcohols (3-hydroxycontinine, Scheme 11.13), aromatic or aliphatic amines (nicotine, cotinine, Scheme 11.13), carboxylic acids (acetylsalicylic, Scheme 11.11), and thiols [56] are suitable functional groups for glucuronidation.

While glucuronidation is normally associated with termination of drug activity, morphine-6-glucuronide (Scheme 11.14) is a more potent analgesic than its parent compound. Morphine-3-glucuronide is the major metabolite (45–55%); morphine-6-glucuronide is 20 to 30% of that level. Although morphine-3-glucuronide lacks analgesic activity, it antagonizes the respiratory depression induced by morphine and morphine-6-glucuronide. Recognition of the potency of morphine-6-glucuronide has led to its testing as a drug for intravenous administration [57–59].

Drug $N^+$-glucuronides, the quaternary ammonium products from glucuronidation of tertiary amines and pyridines, were recognized as major drug metabolites only after liquid chromatographic–mass spectrometric analytical methods became available [60, 61]. The percentage of the administered dose of nicotine excreted in human urine as nicotine-$N_1$-glucuronide or cotinine-$N_1$-glucuronide, (Schemes 11.13 and 11.14) is 3–5% or 12–20%, respectively [50]. The pharmacological properties of most drug $N^+$-glucuronides have not yet been determined, but the $N^+$-glucuronides of arylamines have carcinogenic properties. In particular, $N^+$-glucuronides formed in the liver can be hydrolyzed in acidic urine to a reactive electrophilic intermediate that attacks the bladder epithelium [62].

### Sulfonation

Sulfonation is catalyzed by sulfotransferases (STs) that metabolize phenols, hydroxylamines, or alcohols to sulfate esters as shown in Scheme 11.15, converting somewhat polar to very polar functionalities that are fully ionized at neutral pH. In humans, the SULT1, SULT2, and SULT4 families contain at least 13 subfamilies [63]. Broadly, the subfamilies are either cytosolic

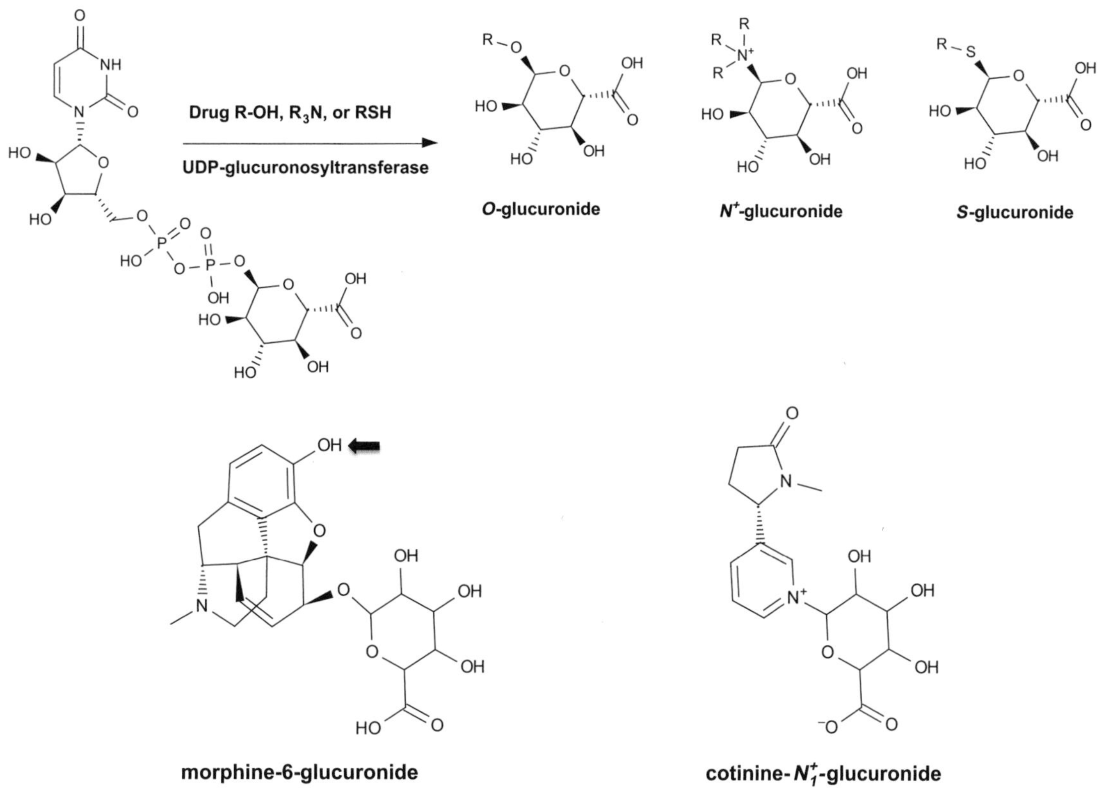

*O*-glucuronide    *N*⁺-glucuronide    *S*-glucuronide

morphine-6-glucuronide    cotinine-*N*₁⁺-glucuronide

**SCHEME 11.14** Glucuronidation of oxygen-, nitrogen-, and sulfur-containing drugs enhances their polarity and water solubility. Morphine-6-glucuronide is an example of an alcohol *O*-glucuronide; cotinine-$N_1^+$-glucuronide is an example of a quaternary amine N-linked glucuronide. The major metabolite of morphine is the phenolic morphine-3-glucuronide, with the position of conjugation indicated by an arrow.

and associated with drug metabolism, or membrane-bound, localized in the Golgi apparatus, and associated with sulfonation of glycoproteins, proteins, and glycosaminoglycans [64]. The STs are widely distributed in human tissues. Eleven cytosolic ST isoforms have been identified and characterized in human tissue that catalyze sulfonation of endogenous phenols, hydroxy steroids, iodothyronines, and catecholamines [63].

By analogy to glucuronidation, sulfonated drug metabolites may be pharmacologically more active than their respective parent drugs. For example, minoxidil (shown in Scheme 11.15), when applied to the scalp for the treatment of baldness, requires bioactivation by STs present in hair follicles [65, 66]. Minoxidil sulfate is a potent vasodilator, apparently because it is a potassium channel agonist, and was initially developed as an antihypertensive agent before its hair-growing properties were noted.

## Acetylation

The acetyl transferase enzymes are cytosolic and found in many tissues, including liver, small intestine, blood, and kidney. Acetylation substrates are aromatic

or aliphatic amines, or hydroxyl or sulfhydryl groups (Scheme 11.16).

The *N*-acetyltransferase (NAT) enzymes have been highly characterized in humans for the historical reason that isoniazid, an NAT substrate, has played a pivotal role in treating patients with tuberculosis. The major route of metabolism of isoniazid is through acetylation (Scheme 11.16).

In treating Caucasian and black patients with isoniazid, it was noted that the half-life of the parent drug was 70 minutes in about one-half of the patients (*rapid acetylators*) and 3 hours in the other half (*slow acetylators*). There are two NAT families of enzymes, NAT1 and NAT2, which are distinguished by their preferential acetylation of *p*-aminosalicylic acid (NAT1) or sulfamethazine (NAT2). As discussed in Chapter 13, isoniazid is a substrate for NAT2, a highly polymorphic enzyme resulting from at least 20 different NAT2 alleles. Slow acetylators are homozygous for the NAT2 slow acetylator allele(s); rapid acetylators are homozygous or heterozygous for the fast NAT2 acetylator allele. There are clinical consequences of fast and slow acetylation from the different blood levels of isoniazid that result from patient

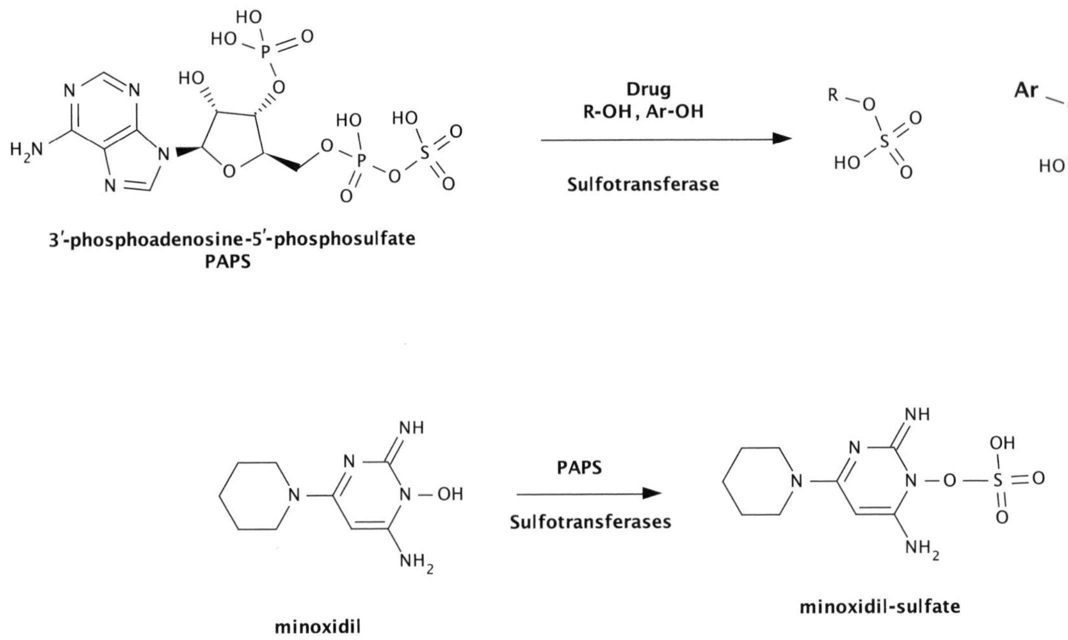

**SCHEME 11.15** Sulfonation requires activated sulfate (PAPS) and one of a family of STs to conjugate with an alcohol, phenol, or aromatic hydroxy function. Minoxidil is an example of a drug activated by sulfonation, as only minoxidil sulfate is taken up into hair follicles.

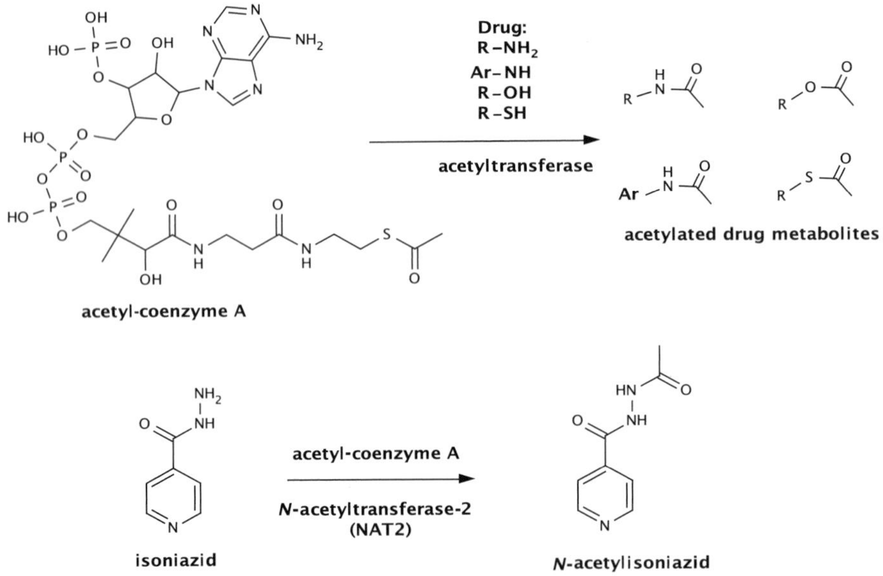

**SCHEME 11.16** Drugs containing primary or secondary aliphatic or aromatic amines, aliphatic alcohols, or thiols are substrates for acetylation catalyzed by a variety of acetyltransferases. Acetylation is a major route of metabolism of isoniazid.

differences in metabolism. Side effects such as peripheral neuropathy [67] and hepatitis [68] are more frequent in slow acetylators.

The Phase II acetylation of aromatic hydroxyl-amines, the products of Phase I metabolism of aromatic amines, constitutes a toxic metabolic pathway that has been implicated in carcinogenesis as illustrated in Scheme 11.17 for PhIP, an aryl amine present in cooked meats. Rapid NAT2 acetylators have been shown to have an increased risk of colon cancer. The mechanism of this toxicity has implicated the intermediacy of the reactive nitrenium ion, which is formed spontaneously by heterolytic cleavage from unstable acetylated, sulfonated, or

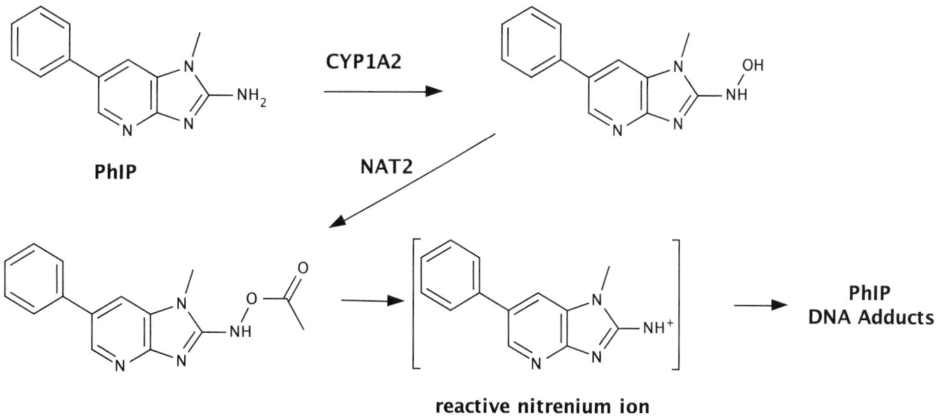

**SCHEME 11.17** PhIP is a food-derived aryl amine, carcinogenic after O-acetylation of its *N*-hydroxy metabolite by NAT2.

other activated aromatic hydroxylamines [69, 70]. Damaging DNA adducts result from nitrenium ion intermediates.

## ADDITIONAL EFFECTS ON DRUG METABOLISM

### Enzyme Induction and Inhibition

The effect of repeated doses of a drug, or of another drug or dietary or environmental constituent on that drug, may be to enhance or inhibit the metabolism of the drug. As discussed in Chapter 15, both enzyme induction and inhibition are important causes of drug interactions. Phenobarbital is prototypical of one general type of inducer; polycyclic aromatic hydrocarbons are representative of another class that affects different CYPs. The mechanism for environmental and drug induction of CYPs involves the intermediacy of ligand-regulated transcription factors. The pregnane X receptor (PXR) and the constitutive androstane receptor (CAR) are both heterodimers with the retinoid X receptor. PXR and CAR are highly expressed in liver and intestine, and seem to have evolved to exhibit protective and non-specific responses to a very wide range of exogenous compounds, as shown in Figure 11.3 [71].

### Species

Different species metabolize drugs to produce varying and characteristic profiles with regard to percentages of metabolite formed in both Phase I and II reactions. This has long been recognized, but it is now known that there is considerable genetic variability in the primary structures of the CYPs and in their regulatory control through DNA- and ligand-binding domains of the PXR and CAR transcription factor receptors. The human and rhesus PXR receptors share 100% homology in their DNA-binding domain, and 95% homology in their ligand-binding domain. In contrast, rats and humans share 96% in their DNA-binding and 76% homology in their ligand-binding domains. The human CAR receptor DNA-binding domain has 66% homology with the human PXR domain and there is only 45% homology in the ligand-binding domains, allowing for considerable diversity in PXR and CAR-mediated responses to different compounds [71]. Metabolism studies conducted in rodents, dogs, monkeys, and other species may be useful in establishing guidelines for likely drug effects in humans, but rarely can be used for predictive interspecies scaling, a topic discussed in Chapter 32.

Guengerich [72] has reviewed several studies of interspecies activities of CYP isoforms. For example, CYP1A2 has been purified and structurally characterized from rats, rabbits, mice, and humans. The different CYP1A2 isoforms catalyze most of the same biotransformations, but there are cases in which the rat and human isoforms differ in substrate activation. Considering that rat and human CYP1A2 are only 75% homologous in amino acid sequence, it is not surprising that their activities differ. Even single amino acid mutation in rat CYP1A2 results in significant changes in catalytic activity. Monkeys lack CYP1A2, a critical issue in the choice of this animal for cancer bioassays. Interspecies variation in the CYP3A subfamilies provides an especially important example because CYP3A4 is involved in the oxidation of 59% of the drugs used today. Humans express CYPs 3A4, 3A5, and 3A7 (the latter in fetal tissue and placenta); rats express CYPs 3A1, 3A2, 3A9, 3A18, and 3A6; rabbits express only CYP3A6. Such genetically

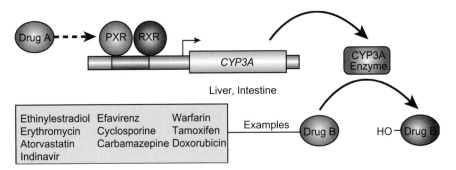

**FIGURE 11.3**  Mechanistic basis of enzyme induction resulting from drug–drug interactions. The orphan nuclear pregnane X receptor (PXR) is a transcription factor that forms a heterodimer with the nuclear retinoid X receptor (RXR) to regulate expression of the CYP3A gene. Drug A binds to PXR and induces expression of the CYP3A enzyme, thereby accelerating metabolism of drug B. Reproduced with permission from Wilson TM, Kliewer SA. Nat Rev Drug Discov 2002;1:259–66 [71].

determined enzyme differences are reflected in other drug-metabolizing enzymes and in their responses to inducers and inhibitors, further complicating extrapolation of drug metabolism between species [73–75].

There are two emerging animal models that better replicate human drug metabolism – transgenic humanized mice, as reviewed by Cheung *et al.* [76], and chimeric mice with humanized liver, as reviewed by Katoh *et al.* [77]. Transgenic humanized mice, particularly when developed in mice with genetically knocked-out mouse drug-metabolizing enzymes [78], offer the prospect of stable lines of laboratory animal models that express common human CYPs (e.g., CYP1A1/CYP1A2, CYP2E1, CYP2D6, CYP3A4, CYP3A7) which exhibit catalytic activities at levels comparable to those measured in human tissues. The human PXR ligand-activated nuclear receptor and the human peroxisome proliferator (PPAR-alpha) have similarly been expressed in transgenic mice, enabling the observation of drug–drug interactions that otherwise could not be directly studied in laboratory animals [76]. Transgenic humanized mice express the humanized genes in intestine as well as liver, making them suitable for certain additional pharmacokinetic studies.

The development of chimeric mice, in which mouse liver has been populated with human hepatocytes thereby replacing more than 90% of mouse liver, effectively introduces all the human drug-metabolizing enzymes that are contained within the human donor hepatocytes. The resulting animals exhibit a humanized profile of drug metabolism (Phase I and Phase II enzymes), induction and inhibition of liver drug-metabolizing enzymes, making them potentially useful for assessing drug interactions and liver metabolism *in vivo* [77]. In contrast to transgenic mice that can be bred and widely distributed, the availability of chimeric mice is constrained because they must be generated *de novo*. In addition, because they reflect the variability inherent in hepatocytes from a single human donor, comprehensive drug metabolism assessment would require testing in a population of chimeric mice generated from different human donors.

## Sex

The effects of sex on drug disposition and pharmacokinetics have been incompletely evaluated but may be significant. In addition, the contribution of sex differences is sometimes difficult to separate from the major complicating effects of dietary and environmental inducers and inhibitors on drug-metabolizing enzymes. Sex differences in drug metabolism are considered in detail in Chapter 23.

## Age

The effects of age on drug metabolism are discussed in specific chapters dealing with pediatric (Chapter 25) and geriatric (Chapter 26) clinical pharmacology. The most significant age differences are expressed developmentally in that drug-metabolizing enzyme systems frequently are immature in neonates. An important example of this is provided by UDP-glucuronosyltransferase. Particularly in premature infants, hepatic UDP-glucuronosyltransferase activity is markedly decreased and does not reach adult levels until 14 weeks after birth [79]. This results in increased serum levels of unconjugated bilirubin and a greater risk of potentially fatal kernicterus, which is likely when the serum bilirubin levels exceed 30 mg/dL. Low conjugation capacity can be exacerbated by concurrent therapy with sulfonamides, which compete with bilirubin for albumin binding, and can be ameliorated either by prenatal therapy of the mother or by postnatal therapy of the infant with phenobarbital to stimulate the gene transcription of CYPs and UDP-glucuronosyltransferase. However, phenobarbital therapy is no longer favored as a pharmacological approach to this problem because prenatal therapy with phenobarbital results in a significant decrease in prothrombin levels and because postnatal phototherapy is much more effective [80, 81].

# REFERENCES

[1] Williams RT. Detoxication mechanisms. The metabolism and detoxication of drugs, toxic substances and other organic compounds. 2nd ed. London: Chapman and Hall Ltd; 1959.

[2] Holtzman JL. The role of covalent binding to microsomal proteins in the hepatotoxicity of acetaminophen. Drug Metab Rev 1995;27:277–97.

[3] Nelson SD. Mechanisms of the formation and disposition of reactive metabolites that can cause acute liver injury. Drug Metab Rev 1995;27:147–77.

[4] Rumack BH. Acetaminophen overdose. Am J Med 1983; 75:104–12.

[5] Chen C, Krausz KW, Idle JR, Gonzalez FJ. Identification of novel toxicity-associated metabolites by metabolomics and mass isotopomer analysis of acetaminophen metabolism in wild-type and Cyp2e1-null mice. J Biol Chem 2008;283: 4543–59.

[6] Mautz FR. Reduction of cardiac irritability by the epicardial and systemic administration of drugs as a protection in cardiac surgery. J Thoracic Surg 1936;5:612.

[7] Mark LC, Kayden HJ, Steele JM, Cooper JR, Berlin I, Rovenstine EA, et al. The physiological disposition and cardiac effects of procaine amide. J Pharmacol Exp Ther 1951;102:5–15.

[8] Atkinson AJJ, Ruo TI, Piergies AA. Comparison of the pharmacokinetic and pharmacodynamic properties of procainamide and N-acetylprocainamide. Angiology 1988;39:655–67.

[9] Nassar AF. Drug metabolism handbook: Concepts and applications. Hoboken, NJ: Wiley; 2009.

[10] Baselt RC. Disposition of toxic drugs and chemicals in man. 9th ed. Foster City, CA: Biomedical Publications; 2011.

[11] Rendic S. Summary of information on human CYP enzymes: Human P450 metabolism data. Drug Metab Rev 2002;34:83–448.

[12] Rendic S, Di Carlo FJ. Human cytochrome P450 enzymes: A status report summarizing their reactions, substrates, inducers, and inhibitors. Drug Metab Rev 1997;29:413–580.

[13] Czekaj P, Wiaderkiewicz A, Florek E, Wiaderkiewicz R. Tobacco smoke-dependent changes in cytochrome P450 1A1, 1A2, and 2E1 protein expressions in fetuses, newborns, pregnant rats, and human placenta. Arch Toxicol 2005;79:13–24.

[14] Lieber CS. Cytochrome P-4502E1: Its physiological and pathological role. Physiol Rev 1997;77:517–44.

[15] Guengerich FP, Rendic S. Update information on drug metabolism systems – 2009. Part I. Curr Drug Metab 2010;11:1–3.

[16] Rendic S, Guengerich FP. Update information on drug metabolism systems – 2009, Part II: Summary of information on the effects of diseases and environmental factors on human cytochrome P450 (CYP) enzymes and transporters. Curr Drug Metab 2010;11:4–84.

[17] Bailey DG, Malcolm J, Arnold O, Spence JD. Grapefruit juice–drug interactions. Br J Clin Pharmacol 1998;46:101–10.

[18] Lown KS, Bailey DG, Fontana RJ, Janardan SK, Adair CH, Fortlage LA, et al. Grapefruit juice increases felodipine oral availability in humans by decreasing intestinal CYP3A protein expression. J Clin Invest 1997;99:2545–53.

[19] Takanaga H, Ohnishi A, Murakami H, Matsuo H, Higuchi S, Urae A, et al. Relationship between time after intake of grapefruit juice and the effect on pharmacokinetics and pharmacodynamics of nisoldipine in healthy subjects. Clin Pharmacol Ther 2000;67:201–14.

[20] Malhotra S, Bailey DG, Paine MF, Watkins PB. Seville orange juice–felodipine interaction: Comparison with dilute grapefruit juice and involvement of furocoumarins. Clin Pharmacol Ther 2001;69:14–23.

[21] Honda Y, Ushigome F, Koyabu N, Morimoto S, Shoyama Y, Uchiumi T, et al. Effects of grapefruit juice and orange juice components on P-glycoprotein- and MRP2-mediated drug efflux. Br J Pharmacol 2004;143:856–64.

[22] Bailey DG, Dresser GK. Interactions between grapefruit juice and cardiovascular drugs. Am J Cardiovasc Drugs 2004;4:281–97.

[23] Guengerich FP. Common and uncommon cytochrome P450 reactions related to metabolism and chemical toxicity. Chem Res Toxicol 2001;14:611–50.

[24] Guengerich FP. Mechanisms of cytochrome P450 substrate oxidation: MiniReview. J Biochem Mol Toxicol 2007;21:163–8.

[25] Hamman MA, Thompson GA, Hall SD. Regioselective and stereoselective metabolism of ibuprofen by human cytochrome P450 2C. Biochem Pharmacol 1997;54:33–41.

[26] Davies NM. Clinical pharmacokinetics of ibuprofen. The first 30 years. Clin Pharmacokinet 1998;34:101–54.

[27] Daly JW, Jerina DM, Witkop B. Arene oxides and the NIH shift: The metabolism, toxicity and carcinogenicity of aromatic compounds. Experientia 1972;28:1129–49.

[28] Komatsu T, Yamazaki H, Asahi S, Gillam EM, Guengerich FP, Nakajima M, et al. Formation of a dihydroxy metabolite of phenytoin in human liver microsomes/cytosol: Roles of cytochromes P450 2C9, 2C19, and 3A4. Drug Metab Dispos 2000;28:1361–8.

[29] Billings RE, Fischer LJ. Oxygen-18 incorporation studies of the metabolism of phenytoin to the catechol. Drug Metab Dispos 1985;13:312–7.

[30] Lu W, Uetrecht JP. Peroxidase-mediated bioactivation of hydroxylated metabolites of carbamazepine and phenytoin. Drug Metab Dispos 2008;36:1624–36.

[31] Munns AJ, De Voss JJ, Hooper WD, Dickinson RG, Gillam EM. Bioactivation of phenytoin by human cytochrome P450: Characterization of the mechanism and targets of covalent adduct formation. Chem Res Toxicol 1997;10:1049–58.

[32] Li XQ, Björkman A, Andersson TB, Ridderström M, Masimirembwa CM. Amodiaquine clearance and its metabolism to N-desethylamodiaquine is mediated by CYP2C8: A new high affinity and turnover enzyme-specific probe substrate. J Pharmacol Exp Ther 2002;300:399–407.

[33] Walsky RL, Obach RS. Validated assays for human cytochrome P450 activities. Drug Metab Dispos 2004;32:647–60.

[34] Guengerich FP, Yun CH, Macdonald TL. Evidence for a 1-electron oxidation mechanism in N-dealkylation of N,N-dialkylanilines by cytochrome P450 2B1. Kinetic hydrogen isotope effects, linear free energy relationships, comparisons with horseradish peroxidase, and studies with oxygen surrogates. J Biol Chem 1996;271:27321–9.

[35] Buehler BA, Rao V, Finnell RH. Biochemical and molecular teratology of fetal hydantoin syndrome. Neurol Clin 1994; 12:741–8.

[36] Kitteringham NR, Davis C, Howard N, Pirmohamed M, Park BK. Interindividual and interspecies variation in hepatic microsomal epoxide hydrolase activity: Studies with cis-stilbene oxide, carbamazepine 10, 11-epoxide and naphthalene. J Pharmacol Exp Ther 1996;278:1018–27.

[37] Martz F, Failinger C, Blake DA. Phenytoin teratogenesis: Correlation between embryopathic effect and covalent binding of putative arene oxide metabolite in gestational tissue. J Pharmacol Exp Ther 1977;203:231–9.

[38] Gaedigk A, Leeder JS, Grant DM. Tissue-specific expression and alternative splicing of human microsomal epoxide hydrolase. DNA Cell Biol 1997;16:1257–66.

[39] Liang SH, Hassett C, Omiecinski CJ. Alternative promoters determine tissue-specific expression profiles of the human microsomal epoxide hydrolase gene (EPHX1). Mol Pharmacol 2005;67:220–30.

[40] Winter HR, Wang Y, Unadkat JD. CYP2C8/9 mediate dapsone N-hydroxylation at clinical concentrations of dapsone. Drug Metab Dispos 2000;28:865–8.

[41] Bordin L, Fiore C, Zen F, Coleman MD, Ragazzi E, Clari G. Dapsone hydroxylamine induces premature removal of human erythrocytes by membrane reorganization and antibody binding. Br J Pharmacol 2010;161:1186–99.

[42] Wojcikowski J, Boksa J, Daniel WA. Main contribution of the cytochrome P450 isoenzyme 1A2 (CYP1A2) to N-demethylation and 5-sulfoxidation of the phenothiazine neuroleptic chlorpromazine in human liver – a comparison with other phenothiazines. Biochem Pharmacol 2010;80:1252–9.

[43] Hutt AJ, Caldwell J, Smith RL. The metabolism of [carboxyl-$^{14}$C]aspirin in man. Xenobiotica 1982;12:601–10.

[44] van Miert AS. The sulfonamide–diaminopyrimidine story. J Vet Pharmacol Ther 1994;17:309–16.

[45] Saha JR, Butler VPJ, Neu HC, Lindenbaum J. Digoxin-inactivating bacteria: Identification in human gut flora. Science 1983;220:325–7.

[46] Bizjak ED, Mauro VF. Digoxin–macrolide drug interaction. Ann Pharmacother 1997;31:1077–9.

[47] Cashman JR. Human flavin-containing monooxygenase (form 3): Polymorphisms and variations in chemical metabolism. Pharmacogenomics 2002;3:325–39.

[48] Krueger SK, Williams DE. Mammalian flavin-containing monooxygenases: Structure/function, genetic polymorphisms and role in drug metabolism. Pharmacol Ther 2005;106:357–87.

[49] Hodgson E, Rose RL, Cao Y, Dehal SS, Kupfer D. Flavin-containing monooxygenase isoform specificity for the N-oxidation of tamoxifen determined by product measurement and NADPH oxidation. J Biochem Mol Toxicol 2000;14:118–20.

[50] Tricker AR. Nicotine metabolism, human drug metabolism polymorphisms, and smoking behaviour. Toxicology 2003; 183:151–73.

[51] Park SB, Jacob Pr, Benowitz NL, Cashman JR. Stereoselective metabolism of (S)-(−)-nicotine in humans: formation of trans-(S)-(−)-nicotine N-1'-oxide. Chem Res Toxicol 1993;6:880–8.

[52] Youdim M, Edmondson D, Tipton K. The therapeutic potential of monoamine oxidase inhibitors. Nat Rev Neurosci 2006;7: 295–309.

[53] Šebela M, Tylichová M, Peč P. Inhibition of diamine oxidases and polyamine oxidases by diamine-based compounds. J Neural Transm 2007;114:793–8.

[54] Radominska-Pandya A, Bratton S, Little JM. A historical overview of the heterologous expression of mammalian UDP-glucuronosyltransferase isoforms over the past twenty years. Curr Drug Metab 2005;6:141–60.

[55] Wells PG, Mackenzie PI, Chowdhury JR, Guillemette C, Gregory PA, Ishii Y, et al. Glucuronidation and the UDP-glucuronosyltransferases in health and disease. Drug Metab Dispos 2004;32:281–90.

[56] Buchheit D, Schmitt EI, Bischoff D, Ebner T, Bureik M. S-Glucuronidation of 7-mercapto-4-methylcoumarin by human UDP glycosyltransferases in genetically engineered fission yeast cells. Biol Chem 2011;392:1089–95.

[57] Smith TW, Binning AR, Dahan A. Efficacy and safety of morphine-6-glucuronide (M6G) for postoperative pain relief: A randomized, double-blind study. Eur J Pain 2009;13:293–9.

[58] Christrup LL, Sjøgren P, Jensen NH, Banning AM, Elbaek K, Ersbøll AK. Steady-state kinetics and dynamics of morphine in cancer patients: Is sedation related to the absorption rate of morphine? J Pain Symptom Manage 1999;18:164–73.

[59] Romberg R, Olofsen E, Sarton E, den Hartigh J, Taschner PE, Dahan A. Pharmacokinetic–pharmacodynamic modeling of morphine-6-glucuronide-induced analgesia in healthy volunteers: Absence of sex differences. Anesthesiology 2004;100: 120–33.

[60] Hawes EM. N+-glucuronidation, a common pathway in human metabolism of drugs with a tertiary amine group. Drug Metab Dispos 1998;26:830–7.

[61] Ketola RA, Hakala KS. Direct analysis of glucuronides with liquid chromatography-mass spectrometric techniques and methods. Curr Drug Metab 2010;11:561–82.

[62] Al-Zoughool M, Succop P, Desai P, Vietas J, Talaska G. Effect of N-glucuronidation on urinary bladder genotoxicity of 4-aminobiphenyl in male and female mice. Environ Toxicol Pharmacol 2006;22:153–9.

[63] Gamage N, Barnett A, Hempel N, Duggleby RG, Windmill KF, Martin JL, et al. Human sulfotransferases and their role in chemical metabolism. Toxicol Sci 2006;90:5–22.

[64] Kauffman FC. Sulfonation in pharmacology and toxicology. Drug Metab Rev 2004;36:823–43.

[65] Baker CA, Uno H, Johnson GA. Minoxidil sulfation in the hair follicle. Skin Pharmacol 1994;7:335–9.

[66] Buhl AE, Waldon DJ, Baker CA, Johnson GA. Minoxidil sulfate is the active metabolite that stimulates hair follicles. J Invest Dermatol 1990;95:553–7.

[67] Holdiness MR. Neurological manifestations and toxicities of the antituberculosis drugs. A review. Med Toxicol 1987; 2:33–51.

[68] Dickinson DS, Bailey WC, Hirschowitz BI, Soong SJ, Eidus L, Hodgkin MM. Risk factors for isoniazid (NIH)-induced liver dysfunction. J Clin Gastroenterol 1981;3:271–9.

[69] Cui L, Sun HL, Wishnok JS, Tannenbaum SR, Skipper PL. Identification of adducts formed by reaction of N-acetoxy-3,5-dimethylaniline with DNA. Chem Res Toxicol 2007;20:1730–6.

[70] Kim D, Guengerich FP. Cytochrome P450 activation of arylamines and heterocyclic amines. Annu Rev Pharmacol Toxicol 2005;45:27–49.

[71] Wilson TM, Kliewer SA. PXR, CAR and drug metabolism. Nat Rev Drug Discov 2002;1:259–66.

[72] Guengerich FP. Comparisons of catalytic selectivity of cytochrome P450 subfamily enzymes from different species. Chem Biol Interact 1997;106:161–82.

[73] Bogaards JJ, Bertrand M, Jackson P, Oudshoorn MJ, Weaver RJ, van Bladeren PJ, et al. Determining the best animal model for human cytochrome P450 activities: A comparison of mouse, rat, rabbit, dog, micropig, monkey and man. Xenobiotica 2000;30:1131–52.

[74] Skaanild MT. Porcine cytochrome P450 and metabolism. Curr Pharm Des 2006;12:1421–7.

[75] Soucek P, Zuber R, Anzenbacherova E, Anzenbacher P, Guengerich FP. Minipig cytochrome P450 3A, 2A and 2C enzymes have similar properties to human analogs. BMC Pharmacol 2001;1:11.

[76] Cheung C, Gonzalez FJ. Humanized mouse lines and their application for prediction of human drug metabolism and toxicological risk assessment. J Pharmacol Exp Ther 2008; 327:288–99.

[77] Katoh M, Tateno C, Yoshizato K, Yokoi T. Chimeric mice with humanized liver. Toxicology 2008;246:9–17.

[78] Scheer N, Kapelyukh Y, McEwan J, Beuger V, Stanley L, Rode A, et al. Modeling human cytochrome P450 2D6 metabolism and drug–drug interaction by a novel panel of knockout and humanized mouse lines. Mol Pharmacol 2012;81:63–72.

[79] Gourley GR. Bilirubin metabolism and kernicterus. Adv Pediatr 1997;44:173–229.

[80] Bhutani V, Maisels M, Stark A, Buonocore G. Management of jaundice and prevention of severe neonatal hyperbilirubinemia in infants ≥ 35 weeks gestation. Neonatology 2008; 94:63–7.

[81] Rubaltelli FF. Current drug treatment options in neonatal hyperbilirubinaemia and the prevention of kernicterus. Drugs 1998;56:23–30.

[82] Snyder R. Cytochrome P450, the oxygen-activating enzyme in xenobiotic metabolism. Toxicol Sci 2000;58:3–4.

# 12

# Methods of Analysis of Drugs and Drug Metabolites

Sanford P. Markey

*Laboratory of Neurotoxicology, National Institute of Mental Health, National Institutes of Health, Bethesda, MD 20892*

## INTRODUCTION

Pharmacokinetics requires the determination of concentrations of a drug, its metabolite(s), or an endogenous targeted substance in physiological fluids or tissues, with respect to time. These analytical tasks have stimulated the field of analytical chemistry to devise technologies that are appropriately sensitive, precise, accurate, and matched to the demands for speed and automation – important factors in research and clinical chemistry. During the past decade, the principle determinant influencing the choice of competing analytical technologies has been speed – the coupled need to reduce both the time required for assay development and the assay cycle time for large numbers of samples. As a result, instrumentation that can measure drug concentrations in blood, tissue, and urine with minimal chemical treatment has emerged, and will be discussed in this chapter using recently published examples.

Several terms used frequently in analytical laboratories have significant and specific definitions that are important in the discussion of analytical assays. The *limit of detection* (LOD) is the minimum amount or concentration that can be detected at a defined signal-to-noise ratio (usually 3/1). The *lower limit of quantification* (LLOQ) is the analyte amount or concentration required to give an acceptable level of confidence in the measured analyte quantity, usually 3-fold the limit of detection, or 10-fold background noise. *Sensitivity* of a measurement is the minimum detectable change that can be observed in a specified range. For example, a 1-pg sensitivity may be measured for a pure chemical standard, but in the presence of 1000 pg, the assay

sensitivity is the ability to distinguish between 999, 1000, or 1001 pg. *Selectivity* of an assay is the ability of the technique to maintain a limit of detection independent of the sample's matrix. Phrased another way, selectivity is the ability of an analytical method to differentiate and quantify the analyte in the presence of other components in the sample. Thus, a highly selective assay will not be affected by the presence or type of physiological fluid. *Accuracy* of a method is the ability to measure the true concentration of an analyte, whereas *precision* is the ability to repeat the measurement of the same sample with low variance.

*Reproducibility* differs from precision, connoting variability in single measurements of a series of identical samples as compared to repeated measurements of the same sample. The US Food and Drug Administration and the corresponding European agencies have recognized the need to establish standardized definitions and practices for analytical methods. There are several Internet sites containing documentation describing terms and practices consistent with regulatory agency guidelines (for example, www.fda.gov/cder/guidance/, and www.nmschembio.org.uk/Index.aspx). The FDA produced a useful reference defining standard nomenclature and acceptable practices for bioanalytical method development in 2001 [1], and the examples chosen here are consistent with that documentation.

## CHOICE OF ANALYTICAL METHODOLOGY

The types of information required largely determine the choices of analytical methodology available.

Pharmacokinetic studies for new chemical entities require determinations of the administered drug and its metabolites. Selective techniques capable of distinguishing between parent drug and metabolites are necessary. For some marketed drugs, good medical practice requires measurements to determine whether patient blood concentrations are within the desired therapeutic index. Instrumentation and immunoassay kits are commercially available for highly prescribed medications with narrow therapeutic indices, as well as for drugs of abuse.

The scale of a planned pharmacokinetic study further determines the assay methodologies to be considered. For a typical pharmacokinetic study of a new chemical entity, the analyst must choose methods suitable for analyzing at least 30–50 samples/patient plus 10–15 standards and procedural blanks. Quality control measures may require an additional 10–15 samples containing pooled and previously analyzed samples that permit assessment of run-to-run reproducibility. To maximize instrumental efficiency, analysts commonly choose to process more than a single patient's samples at one time, resulting in runs usually containing 100–600 patient samples plus standards and quality control samples. Standard curves are determinations of instrument response to different known concentrations of analyte, and are prepared as quality control measures before and after each group of patient samples is analyzed. Highly automated, rugged, and dependable instrumentation is critical because analyses must continue without interruption until the entire sample set has been analyzed. If the assay cycle time is short (few seconds/sample), the instrumentation requires stability of operation over only 5–30 minutes. However, when assays involve multiple stages, such as extraction and chromatographic separation, assay cycle time is more typically 5–30 minutes/sample. The resulting requirement for more than 3 days of instrumental operation may introduce conditions and costs that then serve to limit and define the study protocol. When possible, methods that are selective and sensitive and that do not require separation or chemical reactions are chosen, because time and cost clearly are critical factors. Early in the drug discovery process, any conceivable and accessible analytical method may be chosen. After the potential for commercial development has been demonstrated, time and effort can be directed toward developing simpler and more cost-effective analytical methods that eventually can be marketed as kits for therapeutic drug monitoring.

Over several decades, the pharmaceutical industry research laboratories involved in evaluating new agents have shifted their emphasis from predominantly using ultraviolet (UV) detection to tandem mass spectrometric (MS/MS) detectors with ultra high performance liquid chromatography (LC) separations. The driving force for the utilization of this more expensive instrumentation has been the need to decrease the time allotted for quantitative assay method development, while enhancing the analytical specificity for multiple targets and decreasing the cycle time for analyses. Improvements in mass spectrometric instrumentation have now made LC/MS/MS routine and widely available. The required assay limit of quantification has remained relatively constant for some classes of drugs, typically in the nanogram-to-microgram per milliliter range, but newer drugs are designed to be more selective to minimize side effects, dropping therapeutic indices to picogram per milliliter. Once new drugs have passed through the initial stages of development, then the market for therapeutic drug monitoring dictates that more robust and less expensive technologies be utilized, amenable to instrumentation accessible to hospital clinical chemistry laboratories. Consequently, analytical kits sold for drug monitoring are likely to be based upon immunoassay methodologies. The emerging development of chip-based microanalytical methods suggests that instrumentation for therapeutic drug development and monitoring will continue to evolve but will be based on many of these same separation and spectroscopic principles.

## PRINCIPLES OF ANALYSIS

### Chromatographic Separations

*Chromatography* refers to the separation of materials using their relative solubility and absorption differences in two immiscible phases, one stationary and the other mobile. The defining work of Mikhail Tswett in the early 1900s demonstrated the separation of colored plant pigments on a carbohydrate powder through which hydrocarbon solvents were passed, and he coined the term "chromatography" to describe this phenomenon.

Modern chromatographic science has refined these basic principles in *high pressure liquid chromatography* (HPLC) and ultra-HPLC (UHPLC) [2]. A schematic outline of an HPLC instrument is shown in Figure 12.1. Modern HPLC systems are designed to make separations rapid, reproducible, and sensitive. Particulate adsorption material that is packed in a chromatographic column is engineered to have small, uniform, and rigid (non-compressible) particles, with a size of 3 or 5 μm for HPLC, and 1–2 μm for UHPLC. Columns of 1–5 mm diameter and 5–15 cm long exhibit sufficient

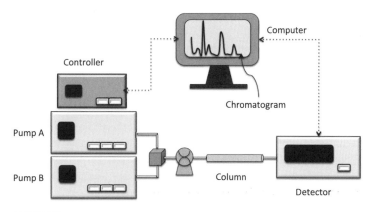

**FIGURE 12.1**   Schematic of HPLC system showing component modules.

resolution to effect useful separations. Columns of such length packed with small particles require high pressure (thousands of pounds per square inch or hundreds of atmospheres; for UHPLC, thousands of atmospheres) to force solvent to flow from 100 nL/min to 1.0 mL/min, requiring inert, precision machined, high-pressure fittings and materials. Pumps are designed to deliver precisely metered, pulseless flow of the mobile phase, composed of either organic and/or aqueous solutions. Pumps are controlled electronically so that a gradient of the mobile-phase solvents from the pumps can be continuously programmed. The polarity, the pH, or the ionic concentration differs in the solutions that are pumped from solvent reservoirs into a mixing chamber and then directed into the column. During an analytical run, the mobile phase can be varied so that materials in a mixture partition with respect to solubility in the mobile phase and adsorption on the stationary phase. When a component is more soluble in the mobile phase than in the film on the particle, it will elute from the column and be detected with respect to a characteristic chemical property, such as UV absorption.

The popularity and acceptance of HPLC and UHPLC in clinical assays is due to the versatility and wide applicability of the methodology. Most pharmaceuticals are small molecules ($< 1000$ Da) with some lipid solubility. They commonly share the property that they adsorb to silica particles coated with stable organic hydrocarbon films (C18, typically) and can then be eluted when the organic content of the mobile phase is increased. Consequently, a single analytical system can be used for many types of analyses, tailored to each by changing the solvents and gradients. The reproducibility of these separations can be rigorously controlled due to extensive engineering of all of the components in these systems. Reproducibility is especially dependent upon consistent gradient elution and establishing equilibrium

conditions before each run. The most reproducible HPLC separations, termed *isocratic*, use a single solvent during the analysis. However, the complexity of most biological fluids necessitates mobile phase gradient programming to accomplish the desired separations and cleanse the column of adsorbed components from each injected sample. Recently, UHPLC has largely replaced HPLC due to the development of highly reproducible columns and well-controlled pumping systems that produce fast, consistent separations and lower cycle times (1–2 min) for analytical separations.

## Absorption and Emission Spectroscopy

Spectroscopy is the measurement of electromagnetic radiation absorbed, scattered, or emitted by chemical species. Because different chemical species and electromagnetic radiation interact in characteristic ways, it is possible to tailor instrumentation to detect these interactions specifically and quantitatively. A simple absorption spectrophotometer (depicted schematically in Figure 12.2) contains components that are common to many spectroscopic devices, and illustrates many of the basic principles of instrumentation found in analytical biochemistry.

A light source produces radiation over the wavelength region where absorption is to be studied. For the visible spectrum, a source producing radiation between 380 and 780 nm is required; for ultraviolet radiation, 160–400 nm is required. Both can be supplied by hydrogen or deuterium discharge lamps combined with incandescent lamps. A high-quality light source combines brightness with stability to produce a constant source of radiant energy. The monochromator is a wavelength selector (prism or grating), separating the discrete component energies of the light source. The quality of a monochromator is related to its ability to resolve radiation in defined

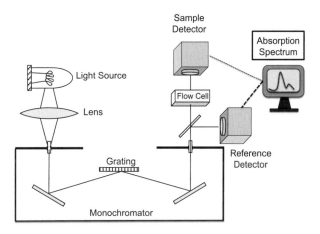

**FIGURE 12.2** Schematic of the components of an absorption spectrophotometer.

wavelengths without loss of intensity. An inexpensive substitute for a monochromator is a filter that transmits a fixed, discrete band of energy. When a discrete wavelength is passed through a solvent or through solvent containing dissolved sample, some of the radiant energy is absorbed, depending upon the chemical structure of the sample. Colored substances, such as hemoglobin, absorb in the visible region. Colorless proteins containing aromatic amino acids absorb UV light at 280 nm; all proteins absorb UV light at 214 nm due to the amide function. Many carbohydrates and lipids do not absorb light in the UV or visible region and are consequently transparent. The absorption characteristics of each chemical structure can be predicted based upon the presence or absence of component functional groups, such as aromatic, unsaturated, and conjugated groups.

The quantity of absorbed energy is proportional to the concentration of the sample, the molar absorptivity of the sample and its solvent, and the distance or path length of the sample container or cell. Molar absorptivity is an expression of the intensity of absorbance of a compound at a given wavelength relative to its molar concentration. The light transmitted through the sample or solvent cell is directed onto a photosensitive detector, converted to an electronic signal, and sent through amplifiers to a recorder or computer. Most spectrophotometers contain optics designed so that the signal from light absorbed by the solvent is compared with and subtracted from the signal from the light absorbed by the sample in an equal quantity of solvent.

The absorbance due to spectrophotometric analysis of a molecular compound in a transparent solvent is termed *optical density*. The measurement of the optical density of a sample at varying wavelengths is the *absorbance spectrum*. The absorbance spectrum of a drug

may not be very different from absorbance spectra of many of the common metabolic intermediates in cellular metabolism. Because endogenous cellular intermediates are present typically in $10^3$–$10^6$ greater concentrations than drugs (typically nanomolar to micromolar), it is usually not possible to use absorbance spectrophotometry alone to detect differences between drug-treated and untreated fluids. However, absorbance spectrophotometers, particularly in the ultraviolet range, are popular detectors for HPLC. For many drugs, the separation power of HPLC may provide sufficient discrimination for quantifying parent drug and metabolites, as illustrated later in this chapter for topically applied moxifloxacin measured within aqueous humor.

Some compounds emit light at characteristic frequencies when radiation of a particular energy is absorbed. The resulting *emission spectrum* is significantly more unique than is an absorbance spectrum. Consequently, the measurement of emitted (fluorescent or phosphorescent) light can frequently be used for sensitive measurements of trace amounts of naturally luminescent compounds. The instrumentation for emission spectrophotometry is similar to absorbance instrumentation in the selection of monochromatic radiation to pass through the sample. Subsequently, a second monochromator or filter is used to collect and separate the radiation emitted prior to detection. Drugs that are naturally fluorescent may be candidates for direct fluorescent assay, but frequently a specific separation, such as HPLC, precedes fluorescent detection in order to lower interference from background. A further way to enhance selectivity is to measure the absorption and emission of polarized light. This technique is appropriate for assaying large molecules with restricted rotational movements, such as antigen–antibody complexes. An antigen, such as a drug, can be labeled with a fluorescent tag, and the fluorescent emission of polarized light is measured in a competitive antibody-binding assay, as described for cyclosporine later in this chapter.

## Immunoaffinity Assays

Antibodies created by the immune response system can be harvested as analytical reagents exhibiting unique specificity for molecular recognition. Antibodies are proteins that exhibit high affinity toward a specific antigen, such as a particular amino acid sequence or chemical structure. The science of generating antibodies to low molecular weight drugs as antigens is highly advanced, beyond the scope of this chapter. In general, drugs are covalently bound to multiple sites on a large carrier protein, and antibodies that recognize the drug functionality are purified. An expanding library of antibodies is commercially available. Additionally, there are commercial services that will generate custom poly- or monoclonal antibodies to any drug or protein.

The analytical use of antibodies is predicated on their specificity and affinity with regard to binding a targeted analyte in the presence of a complex mixture such as serum. This affinity interaction contrasts with chromatographic media, which bind and release components with respect to general physicochemical parameters, such as acidity, size, and lipid solubility. The antibody–antigen interaction is analogous to the selectivity of a molecular lock-and-key, in contrast to the general non-specific interactions of chromatography. The epitope (or key-like) region of an antigen that binds to an antibody can be exquisitely specific. Monoclonal antibodies recognize a single epitope; polyclonal antibodies recognize multiple epitopes. Both types of antibodies are likely to recognize or *cross-react* with metabolites or congeners of an antigen with unpredictable (but reproducible) affinity. Mass production of purified mono- and polyclonal antibodies as reagents affords materials that are used routinely to recognize and separate targeted analytes. Antibodies can be bound to films, papers, surfaces, or chromatographic supports. There are inherent variations in the affinities and properties of antibodies. Consequently, cost and availability of antibody materials are directly related to the degree to which they have been pretested and characterized.

Quantification requires measurement of the extent of antibody–antigen interaction, and the assessment of the amount of bound vs free antigen. Immunoaffinity assays must be coupled with colorimetric, spectroscopic or radiometric detection in order to create an output signal. An assay may incorporate a step to separate the antibody–ligand complex (heterogeneous assay) or may entail direct detection of the extent of antigen–antibody complex formation (homogeneous assay). The latter type of assay is particularly popular in clinical chemistry because of its inherent simplicity. Homogeneous immunoassays may use a marker-labeled antigen (for example, a fluorescent tag on a target analyte drug) to indicate whether binding has decreased or increased, directly reflecting the bound/ free ratio of the drug. Examples of immunoaffinity-based assays are discussed later in this chapter using cyclosporine as a target analyte.

Immunoaffinity-based assays are routinely developed for new biologicals and products of the biotechnology industry as part of their characterization as new agents. In contrast, assays used for pharmacokinetic studies of new chemically synthesized entities are less likely to be immunoaffinity based because they are required to measure accurately the concentration of the administered parent drug without cross-reactivity from drug metabolites that are structurally very similar but exhibit different pharmacological activity. In addition, determination of the structures of these metabolites and, commonly, the measurement of their concentrations is a key part of the analytical requirement associated with the development of chemically synthesized drugs. So immunoaffinity assays for these drugs cannot be interpreted without prior knowledge of their metabolic fate, found by using an assay that is drug and metabolite specific.

## Mass Spectrometry

The analysis of the mass of an organic compound provides information on its component elements and their arrangement. For example, the mass spectrum of water, $H_2O$, in Figure 12.3A illustrates several characteristics of such data. The bar graph in the figure plots the mass-to-charge ratio ($m/z$) on the $x$-axis, and relative ion intensity on the $y$-axis. Water, composed

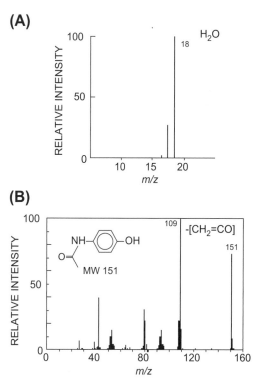

**FIGURE 12.3** Electron ionization mass spectra of water (A) and acetaminophen (B). The intensities are normalized with respect to the predominant ion (base peak), which in the case of water is also the molecular ion with mass/charge ($m/z$).

only of oxygen (16 Da) and two atoms of hydrogen (1 Da), has a molecular weight of 18 Da. In this mass spectrum, $m/z$ 18 is not only the *molecular ion* but also the strongest signal or *base peak*. There are signals seen for unpaired (odd) electron fragment ions containing the components $O^{+\cdot}$ at $m/z$ 16, and $OH^{+\cdot}$ at $m/z$ 17, as well as $HOH^+$. There are no signals at other $m/z$, such as 12, 13, 14, 20, or 21, because elements with those masses are not present. To generalize, mass spectra can be interpreted by a simple arithmetic accounting of elemental constituents.

The same principles of analysis can be applied to the mass spectra of more complex organic molecules. For example, the electron ionization mass spectrum of acetaminophen is shown in Figure 12.3B. A molecular ion is seen for the total assembly of all of the elements $C_8H_9NO_2$ at $m/z$ 151. The strongest signal at $m/z$ 109 derives from the loss of ketene ($CH_2C{=}O$) as a stable neutral from the ionized molecule. The remainder of the fragmentation pattern reveals characteristics of a molecule's architecture, such as the presence of an acetyl function. The interpretation of electron ionization mass spectra can in this way provide rich substructural information.

How mass spectra are produced largely determines the kind of information in the spectra [3]. Mass spectrometry differs from absorbance or emission spectroscopy in that it is a destructive technique, consuming sample used during the measurement process. Mass spectrometry is also a very sensitive technique, requiring as little as a few attomoles ($10^{-18}$ moles or $10^5$ molecules) in the best cases, but more typically needing from 1 to ~10 femtomoles ($10^{-15}$ moles) for the routine quantitative analyses common in the pharmaceutical industry. Accelerator mass spectrometry (AMS) is an alternative technology of particular value to human pharmacokinetic assays because of its high sensitivity. It is discussed separately because it is based on very different principles and instrumentation than those found in typical pharmacology laboratories.

From the overview outline in Figure 12.4, there are several integral components that comprise every mass spectrometer. First, all substances must be ionized in order to be mass analyzed. Neutral molecules must be positively or negatively charged so that electric and magnetic fields can affect the motion of the resulting ions. Second, the ions must enter a mass analyzer in a vacuum chamber maintained at a pressure sufficiently low as to permit ions to travel without interacting with other molecules or ions. Third, there must be a means of ion detection capable of converting the separated ions into electronic signals. Fourth, there

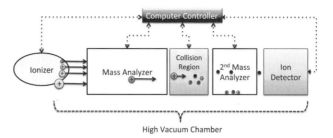

**FIGURE 12.4** Mass spectrometer component overview (note that ion cyclotron resonance and orbitrap instruments combine mass separation and ion detection)

must be controlling electronics, usually integrated with a computer, to regulate the ionization, mass analysis, ion detection, and vacuum systems, and to record and process ion signals.

### Ionization

There are efficient ionization methods for producing ions *in vacuo* of organic compounds of any size or complexity from gases, liquids or solids. Figures 12.5A–C picture three common mechanisms – electron ionization, electrospray ionization, and matrix assisted laser desorption ionization (MALDI) – that are widely used by investigators in clinical pharmacology.

Electron ionization of neutral organic molecules in the vapor phase occurs when electrons emitted from a heated filament remove an electron from the molecule. The resultant odd-electron ions are focused and accelerated into a mass analyzer by electric fields. Electron ionization and a closely related method, chemical ionization, were the principal methods used in clinical pharmacology until around 1990.

However, because most drugs are studied in biological fluids or solubilized extracts of tissues, electrospray ionization has largely replaced electron ionization as the principle method of ionization used in clinical pharmacology. Electrospray ionization of neutral organic molecules in liquid solutions occurs when liquids flow through a conductive needle bearing several thousand volts at atmospheric pressure. The emerging liquid forms a sharp cone, with microdroplets of ion clusters bearing multiple charges and attached solvent molecules. A gas stream dries the clusters and the resulting desolvated singly and multiply charged ions are electronically guided into the vacuum system of the mass analyzer.

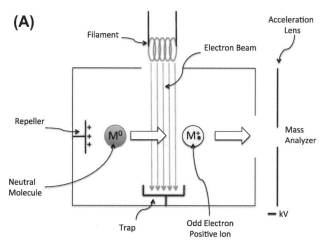

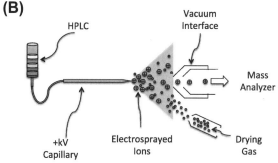

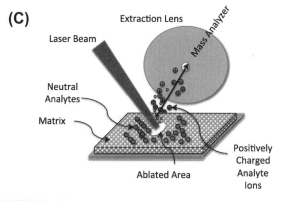

**FIGURE 12.5** Schematic representations of (A) an electron ionization source, (B) an electrospray ionization source, and (C) and a matrix assisted laser desorption ionization (MALDI) source.

MALDI analysis of molecules on specially prepared surfaces provides an alternative soft ionization method of obtaining mass selective information that is location specific, and has become a powerful alternative tool of increasing value in the investigation of new drugs. A directed laser ablates a plume of neutral and ionized species from the surface in a high vacuum chamber. The plume is sampled by ion lenses, and

protonated or cation-attached to Na$^+$ or K$^+$, then extracted into the mass analyzer.

## Mass Analysis

Following ionization, the charged molecular, cluster or fragment ions are accelerated and focused into a mass analyzer. The type of mass analyzer influences the range and quality of the mass spectrum. Some analyzers have a limited mass/charge detection range (for example, $m/z$ 0 to 1000, or 0 to 100,000). Others have limited resolution of $m/z$ (for example, the ability to resolve the difference between $m/z$ 1000 and 1001 in low-resolution mass spectrometry compared to the difference between $m/z$ 1001.000 and 1001.010 in high-resolution mass spectrometry). The first application of mass analysis to pharmacology used magnetic sector mass analyzers in the identification of metabolites of chlorpromazine [4]. This work introduced the concept of *selected ion monitoring* (then termed "mass fragmentography"), a technique of alternating between preselected ions of interest, thereby enhancing sensitivity and making the mass spectrometer a sophisticated gas chromatographic detector. The principles of online chromatography and selected ion monitoring are integral in all modern mass spectrometric instrumentation. Currently, the most commonly used mass analyzers in pharmacology include time-of-flight, quadrupole, and linear ion traps, which are illustrated in Figures 12.6A–C.

The time-of-flight (TOF) mass analyzer (Figure 12.6A) separates ions by accelerating a pulse of ions in vacuum and then measuring their time of arrival at a detector. Because all ions are given the same initial kinetic energy, lighter ions arrive at the detector faster than heavier ions. All ions from a single pulse are analyzed, so there is, in theory, no upper $m/z$ limit on TOF analyzers. Resolution is a function of flight path length and initial position in the beam of pulsed ions. The inherent simplicity, speed (or duty cycle), and mass range of TOF analyzers have resulted in low-cost, high-performance instrumentation for routine analyses.

A quadrupole mass analyzer (Figure 12.6B) separates or filters ions using radio-frequency alternating voltages at a constant direct current potential on paired cylindrical or hyperbolic rods. A continuous beam of ions enters the alternating field region at low energy. Resonant positive ions of a particular $m/z$ ratio traverse the field region through to the detector, oscillating first to poles of negative charge and then, when the field alternates, being drawn toward to the opposite pair of rods. Non-resonant ions collide with the surface of the rods and do not reach the detector.

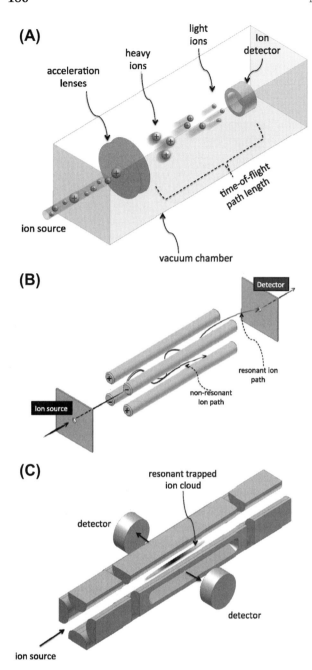

**FIGURE 12.6** Schematic representations of three principles of mass analyzers: (A) Time-of-flight, in which lower *m/z* ions traverse faster than higher *m/z* ions over a fixed path length; (B) quadrupole mass filter, in which potentials on the quadrupole assembly alternate at radiofrequencies to create fields allowing resonant ions of defined *m/z* to traverse to the ion detector, filtering the non-resonant ions; and (C) linear quadrupole mass storage/filter, in which two short quadrupole assemblies are used to guide and constrain selected ions in a central quadrupole assembly, and pulse the accumulated axially resonant ions to detectors through slits in the sides of that center quadrupole. Figures provided by Victoria Pai, Potomac, MD.

Quadrupole mass filters are designed to filter limited *m/z* ranges, typically *m/z* 10 to 2000 for organic ion analysis. Quadrupole analyzers are widely used in clinical pharmacology, especially with electrospray ionization.

A linear quadrupole ion trap mass analyzer (Figure 12.6C) collects ions in stable trajectories using one set of quadrupole rods to confine ions radially, and two additional sets to confine the ions axially. The linear ion trap has replaced the three-dimensional cylindrical ion trap and is now widely used, either separately or as an element in tandem mass spectrometer configurations, due to its power to accumulate and pulse stored ions as described below.

High-resolution mass analysis began in the 1940s with electrical and magnetic sector mass analyzers that utilized conventional electron multiplier ion detectors, but is increasingly the domain of instrumentation that senses ion oscillation, and then converts the resulting frequency measurements to mass using Fourier transforms. An ion cyclotron resonance spectrometer operated in a high field superconducting magnet was invented in 1974 [5], and was the first type of high-resolution instrument to gain wide acceptance in analytical mass spectrometry. However, its requirement for a specialized laboratory environment limited its deployment in pharmacology to academic centers and pharmaceutical company central analytical facilities. The orbitrap mass analyzer was invented in 2000 [6] and uses only electrical fields to cycle ions around an inner electrode, so its lower cost and smaller footprint has made it more widely accessible to pharmacology laboratories.

### Tandem Mass Analysis

Permutation of ionization and mass analyzer alternatives presents many instrument configurations to prospective users, and there continues to be significant instrumentation development leading to new capabilities with different configurations. Consequently, no single ionizer/mass analyzer combination dominates the clinical pharmacology laboratory. However, tandem mass analysis may be the deciding factor in instrument selection. Tandem mass analysis, termed MS/MS, entails the separation of a mass resolved ion beam, its subsequent fragmentation in an ion collision chamber, and further mass analysis to provide mass spectra of these fragment ions. The relationship between the primary ion beam mass spectrum (MS1) and a second stage of analysis (MS2 spectrum) is illustrated in Figure 12.7. In tandem instruments, primary MS1 spectra are acquired in milliseconds, and MS2 spectra are acquired either continuously (TOF

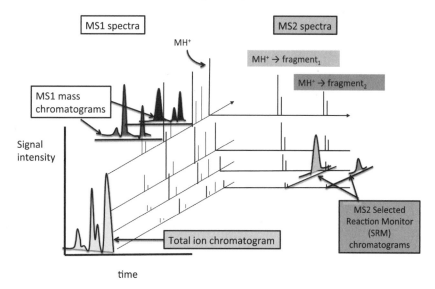

**FIGURE 12.7** The relationship of MS1 and MS2 data from tandem mass spectrometric analyses results in time-dependent three-dimensional arrays of intensity and *m/z* data that can be queried effectively with software to produce chromatograms yielding total ion, MS1 (mass chromatogram) or MS2 (selected reaction monitor) plots.

instruments), or for milliseconds using data-dependent *m/z* selection. When surveying samples of unknown composition, MS1 and MS2 analyses are automated. The stored digital files are subsequently analyzed as a multidimensional data array composed of MS1 mass spectra and chromatograms, and MS2 spectra or their *selected reaction monitoring* (SRM) chromatograms as illustrated in Figure 12.7. Some of the most common tandem mass analyzer configurations are quadrupole–quadrupole–quadrupole (qqq), quadrupole–quadrupole–TOF (qqTOF), TOF/TOF, and linear trap quadrupoles with Fourier transform orbitrap mass analyzers. The qqq configuration is illustrated in Figure 12.8, and is widely used in quantitative pharmacology.

MS/MS analysis significantly increases the selectivity of analytical mass spectrometry by requiring not only that a specific *m/z* is characteristic of a compound, but also that specific *m/z* fragments be present in a characteristic pattern to yield a second product ion. For example, in Figure 12.3B, the primary mass spectrum of acetaminophen is characterized by *m/z* 151 as a base peak with a significant fragment ion at *m/z* 109 which derived from that molecular species. Thus, in a chromatography-MS/MS analysis, an instrument could be set to pass *m/z* 151 in a first stage of analysis and *m/z* 109 in the second stage. The result would be a time-varying signal representing only ions of *m/z* 109 that derived from *m/z* 151, a very stringent criterion for mass detection. Consequently, this particular signal would be detected only when acetaminophen eluted from the chromatograph. Because the chemical background is reduced, MS/MS analyses also frequently have enhanced sensitivity and selectivity when compared to MS analyses.

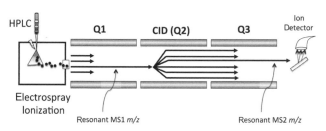

**FIGURE 12.8** HPLC-electrospray ionization-triple quadrupole mass spectrometer configuration used commonly in quantitative studies in clinical pharmacology. HPLC separated components are ionized and vaporized in a high-voltage spray; ions separated by *m/z* in the first quadrupole region (Q1) are collisional dissociated to fragments in the second quadrupole (Q2) and mass analyzed by scanning the third quadrupole (Q3). Resonant ions emerge from Q3 into an electron multiplier detector.

## Accelerator Mass Spectrometry

Over the past 20 years, a new and distinct form of mass spectrometry analysis has been developed that has unique pharmacologic applications. Accelerator mass spectrometry (AMS) is a sensitive and specialized type of mass analysis, capable of detecting amounts of isotope-labeled drugs that are below levels required for either pharmacological effects ($<1\%$, typically 100 µg or less) or conventional scintillation-counter detection, which for an emission rate of one disintegration per second requires $4.3 \times 10^9$ radioactive $^{14}C$ atoms. Because only approximately 1000 $^{14}C$ atoms are required for an accurate AMS measurement, this represents a million-fold sensitivity enhancement compared to scintillation-counter detection. Unlike the conventional organic mass spectrometry analyses described previously, AMS measures not molecules or their structural fragments, but the negatively charged $^{12}C$, $^{13}C$, and $^{14}C$ atoms generated by the complete combustion of an analyte to $CO_2$, followed by its reduction to carbon (graphite). Negative ions sputtered from the graphitized sample are highly accelerated (millions of volts) toward a collision cell, where they are converted to positive ions through a charge-stripping process, and pass through a high-energy analyzing magnet to a Faraday cup detector, where their current can be accurately and precisely determined. The facilities for AMS were developed in national accelerator laboratories and physics departments, but are now commercially available. The basic instrumentation cost remains beyond the resources of individual laboratories or most pharmaceutical research companies. However, good laboratory practice-compliant contracting companies, consortia, and publicly financed facilities offer services for ultrasensitive detection consistent with pharmacokinetic analyses.

## EXAMPLES OF CURRENT ASSAY METHODS

### UHPLC-UV Assays of New Chemical Entities

When beginning investigation of new chemical entities, robust, reproducible quantitative assays are required. It is expected that the developed analytical assays will be scaled to be suitable for thousands of samples, and will be able to accommodate clinical pharmacokinetic studies. Selection of a suitable assay method begins with consideration of chemical characteristics of the drug, and the determination of the likely range of blood and tissue concentration required for pharmacological effect. For chromatographic assays, the analyst then characterizes the chromatography of the analytes, choosing column materials and eluents either recommended for structurally similar compounds or broadly applicable in pharmacology. For example, moxifloxacin (see Figure 12.9) is a fluoroquinolone broad-spectrum antibiotic useful in the treatment of ocular infections. Consequently, an assay was required for the analysis of moxifloxacin in aqueous humor [7]. Moxifloxacin

has ultraviolet absorption maxima at 290 (major) and 340 (minor) nm, due to its aromatic ring and conjugated side chains and atoms, so the investigators selected UHPLC, reasoning that moxifloxacin's ultraviolet absorption could provide sufficient selectivity for the desired pharmacokinetic assays of aqueous humor samples obtained after the drug was administered in solution or with negative- or positive-charged nanoparticles. Chromatographic conditions were required that provided retention and elution of moxifloxacin with symmetrical peak shape and separation. In this case, the investigators used a C18 (bridged ethyl hybrid) reverse phase column (50-mm length × 2.1-mm diameter, with 1.7-µm particles) with a linear gradient in mobile phase composition programmed from 20 to 30% acetonitrile with respect to 0.1% aqueous trifluoroacetic acid, at a constant optimized 50°C. For a specific analyte, the choice of parameters results from iterative trials, with the objective of improving chromatographic separation and peak shape sufficiently to enable quantitative measurement in the biological fluid being sampled. Moxifloxacin has three amines and one carboxylic acid, and, as a result, may chromatograph inconsistently as either a neutral or a cationic species unless pH and ion pairing are controlled. The choice of trifluoracetic acid in the mobile phase ensures ion pairing and pH control, resulting in sharp, symmetrical chromatographic peaks (Figure 12.9).

Direct injection of biological fluids into chromatographic columns is possible, but to preserve the life of the column some type of solvent extraction or pre-filtration is recommended to remove cellular debris or particulate material. After obtaining satisfactory chromatograms of pure analyte, the analyst adds the same quantity of analyte to a blank biological fluid to determine the chromatography and background in the presence of the biological matrix. The chromatographic profile of the biological fluid with and without added analyte standards will determine the necessity for alternative chromatographic conditions, column selection and sample cleanup. For moxifloxacin, 50 µL of aqueous humor was added to 100 µL of acetonitrile, vortex mixed, and the resulting solution filtered through 0.22-µm nylon prior to injection of 5 µL of solution into the UHPLC. This simple sample pretreatment was sufficient for reproducible analyses with detection limits of 0.75 ng/mL and a limit of quantification of 2.5 ng/mL. The UHPLC-UV assay was used to characterize pharmacokinetic profiles of moxifloxacin in rabbit aqueous humor after topical application of drug absorbed to cationic or anionic nanoparticles (CNP, ANP) (Figure 12.9).

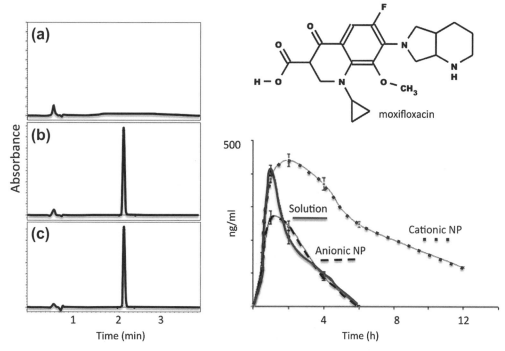

**FIGURE 12.9** *(Upper right)* Structure of moxifloxacin; *(lower right)* concentration vs time curves for three preparations of moxifloxacin (solution, cationic and anionic nanoparticle); *(left)* UHPLC traces showing untreated aqueous humor (a), 400-ng/ml moxifloxacin in aqueous humor (b), and 1 h after cationic moxifloxacin nanoparticle (c). Reproduced with permission from Jain GK, Jain N, Pathan SA. *et al.* J Pharm Biomed Anal 2010;52:110–3 [7].

## UHPLC-MS/MS Assays of New Chemical Entities

An example of a current UHPLC-MS/MS assay is provided by vorapaxar, an orally active antithrombotic agent (Figure 12.10). Its electrospray ionization mass spectrum exhibits a prominent MH+ ion at *m/z* 493, and, when analyzed by MS/MS, loses 46 Da to form a stable *m/z* 447 fragment (Figure 12.10). Tama *et al.* [8] evaluated sample enrichment of vorapaxar from human plasma using solid phase extraction cartridges, but preferred simple protein removal by diluting 100 µL plasma with 500 µL acetonitrile:acetone (95 : 5, v : v) and vortex mixing, followed by refrigeration to precipitate proteins, centrifugation, and, finally, transfer of 200 µL to a fresh well. This procedure was adapted to robotic systems, enabling analysts to scale procedures to automated 96-well plates. A 10-µL aliquot was injected for the UHPLC-MS/MS method that was validated over a concentration range of 1.00–1000 ng/mL. As expected when only protein precipitation was used for sample cleanup, there were copious quantities of potentially interfering phospholipids in each plasma extract. However, the phospholipids were eluted, and a cycle time of 3 minutes/injection was achieved by programming the UHPLC

mobile phase to elute vorapaxar at 1.5 min, and ramping to 98% acetonitrile : methanol : acetic acid (70 : 30 : 0.1, v : v : v) and holding for 1 minute.

Quantitative assays require the analyst to select appropriate compounds to serve as internal standards. A fixed quantity of an internal standard is added to each sample so that the intensity of the signals from the analyte from each sample can be normalized to those from the internal standard and compared to samples analyzed during the same run or from another analytical set on another date. Stable isotope-labeled internal standards result in the generation of linear standard curves, with proportional increases in the ratio of analyte to internal standard with increasing mass of analyte. Data from the standard curve prepared for each sample set are used to convert relative signal response to absolute concentration data. For vorapaxar assays, the investigators had synthesized $^{13}C_6$-(phenyl)-labeled-vorapaxar. A set of 10 different known concentrations of vorapaxar was prepared to construct standard curves covering the sample concentration range of measurement (1–1000 ng/mL).

Stable isotope-labeled internal standards have long been accepted as ideal benchmarks for ratio measurement in mass spectrometry because they

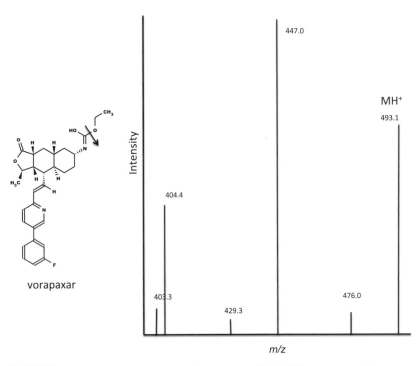

**FIGURE 12.10**  Chemical structure of vorapaxar and the MS2 spectrum of its protonated molecular ion at *m/z* 493. The base peak at *m/z* 447 corresponds to the likely fragmentation of ethanol with a hydrogen atom transfer as indicated in the structure. The internal standard for quantification was vorapaxar labeled with $^{13}C_6$ in the phenyl ring. Reproduced with permission from Tama CI, Shen JX, Schiller JE. J Pharm Biomed Anal 2011;55:349–59 [8].

are not readily separable from their isotopomers, assuming they have been thoroughly mixed and integrated into the fluid being analyzed. Importantly for a substance like vorapaxar, its internal standard differs only in the substitution of $^{13}C_6$ atoms on a phenyl ring, and is identical at all seven stereogenic centers. There are many stable isotope-labeled reagents commercially available, allowing analysts to incorporate $^{13}C$, $^{15}N$, $^{18}O$, and $^2H$ (deuterium) into target analytes to custom-synthesize internal standards without incurring excessive cost. However, caution may need to be exercised with deuterium-labeled standards. Because deuterium is less polar than hydrogen, there may not be co-elution of isotopomers on HPLC, necessitating adjustment during peak area and quantification calculations.

An example of the SRM vorapaxar chromatograms on a triple quadrupole (QQQ) instrument is shown in Figure 12.11. The upper trace was generated by isolation of the protonated $^{13}C_6$ isotope-labeled molecular ion (*m/z* 499) at unit mass resolution in Q1 (or MS1), collisional dissociating to cause fragmentation in Q2, and monitoring the fragment ion *m/z* 453 in Q3 (MS2). The lower trace shows the isolation of MH+ (*m/z* 493) from unlabeled vorapaxar and measuring its

fragmentation to *m/z* 447 at a concentration of 1 ng/mL (LLOQ). Note that both traces superimpose signals recorded, 270 injections apart, indicating the high quality of the signal/noise, reproducibility, and stability of the analyses. The lack of appreciable chemical background at the LLOQ is an impressive characteristic of the high degree of selectivity associated with UHPLC-SRM assays, and a major reason for their wide acceptance for pharmacokinetic studies. Tama *et al.* (personal communication) used this UHPLC-MS/MS assay to analyze over 13,000 samples in approximately 12 different clinical studies of vorapaxar between 2006 and 2011.

## HPLC/MS/MS Quantitative Assays of Cytochrome P450 Enzyme Activity

Knowledge of potential drug–drug interactions has led to a need to assay specific cytochrome P450 (CYP) enzyme activities to determine whether new drug entities have drug-metabolizing enzyme inhibitory properties. Enzyme activity measurements require kinetic assays that will remain highly specific in the presence of the new drug entities that are being evaluated. Each CYP enzyme can be distinguished by

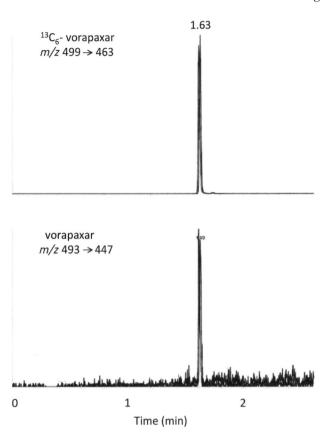

1.63

$^{13}C_6$- vorapaxar
m/z 499 → 463

vorapaxar
m/z 493 → 447

0                    1                    2

Time (min)

**FIGURE 12.11** Superimposition of two traces of vorapaxar chromatograms 270 injections apart in a clinical study analytical run. Upper panel chromatogram is from the labeled internal standard; lower traces are vorapaxar at 1 ng/mL concentration, the LLOQ. Reproduced with permission from Tama CI, Shen JX, Schiller JE. J Pharm Biomed Anal 2011;55:349–59 [8].

a characteristic marker substrate, a compound whose metabolism has been demonstrated to correlate with the concentration of the CYP enzyme protein. That requirement led Walsky and Obach [9] to develop a panel of 12 validated LC/MS/MS assays for 10 of the human CYP enzymes most commonly involved in drug metabolism. The assay of CYP 2B6 activity is described in some detail because it illustrates the principles applied to the separation and analytical steps common to all of the assays. Bupropion hydroxylation is a selective *in vitro* indicator of CYP 2B6 activity [10, 11].

For the enzyme assay, bupropion is added to pooled liver microsomes and incubated for 20 minutes. Incubations are terminated by the addition of an acidic solution containing a fixed quantity of the deuterium-labeled internal standard $^2H_6$-hydroxybupropion. The incubation mixture and appropriate standard curve and control samples are filtered and stored in 96-well plates for automated LC/MS/MS analyses. Once loaded into the LC/MS injection system, the analyses

proceed completely unattended in an automated sequence. HPLC analyses are performed on a short 30-mm reverse phase column with a 3-minute gradient elution to facilitate rapid analytical cycle times. The eluent from the HPLC is diverted to waste except during a time interval bracketing analyte elution. The eluent then is connected to an electrospray needle and the ionized (protonated) analyte and internal standard are transmitted into a triple quadrupole mass analyzer [9]. At a millisecond frequency, preselected ions are alternatively transmitted from the first quadrupole, into a second quadrupole collision chamber, and the resulting fragment ions mass separated and detected in the third quadrupole region. In the case of hydroxybupropion and its isotopomer internal standard, the protonated molecular species at m/z 256 and 262 (Figure 12.12) are alternatively selected and fragmented (Figure 12.13) many times per second. Both hydroxybupropion and its internal standard are collision induced to fragment in the second quadrupole chamber. The characteristic chlorophenylacetyl fragments at m/z 139 are produced and are mass separated from other fragments in third quadrupole. The resulting selected reaction monitoring data can be displayed in a chromatogram format (Figure 12.14). Facile quantification is possible by measuring the ratio of the relative intensity of the signal from unlabeled hydroxybupropion (area = 628) to that from its deuterated isotopomer (area = 96,538). The resulting data are used to construct kinetic profiles. CYP 2B6 was determined to exhibit a $K_m$ of $81.7 \pm 1.3$ and $V_{max}$ of $413 \pm 2$ pmol/mg/min for microsomes pooled from 54 human livers.

Adding varying concentrations of other drug entities to the bupropion assay permits the measurement of their potential inhibitory properties on CYP 2B6 [12]. The investigators surveyed 227 of the most commonly prescribed agents at 7 concentrations (0–30 μM), and found 30 drugs that demonstrated 50% or greater inhibition at 30 μM, 6 of which had an $IC_{50}$ less than 1 μM. The HPLC/MS/MS assays of other CYP enzymes are very similar in principle and use the identical instrumentation but employ different internal standards. As a consequence of the high degree of specificity of MS/MS selected reaction monitoring, batteries of CYP assays can be robotically programmed for high throughput with little additional manpower.

## HPLC/UV and Immunoassays of Cyclosporine: Assays for Therapeutic Drug Monitoring

Cyclosporine (cyclosporine A) is a potent and widely used immunosuppressive agent with a narrow

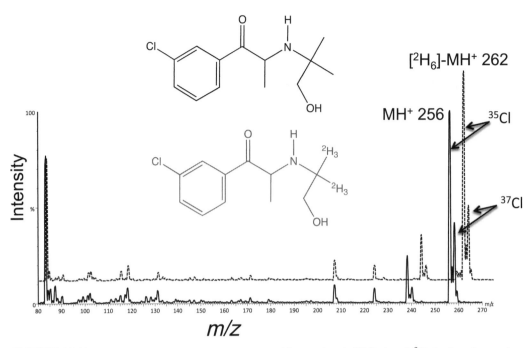

**FIGURE 12.12** Electrospray ionization mass spectra of bupropion *(solid line)* and $^2$H$_6$-hydroxybupropion *(dotted line)*. Note that the protonated molecular ions (MH$^+$ at m/z 256, 262) exhibit characteristic 25% chlorine isotope peaks at m/z 258, 264. The natural abundance of $^{35}$Cl and $^{37}$Cl is reflected also in the MH$^+$-H$_2$O ions at m/z 238 and 244. Data provided by R.L. Walsky and R.S. Obach, Pfizer, New York, NY.

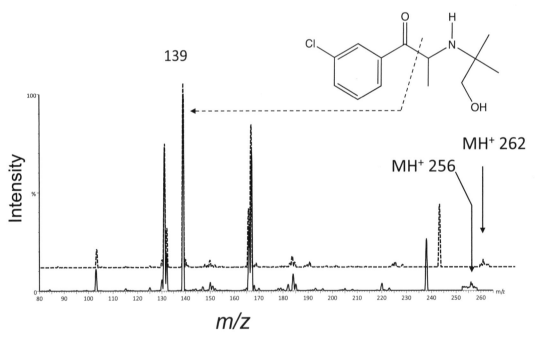

**FIGURE 12.13** Collisional induced MS/MS spectra of the MH$^+$ ions at m/z 256 and 262 of hydroxybupropion *(solid line)* and $^2$H$_6$-hydroxybupropion *(dotted line)*. Note that the fragment ions do not display the characteristic chlorine isotope pattern because only the higher abundance $^{35}$Cl species was selected for MS/MS. The origin of fragments at m/z 167 and 139 is shown; neither retains deuterium atoms present in the internal standard. Data provided by R.L. Walsky and R.S. Obach, Pfizer, New York, NY.

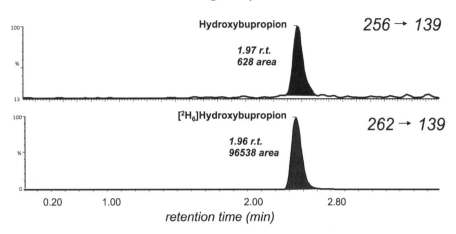

**FIGURE 12.14** Selected reaction chromatograms reflecting the intensity of the transitions *m/z* 256 to 139 and 262 to 139. Note that the peak profiles are free from interference, indicating the specificity and selectivity of the measurement. The internal standard signal is ~153 times the intensity of hydroxybupropion. Data provided by R.L. Walsky and R.S. Obach, Pfizer, New York, NY.

therapeutic index. As a consequence, there is ongoing competition to develop rapid and accurate assays for therapeutic monitoring of transplant patients treated with this drug. This competition produced the refinement and automation of the reference HPLC/UV methods initially developed for cyclosporine, as well as the development of faster, automated assays suitable for use in hospital clinical laboratories. Consideration of the chromatographic and immunoassay methods developed for cyclosporine offers an opportunity to review the process of clinical assay development and maturation. When developing new chemical entities, pharmaceutical researchers pay a premium for the speed of assay development and an assurance of assay selectivity. However, for marketed drugs, clinical laboratories require reliable and accurate assays that are less expensive and less demanding of sophisticated equipment and operator skill.

Cyclosporine is a hydrophobic cyclic peptide of fungal origin and is composed of 11 amino acid residues. The structure of cyclosporine shows that all of the constituent amino acids are aliphatic (Figure 12.15). UV absorbance at 210 nm is due to the amide bonds in the molecule and is consequently not as intense or distinctive as that of many drugs containing aromatic rings. Development of cyclosporine as a pharmaceutical occurred in the 1970s, a period when HPLC/UV, but not LC/MS, methods were available. Consequently, HPLC/UV was the initial benchmark clinical chemical assay method for cylcosporine, and was verified subsequently by comparison with newer LC/MS/MS methods [13, 14].

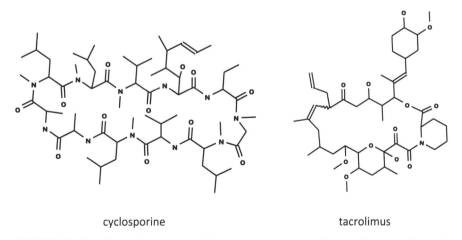

cyclosporine                    tacrolimus

**FIGURE 12.15** Chemical structures of the immunosuppressive drugs cyclosporine *(left)* and tacrolimus *(right)*.

HPLC/UV methods for cyclosporine analyses use whole blood samples with cyclosporine D added as an internal standard [15, 16]. Patient blood samples are diluted with a solution of the internal standard in organic solvents to effect cell lysis, dissociation, and solubilization of the cyclosporine. After centrifugation, the analytes in the supernatant are adsorbed on a solid-phase extraction cartridge, washed, and eluted. Interfering lipids are removed from the eluent by extraction with a hydrocarbon solvent, and the sample is separated on a reverse-phase column at 70°C using isocratic conditions, monitoring UV absorbance at 210 nm. Isocratic elution conditions facilitate faster analytical runs because, as previously noted, there is no time required for resetting gradients and stabilizing the chromatographic conditions. One sample requires 5–15 minutes of chromatography time. The LLOQ of the HPLC/UV method is ~20–45 µg/L, which is acceptable because the therapeutic range is 80–300 µg/L. Cyclosporine HPLC/UV assay methods have been optimized in a variety of research and commercial laboratories. It is possible for future improvements to be made in sample processing, but this assay represents state-of-the-art HPLC/UV analyses in the mid-1990s [15, 16].

Currently, there are several commercial and widely used immunoassays for cyclosporine measurement. Fluorescence polarization immunoassay (FPIA) is one popular technique, typical of a homogeneous immunoassay, and instructive with regard to its principles and limitations. FPIA instrumentation uses a polarized light source to excite emission by a fluorescein-tagged antigen, and quantitation is based on the difference in polarized light emission by antibody-bound and free fluorescent antigen [17, 18]. Because cyclosporine is not fluorescent, the assay is based on competition for binding to a monoclonal antibody between cyclosporine in patient blood samples and a fluorescein-tagged cyclosporine reagent. The degree of polarization of the emitted light depends on the percentage of molecules that are fixed or highly oriented. In the absence of available antibody, the fluorescein-tagged cyclosporine is randomly oriented in solution, whereas binding to a macromolecule has the effect of slowing random molecular motion in solutions. Thus, bound fluorescein-tagged cyclosporine–antibody complexes are preferentially excited because they retain greater orientation to the plane of the incident polarized light and emit this light more efficiently than free fluorescein-tagged cyclosporine. By competing with free fluorescein-tagged cyclosporine for antibody complex formation, cyclosporine present in patient blood samples reduces the emission of polarized light and enables the FPIA assay to measure the bound/free ratio of fluorescein-tagged cyclosporine directly and, by reference to a standard curve, the cyclosporine concentration in the blood sample.

FPIA is not affected by background light interference, but is affected by cyclosporine metabolites that cross-react with the antibody. FPIA instrumentation can, in principle, be adapted to quantify any drug for which a fluorescein-tagged analog and specific antibodies can be prepared. The instrumentation is highly automated and designed for routine use in hospital clinical laboratories. Unattended assay of a single sample requires 14 minutes, but most of the time is required for incubation, so analysis of a full carousel of 20 samples requires only 19 minutes. The LLOQ for FPIA assays of cyclosporine is 25 µg/L.

Several enzyme immunoassays (EIAs) are also popular commercial clinical assays with cyclosporine measurement capability [e.g., Enzyme Monitored (Multiplied) Immunoassay Technique (EMIT™), Cloned Enzyme Donor Immunoassay (CEDIA™)]. All homogeneous EIAs are competitive immunoassays in which enzyme-labeled antigen competes with sample antigen for a limited quantity of antibody binding sites. The resulting enzyme-labeled antigen–antibody bound complex exhibits a change in its rate of enzymatic action in comparison with free enzyme-labeled antigen. A kinetic measurement of the rate of reaction corresponds to determination of bound/free antigen, and consequently permits the drug present in the sample to be measured. The reagents for the cyclosporine EMIT assay use cyclosporine linked to recombinant glucose-6-phosphate dehydrogenase. The active enzyme converts bacterial coenzyme $NAD^+$ to NADH, resulting in a change of UV absorbance. Enzyme activity is decreased when added monoclonal antibody binds to the cyclosporine-linked enzyme. Highest enzyme activity corresponds to the occupation of all antibody sites by high levels of cyclosporine in the blood sample.

The reagents for CEDIA detect the association of two cloned fragments of β-galactosidase, an enzyme that catalyzes the hydrolysis of a chlorophenol-β-galactopyranoside to generate a product detected by UV absorbance at 570 nm. One cloned fragment of the β-galactosidase is linked to cyclosporine. When a monoclonal antibody to cyclosporine is added, competition is established between the cyclosporine in the blood sample and the cyclosporine-linked to the β-galactosidase fragment. Higher enzyme activity correlates with higher concentrations of cyclosporine in patient blood. Both EMIT and CEDIA assays are kinetic measurements that are performed in clinical autoanalyzers, much like the FPIA assay previously described.

In addition to the FPIA, EMIT, and CEDIA methods, several other commercial homogeneous immunoassays have been developed for cyclosporine quantification. Each manufacturer develops and controls the distribution of their antibodies and labeled cyclosporine antigens that define the quantitative response characteristics of their assay kits. Polyclonal antibodies are raised in animals and recognize cyclosporine through a variety of epitope sites; monoclonal antibodies are more specific with regard to structural epitope selection. However, more than 30 cyclosporine metabolites have been characterized, and many of them exhibit cross-reactivity (i.e., high affinity) toward poly- and monoclonal antibodies. As a consequence, most of the immunoassays report values that are elevated in comparison to the HPLC/UV or LC/MS/MS reference data. This has led to considerable debate and discussion in the clinical chemistry community with regard to methods for the analysis of cyclosporine and interpretation of the resulting data [19]. Several LC/MS/MS methods have been proposed as suitable alternatives in routine clinical chemistry environments, and one of these is discussed with respect to dried blood spot analyses. To some extent, the higher capital cost of LC/MS/MS equipment is offset by lower reagent expenditures and applicability to multiple clinical drug assays.

## Dried Blood Spot Analyses: New Chemical Entities and Cyclosporine

Methods for chemical analyses of biofluids are highly dependent on the availability of sample material and its successful transfer to the analytical laboratory. Dried blood spots have been used to screen newborns for inborn errors of metabolism since the 1960s [20], and occasionally to analyze samples for pharmacokinetic studies or target analytes [21, 22]. However, most pharmacokinetic studies and clinical assays have required measured aliquots of blood (or serum or plasma) and the accompanying cost associated with sample collection and proper temperature maintenance for storage and shipping. Barfield et al. [23] demonstrated that dried 15-μL blood spots were suitable for repeated collection of dog blood for a toxicokinetic analysis of acetaminophen. Subsequently, Spooner et al. [24] used LC/MS/MS to validate dried blood spot technology as a quantitative analytical resource for pharmacokinetic studies, and noted that there were multiple prior reports of this use in the pharmacology literature. Using acetaminophen as a test molecule, they determined the influences of the volume of blood spotted, the device used for spotting, the whole blood

temperature, and analyte stability within the dried blood spot in comparison to stability of analyte and metabolites in whole blood, and found the collection medium to be very satisfactory. Compared to liquid matrices, dried blood spot technology was found by Bowen et al. [25] to minimize photodegradation for the light-sensitive compounds nifedipine and omeprazole. Dried blood spot technology also has been developed for UHPLC/MS/MS analyses of the NCE peptide Exendin-4 [26].

Hinchliffe et al. [27] described an assay for UHPLC/MS/MS measurement of cyclosporine and tacrolimus (Figure 12.15) that exemplifies many of the approaches described in this chapter. While assay methods had been reported previously for each immunosuppression agent, these investigators sought to quantify both cyclosporine and tacrolimus on a single analytical platform because their clinical laboratory handles patient samples from multiple transplant departments. They prepared calibration standards and quality control samples by spiking whole blood with pure cyclosporine and tacrolimus, then diluted them with whole blood to give a range of concentrations prior to spotting 25 μL aliquots onto cards selected for dried blood spot collection. Discs of 6 mm diameter were punched from the dried blood spot cards using a stationery paper hole punch, placed into 96-well plates, and ultrasonically extracted using hot methanol in the presence of added internal standards. UHPLC was performed using a fast gradient with an analytical cycle of 3 minutes. A triple quadrupole mass spectrometer was used to monitor selected molecular transitions characteristic of cyclosporine A, its $^2H_{12}$-internal standard, tacrolimus, and its internal standard, ascomycin. The LLOQ for cyclosporine was 8.5 μg/L (linear range 0–1500) and that for tacrolimus was 2.3 μg/L (linear range 0–50). The dried blood spot based assay yielded results comparable to the standard whole blood LC/MS/MS cyclosporine assay. The advantage of this approach was that it allowed simultaneous measurement of cyclosporine A and tacrolimus from fingerprick capillary blood samples from transplant recipients in any community.

## Accelerator Mass Spectrometry Assay: Microdosing in Early Drug Development

Microdosing, or the administration of sub-pharmacological doses of new chemical entities, is a promising technique for obtaining human pharmacokinetic information early in the drug development process [28]. Because extensive animal testing frequently fails to predict human pharmacokinetics in candidate drugs [29], a method for early assessment of human pharmacokinetic parameters could markedly facilitate successful drug development. Sandu *et al.* [30] explored the microdosing strategy in dogs to provide data as to the equivalence of kinetics across sub-pharmacological and pharmacological dose ranges for an antiviral nucleoside analog (Compound A, Figure 12.16).

LC/MS/MS assay methods were employed to determine the pharmacokinetics of [14]C-labeled Compound A in male beagle dogs. A triple quadrupole mass spectrometer was used to monitor the $m/z$ 281 to 135 transition for Compound A, and the $m/z$ 267 to 135 transition for its desmethyl homolog, used as an internal standard. The assay was linear over the range 2–2000 ng/mL plasma, with a LLOQ of 2 ng/mL; assay accuracy and precision (% CV) ranged from 95.5 to 102.3% and 2.1 to 7.2%, respectively.

AMS assays were conducted at the Lawrence Livermore National Laboratory Resource for Biomedical Accelerator Mass Spectrometry, which was remote from the site of the animal experiments (Merck Research Laboratories, NJ). Samples were therefore shipped frozen, and converted to elemental carbon in a two-step process. First, samples were oxidized to $CO_2$ in individual sealed tubes, followed by reduction onto approximately 10 mg of iron. The process requires approximately 10 µL plasma (400 µg carbon), but the exact amount was not important since it is only the precise isotopic ratio that is needed for accurate quantification. Each sample was measured to > 15,000 [14]C counts between three and seven times to achieve the requisite precision. The isotope ratio was derived by comparing the measured isotope ratio to that of the calibration standards. AMS-derived [14]C concentrations, which include parent compound as well as metabolites, were converted to nanogram equivalents of Compound A per milliliter (ng Eq/ml) using the specific activity of the dosed compound.

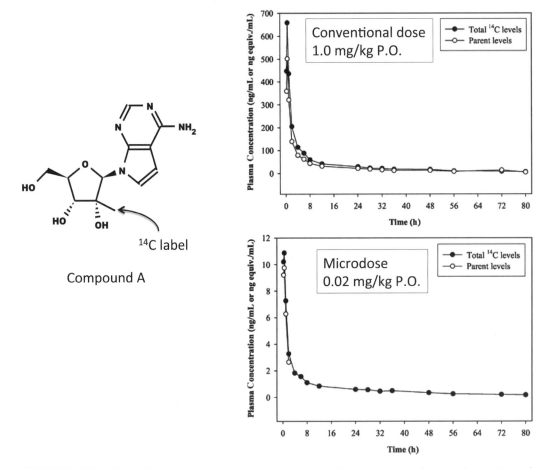

**FIGURE 12.16** *(Left)* Chemical structure of nucleoside analog Compound A indicating the position of a carbon-14 label; *(right)* mean plasma concentration–time profiles of parent levels of Compound A (ng/ml; ○) and total 14C levels (ng Eq/ml; ●) after oral administration of *(upper panel)* 1.0 mg/kg dose or *(lower panel)* 0.02 mg/kg (~100 nCi) [14C]Compound A to dogs (*n* = 2). Reproduced with permission from Sandhu P, Vogel JS, Rose M. *et al.* Drug Metab Dispos 2004;32:1254–9 [30].

Beagles were injected with ~100 nCi [14]C-labeled Compound A in either a pharmacological dose (1 mg/kg oral, 0.4 mg/kg IV ) or a microdose (0.02 mg/kg, oral and IV). The resulting plasma-concentration vs time curves for the oral doses are shown in Figure 12.16. Plasma concentrations after the pharmacological dose were readily measured for 80 hours after the dose using LC/MS/MS and AMS, and the curves for the parent compound and total [14]C were identical. The curve for the microdose (1/50th of the pharmacological dose) determined by AMS was identical to the curve for the larger dose. However, the LLOQ of the LC/MS/MS assay did not allow measurement of plasma concentrations of parent drug beyond the 2-hour time point for microdose administration, demonstrating the potential of AMS to significantly enhance the sensitivity of these measurements. For compounds that are extensively metabolized it would be necessary to fractionate the metabolites on HPLC prior to AMS, but for Compound A the total radioactivity determination accurately reflects the concentration.

A consortium of European laboratories (EUMAPP) selected seven compounds problematic for traditional pK predictive models to test human microdose and pharmacological dose pharmacokinetic results (www.eumapp.com/) [28]. EUMAPP's summary concluded that "Intravenous microdose data predicted $t_{1/2}$, $CL$ and $V_d$ very well. Oral dose data did not scale as well as the intravenous dose but, in general, the data

obtained would have been useful in the selection of drug candidates for further development (or dropped from the development pipeline)." A further advantage of this approach is that the doses of radioactivity required for AMS studies for human microdosing would generally be below those requiring regulatory approval, since the ionizing radiation is lower than expected from the background environment. Thus, it seems likely that AMS assays will be more routinely deployed in clinical pharmacology.

## Imaging Mass Spectrometry

The combination of newer soft ionization techniques, particularly MALDI and faster mass spectrometers, has allowed the development of Imaging Mass Spectrometry (IMS). MALDI-IMS is a powerful tool for clinical pharmacology research, as it allows spatial mass analysis of tissue or cellular samples. Autoradiography is a well established technique in drug distribution studies, but it requires radiolabeled substances. In contrast, MALDI-IMS provides a visual record of drug and metabolite distribution without the need for radiolabeling [31–33]. Molecular masses from 400 Da to 80 kDa can be measured with lateral resolutions approaching 10 μm.

The schematic workflow for drug distribution and metabolite analysis by IMS is shown in Figure 12.17. Fresh frozen or, if appropriate, formalin-fixed paraffin-embedded tissue is cut and mounted on

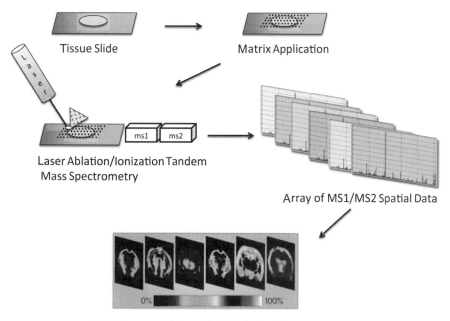

**FIGURE 12.17** Workflow for imaging mass spectrometry (IMS).

a conductive target. Matrix (e.g., cyano-4-hydroxycinnamic acid) is applied in an ordered array across the tissue, and a laser directed at the *x,y*-coordinate array. Ions can be analyzed in a variety of MS/MS instrumentation configurations, and the data from the resulting MS1 or MS2 spectra visualized as images with respect to each *m/z* and color-scaled intensity parameters.

Two examples of IMS are instructive. Whole-body distributions of olanzapine and its desmethyl and 2-hydroxy metabolites in 10-week-old rats were reported from the Caprioli laboratory, which has pioneered IMS [34]. Color images demonstrate that when metabolism information is known, MALDI-IMS can reveal drug metabolite distribution with a high degree of specificity. The same sample can be reanalyzed with respect to other characteristic ions and their transitions. Also, the data from multiple samples can be used to characterize differential kinetics of distribution, as evidenced in a second example [35]. MALDI-IMS was used to determine the distribution of moxifloxacin (SRM recording MH+ *m/z* 402 to *m/z* 385) in tuberculosis-infected rabbit lungs and granulomatous lesions over a period of 5 hours (Figure 12.18). Initially the moxafloxacin distributes throughout the tissue, but at

1.5 hours there was preferential accumulation of the compound in the large granulomas.

There are many technical aspects not detailed in this introduction to IMS technology. The specific techniques are likely to change in this rapidly developing field, but spatial sampling of molecular concentrations in biological tissues with mass analysis characterization is likely to be a useful analytical tool in future pharmacological research.

## ASSAY SELECTION

Liquid chromatographic separations are well suited for pharmacokinetic studies, because the same physicochemical characteristics that are required for drug bioavailability (solubility, polarity, chemical stability) are appropriate for liquid chromatography. The selectivity of detection and not the detector sensitivity (UV absorbance, fluorescence, mass, or mass-to-mass fragment, or radioactive element) in the presence of a biological fluid or tissue defines assay LLOQ. FPIA and similar assays that can be automated in clinical laboratories are generally preferred for therapeutic drug monitoring. The general

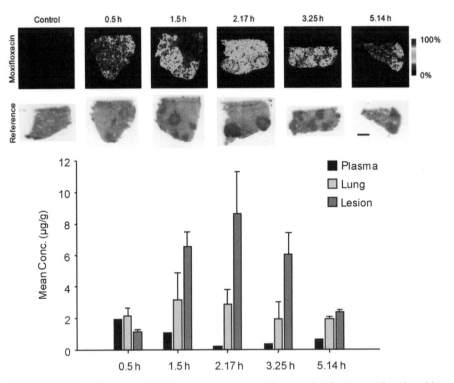

**FIGURE 12.18**  *(Upper panel)* MS images showing moxifloxacin distributions within the rabbit lung biopsy sections at a defined range of post-dose times. A subsequent H&E stained reference tissue section is displayed below these images. Grayscale was derived from the original published color images. Scale bar = 5 mm. *(Lower panel)* Graph showing the concentrations of moxifloxacin in plasma, lung, and granuloma lesion tissues at a range of time points post-dose. Reproduced with permission from Prideaux B, Dartois V, Staab D *et al. Anal Chem* 2011;83:2112–8 [35] .

applicability of LC/MS/MS recommends its consideration as the primary assay method for new chemical entities, but it may also be increasingly applied in therapeutic drug monitoring. The recommendation for new chemical entities is based on the simplicity and ease with which assays can be developed for diverse types of analytes using a single analytical LC/MS/MS platform. LC/MS/MS procedures also can be easily modified to include the metabolites in the analyses, simply by adding other target masses and their mass fragmentation.

## REFERENCES

[1] CDER. Guidance for industry: Bioanalytical method validation. Rockville, MD: FDA. Internet at, www.fda.gov/downloads/Drugs/GuidanceComplianceRegulatoryInformation/Guidances/UCM070107.pdf.; 2001.

[2] Jorgenson J. Capillary liquid chromatography at ultrahigh pressures. Annu Rev Analytic Chem 2010;3:129–50.

[3] Watson JT, Sparkman OD. Introduction to mass spectrometry: Instrumentation, applications, and strategies for data interpretation. Hoboken, NJ: Wiley; 2007.

[4] Hammar C, Holmstedt B, Ryhage R. Mass fragmentography identification of chlorpromazine and its metabolites in human blood by a new method. Analytic Biochem 1968;25:532–48.

[5] Comisarow MB, Marshall AG. The early development of Fourier transform ion cyclotron resonance (FT-ICR) spectroscopy. J Mass Spectrom 1996;31:581–5.

[6] Hu Q, Noll RJ, Li H, Makarov A, Hardman M, Graham Cooks R. The orbitrap: A new mass spectrometer. J Mass Spectrom 2005;40:430–43.

[7] Jain GK, Jain N, Pathan SA, Akhter S, Talegaonkar S, Chander P, et al. Ultra high-pressure liquid chromatographic assay of moxifloxacin in rabbit aqueous humor after topical instillation of moxifloxacin nanoparticles. J Pharm Biomed Anal 2010;52:110–3.

[8] Tama CI, Shen JX, Schiller JE, Hayes RN, Clement RP. Determination of a novel thrombin receptor antagonist (SCH 530348) in human plasma: Evaluation of Ultra Performance Liquid Chromatography-tandem mass spectrometry for routine bioanalytical analysis. J Pharm Biomed Anal 2011; 55:349–59.

[9] Walsky RL, Obach RS. Validated assays for human cytochrome P450 activities. Drug Metab Dispos 2004;32:647–60.

[10] Faucette SR, Hawke RL, Lecluyse EL, Shord SS, Yan B, Laetham RM, et al. Validation of bupropion hydroxylation as a selective marker of human cytochrome P450 2B6 catalytic activity. Drug Metab Dispos 2000;28:1222–30.

[11] Hesse LM, Venkatakrishnan K, Court MH, von Moltke LL, Duan SX, Shader RI, et al. CYP2B6 mediates the *in vitro* hydroxylation of bupropion: Potential drug interactions with other antidepressants. Drug Metab Dispos 2000;28:1176–83.

[12] Walsky RL, Astuccio AV, Obach RS. Evaluation of 227 drugs for *in vitro* inhibition of cytochrome P450 2B6. J Clin Pharmacol 2006;46:1426–38.

[13] Oellerich M, Armstrong VW, Schutz E, Shaw LM. Therapeutic drug monitoring of cyclosporine and tacrolimus. Update on Lake Louise Consensus Conference on cyclosporin and tacrolimus. Clin Biochem 1998;31:309–16.

[14] Simpson J, Zhang Q, Ozaeta P, Aboleneen H. A specific method for the measurement of cyclosporin A in human whole blood by liquid chromatography-tandem mass spectrometry. Ther Drug Monit 1998;20:294–300.

[15] McBride JH, Kim SS, Rodgerson DO, Reyes AF, Ota MK. Measurement of cyclosporine by liquid chromatography and three immunoassays in blood from liver, cardiac, and renal transplant recipients. Clin Chem 1992;38:2300–6.

[16] Salm P, Norris RL, Taylor PJ, Davis DE, Ravenscroft PJ. A reliable high-performance liquid chromatography assay for high-throughput routine cyclosporin A monitoring in whole blood. Ther Drug Monit 1993;15:65–9.

[17] Diamandis EP, Christopoulos TK. Immunoassay. San Diego, CA: Academic Press; 1996.

[18] Price CP, Newman DJ. Principles and practice of immunoassay. 2nd ed. London: Macmillan; 1997.

[19] Jorga A, Holt DW, Johnston A. Therapeutic drug monitoring of cyclosporine. Transplant Proc 2004;36:396S–403S.

[20] Guthrie R, Susi A. A simple phenylalanine method for detecting phenylketonuria in large populations of newborn infants. Pediatrics 1963;32:338–43.

[21] Hibberd SG, Alveyn C, Coombes EJ, Holgate ST. Acute and chronic pharmacokinetics of asymmetrical doses of slow release choline theophyllinate in asthma. Br J Clin Pharmacol 1986;22:337–41.

[22] Oliveira EJ, Watson DG, Morton NS. A simple microanalytical technique for the determination of paracetamol and its main metabolites in blood spots. J Pharm Biomed Anal 2002;29:803–9.

[23] Barfield M, Spooner N, Lad R, Parry S, Fowles S. Application of dried blood spots combined with HPLC-MS/MS for the quantification of acetaminophen in toxicokinetic studies. J Chromatogr B Analyt Technol Biomed Life Sci 2008;870:32–7.

[24] Spooner N, Lad R, Barfield M. Dried blood spots as a sample collection technique for the determination of pharmacokinetics in clinical studies: Considerations for the validation of a quantitative bioanalytical method. Analytical Chemistry 2009;81:1557–63.

[25] Bowen CL, Hemberger MD, Kehler JR, Evans CA. Utility of dried blood spot sampling and storage for increased stability of photosensitive compounds. Bioanalysis 2010;2:1823–8.

[26] Kehler JR, Bowen CL, Boram SL, Evans CA. Application of DBS for quantitative assessment of the peptide Exendin-4; comparison of plasma and DBS method by UHPLC-MS/MS. Bioanalysis 2010;2:1461–8.

[27] Hinchliffe E, Adaway JE, Keevil BG. Simultaneous measurement of cyclosporin A and tacrolimus from dried blood spots by ultra high performance liquid chromatography tandem mass spectrometry. J Chromatogr B Analyt Technol Biomed Life Sci 2012;883–884:102–7.

[28] Stenstrom K, Sydoff M, Mattsson S. Microdosing for early biokinetic studies in humans. Radiat Prot Dosimetry 2010;139:348–52.

[29] Dimasi JA. Risks in new drug development: Approval success rates for investigational drugs. Clin Pharmacol Ther 2001;69:297–307.

[30] Sandhu P, Vogel JS, Rose M, Ubick EA, Brunner JE, Wallace MA, et al. Evaluation of microdosing strategies for studies in preclinical drug development: Demonstration of linear pharmacokinetics in dogs of a nucleoside analog over a 50-fold dose range. Drug Metab Dispos 2004;32:1254–9.

[31] Esquenazi E, Yang YL, Watrous J, Gerwick WH, Dorrestein PC. Imaging mass spectrometry of natural products. Nat Prod Rep 2009;26:1521–34.

[32] Seeley EH, Schwamborn K, Caprioli RM. Imaging of intact tissue sections: Moving beyond the microscope. J Biol Chem 2011;286:25459–66.

[33] Solon EG, Schweitzer A, Stoeckli M, Prideaux B. Autoradiography, MALDI-MS, and SIMS-MS imaging in pharmaceutical discovery and development. AAPS J 2010;12:11–26.

[34] Khatib-Shahidi S, Andersson M, Herman JL, Gillespie TA, Caprioli RM. Direct molecular analysis of whole-body animal tissue sections by imaging MALDI mass spectrometry. Anal Chem 2006;78:6448–56.

[35] Prideaux B, Dartois V, Staab D, Weiner DM, Goh A, Via LE, et al. High-sensitivity MALDI-MRM-MS imaging of moxifloxacin distribution in tuberculosis-infected rabbit lungs and granulomatous lesions. Anal Chem 2011;83:2112–8.

# 13

# Clinical Pharmacogenetics

**David A. Flockhart[1] and Shiew-Mei Huang[2]**

[1]*Division of Clinical Pharmacology, Indiana University School of Medicine, Indianapolis, IN 46250*
[2]*Office of Clinical Pharmacology, Office of Translational Sciences, Center for Drug Evaluation and Research, US Food and Drug Administration, Silver Spring, MD 20993*

## INTRODUCTION

The juxtaposition in time of the sequencing of the entire human genome and of the realization that medication errors constitute one of the leading causes of death in the United States [1] has led many to believe that pharmacogenetics may be able to improve pharmacotherapy. As a result, a fairly uncritical series of hopes and predictions have led not only physicians and scientists but also venture capitalists and Wall Street to believe that genomics will lead to a new era of "personalized medicine". If this is to occur, it will require a series of accurate and reliable genetic tests that allow physicians to predict clinically relevant outcomes with confidence. Genomic education for healthcare professionals is a critical first step towards the integration of genomic discoveries into clinical application [2]. In addition, if medicine is to become more effective and efficient in its delivery by becoming more personalized, further consideration needs to be given regarding the evidence required to support the "clinical utility" of various genomic tests ([3] and references therein) and the means for developing these genomic and other biomarkers in a way that facilitates their reliable clinical implementation [4, 5]. This short summary of the state of pharmacogenetics is intended as an introduction to the field, using pertinent examples to emphasize important concepts of the discipline, which we hope will transcend the moment and serve as a useful group of principles with which to evaluate and follow this rapidly evolving field.

It is particularly important to realize that the huge amount of media, Internet, and marketing hyperbole surrounding pharmacogenomics at this time should be greeted with a healthy dose of scientific skepticism. First, we must note that pharmacogenetics is *not* a new discipline. The coalition of the science of genetics, founded by the work of an Austrian Monk, Gregor Mendel, with peas, and the ancient science of pharmacology did not occur until the twentieth century, but it was early in that century. After the rediscovery of the Mendelian laws of genetics at the dawn of the twentieth century, some connection with the ancient science of pharmacology would seem inevitable, and indeed a series of investigators contributed important observations that named and then laid the foundations of the field (Table 13.1) [6]. These rested in part in genetics and in part in pharmacology.

In the area of genetics, the separate observations of Hardy and Weinberg that resulted in the Hardy-Weinberg law are particularly pertinent to modern pharmacogenetics. This law states that when an allele with a single change in it is distributed at equilibrium in a population, the incidences $p$ and $q$ of the two resulting alleles will result in a genotype incidence that can be represented by the following equation:

$$p^2 + 2\,pq + q^2 = 1$$

Two important predictions follow:

1. The incidence of heterozygotes (2 $pq$) and of the homozygous q genotype ($q^2$) can be predicted if the

**TABLE 13.1   The Early History of Pharmacogenetics**

| | |
|---|---|
| 1932 | First inherited difference in a response to a chemical — inability to taste phenythiourea |
| World War II | Hemolysis in African American soldiers treated with primaquine highlights importance of genetic deficiency of glucose-6-phosphate dehydrogenase |
| 1957 | Motulsky proposes that "inheritance might explain many individual differences in the efficacy of drugs and in the occurrence of adverse drug reactions" |
| 1959 | Vogel publishes "Pharmacogenetics: The role of genetics in drug response" |
| 1959 | Genetic polymorphism found to influence isoniazid blood concentrations |
| 1964 | Genetic differences found in ethanol metabolism |
| 1977 | CYP2D6 polymorphism identified by Mahgoub *et al.* and Eichelbaum |

incidence of the homozygous p genotype ($p^2$) is known.

2. If this equation accurately predicts the incidence of genotypes and alleles, then we are dealing with a single change that results in two alleles and two resultant phenotypes. If genotypes are present in a population in disequilibrium with this law, the influence of population concentrating factors or environment must be invoked, and a pure genetic etiology is inadequate.

In the area of pharmacology, the identification of the series of proteins in the familiar pharmacologic cascade essentially identified not only a series of targets for drugs, but also a series of genetic "targets" that might contribute to interindividual variability in drug response. The proteins involved turned out to be diverse in structure, function, and location, ranging from those that control and facilitate drug absorption, through the enzymes in the gastrointestinal tract and liver that influence drug elimination, to molecules involved in the complex series of interactions that occur during and after the interaction between drugs and cellular receptor molecules. Along the way, the complexity of human response to exogenous xenobiotics was constantly re-emphasized. The complexity was then exploited to the benefit of patients, as demonstrated by the early work on propranolol, the first β-adrenoreceptor blocker, and cimetidine, the first $H_2$-receptor blocker. Subsequent work demonstrated the involvement of multiple intracellular proteins in the second messenger response proposed by Earl

Sutherland, and in the responses to steroids and other exogenous molecules that have intranuclear sites of action. The twentieth century in pharmacology therefore laid the ground for work in the twenty-first century, which will involve the study of genetic changes in this cascade of important proteins, even as genetic information itself leads to the identification of a large number of new protein and genetic drug targets.

## HIERARCHY OF PHARMACOGENETIC INFORMATION

An important second principle of modern pharmacogenetics is illustrated in Figure 13.1, in which the hierarchy of useful information from

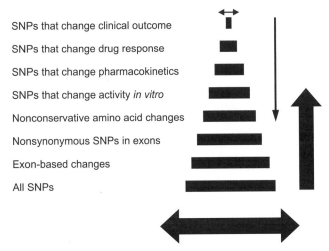

SNPs that change clinical outcome

SNPs that change drug response

SNPs that change pharmacokinetics

SNPs that change activity *in vitro*

Nonconservative amino acid changes

Nonsynonymous SNPs in exons

Exon-based changes

All SNPs

**FIGURE 13.1**   The hierarchy of pharmacogenetic information from single nucleotide polymorphisms (SNPs). The size of the bar at each level of the pyramid represents an approximation of the number of SNPs in each category. At the base is the total number of SNPs, estimated to be somewhere between 20 million and 80 million. Most of these are not in exons, the expressed sequences that code for proteins, and so the second level is much smaller, in the 300,000 range. Exon-based changes are more likely to result in a clinical effect, but there are good examples of intronic changes and promoter variants that result in important, expressed changes. Nonsynonymous SNPs are those that result in a change in amino acid, and the number of these that are non-conservative, and therefore have a greater chance of changing the structure or activity of the protein domain they code for, is even smaller. Through a wide range of techniques, laboratory scientists are expressing these variants and testing whether they change activity *in vitro*, and it is clear that most do not, so the number of SNPs at this level of the hierarchy shrinks further. SNPs that result in statistically significant changes in pharmacokinetics due to changes in receptors, transporters, or drug-metabolizing enzymes that are rate limiting are well described, but few and far between. Very few of these result in clinically significant changes in drug response, and even fewer could be measured by the epidemiologists and managers that measure aggregate clinical outcomes.

pharmacogenetic studies is shown. Although this figure depicts an information hierarchy for single nucleotide polymorphisms (SNPs), a similar hierarchy could equally well be constructed for deletions, insertions, duplications, splice variants, copy number polymorphisms, or genetic mutations in general. There is a large amount of research activity at the base of this pyramid at the moment, and available information about the presence, incidence, and validity of individual SNPs is large and rapidly expanding as the result of the work of the SNP consortium, the Human Genome Project, and a large number of individual scientists. As we ascend the pyramid toward increasingly functional data, the pyramid becomes dramatically thinner as the databases containing data about non-synonymous SNPs, non-conservative amino acid changes, and SNPs that change activity *in vitro*, clinical pharmacokinetics, drug response, or finally clinically

important outcomes are progressively smaller. The number of SNPs that have been clearly shown to bring about clinically important outcomes is indeed small, and this is reflected in the fact that few pharmacogenetic tests are routinely available to physicians, although a number have become available in the past 5 years (Tables 13.2 and 13.3).

Figure 13.1 also makes clear the long scientific route from the discovery of an individual SNP to the actual demonstration of a clinically important outcome. This is particularly pertinent in view of the simple fact that the vast majority of individual polymorphisms in human DNA likely have no dynamic consequence. A lot of work in the laboratories of molecular biologists and geneticists can therefore be expended to little avail. As a result, a number of clinical pharmacologists and scientists with expertise in pharmacology, genetics, and medicine have elected to start at the other end – the top

**TABLE 13.2   Examples of Marketed Genomic Tests and Their Applications**

| Genes | Example of FDA Cleared/Approved Tests[a] (manufacturers) or Laboratory Developed Tests (LDT) | Example applications (Drugs)[b] |
|---|---|---|
| CYP2D6 | Roche AmpliChip CYP450 | Atomoxetine: Indicate that tests are available for PMs<br>Tetrabenazine: Suggest genotying if patients require more than 50-mg dose<br>Codeine: Warn about UMs |
| CYP2C9/VKORC1 | Esensor warfarin sensitivity saliva test (Genmark)<br>EQ-PRC LC warfarin genotyping kit (Trimgen)<br>Esensor Warfarin Sensitivity Test (Osmetech);<br>INFINITI 2C9 &VKORC1 Multiplex assay (Autogenomics);<br>Rapid Genotyping Assay (Paragondx)<br>Verigene Warfarin Metabolism Nucleic Acid Test (Nanosphere) | Warfarin: Provided a dose schedule |
| CYP2C19 | AmpliChip CYP450 (Roche);<br>INFINITY CYP2C19 Assay (Autogenomics) | Clopidogrel: Contains a BlackBox Warning about use in PMs and indicates that alternative treatment or treatment strategies are available |
| TPMT | LDT | Mercaptopurine: Indicates dose reduction for PMs |
| UGT1A1 | TWT Invader UGT1A1 Molecular Assay | Irinotecan: Label recommends dose reduction for … homozygous for the UGT1A1*28 allele |
| HER 2/neu | Vysis PathVysion HER-2 DNA Probe Kit | Trastuzumab: Label mentions the test and describes available tests |
| HLA-B | LDT | Carbamazepine: Contains a Boxed Warning about TEN and SJS in Asian patients with HLA-B*1502<br>Abacavir: Contains a Boxed Warning that "Patients who carry the HLA-B*5701 allele are at high risk for experiencing a hypersensitivity reaction" |
| KRAS | LDT | Cetuximab label did not recommend the use in patients whose tumors had KRAS mutations in codon 12 or 13<br>Panitumumab: Similar labeling as cetuximab |

[a]See the following website for updated information on FDA cleared or approved tests: http://www.accessdata.fda.gov/scripts/cdrh/cfdocs/cfPMN/pmn.cfm

[b]See the following website for updated information on FDA approved drug labeling, http://www.accessdata.fda.gov/scripts/cder/drugsatfda

**TABLE 13.3**   Three Ranges of Expected Maintenance Warfarin Daily Doses Based on CYP2C9 and VKORC1 Genotype[a,b]

| VKORC1 | CYP2C9 | | | | | |
|---|---|---|---|---|---|---|
|  | *1/*1 | *1/*2 | *1/*3 | *2/*2 | *2/*3 | *3/*3 |
| GG | 5–7 mg | 5–7 mg | 3–4 mg | 3–4 mg | 3–4 mg | 0.5–2 mg |
| AG | 5–7 mg | 3–4 mg | 3–4 mg | 3–4 mg | 0.5–2 mg | 0.5–2 mg |
| AA | 3–4 mg | 3–4 mg | 0.5–2 mg | 0.5–2 mg | 0.5–2 mg | 0.5–2 mg |

[a]Ranges are derived from multiple published clinical studies. VKORC1 −1639G>A (rs99232331) variant is used in this table. Other co-inherited VKORC1 variants may also be important determinants of warfarin dose.

[b]See the following website for updated information on FDA approved drug labeling, http://www.accessdata. fda.gov/scripts/cder/drugsatfda/

of the pyramid. By searching for outliers in populations that demonstrate aberrant clinical responses and by focusing on these polymorphisms, they hope to elicit valuable genetic, mechanistic, and clinical lessons. This approach has already borne considerable fruit, as illustrated later in this chapter. It is important to note that these approaches have tended to be most successful when collaborative groups of physicians, pharmacologists, bioinformatics experts, statisticians and epidemiologists, molecular biologists, and geneticists have been able to form translational teams to carry research from the clinic to the laboratory and back.

It is possible for scientists who study specific drug responses to place the phenomena that they study at individual levels within this hierarchy of information. For example, the cytochrome P450 and some Phase II conjugation enzymes present in the human liver and gastrointestinal tract have a long pharmacogenetic history, and genetic variants in some of these enzymes

can be placed at present in the top two levels of the hierarchy. Of course, there are many individual SNPs in the genes corresponding to these enzymes that have no functional consequence, and these remain in the bottom level. In contrast, the majority of the information available at present about drug receptors, transporters, or ketoreductases occupies the lower few levels of the pyramid, although this is rapidly changing, and a number of transporter variants of clinical importance have already been reported.

For obvious reasons, we have more information about drug responses that are easy to measure. Genetic changes which result in changes in plasma concentrations of drugs that can be measured easily are relatively amenable to study by analytical chemists and clinical pharmacokineticists, whereas genetic polymorphisms in receptors that might influence drug response require careful clinical pharmacologic studies. These simple observations emphasize the need for a qualified cadre of

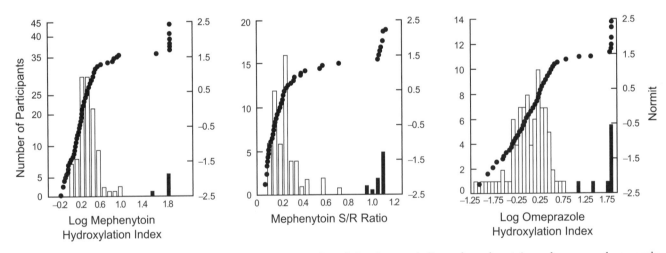

**FIGURE 13.2**  Normit plots (●) of CYP2C19 activity as indicated by the metabolism of mephenytoin and omeprazole as probe drugs. Comparisons for a population of 142 subjects are shown based on log hydroxylation indices for mephenytoin [$\log_{10}$(μmole S-phenytoin given/μmole 4′-hydroxymephenytoin recovered in urine)], and omeprazole [$\log_{10}$(omeprazole/5′-hydroxyomeprazole)], and the ratio of S-mephenytoin/R-mephenytoin recovered in urine. In the histograms, rapid metabolizers are represented by lightly shaded bars and slow metabolizers by solid bars. The same seven individuals were identified by all three methods as poor CYP2C19 metabolizers. Reproduced with permission from Balian JD, Sukhova N, Harris JW *et al. Clin Pharmacol Ther* 1998;57:662–9 [7].

clinical pharmacologists in the field of pharmacogenetics and translational medicine to effectively exploit the huge amount of information made available by the sequencing of the human genome, and perhaps explain also the already apparent concentration of contributions from clinical pharmacologists to the field.

## IDENTIFICATION AND SELECTION OF OUTLIERS IN A POPULATION

Figure 13.2 illustrates one useful means of identifying population outliers that allows investigators to focus on these individuals and take information from the top of the hierarchy of information presented in Figure 13.1 and apply it fairly quickly to questions of clinical relevance. Figure 13.2 contains both histograms and Normit plots that illustrate the range of metabolic capacities for CYP2C19 in a population. A Normit plot is essentially a means of describing this range as a cumulative distribution in units of standard deviation from the mean. The cumulative plot of a pure normal distribution will be a straight line, the slope of which is determined by the variance of the distribution. In other words, the steeper the slope, the more tightly the group would be distributed around the mean, whereas a more shallow slope would indicate a more broadly distributed group. The value of this analysis to pharmacogeneticists is that changes in the slope of the line indicate a *new* distribution, and if this different population represents more than 1% of the total, it can reasonably be expected to be genetically stable, and to be termed a *polymorphism*. In the case illustrated, the six subjects on the right were all shown to possess, in both the alleles coding for CYP2C19, a SNP that was subsequently shown to render the enzyme inactive [7]. Figure 13.2 also illustrates the important point that a number of probes can be developed to determine the *phenotype* that results from the expression of such a *genotype*. In this case, the study was carried out to demonstrate the utility of a single dose of the proton pump inhibitor omeprazole to serve as a probe for the genetic polymorphism in CYP2C19. As summarized in Table 13.4, ideal characteristics of probes for phenotyping include specificity

**TABLE 13.4** **Properties of an Ideal Probe for Phenotyping**

- Specific for the pharmacogenetic trait in question
- Sensitive
- Simple to administer
- Inexpensive
- Easy to assay
- Clinical benign

for the trait in question, sensitivity and ease of available assays, and, most important, the requirement that they be clinically benign so that they can be tested in large numbers of people without risk. The absence of some of these characteristics in many probes and the difficulty in finding ideal probes are some of the most significant impediments to progress in developing clinically useful pharmacogenetic tests, and are a key issue that critical scientific evaluators should address. In all pharmacogenomic research, the quality of the phenotype is salient.

Upon the identification of an outlier phenotype such as this, the logical next step is a valid demonstration that it can be explained by a genetic change. Family and twin studies are a valuable means of confirming this, and have been the standard in the field since the days of Mendel. These remain an important part of any genetic association study, but they are now being replaced by genetic tests that are able to define changes at specific loci and to test for their presence in broad, unrelated groups of people.

The clinical relevance of the CYP2C19 polymorphism, primarily present in Asian populations [8], has been studied by a number of investigators, who have shown that the cure rate for *Helicobacter pylori* infection is greater in patients who are genetic poor metabolizers of CYP2C9 substrates [9]. When given omeprazole doses of 20 mg/day for 4 weeks, these individuals have areas under their omeprazole plasma-concentrations vs time curves (*AUCs*) that are 5- to 10-fold higher than are those of extensive metabolizers [10]. The resultant decreases in gastric acid exposure are associated with a clinically important difference in the response of *H. pylori* to treatment [11]. As illustrated in Figure 13.3, patients with duodenal ulcers who were

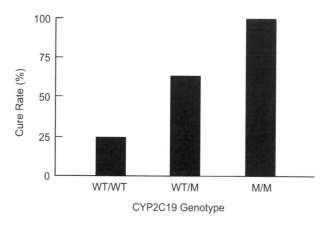

**FIGURE 13.3** Effectiveness of omeprazole and amoxacillin in eradicating *Helicobacter pylori* infection in duodenal ulcer patients with CYP2C19 genotypes (WT, wild type allele; M, mutant allele). Data from Furuta T, Ohashi K, Kamata T *et al*. Ann Intern Med 1998;129:1027–30 [9].

poor metabolizers (PMs) had a 100% cure rate, but extensive metabolizers (EMs) with both alleles active had only a 25% cure rate when treated with an omeprazole dose of 20 mg/day. Despite the apparent importance of these data, it might reasonably be argued that selecting a 40- or 60-mg dose of omeprazole for all patients might result in a uniformly beneficial outcome without the need for pharmacogenetic testing.

CYP2C19 polymorphisms also affect the clinical efficacy of clopidogrel, a widely prescribed antiplatelet drug that is used to prevent restenosis after coronary stunting. Clopidogrel is a *prodrug*, because it requires hepatic metabolism by CYP2C19 in order to generate its pharmacologically active metabolite. Mega *et al.* [12] found that *CYP2C19*2* carriers with one loss-of-function allele of CYP2C19 have reduced concentrations of this active metabolite and correspondingly lower inhibition of platelet inhibition, resulting in a higher rate of stent thrombosis and the primary efficacy outcome of death, non-fatal myocardial infarction, or non-fatal stroke (Figure 13.4) [12]. These investigators subsequently demonstrated that treating *CYP2C19*2* heterozygotes with 225 mg/day clopidogrel could reduce their platelet reactivity to the same level as observed in non-carriers who received the standard 75-mg/day dose of this drug [13]. However, even doses as high as 300 mg/day did not provide *CYP2C19*2* homozygotes with comparable levels of platelet inhibition. A meta-analysis of data from several clinical trials showed that patients with only one variant allele of CYP2C19 have reduced clinical efficacy or increased stent thrombosis during clopidogrel treatment [14].

## EXAMPLES OF IMPORTANT GENETIC POLYMORPHISMS

Pharmacologically significant genetic variation has been described at every point of the cascade leading from the pharmacokinetics of drug absorption to the pharmacodynamics of drug effect (Figure 13.1), in many cases reflecting interindividual differences in proteins involved in the absorption, distribution, elimination, and direct cellular action of drugs.

## Drug Absorption

As discussed in Chapter 14 an elegant series of studies in mice that have the multidrug-resistance gene (MDR) for P-glycoprotein (P-gp) knocked out have clearly demonstrated an important role for this multidrug transporter in the absorption and disposition of a large number of clinically important

medicines [15–17]. The first significant *MDR* mutated allele was shown to change the pharmacokinetics of digoxin in a marked and likely clinically significant manner. Although the importance of P-gp in the disposition of drugs besides digoxin has been recognized, many findings on the effect of *MDR gene* polymorphisms on P-gp substrates have not been consistently reported to date [18]. Many other transporters have been identified more recently (see Chapter 14), but the contribution of their genetic variation to clinical response varies. This may in part relate to the ability of most drugs to employ multiple transporters, to the promiscuous ability of many transporters to interact with a large number of drugs, and to the fact that we have yet to identify a human "knockout" of any transporter.

## Drug Distribution

As discussed in Chapter 17, a recent genome-wide association study showed that a common SNP (c.521T>C) in the solute carrier organic transporter 1B1 (*SLCO1B1*) gene that encodes for the organic anion transporter 1B1 (OATP1B1) protein was associated with an increased incidence of simvastatin-induced myopathy [19]. This same SNP has affected the hepatic uptake of statins and has been associated with altered pharmacokinetics of various statins [20].

## Drug Elimination

### The Aldehyde Dehydrogenase Gene

One of the most well-known polymorphisms relevant to pharmacodynamic response is in the aldehyde dehydrogenase gene (*ALDH2*) [21]. There are 10 human *ALDH* genes and 13 different alleles that result in an autosomal dominant trait that lacks catalytic activity if one subunit of the tetramer is inactive. *ALDH2* deficiency occurs in up to 45% of Chinese, but rarely in Caucasians or Africans, and results in build-up of toxic acetaldehyde and alcohol-related flushing in Asians. Although the genetics of this enzyme and of alcohol metabolism are generally well characterized, a genetic diagnostic test would have little clinical utility because the carriers of the defective alleles are usually acutely aware of it. This illustrates a more widely relevant point in that the *availability of genetic testing methodology does not necessarily mean that it is clinically useful, and the incremental value of any pharmacogenetic test is inversely related to our ability to predict drug response with the clinical tools we already have available.*

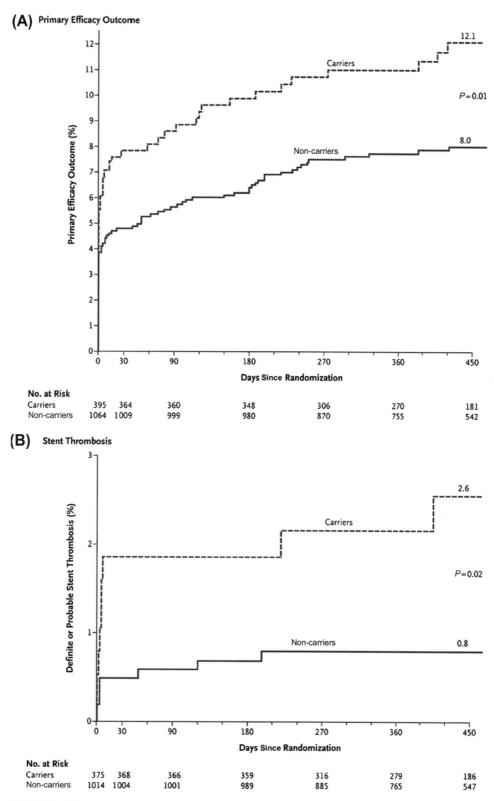

**FIGURE 13.4** Association between status as a carrier of a CYP2C19 reduced-function allele and (A) the primary efficacy outcome or (B) stent thrombosis in subjects receiving clopidogrel. Reproduced with permission from Mega JL, Close S, Wiviott SD *et al.* N Engl J Med 2009;360:354–62 [12].

## The CYP2D6 Polymorphism

No protein involved in drug metabolism or response that has a pharmacogenetic component has been more studied than CYP2D6. In 1977, British investigators described a polymorphism in the hydroxylation of the antihypertensive drug debrisoquine [22, 23]. Independently, Eichelbaum *et al.* [24] showed in Germany that the oxidation of sparteine is also polymorphic. The metabolic ratios (MR = ratio of parent drug/metabolite) of the two drugs were closely correlated, indicating that the same enzyme, now termed CYP2D6, is responsible for the two metabolic reactions [25].

The incidence of PMs of debrisoquine/sparteine now has been investigated in many populations, most of them with a fairly small number of subjects [26]. Bertilsson *et al.* [27] found 69 (6.3%) PMs of debrisoquine among 1011 Swedish Caucasians (Figure 13.5). This incidence is very similar to that found in other European [26] and American [28] Caucasian populations. It was shown that the incidence of PMs among 695 Chinese was only 1.0% using the antimode MR = 12.6 established in Caucasian populations (Figure 13.6) [27]. A similar low incidence of PMs has been shown in Japanese [28] and Koreans [29, 30].

## CYP2D6 Alleles Causing Absent or Decreased Enzyme Activity

The gene encoding the CYP2D6 enzyme is localized on chromosome 22 [31]. Using restriction fragment length polymorphism (RFLP) analysis and the allele-specific polymerase chain reaction (PCR), three major mutant alleles were found in Caucasians [32–35]. These are now termed *CYP2D6*3*, *CYP2D6*4*, and *CYP2D6*5* (Table 13.4) [36]. In Swedish Caucasians, the *CYP2D6*4* allele occurs with a frequency of 22% and accounts for more than 75% of the variant alleles in this population [37]. In contrast, the *CYP2D6*4* allele is almost absent in Chinese, accounting for the lower incidence of PMs in this population compared to 7% in Caucasians [27]. As shown in Table 13.5, the

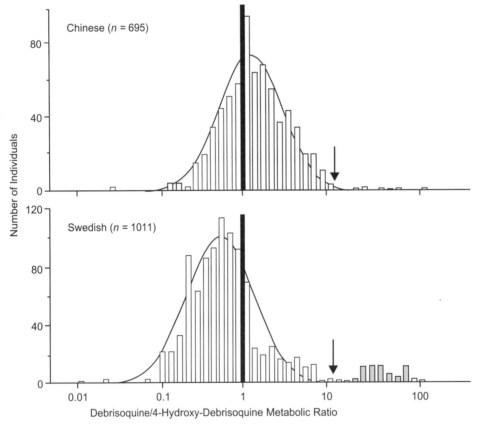

**FIGURE 13.5** Distribution of the urinary debrisoquine/4-hydroxydebrisoquine metabolic ratio (MR) in 695 Chinese and 1011 Swedish healthy subjects. The arrows indicate MR = 2.6, the antimode between EM and PM established in Caucasians. A line is drawn at MR = 1. Most Chinese EM have MR > 1, while most Swedish EM have MR < 1. Reproduced with permission from Bertilsson L, Lou Y-Q, Du Y-L *et al.* Clin Pharmacol Ther 1992;52:388–97 [27].

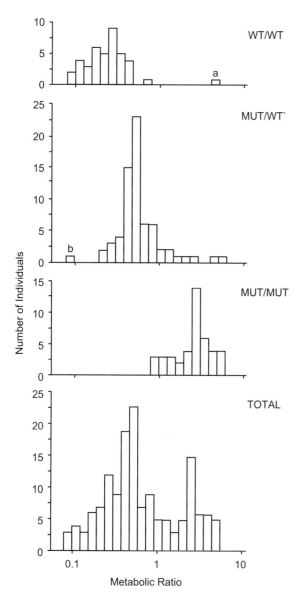

**FIGURE 13.6** Distribution of the debrisoquine MR in three genotype groups related to the *CYP2D6*10* allele in 152 Korean subjects. Wild type (WT) = *CYP2D6*1(or*2)* and mutant (MUT) = *CYP2D6*10*. Reproduced with permission from Roh HK, Dahl ML, Johansson I *et al.* Pharmacogenetics 1996;6:441–7 [30].

occurrence of the gene deletion (*CYP2D6*5*) is very similar, ranging from 4% to 6% in Sweden, China, and Zimbabwe. This indicates that this is a very old mutation, which occurred before the separation of the three major races 100,000–150,000 years ago [38]. It is apparent from Figure 13.5 that the distribution of the MR of Chinese EMs is shifted to the right compared to Swedish EMs (*P* < 0.01) [27]. Most Swedes have MR < 1, whereas the opposite is true for Chinese subjects. This shows that the mean rate of hydroxylation of debrisoquine is lower in Chinese EMs than in Caucasian EMs [27]. This right shift in MR in Asians is

due to the presence of a mutant *CYP2D6*10* allele at the high frequency of 51% in Chinese [39, 40] (Table 13.5). The SNP C188T causes a Pro34Ser amino acid substitution that results in an unstable enzyme with decreased catalytic activity [40]. As shown in Figure 13.6, the presence of this C188T mutation causes a rightward shift in a Korean population [40]. The high frequency of this *CYP2D6*10* allele is similar in Chinese, Japanese, and Koreans.

Masimirembwa *et al.* [41] found a right shift of debrisoquine MR in black Zimbabweans similar to that found in Asians. A variant allele that encodes an enzyme with decreased debrisoquine hydroxylase activity was subsequently identified and named *CYP2D6*17*. Among black Africans, the frequency of this allele was found to be 34% in Zimbabweans [41] (see Table 13.4), 17% in Tanzanians [42], 28% in Ghanaians [43], and 9% in Ethiopians [44]. This and many other studies demonstrate the genetic heterogeneity of different populations in Africa. Wennerholm *et al.* [45] administered four different CYP2D6 substrates on separate occasions to Tanzanians with different genotypes. Subjects with the *CYP2D6*17/*17* genotype had a decreased rate of metabolism of debrisoquine and dextromethorphan, but normal metabolism of codeine and metoprolol. This demonstrates a *population-specific* change in the substrate specificity of the *CYP2D6*17* encoded enzyme [45].

In several studies, a close genotype and phenotype relationship has been demonstrated in Caucasians and Asians [37, 39, 40]. However, in studies in Ethiopia [44], Ghana [43], and Tanzania [42] a lower CYP2D6 activity in relation to genotype has been demonstrated, indicating that in addition to genetic factors, environmental factors such as infections or food intake are of phenotypic importance in Africa. Evidence for an environmental influence on CYP2D6 catalyzed debrisoquine hydroxylation also was demonstrated by comparing Ethiopians living in Ethiopia with those living in Sweden [46].

### Multiple Copies of Genes as a Cause of Increased CYP2D6 Activity

The problem of treating CYP2D6 PMs with various drugs has been extensively discussed [26]. Less attention has been given to patients who are ultra-rapid metabolizers and lie at the other extreme of the MR distribution. Bertilsson *et al.* [47] described a woman with depression who had a debrisoquine MR of 0.07 and had to be treated with 500 mg of nortriptyline daily to achieve a therapeutic response. This is three to five times higher than the recommended dose. The molecular genetic basis for the

**Table 13.5  Frequency of Normal CYP2D6*1 or *2 Alleles and Some Alleles Causing No or Deficient CYP2D6 Activity in Three Different Populations**

| CYP2D6 alleles | Functional mutation | Consequence | Allele frequency (%)[a] | Swedish Chinese | Zimbabwean |
|---|---|---|---|---|---|
| *1 or *2 (wild type) | | | 69 | 43 | 54 |
| *3 (A) | A2637 del | Frame shift | 21 | 0 | 0 |
| *4 (B) | G1934A | Splicing defect | 22 | 0–1 | 2 |
| *5 (D) | Gene deletion | No enzyme | 4 | 6 | 4 |
| *10 (Ch) | C188T | Unstable enzyme | n.d. | 51 | 6 |
| *17 (Z) | C1111T | Reduced affinity | n.d. | n.d. | 34 |

[a]n.d. = not determined.

Data are from Desta Z, Zhao X, Shin JG, Flockhart DA. Clin Pharmacokinet. 2002;41:913–58 [8]; Eichelbaum M, Gross AS. The genetic polymorphism of debrisoquine/sparteine metabolism: Clinical aspects. In: Kalow W, editor. Pharmacogenetics of drug metabolism. New York, NY: Pergamon Press; 1992. pp. 625–48 [26]; Bertilsson L, Lou Y-Q, Du Y-L et al. [erratum in Clin Pharmacol Ther 1994;55:648]. Clin Pharmacol Ther 1992;51:388–97 [27]; Sohn D-R, Shin S-G, Park C-W et al. Br J Clin Pharmacol 1991;32:504–7 [29]; Eichelbaum M, Baur MP, Dengler HJ et al. Br J Clin Pharmacol 1987;23:455–8 [31].

ultrarapid metabolism subsequently was identified both in this patient and in another patient, who had to be treated with megadoses of clomipramine [48]. That same year, a father and his daughter and son with 12 extra copies of the CYP2D6 gene were described [49]. These were the first demonstrations of an inherited amplification of an active gene encoding a drug-metabolizing enzyme.

In Swedish Caucasians the frequency of subjects having multiple copies of genes is about 1% [50], while it is 3.6% in Germany [51], 7–10% in Spain [52, 53], and 10% on Sicily [54]. The frequency is as high as 29% in black Ethiopians [46] and 20% in Saudi Arabians [55]. Thus, there is a European–African north–south gradient in the incidence of CYP2D6 gene duplication. However, there are now well-documented examples of duplicated CYP2D6*1 and CYP2D6*4 variant genes, making the important point that not all multiple copies are functional [51].

In terms of the clinical relevance of these variants, Kawanishi et al. [56] studied 81 depressed patients who failed to respond to antidepressant drugs that are CYP2D6 substrates and found that 8 of them had a gene duplication. This is a significantly higher frequency than the 1% found in healthy Swedish subjects by Dahl et al. [50], and suggests that ultrarapid drug metabolism resulting from CYP2D6 gene duplication is a possible factor responsible for the lack of therapeutic response in some depressed patients. A recent case of infant mortality appears to be the result of the CYP2D6 ultrarapid metabolizer genotype [57]. Although codeine has been used safely for many years in many people, including nursing mothers, a healthy 13-day-old baby died from morphine poisoning. After finding high concentrations of morphine in the baby's blood, genetic analysis of the baby's mother, who had

only been taking the usual dose of codeine, showed that she was an ultrarapid metabolizer of this CYP2D6 substrate. Resulting high concentrations of morphine in a breastfed infant, along with the reduced ability of the infant to further metabolize and eliminate morphine, thus can result in life-threatening toxicity. Recent studies have shown that a combination of the CYP2D6 ultrarapid metabolizer and UGT2B7*2*2 genotype may also predispose to life-threatening CNS depression after codeine administration [58].

### Metabolism of CYP2D6 Drug Substrates in Relation to Genotypes

Although CYP2D6 represents a relatively small proportion of the immunoblottable CYP450 protein in human livers, it is clear that it is responsible for the metabolism of a relatively large number of important medicines [39]. Since the discovery of the CYP2D6 polymorphism in the 1970s, almost 100 drugs have been shown to be substrates of this enzyme. Drugs that are CYP2D6 substrates are all lipophilic bases, and some of these are shown in Table 13.6. Both in vitro and in vivo techniques may be employed to study whether or not a drug is metabolized by CYP2D6. In vivo studies need to be performed to establish the quantitative importance of this enzyme for the total metabolism of the drug. We illustrate here some of the key principles involved in the study of this important enzyme, using the examples of the anti-estrogen tamoxifen and the tricyclic antidepressant nortriptyline.

### Tamoxifen

Tamoxifen is an excellent example of a prodrug, whose conversion to its active metabolite [59] is

**TABLE 13.6    Some Drugs Whose Metabolism is Catalyzed by the CYP2D6 Enzyme**

| β-Adrenoceptor blockers | Antidepressants | Neuroleptics | Miscellaneous |
|---|---|---|---|
| Metoprolol | Amitriptyline | Haloperidol | Atomoxetine |
| Nebivolol | Clomipramine | Perphenazine | Codeine |
| Propranolol | Desipramine | Risperidone | Debrisoquine |
| Timolol | Fluoxetine | Thioridazine | Dextromethorphan |
| | Imipramine | Zuclopenthixol | Phenformin |
| | Mianserin | | Tamoxifen |
| | Nortriptyline | | Tetrabenazine |
| | Paroxetine | | Tolterodine |
| | Venafaxine | | Tramadol |

mediated almost exclusively by a genetically polymorphic enzyme. In this case, the metabolite, endoxifen, was first shown by Desta *et al.* [60] to be generated from *N*-desmethyl tamoxifen *in vitro*, almost exclusively by CYP2D6. Subsequent studies conducted by the Consortium on Breast Cancer Pharmacogenomics [61], and then confirmed by a large number of investigators in every major population around the world, showed that breast cancer patients treated with standard tamoxifen doses had serum endoxifen concentrations that were consistently associated with CYP2D6 genotype and that were invariably lower in poor metabolizers [62, 63]. These data generated a large number of important hypotheses to be tested. These included the possibility that (1) tamoxifen efficacy is associated with *CYP2D6* genotype in any of the settings in which the drug is used; (2) that *CYP2D6* genotype might be used to identify patients who would benefit most from tamoxifen treatment; (3) that tamoxifen toxicity is similarly associated with *CYP2D6* genotype; (4) that drugs which inhibit CYP2D6, such as the selective serotonin reuptake inhibitor antidepressants, commonly taken by patients with breast cancer to treat depression or hot flashes, might reduce tamoxifen efficacy; and (5) that these pharmacogenetic concerns might be avoided entirely by developing endoxifen itself, as a so-called *improved chemical entity*, to replace tamoxifen as an endocrine therapy for breast cancer patients. All of these possibilities are the subject of ongoing investigation, including the last, and endoxifen is the subject of ongoing Phase II trials being carried out at the National Cancer Institute and by a number of other sponsors.

A large number of studies have now been carried out to test whether *CYP2D6* genotype could be used to predict either tamoxifen efficacy or toxicity of tamoxifen. Since it would now be unethical to conduct placebo-controlled trials of tamoxifen in breast cancer

patients, a large number of retrospective association studies have been conducted within trials where tamoxifen has been compared to aromatase inhibitor drugs, which are an important therapeutic alternative to tamoxifen. A large number of "banking" studies also have been conducted in which DNA samples from tamoxifen-treated patients were retrospectively tested for associations between efficacy and *CYP2D6* genotype. However, no clear, consistent association has been identified at this point that stands up to the test of reproducibility [64–66], and it is unlikely that, in this context, widespread CYP2D6 testing will be introduced in the foreseeable future. On the other hand, it remains possible that as yet undefined groups of breast cancer patients might benefit from broader pharmacogenomic testing. This possibility is emphasized by the recent demonstration that tamoxifen metabolites can also act as aromatase inhibitors, and that aromatase genotype might affect the drug's overall efficacy [67, 68]. In addition, genome-wide association studies based on tamoxifen and aromatase inhibitor trials have brought forth the possible involvement of heretofore unrecognized genes. These include the *BRCA* gene, which may be important in the tamoxifen therapy setting, and the *TCL1A* gene [69]. These findings now serve as an important addition to early discoveries of associations that link estrogen-receptor and aromatase [70] polymorphisms with tamoxifen efficacy and toxicity outcomes, and illustrate the important principle that *a full understanding of drug effect eludes us in many situations, and studies designed using single candidate gene approaches may miss important associations.*

### Nortriptyline

Nortriptyline was one of the first clinically important drugs to be shown to be metabolized by

CYP2D6 [71, 72]. These early studies, prior to the era of genotyping, were performed in phenotyped panels of healthy subjects and the results subsequently were confirmed in patient studies as well as *in vitro*, using human liver microsomes and expressed enzymes. Dalén *et al.* [73] administered nortriptyline as a single oral dose to 21 healthy Swedish Caucasian subjects with different genotypes. As seen in the left panel of Figure 13.7, plasma concentrations of nortriptyline were higher in subjects with the *CYP2D6*4/*4* genotype (no functional genes) than in those with one to three functional genes (gene duplication). The plasma concentrations of the nortriptyline metabolite, 10-hydroxynortriptyline, show the opposite pattern – that is, the lowest concentrations were measured in the PMs (Figure 13.8, right panel). This study clearly shows the impact on nortriptyline metabolism of the detrimental *CYP2D6*4* allele as well as of *CYP2D6*2* gene duplication/amplification [73].

A relationship between CYP2D6 genotype and steady-state plasma concentrations of nortriptyline and its hydroxy metabolite also was shown in Swedish depressed patients [74], and in Chinese subjects living in Sweden. Morita *et al.* [75] correlated the *CYP2D6*10* allele with steady-state plasma levels of nortriptyline and its metabolites in Japanese depressed patients. These authors concluded that the Asian *CYP2D6*10* allele encodes an enzyme with decreased nortriptyline-metabolizing activity.

However, this effect is less pronounced than is the effect of the Caucasian-specific *CYP2D6*4* allele, which encodes no enzyme at all. Although CYP2D6 genotyping may eventually find clinical use as a tool to predict proper dosing of drugs such as nortriptyline in individual patients, it must, however, be remembered that there are population-specific alleles.

### Other Drugs

Another class of CYP2D6-metabolized drugs consists of all the β-adrenoreceptor blockers that undergo metabolism, including propranolol [76], metoprolol [77], carvedilol [78], and timolol [79]. While few studies of patient response are available, an elegant clinical pharmacologic study has demonstrated lower resting heart rates in timolol-treated PMs [80]. On the other hand, a key principle is illustrated by studies demonstrating that altered pharmacokinetics of propranolol in Chinese were *not* accompanied by the expected pharmacodynamic changes [80]. In this case, increased concentrations in PMs apparently were offset by changes in pharmacodynamic responsiveness.

Lastly, an important lesson that has been learned from research on CYP2D6 is that many, but not all, genetic polymorphisms can be mimicked by drug interactions. Not only is codeine metabolism by CYP2D6 potently inhibited by quinidine [81], but the inhibition of this enzyme by commonly prescribed

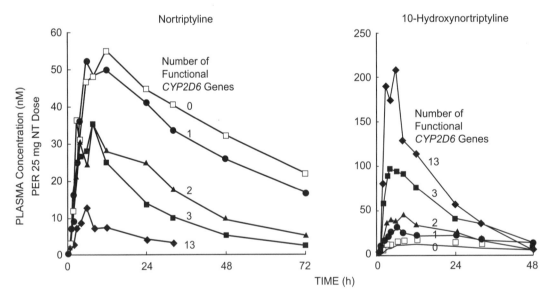

**FIGURE 13.7** Mean plasma concentrations of nortriptyline (NT) (*left*) and 10-hydroxynortriptyline (*right*) in different genotype groups after a single oral dose of nortriptyline. The numerals close to the curves represent the number of functional *CYP2D6* genes in each genotype group. In groups with 0–3 functional genes, there were 5 subjects in each group. There was only one subject with 13 functional genes. Reproduced with permission from Dalén P, Dahl, M-L, Ruiz, MLB *et al.* Clin Pharmacol Ther 1998;63:444–52 [73].

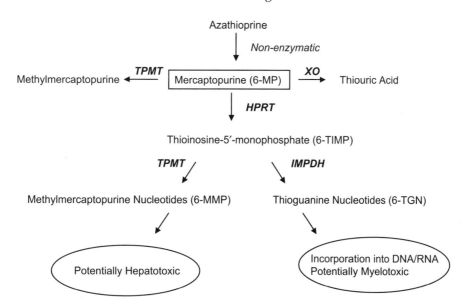

**FIGURE 13.8** Thiopurine metabolic pathways. TPMT, thiopurine methyltransferase; XO, xanthineoxidase; HPRT, hypoxanthine guanine phosphoribosyltransferase; IMPDH, inosine monophosphate dehydrogenase.

drugs such as fluoxetine [82], paroxetine [83, 84], and the majority of antipsychotic drugs [85], including haloperidol [86], is well described. These interactions are likely clinically relevant and more prevalent in many circumstances than the PM genotype [87]. Of note, the ultrarapid metabolizer phenotype of CYP2D6 has not at present been shown to be mimicked by a drug interaction, and the rare reports of effects of metabolic inducers on CYP2D6 activity are unclear, and appear modest at best [88].

*The Thiopurine S-Methyltransferase Polymorphism*

One of the most developed examples of clinical pharmacogenomics involves the polymorphism of thiopurine *S*-methyltransferase (TPMT). This is a cytosolic enzyme whose precise physiological role is unknown. It catalyzes the S-methylation of the thiopurine agents azathioprine, 6-mercaptopurine, and 6-thioguanine using *S*-adenosylmethionine as a methyl donor [89]. Originally found in the kidney and liver of rats and mice, it was subsequently shown to be present in most tissues, including blood cells [90]. Due to its good correlation with TPMT activity in other tissues, TPMT activity is measured clinically in easily obtained erythrocytes [90]. TPMT activity is polymorphic, and a trimodal distribution has been demonstrated in Caucasians [90]. About one subject in 300 is homozygous for a defective *TPMT* allele, with very low or absent enzyme activity. Eleven percent of subjects are heterozygous with an intermediate activity [90]. The frequency with which TPMT activity is lost varies in

different populations, and has been reported to be as low as 0.006–0.04% in Asian populations, in contrast to the frequency of 0.3% in Caucasians [91].

The *TPMT* gene is located on chromosome 6 and includes 10 exons [92]. *TPMT*3A*, the most common mutated allele, contains two point mutations in exons 7 (G460A and Ala154Thr) and 10 (A719G and Tyr240Lys). Two other alleles contain a single mutation, the first SNP (*TPMT*3B*) and the second SNP (*TPMT*3C*) [92]. Aarbakke *et al.* [93] have reviewed the variant alleles of the *TPMT* gene and the relationship to TPMT deficiency. In Caucasians, *TPMT*3A* accounts for about 85% of mutated alleles, and in such populations the analysis of the known alleles may predict the TPMT activity phenotype. In a Korean population, *TPMT*3A* was absent and the most common allele was *TPMT*3C* [94, 95]. However, early investigations focused on allele-specific screening for only four alleles, namely *TPMT*2*, *TPMT*3A*, *TPMT*3B*, and *TPMT*3C* [95]. Due to the limited scope of the screening used in the majority of studies investigating ethnic-specific *TPMT* allele frequencies, continued studies in different populations involving full-gene sequencing or similar techniques seem necessary [96]. Otherwise, selecting only those alleles that are more frequent in a single population may result in important alleles being overlooked in other populations.

Azathioprine and 6-mercaptopurine are immunosuppressants that are used to treat patients with several conditions, including immunological disorders, and to prevent acute rejection in transplant recipients. In Europe, azathioprine, the precursor of

6-mercaptopurine, has been the thiopurine of choice in inflammatory bowel disease, whereas in parts of North America 6-mercaptopurine is more commonly used. 6-Mercaptopurine also is commonly used in acute lymphoblastic leukemia of childhood [97]. Azathioprine is an imidazole derivative of 6-mercaptopurine and is metabolized non-enzymatically to 6-mercaptopurine, as shown in Figure 13.8. As seen in this figure, 6-mercaptopurine is metabolized by several pathways, one of which is catalyzed by TPMT and leads to inactive methyl-thiopurine metabolites. Other pathways are catalyzed by several other enzymes and lead to pharmacologically active thioguanine nucleotides (6-TGNs). The resulting 6-TGNs act as purine antagonists through their incorporation into DNA and subsequent prevention of DNA replication. The reduction in DNA replication suppresses various immunological functions in lymphocytes, T cells, and plasma cells [97]. Numerous studies have shown that TPMT-deficient patients are at very high risk of developing severe hematopoietic toxicity if treated with conventional thiopurine doses [98]. High concentrations of 6-TGNs in patients with low TPMT activity may cause toxicity and bone marrow suppression. On the other hand, low concentrations in patients with high TPMT activity may increase the risk of therapeutic failure and also of liver toxicity, due to the accumulation of other metabolites such as 6-methylmercaptopurine nucleotides (Figure 13.8). Other less serious azathioprine side effects are gastrointestinal symptoms, such as nausea and vomiting, representing azathioprine intolerance that is not clearly associated with TPMT activity or metabolite levels.

An important goal of thiopurine therapy is to provide the intended treatment effect while avoiding adverse effects. In this regard, several studies have shown a relationship between therapeutic effects and TPMT activity or 6-TGN concentrations in red blood cells. However, more clinical studies are needed to establish therapeutic concentration ranges for the various conditions in which these drugs are used. So far, most drug-effect studies are focused on 6-TGN concentrations. However, other enzymes and metabolites are also involved in the complex metabolism of thiopurines. Thus, there could be as yet unknown factors involved in the metabolism and action of thiopurine drugs that might also have a significant correlation with treatment outcome. Possible pharmacogenetic factors include polymorphisms in CYP2C9, CYP2C19, and CYP2D6 that could reasonably be investigated in further studies.

Because it has been conclusively demonstrated that low TPMT activity due to TPMT polymorphism can lead to severe myelosuppression in patients treated with thiopurines, and a number of studies have shown pretreatment TPMT-status testing is a cost-effective and reliable way of predicting life-threatening bone marrow toxicity, we are among the many authors who believe that TPMT *phenotype* status testing should be incorporated in routine clinical practice and used to adjust dosing in order to avoid severe adverse drug reactions in patients identified with intermediate as well as low to absent TPMT activity. Although the pretreatment TPMT status of patients can be measured by phenotype or genotype testing, the clinical utility of measuring *TPMT* genotype is uncertain in view of the difficulties involved in interpreting the consequences of novel polymorphism detection and the chance of missing clinically relevant allelic variation in different racial groups. Furthermore, standard genotyping techniques cannot, as yet, predict those individuals with very high TPMT activities who may not respond to standard doses of azathioprine or 6-mercaptopurine. Thus, despite its clinical importance, pharmacogenetic testing for this polymorphism remains problematic, since a large number of alleles must be tested, genetic haplotype identification is difficult, and phenotypic measurements that quantify the enzyme in erythrocytes remain more useful than genetic tests.

### N-Acetyltransferase 2

In marked contrast to the data on genetic changes in thiopurine methyltransferase, mutations in *N*-acetyltransferase 2 (*NAT-2*) are very common, but have little clinical significance [21]. *NAT-2* can therefore be placed on the pyramid of genetic information at a point where clear pharmacokinetic changes have been noted, but important pharmacodynamic consequences have not yet been demonstrated. In addition, as with *CYP2D6*, it is clear that a large number of mutations, and at least 17 different alleles, contribute to this change in activity [99]. The slow-acetylator phenotype is present in roughly 50% of Caucasian and African populations studied, but in as few 10% of Japanese and as many as 80% of Egyptians [100, 101]. Woosley *et al.* [102] demonstrated that slow acetylators develop positive antinuclear antibody (ANA) titers and procainamide-induced lupus more quickly than rapid acetylators. However, this finding did not lead to widespread phenotypic or genetic testing, because all patients will develop positive ANA titers after 1 year of procainamide therapy and almost a third will have developed arthralgias and/or a skin rash [103]. Although a number of studies have attempted to associate this polymorphism with the risk for xenobiotic-induced bladder, colorectal [104], or breast cancer

[105], there are at present no compelling data that warrant phenotypic testing for this polymorphism in order to improve treatment with any medicine, much less a genetic test that would have to accurately identify such a large number of alleles.

## Mutations that Influence Drug Receptors

### $\beta_2$-Adrenoreceptor Mutations in Asthma

Since the first descriptions of genetic polymorphisms in the $\beta_2$-adrenoreceptor ($\beta_2$AR) that may play a pathogenic role in the development of asthma [106, 107], a number of investigators have shown an association between these mutations and patient response to treatment for this disease. A number of missense mutations within the coding region of the $\beta_2$AR gene on chromosome 5q31 have been identified in humans. In studies utilizing site-directed mutagenesis and recombinant expression, three loci at amino acid positions 16, 27, and 164 have been found to significantly alter *in vitro* receptor function. The Thr164Ile mutation displays altered coupling to adenylyl cyclase, the Arg16Gly mutation displays enhanced agonist-promoted downregulation, and the Gln27Glu form is resistant to downregulation [107]. The frequencies of these various $\beta_2$AR mutations are not different in asthmatic than in normal populations, but Lima *et al.* [108] have shown that the albuterol-evoked increase in forced expiratory volume in 1 second ($FEV_1$) was higher and bronchodilatory response was more rapid in Arg16 homozygotes than in a cohort of carriers of the Gly16 variant. In addition, an association has been demonstrated between the same $\beta_2$AR polymorphism and susceptibility to bronchodilator desensitization in moderately severe stable asthmatics. Although these data are compelling, careful studies have concluded that the $\beta_2$AR genotype is not a major determinant of fatal or near-fatal asthma [109], and widespread testing of asthmatic patients for the presence of genetic polymorphisms in the $\beta_2$AR is not yet routinely carried out. Nevertheless, a number of other potential target proteins may alter the susceptibility and response of asthmatic patients, including histamine N-methyltransferase [110] and the lipoxygenase system, and further developments in the genetics of asthma pharmacotherapy seem likely.

### Mutations in Endothelial Nitric Oxide Synthase

An association has been made between cardiovascular disease and specific mutations in endothelial nitric oxide synthase (e-NOS), the enzyme that creates nitric oxide via the conversion of citrulline to arginine in endothelial cells and in platelets [111]. A firmer understanding of the mechanism of this effect has been provided by a series of careful studies of forearm vascular vasodilation conducted by Abernethy and Babaoglu [112], who showed that acetylcholine, but not nitroprusside-mediated vasodilation, was compromised by the Glu298Asp mutation in this enzyme. These results demonstrate the value of careful clinical pharmacologic studies in confirming a pharmacological consequence of a polymorphism that otherwise would only have had an association with cardiovascular disease. The implications of these findings for patients with hypertension, congestive heart failure, and a variety of other disorders are clear issues for future investigation.

### Somatic Mutations in the Epidermal Growth Factor Receptor in Tumors

From the perspective of medical practitioners and most patients, the treatment of non-small-cell lung cancer has not significantly advanced over the past 25 years. The advent of treatment with the tyrosine kinase inhibitor gefitinib brought a new approach, but it was clear from the start that only a few patients appeared to benefit. Subsequently, somatic mutations in the epidermal growth factor receptor (EGFR) were discovered that appear to identify a subpopulation of patients who respond well to this drug [113]. These mutations entail a "gain of function" within the tumors of these patients that appear to *enhance* their responsiveness to gefitinib. Further studies are ongoing that have been designed to replicate these data in larger populations, and to refine the genetic signature of "responder" tumors. The identification of this subset of responder patients with these mutations represents an important conceptual advance from the usual assumption that all mutations are inevitably deleterious, and also directly challenges the traditional paradigm that a drug should be effective in all patients with a given diagnosis in order to be useful.

Recent retrospective studies on cetuximab, a monoclonal antibody targeted against EGFR, have shown that patients with tumors bearing an activating variant in exon 2 of KRAS, a gene that links EGFR activation with downstream events that regulate cell growth, proliferation, and survival (Figure 13.9), have not benefited from cetuximab treatment [114]. Therefore, following an intense public discussion at an FDA Advisory Committee Meeting [115, 116], the FDA revised the indication section of the cetuximab (Erbitux®) labeling to include the warning that "Erbitux is not recommended for the treatment of colorectal cancer with these mutations". Similar

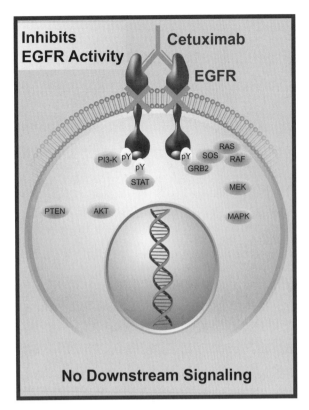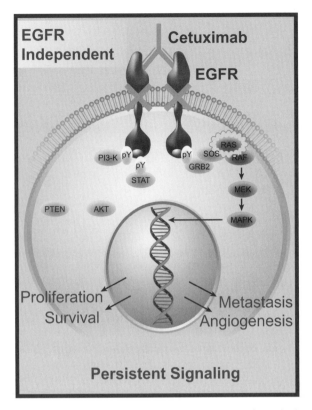

**FIGURE 13.9**    The role of *KRAS* status and cetuximab activity in colorectal cancer. In the wild-type state of *KRAS* (*left panel*), the binding of cetuximab to EGFR can shut down the receptor-mediated signaling. In the variant *KRAS* state (*right panel*), the system is in an active state and not responsive to cetuximab and there is persistent signaling. Modified from Youssoufian H. Oncologic Drugs Advisory Committee Hearing, December 16, 2008 [116]. (Internet at, www.fda.gov/ohrms/dockets/ac/08/slides/2008-4409s1-04-ImClone.pdf.)

wording also appears in the labeling of the EGFR-blocker, panitumumab (Table 13.2). However, there are still patients with wild type *KRAS* who do not respond to EGFR-blocking drugs, so additional genomic or other biomarkers are needed to select only those patients who would benefit from treatment with these drugs.

## Combined Variants in Drug Metabolism and Receptor Genes: The Value of Drug Pathway Analysis

Each drug has a pharmacokinetic pathway of absorption, distribution, metabolism, and excretion that is ultimately linked to an effect pathway involving receptor targets and downstream signaling systems. As in the example of cetuximab and the EGFR pathway, it is clearly possible that many of the proteins in these pathways may be genetically polymorphic. It also is instructive to examine the situation in which patient response is affected by variants in a gene involved in drug *metabolism and transport* and also by variants in a *receptor*. In this situation, consideration of the combination of both these factors provides greater predictive power than when either is considered alone.

Warfarin is a commonly used anticoagulant that requires careful clinical management to balance the risks of over-anticoagulation and bleeding with those of under-anticoagulation and clotting. In a series of well designed studies, Rettie *et al.* [117] first showed that CYP2C9 is the principal enzyme involved in the metabolism of (*S*)-warfarin, the active stereoisomer of warfarin. Two relatively common variant forms with reduced metabolic activity have been identified: *CYP2C9*2* and *CYP2C9*3* [118]. Patients with these genetic variants require lower maintenance doses of warfarin, and these investigators subsequently showed a direct association between CYP2C9 genotype and anticoagulation status or bleeding risk [119]. Finally, employing knowledge of the pathway of warfarin's action via Vitamin K carboxylase (VKOR), these authors showed, first in a test population and then in a validation population of 400 patients at a different medical center, that predictions of patient response based on identification of variants in VKOR combined with those in CYP2C9 were more powerful than when only a single variant was used [120].

**TABLE 13.7 Key Pharmacogenetic Principles**

- The excessive initial hyperbole surrounding many pharmacogenetics studies before they are replicated has resulted in an inappropriately high level of expectation of clinically meaningful results in the near term, and may have impeded researchers who wish to replicate the data in other populations
- There are now well-documented examples of duplicated CYP2D6*1 and CYP2D6*4 genes, making the important point that not all multiple copies are functional
- Pharmacogenetic testing is of most clinical value when there is great variability in drug effect
- Variants in genes involved in drug metabolism and transport may be combined with variants in a receptor, and this approach may provide more predictive power than when either is considered alone
- A full understanding of drug effect eludes us in many situations, and studies designed using single candidate gene approaches may miss important associations
- It is critically important to replicate pharmacogenetic findings in relatively large datasets consisting of patients in real clinical practice

A final key pharmacogenetic principle made clear by these studies is the crucial importance of replicating pharmacogenetic findings in relatively large datasets consisting of patients in real clinical practice. This is related to the very first pharmacogenetic principle described in this chapter; namely, that the excessive initial hyperbole surrounding many pharmacogenetics studies before they are replicated has resulted in an inappropriately high level of expectation of clinically meaningful results in the near term, and may have impeded researchers who wish to replicate the data in other populations (Table 13.7).

## CONCLUSIONS AND FUTURE DIRECTIONS

There are many potential pitfalls that lie in the way of researchers on the route from the discovery of a mutation in human DNA that codes for a pharmacologically important protein, to the development of a clinically useful pharmacogenetic test. Very few such tests have been developed and included in drug labeling as yet, but a considerable number seem likely to be found useful over the next decade in guiding the treatment of patients with cancer, asthma, depression, hypertension, and pain. It is evident that the future evolution of pharmacogenomic tests as clinically useful biomarkers will require the iterative process of analytical validation and context-specific clinical qualification that is described in Chapter 18, as their use is first assessed in relatively small laboratory-based studies in clinical research settings and then expanded into more general clinical practice.

The technical reliability of DNA testing in terms of intra- and interday variability and the robustness of assays when applied to multiple DNA samples will have to be demonstrated almost more carefully than would be required for routine serum chemistries or hematology assays. This is because there are significant societal pressures that insist upon the accuracy of a diagnostic test that informs a physician and a patient about an individual's genetic makeup. However, the requirement for robust tests has not prevented any other technology from entering clinical practice, and already a number of validated array-based genetic tests are available that are able to diagnose genotypes simultaneously at a relatively large number of loci.

The evidence supporting the clinical utility of any test will necessarily be diverse, and will not universally consist of data generated from randomized clinical trials. This is clear already, since the cost, time, and lack of generalizability of randomized clinical trials limit their usefulness in this context. Alternative and credible study designs will inevitably be required to make possible the rapid translation of new tests and their associated drugs into practice. Indeed, there are many complementary sources of evidence (mechanistic, pharmacological, and observational studies) that can all contribute to establishing clinical utility [121]. The aggregate of this diverse evidence, rather than the results of single studies or randomized clinical trials, will be required by regulatory agencies, learned societies, and healthcare reimbursement agencies to provide guidances and guidelines that allow approval and access to appropriately characterized groups of patients.

When these barriers are overcome, it seems very likely that the practice of medicine will evolve so that individual patients can be treated for their diseases with appropriately individualized doses of medicines, or indeed different medicines directed at specific therapeutic targets, based on their genotype or phenotype. However, as noted earlier, genomic education is key to the successful clinical implementation of personalized medicine. Understanding of the clinical utility of genomic tests is critical for their practical use, and various consortia have been formed with the aim of providing evidence-based decision-making in the use of pharmacogenetic/genomic tests

These consortia include the recently established Clinical Pharmacogenetic Implementation Consortium (CPIC), which has published guidelines for the use of specific tests with individual drug therapies, including tests for variants of TPMT (for azathioprine, mercaptopurine), CYP2C19 (for clopidogrel), CYP2C9, and VKORC1 (for warfarin) [122].

## REFERENCES

[1] Kohn LT, Corrigan JM, Donaldson MS, editors. Committee on Quality of Health Care in America. To err is human: Building a safer health system. Washington, DC: National Academy Press; 1999.

[2] Feero WG, Green ED. Genomic education for healthcare professionals in the 21st century. JAMA 2011;306:989–90.

[3] Lesko LJ, Zineh I, Huang S-M. What is clinical utility and why should we care? Clin Pharmacol Ther 2010;88:729–33.

[4] Zineh I, Huang S-M. Biomarkers in drug development and regulation: A paradigm for clinical implementation of personalized medicine. Biomarker Med 2011;5:705–13.

[5] Hamburg MA, Collins FS. The path to personalized medicine. N Engl J Med 2010;363:301–4.

[6] Nebert DW. Pharmacogenetics: 65 candles on the cake. Pharmacogenetics 1997;7:435–40.

[7] Balian JD, Sukhova N, Harris JW, Hewett J, Pickle L, Goldstein JA, et al. The hydroxylation of omeprazole correlates with S-mephenytoin metabolism: A population study. Clin Pharmacol Ther 1995;57:662–9.

[8] Desta Z, Zhao X, Shin JG, Flockhart DA. Clinical significance of the cytochrome P450 2C19 polymorphism. Clin Pharmacokinet 2002;41:913–58.

[9] Furuta T, Ohashi K, Kamata T, Takashiima M, Kosuge K, Kawasaki T, et al. Effect of genetic differences in omeprazole metabolism on cure rates for Helicobacter pylori infection and peptic ulcer. Ann Intern Med 1998;129:1027–30.

[10] Andersson T, Regardh CG, Lou YC, Zhang Y, Dahl M-L, Bertilsson L. Polymorphic hydroxylation of S-mephenytoin and omeprazole metabolism in Caucasian and Chinese subjects. Pharmacogenetics 1992;2:25–31.

[11] Furuta T, Ohashi K, Kosuge K, Zhao XJ, Takashima M, Kimura M, et al. CYP2C19 genotype status and effect of omeprazole on intragastric pH in humans. Clin Pharmacol Ther 1999;65:552–61.

[12] Mega JL, Close S, Wiviott SD, Shen L, Hockett RD, Brandt JT, et al. Cytochrome P-450 polymorphisms and response to clopidogrel. N Engl J Med 2009;360:354–62.

[13] Mega JL, Hochholzer W, Frelinger III AL, Kluk MJ, Angiolillo DJ, Kereiakes DJ, et al. Dosing clopidogrel based on CYP2C19 genotype and the effect on platelet reactivity in patients with stable cardiovascular disease. JAMA 2011;306:2221–8.

[14] Mega JL, Simon T, Collet JP, Anderson JL, Antman EM, Bliden K, et al. Reduced-function CYP2C19 genotype and risk of adverse clinical outcomes among patients treated with clopidogrel predominantly for PCI: A meta-analysis. JAMA 2010;04:1821–30.

[15] Schinkel AH, Smit JJ, van Tellingen O, Beijnen JH, Wagenaar E, van Deemter L, et al. Disruption of the mouse mdr1a P-glycoprotein gene leads to a deficiency in the blood–brain barrier and to increase sensitivity to drugs. Cell 1994;77:491–502.

[16] Schinkel AH, Wagenaar E, Mol CAM, van Deemter L. P-Glycoprotein in the blood–brain barrier of mice influences the brain penetration and pharmacological activity of many drugs. J Clin Invest 1996;97:2517–24.

[17] van Asperen J, Schinkel AH, Beijnen JH, Nooijen WJ, Borst P, van Telligen O. Altered pharmacokinetics of vinblastine in Mdr1a P-glycoprotein-deficient mice. J Natl Cancer Inst 1996;88:994–9.

[18] International Transporter Consortium, Giacomini KM, Huang S-M, Tweedie DJ, Benet LZ, Brouwer KL, et al. Membrane transporters in drug development. Nat Rev Drug Disc 2010;9:215–36.

[19] Link E, Parish S, Armitage J, Bowman L, Heath S, Matsuda F, et al. SLCO1B1 variants and statin-induced myopathy–a genomewide study. N Engl J Med 2008;359:789–99.

[20] Niemi M. Transporter pharmacogenetics and statin toxicity. Clin Pharmacol Ther 2010;87:130–3.

[21] Kalow W, Bertilsson L. Interethnic factors affecting drug metabolism. Adv Drug Res 1994;25:1–53.

[22] Mahgoub A, Idle JR, Dring LG, Lancaster R, Smith RL. Polymorphic hydroxylation of debrisoquine in man. Lancet 1977;2:584–6.

[23] Tucker GT, Silas JH, Iyun AO, Lennard MS, Smith AJ. Polymorphic hydroxylation of debrisoquine in man. Lancet 1977;2:718.

[24] Eichelbaum M, Spannbrucker N, Steincke B, Dengler HJ. Defective N-oxidation of sparteine in man: A new pharmacogenetic defect. Eur J Clin Pharmacol 1979;16:183–7.

[25] Eichelbaum M, Bertilsson L, Säwe J, Zekorn C. Polymorphic oxidation of sparteine and debrisoquine: Related pharmacogenetic entities. Clin Pharmacol Ther 1982;31:184–6.

[26] Eichelbaum M, Gross AS. The genetic polymorphism of debrisoquine/sparteine metabolism: Clinical aspects. In: Kalow W, editor. Pharmacogenetics of drug metabolism. New York, NY: Pergamon Press; 1992. p. 625–48.

[27] Bertilsson L, Lou Y-Q, Du Y-L, Liu Y, Kuang T-Y, Liao X-M, et al. Pronounced differences between native Chinese and Swedish populations in the polymorphic hydroxylations of debrisoquin and S-mephenytoin [erratum in Clin Pharmacol Ther 1994;55:648]. Clin Pharmacol Ther 1992;51:388–97.

[28] Nakamura K, Goto F, Ray WA, McAllister CB, Jacqz E, Wilkinson GR, et al. Interethnic differences in genetic polymorphism of debrisoquin and mephenytoin hydroxylation between Japanese and Caucasian populations. Clin Pharmacol Ther 1985;38:402–8.

[29] Sohn D-R, Shin S-G, Park C-W, Kusaka M, Chiba K, Ishizaki T. Metoprolol oxidation polymorphism in a Korean population: Comparison with native Japanese and Chinese populations. Br J Clin Pharmacol 1991;32:504–7.

[30] Roh HK, Dahl ML, Johansson I, Ingelman-Sundberg M, Cha YN, Bertilsson L. Debrisoquine and S-mephenytoin hydroxylation phenotypes and genotypes in a Korean population. Pharmacogenetics 1996;6:441–7.

[31] Eichelbaum M, Baur MP, Dengler HJ, Osikowska-Evers BO, Tieves G, Zekorn C, et al. Chromosomal assignment of human cytochrome P450 (debrisoquine/sparteine type) to chromosome 22. Br J Clin Pharmacol 1987;23:455–8.

[32] Gonzalez FJ, Skoda RC, Kimura S, Umeno M, Zanger UM, Nebert DW, et al. Characterization of the common genetic defect in humans deficient in debrisoquine metabolism. Nature 1988;331:442–6.

[33] Gaedigk A, Blum M, Gaedigk R, Eichelbaum M, Meyer UA. Deletion of the entire cytochrome P450 CYP2D6 gene as a cause of impaired drug metabolism in poor metabolizers of the debrisoquine/sparteine polymorphism. Am J Hum Genet 1991;48:943–50.

[34] Heim M, Meyer UA. Genotyping of poor metabolisers of debrisoquine by allele-specific PCR amplification [see comments]. Lancet 1990;336:529–32.

[35] Heim M, Meyer UA. Evolution of a highly polymorphic human cytochrome P450 gene cluster: CYP2D6. Genomics 1992;14:49–58.

[36] Daly AK, Brockmoller J, Broly F, Eichelbaum M, Evans WE, Gonzalez FJ, et al. Nomenclature for human CYP2D6 alleles. Pharmacogenetics 1996;6:193–201.

[37] Dahl M-L, Johansson I, Palmertz MP, Ingelman-Sundberg M, Sjöqvist F. Analysis of the *CYP2D6* gene in relation to debrisoquin and desipramine hydroxylation in a Swedish population. Clin Pharmacol Ther 1992;51:12–7.

[38] Bertilsson L, Dahl M-L, Dalén P, Al-Sjurbaji A. Molecular genetics of CYP2D6: Clinical relevance with focus on psychotropic drugs. Br J Clin Pharmacol 2002;54:111–38.

[39] Wang S-L, Huang J-D, Lai M-D, Liu B-H, Lai M-L. Molecular basis of genetic variation in debrisoquine hydroxylation in Chinese subjects: Polymorphism in RFLP and DNA sequence of *CYP2D6*. Clin Pharmacol Ther 1993;53:410–8.

[40] Johansson I, Oscarson M, Yue QY, Bertilsson L, Sjöqvist F, Ingelman-Sundberg M. Genetic analysis of the Chinese chromosome P4502D locus: Characterization of variant CYP2D6 genes present in subjects with diminished capacity for debrisoquine hydroxylation. Mol Pharmacol 1994;46:452–9.

[41] Masimirembwa C, Hasler JA, Bertilsson L, Johansson I, Ekberg O, Ingelman-Sundberg M. Phenotype and genotype analysis of debrisoquine hydroxylase (CYP2D6) in a black Zimbabwean population. Reduced enzyme activity and evaluation of metabolic correlation of CYP2D6 probe drugs. Eur J Clin Pharmacol 1996;51:117–22.

[42] Wennerholm A, Johansson I, Massele AY, Jande M, Alm C, Aden-Abdi Y, et al. Decreased capacity for debrisoquine metabolism among black Tanzanians: Analyses of the CYP2D6 genotype and phenotype. Pharmacogenetics 1999;9:707–14.

[43] Griese EU, Asante-Poku S, Ofori-Adjei D, Mikus G, Eichelbaum M. Analysis of the *CYP2D6* mutations and their consequences for enzyme function in a West African population. Pharmacogenetics 1999;9:715–23.

[44] Aklillu E, Persson I, Bertilsson L, Johansson I, Rodrigues F, Ingelman-Sundberg M. Frequent distribution of ultrarapid metabolizers of debrisoquine in an Ethiopian population carrying duplicated and multiduplicated functional *CYP2D6* alleles. J Pharmacol Exp Ther 1996;278:441–6.

[45] Wennerholm A, Dandara C, Sayi J, Svennson J-O, Aden Abdi Y, Ingeman-Sundberg M, et al. The African-specific *CYP2D6*17* allele encodes an enzyme with changed substrate specificity. Clin Pharmacol Ther 2002;71:77–88.

[46] Aklillu E, Herrlin K, Gustafsson LL, Bertilsson L, Ingelman-Sundberg M. Evidence for environmental influence on CYP2D6-catalysed debrisoquine hydroxylation as demonstrated by phenotyping and genotyping of Ethiopians living in Ethiopia or in Sweden. Pharmacogenetics 2002;12:375–83.

[47] Bertilsson L, Åberg-Wistedt A, Gustafsson LL, Nordin C. Extremely rapid hydroxylation of debrisoquine: A case report with implication for treatment with nortryptyline and other tricyclic antidepressants. Ther Drug Monitor 1985;7:478–80.

[48] Bertilsson L, Dahl M-L, Sjöqvist F, Åberg-Wistedt A, Humble M, Johansson I, et al. Molecular basis for rational megaprescribing in ultrarapid hydroxylators of debrisoquine. Lancet 1993;341:63.

[49] Johansson I, Lundqvist E, Bertilsson L, Dahl M-L, Sjöqvist F, Ingelman-Sundberg M. Inherited amplification of an active gene in the cytochrome P450 CYP2D6 locus as a cause of ultrarapid metabolism of debrisoquine. Proc Natl Acad Sci USA 1993;90:11825–9.

[50] Dahl M-L, Johansson I, Bertilsson L, Ingelman-Sundberg M, Sjöqvist F. Ultrarapid hydroxylation of debrisoquine in a Swedish population: Analysis of the molecular genetic basis. J Pharmacol Exp Ther 1995;274:516–20.

[51] Sachse C, Brockmoller J, Bauer S, Roots I. Cytochrome P450 2D6 variants in a Caucasian population: Allele frequencies and phenotypic consequences. Am J Hum Genet 1997;60:284–95.

[52] Bernal ML, Sinues B, Johansson I, McLellan RA, Wennerholm A, Dahl M-L, et al. Ten percent of North Spanish individuals carry duplicated or triplicated *CYP2D6* genes associated with ultrarapid metabolism of debrisoquine. Pharmacogenetics 1999;9:657–60.

[53] Agúndez JAG, Ledesma MC, Ladero JM, Benitez J. Prevalence of *CYP2D6* gene duplication and its repercussion on the oxidative phenotype in a white population. Clin Pharmacol Ther 1995;57:265–9.

[54] Scordo MG, Spina E, Facciola G, Avenoso A, Johansson I, Dahl M-L. Cytochrome P450 2D6 genotype and steady state plasma levels of risperidone and 9-hydroxy-risperidone. Psychopharmacology 1999;147:300–5.

[55] McLellan RA, Oscarson M, Seidegard J, Evans DA, Ingelman-Sundberg M. Frequent occurrence of *CYP2D6* gene duplication in Saudi Arabians. Pharmacogenetics 1997;7:187–91.

[56] Kawanishi C, Lundgren S, Ågren H, Bertilsson L. Increased incidence of *CYP2D6* gene duplication in patients with persistent mood disorders: Ultrarapid metabolism of antidepressants as a cause of non response. A pilot study. Eur J Clin Pharmacol 2004;59:803–7.

[57] Koren G, Cairns J, Gaedigk A, Leeder SJ. Pharmacogenetics of morphine poisoning in a breastfed neonate of a codeine-prescribed mother. Lancet 2006;368:704.

[58] Madadi P, Ross CJ, Hayden MR, Carleton BC, Gaedigk A, Leeder JS, et al. Pharmacogenetics of neonatal opioid toxicity following maternal use of codeine during breastfeeding: A case–control study. Clin Pharmacol Ther 2009;85:31–5.

[59] Johnson MD, Zuo H, Lee KH, Trebley JP, Rae JM, Weatherman RV, et al. Pharmacological characterization of 4-hydroxy-N-desmethyl tamoxifen, a novel active metabolite of tamoxifen. Breast Cancer Res Treat 2004;85:151–9.

[60] Desta Z, Ward BA, Soukhova NV, Flockhart DA. Comprehensive evaluation of tamoxifen sequential biotransformation by the human cytochrome P450 system *in vitro*: Prominent roles for CYP3A and CYP2D6. J Pharmacol Exp Ther 2004;310:1062–75.

[61] Jin Y, Desta Z, Stearns V, Ward B, Ho H, Lee KH, et al. CYP2D6 genotype, antidepressant use, and tamoxifen metabolism during adjuvant breast cancer treatment. J Natl Cancer Inst 2005;97:30–9.

[62] Kiyotani K, Mushiroda T, Imamura CK, Tanigawara Y, Hosono N, Kubo M, et al. Dose-adjustment study of tamoxifen based on CYP2D6 genotypes in Japanese breast cancer patients. Breast Cancer Res Treat 2012;131:137–45.

[63] Barginear MF, Jaremko M, Peter I, Yu C, Kasai Y, Kemeny M, et al. Increasing tamoxifen dose in breast cancer patients based on CYP2D6 genotypes and endoxifen levels: Effect on active metabolite isomers and the antiestrogenic activity score. Clin Pharmacol Ther 2011;90:605–11.

[64] Henry NL, Hayes DF, Rae JM. CYP2D6 testing for breast cancer patients: Is there more to the story? Oncology (Williston Park) 2009;23. 1236, 1243, 1249.

[65] Del Re M, Michelucci A, Simi P, Danesi R. Pharmacogenetics of anti-estrogen treatment of breast cancer. Cancer Treat Rev (in press) [Epub ahead of print Sep 12, 2011].

[66] Woods B, Veenstra D, Hawkins N. Prioritizing pharmacogenetic research: A value of information analysis of CYP2D6 testing to guide breast cancer treatment. Value Health (in press). [Epub ahead of print Nov 12, 2011].

[67] Lu WJ, Xu C, Pei Z, Mayhoub AS, Cushman M, Flockhart DA. The tamoxifen metabolite norendoxifen is a potent and selective inhibitor of aromatase (CYP19) and a potential lead compound for novel therapeutic agents. Breast Cancer Res Treat (in press) [Epub ahead of print Aug 4, 2011].

[68] Lu WJ, Desta Z, Flockhart DA. Tamoxifen metabolites as active inhibitors of aromatase in the treatment of breast cancer. Breast Cancer Res Treat 2012;131:473–81.

[69] Ingle JN, Schaid DJ, Goss PE, Liu M, Mushiroda T, Chapman JA, et al. Genome-wide associations and functional genomic studies of musculoskeletal adverse events in women receiving aromatase inhibitors. J Clin Oncol 2010;28:4674–82.

[70] Wang L, Ellsworth KA, Moon I, Pelleymounter LL, Eckloff BW, Martin YN, et al. Functional genetic polymorphisms in the aromatase gene *CYP19* vary the response of breast cancer patients to neoadjuvant therapy with aromatase inhibitors. Cancer Res. 2010;70:319–28.

[71] Bertilsson L, Eichelbaum M, Mellström B, Säwe J, Schulz H-U, Sjöqvist F. Nortryptyline and antipyrine clearance in relation to debrisoquine hydroxylation in man. Life Sci 1980;27:1673–7.

[72] Mellström B, Bertilsson L, Säwe J, Schulz H-U, Sjöqvist F. E- and Z-10-hydroxylation of nortryptyline: relationship to polymorphic debrisoquine hydroxylation. Clin Pharmacol Ther 1991;30:189–93.

[73] Dalén P, Dahl M-L, Ruiz MLB, Nordin J, Eng R, Bertilsson L. 10-hydroxylation of nortriptyline in white persons with 0, 1, 2, 3, and 13 functional CYPD6 genes. Clin Pharmacol Ther 1998;63:444–52.

[74] Dahl M-L, Bertilsson L, Nordin C. Steady state plasma levels of nortriptyline and its 10-hydroxy metabolite: relationship to the CYP2D6 genotype. Psychopharmacology 1996;123:315–9.

[75] Morita S, Shimoda K, Someya T, Yoshimura Y, Kamijima K, Kato N. Steady state plasma levels of nortriptyline and its hydroxylated metabolites in Japanese patients: Impact of CYP2D6 genotype on the hydroxylation of nortriptyline. J Clin Psychopharmacol 2000;20:141–9.

[76] Ward SA, Walle T, Walle UK, Wilkinson GR, Branch RA. Propanolol's metabolism is determined by both mephenytoin and debrisoquin hydroxylase activities. Clin Pharmacol Ther 1989;45:72–9.

[77] Johnson JA, Burlew BS. Metoprolol metabolism via cytochrome P450 2D6 in ethnic populations. Drug Metab Dispos 1996;24:350–5.

[78] Zhou HH, Wood AJ. Stereoselective disposition of carvedilol is determined by CYP2D6. Clin Pharmacol Ther 1995;57:518–24.

[79] McGourty JC, Silas JH, Fleming JJ, McBurney A, Ward JW. Pharmacokinetics and beta-blocking effects of timolol in poor and extensive metabolizers of debrisoquin. Clin Pharmacol Ther 1985;38:409–13.

[80] Zhou HH, Koshakji RP, Silberstein DJ, Wilkinson GR, Wood AJ. Racial differences in drug response: Altered sensitivity to and clearance of propanolol in men of Chinese descent as compared with American whites. N Engl J Med 1989;320:565–70.

[81] Caraco Y, Sheller J, Wood AJ. Impact of ethnic origin and quinidine coadministration on codeine's disposition and pharmacodynamic effects. J Pharmacol Exp Ther 1999;290:413–22.

[82] Otton SV, Wu D, Joffe RT, Cheung SW, Sellers EM. Inhibition by fluoxetine of cytochrome P450 2D6 activity. Clin Pharmacol Ther 1993;53:401–9.

[83] Sindrup SH, Brøsen K, Gram LF, Hallas J, Skjelbo E, Allen A, et al. The relationship between paroxetine and the sparteine oxidation polymorphism. Clin Pharmacol Ther 1992;51:278–87.

[84] Alderman J, Preskorn SH, Greenblatt DJ, Harrison W, Penenberg D, Allison J, et al. Desipramine pharmacokinetics when coadministered with paroxetine or sertraline in extensive metabolizers. J Clin Psychopharmacol 1997;17:284–91.

[85] Shin J-G, Soukhova N, Flockhart DA. Effect of antipsychotic drugs on human liver cytochrome P-450 (CYP) isoforms in vitro: Preferential inhibition of CYP2D6. Drug Metab Dispos 1999;27:1078–84.

[86] Ereshefsky L. Pharmacokinetics and drug interactions: Update for new antipsychotics [see comments]. J Clin Psychiatry 1996;57(Suppl. 11):12–25.

[87] Goff DC, Midha KK, Brotman AW, Waites M, Baldessarini RJ. Elevation of plasma concentrations of haloperidol after the addition of fluoxetine. Am J Psychiatry 1991;148:790–2.

[88] Dilger K, Greiner B, Fromm MF, Hofmann U, Kroemer HK, Eichelbaum M. Consequences of rifampicin treatment on propafenone disposition in extensive and poor metabolizers of CYP2D6. Pharmacogenetics 1999;9:551–9.

[89] Krynetski EY, Tai HL, Yates CR, Fessing MY, Loennechen T. Schuetz JD et al. Genetic polymorphism of thiopurine S-methyltransferase: Clinical importance and molecular mechanisms. Pharmacogenetics 1996;6:279–90.

[90] Weinshilboum RM, Sladek SL. Mercaptopurine pharmacogenetics: Monogenic inheritance of erythrocyte thiopurine methyltranferase activity. Am J Hum Genet 1980;32:651–62.

[91] Yates CR, Krynetski EY, Loennechen T, Fessing MY, Tai HL, Pui CH, et al. Molecular diagnosis of thiopurine S-methyltransferase deficiency: Genetic basis for azathioprine and mercaptopurine intolerance. Ann Intern Med 1997;126:608–14.

[92] Szumlanski C, Otterness D, Her C, Lee D, Brandriff B, Kelsell D, et al. Thiopurine methyltransferase pharmacogenetics: Human gene cloning and characterization of a common polymorphism. DNA Cell Biol 1996;15:17–30.

[93] Aarbakke J, Janka-Schaub G, Elion GB. Thiopurine biology and pharmacology. Trends Pharmacol Sci 1997;18:3–7.

[94] Lennard L. Clinical implications of thiopurine methyltransferase – optimization of drug dosage and potential drug interactions. Ther Drug Monitor 1998;20:527–31.

[95] Otterness D, Szumlanski C, Lennard L, Klemetsdal B, Aarbakke J, Park-Hah JO, et al. Human thiopurine methyltransferase pharmacogenetics: Gene sequence polymorphisms. Clin Pharmacol Ther 1997;62:60–73.

[96] Van Aken J, Schmedders M, Feuerstein G, Kollek R. Prospects and limits of pharmacogenetics: The thiopurine methyltransferase (TPMT) experience. Am J Pharmacogenomics 2003;3:149–55.

[97] Baker DE. Pharmacogenomics of azathioprine and 6-mercaptopurine in gastroenterologic therapy. Rev Gastroenterol Disord 2003;3:150–7.

[98] McLeod HL, Yu J. Cancer Pharmacogenomics: SNPs, chips and the individual patient. Cancer Invest 2003;21:630–40.

[99] Agúndez JAG, Olivera M, Martinez C, Ladero JM, Benitez J. Identification and prevalence study of 17 allelic variants of the human NAT2 gene in a white population. Pharmacogenetics 1996;6:423–8.

[100] Lin HJ, Han CY, Lin BK, Hardy S. Ethnic distribution of slow acetylator mutations in the polymorphic N-acetyltransferase (NAT2) gene. Pharmacogenetics 1994;4:125–34.

[101] Lin HJ, Han CY, Lin BK, Hardy S. Slow acetylator mutations in the human polymorphic N-acetyltransferase gene in 786 Asians, blacks, Hispanics, and whites: Application to metabolic epidemiology. Am J Hum Genet 1993;52:827–34.

[102] Woosley RL, Drayer DE, Reidenberg MM, Nies AS, Carr K, Oates JA. Effect of acetylator phenotype on the rate at which procainamide induces antinuclear antibodies and the lupus syndrome. N Engl J Med 1978;298:1157–9.

[103] Kosowsky BD, Taylor J, Lown B, Ritchie RF. Long-term use of procaine amide following acute myocardial infarction. Circulation 1973;47:1204–10.

[104] Lee EJ, Zhao B, Seow-Choen F. Relationship between polymorphism of N-acetyltransferase gene and susceptibility to colorectal carcinoma in a Chinese population. Pharmacogenetics 1998;8:513–7.

[105] Ambrosone CB, Freudenheim JL, Graham S, Marshall JR, Vena JE, Brasure JR, et al. Cigarette smoking, N-acetyltransferase 2 genetic polymorphisms, and breast cancer risk. JAMA 1996;276:1494–501.

[106] Reihsaus E, Innis M, MacIntyre N, Liggett SB. Mutations in the gene encoding for the β2-adrenergic receptor in normal and asthmatic subjects. Am J Respir Cell Mol Biol 1993;8:334–9.

[107] Liggett SB. Polymorphisms of the β2-adrenergic receptor and asthma. Am J Respir Crit Care Med 1997;156:S156–62.

[108] Lima JJ, Thomason DB, Mohamed MHN, Eberle LV, Self TH, Johnson JA. Impact of genetic polymorphisms of the β2-adrenergic receptor on albuterol bronchodilator pharmacodynamics. Clin Pharmacol Ther 1999;65:519–25.

[109] Weir TD, Mallek N, Sandford AJ, Bai TR, Awadh N, Fitzgerald JM, et al. β2-Adrenergic receptor haplotypes in mild, moderate and fatal/near fatal asthma. Am J Respir Crit Care Med 1998;158:787–91.

[110] Preuss CV, Wood TC, Szumlanski CL, Raftogianis RB, Otterness DM, Girard B, et al. Human histamine

*N*-methyltransferase pharmacogenetics: Common genetic polymorphisms that alter activity. Mol Pharmacol 1998;53:708–17.

[111] Hibi K, Ishigami T, Tamura K, Mizushima S, Nyui N, Fujita T, et al. Endothelial nitric oxide synthase gene polymorphism and acute myocardial infarction. Hypertension 1998;32:521–6.

[112] Abernethy DR, Babaoglu MO. Polymorphic variant of endothelial nitric oxide synthase (eNOS) markedly impairs endothelium-dependent vascular relaxation [abstract]. Clin Pharmacol Ther 2000;67:141.

[113] Lynch TJ, Bell DW, Sordella R, Gurubhagavatula S, Okimoto RA, Brannigan BW, et al. Activating mutations in the epidermal growth factor receptor underlying responsiveness of non-small-cell lung cancer to gefitinib. N Engl J Med 2004;350:2129–39.

[114] Karapetis CS, Khambata-Ford S, Jonker DJ, O'Callaghan CJ, Tu D, Tebutt NC, et al. *K-ras* mutations and benefit from cetuximab in advanced colorectal cancer. N Engl J Med 2008;359:1757–65.

[115] U.S. Food and Drug Administration. December 16, 2008 FDA CDER Oncologic Drugs Advisory Committee. CDER 2008 Meeting Documents. Silver Spring, MD: FDA (Internet at, www.fda.gov/ohrms/dockets/ac/cder08.html#OncologicDrugs; 2008.)

[116] Youssoufian H. Oncologic Drugs Advisory Committee Hearing, December 16, 2008. Internet at, www.fda.gov/ohrms/dockets/ac/08/slides/2008-4409s1-04-ImClone.pdf.

[117] Rettie AE, Eddy AC, Heimark LD, Gibaldi M, Trager WF. Characteristics of warfarin hydroxylation catalyzed by human liver microsomes. Drug Metab Dispos 1989;17:265–70.

[118] Rettie AE, Wienkers LC, Gonzalez FJ, Trager WF, Korzekwa KR. Impaired (*S*)-warfarin metabolism catalysed by the R144C allelic variant of CYP2C9. Pharmacogenetics 1994;4:39–42.

[119] Higashi MK, Veenstra DL, Kondo LM, Wittkowsky AK, Srinouanprachanh SL, Farin FM, et al. Association between CYP2C9 genetic variants and anticoagulation-related outcomes during warfarin therapy. JAMA 2002;287:1690–8.

[120] Rieder MJ, Reiner AP, Gage BF, Nickerson DA, Eby CS, McLeod HL, et al. Effect of *VKORC1* haplotypes on transcriptional regulation and warfarin dose. N Engl J Med 2005;352:2285–93.

[121] Woodcock J. Assessing the clinical utility of diagnostics used in drug therapy. Clin Pharmacol Ther 2010;88:765–73.

[122] Relling MV, Klein TE. CPIC: Clinical Pharmacogenetics Implementation Consortium of the Pharmacogenomics Research Network. Clin Pharmacol Ther 2011;89:464–7.

# 14

# Mechanisms and Genetics of Drug Transport

**Joseph A. Ware[1], Lei Zhang[2] and Shiew-Mei Huang[2]**

[1]*Clinical Pharmacology, Genentech Research and Early Development, South San Francisco, CA 94080*
[2]*Office of Clinical Pharmacology, Office of Translational Sciences, Center for Drug Evaluation and Research, US Food and Drug Administration, Silver Spring, MD 20993*

## INTRODUCTION

The processes of drug absorption, distribution, metabolism, and excretion (ADME) include transport steps that are mediated by membrane-bound carriers or transporters. Over 400 membrane transporters have been annotated in the human genome, belonging to two major superfamilies: ATP-Binding Cassette (ABC) and Solute Carrier (SLC). Most of the membrane transporters have been cloned, characterized, and localized to tissues and polarized cellular membrane domains (apical or basolateral) in the human body. The physiological roles of transporters include supplying nutrients, removing waste products, maintenance of cell homeostasis, signal transduction, energy transduction, maintain cell motility, etc. Although more than 400 transporters are identified, only approximately 30 transporters are known to be important for drug transport. Numerous preclinical and clinical studies now suggest that drug transport is an important determinant of drug pharmacokinetics (PK) and pharmacodynamics (PD) because transport mechanisms control the access of many drugs to various tissues and to their site of action. In some instances, membrane transporters may represent the rate-limiting step in the processes of drug absorption, distribution, and elimination, and are involved in many drug–drug interactions (Chapter 15). There is growing appreciation of the importance of understanding the impact of membrane transporters on drug development and of their role in determining drug efficacy and toxicity outcomes (Table 14.1).

A recent White Paper from the International Transporter Consortium [1] from a DIA–FDA Critical Path Initiative [2]-sponsored transporter workshop [3] provided an overview of key transporters that play a role in drug absorption and disposition, and clinical drug interactions, and described examples of various technologies used in the study of drug transporter-based interactions, including computational methods for constructing models to predict drug transporter interactions. Furthermore, it provided criteria based on *in vitro* assessment along with decision trees that can be used by drug development and regulatory scientists to decide if clinical studies of transporter-mediated drug–drug interaction are warranted. This is a prime example that illustrates how government, industry, and academic scientists have collaborated to develop and apply innovative, predictive tools to enhance the safety and efficacy of medical therapies. The incorporation of these new scientific advances in drug development [4, 5] and their rapid regulatory adoption [6] are both critical to the development of novel medical products.

## MECHANISMS OF TRANSPORT ACROSS BIOLOGICAL MEMBRANES

After oral administration, there are multiple membrane barriers that a drug must traverse to reach its cellular target. Research over the past several years has defined several mechanisms by which drugs are

**TABLE 14.1    Influence of Membrane Transporters in Drug Development**

| Area of research | Phase of drug development | Comments and examples *Impact if ignored* |
|---|---|---|
| ADME | All | Active transport impacts the absorption, distribution, metabolism, and excretion of many NMEs and drugs. Inclusion or exclusion of NME or drug from target tissues may greatly influence pharmacology. Representative examples include: <br> • Role of P-gp (ABCB1) at the blood–brain barrier <br> • Role of BCRP (ABCG2) in the absorption of topotecan <br> • Role of OATP1B1 and/or OATP1B3 in hepatic uptake and skeletal muscle toxicity <br> • Role of OATs/OCTs in renal elimination and clearance. <br> *Failure to understand the interplay between membrane transporters during drug development limits scope and accuracy of PK prediction, efficacy and/or toxicity.* |
| ADMET | Development | Altered hepatic uptake, metabolism, and efflux of bilirubin and thyroxine yield significant alteration in hepato-biliary homeostasis. <br> *Failure to deconvolute the complex interdependence of metabolism and transport with toxicological observations may delay candidate selection and/or lead to premature project termination.* |
| ADMET | Development | Cross-species comparison(s) of drug transport expression is not considered in the preclinical ADME or toxicology plan. Targeted *in vivo* and *in vitro* studies are needed to define transport properties of many preclinical species. <br> *Failure to understand interspecies differences in drug transport may delay drug development.* |
| Clinical pharmacology | Registration and planning | Global regulatory agencies and sponsors now recognize the potential involvement of drug transport in DDIs and expect sponsors to address potential transport-mediated interactions within their clinical pharmacology plan. <br> Target distribution and imaging studies may be strongly influenced by drug transporters. <br> *Failure to predict and define mechanism(s) of DDI may result in delayed registration, labeling changes of registered compound, loss of competitive marketing advantage, and/or drug withdrawal.* |
| Clinical pharmacology | All | Genetic polymorphism(s) of drug transporters is an emerging area of personalized drug therapy, requiring: <br> • Association studies with efficacy and/or toxicity <br> • Association studies with ADME. <br> *Failure to understand intersubject and ethnic variability in drug transporters may delay optimal regimen design.* |

ADME = absorption, distribution, metabolism, and excretion. ADMET = ADME + toxicity, DDI = drug-drug interaction, NME = new molecular entity.

transported across biological membranes (see Figure 14.1). Some drugs cross membranes by simple diffusion, by either a paracellular or a transcellular mechanism. Their transfer obeys Fick's law of diffusion, and is driven by the cross-membrane concentration gradient. As described in Chapter 3, factors that can affect simple diffusion include molecular weight, charge and polarity, and lipophilicity (e.g., octanol : buffer partition ratio). However, other drugs are assisted by carrier proteins, known as transporters, that help them cross membranes. This process, called *carrier-mediated* transport, can be either facilitated (passive) or active. Mechanistically, the molecule binds to the transporter, is translocated across the membrane, and is then released on the other side of the membrane. The process is usually specific, saturable, inhibitable, and temperature sensitive. Carrier-mediated transport processes are categorized as follows:

1. Facilitated passive diffusion (driven by a concentration gradient)
2. Active transport (i.e., via energy linked transporters)
   a. Primary active
   b. Secondary active
      i. Symport (Co-transporters)
      ii. Antiport (Exchangers).

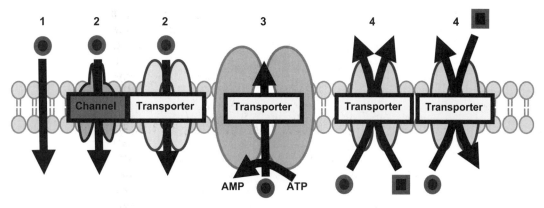

**FIGURE 14.1** Energy-based classification of drug transport across membranes. 1. Simple diffusion; 2. Facilitated diffusion; 3. Primary active transport; 4. Secondary active transport. Note that two arrows in the same direction show a symport or co-transport process, while two arrows in opposite directions show an antiport or exchange process. (The authors acknowledged Dr. Naoki Ishiguro, Boehringer Ingelheim, for this figure).

Facilitative transporters are not energy dependent and are termed uniporters in that they move a single class of substrate down a concentration gradient. Examples of facilitative transporters in the SLC family are the organic anion transporting polypeptides (OATPs), the organic cation transporters (OCT), and the organic anion transporters (OAT). Active transporters that move solutes against a concentration gradient are energy dependent. Primary active transporters generate energy themselves (e.g., by ATP hydrolysis) and include transporters in the ABC families, such as P-gp (P-glycoprotein) and BCRP (Breast Cancer Resistance Protein). Secondary active transporters utilize energy stored in a voltage and ion gradient that is generated by a primary active transporter (e.g., $Na^+/K^+$-ATPase). Symporters, such as the $Na^+$-glucose transporter, transport molecules against a concentration gradient in the same direction as ions. Antiporters or counterporters, such as the $Na^+/H^+$-exchanger, transport molecules against a concentration gradient in the opposite direction to the ion.

## NOMENCLATURE, GENETIC CLASSIFICATION, AND FUNCTION OF SELECTED MEMBRANE TRANSPORTERS

The physiological or pharmacological functions of a substantial number of transporters have been defined in various tissues, and have been associated with specific genes, mRNA, and deduced protein sequences. However, relatively few have been isolated and fully characterized biochemically. The ABC superfamily includes about 50 transporters that contain an ATP-binding cassette and function as "primary" active transporters. Their Human Genome Organization (HUGO) [7] nomenclature begins with

"ABC", which is followed by a letter and a number. For example, P-gp is ABCB1, BCRP is ABCG2, MRP2 (Multidrug-Resistance Related Protein 2) is ABCC2. The SLC superfamily contains more transporters than the ABC superfamily, and includes more than 350 transporters and 50 families. They are either facilitated passive transporters, or active transporters that rely on a secondary energy source ("secondary" active). A transporter is assigned to a specific SLC family if it has at least 20–25% amino acid sequence identity to other members of that family [8]. Most of their HUGO nomenclature begins with SLC, followed by a number, a letter, and another number, with an exception being the OATPs (SLC family 21). For example, OCT2 is SLC22A2 and OAT1 is SLC22A6. For organic anion transporting polypeptides, the HUGO nomenclature begins with SLCO (solute carrier organic anion transporter family), followed by a family number, subfamily letter, and member number (e.g., 1A2, 1B1). For example, OATP1A2 is SLCO1A2 (also known as SLC21A3) and OATP1B1 is SLCO1B1 (also known as SLC21A6). Table 14.2 provides a partial listing of membrane transporter families.

### The ATP-Binding Cassette (ABC) Superfamily

ABC transporters, such as P-gp, BCRP and MRP, are expressed in multiple tissues, including intestine, liver, kidney and brain.

#### P-glycoprotein

The most extensively studied drug transporter of the ABC superfamily is P-glycoprotein (P-gp, *ABCB1*), a member of the multidrug resistance (MDR) family of transporters and the product of the multidrug resistance 1 (*ABCB1*) gene [9]. P-gp mediates the ATP-

**TABLE 14.2   Selected Transporter-Mediated Clinical Significant Drug–Drug Interactions[a]**

| Gene | Aliases[b] | Tissue | Function | Interacting Drug | Substrate (Affected Drug) | Changes in Substrate Plasma AUC (AUC ratios) |
|---|---|---|---|---|---|---|
| *ABC Transporters of clinical importance in the absorption, disposition, and excretion of drugs* | | | | | | |
| *ABCB1* | P-gp, MDR1 | Intestinal enterocyte, kidney proximal tubule, hepatocyte (canalicular), brain endothelia | Efflux | Dronedarone | Digoxin | 2.6-fold |
| | | | | Quinidine | Digoxin | 1.7-fold |
| | | | | Ranolazine | Digoxin | 1.6-fold |
| | | | | Tipranavir/ ritonavir | Loperamide | 0.5-fold |
| | | | | Tipranavir/ ritonavir | Saquinavir/ ritonavir | 0.2-fold |
| *ABCG2* | BCRP | Intestinal enterocyte, hepatocyte (canalicular), kidney proximal tubule, brain endothelia, placenta, stem cells, mammary gland (lactating) | Efflux | GF120918 | Topotecan | 2.4-fold |
| *SLC Transporters of clinical importance in the disposition and excretion of drugs* | | | | | | |
| *SLCO1B1* | OATP1B1 OATP-C OATP2 LST-1 | Hepatocyte (sinusoidal) | Hepatocyte (sinusoidal) | Lopinavir/ ritonavir | Bosentan | 5- to 48-fold[c] |
| | | | | Cyclosporine | Pravastatin | 9.9-fold |
| | | | | Rifampin (single dose) | Glyburide | 2.3-fold |
| *SLCO1B3* | OATP1B3, OATP-8 | Hepatocyte (sinusoidal) | Uptake | Cyclosporine | Rosuvastatin | 7.1- fold[d] |
| | | | | Cyclosporine | Pitavastatin | 4.6-fold[e] |
| | | | | Lopinavir/ ritonavir | Rosuvastatin | 2.1-fold[e] |
| *SLC22A2* | OCT2 | Kidney proximal tubule | Uptake | Cimetidine | Dofetilide | 1.5-fold |
| | | | | Cimetidine | Pindolol | 1.5-fold |
| | | | | Cimetidine | Metformin | 1.4-fold[f] |
| *SLC22A6* | OAT1 | Kidney proximal tubule, placenta | Uptake | Probenecid | Cephradin | 3.6-fold |
| | | | | Probenecid | Cidofovir | 1.5-fold |
| | | | | Probenecid | Acyclovir | 1.4-fold |
| *SLC22A8* | OAT3 | Kidney proximal tubule, choroid plexus, brain endothelia | Uptake | Probenecid | Furosemide | 2.9-fold[g] |

[a]Abbreviations: BCRP, breast cancer resistance protein; P-gp, p-glycoprotein; MDR, multidrug resistance; LST, liver-specific transporters; OATP, organic anion transporting polypeptide; OCT, organic cation transporter; OAT, organic anion transporter.

[b]Implicated transporter refers to the likely transporter; however, because the studies are *in vivo*, it is not possible to assign definitively specific transporters to these interactions.

[c]Minimum pre-dose plasma level ($C_{trough}$) data from Day 4 (48-fold), Day 10 (5-fold) after co-administration.

[d]Interaction could be partly mediated by BCRP.

[e]Interaction could be partly mediated by OATP1B1.

[f]Interaction could be partly mediated by MATE-1/MATE-2K.

[g]Interaction could be partly mediated by OAT1.

Reproduced from the FDA Drug Interaction Website (Internet at, www.fda.gov/Drugs/DevelopmentApprovalProcess/Development Resources/DrugInteractionsLabeling/ucm093664.htm#transporter.)

dependent export of drugs from cells and has a wide tissue expression, being expressed in the luminal membrane of the small intestine and blood–brain barrier, and in the apical membranes of excretory cells such as hepatocytes and kidney proximal tubule epithelia. P-gp plays an important role in the intestinal absorption and in the biliary and urinary excretion of drugs, but also limits the central nervous system (CNS) entry of various drugs. The level of expression and functionality of P-gp can be modulated by inhibition and induction, which can affect the PK, efficacy, and safety of P-gp substrate drugs [10–15].

Initially discovered as a result of its interaction with multiple anticancer drugs, P-gp is responsible for the efflux across biological membranes of a broad range of different drugs. Digoxin is a particularly relevant substrate of P-gp because of its narrow therapeutic range (see Table 14.2). Because many drugs are inhibitors of P-gp, their co-administration may cause a two- to three-fold increase in systemic exposure to P-gp substrates such as digoxin or fexofenadine. However, not all potent *in vitro* inhibitors of P-gp produce clinically meaningful changes in the PK of digoxin or other P-gp substrates, and changes in tissue exposure to these substrates may not be detected by monitoring their plasma concentrations [16]. Potent P-gp inhibitors include itraconazole and dronederone. Many drugs have been identified as substrates and/or inhibitors of P-gp (Table 14.3) [3, 17].

## Multidrug-Resistance Related Protein

The multidrug-resistance related protein (MRP, *ABCC*) family of transporters is closely related and structurally similar to the MDR family. MRP transporters constitute 9 members of the ATP-binding cassette C subfamily (*ABCC1–6, 10–12*). Other transporters in the ABCC subfamily are the cystic fibrosis transmembrane conductance regulator (*ABCC7*) and two sulfonylurea receptor isoforms (*ABCC8* and *-9*) [18, 19]. Cloning, functional characterization, and cellular localization of most MRP subfamily members have identified them as ATP-dependent efflux pumps that transport a broad spectrum of endogenous and xenobiotic anionic substances across cellular plasma membranes [18, 19].

MRP1 (*ABCC1*), MRP2 (*ABCC2*), and MRP4 (*ABCC4*) have been the most widely studied members of the MRP family in the context of PK and drug response. MRP1 was initially identified in lung cells which were known to not express P-gp, and pumps anionic compounds, in contrast to the cations pumped by P-gp [20]. Substrates for MRP1 include anionic natural products; glutathione, glucuronosyl, and sulfate conjugates; and, in some cases, neutral molecules coupled to glutathione transport without

**TABLE 14.3  Partial List of Drugs that are Substrates, Inhibitors or Inducers of Transporters**[a]

| Transporter | Substrate | Inhibitor |
|---|---|---|
| **ABC Transporters** | | |
| P-gp | Aliskiren, ambrisentan, *bocepravir, cabazitaxel*, colchicine, *crizotinib, cyclosporine*, dabigatran extile, *eribulin, everolimus*, ezogabine (metabolite), fexofenadine, fidaxomicin, *lapatinib, maraviroc, nilotinib*, pazopanib, posaconazole, propranolol, *ranolazine*, rivaroxaban, saxagliptin, silodosin, sirolimus, sitagliptin, *ticagrelor, tipranavir*[b], *tolvaptan*, topotecan, *vemurafenib* | *Boceprevir, cabazitaxel*, clarithromycin, conivaptan, *crizotinib, cyclosporine*, dronedarone, etravirine, *eribulin, everolimus, lapatinib, maraviroc, nilotinib*, paliperidone, *ranolazine*, sorafenib, *ticagrelor, tipranavir*[b], *tolvaptan, vemurafenib* |
| BCRP | *Eltrombopag, lapatinib*, pazopanib, pralatrexate, topotecan | Cabazitaxel, *eltrombopag, lapatinib* |
| MRP2 | Mycophenolate, *pralatrexate*, valsartan | *Pralatrexate* |
| **SLC Transporters** | | |
| OATP1B1 | Ambrisentan, atorvastatin, valsartan | Cyclosporine[c], dronedarone, eltrombopag[d], lapatinib, panzopanib, telithromycin |
| OATP1B3 | Ambrisentan | Dronedarone, telithromycin |
| OAT3 | Sitagliptin | Dronedarone |
| OCT2 | Metformin, gabapentin, pramipexole, varenicline | Dronedarone, vandetanib |

Abbreviations: P-gp, P-glycoprotein; BCRP, breast cancer resistance protein; MRP, multidrug resistance associated protein; OATP, organic anion transporting polypeptide; OAT, organic anion transporter; OCT, organic cation transporter. Note that when the drug names are italicized and emboldened, they are both substrates and inhibitors.

[a]Based on *in vitro* or *in vivo* data as stated in the current FDA labeling (updated from Huang S-M, Zhang L, Giacomini KM. Clin Pharmacol Ther 2010;87:32–6 [3]). For additional substrates or inhibitors that are not included in FDA labeling, refer to FDA drug development and drug interaction website (Internet at, www.fda.gov/Drugs/DevelopmentApprovalProcess/DevelopmentResources/DrugInteractionsLabeling/ucm080499.htm), UCSF-FDA transporter database (Internet at, http://bts.ucsf.edu/fdatransportal/), and University of Washington Drug Interaction Database (UW-DIDB) (Internet at, www.druginteractioninfo.org).

[b]Tipranavir is also a P-gp inducer.

[c]Cyclosporine is stated as an inhibitor in the labeling for other drugs.

[d]In eltrombopag labeling, the following were mentioned as OATP1B1 substrates: benzylpenicillin, atorvastatin, fluvastatin, pravastatin, rosuvastatin, methotrexate, nateglinide, repaglinide, rifampin.

conjugation. MRP2 (*ABCC2*) is similar to MRP1 except in its tissue distribution and localization. It is expressed on the canalicular membrane of hepatocytes, and was formerly known as the canalicular multispecific organic anion transporter (cMOAT). The hepatobiliary and renal elimination of many drugs and their metabolites is mediated by MRP2 in the hepatocyte canalicular membrane and by MRP4 as well as MRP2 in the luminal membrane of proximal renal tubules. Therefore, inhibition of these efflux pumps affects PK unless compensation is provided by other ATP-dependent efflux pumps with overlapping substrate specificities. Genetic mutations in MRP2 cause Dubin-Johnson syndrome, a disease characterized by hyperbilirubinemia resulting from reduced transport of conjugated bilirubin into bile [21]. MRP3 has been recently shown to transport phenolic glucuronide conjugates of acetaminophen, etoposide, methotrexate, and morphine from the apical surface of hepatocytes into blood [22]. MRP4 (*ABCC4*) has been shown to transport a number of endogenous substrates, such as eicosanoids, urate, conjugated steroids, folate, bile acids, and glutathione, as well as many drug substrates, including cephalosporines, methotrexate, and nucleotide analog reverse transcriptase inhibitors [23, 24].

### Breast Cancer Resistance Protein

Breast cancer resistance protein (BCRP, *ABCG2*) is a "half ABC transporter" consisting of 655 amino acids and 6 transmembrane domains [25]. BCRP was identified originally as a determinant of *in vitro* multidrug resistance in cancer cell lines [26, 27]. Similar to P-gp, BCRP is expressed in the gastrointestinal tract, liver, kidney, brain endothelium, mammary tissue, testis, and placenta. It has a role in limiting the oral bioavailability and transport of substrates across the blood–brain barrier, blood–testis barrier, and maternal–fetal barrier [28, 29]. Similar to P-gp, BCRP has a wide variety of substrates and inhibitors. Although there is considerable overlap between BCRP and P-gp substrates and inhibitors, a quantitative structure–activity relationship (QSAR) analysis has been used to identify key structural elements that enable a molecule to interact with BCRP or P-gp and is thus able to differentiate some substrates and inhibitors of BCRP from those of P-gp [1, 30, 31].

BCRP function can contribute to variable bioavailability, exposure, and pharmacological response to BCRP substrate drugs. The most significant clinical effects are likely to be for drugs that have a low bioavailability and a narrow therapeutic range. Recent clinical studies also have demonstrated that patients with reduced BCRP expression levels, correlating with the Q141K (*ABCG2* c.421C>A) variant, are at increased risk for gefitinib-induced diarrhea [32] and have altered PK of irinotecan, rosuvastatin, sulfasalazine and topotecan [33–37]. Based on *in vitro* data, several drugs (e.g., eltrombopag, lapatinib, pazopanib, sulfasalazine, and topotecan) have been found to be substrates while eltrombopag, GF-120918, and lapatinib are inhibitors of BCRP (Table 14.3). A clinical study has shown that eltormbopag increased rosuvastatin exposure by approximately two-fold [38], possibly due to inhibition of BCRP and OATP1B1. Exposure to sulfasalazine administered as an immediate release oral formulation (suspension or tablet) was significantly increased in healthy volunteers with one or more *ABCG2* variants [39, 40]. These findings were consistent with studies in *Bcrp1*$^{-/-}$ mice that also demonstrated increased oral bioavailability and reduced systemic clearance of sulfasalazine [41]. However, another study in humans failed to show an effect of the *ABCG2* c.421C>A polymorphism on plasma exposure when a delayed release formulation (enteric-coated tablets) of sulfasalazine was administered [42]. A PK interaction study by Kusuhara *et al.* [43] in healthy subjects evaluated the impact of curcumin as an *in vivo* inhibitor of BCRP and found that curcumin could increase sulfasalazine exposure 2.0- and 3.2-fold after administration of 100 μg and 2 g of sulfasalazine, respectively. These authors reported that curcumin is a useful inhibitor of BCRP *in vitro* and *in vivo*, but further work is needed to validate the utility of sulfasalazine as an *in vivo* probe of BCRP. The same authors reported that sulfasalazine uptake and efflux in the small intestine is dose dependent and is mediated by OATP2B1, which functions as a high-affinity, low-capacity uptake transporter, as well as by BCRP [43].

### Bile Salt Export Pump

Enterohepatic circulation of bile acids is mediated by specific transporters in the hepatocytes and enterocytes [19]. Bile salt export pump (BSEP, *ABCB11*) is a transporter that is expressed exclusively on the canalicular side of hepatocytes and is involved in the biliary efflux of monovalent bile acids, whereas MRP2 exports divalent and sulfated and/or glucuronidated bile acids and other conjugated anions including Phase II drug metabolites. Although BSEP primarily transports bile acids, it can also transport drugs such as pravastatin [44]. A number of BSEP inhibitors have been identified (e.g., cyclosporine A, rifampicin, glibenclamide) [45].

Altered expression or function of bile-acid transporters can be either a cause or a consequence of cholestasis. Progressive familial intrahepatic cholestasis type 2 (PFIC2) is caused by mutations in the *ABCB11* gene, which encodes BSEP [46, 47]. Mutations in the *ABCB11* gene can lead to a rapid progressive hepatic dysfunction in early infancy. In such patients, the biliary bile salt levels can be reduced to less than 1% of that in normal subjects. These defects or inhibition of BSEP may contribute to certain types of drug-induced cholestasis or other liver injury [48, 49], but further research is needed to determine how drugs can be studied early in their development to assess their BSEP-related safety liabilities [50].

## Solute Carriers (SLCs)

### Organic Anion Transporting Polypeptides

Organic Anion Transporting Polypeptides (OATPs, *SLCOs*) represent a family of important membrane transport proteins within the solute carrier (SLC) superfamily that mediate the sodium-independent transport of a diverse range of amphiphilic organic compounds [51–56]. These include bile acids, steroid conjugates, thyroid hormones, anionic peptides, and drugs. OATP1B1 and OATP1B3 are the major OATPs expressed on the sinusoidal side of hepatocytes and they function as uptake transporters, transporting molecules from blood into hepatoctyes. OATP2B1 is expressed in both the liver and the intestine, whereas OATP1A2 is expressed only in the intestine.

Link *et al.* [57] conducted a genome-wide association study (GWAS) of patients with simvastatin-induced myopathy and demonstrated that polymorphisms in the *SLCO1B1* gene that encodes for OATP1B1 play an important role in predisposing individuals to simvastatin-induced myopathy (see Chapter 17). In addition, clinically relevant drug interactions have been noted for certain OATPs, such as OATP1B1 and OATP1B3 (Table 14.2). Inhibition of OATP1B1-mediated hepatic uptake appears to have contributed to the significant increase in the concentration of statins in blood after cyclosporine administration [58–60]. Because cyclosporine is an inhibitor of multiple transporters, including OATP1B1 and BCRP, inhibition of either BCRP or OATP1B1 may have contributed to the interaction between cyclosporine and rosuvastatin [61, 62]. Drugs such as ambrisentan are substrates for OATP1B1 and OATP1B3, and eltrombopag is an inhibitor of OATP1B1 (Table 14.3) [38].

### Organ Cation and Organ Anion Transporters

A distinct family of proteins within the SLC superfamily is encoded by 22 genes of the human SLC22A family, and includes the electrogenic organic cation transporters (OCTs) (isoforms 1–3) and the organic anion transporters (OATs) (significant isoforms in humans include OAT1–4 and 7, and URAT1) [8, 63, 64]. Various compounds interact with human OCTs and OATs [65, 66]. OCTs transport relatively hydrophilic, low molecular mass organic cations including metformin (Table 14.3). Properties of inhibitors of OCT1 and OCT2 have been identified and include a net positive charge and high lipophilicity [67–69]. OCT1 is mainly expressed in human liver (sinusoidal) while OCT2 is mainly expressed in human kidney (basolateral). OAT1, OAT3 and OAT4 mediate exchange of intracellular 2-oxoglutarate for extracellular substrates [70]. OAT1 and OAT3 mediate the basolateral entry step in renal secretion of different structural classes of monovalent and selected divalent anions that are less than 500 Da (type I organic anions) [71]. In addition OAT3 can also transport some positively charged drugs, such as cimetidine.

### Multidrug and Toxin Extrusion Transporters

The multidrug and toxin extrusion transporter MATE1 (*SLC47A1*) is expressed in both kidney and liver cells at the apical side of the cell membrane, whereas MATE2-K (*SLC47A2*) is mainly expressed in the kidney (Figure 14.2) [1, 72–74]. In 2005, Otsuka *et al.* [74] identified and functionally characterized the human $H^+$/organic cation antiporter MATE1 and Masuda *et al.* [73] characterized a paralog, MATE2, the following year. Two isoforms of MATE2 have been identified, one of which, MATE2-K, has been characterized as a membrane transporter in the kidney [73]. Various drugs, including metformin, as well as endogenous substances such as guanidine, have been shown to be substrates of MATE1 [74]. MATE2-K, like MATE1, appears to transport an array of structurally diverse compounds, including many cationic drugs and endogenous compounds [75]. Recently, Komatsu *et al.* [76] characterized isoform 1 of MATE2 (NP_690872) and showed that both human MATE2 (isoform 1) and MATE2-K (isoform 2): (1) operate in the kidney as electroneutral $H^+$/organic cation exchangers; (2) express and localize in the kidney, with MATE2-K being slightly more abundant than MATE2; (3) transport tetraethyl ammonium (TEA); and (4) have similar inhibitor specificities. Since some substrates (e.g., metaformin) or inhibitors (e.g., cimetidine) recognized by OCT2

**(A)** **Intestinal epithelia**

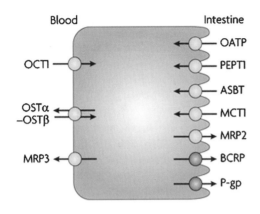

**(B)** **Hepatocytes**

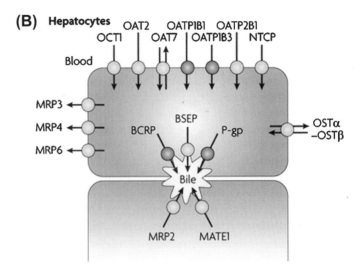

**(C)** **Kidney proximal tubules**

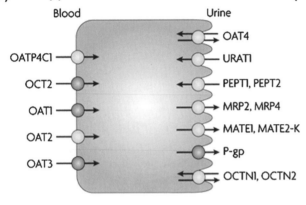

**(D)** **Blood–brain barrier**

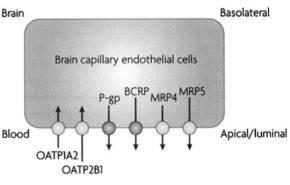

**Nature Reviews** | Drug Discovery

**FIGURE 14.2**    Selected human transport proteins for drugs and endogenous substances. Transporters in plasma membrane domains of (A) intestinal epithelia, (B) hepatocytes, (C) kidney proximal tubules, and (D) blood–brain barrier. Reproduced with permission from the Nature Publishing Group and corresponding authors, Giacomini KM, Huang SM, Tweedie DJ *et al.* Nat Rev Drug Discov 2010;9:215–36 [1]. Refer to Reference [1] for abbreviations of transporters listed in the figure.

are also recognized by MATEs [75], MATEs may act in concert with OCT2 to mediate the excretion of some drugs [77, 78].

## ROLE OF TRANSPORTERS IN PHARMACOKINETICS AND DRUG ACTION

There is increasing recognition of the important roles played by membrane transporters in the processes of drug absorption, distribution, and elimination. This is particularly true with respect to the barrier and drug-eliminating functions of gastrointestinal epithelial cells (enterocytes), hepatocytes, and renal tubule cells. Figure 14.2 indicates some of the

known membrane transport systems that are expressed in various body tissues [1].

## Role of Membrane Transport in the Intestine

As discussed in Chapter 4, factors affecting the absorption of orally administered drugs include the physicochemical (e.g., lipophilicity, solubility, etc.) and pharmaceutical (e.g., dissolution and dosage forms) properties of the drug, as well as physiological factors (e.g., gastric emptying rate, intestine motility, metabolizing enzymes and transporters in the intestine). Transporters can either facilitate the absorption of a drug (e.g., absorptive transporters such as peptide transporters or OATP transporters) or limit its oral absorption (e.g., efflux transporters such as P-gp, BCRP, and MRP).

### Absorptive (Uptake) Transporters

As described in Chapter 4, oligopeptide and monocarboxylic acid transporters facilitate the absorption of certain drugs, and these natural transport pathways have been exploited to enhance the bioavailability of some drugs. For example, the usefulness of acyclovir is limited by its poor bioavailability. However, valacyclovir is an amino acid ester of acyclovir (acyclovir conjugated with valine) and is a substrate for the PEPT1 transporter [79]. Consequently, the oral bioavailability of valacyclovir is three- to five-fold that of acyclovir in human subjects and, because it is readily hydrolyzed after absorption to release acyclovir, it functions as a useful prodrug for acyclovir [80]. This example represents a drug delivery strategy in which the absorption of an active drug can be significantly improved by coupling it with an amino acid that enables it to be transported by PEPT1.

Members of the OATP family, such as OATP1A2 and OATP2B1, have been identified as playing a role in the absorption of drugs such as fexofenadine. *In vitro* studies have shown that grapefruit juice inhibits OATP1A2-mediated fexofenadine uptake, presumably accounting for the clinical observation that grapefruit juice decreases fexofenadine exposure by three- to four-fold without changing its renal clearance [81].

### Efflux Transporters

In contrast to absorptive transporters, efflux transporters such as P-gp and BCRP limit the intestinal absorption of drugs that are their substrates, and

inhibition of these transporters has been shown to significantly increase systemic exposure to these drugs (Table 14.2). The impact of P-gp or BCRP on intestinal drug absorption is responsible for reducing the bioavailability of drugs such as digoxin, topotecan, and sulfasalazine. Consequently, the bioavailability of these drugs is enhanced when they are co-administered with a P-gp inhibitor (e.g., quinidine's interaction with digoxin [82]) or a BCRP inhibitor (e.g. GF120918's interaction with topotecan, shown in Figure 14.3 [83]).

## Metabolism and Transport Interplay

Drugs that are substrates, inhibitors, or inducers of cytochrome P450 (CYP) or Phase II enzymes can also be substrates, inhibitors, or inducers of transporters. The effect on drug metabolism of interactions that modify transporter activity is based on the location of the transporters, and may either enhance or reduce the access of drugs to the intracellular space where metabolism occurs [84–86]. The impact of this interplay between drug transporters and metabolizing enzymes has been demonstrated in both animal and human studies [84, 87]. As discussed in Chapters 4 and 15, both P-gp and CYP3A4 are co-localized in intestinal enterocytes and may limit bioavailability either by intestinal first-pass metabolism by CYP3A4 or by P-gp-mediated efflux. Many of the substrates for CYP3A4 are also substrates for P-gp, so that many CYP3A4 substrates may also be competing for transport by P-gp.

Figure 14.4 illustrates the overlap between CYP3A and P-gp inhibitors and indicates their relative potency [88]. Although many CYP3A inhibitors are also P-gp

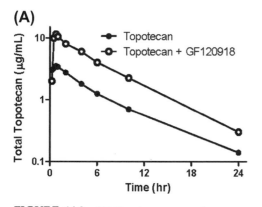
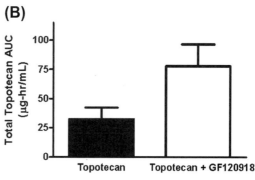

**FIGURE 14.3** (A) Topotecan mean plasma-concentration vs time profile demonstrating the influence of breast cancer resistance protein (BCRP) on the bioavailability of topotecan after an oral topotecan dose of 1.0 mg/m$^2$ alone (●) and together with a 1000-mg oral dose of the BCRP inhibitor GF120918 (○). (B) Area under plasma-concentration vs time curve (*AUC*) of topotecan (*closed bar*) and topotecan plus BCRP inhibitor GF120918 (*open bar*) demonstrates a significant increase in topotecan exposure ($n = 8$ patients, $P = 0.008$). Based on data from Kruijtzer CM Beijnen JH, Rosing H. *et al.* J Clin Oncol 2002;20:2943–50 [83].

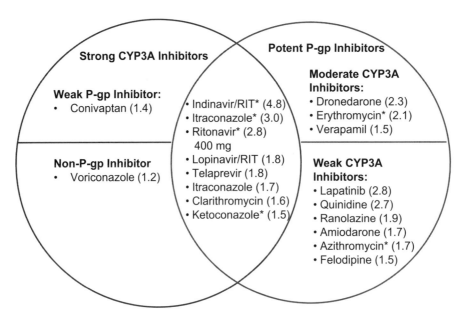

**FIGURE 14.4**   Venn diagram illustrating the overlap between inhibitors of CYP3A and P-gp and their relative potency. The fold increases in the *AUC* of P-gp substrates are provided after the inhibitor drug names by the numbers in parentheses. Digoxin was the substrate drug, except when fexofenadine was used (indicated by an asterisk).  RIT: ritonavir. Adapted from Zhang L, Zhang YD, Huang SM. Mol Pharm 2009;6:1766–74 [88] and US FDA. Drug development and drug interactions: Table of substrates, inhibitors and inducers. (Internet at, www.fda.gov/ Drugs/Development     ApprovalProcess/DevelopmentResources/DrugInteractionsLabeling/ ucm093664.htm#PgpTransport.)

inhibitors, a strong CYP3A inhibitor does not necessarily cause a large increase in exposure of a P-gp substrate, such as digoxin or fexofenadine. Thus, the area under the plasma-level vs time curve (*AUC*) of digoxin, a P-gp substrate, was significantly increased when it was co-administered with some strong CYP3A inhibitors, such as itraconazole, clarithromycin, ketoconazole, but not when it was given with other strong CYP3A inhibitors, such as voriconazole. Similarly, some P-gp inhibitors, such as amiodarone and quinidine, increased digoxin *AUC* significantly and yet are weak CYP3A inhibitors. In many cases, known inhibitors of either CYP3A or P-gp have not been tested for their respective potency for the other entity, so it may be difficult to generalize interaction data generated from studies using these inhibitors to drugs that are substrates for both CYP3A and P-gp. For example, the net effect of tipranavir/ritonavir on the oral bioavailability and plasma concentrations of drugs that are dual substrates of CYP 3A and P-gp will vary depending on the relative affinity of the co-administered drugs for CYP3A and P-gp, and the extent of intestinal first-pass metabolism/efflux [38, 88].

## Role of Membrane Transporters in Drug Distribution

Transporters are expressed in varying abundance in all tissues in the body where they govern the access of molecules to cells or their exit from cells, thereby controlling the overall distribution of drugs to their intracellular site of action. For this reason, intracellular concentrations of drugs can in some cases change drastically enough to affect the efficacy or safety of a drug without this being reflected in the drug's *AUC*. Many tissues express the same drug export pumps that occur in the barrier epithelial tissues (e.g., P-gp, MRP, BCRP), and these may be important in normal tissues, as well as in drug-resistant cancers.

Transporters are also critical to target tissue uptake of drugs from the extravascular space. As discussed in Chapter 3, transport of drugs between the vascular and extravascular spaces, except in capillaries with tight junctions, is probably by non-mediated diffusion and bulk flow. Transporters play a critical role in the function of capillary endothelium, where they contribute to the blood–brain, blood–germinal epithelium (blood–testis and blood–ovary), and blood–placental barriers. Endothelial cells in each of these tissues express high levels of P-gp and BCRP. However, specific transporters also are necessary for many drugs to enter target cells and to be transported to their subcellular sites of action. Specific examples include the nucleotide transporter family responsible for antiviral and anticancer drug uptake [89], and the reduced folate carrier which is essential for methotrexate uptake [90].

### Blood–Brain Barrier and Blood-Cerebrospinal Fluid Barrier

The blood–brain barrier results from the formation of tight junctions between brain endothelial cells, and is enhanced by the action of a number of transporters (Figure 14.2D) [1, 91]. The blood-cerebrospinal fluid (CSF) barrier is formed by epithelial cells of the choroid plexus, and tight junctions limit drug transfer between blood and CSF [91]. P-gp is the best studied of these and is located on the apical surface of choroid plexus cells, analogous to its location in other tissues. However, choroid plexus cells also have been shown to express MRP on their basolateral surface, consistent with a brain-protective role for this transport protein [92]. In addition, several other blood–brain barrier and choroid plexus transporters have been recognized, including BCRP, OATP1A2, OATP2B1, MRP4, and MRP5 [1, 93, 94]. OCTs on the apical surface of the choroid plexus appear to serve as efflux transporters, taking organic cations from the cerebrospinal fluid into epithelial cells. OCT3 is expressed at high levels in brain [94] and has been shown to transport cimetidine, amphetamine, and methamphetamine, as well as serotonin and dopamine [95, 96].

The importance of P-gp in the blood–brain barrier was revealed by a laboratory incident in which ivermectin, routinely used in rodent facilities to control parasitic worms, was administered to *abcb1a/b* knockout mice. The day after one mouse colony was given standard ivermectin treatment, all of the homozygous *abcb1a/b* knockout mice were found dead, and ivermectin levels were 100-fold higher in their brains than in the brains of wild-type mice [97]. The clinical significance of P-gp in preventing the central nervous system (CNS) effects of loperamide was demonstrated in a study in which it was shown that co-administration of quinidine not only increased loperamide plasma concentrations but also resulted in a depressed respiratory response to carbon dioxide rebreathing that was not seen when loperamide was given by itself [98]. P-gp may contribute to resistance to peptidomimetic HIV protease inhibitors (e.g., indinavir, saquinavir, and nelfinavir) in AIDS patients because it limits the access of these P-gp substrates to HIV within the CNS [99, 100].

### Placenta

BCRP (*ABCG2*) was originally identified in human placenta [101], and may function in the human placenta to protect the fetus or to transport steroid hormones produced in the placenta. Specifically, estrogen sulfate ($E_1S$) and dehydroepiandrosterone sulfate (DHEAS) are among the major estrogens produced and secreted by the placenta and are shown to be substrates for BCRP. Given its high expression in the syncytiotrophoblast near the apical surface at the chorionic villus, BCRP may help form the barrier between the maternal and fetal circulation systems and thus protect the fetus from endogenous and exogenous toxins.

### Hepatocytes

From Figure 14.2B [1], it is clear that many uptake transporters govern the entry and exit of drugs to and from the liver. OATP1B1, OATP1B3, OATP2B1, NTCP, OAT2, OAT7 and OCT1 are examples of uptake transporters, while MRP3, MRP4, and MRP6 are efflux transporters located in the basolateral (sinusoidal) membrane. On the apical (canalicular) side, P-gp, BSEP, BCRP, MRP2, and MATE-1 are efflux transporters, which govern the secretion of drugs in the bile. Lapatinib is a substrate for efflux transporters P-gp and BCRP (Tables 14.2 and 14.3) [38]. Rosuvastatin is a substrate for both BCRP and OATP1B1 [102], while pravastatin is a substrate for OATP1B1 and MRP2 [103]. As there are multiple pathways for clearance of these drugs, evaluation of a transporter's effect on a drug's plasma and tissues levels and its safety and efficacy needs to consider the multiple transport and enzymatic pathways that are involved in a drug's clearance.

Various recent clinical studies have evaluated the role of P-gp, OATP1B1, and BCRP in a drug's ADME and clinical response. As mentioned earlier, a GWAS study demonstrated that decreased OATP1B1 activity due to the presence of a genetic variant was associated with increased incidence of myopathy in patients taking 40 or 80 mg of simvastatin (Table 14.4) [57]. Similarly, Maeda *et al.* [104] used a micro-dosing approach to demonstrate that OATP1B1 (and not CYP3A) was the rate-determining process in the hepatic clearance of another statin, atorvastatin. However, OATP1B1 appeared to have played a small role in the LDL-cholesterol lowering effect of either rosuvastatin [105] or simvastatin [57].

Sugiyama's laboratory [103] has delineated how the activities of different transporters located in hepatocytes may have different effects on the plasma or tissue levels of a drug. As shown in Figure 14.5, a sensitivity analysis showed that decreased activity of OATP1B1, which governs the entry of pravastatin to the liver, could result in an increased plasma level of pravastatin that could lead to increased adverse events. On the other hand, an increase in MRP2

**TABLE 14.4   Association of Transporter Gene Polymorphisms with Drug PK and/or Clinical Responses[a]**

| Transporter | Model drugs or substrates | Outcome measures | Study results | Ref(s) |
|---|---|---|---|---|
| P-gp | Digoxin | Pharmacokinetics | TT homozygous C3435 associated with higher plasma concentrations | [124] |
| | Fexofenadine | Pharmacokinetics | TT homozygous C3435 associated with lower plasma concentrations | [126] |
| | Nelfinavir, efavirenz | Pharmacokinetics and immune recovery | TT homozygous C3435 associated with lower plasma concentrations, and greater rise in CD4 responses | [123] |
| | Anti-epileptic drugs | Clinical response | CC homozygous C3435 associated with drug-resistant epilepsy | [131] |
| BCRP | Rosuvastatin, atorvastatin, sulfasalazine | Pharmacokinetics | c.421AA with higher $AUC$ and $C_{max}$ | [39, 40, 61, 133] |
| BSEP | Bile acid | Clinical observations | C1331T associated with drug-induced cholestasis | [127] |
| MRP2 | Methotrexate | Pharmacokinetics and clinical response | 412A>G associated with impaired renal elimination and renal toxicity | [125] |
| | Platinum-based therapy | Pharmacokinetics | C-24T associated with increased platinum-based chemotherapy response in 113 advanced non-small cell lung cancer patients | [132] |
| OATP1B1 | Pravastatin | Pharmacokinetics | *15 lower clearance | [128] |
| | Simvastatin | Clinical response | c.521T>C associated with higher incidence of myopathy | [57] |
| | Pitavastatin | Clinical response | SLCO521T>C and 388A>G unrelated to lipid-lowering effect in Chinese patients | [138] |
| OATP1A2 | Imatinib | Pharmacokinetics | Neither 38T>C nor 516A>C was associated with the steady-state levels in 94 white patients | [122] |
| | Imatinib | Pharmacokinetics | −360GG associated with higher clearance than GA and AA in CML patients | [134] |
| MATE2-K | Metformin | Clinical response | Homozygous for g.−130A associated with poorer response | [77] |
| OCT1 | Metformin | Pharmacokinetics and biomarkers | Reduced function alleles associated with higher plasma levels and lower glucose tolerance test | [129, 130] |
| | Tramadol | Pharmacokinetics and biomarkers | Active alleles associated with decreased *O*-desmethyl metabolite of tramadol and decreased pupil diameter | [115] |
| OCT2 | Metformin | Pharmacokinetics | Variant alleles associated with renal clearance and net secretion | [121] |

[a]Abbreviations: ABCB1, ATP-binding cassette family (ABC); B1, multi-drug resistance (MDR1), a human gene that encodes P-glycoprotein; MRP, multidrug resistance protein; OATP-1B1, organic anion transporting peptide 1B1.

activity, which is one of the pathways responsible for pravastatin's excretion into the bile, could result in decreased levels of pravastatin at its site of action in the liver, thereby diminishing its clinical efficacy while not affecting its plasma level. This sensitivity analysis used a systems approach based on physiologically-based pharmacokinetic (PBPK) modeling, and is a useful approach for providing hypotheses for further evaluation or for interpreting laboratory or clinical observations related to the complex interplay of various elimination pathways, including transporters [103, 106–108].

## Role of Membrane Transporters in Renal Drug Elimination

Many drugs are eliminated via the kidneys, either unchanged or after biotransformation into more polar metabolites. It is generally accepted that smaller and more hydrophilic (anionic or cationic) drugs are

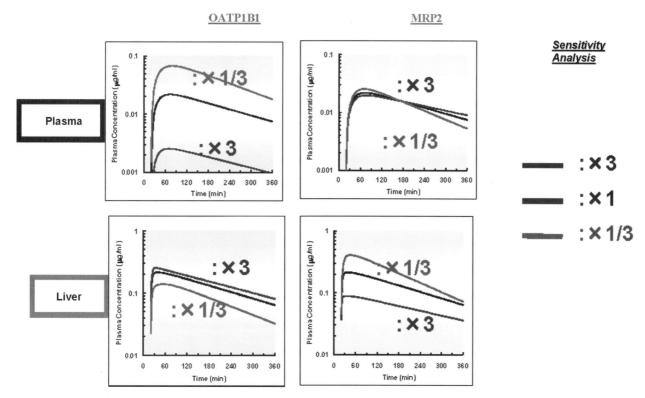

**FIGURE 14.5** Sensitivity analysis using physiologically-based PK modeling to predict the effect of increases and decreases in the activity (1/3, 1, or 3× normal activity) of OATP1B1-mediated hepatic uptake and MRP2-mediated biliary excretion on plasma and liver concentrations of pravastatin. Modified from Watanabe T, Kusuhara H, Maeda K *et al*. J Pharmacol Exp Ther 2009;328:652–62 [103].

eliminated by the kidney, whereas bulkier and more hydrophobic drugs are eliminated by the liver [63, 109, 110]. After filtration at the glomerulus, drugs pass through renal tubules that are the site of active drug secretion and reabsorption by various transporters. As discussed in Chapter 5, only the drug not bound to plasma proteins is filtered at the glomerulus, so an indicator of net tubular secretion or reabsorption can be obtained by comparing a drug's renal clearance ($CL_R$) with its glomerular filtration rate ($f_u$*GFR, where $f_u$ is the fraction free in plasma and GFR is the glomerular filtration rate). If $CL_R \neq f_u$*GFR, then there is either net secretion or reabsorption and transporter involvement ($CL_R$ could also equal $f_u$*GFR in the unlikely event that both the secretion and reabsorption processes canceled each other out).

Various transporters are responsible for tubular secretion and reabsorption of drugs (Figure 14.2C) [1, 65, 110]. P-gp expressed in the kidney is responsible for secretion of digoxin and other large neutral compounds. In addition to P-gp, OCT2, MATE2-K, OAT1 and OAT3 are the major transporters for drugs in human kidneys. Competitive inhibition of renal drug transporters can lead to changes in drug excretion, and to enhanced or reduced systemic exposure. OCT2 is responsible for the renal secretion of

cytostatic (e.g., cisplatin and oxaliplatin) [111–113], and antiretroviral agents [114]. Both OCT2 inhibition and genetic polymorphisms have been shown to affect the PK of these drugs [115]. Recent studies have shown that MATEs, and not OCT2, is the rate-determining process in metformin renal elimination [77, 78].

### Renal Transporters and Nephrotoxicity

OATs are involved in the development of organ-specific toxicity for some drugs and their metabolites [116]. For example, OATs are responsible for the high renal tubular accumulation of antiviral drugs such as adefovir and cidofovir that is responsible for their nephrotoxicity [117, 118]. This nephrotoxicity can be reduced by co-administering OAT inhibitors, such as probenicid, that can inhibit the tubular accumulation of cidofovir and thus reduce its potential risk. For this reason, probenicid is now recommended in the cidofovir label as a nephroprotectant [38].

## Transporter-Mediated Drug–Drug Interactions

Although animal models and whole cell systems, such as liver slices, have been used to evaluate transporter-mediated drug–drug interactions, a White Paper published by the International Transporter Consortium [1] and a recently published FDA drug interaction guidance [119] both have recommended the use of *in vitro* models (e.g., membrane vesicles, oocytes, cell lines, single or double transfected cell-lines, and hepatocytes) to determine a drug's potential as a substrate or inhibitor of several major transporters (P-gp, BCRP, OATP1B1, OATP1B3, OCT2, OAT1 and OAT3). Figure 14.6 shows a decision tree that can be used to determine if a drug is a substrate of OATP1B1 and what *in vitro* results may warrant further *in vivo* drug interaction studies [1, 119]. This approach can assist the pharmaceutical industry in identifying potentially important interactions earlier during drug development and help prioritize the human studies that may be informative.

## PHARMACOGENETICS AND PHARMACOGENOMICS OF MEMBRANE TRANSPORT

Genetic variants in many transporters have been identified and functionally characterized in a number of studies ([120] and references therein). Comparative studies in subjects with various transporter genotypes have helped to determine the relative contribution of the transporter in a drug's PK, even when a specific inhibitor drug was not available. Many techniques, including GWAS and candidate gene approaches, were used to evaluate the associations of SNPs of transporter genes, and clinical phenotypes were related to drug concentrations in plasma and tissue, and drug efficacy and safety. Table 14.4 shows the correlations that were made for selected substrates of

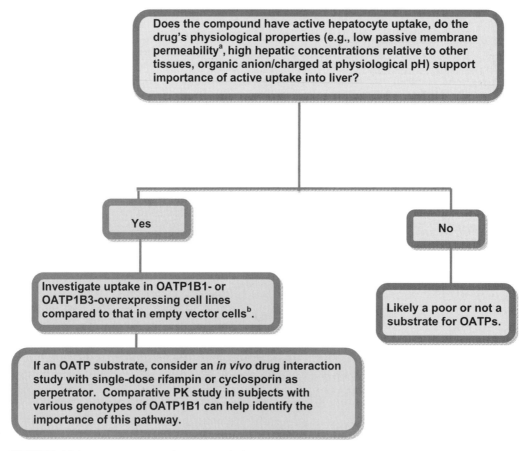

**FIGURE 14.6** Decision tree to determine whether an investigational drug is a substrate for OATP1B1 or OATP1B3 and when an *in vivo* clinical study is needed. [a]Low permeability needs to be defined based on standards, such as those specified in the biopharmaceutics classification system; [b] The following criteria suggest the investigational drug is a substrate of OATP1B1 or OATP1B3: uptake in OATP1B1- or OATP1B3-transfected cells greater than two-fold of that in empty vector transfected cells and inhibitable by a known inhibitor. Reproduced from CDER Drug interaction studies – Study design, data analysis, implications for dosing and labeling recommendations. Draft Guidance for Industry, Silver Spring, MD: FDA; February 2012. (Internet at, www.fda. gov/downloads/Drugs/Guidance ComplianceRegulatoryInformation/Guidances/UCM292362.pdf [119].)

P-gp, BCRP, BSEP, MRP2, OATP1B1, OATP1A2, MATE2-K, OCT1, and OCT2 between genetic variants of these transporters and altered drug PK and/or clinical response [57, 61, 77, 102, 115, 121–134]. Although many of these studies were exploratory and were conducted in small human studies with limited numbers of subjects (10–30/arm), some were case studies selected from cohorts of patients in large clinical trials, such as the study on simvastatin and OATP1B1 [57]. The correlations of *SLCO1B1* variants and adverse events (e.g., myopathy) in patients taking 80 or 40 mg of simvastatin for up to 6 years are discussed extensively in Chapter 17, and illustrate how GWAS has identified a clear contribution of transporter genetics to the variability of a drug response.

Further studies are ongoing to evaluate how the genetics of OATP1B1 and other transporters may affect the clinical efficacy (e.g., LDL-cholesterol lowering effect) of statins and will shed some light on how variation in the activity of efflux transporters (e.g., BCRP, MRP) and uptake transporters (e.g., OATP1B1) may affect the efficacy and safety of statin drugs. The research data on how variants of OATP1A2 affect the absorption of imatinib (Table 14.4) also is of interest, and may warrant additional research to determine how polymorphism of this transporter affects the absorption, systemic exposure, and clinical response of other orally administered OATP1A2 substrate drugs. Polymorphisms in MRP2, MRP4, MRP7, P-gp, OAT1, and OAT4 and their individual associations with drug response are discussed in detail in Chapter 17, using tenofavir and the renal toxicity associated with its use as an example.

Because alterations in P-gp function can affect drug absorption and bioavailability, drug distribution to the brain and other tissues, and drug elimination, drugs

**TABLE 14.5  Allele Frequency of the Most Common Non-synonymous Variants for African Americans, European Americans and Asians[a]**

| Protein name | African Americans (%) | European Americans (%) | Asians (%) |
|---|---|---|---|
| **ABC Transporters** | | | |
| P-gp | Ser1141Thr (11.1) | Ala893Ser (43.8) | Ala893Ser (45.0) |
| BSEP | Ala444Val (47.0) | Ala444Val (42.9) | Ala444Val (33.3) |
| MRP1[a] | Cys1047Ser (4.5) | Val353Met (0.5) | None |
| MRP2 | Cys1515Tyr (19.6) | Val417Ile (17.0) | Val417Ile (11.7) |
| MRP3 | Pro920Ser (11.3) | Ser346Phe (2.5) | Gly11Asp (0.8) |
| MRP4 | Lys304Asn (18.1) | Lys304Asn (8.7) | Lys304Asn (22.5) |
| MRP6 | Val614Ala (41.2) | Val614Ala (41.9) | Val614Ala (14.2) |
| BCRP | Val12Met (7.7) | Gln141Lys (8.1) | Gln141Lys (40.8) |
| **SLC Transporters** | | | |
| OCT1 | Val408Met (26.5) | Val408Met (40.2) | Val408Met (23.8) |
| OCT2 | Ala270Ser (11.0) | Ala270Ser (15.8) | Ala270Ser (8.6) |
| OAT1 | Arg50His (3.2) | Ile226Thr (0.6) | None |
| OAT2 | Thr110Ile (2.3) | Arg227His (0.8) | None |
| OAT3 | Val281Ala (6.0) | Val448Ile (1.3) | Ile305Phe (3.5) |
| OAT4 | Arg121Cys (2.3) | Arg48STOP (2.3) | None |
| URAT1 | Thr542LysfsX13 (1.5) | None | Arg342His (0.8) |
| OATP1A2 | Thr668Ser (4.4) | Ile13Thr (16.3) | Ile281Val (0.8) |
| OATP1B1 | Asp130Asn (27.2) | Asn130Asp (44.1) | Asp130Asn (19.9) |
| OATP1B3 | Met233Ile (42.0) | Ala112Ser (19.0) | Ala112Ser (32.0) |
| | | Ile233Met (19.0) | Ile233Met (32.0) |
| OATP2B1 | Ser486Phe (40.5) | Arg312Gln (10.8) | Arg312Gln (38.9) |
| MATE1 | Val338Ile (5.1) | None | Val480Met (0.8) |
| MATE2-K | Pro162Leu (5.6) | Gly429Arg (0.9) | None |

[a]Abbreviations: BCRP, breast cancer resistance protein; BSEP, bile salt export pump; MATE, multidrug and toxin extrusion; MRP, multidrug resistance-associated protein; OAT, organic anion transporter; OATP, organic anion transporting polypeptide; OCT, organic cation transporter; OCTN, novel organic cation transporter; P-gp, P-glycoprotein; URAT1, urate anion exchanger 1.

Modified from Cropp CD, Yee SW, Giacomini KM. Clin Pharmacol Ther 2008;84:412–6 [135].

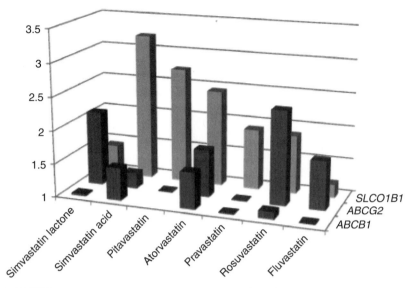

**FIGURE 14.7** Effects of *SLCO1B1*, *ABCG2*, and *ABCB1* genotypes on systemic exposure to various statins. Data are shown as multiples of *AUC* increase by *SLCO1B1* c.521CC, *ABCG2* c.421AA, and *ABCB1* c.1236TT-c.2677TT-c.3435TT genotype as compared with the reference genotype (c.521TT, c.421CC, and c.1236CC-c.2677GG-c.3435CC, respectively). Weighted mean values from various studies are shown for pitavastatin, rosuvastatin, and pravastatin. Reproduced with permission from Niemi M. Clin Pharmacol Ther 2010;87:130–3 [102].

are now routinely tested during their development to ascertain whether they are substrates, inhibitors, or inducers of P-gp. However, studies of genetic differences in P-gp expression have not provided consistent results [10]. For example, although higher drug concentrations of one P-gp substrate, digoxin, were found in individuals with the TT homogyzous C3435T variant of the *ABCB1* gene, lower concentrations of other P-gp substrates, fexofenadine, nelfinavir, and efavirenz, were found to be associated with this genotype (Table 14.4). This discrepancy possibly reflects different degrees of P-gp contribution to the overall PK of these drugs, as they are also substrates of other transporters and enzymes. In addition, other studies showed only modest effect of *ABCB1* polymorphism on the PK of various P-gp substrate drugs. For the above reasons, *ABCB1* genetic testing has not been recommended in any drug label, and tests for its clinical use are not widely available.

## Race/Ethnic Differences in Transporter Genes

As discussed in Chapter 13, there are significant differences in the frequencies of some variant alleles in genes encoding metabolizing enzymes in different race/ethnic groups. Similarly, significant differences in frequencies of various alleles in genes encoding transporters exist in different race/ethnic groups. Table 14.5 lists the distribution of various alleles in

different populations for ABCB1, ABCG2, and SLCO1B1 [135–137]. As shown in Figure 14.7, statin plasma levels are variably affected by the genetics of P-gp, BCRP, and OATP1B1 (102).

The relative contributions of these transporters to each statin's PK and the ethnic distribution of the critical variant alleles may be one of the key factors determining the relative efficacy and safety profile of these statins in different race/ethnic groups. For example, Tomlinson *et al.* [133] studied 305 Chinese patients and found that the ABCG2 (C.421C>A) variant appeared to increase the LDL-cholesterol lowering effect of rosuvastatin. This drug had a 6.9% greater effect in reducing LDL-cholesterol in C.421AA variants than in C.421CC genotypes – an effect equivalent to doubling the dose in C.421CC patients (Table 14.4). On the other hand, based on evaluation of SLCO521T>C and 388A>G, OATP1B1 genetics appeared to be unrelated to the lipid-lowering effect of another statin drug, pitavastatin, in 140 Chinese patients (Table 14.4) [138].

## CONCLUSIONS AND FUTURE PERSPECTIVES

Drug-metabolizing enzymes and transporters work in concert, participating together in the absorption, distribution, metabolism, and excretion of many

**TABLE 14.6 Recommendations for Conduct of Future Association Studies**

1. Conduct *in vitro* studies to evaluate if a drug is a substrate, inhibitor, and/or inducer of key metabolizing enzymes and transporters; such studies are critical in providing basic data that will help the design and interpretation of *in vivo* human studies.
2. Develop needed technology platforms and tools to characterize the contribution of established and evolving allelic variations of metabolism and transporter genes to better understand the genomic basis for individual variability in plasma levels and response to interacting drugs.
3. Conduct correlation studies with well characterized *in vivo* phenotypes in order to enhance the interpretability of study results.
4. Design studies that consider multiple drug-metabolizing enzymes and transporters and that have the potential to differentiate the impact of rate-limiting transporters for drugs that are substrates for multiple transporters that govern their uptake and efflux into and out of key eliminating organs (e.g., design studies to differentiate between the contributions of MATE2-K and OCT2 to metformin elimination).
5. Conduct studies that enroll a sufficient number of subjects with major variant alleles representative of various race/ethnic groups.
6. Evaluate genetic association data along with drug–drug interaction data (i.e., the evaluation of comparative PK in subgroups genetically defined as high or low expressors) to provide crucial information on potential drug–drug interactions (e.g., clopidogrel genetic study results informed the CYP2C19 interaction possibility).
7. Apply a systems biology approach that incorporates all data (*in vitro* and *in vivo* human studies) to improve understanding of the interplay among metabolizing enzymes and transporters (e.g., metabolism/transport, transporter/transporter, and/or metabolism/transport/orphan nuclear receptor interplay) and other patient factors (age, race, sex, organ impairment, disease, etc).

drugs. It is therefore important to understand how each of the processes alone and in combination contributes to individual variability in drug exposure and clinical response. Association studies linking genetics to drug exposure and clinical response have been increasingly conducted, and are critical to elucidating the basis underlying variation in the response of individuals to drug treatments. Based on cumulative evidence, genetic tests of enzyme polymorphisms are now available to help determine the initial dose of warfarin (*CYP2C9* and *VKORC1*), to suggest treatment alternatives to clopidogrel (*CYP2C19*), and to determine whether a high dose of tetrabenazine can be given (*CYP2D6*) (see Chapter 13). Although transporter–genetic association studies have not yet resulted in direct, clinically actionable recommendations, the results of many of the studies summarized in Table 14.4 have helped to:

1. Elucidate the role of specific transporters in a drug elimination clearance pathway (e.g., OATP1B1 and plasma levels of atorvastatin)
2. Explain variability in PK, PD, and drug response and clarify the role of one transporter vs the other (e.g., OATP1B1 and simvastatin-induced myopathy; BCRP and the cholesterol lowering effect of rosuvastatin; the relative contribution of MATE2-K vs OCT2 to metformin elimination)
3. Suggest a toxicity mechanism (e.g., BSEP and troglitazone liver toxicity) [49]
4. Provide data and input for a systems biology approach to analyzing complex pathways (e.g., differential roles of OATP1B1 and MRP2 in pravastatin's levels in plasma and in liver cells that may link to pravastatin's adverse reactions and cholesterol-lowering effect [103]; OATP1B1 and

increased levels of repaglinide in renal impairment [139]).

Table 14.6 enumerates considerations to improve the outcomes of association studies.

In its initial workshop, the International Transporter Consortium identified key transporters that warrant early evaluation in future clinical pharmacology studies, including P-gp, BCRP, OATP1B1/1B3, OAT1, OAT3, and OCT2 [1, 3, 6]. In a subsequent workshop, the Consortium continued to evaluate the suitability of various *in vitro*, *in vivo*, and *in silico* methods in studying the abovementioned key transporters and additional, emerging transporters (e.g., BSEP, MRPs, MATEs) [140].

## REFERENCES

[1] Giacomini KM, Huang SM, Tweedie DJ, Benet LZ, Brouwer KL, Chu X, et al. Membrane transporters in drug development. Nat Rev Drug Discov 2010;9:215–36.
[2] US Food and Drug Administration. Innovation or stagnation: Challenge and opportunity on the critical path to new medical products. Reports. Rockville, MD: FDA (Internet at, http://www.fda.gov/ScienceResearch/SpecialTopics/CriticalPathInitiative/CriticalPathOpportunitiesReports/ucm077262.htm; 2004).
[3] Huang SM, Zhang L, Giacomini KM. The International Transporter Consortium: A collaborative group of scientists from academia, industry, and the FDA. Clin Pharmacol Ther 2010;87:32–6.
[4] US Food and Drug Administration. Driving biomedical innovation: Initiatives for improving products for patients. Reports. Silver Spring, MD: FDA (Internet at, www.fda.gov/AboutFDA/ReportsManualsForms/Reports/ucm274333.htm; October 2011).
[5] US Food and Drug Administration. Advancing regulatory science at FDA. Strategic Plan. Silver Spring, MD: FDA (Internet at, www.fda.gov/downloads/ScienceResearch/SpecialTopics/RegulatoryScience/UCM268225.pdf; August 2011).

[6] Huang SM, Woodcock J. Transporters in drug development: Advancing on the critical path. Nat Rev Drug Discov 2010;9:175–6.

[7] Povey S, Lovering R, Bruford E, Wright M, Lush M, Wain H. The HUGO Gene Nomenclature Committee (HGNC). Hum Genet 2001;109:678–80.

[8] Hediger MA, Romero MF, Peng JB, Rolfs A, Takanaga H, Bruford EA. The ABCs of solute carriers: Physiological, pathological and therapeutic implications of human membrane transport proteins. Introduction. Pflugers Arch 2004;447:465–8.

[9] Schinkel AH, Jonker JW. Mammalian drug efflux transporters of the ATP binding cassette (ABC) family: An overview. Adv Drug Deliv Rev 2003;55:3–29.

[10] Chinn LW, Kroetz DL. ABCB1 pharmacogenetics: Progress, pitfalls, and promise. Clin Pharmacol Ther 2007;81:265–9.

[11] Choudhuri S, Klaassen CD. Structure, function, expression, genomic organization, and single nucleotide polymorphisms of human ABCB1 (MDR1), ABCC (MRP), and ABCG2 (BCRP) efflux transporters. Intl J Toxicol 2006; 25:231–59.

[12] Kimura Y, Morita SY, Matsuo M, Ueda K. Mechanism of multidrug recognition by MDR1/ABCB1. Cancer Sci 2007;98:1303–10.

[13] Miller DS, Bauer B, Hartz AM. Modulation of P-glycoprotein at the blood–brain barrier: Opportunities to improve central nervous system pharmacotherapy. Pharmacol Rev 2008;60:196–209.

[14] Raub TJ. P-glycoprotein recognition of substrates and circumvention through rational drug design. Mol Pharm 2006;3:3–25.

[15] Zhou SF. Structure, function and regulation of P-glycoprotein and its clinical relevance in drug disposition. Xenobiotica 2008;38:802–32.

[16] Fenner K, Troutman M, Kempshall S, Cook J, Ware J, Smith D, et al. Drug–drug interactions mediated through P-glycoprotein: Clinical relevance and *in vitro–in vivo* correlation using digoxin as a probe drug. Clin Pharmacol Ther 2009;85:173–81.

[17] Agarwal S, Zhang L, Huang S-M. Relevance and value of *in vitro* P-gp inhibition data for new molecular entities. Clin Pharm Ther 2011;89(Suppl. 1): S40 (Abstract).

[18] Keppler D. Multidrug resistance proteins (MRPs, ABCCs): Importance for pathophysiology and drug therapy. Handb Exp Pharmacol 2011;201:299–323.

[19] Klaassen CD, Aleksunes LM. Xenobiotic, bile acid, and cholesterol transporters: Function and regulation. Pharmacol Rev 2010;62:1–96.

[20] Cole SP, Bhardwaj G, Gerlach JH, Mackie JE, Grant CE, Almquist KC, et al. Overexpression of a transporter gene in a multidrug-resistant human lung cancer cell line. Science 1992;258:1650–4.

[21] Paulusma CC, Kool M, Bosma PJ, Scheffer GL, ter BF, Scheper RJ, et al. A mutation in the human canalicular multispecific organic anion transporter gene causes the Dubin-Johnson syndrome. Hepatology 1997;25:1539–42.

[22] Zelcer N, van de Wetering K, Hillebrand M, Sarton E, Kuil A, Wielinga PR, et al. Mice lacking multidrug resistance protein 3 show altered morphine pharmacokinetics and morphine-6-glucuronide antinociception. Proc Natl Acad Sci USA 2005;102:7274–9.

[23] Schuetz JD, Connelly MC, Sun D, Paibir SG, Flynn PM, Srinivas RV, et al. MRP4: A previously unidentified factor in resistance to nucleoside-based antiviral drugs. Nat Med 1999;5:1048–51.

[24] Russel FG, Koenderink JB, Masereeuw R. Multidrug resistance protein 4 (MRP4/ABCC4): A versatile efflux transporter for drugs and signalling molecules. Trends Pharmacol Sci 2008;29:200–7.

[25] Wakabayashi K, Tamura A, Saito H, Onishi Y, Ishikawa T. Human ABC transporter ABCG2 in xenobiotic protection and redox biology. Drug Metab Rev 2006;38:371–91.

[26] Doyle LA, Yang W, Abruzzo LV, Krogmann T, Gao Y, Rishi AK, et al. A multidrug resistance transporter from human MCF-7 breast cancer cells. Proc Natl Acad Sci USA 1998;95:15665–70.

[27] Robey RW, To KK, Polgar O, Dohse M, Fetsch P, Dean M, et al. ABCG2: a perspective. Adv Drug Deliv Rev 2009;61:3–13.

[28] van Herwaarden AE, Schinkel AH. The function of breast cancer resistance protein in epithelial barriers, stem cells and milk secretion of drugs and xenotoxins. Trends Pharmacol Sci 2006;27:10–6.

[29] Vlaming ML, Lagas JS, Schinkel AH. Physiological and pharmacological roles of ABCG2 (BCRP): Recent findings in Abcg2 knockout mice. Adv Drug Deliv Rev 2009;61:14–25.

[30] Ishikawa T, Sakurai A, Hirano H, Lezhava A, Sakurai M, Hayashizaki Y. Emerging new technologies in pharmacogenomics: Rapid SNP detection, molecular dynamic simulation, and QSAR analysis methods to validate clinically important genetic variants of human ABC Transporter ABCB1 (P-gp/MDR1). Pharmacol Ther 2010;126:69–81.

[31] Saito H, Hirano H, Nakagawa H, Fukami T, Oosumi K, Murakami K, et al. A new strategy of high-speed screening and quantitative structure–activity relationship analysis to evaluate human ATP-binding cassette transporter ABCG2–drug interactions. J Pharmacol Exp Ther 2006;317:1114–24.

[32] Cusatis G, Gregorc V, Li J, Spreafico A, Ingersoll RG, Verweij J, et al. Pharmacogenetics of ABCG2 and adverse reactions to gefitinib. J Natl Cancer Inst 2006;98:1739–42.

[33] Cusatis G, Sparreboom A. Pharmacogenomic importance of ABCG2. Pharmacogenomics 2008;9:1005–9.

[34] Morisaki K, Robey RW, Ozvegy-Laczka C, Honjo Y, Polgar O, Steadman K, et al. Single nucleotide polymorphisms modify the transporter activity of ABCG2. Cancer Chemother Pharmacol 2005;56:161–72.

[35] Yamasaki Y, Ieiri I, Kusuhara H, Sasaki T, Kimura M, Tabuchi H, et al. Pharmacogenetic characterization of sulfasalazine disposition based on NAT2 and ABCG2 (BCRP) gene polymorphisms in humans. Clin Pharmacol Ther 2008;84:95–103.

[36] Zhang W, Yu BN, He YJ, Fan L, Li Q, Liu ZQ, et al. Role of BCRP 421C>A polymorphism on rosuvastatin pharmacokinetics in healthy Chinese males. Clin Chim Acta 2006;373:99–103.

[37] Polgar O, Robey RW, Bates SE. ABCG2: structure, function and role in drug response. Expert Opin Drug Metab Toxicol 2008;4:1–15.

[38] CDER. Drugs@FDA. Silver Spring, MD; FDA. (Internet at, www.accessdata.fda.gov/scripts/cder/drugsatfda/index.cfm.)

[39] Urquhart BL, Ware JA, Tirona RG, Ho RH, Leake BF, Schwarz UI, et al. Breast cancer resistance protein (ABCG2) and drug disposition: Intestinal expression, polymorphisms and sulfasalazine as an *in vivo* probe. Pharmacogenet Genomics 2008;18:439–48.

[40] Yamasaki Y, Ieiri I, Kusuhara H, Sasaki T, Kimura M, Tabuchi H, et al. Pharmacogenetic characterization of sulfasalazine disposition based on NAT2 and ABCG2 (BCRP) gene polymorphisms in humans. Clin Pharmacol Ther 2008;84:95–103.

[41] Zaher H, Khan AA, Palandra J, Brayman TG, Yu L, Ware JA. Breast cancer resistance protein (Bcrp/abcg2) is a major determinant of sulfasalazine absorption and elimination in the mouse. Mol Pharm 2006;3:55–61.

[42] Adkison KK, Vaidya SS, Lee DY, Koo SH, Li L, Mehta AA, et al. Oral sulfasalazine as a clinical BCRP probe substrate: Pharmacokinetic effects of genetic variation (C421A) and pantoprazole coadministration. J Pharm Sci 2010;99:1046–62.

[43] Kusuhara H, Furuie H, Inano A, Sunagawa A, Yamada S, Wu C, et al. Pharmacokinetic interaction study of sulfasalazine in healthy subjects and the impact of curcumin as an *in vivo* inhibitor of BCRP. Br J Pharmacol 2012. E-Pub, PMID: 22300367.

[44] Hirano M, Maeda K, Hayashi H, Kusuhara H, Sugiyama Y. Bile salt export pump (BSEP/ABCB11) can transport a nonbile

acid substrate, pravastatin. J Pharmacol Exp Ther 2005;314:876–82.

[45] Byrne JA, Strautnieks SS, Mieli-Vergani G, Higgins CF, Linton KJ, Thompson RJ. The human bile salt export pump: Characterization of substrate specificity and identification of inhibitors. Gastroenterology 2002;123:1649–58.

[46] Jansen PL, Strautnieks SS, Jacquemin E, Hadchouel M, Sokal EM, Hooiveld GJ, et al. Hepatocanalicular bile salt export pump deficiency in patients with progressive familial intrahepatic cholestasis. Gastroenterology 1999;117:1370–9.

[47] Strautnieks SS, Bull LN, Knisely AS, Kocoshis SA, Dahl N, Arnell H, et al. A gene encoding a liver-specific ABC transporter is mutated in progressive familial intrahepatic cholestasis. Nat Genet 1998;20:233–8.

[48] Noe J, Kullak-Ublick GA, Jochum W, Stieger B, Kerb R, Haberl M, et al. Impaired expression and function of the bile salt export pump due to three novel ABCB11 mutations in intrahepatic cholestasis. J Hepatol 2005;43:536–43.

[49] Ogimura E, Sekine S, Horie T. Bile salt export pump inhibitors are associated with bile acid-dependent drug-induced toxicity in sandwich-cultured hepatocytes. Biochem Biophys Res Commun 2011;416:313–7.

[50] Morgan RE, Trauner M, van Staden CJ, Lee PH, Ramachandran B, Eschenberg M, et al. Interference with bile salt export pump function is a susceptibility factor for human liver injury in drug development. Toxicol Sci 2010;118:485–500.

[51] Nakanishi T, Tamai I. Genetic polymorphisms of OATP transporters and their impact on intestinal absorption and hepatic disposition of drugs. Drug Metab Pharmacokinet 2012;27:106–21.

[52] König J. Uptake transporters of the human OATP family: Molecular characteristics, substrates, their role in drug–drug interactions, and functional consequences of polymorphisms. Handb Exp Pharmacol 2011;201:1–28.

[53] Fahrmayr C, Fromm MF, König J. Hepatic OATP and OCT uptake transporters: Their role for drug–drug interactions and pharmacogenetic aspects. Drug Metab Rev 2010;42:380–401.

[54] Kalliokoski A, Niemi M. Impact of OATP transporters on pharmacokinetics. Br J Pharmacol 2009;158:693–705.

[55] Hagenbuch B, Gui C. Xenobiotic transporters of the human organic anion transporting polypeptides (OATP) family. Xenobiotica 2008;38:778–801.

[56] Kim RB. Organic anion-transporting polypeptide (OATP) transporter family and drug disposition. Eur J Clin Invest 2003;33(Suppl. 2):1–5.

[57] Link E, Parish S, Armitage J, Bowman L, Heath S, Matsuda F, et al. SLCO1B1 variants and statin-induced myopathy–a genomewide study. N Engl J Med 2008;359:789–99.

[58] Neuvonen PJ, Niemi M, Backman JT. Drug interactions with lipid-lowering drugs: Mechanisms and clinical relevance. Clin Pharmacol Ther 2006;80:565–81.

[59] Shitara Y, Itoh T, Sato H, Li AP, Sugiyama Y. Inhibition of transporter-mediated hepatic uptake as a mechanism for drug–drug interaction between cerivastatin and cyclosporin A. J Pharmacol Exp Ther 2003;304:610–6.

[60] Simonson SG, Raza A, Martin PD, Mitchell PD, Jarcho JA, Brown CD, et al. Rosuvastatin pharmacokinetics in heart transplant recipients administered an antirejection regimen including cyclosporine. Clin Pharmacol Ther 2004;76:167–77.

[61] Keskitalo JE, Zolk O, Fromm MF, Kurkinen KJ, Neuvonen PJ, Niemi M. ABCG2 polymorphism markedly affects the pharmacokinetics of atorvastatin and rosuvastatin. Clin Pharmacol Ther 2009;86:197–203.

[62] Xia CQ, Liu N, Miwa GT, Gan LS. Interactions of cyclosporin A with breast cancer resistance protein. Drug Metab Dispos 2007;35:576–82.

[63] Koepsell H, Lips K, Volk C. Polyspecific organic cation transporters: Structure, function, physiological roles, and biopharmaceutical implications. Pharm Res 2007;24:1227–51.

[64] Koepsell H, Endou H. The SLC22 drug transporter family. Pflugers Arch 2004;447:666–76.

[65] Li M, Anderson GD, Wang J. Drug–drug interactions involving membrane transporters in the human kidney. Expert Opin Drug Metab Toxicol 2006;2:505–32.

[66] Dresser MJ, Zhang L, Giacomini KM. Molecular and functional characteristics of cloned human organic cation transporters. Pharm Biotechnol 1999;12:441–69.

[67] Ahlin G, Karlsson J, Pedersen JM, Gustavsson L, Larsson R, Matsson P, et al. Structural requirements for drug inhibition of the liver-specific human organic cation transport protein 1. J Med Chem 2008;51:5932–42.

[68] Zhang L, Gorset W, Dresser MJ, Giacomini KM. The interaction of n-tetraalkylammonium compounds with a human organic cation transporter, hOCT1. J Pharmacol Exp Ther 1999;288:1192–8.

[69] Urban TJ, Giacomini KM. Organic cation transporters. In: You G, Morris M, editors. Drug transporters: Molecular characterization and role in drug disposition. Hoboken, NJ: John Wiley & Sons, Inc.; 2007. p. 11–33.

[70] Rizwan AN, Burckhardt G. Organic anion transporters of the SLC22 family: Biopharmaceutical, physiological, and pathological roles. Pharm Res 2007;24:450–70.

[71] Wright SH. Role of organic cation transporters in the renal handling of therapeutic agents and xenobiotics. Toxicol Appl Pharmacol 2005;204:309–19.

[72] Damme K, Nies AT, Schaeffeler E, Schwab M, Mammalian MATE. (SLC47A) transport proteins: Impact on efflux of endogenous substrates and xenobiotics. Drug Metab Rev 2011;43:499–523.

[73] Masuda S, Terada T, Yonezawa A, Tanihara Y, Kishimoto K, Katsura T, et al. Identification and functional characterization of a new human kidney-specific H+/organic cation antiporter, kidney-specific multidrug and toxin extrusion 2. J Am Soc Nephrol 2006;17:2127–35.

[74] Otsuka M, Matsumoto T, Morimoto R, Arioka S, Omote H, Moriyama Y. A human transporter protein that mediates the final excretion step for toxic organic cations. Proc Natl Acad Sci USA 2005;102:17923–8.

[75] Tanihara Y, Masuda S, Sato T, Katsura T, Ogawa O, Inui K. Substrate specificity of MATE1 and MATE2-K, human multidrug and toxin extrusions/H(+)-organic cation antiporters. Biochem Pharmacol 2007;74:359–71.

[76] Komatsu T, Hiasa M, Miyaji T, Kanamoto T, Matsumoto T, Otsuka M, et al. Characterization of the human MATE2 proton-coupled polyspecific organic cation exporter. Intl J Biochem Cell Biol 2011;43:913–8.

[77] Choi JH, Yee SW, Ramirez AH, Morrissey KM, Jang GH, Joski PJ, et al. A common 5′-UTR variant in MATE2-K is associated with poor response to metformin. Clin Pharmacol Ther 2011;90:674–84.

[78] Kusuhara H, Ito S, Kumagai Y, Jiang M, Shiroshita T, Moriyama Y, et al. Effects of a MATE protein inhibitor, pyrimethamine, on the renal elimination of metformin at oral microdose and at therapeutic dose in healthy subjects. Clin Pharmacol Ther 2011;89:837–44.

[79] Balimane PV, Tamai I, Guo A, Nakanishi T, Kitada H, Leibach FH, et al. Direct evidence for peptide transporter (PepT1)-mediated uptake of a nonpeptide prodrug, valacyclovir. Biochem Biophys Res Commun 1998;250:246–51.

[80] Li F, Maag H, Alfredson T. Prodrugs of nucleoside analogues for improved oral absorption and tissue targeting. J Pharm Sci 2008;97:1109–34.

[81] Dresser GK, Bailey DG, Leake BF, Schwarz UI, Dawson PA, Freeman DJ, et al. Fruit juices inhibit organic anion transporting polypeptide-mediated drug uptake to decrease the oral availability of fexofenadine. Clin Pharmacol Ther 2002;71:11–20.

[82] Fromm MF, Kim RB, Stein CM, Wilkinson GR, Roden DM. Inhibition of P-glycoprotein-mediated drug transport: A

unifying mechanism to explain the interaction between digoxin and quinidine. Circulation 1999;99:552–7.

[83] Kruijtzer CM, Beijnen JH, Rosing H, ten Bokkel Huinink WW, Schot M, Jewell RC, et al. Increased oral bioavailability of topotecan in combination with the breast cancer resistance protein and P-glycoprotein inhibitor GF120918. J Clin Oncol 2002;20:2943–50.

[84] Benet LZ. The drug transporter–metabolism alliance: Uncovering and defining the interplay. Mol Pharm 2009;6:1631–43.

[85] Tachibana T, Kato M, Takano J, Sugiyama Y. Predicting drug–drug interactions involving the inhibition of intestinal CYP3A4 and P-glycoprotein. Curr Drug Metab 2010;11:762–77.

[86] Zhang L, Zhang Y, Zhao P, Huang SM. Predicting drug–drug interactions: An FDA perspective. AAPS J 2009;11:300–6.

[87] Benet LZ, Cummins CL, Wu CY. Unmasking the dynamic interplay between efflux transporters and metabolic enzymes. Intl J Pharm 2004;277:3–9.

[88] Zhang L, Zhang YD, Huang SM. Scientific and regulatory perspectives on metabolizing enzyme–transporter interplay and its role in drug interactions – challenges in predicting drug interactions. Mol Pharm 2009;6:1766–74.

[89] Cass C. Neucleoside transport. In: Georgopapadakou N, editor. New York, NY: Marcel Dekker, Inc; 1995. p. 408–51.

[90] Rothem L, Ifergan I, Kaufman Y, Priest DG, Jansen G, Assaraf YG. Resistance to multiple novel antifolates is mediated via defective drug transport resulting from clustered mutations in the reduced folate carrier gene in human leukaemia cell lines. Biochem J 2002;367:741–50.

[91] Davson H, Segal M, editors. Physiology of the CSF and blood–brain barriers. Boca Ration, FL: CRC Press; 1996.

[92] Rao VV, Dahlheimer JL, Bardgett ME, Snyder AZ, Finch RA, Sartorelli AC, et al. Choroid plexus epithelial expression of MDR1 P glycoprotein and multidrug resistance-associated protein contribute to the blood–cerebrospinal fluid drug-permeability barrier. Proc Natl Acad Sci USA 1999;96:3900–5.

[93] Golden PL, Pollack GM. Blood–brain barrier efflux transport. J Pharm Sci 2003;92:1739–53.

[94] UCSF-FDA TransPortal (Internet at, http://bts.ucsf.edu/fdatransportal/; 2012).

[95] Nies AT, Koepsell H, Damme K, Schwab M. Organic cation transporters (OCTs, MATEs), *in vitro* and *in vivo* evidence for the importance in drug therapy. Handb Exp Pharmacol 2011;201:105–67.

[96] Kusuhara H, Sugiyama Y. Efflux transport systems for organic anions and cations at the blood–CSF barrier. Adv Drug Deliv Rev 2004;56:1741–63.

[97] Schinkel AH, Smit JJ, van TO, Beijnen JH, Wagenaar E, van DL, et al. Disruption of the mouse mdr1a P-glycoprotein gene leads to a deficiency in the blood–brain barrier and to increased sensitivity to drugs. Cell 1994;77:491–502.

[98] Sadeque AJ, Wandel C, He H, Shah S, Wood AJ. Increased drug delivery to the brain by P-glycoprotein inhibition. Clin Pharmacol Ther 2000;68:231–7.

[99] Fromm MF. P-glycoprotein: A defense mechanism limiting oral bioavailability and CNS accumulation of drugs. Intl J Clin Pharmacol Ther 2000;38:69–74.

[100] Kim RB. Drug transporters in HIV therapy. Top HIV Med 2003;11:136–9.

[101] Allikmets R, Schriml LM, Hutchinson A, Romano-Spica V, Dean M. A human placenta-specific ATP-binding cassette gene (ABCP) on chromosome 4q22 that is involved in multidrug resistance. Cancer Res 1998;58:5337–9.

[102] Niemi M. Transporter pharmacogenetics and statin toxicity. Clin Pharmacol Ther 2010;87:130–3.

[103] Watanabe T, Kusuhara H, Maeda K, Shitara Y, Sugiyama Y. Physiologically based pharmacokinetic modeling to predict transporter-mediated clearance and distribution of pravastatin in humans. J Pharmacol Exp Ther 2009;328:652–62.

[104] Maeda K, Ikeda Y, Fujita T, Yoshida K, Azuma Y, Haruyama Y, et al. Identification of the rate-determining process in the hepatic clearance of atorvastatin in a clinical cassette microdosing study. Clin Pharmacol Ther 2011;90:575–81.

[105] Bailey KM, Romaine SP, Jackson BM, Farrin AJ, Efthymiou M, Barth JH, et al. Hepatic metabolism and transporter gene variants enhance response to rosuvastatin in patients with acute myocardial infarction: The GEOSTAT-1 Study. Circ Cardiovasc Genet 2010;3:276–85.

[106] Huang SM, Rowland M. The role of physiologically based pharmacokinetic modeling in regulatory review. Clin Pharmacol Ther 2012;91:542–9.

[107] Zhang L, Huang SM, Lesko LJ. Transporter-mediated drug–drug interactions. Clin Pharmacol Ther 2011;89:481–4.

[108] Shitara Y, Horie T, Sugiyama Y. Transporters as a determinant of drug clearance and tissue distribution. Eur J Pharm Sci 2006;27:425–46.

[109] Meier PJ, Eckhardt U, Schroeder A, Hagenbuch B, Stieger B. Substrate specificity of sinusoidal bile acid and organic anion uptake systems in rat and human liver. Hepatology 1997;26:1667–77.

[110] Dresser MJ, Leabman MK, Giacomini KM. Transporters involved in the elimination of drugs in the kidney: Organic anion transporters and organic cation transporters. J Pharm Sci 2001;90:397–421.

[111] Filipski KK, Mathijssen RH, Mikkelsen TS, Schinkel AH, Sparreboom A. Contribution of organic cation transporter 2 (OCT2) to cisplatin-induced nephrotoxicity. Clin Pharmacol Ther 2009;86:396–402.

[112] Filipski KK, Loos WJ, Verweij J, Sparreboom A. Interaction of cisplatin with the human organic cation transporter 2. Clin Cancer Res 2008;14:3875–80.

[113] Zhang S, Lovejoy KS, Shima JE, Lagpacan LL, Shu Y, Lapuk A, et al. Organic cation transporters are determinants of oxaliplatin cytotoxicity. Cancer Res 2006;66:8847–57.

[114] Jung N, Lehmann C, Rubbert A, Knispel M, Hartmann P, van Lunzen J, et al. Relevance of the organic cation transporters 1 and 2 for antiretroviral drug therapy in human immunodeficiency virus infection. Drug Metab Dispos 2008;36:1616–23.

[115] Tzvetkov MV, Vormfelde SV, Balen D, Meineke I, Schmidt T, Sehrt D, et al. The effects of genetic polymorphisms in the organic cation transporters OCT1, OCT2, and OCT3 on the renal clearance of metformin. Clin Pharmacol Ther 2009;86:299–306.

[116] Hagos Y, Wolff NA. Assessment of the role of renal organic anion transporters in drug-induced nephrotoxicity. Toxins (Basel) 2010;2:2055–82.

[117] You G. Structure, function, and regulation of renal organic anion transporters. Med Res Rev 2002;22:602–16.

[118] Ho ES, Lin DC, Mendel DB, Cihlar T. Cytotoxicity of antiviral nucleotides adefovir and cidofovir is induced by the expression of human renal organic anion transporter 1. J Am Soc Nephrol 2000;11:383–93.

[119] CDER. Drug interaction studies – Study design, data analysis, implications for dosing, and labeling recommendations. Draft guidance for industry. Silver Spring, MD: FDA (Internet at, www.fda.gov/downloads/Drugs/Guidance ComplianceRegulatoryInformation/Guidances/UCM292362. pdf; 2012).

[120] Yee SW, Chen L, Giacomini KM. Pharmacogenomics of membrane transporters: Past, present and future. Pharmacogenomics 2010;11:475–9.

[121] Chen Y, Li S, Brown C, Cheatham S, Castro RA, Leabman MK, et al. Effect of genetic variation in the organic cation transporter 2 on the renal elimination of metformin. Pharmacogenet Genomics 2009;19:497–504.

[122] Eechoute K, Franke RM, Loos WJ, Scherkenbach LA, Boere I, Verweij J, et al. Environmental and genetic factors affecting transport of imatinib by OATP1A2. Clin Pharmacol Ther 2011;89:816–20.

[123] Fellay J, Marzolini C, Meaden ER, Back DJ, Buclin T, Chave JP, et al. Response to antiretroviral treatment in HIV-1-infected individuals with allelic variants of the multidrug resistance transporter 1: A pharmacogenetics study. Lancet 2002;359:30–6.

[124] Hoffmeyer S, Burk O, von RO, Arnold HP, Brockmoller J, Johne A, et al. Functional polymorphisms of the human multidrug-resistance gene: Multiple sequence variations and correlation of one allele with P-glycoprotein expression and activity *in vivo*. Proc Natl Acad Sci USA 2000;97:3473–8.

[125] Hulot JS, Villard E, Maguy A, Morel V, Mir L, Tostivint I, et al. A mutation in the drug transporter gene ABCC2 associated with impaired methotrexate elimination. Pharmacogenet Genomics 2005;15:277–85.

[126] Kim RB, Leake BF, Choo EF, Dresser GK, Kubba SV, Schwarz UI, et al. Identification of functionally variant MDR1 alleles among European Americans and African Americans. Clin Pharmacol Ther 2001;70:189–99.

[127] Lang C, Meier Y, Stieger B, Beuers U, Lang T, Kerb R, et al. Mutations and polymorphisms in the bile salt export pump and the multidrug resistance protein 3 associated with drug-induced liver injury. Pharmacogenet Genomics 2007;17:47–60.

[128] Nishizato Y, Ieiri I, Suzuki H, Kimura M, Kawabata K, Hirota T, et al. Polymorphisms of OATP-C (SLC21A6) and OAT3 (SLC22A8) genes: Consequences for pravastatin pharmacokinetics. Clin Pharmacol Ther 2003;73:554–65.

[129] Shu Y, Sheardown SA, Brown C, Owen RP, Zhang S, Castro RA, et al. Effect of genetic variation in the organic cation transporter 1 (OCT1) on metformin action. J Clin Invest 2007;117:1422–31.

[130] Shu Y, Brown C, Castro RA, Shi RJ, Lin ET, Owen RP, et al. Effect of genetic variation in the organic cation transporter 1, OCT1, on metformin pharmacokinetics. Clin Pharmacol Ther 2008;83:273–80.

[131] Siddiqui A, Kerb R, Weale ME, Brinkmann U, Smith A, Goldstein DB, et al. Association of multidrug resistance in epilepsy with a polymorphism in the drug-transporter gene ABCB1. N Engl J Med 2003;348:1442–8.

[132] Sun N, Sun X, Chen B, Cheng H, Feng J, Cheng L, et al. MRP2 and GSTP1 polymorphisms and chemotherapy response in advanced non-small cell lung cancer. Cancer Chemother Pharmacol 2010;65:437–46.

[133] Tomlinson B, Hu M, Lee VW, Lui SS, Chu TT, Poon EW, et al. ABCG2 polymorphism is associated with the low-density lipoprotein cholesterol response to rosuvastatin. Clin Pharmacol Ther 2010;87:558–62.

[134] Yamakawa Y, Hamada A, Shuto T, Yuki M, Uchida T, Kai H, et al. Pharmacokinetic impact of SLCO1A2 polymorphisms on imatinib disposition in patients with chronic myeloid leukemia. Clin Pharmacol Ther 2011;90:157–63.

[135] Cropp CD, Yee SW, Giacomini KM. Genetic variation in drug transporters in ethnic populations. Clin Pharmacol Ther 2008;84:412–6.

[136] Kroetz DL, Yee SW, Giacomini KM. The pharmacogenomics of membrane transporters project: Research at the interface of genomics and transporter pharmacology. Clin Pharmacol Ther 2010;87:109–16.

[137] Yasuda SU, Zhang L, Huang SM. The role of ethnicity in variability in response to drugs: Focus on clinical pharmacology studies. Clin Pharmacol Ther 2008;84:417–23.

[138] Yang GP, Yuan H, Tang B, Zhang W, Wang LS, Huang ZJ, et al. Lack of effect of genetic polymorphisms of SLCO1B1 on the lipid-lowering response to pitavastatin in Chinese patients. Acta Pharmacol Sin 2010;31:382–6.

[139] Zhao P, Vieira ML, Grillo JA, Song P, Wu TC, Zheng JH, et al. Evaluation of exposure change of nonrenally eliminated drugs in patients with chronic kidney disease using physiologically based pharmacokinetic modeling and simulation. J Clin Pharmacol 2012;52(Suppl. 1):91S–108S.

[140] The International Transporter Consortium Workshop Two (ITCW2). Membrane transporters in drug development: Best practices and future. National Harbor, MD (Internet at www.ascpt.org/2012AnnualMeeting/ScientificPreconferences/InternationalTransporterConsortiumWorkshopTwo/tabid/8208/Default.aspx; 2012).

# 15

# Drug Interactions

Sarah Robertson[1], Scott R. Penzak[2] and Shiew-Mei Huang[1]

[1]Office of Clinical Pharmacology, Office of Translational Sciences, Center for Drug Evaluation and Research, US Food and Drug Administration, Silver Spring, MD 20993
[2]Clinical Research Center, Department of Pharmacy, National Institutes of Health, Bethesda, MD 20892

## INTRODUCTION

A drug–drug interaction (DDI) can result from changes in the pharmacokinetics (PK) of a drug or its metabolites due to alteration in absorption, distribution, metabolism or excretion, or as a result of amplification or disruption of a pharmacodynamic (PD) effect. In either case, both the efficacy and safety implications of the DDI are important considerations. This chapter will focus primarily on PK interactions between two drugs, though certainly PD interactions are an important consideration for many classes of drugs. For example, one well-documented PD interaction is that between phosphodiesterase inhibitors, commonly used agents for erectile dysfunction, and nitrates, the combination of which may result in severe hypotension due to excessive accumulation of cyclic guanosine monophosphate (cGMP) [1].

During the clinical development of a new drug much emphasis is placed on characterizing the DDI potential, both for the drug to be acted upon (i.e. "victim") and for the drug to affect other drugs (i.e. "perpetrator"). Early characterization of a drug's route of elimination, including its specificity for transporters and metabolizing enzymes, as well as its potential to modulate (induce or inhibit) transporters and enzymes, is critical for evaluating the need for *in vivo* drug interaction studies. A well thought-out development program can often fully address the DDI potential of a new drug and require a minimal number of studies, if the studies are conceptualized and designed well. The advancement of modeling techniques in recent years, specifically physiologically-based pharmacokinetic (PBPK) modeling, has added another approach for characterizing a drug's interaction potential without extensive *in vivo* studies.

This chapter will outline the different types or mechanisms of PK-mediated DDIs and provide examples that focus on the more clinically relevant DDI types. In addition, *in vitro* techniques and modeling approaches utilized in the prediction of drug interactions will be described. Finally, this chapter will also address the implications of DDIs in product labeling.

## MECHANISMS OF DRUG INTERACTIONS

### Interactions Affecting Drug Absorption

Interactions affecting drug absorption may result in changes in the *rate* of absorption, the *extent* of absorption, or a combination of both. Interactions resulting in a reduced rate of absorption are not typically clinically important for maintenance medications, as long as the total amount of drug absorbed is not affected. On the other hand, for acutely administered medications, such as sedative-hypnotics or analgesics, a reduction in the rate of absorption may cause an unacceptable delay in the onset of the drug's pharmacologic effect. The extent to which a drug is absorbed can be affected by changes in gastrointestinal (GI) motility, GI pH, intestinal cytochrome P450 (CYP) enzyme and transport protein activity, and drug chelation in the gut.

As described in Chapter 4, medications that alter GI motility can affect drug absorption by changing the rate at which drugs are transported into and through the small intestine, the primary site of absorption for most drugs. The prokinetic agent metoclopramide, for instance, increases the rate of drug transport through the gut, thereby increasing the rate of absorption for certain drugs and also altering the extent of absorption in some cases. For instance, despite no change in cyclosporine elimination, the mean area under the plasma-concentration vs time curve (*AUC*) and maximum serum concentration ($C_{max}$) of cyclosporine increased by 22% and 46%, respectively, when it was given with metoclopramide to 14 kidney transplant patients [2].

For some drugs, absorption is limited by a compound's solubility, with dissolution being highly dependent on gastric pH. The antiretroviral agent didanosine, for example, is an acid-labile compound, originally formulated as a buffered preparation to improve its bioavailability. Other medications, such as atazanavir and certain azole antifungals (particularly itraconazole and ketoconazole), require an acidic environment for adequate absorption [3–5]. As such, these medications should be administered 2 hours before or 1 hour after antacids or buffered drugs. Likewise, proton-pump inhibitors and $H_2$-receptor antagonists markedly reduce the absorption and plasma concentration of these agents [3–5]. The bioavailability of itraconazole has been shown to improve when it is administered with a cola beverage in patients being treated with an $H_2$-receptor antagonist [6].

Drug absorption may also be limited by the formation of insoluble complexes that result when certain drugs are exposed to di- and trivalent cations in the GI tract. Quinolone antibiotics chelate with co-administered magnesium, aluminum, calcium, and iron-containing products, significantly limiting quinolone absorption [7]. Ciprofloxacin absorption was shown to decrease by 50–75% when administered within 2 hours of aluminum hydroxide or calcium carbonate tablets [8]. Additionally, tetracycline antibiotics have long been known to complex with antacids and iron in the gut [9, 10]. Adsorbents, such as the cholesterol-lowering anionic exchange resin cholestyramine, bind multiple medications when co-administered [11]. However, dosing separation improves the bioavailability of co-administered medications.

## Interactions Affecting Drug Distribution

Theoretically, drugs that are highly protein bound (> 90%) may displace other highly protein-bound drugs from binding sites, thereby increasing the magnitude of biologically active free drug. This mechanism of interaction is considered to be significant only for drugs that are highly protein bound, and have a narrow therapeutic index and a small volume of distribution. In reality, there are very few clinically relevant interactions that result from disruption of protein binding [12]. Warfarin, a restrictively eliminated drug that is bound extensively to plasma albumin (> 97%), is the most commonly reported victim of this purported mechanism of interaction. Warfarin may be displaced by acidic compounds that are also highly bound to albumin, such as valproic acid, resulting in transient increases in free warfarin and rapid increases in INR [13, 14]. However, as concentrations of free warfarin increase, the drug is eliminated more rapidly from the body; hence, the resulting effect is often transient (see Chapter 7, Figure 7.2). Thus for restrictively metabolized drugs, as the fraction of unbound drug increases due to displacement from protein binding sites, elimination of unbound drug increases to return unbound concentrations to their previous levels. As discussed in Chapters 5 and 7, non-restrictively metabolized drugs rely primarily on hepatic blood flow for their elimination; thus, increases in the fraction of unbound drug do not result in immediate compensatory elimination of unbound drug.

Inhibition of certain transporters may limit the distribution of a drug to its site(s) of action. Examples include inhibition of P-glycoprotein (P-gp) that limits drug distribution across the blood–brain barrier, or inhibition of organic anion transporting polypeptides (OATPs) OATP1B1 and OATP1B3 that limits drug distribution to the liver. HMG-CoA reductase inhibitors ("statins") act by reducing hepatic cholesterol synthesis. Since OATP1B1 is the primary transporter responsible for the hepatic uptake of most statins, concomitant administration with drugs that inhibit OATP1B1, such as cyclosporine and HIV protease inhibitors, may result in loss of statin efficacy, despite an increase in statin plasma concentrations [15]. Compounds that inhibit OATP1B1 may also inhibit breast cancer resistance protein (BCRP), an important transporter for the oral absorption and biliary elimination of statins, thus further confounding the disposition of statins [16].

## Interactions Affecting Drug Metabolism

As described in Chapter 11, drug metabolism is comprised of two distinct mechanisms of biochemical processing: Phase I and Phase II. Phase I is a chemical modification of the drug, typically by oxidation, hydrolysis or reduction reactions, performed primarily by members of the CYP enzyme family [17]. Phase II metabolism entails conjugation of the drug or Phase I product with endogenous compounds by reactions such as glucuronidation, sulfation, methylation, acetylation, and glycine conjugation. Modulation of CYP-mediated metabolism, by either enzyme inhibition or enzyme induction, has traditionally been recognized as the primary mechanism by which one drug interacts with another. However, modulation of Phase II metabolizing enzymes, such as UDP-glucuronosyl transferase (UGT) enzymes, is also an important source of potentially significant interactions. The impact of simultaneous enzyme and transporter-mediated interactions has recently received greater attention. As will be described more fully in the subsequent section on drug transporters, interactions resulting from complex enzyme–transporter interplay are common for many classes of drugs, and certain transporters are commonly co-inhibited in parallel with certain P450 enzymes, such as P-gp and CYP3A4.

### Enzyme Inhibition

Inhibition of enzyme activity is a common mechanism of clinically significant DDIs. Enzyme inhibition decreases the rate of drug metabolism, thereby increasing the amount of drug in the body, leading to accumulation and potential toxicity. Enzyme inhibition may be described by its reversibility, ranging from rapidly reversible to irreversible. Interactions due to reversible metabolic inhibition can be further categorized into competitive, non-competitive, or uncompetitive mechanisms.

In *reversible inhibition*, enzymatic activity is regained by the systemic elimination of inhibitor, such that the time to enzyme recovery is dependent on the elimination half-life of the inhibitor. *Competitive inhibition* is characterized by competition between substrate and inhibitor for the enzyme's active site. Competition for enzyme binding can be overcome by increasing the concentration of substrate, thereby sustaining the velocity of the enzymatic reaction despite the presence of an inhibitor [18, 19]. In contrast, *non-competitive inhibition* cannot be overcome by increased substrate concentration. In non-competitive inhibition the inhibitor binds to a separate site on the enzyme, rendering the enzyme–substrate complex non-functional [18, 19]. *Uncompetitive inhibition* results when the inhibitor binds only to the substrate–enzyme complex. From a clinical standpoint uncompetitive inhibition is rare, since saturation of enzyme with substrate is not common *in vivo*. Further, uncompetitive inhibition is clinically insignificant when the substrate concentration is well below the reaction's $K_m$ [18]. The following equations describe reversible inhibition mechanisms, where [$I$] and [$S$] are the respective

concentrations of inhibitor and substrate, $K_i$ is the inhibitory constant, and $K_m$ is the Michaelis–Menten constant for substrate metabolism by the enzyme:

Competitive inhibition:

$$\% \text{ inhibition} = \frac{\dfrac{[I]}{K_i}}{1 + \dfrac{[I]}{K_i} + \dfrac{[S]}{K_m}}$$

Non-competitive inhibition:

$$\% \text{ inhibition} = \frac{\dfrac{[I]}{K_i}}{1 + \dfrac{[I]}{K_i}}$$

Uncompetitive inhibition:

$$\% \text{ inhibition} = \frac{\dfrac{[I]}{K_i}}{1 + \dfrac{[I]}{K_i} + \dfrac{K_m}{[S]}}$$

*Irreversible* or *quasi-irreversible inhibition* occurs when either the parent compound or a metabolic intermediate binds to the reduced ferrous heme portion of the P450 enzyme, thereby inactivating it [19]. In *irreversible inhibition*, or "suicide inhibition", the intermediate forms a covalent bond with the CYP protein or its heme component, causing permanent inactivation. In *quasi-irreversible* inhibition, the intermediate is so tightly bound to the heme portion of the enzyme that it is practically irreversibly bound. As such, quasi-irreversible and irreversible mechanisms of inhibition are indistinguishable *in vivo* [19]. In irreversible inhibition, also referred to as "mechanism-based inhibition" or "time-dependent inhibition", the time to metabolic recovery is dependent upon the synthesis of new enzyme, rather than upon the dissociation and elimination of the inhibitor, as in the case of reversible inhibition. Examples of irreversible inhibitors include the macrolide antibiotics erythromycin and clarithromycin, and the HIV protease inhibitors. Potent inhibitors of CYP enzymes are typically lipophilic compounds, and often include an N-containing heterocycle, such as a pyridine, imidazole, or triazole functional group [19]. The azole antifungal ketoconazole is a classic example of a potent CYP3A4 inhibitor with a sterically-available nitrogen group.

Drugs are often categorized by the potency of their inhibition of CYP450 enzymes. Strong inhibitors are classified as drugs that increase the *AUC* of a sensitive substrate *in vivo* by $\geq 5$-fold, moderate inhibitors increase the *AUC* of a sensitive substrate by $\geq 2$-fold but $< 5$-fold, and weak inhibitors increase the *AUC* of a sensitive substrate by $\geq 1.25$-fold but $< 2$-fold [20]. Table 15.1 contains a partial list of some strong, moderate, and weak inhibitors of the more clinically relevant CYP450 enzymes [20, 21].

By identifying the metabolic pathways of a drug in the early stage of its development, it is possible to predict which drugs may have the potential to interact *in vivo* prior to conducting clinical investigations. *In vitro* findings of enzyme inhibition may be extrapolated to predict the likelihood of a clinical interaction using estimates of the enzyme-inhibitor dissociation constant ($K_i$) and the maximum plasma concentration of inhibitor achieved *in vivo* (*I*). When the $I/K_i$ ratio exceeds 1 the compound in question is considered to have a high inhibitory risk, while compounds with ratios between 0.1 and 1 are considered to be at medium risk, and those with ratios $< 0.1$ are at low risk [19].

Despite having 10–50% less CYP3A content than the liver, the gut remains an important site for many DDIs [22]. Furanocoumarins in grapefruit juice, for instance, both reversibly and irreversibly inhibit CYP3A4 in the small intestine [23]. Studies with grapefruit juice have shown that it can be classified as a "strong" CYP3A inhibitor when high-dose or double-strength preparations are used, or as a "moderate" CYP3A inhibitor when a lower dose (e.g., single strength) is used [20]. As a result, grapefruit juice in a high enough strength can significantly increase the bioavailability of a number of CYP3A4 substrates, including cyclosporine, midazolam, calcium channel blockers, and certain HMG CoA-reductase inhibitors [23–29]. Other drugs that significantly alter intestinal CYP3A4 metabolism include ketoconazole, itraconazole, erythromycin, cyclosporine, and verapamil [22].

There has been recent interest in the role of UGT enzymes as a source of DDIs. UGT1A1, 1A3, 1A4, 1A6,

**TABLE 15.1    Inhibitors of CYP450 Enzymes[a,b] [20, 21]**

| CYP Enzyme | Strong inhibitors | Moderate inhibitors | Weak inhibitors |
|---|---|---|---|
| CYP1A2 | Ciprofloxacin, enoxacin, fluvoxamine | Methoxsalen, mexiletine, oral contraceptives, phenylpropanolamine, thiabendazole, zileuton | Allopurinol, acyclovir, caffeine, cimetidine, disulfiram, echinacea, famotidine, norfloxacin, propafenone, propranolol, ticlopidine, verapamil |
| CYP2B6 | | | Clopidogrel, ticlopidine, prasugrel |
| CYP2C8 | Gemfibrozil | | Fluvoxamine, ketoconazole, trimethoprim |
| CYP2C9 | | Amiodarone, fluconazole, miconazole, oxandrolone | Capecitabine, cotrimoxazole, estravirine, fluvastatin, fluvoxamine, metronidazole, sulfinpyrazone, tigecycline, voriconazole, zafirlukast |
| CYP2C19 | Fluconazole, fluvoxamine, ticlopidine | Fluoxetine, moclobemide, omeprazole, voriconazole | Armodafinil, carbamazepine, cimetidine, ethinyl estradiol, etravirine, human growth hormone (rhGH), felbamate, ketoconazole |
| CYP3A | Clarithromycin, grapefruit juice (high strength), itraconazole, ketoconazole, lopinavir/ritonavir, nefazodone, posaconazole, ritonavir, saquinavir, telaprevir, telithromycin, voriconazole | Aprepitant, ciprofloxacin, darunavir/ ritonavir, diltiazem, erythromycin, fluconazole, fosamprenavir, grapefruit juice (regular strength), imatinib, verapamil | Alprazolam, amiodarone, amlodipine, atorvastatin, bicalutamide, cilostazol, cimetadine, cyclosporine, fluoxetine, fluvoxamine, ginkgo, goldenseal, isoniazid, nilotinib, oral contraceptives, ranitidine, ranolazine, tipranavir/ ritonavir, zileuton |
| CYP2D6 | Bupropion, fluoxetine, paroxetine, quinidine | Cinacalcet, duloxetine, terbinafine | Amiodarone, celecoxib, cimetidine, desvenlafaxine, diltiazem, diphenhydramine, Echinacea, (5) escitalopram, febuxostat, gefitinib, hydralazine, hydroxychloroquine, imatinib, methadone, oral contraceptives, propafenone, ranitidine, ritonavir, sertraline, telithromycin, verapamil |

[a]Not an exhaustive list.
[b]Strong, moderate and weak inhibitors increase the *AUC* of a sensitive substrate *in vivo* by $\geq 5$-fold, $\geq 2$-fold but $< 5$-fold, and $\geq 1.25$-fold but $< 2$-fold, respectively.

1A8, 1A9, 1A10, 2B4, 2B7, and 2B15 have all been identified as playing a role in drug metabolism [20, 30]. However, compared to P450 enzymes, there are relatively fewer examples of clinically relevant DDIs resulting from inhibition of UGTs. UGT substrates are often metabolized by multiple UGT enzymes and have high $K_m$ values relative to P450 substrates, making them less susceptible to significant increases in exposure [30]. As a result, the magnitude of effect due to UGT inhibition is typically less than encountered with P450 inhibition; most interactions involving UGT enzymes result in a < 2-fold increase in drug exposure, whereas inhibitory interactions involving P450 enzymes commonly result in a > 2-fold increase, with some cases of up to 30-fold or greater increase in drug exposure.

## Enzyme Induction

The molecular mechanisms underlying enzyme induction are more complex than those of inhibition. Simply put, induction results when a series of molecular events leads to enhanced transcription and increased synthesis of drug-metabolizing enzymes, with a resultant augmentation of their catalytic activity. This increase in metabolic activity may increase the intestinal and/or hepatic clearance of substrate drugs, subsequently reducing serum concentrations. Enzyme induction usually results in a loss of pharmacologic activity. However, in some cases induction may lead to the formation of active metabolites or reactive intermediates. Induction of CYP2E1, for instance, leads to the enhanced metabolism of acetaminophen to form the hepatotoxic metabolite, N-acetyl-p-amino-benzoquinone (NAPQI) (see Chapter 11, Scheme 11.4) [31]. Most mechanisms of P450 enzyme induction are mediated by intracellular receptors, including aryl hydrocarbon receptor (AhR), pregnane X receptor (PXR), constitutive androstane receptor (CAR), and peroxisome proliferator activated receptor $\alpha$ (PPAR$\alpha$) [32–36]. One exception is the induction of CYP2E1 by ethanol, by which ethanol stabilizes the enzyme following transcription, with no effect on receptor-mediated activation [37].

The nuclear hormone receptor super-family, which includes CAR, PXR, and PPAR$\alpha$, resides in the nucleus and is activated by a diverse array of endogenous and exogenous ligands. The orphan nuclear receptor PXR mediates the induction of CYP1A2, 2B6, 3A4, 2C8, and 2C9, some Phase II enzymes such as glutathione S-transferases, and ABC transporters including P-gp [38–40]. The nuclear receptor contains two binding domains, one for DNA and one for ligand binding. PXR binds as a heterodimer with the retinoid X receptor (RXR) to the DNA response elements of the regulatory region of CYP3A genes. For full activation

of CYP3A4, a coordinated effort is required between two distinct PXR-response elements on the 5'-end of CYP3A4 [39]. Exogenous and endogenous compounds that bind with varying degrees of affinity to PXR include rifampin, mifepristone, phenobarbital, calcium channel blockers, clotrimazole, steroid hormones, St John's wort, HMG Co-A reductase inhibitors, protease inhibitors, and hyperforin [35, 38].

Unlike PXR, CAR is normally located in the cytosol, translocating to the nucleus in response to activation by ligand binding. Once in the nucleus, CAR forms a heterodimer with RXR$\alpha$, binding to the appropriate response element and activating the transcription of targeted genes. CAR has been identified as a mediator of phenobarbital-type induction of CYP1A2, CYP2B6, CYP3A4, CYP2C8, CYP2C9, and P-gp expression [38, 39]. CAR and PXR appear to be interrelated, in that many compounds interact with both receptors. In addition, certain gene response elements are recognized and activated by both CAR and PXR. However, rifampin has a much greater effect on PXR than on CAR. In addition to their role in CYP induction, CAR and PXR also appear to have a role in the expression of Phase II conjugative enzymes and transport proteins, including P-gp and OATP transport proteins [38, 39].

AhR is the principle mediator of CYP1A1 and 1A2 induction, and also controls expression of glutathione S-transferase, UGT1A1 and BCRP [36, 41]. It binds tightly but non-covalently to the inducing molecule in the cytoplasm, then translocates to the nucleus where it heterodimerizes with the AhR nuclear translocator (Arnt), and finally binds to the xenobiotic or drug response element to regulate gene transcription. Unlike PXR and CAR, endogenous compounds, including steroids, do not appear to interact with AhR. Omeprazole is a prototypical inducer of AhR-mediated activation of CYP1A metabolism [42].

The rifamycins are well-known for their potent and relatively non-specific induction of CYP enzyme activity. Rifampin is frequently utilized as a prototype inducer in DDI studies that seek to evaluate the effects of induction on drugs that are known CYP3A, CYP2B6, CYP2C8, CYP2C9 or CYP2C19 substrates. Table 15.2 lists some of the more common prototypical inducers classified by their potency. Typically in drug development, a substrate for one or more CYP enzymes is studied initially with a potent inducer of the relevant enzyme(s) to characterize the "worst case scenario" for induction effect on the drug. A clinically significant interaction can be ruled out if the study results are negative. However, if the decrease in substrate exposure is significant, additional studies are then conducted with less potent inducers, based on the most likely co-administered drugs. In some cases an increased dose of

TABLE 15.2   Inducers of CYP450 Enzymes[a,b] [20, 142]

| CYP Enzyme | Strong inducers | Moderate inducers | Weak inducers |
|---|---|---|---|
| CYP1A2 | | Montelukast, phenytoin, cigarette smoke | Moricizine, omeprazole, phenobarbital |
| CYP2B6 | | Efavirenz, rifampin | Nevirapine |
| CYP2C8 | | Rifampin | |
| CYP2C9 | | Carbamazepine, rifampin | Aprepitant, bosentan, phenobarbital, St. John's wort |
| CYP2C19 | | Rifampin | Artemisinin |
| CYP3A | Avasimibe, carbamazepine, phenytoin, rifampin, St John's wort | Bosentan, efavirenz, etravirine, modafinil, nafcillin | Aprepitant, armodafinil, Echinacea, pioglitazole, prednisone, refinamide |
| CYP2D6 | None known | None known | None known |

[a]Not an exhaustive list.
[b]Strong, moderate and weak inducers decrease the *AUC* of a sensitive substrate *in vivo* by $\geq 80\%$, 50–80%, and 20–50%, respectively.

the substrate drug can be studied with an inducer to determine an appropriate dose needed to compensate for the inductive effects when co-administration of the combination is deemed clinically important.

Unlike enzyme inhibition, which can manifest itself clinically with as little as a single dose of inhibitor, enzyme induction requires chronic exposure to the inducer, typically for several days or more. For drugs that are mixed inhibitors and inducers of a particular enzyme, significant increases in the concentration of a co-administered substrate may be apparent in the first few days of concomitant dosing, followed by a relative decrease in substrate exposure as induction of metabolizing enzymes kicks in and overcomes the inhibitory effect. This paradigm has been observed for ritonavir when administered at higher doses [43].

## Interactions Involving Drug Transport Proteins

As described in Chapter 14, a variety of efflux and uptake proteins are involved in clinically relevant DDIs. Transport-mediated interactions typically occur when a xenobiotic modulates the function of a particular transporter, thereby altering the absorption and elimination as well as the distribution and tissue-specific drug targeting of co-administered drugs that are transported by these proteins [20]. To date, more than 400 membrane transporters have been identified, yet a relatively small number have compelling evidence for involvement in drug absorption, disposition, and DDIs; these are the transport proteins that will be highlighted in this chapter [44].

Membrane transporters can be classified into two major superfamilies: ATP binding cassette (ABC), and solute carrier (SLC). Selected ABC transporters involved in clinically relevant DDIs include the *ABCB1* and *ABCG2* gene products, P-gp, and BCRP,

respectively. SLC transporters of clinical significance include *SLC01B1* and *SLC1B3*, which encode for OATP1B1 and OATP1B3, respectively; *SLCC22A2*, *SLC22A6*, and *SLC22A8* encode for organic cation transporter (OCT) OCT2, and organic anion transporters (OATs) OAT1 and OAT3, respectively. In addition, members of the multidrug resistance protein (MRP), multidrug and toxin extrusion transporter (MATE), and peptide transporter (PEPT) families are involved in drug transport and also may contribute to DDIs [20, 44].

### P-glycoprotein (P-gp)

P-gp was the first identified and is generally the most well-known of the ABC proteins [45, 46]. It is located on the canalicular surface of hepatocytes, the apical surface of renal tubular epithelial cells, the apical surface of intestinal and placental epithelial cells, and the luminal surface of capillary endothelial cells at the blood–brain barrier [45–49]. P-gp is also present on a number of lymphocyte subsets, including CD4+, CD8+, CD19+, and CD56 NK cells [49]. Due to its presence in various anatomic locations, P-gp is frequently involved in the absorption, distribution, metabolism, and excretion of drugs which are substrates for this protein. Therefore, drug-induced modulation of P-gp activity may affect the absorption and/or distribution of a co-administered substrate medication, resulting in a clinically relevant DDI.

An extensive body of literature describing P-gp's involvement in clinically relevant DDIs has been described over the last decade and a half [50]. In general, P-gp functions to limit systemic drug exposure, excreting drug into the intestinal lumen in the gut, into renal tubules in the kidney, and into bile in the liver. P-gp also limits drug access to the brain and

**TABLE 15.3   Summary of P-Glycoprotein Substrates, Inhibitors, and Inducers [20, 21, 44, 49, 57–59]**

| Substrates | Inhibitors | Inducers |
|---|---|---|
| Amitriptyline | Amiodarone | Amiodarone |
| Amprenavir | Amprenavir | Aunorubicin |
| Atorvastatin | Astemizole | Bromocriptine |
| Cefoperazone | Bepredil | Chlorambucil |
| Chlorambucil | Clarithromycin | Cisplatin D |
| Chlorpromazine | Cortisol | Clotrimazole |
| Cimetidine | Cyclosporine | Colchicine |
| Ciprofloxacin | Diltiazem | Cyclosporine |
| Cisplatin | Dipyridamole | Dexamethasone |
| Clarithromycin | Disulfiram | Diltiazem |
| Colchicine | Erythromycin | Doxorubicine |
| Cyclosporine | Felodipine | Erythromycin |
| Cytarabine | Gf 120918 | Etoposide |
| Daunorubicin | Grapefruit juice | Fluorouracil |
| Dexamethasone | constituents: | Grapefruit juice |
| Digoxin | furanocoumarins | constituents: |
| Docetaxel | and flavonoids | furanocoumarins |
| Domperidone | Imatinab mesylate | and flavonoids |
| Doxorubicin | Indinavir | Hydroxyurea |
| Erythromycin | Ketoconazole | methotrexate |
| Estradiol | Lovastatin | Mitoxantrone |
| Etoposide | Ly 335979 | Indinavir |
| Fentanyl | Nelfinavir | Morphine |
| Fexofenadine | Nicardipine | Nicardipine |
| Fluorouracil | Progesterone | Nifedipine |
| Grepafloxacin | Quinidine | Probenecid |
| Hydroxyurea | Quinine | Rifampin |
| Imatinab Mesylate | Ritonavir | Ritonavir |
| Indinavir | Saquinavir | Saquinavir |
| Iraconazole | Simvastatin | Sirolimus |
| Ivermectin | Sirolimus | St John's wort |
| Lansoprozole | Tacrolimus | Tacrolimus |
| Levofloxacin | Tamoxifen | Tamoxifen |
| Lidocaine | Terfenadine | Verapamil |
| Loperamide | Troleandomycin | Vinblastine |
| Losarten | Itraconazole | Vincristine |
| Methadone | Valspodar (Psc 833) | Yohimbine |
| Methotrexate | Verapamil | |
| Methylprednisolone | Vinblastine | |
| Mitoxantrone | | |
| Morphine | | |
| Nelfinavir | | |
| Norfloxacin | | |
| Nortriptyline | | |
| Omeprazole | | |
| Ondansetron | | |
| Paclitaxel | | |
| Pantoprazole | | |
| Phenytoin | | |
| Pravastatin | | |
| Propranolol | | |
| Quinidine | | |
| Ranitidine | | |
| Rhodamine 123 | | |
| Ritonavir | | |
| Saquinavir | | |
| Tacrolimus | | |
| Talinolol | | |
| Tamoxifen | | |

*(Continued)*

**TABLE 15.3   Summary of P-Glycoprotein Substrates, Inhibitors, and Inducers [20, 21, 44, 49, 57–59]—cont'd**

| Substrates | Inhibitors | Inducers |
|---|---|---|
| Topotecan | | |
| Trimethoprim | | |
| Verapamil | | |
| Vinblastine | | |
| Vincristine | | |

lymphocytes via extrusion [51]. P-gp is relatively non-discriminatory in the types of compounds that it transports; it recognizes and transports drugs, drug conjugates, drug metabolites, and endogenous compounds of various chemical structures and weight [45]. A number of medications that are capable of inhibiting and/or inducing this protein are listed in Table 15.3.

A variety of substrate binding sites are contained within the transmembrane domains of P-gp, and these sites interact differentially with P-gp substrates and inhibitors [52]. Therefore, the propensity of a drug to induce or inhibit P-gp may depend on the specific P-gp substrate that is given concurrently [53]. For example, quercetin and colchicine were both found to enhance the *in vitro* transport of the P-gp substrate rhodamime-123, but, conversely, these drugs inhibited the transport of the P-gp substrate Hoechst 33342 [52]. These data suggest that *in vitro* study results indicating that a drug acts exclusively as a P-gp inhibitor or inducer should be interpreted cautiously when the drug has only been investigated in combination with a single substrate.

### Inhibition of P-gp

The mechanism of P-gp inhibition appears to be complex, involving competition for its drug-binding sites as well as blockade of the ATP hydrolysis that is necessary for its transport function [47]. Examples of clinically significant DDIs involving P-gp inhibition include increased digoxin exposure following administration of the P-gp inhibitors verapamil and quinidine [54, 55]. Administration of quinidine with the P-gp substrate loperamide was found to produce respiratory depression in a group of healthy volunteers, despite no change in plasma loperamide concentrations [56]. The basis for this interaction is that quinidine inhibits P-gp at the blood–brain barrier, resulting in greater CNS penetration of loperamide and potentially serious neurotoxicity. As a result of considerable overlap with CYP3A4, the actual role of P-gp inhibitors in DDIs involving P-gp substrates is unclear. Further, poor differentiation between P-gp inhibition in the intestine and liver makes it difficult to determine the relative contribution of P-gp to a specific DDI.

There has been considerable interest in the potential use of P-gp inhibition to optimize pharmacotherapy with anticancer and antiretroviral agents. Significant efforts have been made to exploit P-gp blockade in an effort to enhance chemotherapy uptake in tumors expressing P-gp-mediated drug resistance, to improve chemotherapy bioavailability, and to increase exposure to tumors protected by the blood–brain barrier. Research is also being directed at using P-gp inhibitors in HIV patients to improve protease inhibitor uptake into T lymphocytes and virologic sanctuaries such as the brain and testes.

### Induction of P-gp

A number of medications have been shown to induce P-gp in both animal and human cell lines (Table 15.3). Preclinical studies have noted that P-gp induction appears to depend on tissue type, the animal model employed, and the dose and duration of the inducing compound [57, 58]. In humans, P-gp induction may occur at a variety of anatomical sites, including the gut, liver, and kidney. In each case, induction of P-gp activity leads to reduced systemic concentrations of the substrate medication. Similar to P-gp inhibition, considerable overlap exists between CYP3A4 and P-gp inducers, including phenytoin, phenobarbital, rifampin, dexamethasone, and St John's wort [49, 59]. This overlap is purported to result from the fact that CYP3A4 and *MDR1* are regulated through similar mechanisms, including PXR activation [60–62]. An in-depth review of PXR-mediated induction of P-gp has been published by Lin and colleagues [47].

### P-gp and Drug Absorption

P-gp is present in high concentrations on the villus tip of the apical membrane of enterocytes, where it extrudes substrates from inside the cell back into the lumen of the intestine [45–47, 49]. A number of preclinical studies using *in vitro* cellular systems and *mdr1* knockout mice that lack ABCB1 and consequently do not express P-gp have documented the involvement of P-gp in drug absorption [63–69]. A consistent finding in these studies is that blockade or absence of intestinal P-gp results in decreased extrusion and increased systemic availability of drugs that are P-gp substrates; this may lead to toxicity or enhanced pharmacologic efficacy. However, as discussed in Chapter 4, this should not be construed to suggest that all P-gp substrates will undergo reduced oral absorption in the presence of a P-gp inhibitor [65, 70]. Due to saturation of intestinal P-gp at clinically relevant doses, numerous drugs that are P-gp substrates exhibit reasonably good

bioavailability. Examples of P-gp substrates with good oral availability include vinblastine, digoxin, ritonavir, etoposide, indinavir, and verapamil [46]. Thus, the importance of intestinal P-gp inhibition as a cause of clinically relevant DDIs tends to be overstated. Drug interactions arising from P-gp inhibition in the intestine are likely to be clinically relevant only for those medications given as small oral doses ($< 50$ mg) or with slow dissolution and/or membrane diffusion rates [46]. Exceptions exist for some drugs that are administered at high ($> 50$ mg) doses, but these drugs typically are poorly soluble in water, large in size ($> 800$ Da), or are prepared in formulations that are slow to dissolve [47]. Examples of such drugs include cyclosporine and paclitaxel, and saquinavir hard-gel capsules [46, 47].

Unlike intestinal P-gp inhibition, which is infrequently the source of clinically significant DDIs, induction of intestinal P-gp has been shown to reduce the bioavailability of P-gp substrates, thereby resulting in clinically relevant DDIs [47]. To illustrate, the impact of the P-gp inducer rifampin on digoxin absorption and disposition was studied in eight healthy subjects following a single IV or oral dose of digoxin, a sensitive P-gp substrate that is not extensively metabolized [71]. When given intravenously, digoxin PK was not significantly altered in the presence of rifampin. However, rifampin coadministration decreased the *AUC* and $C_{max}$ of oral digoxin by 31% and 52%, respectively. Furthermore, biopsies revealed that duodenal P-gp content increased 3.5-fold after rifampin administration, confirming the role of intestinal P-gp induction in this interaction.

### P-gp and Drug Metabolism and Biliary Excretion

In the liver, P-gp is localized at the canalicular (basolateral) membrane of hepatocytes facing the bile duct lumen at the exit site of the cell [46]. P-gp substrates, including drugs, drug conjugates, and drug metabolites, do not encounter P-gp until after they have entered the hepatocyte (via active transport or passive diffusion) and undergone intracellular distribution and possible metabolism [46, 47]. Therefore, when attempting to discern the effect of P-gp on hepatic drug excretion it is imperative to consider additional hepatic processes such as drug uptake, metabolism, and biliary excretion by other transport systems. As a result of P-gp's location in hepatocytes, only drugs that are not appreciably metabolized in the liver yet undergo significant biliary excretion by P-gp will be susceptible to P-gp-mediated DDIs in the liver. The prototypical example of such a compound is digoxin. In humans, approximately 20–25% of an oral digoxin dose is excreted as unchanged drug into bile

[72]. A number of P-gp inhibitors have been shown to increase plasma concentrations of digoxin. Inhibition of hepatic P-gp likely contributes to these interactions, although most data suggest that these interactions occur primarily in the kidney [45, 46].

Fexofenadine is another medication that undergoes minimal metabolism and is transported by P-gp as well as by a variety of other transport proteins [73]. A number of P-gp modulators have been reported to alter fexofenadine PK, presumably due to their influence on P-gp-mediated hepatic transport [74, 75]. In healthy volunteers rifampin reduced the $AUC$ and $C_{max}$ of fexofenadine two- and three-fold, respectively, when single doses of fexofenadine were given prior to and after 6 days of rifampin dosing [74].

Although P-gp modulation in the liver by one drug is capable of altering the PK profile of another, it bears repeating that drugs most likely to be affected by P-gp modulation in the liver are those that do not undergo significant hepatic metabolism, and are largely excreted into the bile. Since few medications meet all of these criteria, P-gp modulation in the liver is not routinely associated with clinically relevant DDIs.

*P-gp and Renal Excretion of Drugs*

In the kidney, P-gp is localized on the apical brush border membrane of renal proximal tubular cells, facing the lumen of the renal tubule [46, 47]. As in the liver, renal P-gp does not encounter substrates until intracellular trafficking is complete; it is at this point compounds are excreted into the urine by P-gp [46, 47]. Drugs that are secreted in the urine unchanged are most likely to undergo altered disposition when renal P-gp is inhibited.

Increased systemic exposure secondary to renal P-gp inhibition may cause a drug to exhibit enhanced pharmacologic activity such as unexpected toxicity or augmented clinical efficacy. To illustrate, it was noted in a preclinical investigation that renal excretion of dicloxacillin and trimethoprim was reduced by the P-gp inhibitors ketoconazole, vinblastine, and cyclosporine, suggesting that augmented P-gp-mediated efflux may be responsible for the increase in renal clearance of these, and possibly other, medications in patients with cystic fibrosis [76]. It has also been suggested that alterations in tubular secretion secondary to P-gp modulation may increase intracellular drug accumulation and augment the nephrotoxic potential of certain medications, such as vancomycin and some cephalosporins [77].

As in the liver, other transport proteins must also be considered when evaluating the potential for P-gp-mediated DDIs in the kidney. This is particularly true since other transporters may be simultaneously upregulated and/or downregulated. In general, inhibition of renal P-gp should be considered a potentially clinically relevant mechanism by which plasma concentrations of renally eliminated P-gp substrates are increased.

*Organic Anion Transporting Polypeptides (OATPs)*

As discussed in Chapter 14, the OATP (SLCO) super-family is expressed in multiple organ systems, although the clinically significant DDIs identified to date occur primarily in the liver. OATP substrates consist of a broad spectrum of endogenous compounds, including bile acids, thyroid hormones, and conjugated steroids, anionic peptides, and many additional xenobiotics, including statins, valsartan, repaglinide, and fexofenadine [44]. A number of clinically relevant DDIs have been identified that involve hepatic OATP1B1 and OATP1B3 [44]. Inhibition of hepatic OATP1B1 (and/or OATP1B3) by cyclosporine has resulted in large increases in pravastatin, rosuvastatin, and pitavastatin $AUC$, ranging from 360% to 890% [78–81]. In addition, single-dose rifampin and multi-dose lopinavir–ritonavir were both shown to increase bosentan $C_{trough}$ by 500% and 4700%, respectively [82]. Finally, single-dose rifampin increased glyburide $AUC$ by 125% and lopinavir–ritonavir increased rosuvastatin $AUC$ by 107% [83].

Fexofenadine is a well-known substrate for OATP transport, though the relative contribution of OATP modulation on DDIs involving this drug is unclear, since it is also a P-gp substrate. The 60–80% reduction in fexofenadine bioavailability that results from orange, apple, and grapefruit juice consumption, however, is likely the result of OATP inhibition rather than P-gp induction [84]. While increased systemic exposure to fexofenadine is not likely to cause serious toxicity, elevated plasma concentrations of other drugs may result in serious, potentially life-threatening toxicities. To this end, OATPs represent an increasingly important group of transport proteins that should be routinely considered as a potential mediator of DDIs, especially in patients taking OATP inhibitors in combination with OATP substrates that have a low therapeutic index.

*Organic Cation Transporters (OCTs)*

OCT proteins are expressed on the basolateral membrane of epithelial cells in the kidney, liver, and intestine, predominantly transporting hydrophilic, low molecular weight organic cations [85]. Cimetidine is a well-described inhibitor of OCT2 and has been associated with reduced clearance of a number of concomitantly administered medications, including metformin, pindolol, and dofetilide [44]. However, it is not clear that OCT-2 is the sole mechanism of these interactions, as cimetidine has also been shown to inhibit renal efflux via inhibition of human multidrug and toxin extrusion transporters, MATE-1 and MATE-2K [86, 87]. In addition, the magnitude of these interactions is quite low in comparison to OATP inhibitory interactions described above. For example, reductions in clearance due to cimetidine ranged between 27% and 34% [44]. Cetirizine also has been noted to inhibit OCT, as evidenced by a 41% decrease in pilsicainide clearance [88].

### Organic Anion Transporters (OATs)

OAT proteins are similar in amino acid sequence to OCT proteins, and are expressed in the liver, brain, proximal tubule of the kidney, and placenta. OAT-2 is expressed in the kidney on the basolateral side of the proximal tubule and is involved in the transport of zidovudine, cephalosporins, tetracycline, and salicylates. OAT1 and OAT3 are also located on the basolateral membrane of the proximal tubule and are involved in the transport of cidofovir, cephradine, acyclovir, tenofovir, zidovudine, furosemide, and methotrexate [89–94]. NSAIDS, antitumor drugs, histamine $H_2$ receptor antagonists, prostaglandins, and angiotensin-converting enzyme inhibitors have also been shown to be transported by these OATs [44]. OAT4 is located on the apical side of the proximal tubule, and is involved in the uptake and efflux of compounds such as estrone sulfate and cilastatin [95].

Potentially relevant DDIs have been described for OAT1, which is inhibited by probenecid [44]. For example, cidofovir, furosemide, and acyclovir clearance values were reduced by 32%, 66%, and 32%, respectively, by concurrent probenecid administration [44]. In addition to probenecid, several other therapeutic agents have been associated with inhibition of the OATs. These include pravastatin, cimetidine, cephalosporin antibiotics, thiazide and loop diuretics, acetazolamide, and certain NSAIDs [91, 96–98]. However, the relatively low plasma concentration of most OAT inhibitors, in relation to their $K_i$ values, suggests that many inhibitors identified *in vitro* are not capable of causing clinically significant DDIs [98]. However, probenecid, which has a relatively lower $K_i$ value, is an exception. Probenecid protects against cidofovir-mediated nephrotoxicity by limiting its OAT1-mediated renal transport [99]. Probenecid has also been shown to decrease the cerebrospinal fluid clearance of the OAT substrate zidovudine, thus prolonging its half-life in the brain [100]. Further investigation into human OAT transporters is needed to identify OAT-mediated DDIs that should be avoided or possibly exploited to improve pharmacotherapy.

### Multidrug Resistance Proteins (MRPs)

MRPs (1–12) are contained within the superfamily of mammalian ABC transporters and transport a large number of medications, many of which are also substrates for P-gp [45, 101]. In general, MRPs tend to be widely distributed in a variety of human tissues [102–105]. The majority of published literature with MRPs focuses on their ability to confer multidrug resistance to anticancer compounds.

MRP1 (ABCC1) is localized on the basolateral membrane (tissue side) of epithelial cells in the intestine, liver, brain, lung, peripheral blood mononuclear cells (PBMCs), choroid plexus, CD4+ cells, kidney, testes, and oropharynx [45, 104–107]. In addition to transporting antineoplastic agents, MRP1 also transports organic anions, heavy metals, difloxacin, grepafloxacin, glucuronide conjugates of steroids, leukotrienes and prostaglandins, and several HIV protease inhibitors [108–111]. Several drugs have been shown to inhibit MRP1 *in vitro*, including the HIV protease inhibitors atazanavir, lopinavir, and ritonavir, as well as probenecid [111–113]. Nonetheless, clinically significant DDIs resulting from MRP1 modulation have not been described and further study is required to determine the role of MRP1, alone and in combination with other transporters such as P-gp, in decreasing the therapeutic activity of substrate medications. Once these questions are answered, it is possible that targeted MRP1 inhibition may improve the intracellular penetration of MRP1 substrates. It will also be necessary to determine whether MRP1 inducers, such as rifampin, are capable of reducing the therapeutic efficacy of MRP1 substrates by interfering with their penetration into target cells and sanctuary sites [114–116].

MRP2 (ABCC2; cMOAT) is mainly expressed on the canalicular side of hepatocyes, where it is involved in the excretion of compounds into the bile, and expressed to a lesser degree on the luminal side of kidney proximal tubule cells and enterocytes, the brain, and placenta [115]. Medications transported by MRP2 include cidofovir, adefovir, etoposide, mitoxantrone, and valsartan, among others [44, 105, 117, 118]. A number of MRP2 inhibitors have been identified, including cyclosporine, probenecid, furosemide, cidofovir, and adefovir, as well as the antiretrovirals ritonavir, saquinavir, lamivudine, tenofovir, emtricitabine, nevirapine, efavirenz, abacavir, and delavirdine [44, 50]. Similar to MRP1 and P-gp,

MRP2 is noted for its ability to confer resistance to multiple anticancer agents.

Despite its minimal presence in the kidney, MRP2 has been shown to play a significant role in the renal excretion of some medications [119]. The nucleoside phosphonates cidofovir and adefovir are both inhibitors as well as substrates of MRP2 [118]. Cidofovir and adefovir undergo renal tubular secretion and are associated with nephrotoxicity, particularly at higher doses [118, 120–122]. MRP2 is presumed to mediate the efflux of adefovir and cidofovir from proximal tubule cells [118]. As such, MRP2 inhibition in the kidney may result in reduced efflux of these drugs and increased intracellular accumulation, which may ultimately lead to nephrotoxicity. Conversely, MRP2 induction has the potential to limit accumulation of adefovir and cidofovir in tubular cells, thereby resulting in a nephroprotective effect. Medications that may interact with the nucleoside phosphonates via MRP2 inhibition include probenecid, furosemide, and ritonavir; inducers of MRP2 include indomethacin, sulfinpyrazone, penicillin G, rifampin, and phenobarbital [50]. Other medications that may affect the intracellular accumulation and nephrotoxic potential of cidofovir and adefovir via competition for MRP2-mediated transport include valacyclovir, ganciclovir, and acyclovir [50].

Due to structural differences between MRP2 and MRP4, MRP4 exhibits differences in substrate selectivity. MRP4 is expressed in a variety of tissues, including the kidney, gallbladder, lung, thymus, prostate, tonsil, bladder, lymphocytes, skeletal muscle, pancreas, spleen, testis, ovary, and small intestine [123, 124]. MRP4 is noted for its ability to confer resistance to certain nucleotide and nucleoside analog antiviral medications via enhanced efflux and reduced intracellular accumulation of nucleoside triphosphates [117, 125]. Nucleoside and nucleotide analogs that are transported by MRP4 include abacavir, cidofovir, and a number of anticancer medications [126]. Inhibitors of MRP4 include dipyridamole, MK571, sildenafil, and NSAIDS [50]. Dipyridamole was shown to ameliorate the MRP4-mediated efflux of nucleoside analog triphosphates in MRP4 overexpressing cells, resulting in enhanced antiviral activity of these compounds [127].

### Breast Cancer Resistance Protein (BCRP)

BCRP was originally identified as a multidrug resistance protein in cancer cells. It is expressed in mammary tissue, testis, placenta, and the gastrointestinal tract, kidney, liver, and brain endothelium. BCRP is similar to P-gp in that it acts as an efflux protein that is capable of limiting oral bioavailability and blood–brain transport of selected substrates. BCRP can also limit the passage of substrates across the maternal–fetal and blood–testis barriers; it is also involved in the secretion of riboflavin (vitamin $B_2$) and potentially other vitamins, such as vitamin K and biotin, into breast milk [50].

A number of anticancer compounds, such as mitoxantrone, methotrexate, topotecan, imatinib, and irinotecan, are substrates for BCRP [44]. In addition, statins, sulfate conjugates, folic acid, and porphyrins are also transported by BCRP. Inhibitors of BCRP include estrone, 17β-estradiol, fumitremorgin C (FTC), cimetidine, GF120918, and cyclosporine. In combination with GF120918, topotecan *AUC* was found to be increased by 2.4-fold in patients with cancer [128]. As has been shown with BCRP knockout mice, intestinal BCRP inhibition has the potential to increase the bioavailability of BCRP substrates. However, many substrates for BCRP are also substrates for other transport proteins, such as P-gp and OATP1B1, so it is difficult to isolate the clinical significance of BCRP-mediated DDIs. Nonetheless, research continues to identify additional BCRP inhibitors that might be capable of improving the intestinal absorption of poorly absorbed antineoplastic medications, thereby acting as chemosensitizers in the setting of drug resistance.

### Influence of pH and Renal Blood Flow on Drug Interactions in the Kidney

The pharmacokinetic properties of drugs that are primarily renally excreted may be altered by changes to active transport systems, urinary pH, and renal blood flow. As discussed in Chapter 5, changes in pH alter the ionization of weakly acidic and basic drugs, thereby affecting their degree of passive diffusion. Since most weakly acidic and basic drugs are metabolized to inactive compounds prior to renal excretion, changes in urinary pH do not affect the elimination of most drugs. Exceptions include the acidic compounds phenobarbital, aspirin, and other salicylates, whose serum levels have been demonstrated to decrease with concurrent antacid or sodium bicarbonate administration [129, 130]. Changes in urinary pH have been exploited to increase drug excretion in situations of phenobarbital and salicylate overdose. Inhibition of renal blood flow has also been hypothesized as the mechanism behind the elevated serum lithium levels that have been observed during concurrent NSAID use [12].

## PREDICTING DRUG INTERACTIONS AND PRODUCT LABELING

### *In Vitro* Screening Methods

Characterization of drug interaction potential typically begins early in the development of a new drug, with characterization of its elimination pathways and the use of *in vitro* tools to evaluate the drug's potential to be a substrate, inhibitor or inducer of metabolizing enzymes or transporters. Results of *in vitro* experiments are important for indicating when *in vivo* studies in humans may be necessary to fully define the drug interaction profile of a drug. In many cases, *in vitro* studies can be used to successfully rule out interactions via a particular metabolic or transport pathway, making an *in vivo* DDI study unnecessary. The metabolic profile of a drug is typically defined *in vitro* using recombinantly expressed enzymes, human liver microsomes, freshly isolated or cryopreserved human hepatocytes, or a combination of these methods [131].

In addition to determining which enzymes, if any, are involved in the metabolic turnover of a drug, it is necessary to evaluate the potential for the drug to inhibit or induce metabolic enzymes. Recombinant enzymes, human liver microsomes, and/or fresh hepatocytes are typically used to assess enzyme inhibition and to determine the $K_i$ or $IC_{50}$ value for an inhibitor. *In vitro* inhibition experiments should utilize a validated selective substrate, and should compare the effect of the test compound to that of a well-characterized control inhibitor. Identification of mechanism-based inhibition is achieved by comparing inhibition potential with and without pre-incubation of the test compound.

It is slightly more complicated to evaluate enzyme induction than enzyme inhibition *in vitro*, in that the ligand-activated receptor and the metabolic enzyme must both be present. The primary *in vitro* method used to characterize enzyme induction is by measuring enzyme activity after incubating the drug in a human hepatocyte culture. As with inhibition assays, enzyme activity is determined using specific marker substrates and by comparing the test compound to that of a well-known enzyme inducer. Induction potential may also be assessed using a reporter gene assay and measurement of mRNA levels using RT-PCR. If a drug is both an inducer and inhibitor of an enzyme, induction experiments using hepatocytes may give false negative results. In this case, assessment of induction should include measurement of mRNA levels in addition to evaluation of enzyme activity [20].

## Utility of Physiologically Based Pharmacokinetic (PBPK) Modeling

The decision to conduct an *in vivo* DDI study in humans should be based on quantitative analysis of both *in vitro* and *in vivo* human data. The analysis can be accomplished via various algorithms and models, including basic, mechanistic static, and mechanistic dynamic models, such as PBPK models, as illustrated in Figure 15.1 [132].

The simplest approach is to test the potential for an investigational drug to be an enzyme inhibitor by using a basic model such as $I/K_i$ [133–136]. This model provides a conservative initial estimate and may eliminate the need for later clinical investigations of DDIs if they indicate a low potential for interactions. When the $I/K_i$ value suggests that an interaction potential exists, additional *in vitro* and *in vivo* human data need to be incorporated into more complex models to further investigate the DDI potential and determine the need to conduct a clinical study [20].

Mechanistic static models incorporate detailed drug disposition and drug interaction mechanisms for both drugs in an interaction [137]. For example, parameters such as bioavailability and fractional metabolism data (e.g., "$f_m$" by specific CYP enzymes) for substrate drugs and $K_i$ for inhibitors are incorporated into these models [20]. PBPK models are even more complex than static models in that they integrate system-dependent parameters (e.g., organ blood flow rates, protein contents, and enzyme and transporter activities) with detailed drug-dependent PK parameters (Figure 15.1). When appropriately constructed, PBPK models offer the following advantages over static models:

1. A PBPK model allows the investigation of the effect of an interacting drug on the entire PK profile of the substrate.
2. A PBPK model incorporates concurrent mechanisms of DDIs, such as simultaneous induction and inhibition, the effect of inhibitory metabolites, etc.
3. A PBPK model provides insight into the causes of uncertainty and variability.
4. A PBPK model can be used to investigate DDIs in the presence of multiple intrinsic and/or extrinsic factors.

These features make PBPK models a useful option to (1) design optimal clinical DDI studies and (2) quantitatively predict the magnitude of a DDI in various clinical situations, including multiple concurrent patient factors, such as renal impairment and/or genetic variations in specific metabolizing enzymes or

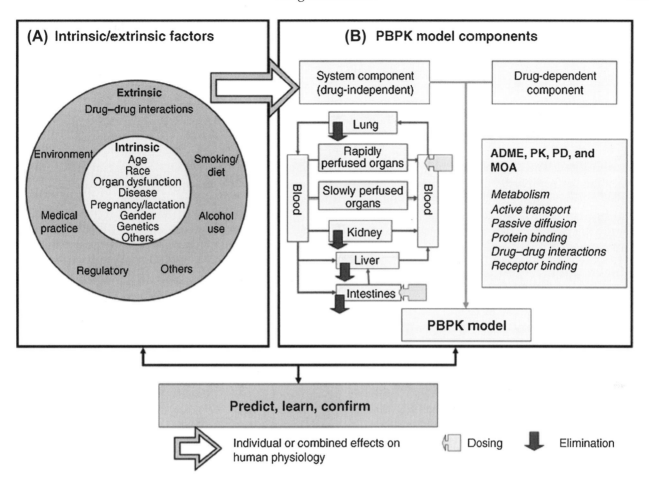

The degree of complexity of the PBPK model can vary according to the need.

**FIGURE 15.1** (A) Intrinsic and extrinsic patient factors that can affect drug exposure and response. (B) Drug-dependent components and drug-independent (system) components of the PBPK model that can act individually or in combination to affect drug exposure. ADME, absorption, distribution, metabolism, and excretion; MOA, mechanism of action; PD, pharmacodynamics; PK, pharmacokinetics. Reproduced with permission from Zhao, P, Zhang L, Grillo JA *et al.* Clin Pharmacol Ther 2011;89:259–67 [132].

transport proteins. Mathematical simulations using population-based, physiological PK/PD models (e.g., PBPK models) that simultaneously integrate various patient-intrinsic and -extrinsic factors can provide an understanding of the potentially complex changes in exposure–response relationships in patients where multiple covariates are present [132].

## Drug Interactions Involving Therapeutic Proteins

As therapeutic proteins do not typically depend on mechanisms of metabolism or transport for clearance, there is less potential for concomitantly administered drugs to affect therapeutic protein disposition or elimination. However, evolving data indicate therapeutic proteins may affect the disposition of other drugs. Exogenously administered immunologic proteins, such

as interferons (IFNs) and interleukins (ILs), may result in changes in the metabolic capacity of the liver that are similar to what has been observed during acute infection or inflammation [138]. It has been demonstrated that cytokines can suppress gene transcription, resulting in downregulation of P450 enzymes [139]. Other mechanisms underlying inflammatory or cytokine-mediated downregulation of P450 may be altered mRNA stability and activation of nitric-oxide synthase to form nitric oxide (NO), a direct enzyme inhibitor. Experiments in mice have also identified inflammatory-mediated changes in the expression and activity of drug transporters, including the downregulation of *mdr1*, *Mrp*, *Bsep*, *Bcrp*, and *Oatp* [139].

In view of the limited ability of *in vitro* experiments to identify cytokine-mediated interactions, *in vivo* DDI studies should be conducted to determine a therapeutic protein's effect on CYP enzymes and transporters. FDA guidance recommends that studies be conducted either with individual marker substrates or by using a cocktail approach [20]. When the therapeutic protein is to be co-administered with a specific small molecule drug as part of combination therapy, both the effect of the therapeutic protein on the small molecule and the effect of the small molecule on the therapeutic protein should be evaluated by *in vivo* studies. Although PBPK modeling may be applied to therapeutic protein–drug interactions to evaluate complex mechanisms and explore the potential for clinically significant interactions, this approach is currently not comprehensive enough to substitute for *in vivo* studies.

## Genetic Variation

As discussed in Chapters 13 and 14, genetic polymorphisms occur in many CYP enzymes and transporters and significantly influence drug metabolism and transport. This genotypic variation also may affect the magnitude of various DDIs. Quinidine, a potent CYP2D6 inhibitor, significantly alters codeine's conversion to morphine via CYP2D6 O-demethylation in CYP2D6 extensive metabolizers. However, the rate of codeine's metabolism is already substantially diminished in genetically poor CYP2D6 metabolizers, so the addition of quinidine does not significantly reduce the rate of conversion to morphine [111]. In another example, rifampin, a potent and broad inducer of CYP450, has been found to have a differential effect on the exposure of the antiretroviral drug efavirenz, which is metabolized chiefly by CYP2B6, depending on patients' genotype. Efavirenz exposure would be expected to decrease dramatically during co-administration with rifampin. However, in patients carrying the *CYP2B6* single nucleotide polymorphism (SNP) 516G>T, which confers reduced CYP2B6 enzyme activity, efavirenz clearance is significantly lower relative to intermediate or normal metabolizer genotypes in the presence of rifampin [140].

In some cases, differences in drug PK among genetically diverse groups of subjects can be used to predict potentially significant DDIs. Clopidogrel, for instance, depends on conversion to an active metabolite by CYP2C19 to exert its activity. In CYP2C19 genetically poor metabolizers, there is decreased active metabolite formation and diminished inhibition of platelet aggregation. A similar decrease in metabolite formation and anticoagulant response occurs when clopidogrel is co-administered with omeprazole, a CYP2C19 inhibitor [141]. Thus, a clinically significant effect in a genetically poor metabolizer population may predict the likelihood for a clinically significant effect in patients who are co-adminstered a drug that inhibits the same pathway.

## Drug Interactions in Product Labeling

Drug interaction information is generally included in the DRUG INTERACTIONS and CLINICAL PHARMACOLOGY sections of the US prescribing information. When DDI information has important implications for the safe and effective use of the drug, it is also often included in varying levels of detail in other sections of the label, such as DOSAGE AND ADMINISTRATION, CONTRAINDICATIONS, WARNINGS AND PRECAUTIONS, or HIGHLIGHTS. The label should include clinically relevant information about metabolic and transport pathways, metabolites, PK and/or PD interactions, and clinical implications of PK and/or PD interactions or genetic polymorphisms of drug-metabolizing enzymes and transporters, if applicable. When relevant, the description of clinical implications should include monitoring and dose adjustment recommendations [20].

Drug interaction information in labeling may not always result from a clinical DDI study. In some cases, *in vitro* studies can rule out a specific type of drug interaction. In other cases, information can be extrapolated from a study conducted with one drug to another drug, when similar results are expected. The following cases illustrate recent labeling examples.

### Case 1

Although prasugrel is not expected to affect CYP2C9 based on *in vitro* data, it has been shown to increase bleeding time when co-administered with warfarin, a CYP2C9 substrate, possibly due to a pharmacodynamic interaction. Warnings about their concomitant use appear in various sections of the prasugrel label (DRUG INTERACTIONS, WARNINGS AND PRECAUTIONS, and PATIENT COUNSELING INFORMATION) to advise about the increased risk of bleeding with concomitant use of prasugrel with warfarin, other oral anticoagulants, chronic use of non-steroidal anti-inflammatory drugs, and fibrinolytic agents [142].

### Case 2

A clinical DDI study showed that plasma concentrations of dasatinib, a CYP3A substrate, were significantly decreased by co-administration of rifampin, a strong CYP3A inducer. The dasatinib label warns about the concomitant use of rifampin and dasatinib, but also includes a list of other CYP3A inducers whose interactions with dasatinib were not evaluated in humans [143]. The recommendation includes suggestions for careful monitoring and increased dosage if an inducer must be co-administered. Similarly, ketoconazole was the only CYP3A inhibitor evaluated in a clinical DDI study with dasatinib, in which a significant increase in plasma dasatinib concentrations was demonstrated. However, the label for dasatinib includes a list of other CYP3A inhibitors that were not evaluated in humans. The DOSAGE AND ADMINISTRATION section of the label recommends the use of an alternate medication with no or minimal enzyme inhibition potential or a decrease in the dasatinib dose if one of these strong inhibitors must be co-administered.

### Case 3

Rivaroxaban was recently approved for the prophylaxis of deep vein thrombosis. It is a substrate for CYP3A4, CYP2J2, P-gp, and BCRP, and also is eliminated renally as unchanged drug [144]. Co-administration of rivaroxaban with ketoconazole or ritonavir, both strong CYP3A and P-gp inhibitors, resulted in a clinically significant, ~2.5-fold increase in rivaroxaban *AUC* and anticoagulation effect (factor Xa inhibition and PT prolongation). However, studies with other inhibitors such as erythromycin and clarithromycin caused only 1.3- and 1.5-fold increases in rivaroxaban *AUC*, respectively, that were not deemed clinically relevant. Further, when rivaroxaban was evaluated in subjects with renal impairment and with $CL_{CR}$ values down to 15 ml/min, the *AUC* was increased 1.4- to 1.6-fold compared to subjects with normal renal function. Thus, it was considered important to address the question of whether a combination of mild-to-moderate renal impairment plus concomitant administration of a mild-to-moderate CYP3A4 inhibitor, each of which by itself would be deemed insignificant, could result in a clinically significant increase in rivaroxaban exposure. This question was answered by PBPK analysis, which indicated that this combination of factors could increase rivaroxaban *AUC* by two-fold or more [145, 146]. Therefore, there was a postmarketing requirement to "perform a clinical trial to evaluate the effect of renal impairment (i.e., mild, moderate, severe) plus the concurrent use of P-gp inhibitors and moderate inhibitors of CYP3A4 on the PK, PD, and safety of rivaroxaban in volunteers so that appropriate dosing recommendations can be developed in these populations". In the meantime, the label indicates:

> Based on simulated pharmacokinetic data, patients with renal impairment receiving XARELTO with drugs that are combined P-gp and weak or moderate

CYP3A4 inhibitors (e.g., erythromycin, azithromycin, diltiazem, verapamil, quinidine, ranolazine, dronedarone, amiodarone, and felodipine) may have significant increases in exposure compared with patients with normal renal function and no inhibitor use, since both pathways of rivaroxaban elimination are affected. Since these increases may increase bleeding risk, use XARELTO in this situation only if the potential benefit justifies the potential risk.

## REFERENCES

[1] Webb DJ, Freestone S, Allen MJ, et al. Sildenafil citrate and blood-pressure-lowering drugs: Results of drug interaction studies with an organic nitrate and a calcium antagonist. Am J Cardiol 1999;83:21C–8C.

[2] Wadhwa NK, Schroeder TJ, O'Flaherty E, et al. The effect of oral metoclopramide on the absorption of cyclosporine. Transplant Proc 1987;19:1730–3.

[3] Reyataz™, atazanavir [package insert]. Princeton, NJ: Bristol-Myers Squibb Company (package insert issued 2/2011).

[4] Van der Meer JWM, Keuning JJ, Scheijgrond HW, et al. The influence of gastric acidity on the bioavailability of ketoconazole. J Antimicrob Chemother 1980;6:552–4.

[5] Sporanox®, itraconazole [package insert]. Titusville, NJ: Janssen Pharmaceutical Products, L.P. (package insert revised 7/2010).

[6] Lange D, Pavao JH, Wu J, Klausner M. Effect of a cola beverage on the bioavailability of itraconazole in the presence of H2 blockers. J Clin Pharmacol 1997;37:535–40.

[7] Polk RE. Drug–drug interactions with ciprofloxacin and other fluoroquinolones. Am J Med 1989;87(Suppl. 5A): 76S–81S.

[8] Nix DE, Watson WA, Lener ME, et al. Effects of aluminum and magnesium antacids and ranitidine on the absorption of ciprofloxacin. Clin Pharmacol Ther 1989;46:700–5.

[9] D'Arcy PF, McElnay JC. Drug–antacid interactions: Assessment of clinical importance. Drug Intell Clin Pharm 1987;21:607–17.

[10] Neuvonen PJ. Interactions with the absorption of tetracyclines. Drugs 1976;11:45–54.

[11] Farmer JA, Gotto Jr AM. Antihyperlipidaemic agents. Drug interactions of clinical significance. Drug Safety 1994;11:201–9.

[12] Stockley IH. General considerations and an outline survey of some basic interaction mechanisms. In: Stockley IH, editor. Stockley's drug interactions. London: Pharmaceutical Press; 2002. p. 1–14.

[13] Panjehshahin MR, Bowmer CJ, Yates MS. Effect of valproic acid, its unsaturated metabolites and some structurally related fatty acids on the binding of warfarin and dansylsarcosine to human albumin. Biochem Pharmacol 1991;41: 1227–33.

[14] Yoon HW, Giraldo EA, Wijdicks EF. Valproic acid and warfarin: An underrecognized drug interaction. Neurocrit Care 2011;15:182–5.

[15] Generaux GT, Bonomo FM, Johnson M, Doan KM. Impact of SLCO1B1 (OATP1B1) and ABCG2 (BCRP) genetic polymorphisms and inhibition on LDL-C lowering and myopathy of statins. Xenobiotica 2011;41:639–51.

[16] Niemi M. Transporter pharmacogenetics and statin toxicity. Clin Pharmacol Ther 2010;87:130–3.

[17] Lewis DF. 57 varieties: The human cytochromes P450. Pharmacogenomics 2004;5:305–18.

[18] Thummel KE, Kunze KL, Shen DD, et al. Metabolically-based drug–drug interactions. principles and mechanisms. In: Levy RH, Thummel KE, Trager WF, editors. Metabolic

drug interactions. Philadelphia, PA: Lippincott Williams & Williams; 2000. p. 3–47.

[19] Bachmann KA, Ring BJ, Wrighton SA. Drug–drug interactions and the cytochromes P450. In: Lee JS, Obach S, Fisher MB, editors. Drug metabolizing enzymes: CYP450 and other enzymes in drug discovery and development. New York, NY: Marcel Dekker, Inc.; 2003. p. 311–36.

[20] CDER, CBER. Drug interaction studies – study design, data analysis, and implications for dosing and labeling, draft guidance for industry. Rockville, MD: FDA (Internet at, www.fda.gov/downloads/Drugs/GuidanceComplianceRegulatory Information/Guidances/UCM072101.pdf; 2006).

[21] FDA Drug Interaction website. Drug Development and Drug Interactions. (Internet at, www.fda.gov/Drugs/DevelopmentApprovalProcess/DevelopmentResources/DrugInteractionsLabeling/ucm080499.htm, accessed 2011.)

[22] Doherty MM, Charman WN. The mucosa of the small intestine. Clin Pharmacokinet 2002;41:235–53.

[23] Kupferschmidt HR, Ha WH, Ziegler PL, et al. Interaction between grapefruit juice and midazolam in humans. Clin Pharmacol Ther 1995;58:20–8.

[24] Lilja JJ, Kivisto KT, Neuvonen PJ. Grapefruit juice–simvastatin interaction: Effect on serum concentrations of simvastatin, simvastatin acid, and HMG-CoA reductase inhibitors. Clin Pharmacol Ther 1998;64:477–83.

[25] Benton RE, Honig PK, Zamani K, et al. Grapefruit juice alters terfenadine pharmacokinetics, resulting in prolongation of repolarization on the electrocardiogram. Clin Pharmacol Ther 1996;59:383–8.

[26] Bailey DG, Spence JD, Munoz C, et al. Interaction of citrus juices with felodipine and nifedipine. Lancet 1991;337:268–9.

[27] Ducharme MP, Warbasse LH, Edwards DJ. Disposition of intravenous and oral cyclosporine after administration with grapefruit juice. Clin Pharmacol Ther 1995;57:485–91.

[28] Kufperschmidt HH, Fattinger KE, Ha HR, et al. Grapefruit juice enhances the bioavailability of the HIV protease inhibitor saquinavir in man. Br J Clin Pharmacol 1998;45:355–9.

[29] Bailey DG, Bend JR, Arnold MO, et al. Erythromycin–felodipine interaction: Magnitude, mechanism and comparison with grapefruit juice. Clin Pharmacol Ther 1996;60:25–33.

[30] Williams JA, Hyland R, Jones BC, et al. Drug–drug interactions for UDP-glucuronosyltransferase substrates: A pharmacokinetic explanation for typically observed low exposure (AUCi/AUC) ratios. Drug Metab Dispos 2004;32:1201–8.

[31] Brackett CC, Bloch JD. Phenytoin as a possible cause of acetaminophen hepatotoxicity: Case report and review of the literature. Pharmacotherapy 2000;20:229–33.

[32] Kliewer SA, Moore JT, Wade L, et al. An orphan nuclear receptor activated by pregnane defines novel steroid signaling pathway. Cell 1998;92:73–82.

[33] Sueyoshi T, Kawamoto T, Zelko I, et al. The repressed nuclear receptor CAR responds to phenobarbital in activating the human CYP2B6 gene. J Biol Chem 1999;274:6043–6.

[34] Lehmann JM, McKee DD, Watson MA, et al. The human orphan nuclear receptor PXR is activated by compounds that regulate CYP3A4 gene expression and cause drug interactions. J Clin Invest 1998;102:1016–23.

[35] Honkakoski P, Sueyoshi T, Negishi M. Drug-activated nuclear receptors CAR and PXR. Ann Med 2003;35:172–82.

[36] Jana S, Paliwal J. Molecular mechanisms of cytochrome P450 induction: Potential for drug–drug interactions. Curr Protein Pept Sci 2007;8:619–28.

[37] Lieber CS. Cytochrome P-4502E1: Its physiological and pathological role. Physiol Rev 1997;77:517–44.

[38] Handschin C, Meyer UA. Induction of drug metabolism: The role of nuclear receptors. Pharmacol Rev 2003;55:649–73.

[39] Christians U. Transport proteins and intestinal metabolism: P-glycoprotein and cytochrome P4503A. Ther Drug Monit 2004;26:104–6.

[40] Zhou SF. Structure, function and regulation of P-glycoprotein and its clinical relevance in drug disposition. Xenobiotica 2008;38:802–32.

[41] Stejskalova L, Dvorak Z, Pavek P. Endogenous and exogenous ligands of aryl hydrocarbon receptor: Current state of art. Curr Drug Metab 2011;12:198–212.

[42] Rhodes SP, Otten JN, Hingorani GP, et al. Simultaneous assessment of cytochrome P450 activity in cultured human hepatocytes for compound-mediated induction of CYP3A4, CYP2B6, and CYP1A2. J Pharmacol Toxicol Methods 2011;63:223–6.

[43] Foisy MM, Yakiwchuk EM, Hughes CA. Induction effects of ritonavir: Implications for drug interactions. Ann Pharmacother 2008;42:1048–59.

[44] The International Transport Consortium. Membrane transporters in drug development. Nat Rev Drug Discov 2010;9:215–36.

[45] Schinkel AH, Jonker JW. Mammalian drug efflux transporters of the ATP binding cassette (ABC) family: An overview. Adv Drug Deliv Rev 2003;55:3–29.

[46] Lin JH. Drug–drug interaction mediated by inhibition and induction of P-glycoprotein. Adv Drug Deliv Rev 2003;55:53–81.

[47] Lin JH, Yamazaki M. Role of P-glycoprotein in pharmacokinetics: Clinical implications. Clin Pharmacokinet 2003;42:59–98.

[48] Ayrton A, Morgan P. Role of transport proteins in drug absorption, distribution and excretion. Xenobiotica 2001;31:469–97.

[49] Matheny CJ, Lamb MW, Brouwer KR, Pollack GM. Pharmacokinetic and pharmacodynamic implications of P-glycoprotein modulation. Pharmacotherapy 2001;21:778–96.

[50] Marzolini C, Battegay M, Back D. Mechanisms of drug interactions 2: Transport proteins. In: Piscitelli SC, Rodvold KA, Pai MP, editors. Drug interactions in infectious diseases. 3rd ed. New York, NY: Humana Press; 2011. p. 43–63.

[51] Rengelshausen J, Goggelmann C, Burhenne J, et al. Contribution of increased oral bioavailability and reduced nonglomerular renal clearance of digoxin to the digoxin–clarithromycin interaction. Br J Clin Pharmacol 2003;56:32–8.

[52] Shapiro AB, Ling V. Positively cooperative sites for drug transport by P-glycoprotein with distinct drug specificities. Eur J Biochem 1997;250:130–7.

[53] Yasuda K, Lan LB, Sanglard D, et al. Interaction of cytochrome P450 3A inhibitors with P-glycoprotein. J Pharmacol Exp Ther 2002;303:323–32.

[54] Mordel A, Halkin H, Zulty L, et al. Quinidine enhances digitalis toxicity at therapeutic serum digoxin levels. Clin Pharmacol Ther 1993;53:457–62.

[55] Verschraagen M, Koks CHW, Schellens JHM, et al. P-glycoprotein system as a determinant of drug interactions: The case of digoxin-verapamil. Pharmacol Res 1999;40:301–6.

[56] Sadeque AJ, Wandel C, He H, Shah S, Wood AJ. Increased drug delivery to the brain by P-glycoprotein inhibition. Clin Pharmacol Ther 2000;68:231–7.

[57] Fardel O, Lecureur V, Guillouzo A. Regulation by dexamethasone of P-glycoprotein expression in cultured rat hepatocytes. FEBS Lett 1993;327:189–93.

[58] Liu J, Brunner LJ. Chronic cyclosporine administration induces renal P-glycoprotein in rats. Eur J Pharmacol 2001;418:127–32.

[59] Patel J, Mitra AK. Strategies to overcome simultaneous P-glycoprotein mediated efflux and CYP3A4 mediated metabolism of drugs. Pharmacogenomics 2001;2:401–15.

[60] Wacher VJ, Wu C-Y, Benet LZ. Overlapping substrate specificities and tissue distribution of cytochrome P450 3A and P-glycoprotein: Implications for drug delivery and activity in cancer chemotherapy. Mol Carcinog 1995;13:129–34.

[61] Synold TW, Dussault I, Forman BM. The orphan nuclear receptor SXR coordinately regulates drug metabolism and efflux. Nature Med 2001;7:584–90.

[62] Geik A, Eichelbaum M, Burk O. Nuclear receptor response elements mediate induction of intestinal MDR1 by rifampin. J Biol Chem 2001;276:14581–7.

[63] Hunter J, Jepson MA, Tsuruo T, et al. Simmons NL, Hirst BH. Functional expression of P-glycoprotein in apical membranes of human intestinal Caco-2 cell layers: Kinetics of vinblastine secretion and interaction with modulators. J Biol Chem 1993;268:14991–7.

[64] Hunter J, Hirst BH, Simmons NL. Drug absorption limited by P-glycoprotein-mediated secretory drug transport in human intestinal epithelial Caco-2 cells. Pharm Res 1993;10:743–9.

[65] Kim RB, Fromm MF, Wandel C, et al. The drug transporter P-glycoprotein limits oral absorption and brain entry of HIV-1 protease inhibitors. J Clin Invest 1998;101:289–94.

[66] Gutmann H, Fricker G, Drewe J, et al. Interactions of HIV protease inhibitors with ATP-dependent drug export proteins. Mol Pharmacol 1999;56:383–9.

[67] Drewe J, Gutmann H, Fricker G, et al. HIV Protease inhibitor ritonavir: A more potent inhibitor of P-glycoprotein than the cyclosporine analogue SDZ PSC 833. Biochem Pharmacol 1999;57:1147–52.

[68] Choo EF, Leake B, Wandel C, et al. Pharmacological inhibition of P-glycoprotein transport enhances the distribution of HIV-1 protease inhibitors into brain and testes. Drug Metab Disposit 2000;28:655–60.

[69] Alsenz J, Steffen H, Alex R. Active apical secretory efflux of HIV protease inhibitors saquinavir and ritonavir in Caco-2 cells. Pharm Res 1998;15:423–8.

[70] Lee CGL, Gottesman MM. HIV protease inhibitors and the MDR1 multidrug transporter. J Clin Invest 1998;101:287–8.

[71] Greiner B, Eichelbaum M, Fritz P, et al. The role of intestinal P-glycoprotein in the interaction of digoxin and rifampin. J Clin Invest 1999;104:147–53.

[72] Mayer U, Wagenaar E, Beijnen JH, et al. Substantial excretion of digoxin via the intestinal mucosa and prevention of long-term digoxin accumulation in the brain by the mdr 1a P-glycoprotein. Br J Pharmacol 1996;119:1038–44.

[73] Ma JD, Tsunoda SM, Bertino Jr JS, et al. Evaluation of in vivo P-glycoprotein phenotyping probes. Clin Pharmacokinet 2010;49:223–37.

[74] Hamman MA, Bruce MA, Haehner-Daniels BD, et al. The effect of rifampin administration on the disposition of fexofenadine. Clin Pharmacol Ther 2001;69:114–21.

[75] Milne RW, Larsen LA, Jorgensen KL, et al. Hepatic disposition of fexofenadine: Influence of the transport inhibitors erythromycin and dibromosulphothalein. Pharm Res 2000;17:1511–5.

[76] Susanto M, Benet LZ. Can the enhanced renal clearance of antibiotics in cystic fibrosis patients be explained by P-glycoprotein transport? Pharm Res 2002;19:457–62.

[77] Fanos V, Cataldi L. Renal transport of antibiotics and nephrotoxicity: A review. J Chemother 2001;13:461–72.

[78] Neuvonen PJ, Niemi M, Backman JT. Drug interactions with lipid-lowering drugs: Mechanisms and clinical relevance. Clin Pharmacol Ther 2006;80:565–81.

[79] Hedman M, Neuvonen PJ, Neuvonen M, et al. Pharmacokinetics and pharmacodynamics of pravastatin in pediatric and adolescent cardiac transplant recipients on a regimen of triple immunosuppression. Clin Pharmacol Ther 2004;75:101–9.

[80] Simonson SG, Raza A, Martin PD, et al. Rosuvastatin pharmacokinetics in heart transplant recipients administered an antirejection regimen including cyclosporine. Clin Pharmacol Ther 2004;76:167–77.

[81] Livalo®, pitavastatin [package insert]. Montgomery, AL: Kowa Pharmaceuticals America, Inc. (package insert revised 8/2011).

[82] Tracleer®, bosentan [package insert]. South San Francisco, CA: Actelion Pharmaceuticals US, Inc. (package insert revised 2/2011).

[83] Kiser JJ, Gerber JG, Predhomme JA, et al. Drug interaction between lopinavir/ritonavir and rosuvastatin in healthy volunteers. J Acquir Immune Defic Syndr 2008;47:570–8.

[84] Dresser GK, Bailey DG, Leake BF, et al. Fruit juices inhibit organic anion transporting polypeptide-mediated drug uptake to decrease the oral availability of fexofenadine. Clin Pharmacol Ther 2002;71:11–20.

[85] Van Cleef GF, Fisher EJ, Polk RE. Drug interaction potential with inhibitors of HIV protease. Pharmacotherapy 1997;42:1553–6.

[86] Matsushima S, Maeda K, Inoue K, et al. The inhibition of human multidrug and toxin extrusion 1 is involved in the drug–drug interaction caused by cimetidine. Drug Metab Dispos 2009;37:555–9.

[87] Ohta KY, Imamura Y, Okudaira N, et al. Functional characterization of multidrug and toxin extrusion protein 1 as a facilitative transporter for fluoroquinolones. J Pharmacol Exp Ther 2009;328:628–34.

[88] Feng B, Obach RS, Burstein AH, et al. Effect of human renal cationic transporter inhibition on the pharmacokinetics of varenicline, a new therapy for smoking cessation: An in vitro–in vivo study. Clin Pharmacol Ther 2008;83:567–76.

[89] Khamdang S, Takeda M, Babu E, et al. Interaction of human and rat organic anion transporter 2 with various cephalosporin antibiotics. Eur J Pharmacol 2003;465:1–7.

[90] Inui K, Masuda S, Saito H. Cellular and molecular aspects of drug transport in the kidney. Kidney Intl 2000;58:944–58.

[91] Cundy KC. Clinical pharmacokinetics of the antiviral nucleotide analogues cidofovir and adefovir. Clin Pharmacokinet 1999;36:127–43.

[92] Takeda M, Khamdang S, Narikawa S, et al. Human organic anion transporters and human organic cation transporters mediate renal antiviral transport. J Pharmacol Exp Ther 2002;300:918–24.

[93] Enomoto A, Takeda M, Shimoda M, et al. Interaction of human organic anion transporters 2 and 4 with organic anion transport inhibitors. J Pharmacol Exp Ther 2002;301:797–802.

[94] Miyazaki H, Sekine T, Endou H. The multispecific organic anion transporter family: Properties and pharmacological significance. Trends Pharmacol Sci 2004;25:654–62.

[95] Khamdang S, Takeda M, Shimoda M, et al. Interactions of human- and rat-organic anion transporters with pravastatin and cimetidine. J Pharmacol Sci 2004;94:197–202.

[96] Uwai Y, Saito H, Hashimoto Y, Inui KI. Interaction and transport of thiazide diuretics, loop diuretics, and acetazolamide via rat renal organic anion transporter rOAT1. J Pharmacol Exp Ther 2000;295:261–5.

[97] Mulato AS, Ho ES, Cihlar T. Nonsteroidal anti-inflammatory drugs efficiently reduce the transport and cytotoxicity of adefovir mediated by the human renal organic anion transportor 1. J Pharmacol Exp Ther 2000;295:10–5.

[98] Shitara Y, Sato H, Sugiyama Y. Evaluation of drug–drug interaction in the hepatobiliary and renal transport of drugs. Annu Rev Pharmacol Toxicol 2005;45:689–723.

[99] Lacy SA, Hitchcock MJM, Lee WA, et al. Effect of oral probenecid coadministration on the chronic toxicity and pharmacokinetics of intravenous cidofovir in cynomolgus monkeys. Toxicol Sci 1998;44:97–106.

[100] Wang Y, Wei Y, Sawchuk RJ. Zidovudine transport within the rabbit brain during intracerebroventricular administration and the effect of probenecid. J Pharm Sci 1997;86:1484–90.

[101] Bart J, Groen HJN, Hendrikse NH, et al. The blood–brain barrier and oncology: New insights into function and modulation. Cancer Treat Rev 2000;26:449–62.

[102] Sugawara I, Kataoka Y, Morishita Y, et al. Tissue distribution of P-glycoprotein encoded by a multidrug-resistant gene as revealed by a monoclonal antibody MRK16. Cancer Res 1988;48:1926–9.

[103] Huai-Yun H, Secrest DT, Mark KS, et al. Expression of multidrug resistance-associated protein (MRP) in brain microvessel endothelial cells. Biochem Biophys Res Commun 1998;243:816–20.

[104] Evers R, Zaman GJ, van Deemter L, et al. Basolateral localization and export activity of the human multidrug resistance-associated protein in polarized pig kidney cells. J Clin Invest 1996;97:1211–8.

[105] Ayrton A, Morgan P. Role of transport proteins in drug absorption, distribution and excretion. Xenobiotica 2001;31:469–97.

[106] Bart J, van der Graff WT, Hollema H, et al. An oncological view of the blood–testes barrier. Lancet Oncol 2002;3:357–63.

[107] Wijnholds J, Scheffer GL, van der Valk M, et al. Multidrug resistance protein 1 protects the oropharyngeal mucosal layer and the testicular tubules against drug-induced damage. J Exp Med 1998;188:797–808.

[108] Shu-Feng Z, Wang Lin-Lin, Di YM, et al. Substrates and inhibitors of human multidrug resistance associated proteins and the implications in drug development. Curr Med Chem 2008;15:1981–2039.

[109] Jones K, Hoggard PG, Sales SD, et al. Differences in the intracellular accumulation of HIV protease inhibitors in vitro and the effect of active transport. AIDS 2001;15:675–81.

[110] Jones K, Bray PG, Khoo SH, et al. P-glycoprotein and transporter MRP1 reduce HIV protease inhibitor uptake in CD4 cells: Potential for accelerated viral drug resistance? AIDS 2001;15:1353–8.

[111] van der Sandt IC, Vos CM, Nabulsi L, et al. Assessment of active transport of HIV protease inhibitors in various cell lines and the in vitro blood–brain barrier. AIDS 2001;15:483–91.

[112] Bierman WF, Scheffer GL, Schoonderwoerd A, et al. Protease inhibitors atazanavir, lopinavir and ritonavir are potent blockers, but poor substrates, of ABC transporters in a broad panel of ABC transporter-overexpressing cell lines. J Antimicrob Chemother 2010;65:1672–80.

[113] Leite DF, Echevarria-Lima J, Calixto JB, Rumjanek VM. Multidrug resistance related protein (ABCC1) and its role on nitrite production by the murine macrophage cell line RAW 264.7. Biochem Pharmacol 2007;73:665–74.

[114] Magnarin M, Morelli M, Rosati A, et al. Induction of proteins involved in multidrug resistance (P-glycoprotein, MRP1, MRP2, LRP) and of CYP 3A4 by rifampicin in LLC-PK1 cells. Eur J Pharmacol 2004;483:19–28.

[115] Tatebe S, Sinicrope FA, Kuo MT. Induction of multidrug resistance proteins MRP1 and MRP3 and gamma-glutamylcysteine synthetase gene expression by nonsteroidal anti-inflammatory drugs in human colon cancer cells. Biochem Biophys Res Commun 2002;290:1427–33.

[116] Lucia MB, Rutella S, Golotta C, et al. Differential induction of P-glycoprotein and MRP by rifamycins in T lymphocytes from HIV-1/tuberculosis co-infected patients. AIDS 2002;16:1563–5.

[117] Kruh GD, Belinsky MG. The MRP family of drug efflux pumps. Oncogene 2003;22:7537–52.

[118] Miller DS. Nucleoside phosphonate interactions with multiple organic anion transporters in renal proximal tubule. J Pharmacol Exp Ther 2001;299:567–74.

[119] Rollot F, Nazal E-M, Chauvelot-Moachon L, et al. Tenofovir-related Fanconi Syndrome with nephrogeneic diabetes insipidus in a patient with acquired immunodeficiency syndrome: The role of lopinavir–ritonavir–didanosine. Clin Infect Dis 2003;37:e174–6.

[120] Lalezari JP, Stagg RJ, Kupperman BD, et al. Intravenous cidofovir for peripheral cytomegalovirus retinitis in patients with AIDS: A randomized controlled trial. Ann Intern Med 1997;126:257–63.

[121] Kahn J, Lagakos S, Wulfsohn M, et al. Efficacy and safety of adefovir dipivoxil with antiretroviral therapy: A randomized controlled trial. JAMA 1999;I:2305–12.

[122] Cundy KC, Petty BG, Flaherty J, et al. Clinical pharmacokinetics of cidofovir in human immunodeficiency virus-infected patients. Antimicrob Agents Chemother 1995;39:1247–52.

[123] Kool M, de Haas GL, Scheffer RJ, et al. Analysis of expression of cMOAT (MRP2), MRP3, MRP4, and MRP5, homologs of the multidrug resistance-associated resistance protein (MRP1), in human cancer cell lines. Cancer Res 1997;57:3537–47.

[124] Lee K, Belinsky MG, Bell DW, et al. Isolation of MOAT-B, a widely expressed multidrug resistance-associated protein/canalicular multispecific organic anion transporter-related transporter. Cancer Res 1998;58:2741–7.

[125] Schuetz JD, Connelly MC, Sun D, et al. MRP4: A previously unidentified factor in resistance to nucleoside-based antiviral drugs. Nature Med 1999;5:1048–51.

[126] Reid G, Wielinga P, Zelcer N, et al. Characterization of the transport of nucleoside analog drugs by the human multidrug resistance proteins MRP4 and MRP5. Mol Pharmacol 2003;63:1094–103.

[127] Fridland A. Effect of multidrug-resistance associated protein 4 on antiviral nucleotide analogs. 8th Conference on Retroviruses and Opportunistic Infections; February 5–8, 2001. Chicago, IL, abstract S2.

[128] Kruijtzer CM, Beijnen JH, Rosing H, et al. Increased oral bioavailability of topotecan in combination with the breast cancer resistance protein and P-glycoprotein inhibitor GF120918. J Clin Oncol 2002;20:2943–50.

[129] Proudfoot AT, Krenzelok EP, Vale JA. Position paper on urine alkalinization. J Toxicol Clin Toxicol 2004;42:1–26.

[130] Hansten PD, Hayton WL. Effect of antacid and ascorbic acid on serum salicylate concentrations. J Clin Pharmacol 1980;20.236–31.

[131] Baranczewski P, Stańczak A, Sundberg K, et al. Introduction to in vitro estimation of metabolic stability and drug interactions of new chemical entities in drug discovery and development. Pharmacol Rep 2006;58:453–72.

[132] Zhao P, Zhang L, Grillo JA, et al. Applications of physiologically based pharmacokinetic (PBPK) modeling and simulation during regulatory review. Clin Pharmacol Ther 2011;89:259–67.

[133] Tucker G, Houston JB, Huang S-M. Optimizing drug development: Strategies to assess drug metabolism/transporter interaction potential – toward a consensus. Clin Pharmacol Ther 2001;70:103–14.

[134] Bjornsson TD, Callaghan JT, Einolf HJ, et al. The conduct of in vitro and in vivo drug–drug interaction studies, a PhRMA perspective. J Clin Pharmacol 2003;43:443–69.

[135] Huang S-M, Temple R, Throckmorton DC, Lesko L. Drug–drug interactions: Study design, data analysis and implications for dosing recommendations. Clin Pharmacol Ther 2007;81:298–304.

[136] Zhang L, Reynolds K, Zhao P, Huang S-M. Drug interactions evaluation: An integrated part of risk assessment of therapeutics. Toxicol Appl Pharmacol 2010;243:134–45.

[137] Fahmi OA, Hurst S, Plowchalk D, et al. Comparison of different algorithms for predicting clinical drug–drug interactions, based on the use of CYP3A4 in vitro data: Predictions of compounds as precipitants of interaction. Drug Metab Dispos 2009;3:1658–66.

[138] Lee JI, Zhang L, Men AY, et al. CYP-mediated drug-therapeutic protein interactions: Clinical findings, proposed mechanisms and regulatory implications. Clin Pharmacokinet 2010;49:295–310.

[139] Morgan ET, Goralski KB, Piquette-Miller M, et al. Regulation of drug-metabolizing enzymes and transporters in

infection, inflammation and cancer. Drug Metab Dispos 2008;36:205–16.

[140] Kwara A, Lartey M, Sagoe KW, et al. Pharmacokinetics of efavirenz when co-administered with rifampin in TB/HIV co-infected patients: Pharmacogenetics effect of CYP2B6 variation. J Clin Pharmacol 2008;48:1032–40.

[141] Ma TKW, Yat-Yin L, Tan VP, et al. Impact of genetic and acquired alteration in cytochrome P450 system on pharmacologic and clinical response to clopidogrel. Pharmacol Ther 2010;125:249–59.

[142] Effient®, prasugrel [package insert]. Indianapolis, IN: Eli Lilly and Co. (package insert revised 9/2011).

[143] Sprycel®, dasatinib [package insert]. Princeton, NJ: Bristol-Myers Squibb Co. (package insert revised 10/2011).

[144] Xarelto®, rivaroxaban [package insert]. Ttusville, NJ: Janssen Pharmaceuticals, Inc. (package insert approved 7/2011).

[145] Grillo JA, Zhao P, Bullock J, Choi Y-M, Booth BP, Lu M, Robie-Suh K, Gil Berglund E, Pang KS, Rahman NA, Zhang L, Lesko LJ, Huang S-M. Utility of a physiologically-based pharmacokinetic (PBPK) modeling approach to quantitatively predict a complex drug-drug-disease interaction scenario with rivaroxaban during the drug review process: implications for clinical practice. Biopharm Drug Disp 2012;33:99–110.

[146] Huang S-M, Rowland M. The Role of Physiologically-Based Pharmacokinetic Modeling in Regulatory Review. Clin Pharmacol Ther 2012 March;91:542–9.

# 16

# Biochemical Mechanisms of Drug Toxicity

Arthur J. Atkinson, Jr.[1] and Sanford P. Markey[2]

[1]*Department of Molecular Pharmacology & Biochemistry, Feinberg School of Medicine, Northwestern University, Chicago, IL 60611*
[2]*Laboratory of Neurotoxicology, National Institute of Mental Health, National Institutes of Health, Bethesda, MD 20892*

## INTRODUCTION

Several attempts have been made to classify different types of adverse drug reactions, and different classifications actually may be appropriate for different purposes. In the classification proposed by Rawlins and Thomas [1], Type A reactions consist of augmented but qualitatively normal pharmacological responses, whereas Type B reactions are those that are qualitatively bizarre. Some Type B reactions represent drug allergy or hypersensitivity, and others were initially labeled idiosyncratic. However, progressively fewer adverse drug reactions are still regarded as simply idiosyncratic as more is learned about their mechanistic basis. In this regard, considerable recent progress has been made in extending our understanding of the causal role that pharmacogenomics plays in adverse drug reactions, and this will be the focus of Chapter 17.

Approximately 70–80% of the adverse drug reactions that occur in clinical practice can be classified as Type A [2]. This category consists of reactions that generally are mediated through pharmacologic receptors and have a pharmacokinetic basis with an obvious dose–response relationship. Hepatotoxic reactions to acetaminophen also have been assigned to this category. However, this and a number of other adverse reactions are mediated by chemically reactive cytotoxic metabolites and deserve separate consideration from a mechanistic standpoint. Allergic or hypersensitivity reactions comprise an additional 6–10% of the adverse drug reactions that are encountered clinically [3], and most of them also entail initial covalent binding of a chemically reactive drug metabolite to an endogenous macromolecule.

This chapter will focus on some representative adverse drug reactions that reflect the chemical reactivity of drugs and metabolites rather than their binding to specific pharmacologic receptors. Although these reactions are commonly thought of as not being dose related, they occur in many cases only after the dose-dependent formation of chemically reactive compounds exceeds a critical threshold that overcomes host detoxification and repair mechanisms. Therefore, it may be possible to minimize the severity or even occurrence of these reactions by prescribing the lowest therapeutically effective drug dose or by co-administering an agent that blocks reactive metabolite formation or bolsters endogenous detoxification mechanisms.

### Drug-Induced Methemoglobinemia

Drug-induced methemoglobinemia is an adverse reaction that has been studied for over 60 years and serves as a paradigm for our understanding of the biochemical mechanism underlying a number of toxic reactions to drugs. Pioneering investigations by Brodie and Axelrod [4] on the metabolism of acetanilide demonstrated that methemoglobin levels following administration of this drug paralleled plasma levels of aniline, suggesting that phenylhydroxylamine was involved in methemoglobin formation (Figure 16.1). These investigators also found that when another metabolite of acetanilide, 4-hydroxyacetanilide, was administered to humans it had analgesic activity that

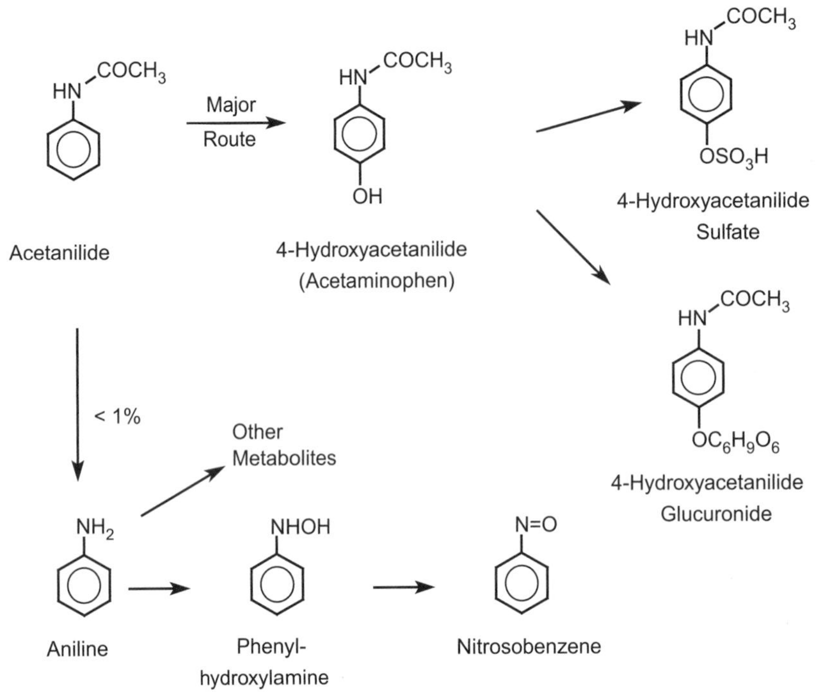

**FIGURE 16.1** Metabolism of acetanilide. The major route of metabolism is via hydroxylation to form 4-hydroxyacetanilide (acetaminophen). Less than 1% is deacetylated to form aniline.

was equal to that of acetanilide, yet did not cause an increase in methemoglobin levels. These findings provided the impetus for the subsequent introduction of this metabolite as the analgesic drug acetaminophen.

In fact, methemoglobin is being formed constantly in normal erythrocytes. In the process of binding oxygen, oxyhemoglobin is converted to a superoxoferriheme ($Fe^{+++}O_2^{\cdot -}$) complex [5, 6]. Although tissue release of oxygen restores heme iron to its ferrous state, some oxygen is dissociated from hemoglobin as superoxide ($O_2^{\cdot -}$), resulting in oxidation of hemoglobin to ferric methemoglobin. The spontaneous formation of methemoglobin is counteracted by the enzymatic reduction of heme iron to the ferrous form so that less than 1% of total hemoglobin normally is present as methemoglobin. However, higher levels of methemoglobinemia are present in individuals with hemoglobin M or other genetically rare hemoglobins that are highly vulnerable to low levels of oxidizing agents. Another rare cause of methemoglobinemia results from a deficiency in NADH-dependent cytochrome $b_5$ methemoglobin reductase (NADH-diaphorase) that normally reduces ferric to ferrous heme.

Drugs and other xenobiotics that cause methemoglobinemia react either stoichiometrically or in a cyclic fashion to convert heme iron from the ferrous to the ferric state. A partial list of these compounds is provided in Table 16.1. Nitrites are representative of stoichiometrically acting compounds. An account of an outbreak of methemoglobinemia that occurred in a cafeteria, where staff had inadvertently placed sodium nitrite in a batch of oatmeal and in a salt shaker, was popularized several years ago in a story entitled *Eleven Blue Men* [7]. Abuse of amyl, butyl and isobutyl nitrates continues to result in a number of fatal episodes of methemoglobinemia [5]. On the other hand, most drugs that cause methemoglobinemia form metabolites that interact in a cyclic fashion to convert hemoglobin to methemoglobin, as shown for

**TABLE 16.1    Partial List of Compounds Producing Methemoglobinemia**

| Stoichimetrically acting | Presumed cyclical mechanism |
| --- | --- |
| Sodium nitrite | Aniline |
| Amyl nitrite | Nitrobenzene |
| Butyl nitrite | Acetanilide |
| Isobutyl nitrite | Phenacetin |
| Nitric oxide | Sulfanilamide |
| Silver nitrate | Sulphamethoxazole |
| | Dapsone |
| | Primaquine |
| | Benzocaine |
| | Prilocaine |
| | Metoclopramide |

Data from Coleman MD, Coleman NA. Drug Saf 1996;14: 394–405 [5].

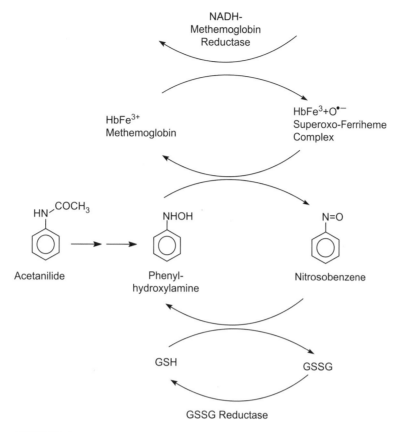

**FIGURE 16.2** Cyclic mechanism by which a single molecule of phenyl-hdroxylamine is able to oxidize several hemoglobin molecules to methemoglobin, thereby overcoming the reductive capacity of NADH-methemoglobin reductase (NADH-diaphorase). Glutathione (GSH) maintains the cycle by reducing nitro-sobenzene back to phenylhdroxylamine, and is itself regenerated from the GSSG dimer by the action of GSSG reductase (also called glutathione reductase).

acetanilide in Figure 16.2. Because less than 1% of an administered acetanilide dose is metabolized to aniline, relatively little methemoglobin would be formed were it not for the fact that phenylhydroxyl-amine is regenerated from nitrosobenzene by the reducing action of cellular glutathione (GSH) [6]. The drugs listed in the right-hand column of Table 16.1 also are presumably converted to hydroxylamine metabo-lites by N-oxidation, as described in Chapter 11. It is not clear why some people are more prone to develop methemoglobinemia than are others. However, it is known that neonates express low levels of functional NADH-diaphorase and are particularly prone to this adverse reaction when treated with methemoglobin-forming drugs [5].

The fact that many of the drugs listed in Table 16.1 incorporate aniline or aniline analogs in their struc-ture is a legacy that, for many drugs, stems from the origin of early pharmaceutical development in the German dye industry. Chloramphenicol, which actu-ally is a natural compound that incorporates

a nitrobenzene moiety (Figure 16.3), causes aplastic anemia in 1 in 20,000 to 40,000 individuals who are treated with this antibiotic [8]. The exact mechanism by which chloramphenicol causes aplastic anemia is unknown but also appears to involve the nitro group,

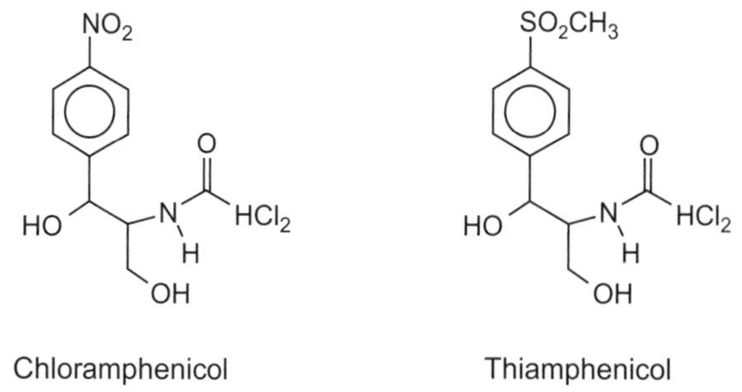

Chloramphenicol                    Thiamphenicol

**FIGURE 16.3** Chemical structures of chloramphenicol and thiamphenicol. Thiamphenicol, in which the nitro group of chlor-amphenicol is replaced by a methylsulfone group, retains antibiotic activity, but does not cause the aplastic anemia that is a major concern with chloramphenicol therapy.

since similar toxicity has not been associated with thiamphenicol, a chloramphenicol analog in which the nitro group is replaced with a methylsulfone group (Figure 16.3).

## The Role of Covalent Binding in Drug Toxicity

As emphasized in Chapter 11, drug-metabolizing enzymes can convert drugs into either inactive, non-toxic compounds or chemically reactive metabolites. With the exception of some anticancer drugs, chemicals directly toxic to tissues are eliminated in the drug development process, so drug toxicity involving covalent binding usually is mediated by chemically reactive metabolites. Although these reactive metabolites can cause toxic reactions by forming covalent linkages with a variety of macromolecules, in many cases they also can be inactivated by further metabolism and excretion, or by binding to GSH or other endogenous scavenger molecules. In these cases, there is a metabolic balance between reactive metabolite formation and elimination that may be altered by genetic factors, or perturbed by disease, environmental factors, or concomitant therapy with other drugs. When the formation of reactive metabolites exceeds a certain threshold, they bind to and inactivate macromolecules that are critical for normal cell development or survival, or form immunogenic protein adducts. In addition, the scavenging process itself can deplete intracellular GSH concentrations and result in increased intracellular oxidative stress. A general scheme for adverse reaction mechanisms of this type is shown in Figure 16.4.

Initial mechanistic understanding of these toxic reactions focused on identification of the reactive metabolite and metabolic pathway involved and the subsequent formation of protein adducts. In some cases, protective mechanisms for scavenging reactive metabolites and metabolite–target protein adducts also were identified. However, more recent investigations have focused on "downstream" events and a central common pathway has been established for some forms of drug-induced liver toxicity [9]. In these reactions, reactive metabolites are scavenged by GSH to the extent that intracellular GSH is depleted, resulting in increased oxidative stress and mitochondrial damage. Cell death by apoptosis then occurs if some mitochondria are left intact and continue to synthesize adenosine triphosphate (ATP). More extensive mitochondrial damage results in ATP depletion and leads to necrotic cell lysis, which in turn induces an inflammatory response (Figure 16.4).

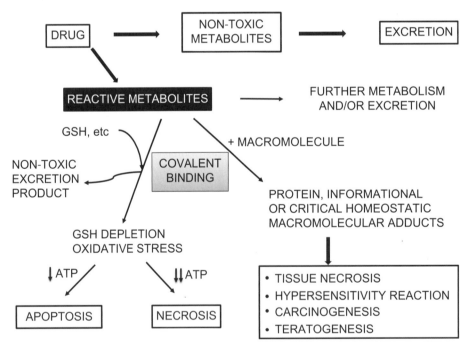

**FIGURE 16.4** General scheme for the role played by reactive drug metabolites in causing a variety of adverse reactions. The reactive metabolites usually account for only a small fraction of total drug metabolism and are too unstable to be chemically isolated and analyzed. In many cases, covalent binding of these metabolites to tissue macromolecules only occurs after their formation exceeds a critical threshold that overcomes host detoxification and repair mechanisms. GSH = glutathione, ATP = adenosine triphosphate.

These reactions are not generally thought of as dose related. However, mass action law considerations dictate that the extent of reactive metabolite formation, and hence adverse reaction risk, will also be a function of drug dosage. It also can be inferred from Figure 16.4 that part of the interindividual variability in incidence of these reactions reflects varying activity in the parallel pathways involved in metabolizing drugs to either non-toxic or reactive metabolites. In some cases, it has been possible to relate the risk of an adverse drug reaction to polymorphic drug-metabolizing phenotype.

# DRUG-INDUCED LIVER TOXICITY

Few areas have been as confusing to clinicians as the perplexing array of adverse drug reactions affecting the liver. Given the central role that the liver plays in drug metabolism, it is not surprising that many drugs are converted to compounds that cause liver damage. In fact, liver injury has been estimated to be the principal safety reason for terminating clinical trials during drug development and for withdrawing marketed drugs [10, 11]. Furthermore, there has been a marked increase in the incidence of some forms of drug-induced liver injury from marketed drugs, and a prospective survey indicated that the percentage of cases of acute liver failure caused by both intentional and unintentional acetaminophen overdose rose from 28% in 1998 to 51% in 2003 [12]. Traditional classifications of drug hepatotoxicity, such as that shown in Table 16.2, have been based on descriptions of

TABLE 16.2  **Classification of Drug-Induced Liver Toxicity**

I. Hepatocellular necrosis
  A. Zonal necrosis ($CCl_4$-type)
  $CCl_4$
  Halogenated benzenes
  Acetaminophen
  B. Viral hepatitis-like (cincophen-type)
  Isoniazid
  Iproniazid
  Halothane
II. Uncomplicated cholestasis (steroid-type)
  Anabolic steroids
  Estrogens
III. Non-specific hepatitis with cholestasis (chlorpromazine-type)
  Phenothiazines
  Isoniazid
  Erythromycin estolate
IV. Drug-induced steatosis
  Tetracycline

observed histopathology rather than on an understanding of the basic mechanism involved [13]. We will focus the discussion here on representative adverse reactions that damage the liver either through covalent binding of a reactive metabolite or through induction of oxidative stress.

## Hepatotoxic Reactions Resulting from Covalent Binding of Reactive Metabolites

A major advance in our understanding of the role of covalent binding of reactive metabolites in causing hepatotoxic drug reactions was provided by Brodie and his co-workers in 1971 [14]. These investigators administered $^{14}C$-labeled bromobenzene to rats and showed that the radioactivity was localized to centrilobular hepatocytes in the region of greatest liver damage and could not be removed from this area by washing the tissue with solvents. Binding did not occur when the bromobenzene was added directly to liver slices *in vitro*, but binding after *in vivo* administration was enhanced when rats were pretreated with phenobarbital and was reduced when they were pretreated with SKF-525A, an inhibitor of drug metabolism. The conclusion was drawn that bromobenzene was being converted to an active arene oxide metabolite that was the proximate hepatotoxin (Figure 16.5). It was subsequently shown that detoxifying enzymes and GSH played an important protective role in removing this arene oxide before it could react covalently with liver macromolecules [15].

### Acetaminophen

A pattern of liver necrosis similar to that caused by bromobenzene is observed in patients who ingest massive doses of acetaminophen (Table 16.2). This toxic reaction also has been produced experimentally in mice and rats and is thought to occur in two phases. An initial metabolic phase in which acetaminophen is converted to a reactive imminoquinone metabolite is followed by an oxidation phase in which an abrupt increase in mitochondrial permeability, termed *mitochondrial permeability transition*, results in hepatocellular necrosis [16, 17].

After therapeutic doses, acetaminophen is primarily converted to inactive glucuronide and sulfate conjugates. However, as shown in Chapter 11, Scheme 11.2, a small amount of acetaminophen is oxidized by CYP2E1, CYP1A2, CYP3A4, and CYP2D6 to *N*-acetyl-*p*-benzoquinone imine (NAPQI) [18], which is chemically reactive and is scavenged by conjugation with GSH [19]. In the setting of an acetaminophen overdose,

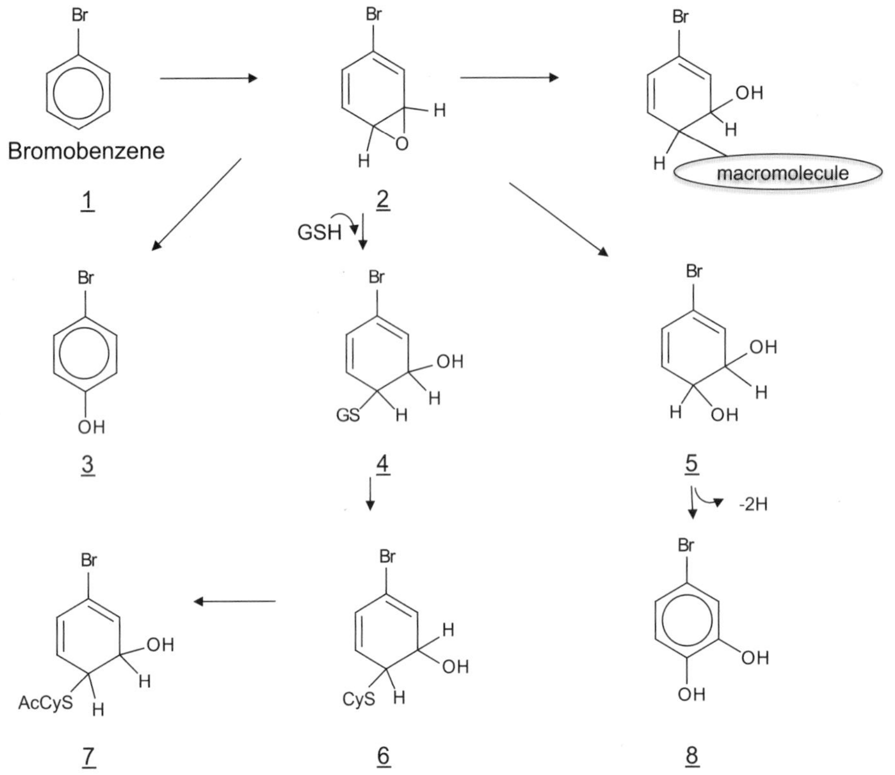

**FIGURE 16.5** Metabolism of bromobenzene (**1**) to a chemically reactive epoxide (arene oxide) metabolite (**2**) that can then either bind covalently to nearby macromolecules, be scavenged by glutathione (GSH) (**4**) and further metabolized (**6**, **7**), or be converted non-enzymatically or by epoxide hydrolase to stable hydroxylated metabolites ( **3**, **5**, **8**).

when NAPQI formation is sufficient to deplete more than 70% of hepatic GSH, excess NAPQI now binds covalently to cysteine residues on proteins [19]. The *in vitro* demonstration that exogenous sulfhydryl donors can minimize NAPQI adduct formation and hepatotoxicity [20] has provided the rationale for the clinical use of *N*-acetylcysteine to treat patients after acetaminophen overdose [21]. Conversely, induction of CYP2E1-mediated NAPQI formation by ethanol explains the increased susceptibility of alcoholic patients to acetaminophen hepatotoxicity [22].

Although there is excellent correlation between the extent of NAPQI adduct formation and the subsequent development of acetaminophen hepatotoxicity, this adduct formation does not appear to be primarily responsible for hepatocellular necrosis. In what was initially regarded as a paradox, Henderson *et al.* [23] found that knockout mice lacking glutathione *S*-transferase Pi (GSTπ) have increased resistance to acetaminophen hepatotoxicity. Even though both the wild-type and knockout mice had similar levels of adduct formation, GSH was only approximately 70% depleted in the knockout mice compared to more than

90% in the wild type mice. In addition, GSH regeneration was found to be more rapid in *GSTπ*-null than in wild-type mice. These findings served to focus attention on hepatoxic mechanisms downstream from GSH depletion rather than on direct binding of NAPQI to cellular proteins [17, 24].

In our current understanding of pathogenesis, GSH depletion leads to hepatotoxicity because it increases hepatocellular oxidative stress, mediated both by the reduction of peroxide by ferrous ions to form highly reactive hydroxyl radicals (Fenton mechanism) and by the formation of peroxynitrites from nitric oxide [17]. A critical step is the release of ferrous iron from damaged lysosomes [24]. Subsequent mitochondrial uptake of ferrous iron results in intramitochondrial formation of reactive species that oxidize critical thiols in pores of the inner mitochondrial membrane, leading to mitochondrial permeability transition and further hepatocellular oxidative stress [16, 25]. After acetaminophen overdose, mitochondrial permeability transition is generally extensive enough to cause mitochondrial ATP depletion so that, as indicated in Figure 16.4, liver cell

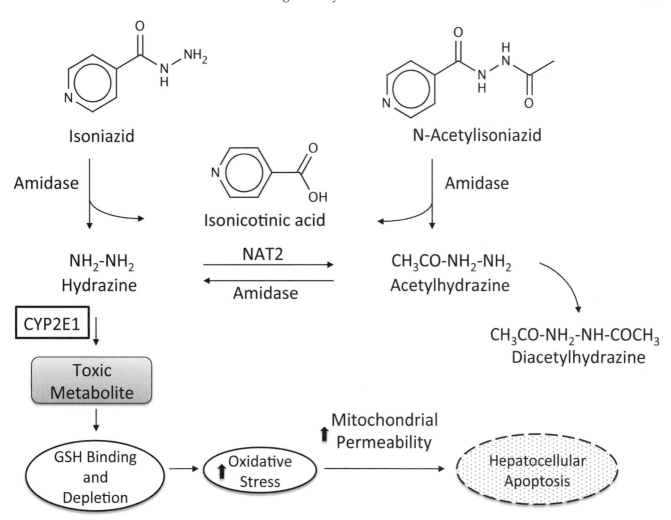

**FIGURE 16.6** Metabolism of isoniazid to hydrazine that is then activated by CYP 2E1 to a chemically reactive metabolite that depletes intracellular GSH, thereby increasing oxidative stress and resulting in mitochondrial permeability transition and hepatocellular apoptosis. N–Acetyltransferase (NAT2) acts at several points in this scheme to reduce hydrazine concentrations. This accounts for the fact that rapid acetylators are less likely than slow acetylators to develop isoniazid-induced hepatitis. On the other hand, chronic alcohol consumption induces CYP 2E1, thereby increasing the extent of toxic metabolite formation from hydrazine and the risk of hepatitis.

death occurs by necrosis and the histological picture is characterized by inflammation [17].

### Isoniazid

The widespread use of isoniazid for treating patients with either active or latent tuberculosis has focused attention on the liver injury caused by this drug. About 20% of patients treated with isoniazid will develop elevated blood concentrations of liver enzymes and bilirubin that subside as treatment is continued [26]. However, clinical hepatitis develops in some patients, and these reactions can prove fatal. Current understanding of the mechanism of isoniazid-induced hepatotoxicity is based on the metabolic

pathways shown in Figure 16.6 [27, 28]. It has been demonstrated in an animal model that hepatotoxicity is correlated with plasma concentrations of hydrazine but not of acetylhydrazine or isoniazid [29], and that pretreatment with an amidase inhibitor can prevent toxicity [28]. *In vitro* studies with hepatocytes have used spin-trapping agents to show that acetylhydrazine is further metabolized to free radical species that decreased intracellular GSH content [30], and further hepatocyte studies have implicated CYP2E1 as the cytochrome P450 isoform responsible for cytotoxic metabolite formation [31]. More recently, Chowdhury *et al.* [32] demonstrated in a mouse model that INH reduced hepatocellular GSH content and thereby resulted in mitochondrial permeability transition with subsequent apoptotic cell death. Direct administration of hydrazine was an even more effective toxicant than INH, and the hepatotoxic effects of INH were enhanced by co-administation of rifampin. However, *in vitro* studies have shown that passive hepatocellular death by necrosis appears to be prominent in some cell lines [33].

A number of features of isoniazid hepatotoxicity can be interpreted by reference to the metabolic scheme shown in Figure 16.6. First, phenotypic slow acetylators are more prone to liver damage than rapid acetylators (Table 16.3) [34]. Not only were hydrazine plasma concentrations higher in slow acetylators than in rapid acetylators treated with isoniazid for 14 days [35], but, in another study, urine excretion of hydrazine was higher in slow than in rapid acetylators, whereas urine excretion of acetylhydrazine and diacetylhydrazine was lower [36]. A study utilizing *NAT2* genotyping confirmed that individuals with slow-acetylator genotypes have a significantly higher risk of developing antituberculosis drug-induced hepatitis than rapid acetylators (OR: 2.87 vs 0.35), and further demonstrated that slow acetylators are more likely to develop severe hepatic injury than are rapid acetylators [37]. Second, it has been shown that patients with wild-type CYP2E1 (CYP2E1 c1/c1) have a higher rate of antituberculosis drug-induced hepatitis than those whose enzyme incorporates the variant c2 allele [38]. Although there was no difference in the basal activity of the CYP2E1 genotypes, isoniazid inhibited CYP2E1 c1/c1 to a lesser extent than enzymes containing the variant allele. Thus, individuals with wild-type CYP2E1 would be expected to have an increased formation rate of the postulated reactive hepatotoxic metabolite. Induction of CYP2E1 by ethyl alcohol also appears to account for the increased incidence of liver damage in alcoholic patients who are treated with isoniazid. In fact, the protective benefit of the rapid acetylator phenotype is no longer apparent in this group of patients [34]. The increased susceptibility of elderly patients to INH hepatotoxicity [39] can also be attributed to the

**TABLE 16.3   Age and Acetylator Phenotype Affect Risk of Isoniazid-Induced Hepatitis[a]**

| Age (years) | Acetylator phenotype | |
| --- | --- | --- |
|  | Fast | Slow |
| < 35 | 3.7% | 13.0% |
| ≥ 35 | 13.2% | 37.0% |

Data from Dickinson DS, Bailey WC, Hirschowitz BI *et al.* J Clin Gastroenterol 1981;3:271–9 [34].

increase in CYP2E1 activity that begins in men at the age of 35 and in women at the age of 50 [40].

## IMMUNOLOGICALLY MEDIATED HEPATOTOXIC REACTIONS

Immune mechanisms also play a prominent role in some hepatotoxic adverse drug reactions. Traditionally, immune-mediated toxicity has been suspected on clinical grounds, such as the presence of fever, rash, an eosinophil response, a delay between exposure to the toxin and the onset of clinical symptoms, and the accelerated recurrence of symptoms and signs of toxicity after readministration of the drug [41]. Recent investigations are beginning to provide a framework for understanding the mechanism of these reactions.

Because a minimum molecular weight of 1000 Da generally is needed for a molecule to elicit an immune response, most drugs elicit immune responses by functioning as haptens. This usually entails initial formation of a chemically reactive metabolite that then binds covalently to macromolecules to form neoantigens (see Figure 16.4). The reactive metabolite may in some cases function as a direct hepatotoxin as well as an immunogen [41, 42]. The enzyme that metabolizes the drug may be among the macromolecular targets and may subsequently be inactivated by the reactive metabolite, a phenomenon referred to as *suicide inhibition*. After the neoantigens are transported to the cell membrane, they are internalized and processed by Kupffer cells for presentation to the immune system [41]. This initiates the formation of antibodies and an incompletely understood cascade of humoral and cellular immune responses that results in hepatocellular damage [43].

### Halothane

Halothane is a volatile general anesthetic that was introduced into the clinical practice of anesthesia in 1956. Shortly after its introduction, two forms of hepatic injury were noted to occur in patients who received halothane anesthesia. A subclinical increase in blood concentration of transaminase enzymes is observed in 20% of patients and has been attributed to lipid peroxidation caused by the free radical formed by reductive metabolism of halothane as shown in Figure 16.7 [44, 45]. The second form of toxicity is a potentially fatal hepatitis-like reaction that is characterized by severe hepatocellular necrosis and is thought to be initiated by the oxidative formation of trifluoroacetyl chloride (Figure 16.7). Fatal hepatic necrosis occurs in only 1 of 35,000 patients exposed to

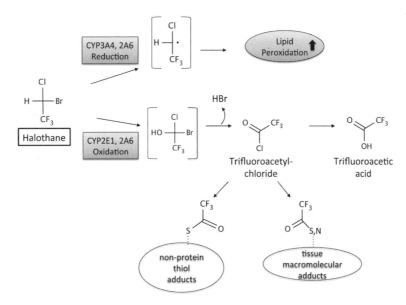

FIGURE 16.7 Oxidation of halothane by CYP2E1 leads to formation of trifluoroacetyl chloride that can be non-enzymatically converted to trifluoroacetic acid, can be scavenged by glutathione, or can bind covalently to tissue macromolecules, thereby causing liver damage. A reductive metabolic pathway generates free radicals that cause lipid peroxidation, but this pathway does not appear to be involved in the pathogenesis of halothane hepatitis.

halothane, but the risk of this adverse event is greater in females and is increased with repeat exposure, obesity, and advancing age [44]. Because the onset of halothane hepatitis is delayed but is more frequent and occurs more rapidly following multiple exposures, and because these patients usually are febrile and demonstrate eosinophilia, this reaction is suspected of having an immunologic basis. This hypothesis is strengthened by the finding that serum from patients with halothane hepatitis contains antibodies that react specifically with the cell membrane of hepatocytes harvested from halothane-anesthetized rabbits, rendering them susceptible to the cytotoxic effects of normal lymphocytes [46].

Satoh *et al.* [47] have further elucidated the mechanism of halothane hepatitis by demonstrating that the reactive acyl chloride metabolite shown in Figure 16.7 binds covalently to the surface membranes of hepatocytes of rats injected with halothane. Among the macromolecular targets of this metabolite is CYP2E1. This is the cytochrome P450 isoform that predominates in forming trifluoroacetyl chloride from halothane, and 45% of patients with halothane hepatitis form autoantibodies against CYP2E1 as well as antibodies against neoantigens formed by this reaction [48]. A number of other macromolecular targets are located in the endoplasmic reticulum where they appear to act as chaperones involved in protein folding [49]. At present, it is not certain that these

antibodies play a pathogenetic role in halothane hepatitis, and it is possible that cell-mediated immune mechanisms might be of greater importance. In that regard, Furst *et al.* [50] have demonstrated in a guinea pig model of halothane hepatitis that Kupffer cells are involved as antigen-presenting cells in initiating a cellular immune response that could account for the observed hepatotoxicity.

It is not clear why so few patients who receive halothane anesthesia are prone to develop hepatitis. Eliasson *et al.* [51] propose that patient risk reflects alterations in the balance between the activity of CYP2E1, which they found to vary by 30-fold in human liver samples, and the protective ability of GSH and other non-protein thiols to scavenge trifluoroacetyl chloride (Figure 16.7). This might explain the increased risk of halothane hepatitis in obese and elderly subjects, who have elevated activities of CYP2E1 [22]. In this regard, Kharasch *et al.* [52] have found that patients treated before halothane anesthesia with disulfiram, a specific CYP2E1 inhibitor, formed less trifluoroacetic acid than those who received no pre-treatment. These investigators demonstrated in subsequent animal studies that disulfiram pre-treatment also reduced formation of trifluoroacetylated protein adducts, lending support to their proposal that a single pre-anesthetic dose of disulfiram might block formation of the neoantigens responsible for immune sensitization and thereby provide effective prophylaxis against halothane hepatitis [45].

## Tienilic Acid

Tienilic acid (ticrynafen) is a uricosuric diuretic that was initially marketed in the United States in 1979. It was withdrawn a few months later because of hepatitis-like adverse reactions which developed in approximately 1 of 1000 patients treated with the drug but were fatal in 10% of the patients who developed overt jaundice [53]. The onset of overt toxicity generally occurred 1–6 months after starting therapy with tienilic acid, and fever, rash, and eosinophilia were reported in some of the patients. These findings led investigators to suspect an immunologic basis for this adverse reaction.

Tienilic acid is metabolized primarily by CYP2C9 to 5-hydroxytienilic acid via electrophilic intermediates that not only bind to and inactivate this microsomal enzyme but also bind to GSH and other intracellular macromolecules (Figure 16.8) [54, 55]. The specificity with which this electrophilic metabolite binds to CYP2C9 was demonstrated by experiments in which site-directed mutagenesis was used to replace serine in the 365th position of CYP2C9 with alanine [56]. The resultant S365A mutant retained the enzymatic ability to hydroxylate tienilic acid without being itself inactivated, strongly suggesting that the serine hydroxyl group is the nucleophilic target for the postulated electrophilic intermediate shown in Figure 16.8. Robin et al. [57] have shown in a rat model that both unaltered CYP2C11, the analog of CYP2C9 in humans, and the CYP2C11 adduct formed after tienilic acid exposure migrate from the endoplasmic reticulum to the plasma membrane by a microtubule-dependent vesicular route. However, plasma membrane expression of the adduct is more prolonged than that of CYP2C11. Despite this difference, Beaune et al. [58] found that the serum of patients with tienilic acid-induced hepatitis contained antibodies that were specifically directed to the CYP2C9 isoenzyme that metabolizes tienilic acid, as well as to the neoantigen formed by the adduct. These antibodies inhibited CYP2C9 function, and a three-site conformational epitope was subsequently identified near the active site of CYP2C9 that reacts with autoantibodies in sera from patients with tienilic acid-induced hepatitis [59].

More recent investigations using intact rat hepatocytes have demonstrated that tienilic acid bioactivation and binding to GSH is extensive enough to result in GSH depletion [55], and that hepatotoxicity was only observed in rats when tienilic acid was co-administered with a GSH synthesis inhibitor [60]. In this latter study, gene expression analysis demonstrated marked upregulation of genes involved in GSH synthesis, reflecting hepatocellular oxidative and/or electrophilic stress even when non-toxic tienilic acid doses were administered. These findings are consistent with the "danger hypothesis", which proposes that not only cell necrosis but even cellular stress can activate antigen-presenting cells and subsequent immune responses [61, 62].

## MECHANISMS OF OTHER DRUG TOXICITIES

Although little is known about the mechanism of many drug toxic reactions, it is likely that covalent binding mediates a large number of them. Small

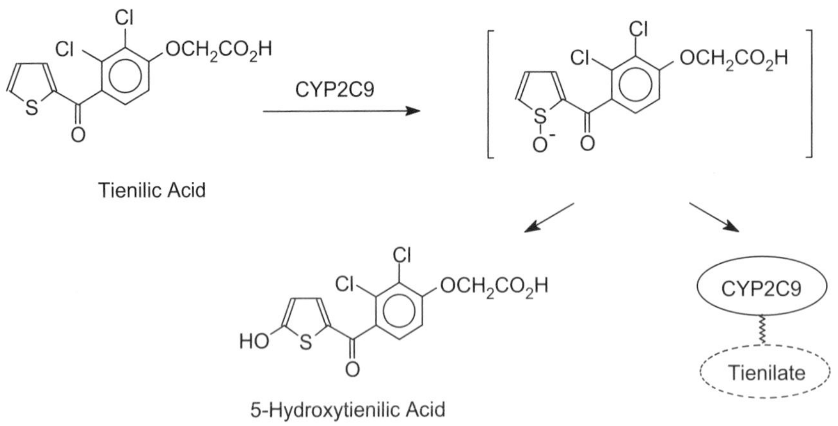

**FIGURE 16.8** Oxidation of tienilic acid by CYP2C9 to an unstable electrophilic thiophene sulfoxide that binds specifically with CYP2C9 to form a haptenic conjugate or reacts with water to form 5-hydroxytienilic acid.

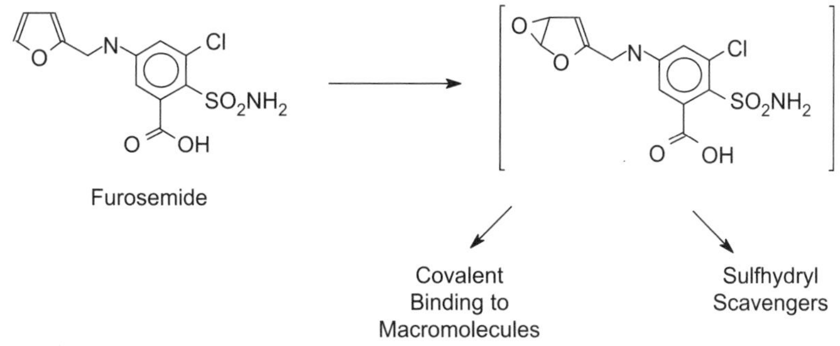

**FIGURE 16.9** Proposed metabolism of furosemide to a chemically reactive furanic epoxide.

alterations in chemical structure also may result in quite different patterns of organ involvement in drug toxic reactions. Mitchell *et al.* [63] have shown that mice treated with large doses of furosemide develop hepatocellular necrosis, presumably due to epoxidation of the furan ring (Figure 16.9). However, these investigators found that furan and several closely related furan congeners also may cause toxic reactions in the kidney and lung, as shown in Table 16.4 [64]. In some cases, the site of toxicity could be shifted from one organ to another by pretreatment with phenobarbital and other agents that alter the activity of drug-metabolizing enzymes. In each case, the presumed reactive metabolite was a furan epoxide analogous to that shown for furosemide in Figure 16.9. Similarly, *in situ* metabolism of acetaminophen by kidney microsomal enzymes occurs by the same pathways shown in Chapter 11, Scheme 11.2 and can cause acute renal tubular necrosis [65].

The skin often is involved in delayed hypersensitivity reactions, either as an isolated target or in conjunction with liver, kidney or other organ involvement. This reaction pattern was first described with anticonvulsant drugs and was initially termed anticonvulsant hypersensitivity syndrome, but as more drugs have been implicated it is now referred to as

Drug Rash with Eosinophilia and Systemic Symptoms (DRESS). A maculopapular erythematous rash is the most common cutaneous manifestation of these reactions, but potentially fatal Stevens-Johnson syndrome and toxic epidermal necrolysis may also occur [66]. Reactive drug metabolites formed by cytochrome P450 enzymes in skin keratinocytes and dendritic cells are thought to play a role in these reactions, but direct drug interactions with T-cell receptors have also been proposed [67]. Danger signals may play a contributory role in some cutaneous reactions, as exemplified by the maculopapular eruption that is estimated to occur in more than 70% of infectious mononucleosis patients who are treated with ampicillin [62, 68]. As will be discussed in Chapter 17, the report that Han Chinese patients homozygous for the *HLA-B*1502* allele are at increased risk of developing Stevens-Johnson syndrome and toxic epidermal necrolysis illustrates the important role that pharmacogenetic factors may play in these adverse reactions [69].

These observations underscore the importance of extrahepatic drug metabolism, because toxic reactions targeting organs other than the liver probably primarily reflect the formation of reactive metabolites in these tissues, rather than the peripheral effects of toxic metabolites formed in the liver. Tissue-specific differences in protective mechanisms may also underlie the organ specificity of some adverse drug reactions. Chemically reactive metabolites not only are involved in the pathogenesis of tissue or organ cytotoxic reactions but also play an important role in mediating adverse drug reactions that have been characterized traditionally as allergic or autoimmune, as well as carcinogenic and teratogenic adverse reactions.

## Systemic Reactions Resulting from Drug Allergy

The important role of immune mechanisms in mediating hepatotoxicity and other organ-specific

**TABLE 16.4 Predominant Sites of Toxicity Caused by Furan Analogs**

| Liver | Kidney | Lung |
|---|---|---|
| Furan | Furan | Ipomeanol |
| Furosemide | 2-Ethyl furan | |
| 2-Furamide | 2,3-Benzofuran | |
| 2-Acetyl furan | 2-Furoic acid | |
| 2-Furfurol | 3-Furoic acid | |
| 2-Ethyl furoate | | |
| 2-Methoxy furan | | |
| Dibenzofuran | | |

Data in mice and rats from Mitchell JR, Potter WZ, Hinson JA, Jollow DJ. Nature 1974;251:508–10 [64].

damage has been appreciated only comparatively recently. However, anaphylaxis and other systemic reactions commonly referred to as drug allergy have traditionally been attributed to covalent binding of a drug or reactive drug metabolite to a protein carrier to form multivalent hapten–carrier complexes that are immunologically competent. Exceptions to this general rule are insulin, dextran, and other macromolecules. In addition, recent studies have focused attention on the ability of radiocontrast media, sulfamethoxazole, and several other low molecular weight drugs to trigger both immediate and delayed hypersensitivity responses by binding non-covalently to the major histocompatibility complex or to T-cell receptors [70].

## Allergic Reactions to Penicillin

Allergic reactions to penicillin are a common cause of allergic drug reactions, and have been reported in various studies to occur in 0.7–8% of patients treated with this drug [71]. As shown in Table 16.5, the spectrum of allergic reactions to penicillin spans all four categories of the Gell and Coombs classification that is described in Chapter 27 [72]. Anaphylaxis is the most serious of these reactions. It occurs in about 0.01% of patients who receive penicillin, and has a fatality rate of 9% [73]. Penicillin-induced cytopenias, interstitial nephritis, and serum sickness reactions occur more frequently with prolonged high-dose therapy [74]. Contact dermatitis occurs primarily after cutaneous exposure to penicillin, but is infrequent in patients since topical penicillin formulations have been discontinued. Consequently, it occurs primarily in nurses, pharmacists, and others whose skin comes in repeated contact with the drug.

Penicillin is unusual in that it forms immunogenic hapten–carrier complexes by binding directly to macromolecules in plasma and on cell surfaces (Figure 16.10). However, even though prior metabolic activation is not required, it has been found that hapten formation is facilitated by one or more low molecular weight serum factors [71]. The penicilloyl–protein conjugate constitutes more than 90% of the haptenic products and is the major antigenic determinant for the formation of penicillin-specific immunoglobulins and T cells [75]. This antigenic determinant is involved in 75% of IgE-mediated allergic reactions and most of the other reactions shown in Table 16.5. Although the minor antigenic determinants are present only in low abundance, they play an important role in some IgE-mediated reactions. The extent of hapten formation and the probability of eliciting a penicillin-specific immune response appear to increase as a function of the cumulative penicillin dose [76]. In one study, 50% of patients who received at least 2 g of penicillin for 10 days had an IgG and/or an IgE antibody response [74].

When initial exposure to penicillin is sufficient to initiate formation of IgE antibodies, re-exposure results in anaphylaxis when the haptenic products that are formed cross-link with the previously formed IgE antibodies that are bound to mast cell FcεR1 receptors, triggering mast-cell activation and release of histamine, leukotriene, and other inflammation mediators [75, 77]. However, the presence of IgE antibodies to penicillin is a necessary but not sufficient indicator that someone is allergic to penicillin, and the activation of CD4$^+$ T cells to differentiate into Th1 and Th2 T-helper cells also plays an important role [77]. Whereas predominance of Th2 cells is associated with anaphylaxis and other immediate hypersensitivity reactions, Th1 responses are associated with delayed hypersensitivity and also appear to suppress both IgE synthesis and Th2 development [75, 78]. The likelihood that haptenic products are formed in everyone

**TABLE 16.5   Representative Immune-Mediated Reactions to Penicillin**

| Gell and Coombs type[a] | Mechanism | Clinical resentation |
|---|---|---|
| I | IgE-mediated | Anaphylaxis<br>Urticaria |
| II | IgG or IgM-mediated, complement-dependent cytolysis | Hemolytic anemia<br>Thrombocytopenia<br>Interstitial nephritis |
| III | Immune complex-mediated, complement-dependent | Serum sickness<br>Drug fever<br>Vasculitis |
| IV | T-cell lymphocyte-mediated | Contact dermatitis<br>Morbilliform skin rash |

[a]Gell PGH, Coombs RRA. Clinical aspects of immunology. Oxford: Blackwell; 1963 [72].

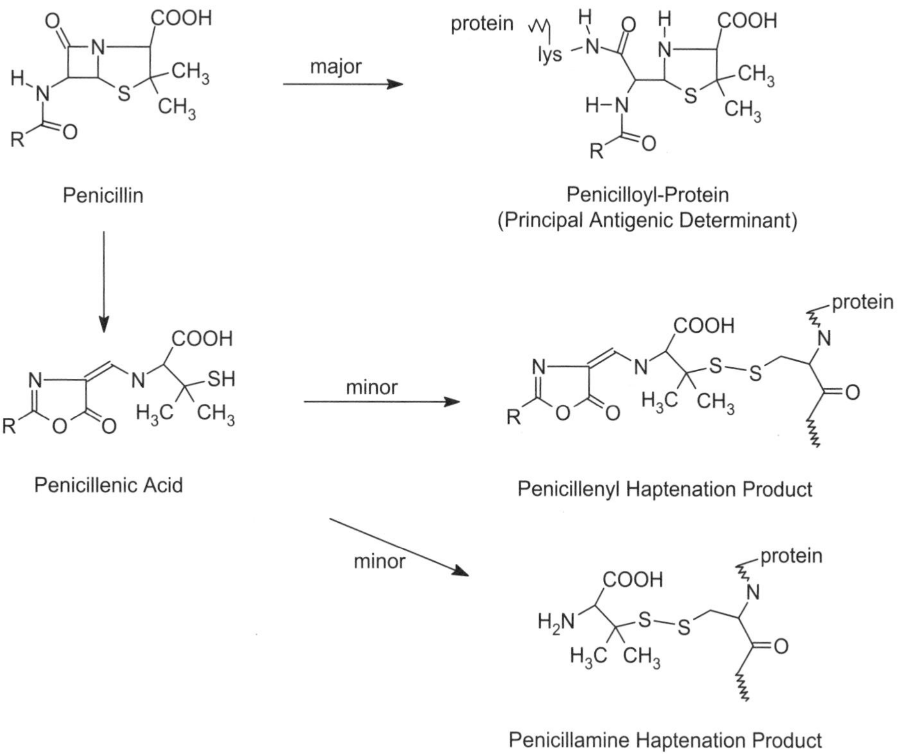

**FIGURE 16.10** Hapten determinants formed by penicillins which contain a β-lactam ring linked to various side chains (R). The primary route of haptenation involves acylation of the ε-amino group of lysine residues of serum or cell surface proteins to form a penicilloyl or major antigenic determinant. Isomerization of penicillin leads to the generation of compounds that form disulfide bonds with the cysteine sulfhydryl groups of proteins. These epitopes are termed minor determinants.

who receives penicillin, and the frequency with which penicillin-specific antibody responses occur, stand in marked contrast to the infrequent occurrence of allergic reactions to this drug and have prompted investigations into possible predisposing genetic risk factors [77, 78].

The cumulative risk of penicillin allergy appears to be related to the persistence of penicillin-specific antibodies, with the half-life of pencilloyl IgE antibodies reported to range from 10 to more than 1000 days [74]. In this regard, dehaptenation was noted to be slower than normal in penicillin-allergic patients [79]. Although it has been found that penicillin-allergic reactions are less common in the young, it is not clear whether youth is an independent protective factor or simply reflects the fact that the young are likely to have had less cumulative exposure to penicillin. Other constitutional or genetic factors are also likely to be important determinants of individual proclivity to develop allergic reactions to penicillin and other drugs.

In clinical practice, both a history of prior penicillin allergy and skin testing can be used to identify individuals at risk for penicillin allergic reactions. These approaches were compared in a National Institute of Allergy and Infectious Diseases-sponsored study of 1539 hospitalized patients in whom penicillin therapy was indicated [80]. Patients received skin tests with both benzylpenicilloyl-octalysine to determine major determinant reactivity, and a minor determinant mixture of benzylpenicillin, benzylpenicilloate, and benzylpenicilloyl-N-propylamine. Of the positive skin test reactors, 84% had major determinant reactivity, and the remaining 16% had positive tests with only the minor determinant mixture. As shown in Table 16.6, most patients with a negative history also had negative skin tests, and none of these patients had an allergic reaction to penicillin. A substantial percentage of patients with a history of penicillin allergy were found to have negative skin tests. Penicillin therapy of patients with a positive or unknown history of penicillin allergy but negative skin tests resulted in a 1.3% incidence of immediate or accelerated IgE-mediated allergic reactions. Most patients with positive skin tests were treated with other antibiotics, but two of the nine individuals who received penicillin had immediate or accelerated allergic reactions and two others developed rashes on days 3 and 9 of penicillin therapy,

**TABLE 16.6 Comparison of Allergy History with Penicillin Skin Test Results**

| Skin test | Allergy history | |
| --- | --- | --- |
| | Positive | Negative |
| Positive | 18% | 4% |
| Negative | 80% | 95% |
| Uninterpretable | 3% | 1% |

Data from Sogn DD, Evans R III, Shepherd GM *et al.* Arch Intern Med 1992;152:1025–32 [80].

respectively. Because primary reliance is placed on history to identify penicillin-allergic individuals, it would appear that those at greatest risk are the 4% of history-negative patients who nonetheless react to skin testing.

### Procainamide-Induced Lupus

Drug-induced lupus differs from classical drug hypersensitivity reactions in that it lacks drug-specific antibodies or T cells, the target autoantigens are not directly affected by the inducing drug, the time-course of development is slower than that of most drug allergies, and reintroduction of the drug does not trigger an accelerated response [81]. Although a number of drugs are capable of inducing a systemic lupus erythematosus-like reaction, procainamide is the most common cause of drug-induced lupus. Kosowski *et al.* [82] found that all patients treated with procainamide for more than a year developed antinuclear antibodies, but that procainamide-induced lupus occurred in slightly less than one-third of those who began therapy. The fact that procainamide contains an aniline moiety, similar to many drugs that cause methemoglobinemia, led to initial speculation that its N-acetylated metabolite (NAPA) might have antiarrhythmic efficacy but would be less likely to cause this adverse effect (Figure 16.11) [83]. This was first demonstrated by switching a patient with procainamide-induced lupus to NAPA, whereupon both the arthralgic symptoms of drug-induce lupus and antinuclear antibody titers returned to normal [84]. Subsequent confirmation was provided by long-term studies in which patients received effective antiarrhythmic therapy with NAPA without developing this reaction [85, 86]. However, the immunologic safety of NAPA is relative rather than absolute, because approximately 3% of an administered NAPA dose is converted to procainamide by deacetylation (Figure 16.11) [87]. In this regard, Kluger *et al.* [85]

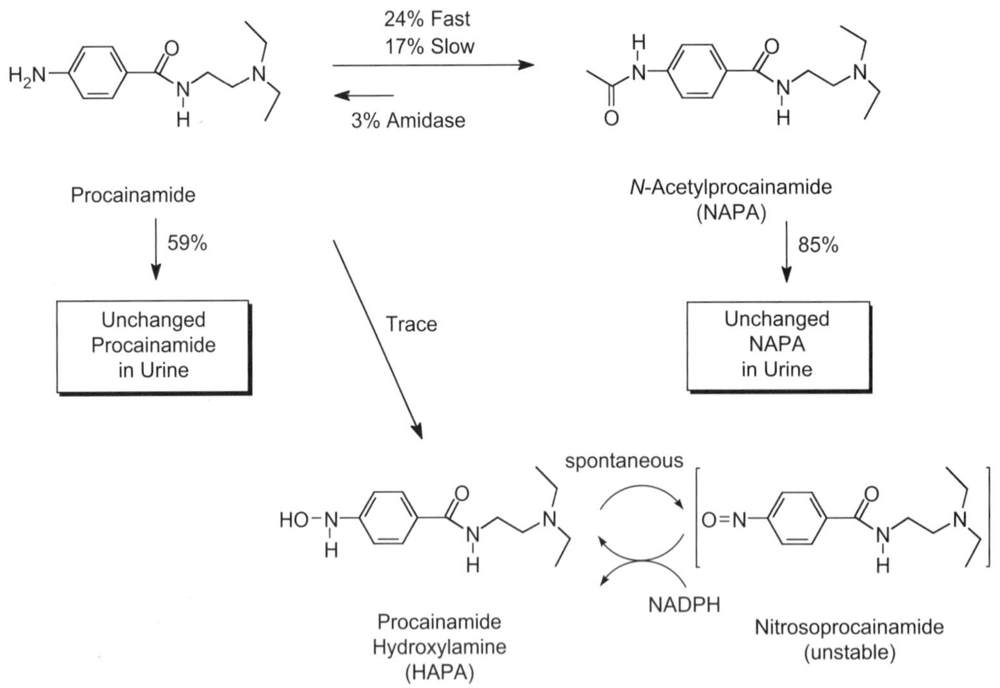

**FIGURE 16.11** Simplified scheme of procainamide metabolism. In subjects with normal kidney function, renal excretion of unchanged drug accounts for more than half the elimination of a procainamide dose, whereas acetylation by NAT2 accounts for only 24% and 17% of elimination in rapid and slow acetylators, respectively. A small amount of procainamide is metabolized to a hydroxylamine, which is in equilibrium with a postulated chemically unstable and reactive nitroso compound.

described a patient who developed drug-induced lupus when treated with NAPA doses sufficient to produce plasma procainamide concentrations of 1.6 μg/mL. The fact that these symptoms subsided when the NAPA dose was reduced so that procainamide levels fell to 0.7 μg/mL suggests that there is a threshold procainamide level that must be exceeded before this toxic reaction occurs.

Uetrecht [88] provided further evidence that the aryl amine group of procainamide is implicated in the development of drug-induced lupus by demonstrating that procainamide is metabolized to a hydroxylamine (HAPA) (Figure 16.11). HAPA is in equilibrium with a chemically unstable nitroso compound that is capable of covalent binding to histones and other proteins and, by rendering them antigenic, may initiate the immune reaction leading to procainamide-induced lupus [89]. Although hepatic CYP2D6 is capable of forming HAPA from procainamide [90], it is likely that the relevant reactive metabolites are generated by myeloperoxidase within activated neutrophiles or monocytes [91]. Uetrecht [92] postulates that these reactive metabolites then activate monocytes, which as precursors of antigen-presenting macrophages cause more generalized immune system activation and autoimmunity.

Two other mechanistic theories also have been proposed. Based on studies in which HAPA but not procainamide prevented the induction of anergy in murine T cells, Kretz-Rommel and Rubin [93] concluded that covalent binding of HAPA to histones does not occur. However, their results support the alternative possibility that the redox cycling of nitrosoprocainamide and HAPA (Figure 16.11) interferes with the redox-linked pathway involved in T-cell activation. Their further investigations with murine thymocytes demonstrated that exposure to HAPA interferes with the positive selection process by which only T cells unresponsive to self antigens emerge during the maturation of thymocytes [94]. Subsequent export of autoreactive T cells from the thymus would then have the potential to break B-cell tolerance and result in systemic autoimmunity [81].

Based on studies in which hydralazine and procainamide were incubated with CD4+ T cells, inhibition of DNA methylation has been proposed as yet another mechanism by which drugs induce autoreactivity [95]. Procainamide was shown to cause DNA hypomethylation by inhibiting DNA methyltransferase. This led to overexpression of lymphocyte function-associated antigen 1 (LFA-1) (also known as CD11a), a member of the integrin family of cell surface receptors, and resulted in the formation of autoreactive T cells [96, 97]. Adoptive transfer of these T cells to syngeneic mice caused an autoimmune reaction that resembled graft-versus-host disease in humans [96]. Mechanistically, the *in vivo* interaction of autoreactive T cells with macrophages is postulated to cause apoptosis with the subsequent release of antigenic nucleosomes that trigger expression of anti-DNA antibodies and overstimulate B cell antibody production [97]. This hypothesis is strengthened by the finding of similar epigenetic functional abnormalities in patients who develop systemic lupus erythematosis [97]. Although adoptive transfer studies demonstrated that NAPA treated CD4+ T cells did not cause an autoimmune reaction [96], a possible role for HAPA has not been incorporated in this hypothesis. However, Rubin [81] proposes that synergism could occur in that autoreactive T cells resulting from HAPA formation might become more aggressively cytotoxic because of LFA-1 overexpression.

## Carcinogenic Reactions to Drugs

It has been realized that chemicals can cause cancer since 1775, when Percival Potts observed a high incidence of scrotal cancer in chimney sweeps [98]. Despite intensive study, much remains to be learned about the mechanistic details of chemical carcinogenesis, of which drug-induced carcinogenesis is a subcategory. Since 1969, the International Agency for Research on Cancer (IARC) has conducted an evaluation of the carcinogenic risk of pharmaceuticals, assigning them to five groups based on the strength of evidence linking compounds to carcinogenesis [99]. Table 16.7 lists pharmaceuticals that are regarded as being either carcinogenic or probably carcinogenic to humans [99, 100]. In addition to these single compounds, combinations of the following are also regarded as carcinogenic: analgesic formulations containing phenacetin, MOPP chemotherapy (nitrogen mustard, vincristine, procarbazine, and prednisone), 8-methyoxypsoralen combined with UVA radiation, and combined or sequential oral contraceptive regimens containing estrogens and progestins.

Chemical carcinogens are generally regarded as being either genotoxic or non-genotoxic, although some carcinogens, such as estrogens, may exert a combination of these effects. Some toxic drugs, such as alkylating agents used in cancer chemotherapy, are directly genotoxic, but others require prior conversion to reactive metabolites. Dioxin and some other non-genotoxic carcinogens appear to activate intracellular receptors, leading to changes in gene expression that result in cancer [101]. Regardless of mechanism, chemical carcinogenesis is a complex process requiring sequential stages of initiation, promotion,

**TABLE 16.7**   IARC List of Carcinogenic and Probably Carcinogenic Pharmaceuticals

| | Carcinogenic | Probably carcinogenic |
|---|---|---|
| **Cytotoxic Drugs** | | |
| | Chlornaphazine | Adriamycin |
| | Myleran | Azacitidine |
| | Chlorambucil | BCNU[a] |
| | Methyl-CCNU[b] | CCNU |
| | Cyclophosphamide | Chlorozotocin |
| | Melphalan | Cisplatin |
| | Thiotepa | Nitrogen mustard |
| | Treosulfan | N-nitroso-N-methylurea |
| | | Procarbazine |
| **Immunosuppressants** | | |
| | Azathioprine | |
| | Cyclosporine | |
| **Hormone Agonists and Antagonists** | | |
| | Diethylstilbestrol | Oxymetholone |
| | Tamoxifen | Testosterone |
| **Other** | | |
| | Arsenic trioxide | Phenacetin |
| | | Chloramphenicol |
| | | 5-Methoxypsoralen |

[a]BCNU, Bis(chloroethyl)nitrosourea.
[b]CCNU, Chloroethyl-cyclohexyl-nitrosourea.
Data from Marselos M, Vainio H. Carcinogenesis 1991;12:1751–66 [99], and White INH. Carcinogenesis 1999;20:1153–60 [100].

and progression [98]. As a result, there is usually a delay of several years between exposure to carcinogens and the appearance of drug-induced cancers.

## Myelodysplastic Syndrome and Secondary Leukemia Following Cancer Chemotherapy

The success of chemotherapeutic regimens for cancer has resulted in an increasing number of patients who develop a secondary myeloid leukemia, but myelodysplastic syndrome also can occur after radiotherapy or immunosuppressive therapy. Data collected from patients who were treated with alkylating agents for Hodgkin's disease, ovarian cancer, and other malignancies provided the initial demonstration that chemotherapy is associated with an excess risk of subsequent treatment-related myelodysplastic syndrome (t-MDS), reflecting impaired cellular maturation of myeloid stem cells and ineffective hematopoiesis, which in some patients progresses to a proliferative phase with the development of acute myeloid leukemia (t-AML) [102, 103]. This risk is greatest in patients more than 40 years old, is greater in males than in females, and is proportionate to the dose and duration of chemotherapy. The risk reaches a peak approximately 5 years after initiating chemotherapy

and persists for up to 10 years. Estimates range from less than 0.3% to 10% for the cumulative 10-year incidence of secondary acute myeloid leukemia in patients who have received chemotherapy for Hodgkin's disease [103]. The World Health Organization (WHO) 2001 classification included two types of t-MDS and t-AML: an alkylating agent/radiation-related type, and a topoisomerase II inhibitor-related type [104].

### T-MDS/T-MDL Following Exposure to Alkylating Agents

Approximately two-thirds of the cases of t-MDS/t-AML that follow exposure to alkylating agents present as t-MDS, and those presenting as t-AML have myelodysplastic features [104]. Alkylation of hematopoietic progenitor cell DNA during chemotherapy with these agents appears to be the genotoxic event that initiates a multistep carcinogenic process by causing genetic mutations that alter cell growth (Figure 16.12). In animal studies, this has been shown to result in a permanent loss of stem-cell reserve and the maintenance of hematopoiesis by a succession of individual stem-cell clones [102]. Following this preliminary clonal restriction, it appears that a chromosomal abnormality develops in a clone that provides it with a selective growth advantage. All together, eight different genetic pathways have been identified in patients who develop t-MDS and t-AML [105]. The most common clonal abnormalities involve losses of part or all of chromosomes 5 or 7 [106]. The most common single abnormality is monosomy 7, followed in frequency by deletion of the long arm of chromosome 5 [del(5q)] and by monosomy 5. More complex karyotypes are associated with abnormalities of chromosome 5 rather than chromosome 7, and include trisomy of chromosome 8 as well as other chromosome deletions. At present it is not clear why only a subset of patients exposed to genotoxic therapy develop t–MDS/t–AML, or how the observed chromosomal changes account for both an increase in hematopoietic cell proliferation and apoptosis that results in the paradoxical combination of normal or increased bone marrow cellularity and pancytopenia that is presented by patients with myelodysplastic syndrome [107].

Multiple genetic mutations are required for the progression of t-MDS to t-AML, and this appears to account for the delay in onset of t-AML that is characteristic of t-MDS/t-AML patients who have previously been exposed to alkylating agents [106]. The mutations involved usually entail either deletion or loss of function of genes that encode hematopoietic transcription factors, or activation of genes that regulate cytokine signaling pathways. In one series of 140

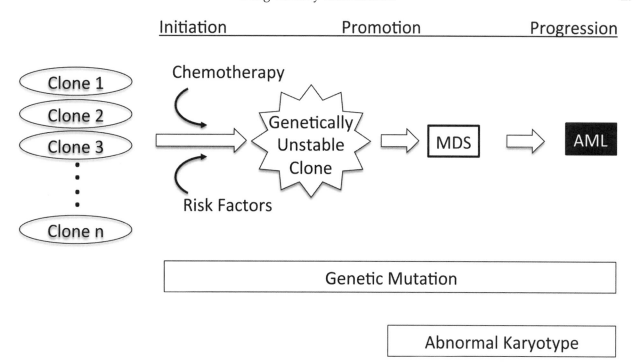

**FIGURE 16.12** Hypothetical scheme for the pathogenesis of secondary myelodysplastic syndrome (MDS) and acute myeloid leukemia (AML) following cancer chemotherapy with alkylating agents.

patients with t-MDS/t-AML, point mutation of *p53*, often with the loss of heterozygosity, was observed most commonly and was primarily related to defects in chromosome 5 and to complex karyotypes with highly rearranged chromosomes [108]. Wild-type *p53* exerts tumor suppressor effects by blocking activation of cyclin–CDK complexes, thus impeding cell cycle progression through G1 by modulating the balance between DNA replication and repair and by binding both to damaged DNA and to transcription repair factors [109]. Loss of these functions presumably mediates progression from t-MDS to t-AML. Point mutations in *AML1* (or *Runx1*), a gene that encodes a core-binding transcription factor that is essential for hematopoiesis, were the second most frequent genetic abnormality detected, and were associated with defects in chromosome 7 [108]. These mutations presumably occur early in the course of t-MDS/t-AML, and progression to t-AML in some patients appears to be associated with concurrent hypermethylation and consequent epigenetic silencing of *p15*, a gene that encodes for a cyclin-dependent kinase [110]. Therapy with decitabine has been effective in treating MDS/AML patients when low doses of this drug are administered, presumably because decitabine is incorporated by MDS and AML cells into newly synthesized DNA and traps DNA methyltransferase, thereby depleting this enzyme and reactivating *p15*

[111]. Mutations in genes that encode for receptor tyrosine kinases also occur frequently in patients with *AML1* point mutations, and may play a role in disease progression from t–MDS to t-AML [108].

*T-MDS and T-MDL following exposure to topoisomerase II inhibitors and anthracyclines*

The second WHO category of treatment-related myeloid neoplasms consists of t-AML following chemotherapy with topoisomerase II-directed epipodophyllotoxins and DNA-intercalating anthracyclines [104]. The onset of leukemia in these patients generally occurs only 2–3 years after chemotherapy, is rarely preceded by MDS, and is associated with balanced chromosomal translocations that are characteristic of the initiating chemotherapeutic agent [103]. These chimeric rearrangements result in production of fusion proteins that cause growth dysregulation and leukemic transformation [109]. The genetic pathway following therapy with epipodophyllotoxins is characterized by balanced translocations to chromosome band 11q23 such that the leukemic proto-oncogene *MLL* (Mixed-Lineage Leukemia gene) at this locus combines with one of a number of partner genes [112]. The fusion proteins thus formed associate stably with menin, the product of the *MEN1* tumor suppressor gene, to inappropriately maintain homeobox (*HOX*) gene function [113]. This hyperexpression of *HOX* function results in leukemogenic transformation [113]. Balanced translocations involving chromosome band 21q22 or 16q22 lead to chimeric rearrangements between the core binding factor genes *AML1* or *CBFβ*, are frequently accompanied by defects in chromosome 7, and are most often associated with previous therapy with anthracyclines [105]. *AML1* forms a heterodimer with *CBFβ* that functions as a transcription factor to regulate the expression of a large number of hemato-poiesis-related genes [114]. Loss of *AML1* function contributes to hematopoietic abnormalities and malignancy in patients with a familial platelet disorder who develop AML, and presumably plays a similar role in this t-AML pathway.

*Risk Factors*

Only a small fraction of chemotherapy-treated patients subsequently develop t–MDS/t-AML, and the risk-determining genetic factors are largely unexplored. The identified risk factors include the magnitude of the chemotherapy dose administered to treat the primary malignancy, individual differences in the metabolism of anticancer drugs, and molecular genetic and biochemical processes relating to carci-nogenic susceptibility and DNA repair [115, 116]. For example, etoposide is metabolized by CYP3A4 to form potentially genotoxic catechol and quinone metabolites, and individuals with the CYP3A4-V polymorphism have a decreased rate of etoposide metabolism that makes them less susceptible to t-AML than individuals with wild-type CYP3A4 [112]. In addition, patients with the inactivating $^{609}C \rightarrow T$ polymorphism in the gene that encodes NAD(P)H:quinone oxidoreductase (NQO1), an enzyme that converts quinones to less toxic hydrox-ymetabolites, are more susceptible t-AML following therapy with alkylating agents, topoisomerase II inhibitors, or radiation [117]. Similarly, patients with hypofunctioning variants of the glutathione *S*-trans-ferase P1 gene (*GSTP1*) have an increased risk of developing t-AML [115]. DNA repair capacity also is genetically determined, and patients deficient in DNA mismatch repair or other repair mechanisms have an increased incidence of t-AML [115].

*Diethylstilbestrol-Induced Vaginal Cancer*

In 1971, Herbst *et al.* [118] reported the unusual occurrence of clear cell adenocarcinoma of the vagina in eight young women. The precipitating factor appeared to be the fact that their mothers had been diagnosed with high-risk pregnancies and had been treated with diethylstilbestrol (DES) in order to prevent spontaneous abortion and premature delivery. Estimates place the incidence of clear cell adenocarci-noma of the vagina at 1.5 per 1000 women who were exposed *in utero* to DES [119].

DES is a non-steroidal estrogen that crosses the placenta and targets intranuclear estrogen receptors that develop in the fetal genital tract early in intra-uterine life. During fetal development, Müllerian-derived columnar epithelium is replaced by a hollow core of squamous epithelium that arises from the vaginal plate [120]. However, neonatal DES exposure leads in mice to persistence of Müllerian-type columnar epithelium in the upper vagina and cervix and subsequent adenosis. DES exerts proliferative effects by binding to the classic estrogen receptor (ER-α), and it has been thought that the carcinogenic effects of DES might be a direct result of its ER-α-mediated activity, its possible non-receptor-mediated genotoxic effects, or both [121].

The pathways of DES metabolism that could lead to potentially genotoxic compounds are partly depicted in Figure 16.13 [122, 123]. It can be seen that redox cycling between the semiquinone and quinone metabolites generates superoxide anion radicals that may cause oxidative damage to DNA and other cellular macromolecules [122]. In addition, chemically reactive semiquinone and diol epoxide metabolites are formed that are capable of forming either stable or depurinating DNA adducts [124]. Stable DNA adducts are formed when reactive metabolites react with exocyclic amino groups on adenine or guanine. De-purinating adducts result when these metabolites bind to the N-3 or N-7 position of adenine, or the N-7 or C-8 position of guanine. The depurinating adducts desta-bilize the glycosidic bond to deoxyribose, spontane-ously releasing the purine base and the metabolite that is bound to it. It is believed that depurinating adducts are the primary culprits that initiate tumorigenesis, and that mutations result from misrepair or mis-replication of the apurinic sites [124]. Stable DNA adducts could also play a role in carcinogenesis by interfering with error-free repair of the apurinic sites. Consistent with the pathogenetic role of impaired DNA repair is the finding that DNA polymerase β mutations were present in a hamster kidney model of DES carcinogenesis [122]. Although specific gene defects have not been identified in DES-induced clear cell adenomas in humans, upregulation of the normal *p53* tumor suppressor gene has been described, and has been attributed to a normal cellular response to persistent DNA damage or genetic instability [125]. However, *p53*-mediated apoptosis was found to be inhibited to at least some extent by overexpression of

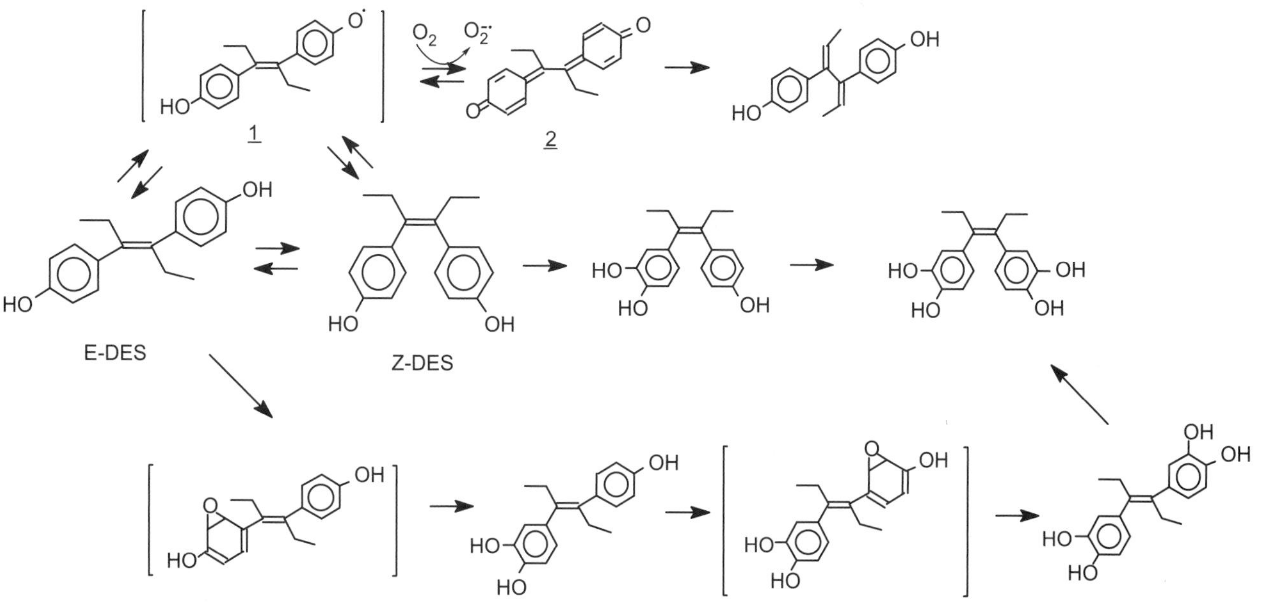

**FIGURE 16.13** Partial scheme for the metabolism of diethylstilbestrol (DES). DES is administered as the *trans* isomer (E-DES) that in solution is in equilibrium with the *cis* isomer (Z-DES). Cytochrome P450 enzymes oxidize E-DES and Z-DES to a postulated chemically reactive semiquinone (**1**) which is further oxidized to a quinone (**2**), thereby generating reactive oxygen species (ROS) that oxidize cellular macromolecules. Redox cycling is perpetuated and ROS formation amplified by cytochrome P450 or cytochrome $b_5$ reductase that reduce the quinone back to the semiquinone. The unstable semiquinone and diol epoxide (**3**) metabolites are presumably those that bind to DNA to form adducts and initiate carcinogenesis.

the proto-oncogene *bcl-2* [126]. In another study, molecular genetic analysis provided evidence of microsatellite instability in all DES-induced and 50% of spontaneous clear cell adenoma tissue samples, again suggesting that defective DNA repair represents a critical molecular feature of this tumor type [127].

On the other hand, observations that neonatal exposure to DES increased the incidence of atypical uterine hyperplasia and cancer in mutant mice that overexpress ER–α, and that squamous metaplasia of the vaginal epithelium was absent in ER–α knockout (αERKO) mice provide unequivocal evidence that ER–α plays an obligatory role in mediating the detrimental effects of DES exposure [121, 128]. DES-treated wild-type but not αERKO mice also demonstrated transient downregulation in the uterine expression of *Wnt7a*, whose gene products regulate tissue patterning during critical periods of reproductive system embryogenesis [128]. So the finding that *Wnt7a*-null mice recapitulate the phenotype seen in DES-treated wild-type mice and develop cervical and/or vaginal adenocarcinomas by 6 months after birth highlights a potentially important downstream event in the estrogen receptor-mediated pathway of DES tumorigenesis [129]. However, these findings do not exclude the possibility that, although DES interactions with

ER–α are required for tumor manifestation, DES genotoxicity initiates tumorigenesis [128].

## Teratogenic Reactions to Drugs

Although the principles of teratogenesis are described more fully in Chapter 24, certain general concepts are central to an understanding of the way in which drugs cause teratogenic adverse reactions. First, teratogens cause a specific abnormality, or pattern of abnormalities, in the fetus, such as phocomelia resulting from maternal therapy with thalidomide [130]. However, even known teratogens will not exert a teratogenic effect unless they are given during the relevant period of fetal organogenesis – generally during the first trimester of pregnancy. In addition, fetal exposure must also exceed a critical threshold for teratogenesis to occur. The level of exposure is not only determined by the rate of drug transfer across the placenta but also by fetal clearance mechanisms [131]. Unfortunately, the ability of the fetal liver to provide teratogenic protection is limited by the facts that the liver does not begin to form until the fourth week of pregnancy, and that smooth endoplasmic reticulum is not detectable in fetal hepatocytes until the twelfth week of pregnancy [132].

Finally, it is likely that genetic factors also determine the outcome of exposure to teratogens.

### The Fetal Hydantoin Syndrome

Hanson *et al.* [133] coined the term "fetal hydantoin syndrome" to describe a pattern of malformations that occurs in epileptic women who are treated with phenytoin during pregnancy. The clinical features of the syndrome include craniofacial anomalies, such as cleft lip or palate; a broad, depressed nasal bridge and inner epicanthic folds; nail and digital hypoplasia; prenatal and postnatal growth retardation; and mental retardation. These authors estimated that about 11% of exposed fetuses have the syndrome with serious sequelae, but that almost three times as many have lesser degrees of impairment. The magnitude and difficulty of this problem are underscored by the estimate that hydantoin therapy is prescribed during 2 per 1000 pregnancies, and by the fact that the risks of untreated epilepsy exceed the teratogenic risk of anticonvulsant therapy.

Phenytoin, phenobarbital, and carbamazepine are teratogenic anticonvulsant drugs that also cause hypersensitivity reactions that include skin rash, fever, and hepatitis [134]. The cytochrome P450-mediated hydroxylation of all three drugs may proceed via the formation of chemically reactive epoxide intermediates (as shown for phenytoin in Chapter 11, Scheme 11.7, Pathway c). A pathogenetic role for phenytoin epoxide is suggested by the finding that the activity of epoxide hydrolase, the enzyme that converts the epoxide to a non-toxic dihydrodiol metabolite, is deficient in lymphocytes from patients with phenytoin-induced hepatotoxic reactions [135]. Covalent binding of phenytoin to rat gingival proteins also suggests that metabolic activation plays a pathogenetic role in the gingival hyperplasia that occurs in 30–70% of patients receiving long-term phenytoin therapy [136].

Martz *et al.* [137] used a mouse model to provide the first evidence that the epoxide metabolite of phenytoin might be similarly implicated in mediating teratogenic reactions to this drug. Pregnant mice were treated with a single dose of phenytoin on gestational day 11. Their fetuses were subsequently found to have a 4% incidence of cleft palate and other anomalies, and inhibition of epoxide hydrolase with trichloropropene oxide resulted in at least a doubling of this incidence. Furthermore, administration of radioactive phenytoin resulted in covalent binding of the radioactivity to gestational tissue macromolecules. By assaying lymphocytes for epoxide hydrolase activity, as had been done for patients with phenytoin hepatotoxicity,

Strickler *et al.* [138] demonstrated that the occurrence of major birth defects, including cleft lip or palate, congenital heart anomalies, and microcephaly, was correlated with subnormal epoxide hydrolase activity. Subsequently, Buehler *et al.* [139] obtained samples of amniocytes at amniocentesis and were able to correlate low amniocyte levels of epoxide hydrolase activity with an increased risk of developing the fetal hydantoin syndrome.

However, Tiboni *et al.* [140] have shown that embryos from pregnant mice pretreated with fluconizole, an inhibitor of phenytoin hydroxylation, had an increased rather than a decreased frequency of cleft palate. This argues against a teratogenic role for the epoxide metabolite of phenytoin and supports an alternative explanation, first proposed by Winn and Wells [141], that phenytoin is bioactivated by embryonic peroxidases to free radical intermediates, which in turn form hydroxyl radicals, superoxide anion, and hydrogen peroxide. Wells *et al.* [142] point out that the developing fetus and embryo have relatively low levels of most CYP enzymes, and that reactive electrophilic phenytoin metabolites formed in the maternal liver are too unstable to be transported across the placenta. On the other hand, embryonic tissues have high levels of enzymes with peroxidase activity that are capable of generating free radical intermediates that can initiate formation of reactive oxygen species (ROS). Thus, Parman *et al.* [143] demonstrated that embryonic prostaglandin H synthase can bioactivate phenytoin to an unstable nitrogen-centered radical that rapidly undergoes ring opening to form more stable carbon-centered radical intermediates (Figure 16.14). This mechanism was extended by Lu and Utrecht [144], who reported that various peroxidases produce free radical intermediates *in vitro* from 4-hydroxyphenytoin as well as from metabolites of carbamazepine, which exhibits similar idiosyncratic drug reactions. The subsequent formation of reactive oxygen species and associated oxidative stress are then believed to exert embryopathic effects by interfering with embryonic signaling pathways or by causing oxidative damage to embryonic DNA and other critical macromolecules, as schematized in Figure 16.15 [142].

One of the most prevalent forms of oxidative DNA damage caused by teratogens is the conversion of guanine to 8-hydroxyguanine, which is in dynamic equilibrium with 7,8-dihydro-8-oxoguanine (8-oxo-G) [142]. During DNA replication, 8-oxo-G is a direct source of A–T transversion mutations and, since guanine is the most easily oxidized natural DNA base, 8-oxo-G is also a commonly used biomarker to indicate the extent of cellular oxidative stress [145].

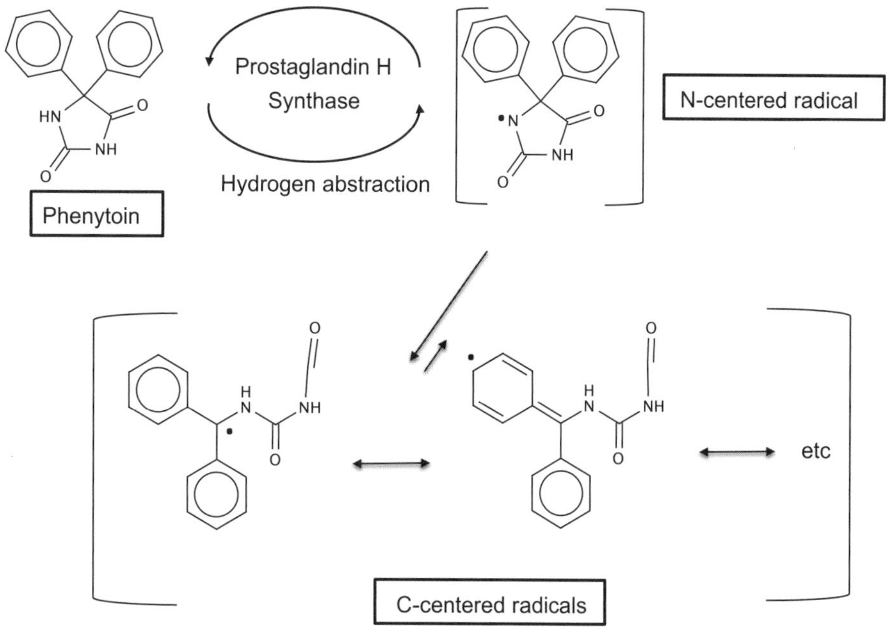

**FIGURE 16.14** Prostaglandin H synthase is postulated to bioactivate phenytoin to an unstable nitrogen-centered (N-centered) radical that then undergoes ring opening to form more stable carbon-centered (C-centered) free radical intermediates. These free radicals in turn generate hydroxyl radicals that alter embryonic signaling pathways and oxidize embryonic DNA, protein, thiol and lipid molecules.

Both phenytoin and thalidomide enhance embryonic and fetal 8-oxo-G levels and also enhance the oxidation of GSH, proteins, and lipids. The recognition and repair of 8-oxo-G DNA damage is mediated in part by p53 and ataxia-telangectasia mutated protein (ATM). During embryogenesis *p53* functions as a teratological suppressor gene, and an increase in embryopathies is observed when *p53*-deficient mice are treated with teratogens [146]. This embryoprotective function is provided by the p53 protein, which performs triage, directing apoptosis when severe DNA damage is detected in cells and DNA repair when damage is less severe. Among other functions, ATM plays an important embryoprotective role by serving as a signal transducer that directs the repair of DNA damage by phosphorylating, and thus activating, p53 and other target proteins. Bhuller and Wells [147] showed that ATM-deficient mice are more sensitive to the embryopathic effects of teratogens and have an increased incidence of spontaneous embryopathies even in the absence of teratogen exposure.

ROS-mediated signal transduction is also thought to play an important role in the causation of phenytoin embryopathies [142]. Phenytoin has been shown in mouse embryo cultures to increase the embryonic levels of both activated Ras protein and embryonic nuclear factor κB (NF-κB) signaling. The significance of this with respect to phenytoin embryopathies has not been demonstrated. However, NF-κB is a redox-sensitive transcription factor that plays a critical role in vertebrate limb outgrowth, and thalidomide-induced ROS are believed to impair NF-κB binding to DNA, resulting in a massive upregulation of apoptosis during embryonic limb development [142, 148]. Knobloch *et al.* [148] have made the important observation that mice appear to be insensitive to thalidomide teratogenesis because they have higher GSH levels than do sensitive species. Similarly, administration of exogenous inhibitors of prostaglandin H synthase and antioxidants, antioxidative enzymes, and free radical spin-trapping agents also has provided embryopathic protection in experimental systems [142]. However, clinical trials have not been conducted yet to evaluate the efficacy of potential embryoprotective agents in women who must take phenytoin and other ROS-forming drugs during pregnancy.

Wells *et al.* [149] recently have concluded that formation of unstable electrophilic and free radical intermediates may both contribute to phenytoin embryopathy, and that neither proposed mechanism is mutually exclusive. They propose that the extent to which each mechanism contributes to embryopathy is

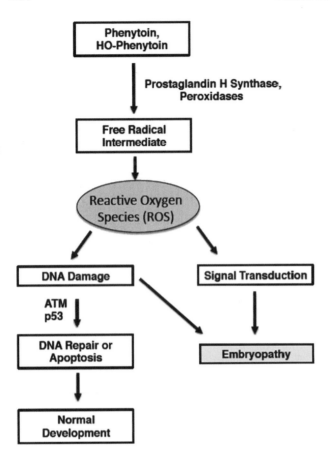

**FIGURE 16.15** Proposed mechanism by which phenytoin is converted to free radical intermediates by prostaglandin H synthase in embryonic/fetal tissues, leading to the formation of reactive oxygen species (ROS). When ROS formation exceeds the capacity of endogenous antioxidant mechanisms, DNA is damaged and normal signal transduction is altered. Causes of embryopathy include these alterations in signal transduction as well as defects in normal antioxidant protective and DNA repair mechanisms. ATM = ataxia-telangectasia mutant protein).

likely to depend on the stage of embryonic development, the concentration of teratogen within the embryo, and the target tissue and cell type, as well as other underlying genetic and environmental factors.

## REFERENCES

[1] Rawlins MD, Thomas SHL. Mechanisms of adverse drug reactions. In: Davies DM, Ferner RE, de Glanville H, editors. Davies's textbook of adverse drug reactions. 5th ed. London: Chapman & Hall Medical; 1998. p. 40–64.

[2] Melmon KL. Preventable drug reactions – causes and cures. New Engl J Med 1971;284:1361–8.

[3] Goldstein RA, Patterson R. Drug allergy: Prevention, diagnosis, and treatment. Ann Intern Med 1984;100:302–3.

[4] Brodie BB, Axelrod J. The fate of acetanilide in man. J Pharmacol Exp Ther 1948;94:29–38.

[5] Coleman MD, Coleman NA. Drug-induced methaemoglobinaemia – treatment issues. Drug Saf 1996;14:394–405.

[6] Coleman MD. Use of *in vitro* methaemoglobin generation to study antioxidant status in diabetic erythrocyte. Biochem Pharmacol 2000;60:1409–16.

[7] Roueché B. The medical detectives. New York, NY: Penguin Books; 1988.

[8] Yunis AA. Chloramphenicol: Relation of structure to activity and toxicity. Annu Rev Pharmacol Toxicol 1988; 28:83–100.

[9] Russmann S, Kullak-Ublick GA, Grattagliano I. Currrent concepts of mechanisms in drug-induced hepatotoxicity. Curr Med Chem 2009;16:3041–53.

[10] Ballet F. Hepatotoxicity in drug development: Detection, significance and solutions. J Hepatol 1997;26(Suppl. 2):26–36.

[11] Temple RJ, Himmel MH. Safety of newly approved drugs: Implications for prescribing. JAMA 2002;287:2273–5.

[12] Larson AM, Polson J, Fontana RJ, Davern TJ, Lalani E, Hynan LS, et al. The Acute Liver Failure Study Group. Acetaminophen-induced acute liver failure: Results of a United States multicenter, prospective study. Hepatology 2005; 42:1364–72.

[13] Popper H, Rubin E, Gardiol D, Schaffer F, Paronetto F. Drug-induced liver disease: A penalty for progress. Arch Intern Med 1965;115:128–36.

[14] Brodie BB, Reid WD, Cho AK, Sipes G, Krishna G, Gillette JR. Possible mechanism of liver necrosis caused by aromatic organic compounds. Proc Natl Acad Sci USA 1971;68:160–4.

[15] Zampaglione N, Jollow DJ, Mitchell JR, Stripp B, Hamrick M, Gillette JR. Role of detoxifying enzymes in bromobenzene-induced liver necrosis. J Pharmacol Exp Ther 1973;187:218–27.

[16] Reid AB, Kurten RC, McCullough SS, Brock RW, Hinson JA. Mechanisms of acetaminophen-induced hepatotoxicity: Role of oxidative stress and mitochondrial permeability transition in freshly isolated mouse hepatocytes. J Pharmacol Exp Ther 2005;312:509–16.

[17] Hinson JA, Roberts DW, James LP. Mechanisms of acetaminophen-induced liver necrosis. Handb Exp Pharmacol 2010;196:369–405.

[18] Zhang J, Huang W, Chua SS, Wei P, Moore DD. Modulation of acetaminophen-induced hepatotoxicity by the xenobiotic receptor CAR. Science 2002;298:422–4.

[19] Mitchell JR, Jollow DJ, Potter WZ, Gillette JR, Brodie BB. Acetaminophen-induced hepatic necrosis. IV. Protective role of glutathione. J Pharmacol Exp Ther 1973;187:211–7.

[20] Mitchell JR, Thorgeirsson SS, Potter WZ, Jollow DJ, Keiser H. Acetaminophen-induced hepatic injury: Protective role of glutathione in man and rationale for therapy. Clin Pharmacol Ther 1974;16:676–84.

[21] Rumack BH. Acetaminophen overdose. Am J Med 1983; 75:104–12.

[22] Cederbaum AI. CYP2E1-biochemical and toxicological aspects and role in alcohol-induced liver injury. Mt Sinai J Med 2006;73:657–72.

[23] Henderson CJ, Wolf CR, Kitteringham N, Powell H, Otto D, Park BK. Increased resistance to acetaminophen hepatotoxicity in mice lacking glutathione S-transferase Pi. Proc Natl Acad Sci USA 2000;97:12741–5.

[24] Kon K, Kim J-S, Uchiyama A, Jaeschke H, Lemasters JJ. Lysosomal iron mobilization and induction of the mitochondrial permeability transition in acetaminophen-induced toxicity to mouse hepatocytes. Toxicol Sci 2010;117:101–8.

[25] Kon K, Ikejima K, Okumura K, Aoyama T, Arai K, Takei Y, et al. Role of apoptosis in acetaminophen hepatotoxicity. J Gastroenterol Hepatol 2007;22:S49–52.

[26] Mitchell JR, Long MW, Thorgeirsson UP, Jollow DJ. Acetylation rates and monthly liver function tests during one year of isoniazid preventive therapy. Chest 1975;68:181–90.

[27] Lauterberg BH, Smith CV, Todd EL, Mitchell JR. Oxidation of hydrazine metabolites formed from isoniazid. Clin Pharmacol Ther 1985;38:566–71.

[28] Sarich TC, Adams SP, Petricca G, Wright JM. Inhibition of isoniazid-induced hepatotoxicity in rabbits by pretreatment

with an amidase inhibitor. J Pharmacol Exp Ther 1999; 289:695–702.

[29] Sarich TC, Youssefi M, Zhou T, Adams SP, Wall RA, Wright JM. Role of hydrazine in the mechanism of isoniazid hepatotoxicity in rabbits. Arch Toxicol 1996;70:835–40.

[30] Albano E, Tomasi A. Spin trapping of free radical intermediates produced during the metabolism of isoniazid and iproniazid in isolated hepatocytes. Biochem Pharmacol 1987; 36:2913–20.

[31] Delaney J, Timbrell JA. Role of cytochrome P450 in hydrazine toxicity in isolated hepatocytes in vitro. Xenobiotica 1995; 25:1399–410.

[32] Chowdhury A, Santra A, Bhattacharjee K, Ghatak S, Saha DR, Dhali GK. Mitochondrial oxidative stress and permeability transition in isoniazid and rifampicin induced liver injury in mice. J Hepatol 2006;45:117–26.

[33] Schwab CE, Tuschl H. In vitro studies on the toxicity of isoniazid in different cell lines. Hum Exp Toxicol 2003;22:607–15.

[34] Dickinson DS, Bailey WC, Hirschowitz BI, Soong S-J, Eidus L, Hodgkin MM. Risk factors for isoniazid (INH)-induced liver dysfunction. J Clin Gastroenterol 1981;3:271–9.

[35] Blair IA, Tinoco RM, Brodie MJ, Care RA, Dollery CT, Timbrell JA, et al. Plasma hydrazine concentrations in man after isoniazid and hydralazine administration. Human Toxicol 1985;4:105–202.

[36] Peretti E, Karlaganis G, Lauterburg BH. Increased urinary excretion of toxic hydrazino metabolites of isoniazid by slow acetylators. Effect of a slow-release preparation of isoniazid. Eur J Clin Pharmacol 1987;33:283–6.

[37] Huang Y-S, Chern H-D, Su W-J, Wu J-C, Lai S-L, Yang S-Y, et al. Polymorphism of the N-acetyltransferase 2 gene as a susceptibility risk factor for antituberculosis drug-induced hepatitis. Hepatology 2002;35:883–9.

[38] Huang Y-S, Chern H-D, Su W-J, Wu J-C, Chang S-C, Chang C-H, et al. Cytochrome P450 2E1 genotype and susceptibility to antituberculosis drug-induced hepatitis. Hepatology 2003;37:924–30.

[39] American Thoracic Society. Treatment of tuberculosis and tuberculosis infection in adults and children. Am Rev Respir Dis 1986;134:355–63.

[40] Bebia Z, Buch SC, Wilson JW, Frye RF, Romkes M, Cecchetti A, et al. Bioequivalence revisited: Influence of age and sex on CYP enzymes. Clin Pharmacol Ther 2004;76:618–27.

[41] Liu Z-X, Kaplowitz N. Immune-mediated drug-induced liver disease. Clin Liver Dis 2002;6:467–86.

[42] Chen M, Gandolfi AJ. Characterization of the humoral immune response and hepatotoxicity after multiple halothane exposures in guinea pigs. Drug Metab Rev 1997;29:103–22.

[43] Adams DH, Ju C, Ramaiah SK, Uetrecht J, Jaeschke H. Mechanisms of immune-mediated liver injury. Toxicol Sci 2010; 115:307–21.

[44] Ray DC, Drummond GB. Halothane hepatitis. Br J Anaesth 1991;67:84–99.

[45] Spracklin DK, Emery ME, Thummel KE, Kharasch ED. Concordance between trifluoroacetic acid and hepatic protein trifluoroacetylation after disulfiram inhibition of halothane metabolism in rats. Acta Anaesthesiol Scand 2003;47:765–70.

[46] Vergani D, Mieli-Vergani G, Alberti A, Neuberger J, Eddleston ALWF, Davis M, et al. Antibodies to the surface of halothane-altered rabbit hepatocytes in patients with severe halothane-associated hepatitis. N Engl J Med 1980;303:66–71.

[47] Satoh H, Fukuda Y, Anderson DK, Ferrans VJ, Gillette JR, Pohl LR. Immunological studies on the mechanism of halothane-induced hepatotoxicity: Immunohistochemical evidence of trifluoroacetylated hepatocytes. J Pharmacol Exp Ther 1985;233:857–62.

[48] Bourdi M, Chen W, Peter RM, Martin JL, Buters JTM, Nelson SD, et al. Human cytochrome P450 2E1 is a major autoantigen associated with halothane hepatitis. Chem Res Toxicol 1996;9:1159–66.

[49] Amouzadeh HR, Bourdi M, Martin JL, Martin BM, Pohl LR. UDP-glucose:glycoprotein glucosyltransferase associates with endoplasmic reticulum chaperones and its activity is decreased in vivo by the inhalation anesthetic halothane. Chem Res Toxicol 1997;10:59–63.

[50] Furst SM, Luedke D, Gaw H-H, Reich R, Gandolfi AJ. Demonstration of a cellular immune response in halothane-exposed guinea pigs. Toxicol Appl Pharmacol 1997;143:245–55.

[51] Eliason E, Gardner I, Hume-Smith H, de Waziers I, Beaune P, Kenna JG. Interindividual variability in P450-dependent generation of neoantigens in halothane hepatitis. Chem Biol Interact 1998;116:123–41.

[52] Karasch ED, Hankins D, Mautz D, Thummel KE. Identification of the enzyme responsible for oxidative halothane metabolism: Implications for prevention of halothane hepatitis. Lancet 1996;347:1367–71.

[53] Zimmerman HJ, Lewis JH, Ishak KG, Maddrey WC. Ticrynafen-associated hepatic injury: Analysis of 340 cases. Hepatology 1984;4:315–23.

[54] López-Garcia MP, Dansette PM, Mansuy D. Thiophene derivatives as new mechanism-based inhibitors of cytochromes P-450: Inactivation of yeast-expressed human liver cytochrome P–450 2C9 by tienilic acid. Biochemistry 1994;33:166–75.

[55] López-Garcia MP, Dansette PM, Coloma J. Kinetics of tienilic acid bioactivation and functional generation of drug-protein adducts in rat hepatocytes. Biochem Pharmacol 2005; 70:1870–82.

[56] Melet A, Assrir N, Jean P, Lopez-Garcia MP, Marques-Soares C, Jaouen M, et al. Substrate selectivity of human cytochrome P450 2C9: Importance of residues 476, 365, and 114 in recognition of diclofenac and sulfaphenazole and in mechanism-based inactivation by tienilic acid. Arch Biochem Biophys 2003;409:80–91.

[57] Robin M-A, Maratrat M, Le Roy M, Le Breton F-P, Bonierbale E, Dansette P, et al. Antigenic targets in tienilic acid hepatitis. Both cytochrome P450 2C11 and 2C11-tienilic acid adducts are transported to the plasma membrane of rat hepatocytes and recognized by human sera. J Clin Invest 1996;98:1471–80.

[58] Beaune P, Dansette PM, Mansuy D, Kiffel L, Finck M, Amar C, et al. Human anti-endoplasmic reticulum autoantibodies appearing in a drug-induced hepatitis are directed against a human liver cytochrome P-450 that hydroxylates the drug. Proc Natl Acad Sci USA 1987;84:551–5.

[59] Lecoeur S, André C, Beaune PH. Tienilic acid-induced hepatitis: Anti-liver and -kidney microsomal type 2 autoantibodies recognize a three-site conformational epitope on cytochrome P4502C9. Mol Pharmacol 1996;50:326–33.

[60] Nishiya T, Mori K, Hattori C, Kai K, Kataoka H, Masubuchi N, et al. The crucial protective role of glutathione against tienilic acid hepatotoxicity in rats. Toxicol Appl Pharmacol 2008;232:280–91.

[61] Matzinger P. The danger model: A renewed sense of self. Science 2002;296:301–5.

[62] Li J, Uetrecht JP. The danger hypothesis applied to idiosyncratic drug reactions. Handb Exp Pharmacol 2010;196: 493–509.

[63] Mitchell JR, Nelson WL, Potter WZ, Sasame HA, Jollow DJ. Metabolic activation of furosemide to a chemically reactive, hepatotoxic metabolite. J Pharmacol Exp Ther 1976;199:41–52.

[64] Mitchell JR, Potter WZ, Hinson JA, Jollow DJ. Hepatic necrosis caused by furosemide. Nature 1974;251:508–10.

[65] McMurtry RJ, Snodgrass WR, Mitchell JR. Renal necrosis, glutathione depletion, and covalent binding after acetaminophen. Toxicol Appl Pharmacol 1978;46:87–100.

[66] Peyrière H, Dereure O, Breton H, Demoly P, Cociglio M, Blayac J-P, et al. The Network of the French Pharmacovigilance Centers. Variability in the clinical pattern of cutaneous side-effects of drugs with systemic symptoms: Does a DRESS syndrome really exist? Br J Dermatol 2006;155:422–8.

[67] Hausmann O, Schnyder B, Pichler WJ. Drug hypersensitivity reactions involving skin. Handb Exp Pharmacol 2010;196: 29–55.

[68] Leung AKC, Rafaat M. Eruption associated with amoxicillin in a patient with infectious mononucleosis. Intl J Dermatol 2003;42:553–5.

[69] Chung W-H, Hung S-I, Hong H-S, Hsih M-S, Yang L-C, Ho H-C, et al. A marker for Stevens-Johnson syndrome. Nature 2004;428:486.

[70] Gerber BO, Pichler WJ. Noncovalent interactions of drugs with immune receptors may mediate drug-induced hypersensitivity reactions. AAPS J 2006;8:E160–5.

[71] DiPiro JT, Adkinson Jr NF, Hamilton RG. Facilitation of penicillin haptenation to serum proteins. Antimicrob Agents Chemother 1993;37:1463–7.

[72] Gell PGH, Coombs RRA. Clinical aspects of immunology. Oxford: Blackwell; 1963.

[73] Saxon A, Beall GN, Rohr AS, Adelman DC. Immediate hypersensitivity reactions to beta-lactam antibiotics. Ann Intern Med 1987;107:204–15.

[74] Adkinson NF. Risk factors for drug allergy. J Allergy Clin Immunol 1984;74:567–72.

[75] Weltzien HU, Padovan E. Molecular features of penicillin allergy. J Invest Dermatol 1998;110:203–6.

[76] Lafaye P, Lapresie C. Fixation of penicilloyl groups to albumin and appearance of anti-penicilloyl antibodies in penicillin-treated patients. J Clin Invest 1988;82:7–12.

[77] Apter AJ, Schelleman H, Walker A, Addya K, Rebbeck T. Clinical and genetic risk factors of self-reported penicillin allergy. J Allergy Clin Immunol 2008;122:152–8.

[78] Gao N, Qiao H-L, Jia L-J, Tian X, Zhang Y- W. Relationships between specific serum IgE, IgG, IFN-γ level and IFN-γ level and IFN-γ, IFNR1 polymorphisms in patients with penicillin allergy. Eur J Clin Pharmacol 2008;64:971–7.

[79] Sullivan TJ. Dehaptenation of albumin substituted with benzylpenicillin G determinants [abstract]. J Allergy Clin Immunol 1988;81:222.

[80] Sogn DD, Evans III R, Shepherd GM, Casale TB, Condemi J, Greenberger PA, et al. Results of the National Institute of Allergy and Infections Diseases Collaborative Clinical Trial to test the predictive value of skin testing with major and minor penicillin derivatives in hospitalized adults. Arch Intern Med 1992;152:1025–32.

[81] Rubin RL. Drug-induced lupus. Toxicology 2005;209:135–47.

[82] Kosowsky BD, Taylor I, Lown B, Ritchie RF. Long-term use of procainamide following acute myocardial infarction. Circulation 1973;47:1204–10.

[83] Drayer DE, Reidenberg MM, Sevy RW. N-Acetylprocainamide: An active metabolite of procainamide. Proc Soc Exp Biol Med 1974;146:358–63.

[84] Stec GP, Lertora JJL, Atkinson AJ Jr, Nevin MJ, Kushner W, Jones C, et al. Remission of procainamide-induced lupus erythematosus with N-acetylprocainamide therapy. Ann Intern Med 1979;90:799–801.

[85] Kluger J, Drayer DE, Reidenberg MM, Lahita R. Acetylprocainamide therapy in patients with previous procainamide-induced lupus syndrome. Ann Intern Med 1981; 95:18–23.

[86] Atkinson AJ Jr, Lertora JJL, Kushner W, Chao GC, Nevin MJ. Efficacy and safety of N-acetylprocainamide in the long-term treatment of patients with ventricular arrhythmias. Clin Pharmacol Ther 1983;33:565–76.

[87] Stec GP, Ruo TI, Thenot J-P, Atkinson AJ Jr, Morita Y, Lertora JJL. Kinetics of N-acetylprocainamide deacetylation. Clin Pharmacol Ther 1980;28:659–66.

[88] Uetrecht JP. Reactivity and possible significance of hydroxylamine and nitroso metabolites of procainamide. J Pharmacol Exp Ther 1985;232:420–5.

[89] Kubicka-Muranyi M, Goebels R, Goebel C, Uetrecht J, Gleichmann E. T lymphocytes ignore procainamide, but respond to its reactive metabolites in peritoneal cells:

Demonstration by the adoptive transfer popliteal lymph node assay. Toxicol Appl Pharmacol 1993;122:88–94.

[90] Lessard É, Hamelin BA, Labbé L, O'Hara G, Bélanger PM, Turgeon J. Involvement of CYP2D6 activity in the N-oxidation of procainamide in man. Pharmacogenetics 1999;9:683–96.

[91] Jiang X, Khursigara G, Rubin RL. Transformation of lupus-inducing drugs to cytotoxic products by activated neutrophils. Science 1994;266:810–3.

[92] Uetrecht J. Current trends in drug-induced autoimmunity. Autoimmunity Rev 2005;4:309–14.

[93] Kretz-Rommel A, Rubin RL. A metabolite of the lupus-inducing drug procainamide prevents anergy induction in T cell clones. J Immunol 1997;158:4465–70.

[94] Kretz-Rommel A, Rubin RL. Disruption of positive selection of thymocytes causes autoimmunity. Nat Med 2000;6:298–305.

[95] Cornacchia E, Golbus J, Maybaum J, Strahler J, Hanash S, Richardson B. Hydralazine and procainamide inhibit T cell DNA methylation and induce autoreactivity. J Immunol 1988;140:2197–200.

[96] Yung R, Chang S, Hemati N, Johnson K, Richardson B. Mechanisms of drug-induced lupus. IV. Comparison of procainamide and hydralazine with analogs in vitro and in vivo. Arthritis Rheum 1997;40:1436–43.

[97] Richardson B. Primer: Epigenetics of autoimmunity Nat Clin Pract Rheumatol 2007;3:521–7.

[98] Graham MA, Riley RJ, Kerr DJ. Drug metabolism in carcinogenesis and cancer chemotherapy. Pharmacol Ther 1991;51:275–89.

[99] Marselos M, Vainio H. Carcinogenic properties of pharmaceutical agents evaluated in the IARC Monographs programme. Carcinogenesis 1991;12:1751–66.

[100] White INH. The tamoxifen dilemma. Carcinogenesis 1999; 20:1153–60.

[101] Green S. Nuclear receptors and chemical carcinogenesis. Trends Pharmacol Sci 1992;13:251–5.

[102] List AF, Jacobs A. Biology and pathogenesis of the myelodysplastic syndromes. Semin Oncol 1992;19:14–24.

[103] Leone G, Mele L, Pulsoni A, Equitani F, Pagano L. The incidence of the secondary leukemias. Haematologica 1999;84:937–45.

[104] Vardiman JW, Harris NL, Brunning RD. The World Health Organization (WHO) classification of the myeloid neoplasms. Blood 2002;100:2292–302.

[105] Pedersen-Bjergaard J, Christiansen DH, Desta F, Andersen MK. Alternative genetic pathways and cooperating genetic abnormalities in the pathogenesis of therapy-related myelodysplasia and acute myeloid leukemia. Leukemia 2006;20:1943–9.

[106] Qian Z, Joslin JM, Tennant TR, Reshmi SC, Young DJ, Stoddart A, et al. Cytogenetic and genetic pathways in therapy-related acute myeloid leukemia. Chem Biol Interact 2010;184:50–7.

[107] Corey SJ, Minden MD, Barber D, Kantarjian H, Wang JCY, Schimmer AD. Myelodysplastic syndromes: The complexity of stem-cell diseases. Nat Rev Cancer 2007;7:118–29.

[108] Pedersen-Bjergaard J, Andersen MK, Andersen MT, Charistiansen DH. Genetics of therapy-related myelodysplasia and acute myeloid leukemia. Leukemia 2008;22:240–8.

[109] Smith MA, McCaffrey RP, Karp JE. The secondary leukemias: Challenges and research directions. J Natl Cancer Inst 1996; 88:407–18.

[110] Christiansen DH, Anderson MK, Pedersen-Bjergaard J. Methylation of p15$^{INK4B}$ is common, is associated with deletion of genes on chromosome arm 7q and predicts a poor prognosis in therapy-related myelodysplasia and acute myeloid leukemia. Leukemia 2003;17:1813–9.

[111] Jabbour E, Issa J-P, Garcia-Manero G, Kantarjian H. Evolution of decitabine development: Accomplishments, ongoing investigations, and future strategies. Cancer 2008;112:2341–51.

[112] Felix CA, Kolaris CP, Osheroff N. Topoisomerase II and the etiology of chromosomal translocations. DNA Repair 2006;5:1093–108.

[113] Yokoyama A, Sommervaille TCP, Smith KS, Rozenblatt-Rosen O, Meyerson M, Cleary ML. The menin tumor suppressor protein is an essential oncogenic cofactor for MLL-associated leukemogenesis. Cell 2005;123:207–18.

[114] Kurokawa M, Hirai H. Role of AML1/Runx1 in the pathogenesis of hematological malignancies. Cancer Sci 2003;94:841–6.

[115] Seedhouse C, Russell N. Advances in the understanding of susceptibility to treatment-related acute myeloid leukemia. Br J Haematol 2007;137:513–29.

[116] Godley LA, Larson RA. Therapy-related myeloid leukemia. Semin Oncol 2008;35:418–29.

[117] Larson RA, Wang Y, Banerjee M, Wiemels J, Hartford C, LeBeau MM, et al. Prevalence of the inactivating $^{609}C \rightarrow T$ polymorphism in the NAD(P)H:quinone oxidoreductase (NQO1) gene in patients with primary and therapy-related myeloid leukemia. Blood 1999;94:803–7.

[118] Herbst AL, Ulfelder H, Poskanzer DC. Adenocarcinoma of the vagina: Association of maternal stilbestrol therapy with tumor appearance in young women. N Engl J Med 1971;284:878–81.

[119] Hatch EE, Palmer JR, Titus-Ernstoff L, Noller KL, Kaufman RH, Mittendorf R, et al. Cancer risk in women exposed to diethylstilbestrol in utero. JAMA 1998;280:630–4.

[120] Herbst AL. Behavior of estrogen-associated female genital tract cancer and its relation to neoplasia following intra-uterine exposure to diethylstilbestrol (DES). Gynecol Oncol 2000;76:147–56.

[121] Dickson RB, Stancel GM. Estrogen receptor-mediated processes in normal and cancer cells. J Natl Cancer Inst Monogr 2000;27:135–45.

[122] Roy D, Palangat M, Chen C-W, Thomas RD, Colerangle J, Atkinson A, et al. Biochemical and molecular changes at the cellular level in response to exposure to environmental estrogen-like chemicals. J Toxicol Environ Health 1997;50:1–29.

[123] Haaf H, Metzler M. In vitro metabolism of diethylstibestrol by hepatic, renal and uterine microsomes of rats and hamsters. Effects of different inducers. Biochem Pharmacol 1985;34:3107–15.

[124] Cavalieri E, Frenkel K, Liehr JG, Rogan E, Roy D. Estrogens as endogenous genotoxic agents – DNA adducts and mutations. J Natl Cancer Inst Monogr 2000;27:75–93.

[125] Waggoner SE, Anderson SM, Luce MC, Takahashi H, Boyd J. p53 Protein expression and gene analysis in clear cell adenocarcinoma of the vagina and cervix. Gynecol Oncol 1996;60:339–44.

[126] Waggoner SE, Baunoch DA, Anderson SA, Leigh F, Zagaja VG. Bcl-2 protein expression associated with resistance to apoptosis in clear cell adencocarcinomas of the vagina and cervix expressing wild-type p53. Ann Surg Oncol 1998;5:544–7.

[127] Boyd J, Takahashi H, Waggoner SE, Jones LA, Hajek RA, Wharton JT, et al. Molecular genetic analysis of clear cell adenocarcinomas of the vagina and cervix associated and unassociated with diethylstilbestrol exposure in utero. Cancer 1996;77:507–13.

[128] Couse JF, Dixon D, Yates M, Moore AB, Ma L, Maas R, et al. Estrogen receptor-α knockout mice exhibit resistance to the developmental effects of neonatal diethylstilbestrol exposure on the female reproductive tract. Dev Biol 2001;238:224–38.

[129] Mericskay M, Carta L, Sassoon D. Dietylstilbestrol exposure in utero: A paradigm for mechanisms leading to adult disease. Birth Defects Res A Mol Teratol 2005;73:133–5.

[130] Taussig HB. A study of the German outbreak of phocomelia: The thalidomide syndrome. JAMA 1962;180:1106–14.

[131] Szeto HH. Maternal–fetal pharmacokinetics: Summary and future directions. NIDA Res Monogr 1995;154:203–7.

[132] Ring JA, Ghabrial H, Ching MS, Smallwood RA, Morgan DJ. Fetal hepatic drug elimination. Pharmacol Ther 1999;84:429–45.

[133] Hanson JW, Myrianthopoulos NC, Harvey MAS, Smith DW. Risks to the offspring of women treated with hydantoin anti-convulsants, with emphasis on the fetal hydantoin syndrome. Pediatr 1976;89:662–8.

[134] Shear NH. Spielberg. Anticonvulsant hypersensitivity syndrome. In vitro assessment of risk. J Clin Invest 1988;82:1826–32.

[135] Spielberg SP, Gordan GB, Blake DA, Goldstein DA, Herlong HF. Predisposition to phenytoin hepatotoxicity assessed in vitro. N Engl J Med 1981;305:722–7.

[136] Wortel JP, Hefferren JJ, Rao GS. Metabolic activation and covalent binding of phenytoin in the rat gingiva. J Periodontal Res 1979;14:178–81.

[137] Martz F, Failinger III C, Blake DA. Phenytoin teratogenesis: Correlation between embryopathic effect and covalent binding of putative arene oxide metabolite in gestational tissue. J Pharmacol Exp Ther 1977;203:231–9.

[138] Strickler SM, Dansky LV, Miller MA, Seni M-H, Andermann E, Spielberg SP. Genetic predisposition to phenytoin-induced birth defects. Lancet 1985;2:746–9.

[139] Buehler BA, Delimont D, van Waes M, Finnell RH. Prenatal prediction of risk of the fetal hydantoin syndrome. N Engl J Med 1990;322:1567–72.

[140] Tiboni GM, Giampietro F, Angelucci S, Moio P, Bellati U, Di Illio C. Additional investigation on the potentiation of phenytoin teratogenicity by fluconazole. Toxicol Lett 2003;145:219–29.

[141] Winn LM, Wells PG. Phenytoin-initiated DNA oxidation in murine embryo culture, and embryo protection by the antioxidative enzymes superoxide dismutase and catalase: Evidence for reactive oxygen species-mediated DNA oxidation in the molecular mechanism of phenytoin teratogenicity. Mol Pharmacol 1995;48:112–20.

[142] Wells PG, McCallum GP, Chen CS, Henderson JT, Lee CJJ, Perstin J, et al. Oxidative stress in developmental origins of disease: Teratogenesis, neurodevelopmental deficits, and cancer. Toxicol Sci 2009;108:4–18.

[143] Parman T, Chen G, Wells PG. Free radical intermediates of phenytoin and related teratogens. J Biol Chem 1998;273:25079–88.

[144] Lu W, Uetrecht JP. Peroxidase-mediated bioactivation of hydroxylated metabolites of carbamazepine and phenytoin. Drug Metab Dispos 2008;36:1624–36.

[145] van Loon B, Markkanen E, Hübscher U. Oxygen as a friend and enemy: How to combat the mutational potential of 8-oxo-guanine. DNA Repair 2010;9:604–16.

[146] Wells PG, Kim PM, Laposa RR, Nicol CJ, Parman T, Winn LM. Oxidative damage in chemical teratogenesis. Mutat Res 1997;396:65–78.

[147] Bhuller Y, Wells PG. A developmental role for ataxia-telangiectasia mutated in protecting the embryo from spontaneous and phenytoin-enhanced embryopathies in culture. Toxicol Sci 2006;93:156–63.

[148] Knobloch J, Reiman K, Klotz L-O, Rüther U. Thalidomide resistance is based on the capacity of the glutathione-dependent antioxidant defense. Mol Pharm 2008;5:1138–44.

[149] Wells PG, McCallum GP, Lam KCH, Henderson JT, Ondovcik SL. Oxidative DNA damage and repair in teratogenesis and neurodevelopmental deficits. Birth Defects Res C Embryo Today 2010;90:103–9.

# Pharmacogenomic Mechanisms of Drug Toxicity

Shiew-Mei Huang[1], Ligong Chen[2] and Kathleen M. Giacomini[2]

[1]*Office of Clinical Pharmacology, Office of Translational Sciences, Center for Drug Evaluation and Research,
US Food and Drug Administration, Silver Spring, MD 20993*
[2]*Department of Bioengineering and Therapeutic Sciences, University of California, San Francisco, CA 94143*

## INTRODUCTION

Many drugs have been discontinued in development or withdrawn from the market after approval because of serious adverse drug reactions (ADRs), including fatalities due to acute liver failure, *torsades de pointes*, rhabdomyolysis, and Stevens-Johnson syndrome [1–3]. For drugs on the market, the spontaneous adverse event reporting, continual monitoring of patient responses, and additional studies conducted postmarketing also can lead to changes in safety labeling [4]. Figure 17.1 shows that between October 2002 and August 2005 a total of 2645 labeling changes were made for 1601 products of New Drug Applications (NDA) and Biologics License Applications (BLA). These labeling changes resulted in either restricted distribution or use with different levels of warnings and precautions in the drug labeling, especially in the first 10 years after their initial approval.

Many ADRs may go unrecognized prior to drug approval due to the limited size and types of patients who have been exposed to the drug during Phase I–III clinical trials. However, with increased understanding of molecular mechanisms, risks for ADRs can be assessed prior to market approval and managed via labeling, education, and/or postmarketing risk evaluation and mitigation strategies established at the time of regulatory approval. The need to collect and store DNA samples in clinical trials to facilitate the identification of genetic basis of ADRs has been emphasized [5–7]. Tetrabenazine is an example of a drug for which a recent pre-market evaluation of genetic effects on

drug toxicity resulted in labeling that described the relation between a patient's CYP2D6 activity and the potential of this drug to prolong the QT interval [8]. Table 17.1 lists examples of FDA-approved drug products that include ethnicity, genetic, and other biomarker information in their labeling [9].

Multiple factors, including both patient-specific factors (such as genetics, race, age) and environmental factors (such as drug–drug interactions), can influence adverse drug response [9]. Understanding the pharmacologic mechanisms of ADRs is therefore critical to provide appropriate treatment decisions for individual patients and to develop safer medications. This chapter will focus on the pharmacogenomic mechanisms that are responsible for a variety of ADRs.

## ADRS WITH A PHARMACOGENOMIC BASIS

ADRs may be related to increased systemic exposure in some patients receiving the same dosage regimens as others. This high exposure can be due to variations in genes that encode metabolizing enzymes (e.g., excessive effect of morphine in infants and breastfeeding mothers of certain genotypes of the drug-metabolizing enzymes CYP2D6 and UGT2B7 who are taking codeine), transporters (e.g., myopathy in patients with certain OATP1B1 genotypes who are treated with simvastatin), or environmental factors such as diet and concomitantly administered drugs that affect drug metabolism and/or transport. In other

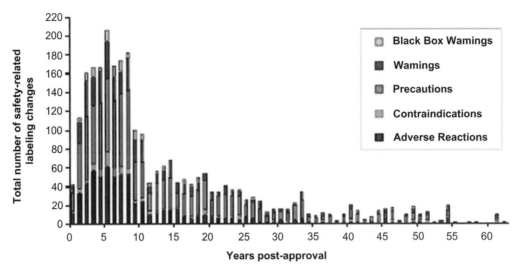

**FIGURE 17.1**    Safety-related labeling changes made between October 2002 and August 2005. (Total of 2645 labeling changes for 1601 NDA and BLA submissions.) Data from T. Mullin, Office and Planning, CDER, FDA, May 2009.

cases, factors other than those affecting the patient's systemic exposure have contributed to ADRs (e.g., time to reach therapeutic ranges of International Normalized Ratio, INR, in patients with certain VKORC1 genotypes who are initiating anticoagulation with warfarin).

For some drugs, the prevalence of certain genotypes in a specific population can explain the different dosing regimens being used in the patient population in certain regions or race and ethnic groups [10]. For example, recent data showing a higher frequency of warfarin-sensitive genotype(s) of *VKORC1* in Asians compared to Caucasians are consistent with the past FDA labeling of warfarin, and practices in some Asian countries based on evidence that Asians need a lower starting dose than Caucasians. Similarly, although Stevens-Johnson syndrome due to the anti-epileptic drug carbamazepine is not completely explained by the presence of HLA-B*1502, ethnic distribution of this allele could explain why the adverse event may be more prevalent in some but not in other populations (Table 17.1).

## Drug Metabolizing Enzyme-Mediated Pharmacogenomic Mechanisms of Drug Toxicity

### Thiopurine Methyltransferase and Thiopurine Myelotoxicity

Azathioprine is used as adjunctive therapy to prevent rejection in renal homotransplantations, and to reduce signs and symptoms in patients with active rheumatoid arthritis. 6-Mercaptopurine (6-MP) is used as part of a combination regimen for maintenance therapy of patients with acute lymphatic (lymphocytic, lymphoblastic) leukemia [11]. Azathioprine is metabolized to 6-MP, which is a substrate of thiopurine methyltransferase (TPMT), a polymorphic enzyme that is responsible for converting 6-MP into the inactive metabolite methyl-6-MP (meMP) (Figure 17.2) [12].

About 10% of Caucasians and African Americans have intermediate TPMT activity and 0.3% of them have low or absent activity. There are several major reduced-function polymorphisms of TPMT. *TPMT*3A* has two base pair changes leading to the amino acid changes Ala154Thr and Tyr240Cys, and is the most common reduced-function polymorphism of *TPMT* in Caucasians. *TPMT*3C* is the most common reduced-function polymorphism in African Americans and has a single amino acid change, Tyr240Cys. The mechanism for the enhanced toxicity of 6-MP in patients with TPMT reduced-function polymorphisms is related to accumulation of bioactive thioguanine nucleotides that cause myelosuppression. Thus, these patients are at increased risk of myelotoxicity if a conventional dose of azathioprine or 6-MP is administered [13, 14].

In July 2003, the FDA Pediatric Subcommittee of the Oncology Drug Advisory Committee (ODAC) discussed TPMT pharmacogenetics and debated whether relabeling 6-MP with genetic information was warranted [15]. Based on the evidence presented, the Subcommittee recommended that the label of 6-MP should be updated with TPMP genetic information. According to the ODAC recommendation, the labels

**TABLE 17.1    Recent FDA Drug Product Labeling Examples That Included Ethnicity or Genetic Information[a]**

| Therapeutic Area | Drug products' generic (brand) names | Ethnicity information | Genetic information[b] |
|---|---|---|---|
| Cardio-renal | Angiotensin II antagonists and ACE inhibitor | Smaller effects in Blacks[c] | Angiotensin II antagonists and ACE inhibitor |
| | Clopidogrel (Plavix) | | Boxed warning for CYP2C19 PM |
| | Isosorbide dinitrate/hydralazine (Bidil) | Indicated for self-identified Blacks | |
| Metabolic | Rosuvastatin (Crestor) | Lower dose for Asians | |
| | Simvastatin (Zocor) | Chinese (on lipid-modifying doses of niacin-containing drugs) not to take 80 mg | |
| Transplant | Azathioprine (Imuran) | | Dose adjustments for TPMT variants |
| | Tacrolimus (Protopic) | Higher dose for Blacks | |
| Oncology | Cetuximab | | Boxed warning for KRAS variants |
| | Dasatinib | | Indicated for Philadelphia chromosome |
| | Erlotinib (Tarceva) | | Different survival and tumor response in EGFR-positive and -negative patients reported |
| | Imatinib | | Indicated for C-kit |
| | Irinotecan (Camptosar) | | Dose reduction for UGT1A1*28 |
| | Lapatinib | | Indicated for HER2 overexpression |
| | 6-Mercaptopurine (Purinethol) | | Dose adjustments for TPMT variants |
| | Nicotinib | | Indicated for Philadelphia chromosome |
| | Panitumumab | | Boxed warning for KRAS variants |
| | Tamoxifen (Nolvadex) | | Estrogen receptor positive more likely to benefit |
| | Trastuzumab (Herceptin) | | Indicated for HER2 overexpression |
| | Vemurafenib (Zelboraf) | | Indicated for BRAF$^{v600E}$ mutation |
| | Crizotinib (Xalkori) | | Indicated for AKL-positive |
| Antiviral | Abacavir | | Boxed warning for HLA-B*5701 |
| | Maraviroc (Selzentry) | | Indicated for CCR5-positive |
| | Oseltamivir (Tamiflu) | Neuropsychiatric events mostly reported in Japan | |
| Pain | Codeine | | Warnings for nursing mothers that CYP2D6 UM metabolized codeine to morphine more rapidly and completely |
| Hematology | Warfarin (Coumadin) | Lower dose for Asians | Lower initial dose for CYP2C9 and VKORC1 sensitive variants |
| Psychopharm | Atomoxetine (Straterra) | | Dosage adjustments for CYP2D6 PM; no drug interactions with strong CYP2D6 inhibitors expected for PM |
| | Thioridazine (Mellaril) | | Contraindication for CYP2D6 PM |

*(Continued)*

**TABLE 17.1   Recent FDA Drug Product Labeling Examples That Included Ethnicity or Genetic Information[a]—cont'd**

| Therapeutic Area | Drug products' generic (brand) names | Ethnicity information | Genetic information[b] |
|---|---|---|---|
| Neuropharm | Carbamazepine (Tegretol) | Boxed warning in Asians with variant alleles of HLA-B*1502 | Boxed warning in Asians with variant alleles of HLA-B*1502 |
| | Tetrabenazine (Xenazine) | | Dose limitation for CYP2D6 PM |

For FDA labeling, see Drugs at the FDA: http://www.accessdata.fda.gov/scripts/cder/drugsatfda/

[a]PM, poor metabolizer; UM, ultra-rapid metabolizer; TPMT, thiopurine methyl transferase; UGT, uridine diphosphate glucuronosyl transferase; HER2, human epidermal growth factor receptor 2; EGFR, epidermal growth factor receptor; CCR5, chemokine (C-C motif) receptor 5; VKORC, vitamin K reductase complex; HLA, human leukocyte antigen; BRAF, B-type Raf kinase; ALK, anaplastic lymphoma kinase.

[b]Genetic information may include information about polymorphisms in germline DNA or mutations and/or expression levels of genes in tumors.

[c]A general statement in the candesartan (Atacand®) labeling.

Modified from Huang SM, Temple R. Clin Pharmacol Ther 2008;84(3):287–94 [9].

for both 6-MP and subsequently, azathioprine were revised to include TPMT genetic information [11]. The current view is that TPMT testing, when combined with other tests and observations, can lead to higher-quality decisions about drug selection and drug dosing that will further decrease the risk of severe and preventable bone-marrow toxicity, yet provide the desired benefit from therapy with these drugs. In addition, a recent survey of TPMT genotyping in patients with acute lymphoblastic leukemia in four European countries (Germany, Ireland, The Netherlands, and the UK) suggested its cost effectiveness in clinical practice [16].

### UGT1A1 and Irinotecan Neutropenia

Irinotecan is an antineoplastic agent of the topoisomerase I inhibitor class that, in combination with 5-fluorouracil and leucovorin, is indicated for first-line therapy of patients with metastatic carcinoma of the colon or rectum. It is also indicated for patients with metastatic carcinoma of the colon or rectum whose

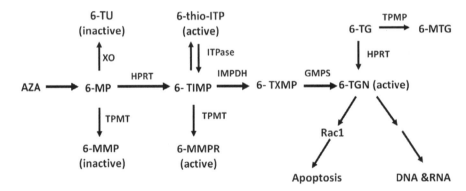

**FIGURE 17.2** Metabolism of thioprines. The prodrug azathioprine (AZA) is converted through a non-enzymatic reaction to 6-mercaptopurine (6-MP). 6-MP then undergoes extensive metabolism through three competing pathways mediated by the following: xanthine oxidase (XO), thiopurine *S*-methyltransferase (TPMT), and hypoxanthine guanine phosphoribosyl transferase (HPRT). The XO-mediated pathway produces inactive metabolite 6-thiouric acid (6-TU). The TPMT-mediated pathway produces a second inactive metabolite 6-methymercaptopurine (6-MMP). The HPRT-mediated pathway produces 6-thioinosine monophosphate (6-TIMP). 6-TIMP can then undergo one of the following: (1) transformation into thioguanine nucleotides (6-TGN) by the inosine-5-monophosphate dehydrogenase (IMPDH) and guanine monophosphate synthetase (GMPS); (2) methylation into 6-methylmercaptopurine ribonucleotides (6-MMPR), by TPMT; (3) phosphorylation to 6-thio-inosine triphosphate (6-thio-ITP). In healthy cells, inosine triphosphatase (ITPase) converts 6-thio-ITP back to 6-TIMP to prevent the accumulation of 6-thio-ITP to toxic levels. AZA can act as an immunosuppressant if 2′-deoxy-6-TGTP is randomly incorporated into DNA and RNA, or, as recent studies suggest, by inhibiting the guanosine triphosphatase Rac1 in T lymphocytes [12, 119, 120].

disease has recurred or progressed following initial fluorouracil-based therapy [11]. Although irinotecan increases survival, it causes severe diarrhea and neutropenia.

Irinotecan is hydrolyzed by carboxylesterase enzymes to its active metabolite, SN-38 (Figure 17.3). UDP-glucuronosyl transferase 1A1 (UGT1A1) is primarily responsible for inactivation of SN-38 [17] and formation of a glucuronide metabolite. *UGT1A1\*28*, a variant allele, is associated with decreased enzyme activity. The variant occurs in the promoter region of the gene and is a variant of TA tandem repeats, which range between five and eight copies. The most common is six TA repeats and the allele, *UGT1A1\*28*, contains seven TA repeats. Reporter assays suggest that the *UGT1A1\*28* allele results in reduced transcription rates of UGTIA1, and therefore a reduced level of the enzyme and consequently reduced function. Because they inactivate SN-38 at a slower rate, patients with *UGT1A1\*28* are at increased risk of neutropenia from irinotecan treatment [18]. Approximately 10% of the North American population is homozygous for the *UGT1A1\*28* allele.

In a study of 66 patients who received irinotecan as a single-agent ($350 \, mg/m^2$ once every 3 weeks), the incidence of grade 4 neutropenia in patients homozygous for the *UGT1A1\*28* allele was 50%, and in patients heterozygous for this allele the incidence was 12.5%. No grade 4 neutropenia was observed in patients homozygous for the wild-type allele (*UGT1A1* 6/6 genotype). In a prospective study to investigate the role of *UGT1A1\*28* polymorphism in the development of toxicity in 250 patients treated with irinotecan ($180 \, mg/m^2$) in combination with infusional 5-FU/LV, the incidence of grade 4 neutropenia in patients homozygous for the *UGT1A1\*28* allele was 4.5%, compared to an incidence of 5.3% in patients heterozygous for this allele [11]. Grade 4 neutropenia was observed in 1.8% of patients homozygous for the wild-type allele [11]. In another study in which 109 patients were treated with irinotecan ($100–125 \, mg/m^2$) in combination with bolus 5-FU/LV, the incidence of grade 4 neutropenia in patients homozygous for the *UGT1A1\*28* allele was 18.2%, and in patients heterozygous for this allele the incidence was 11.1%. Grade 4 neutropenia was observed in 6.8% of patients homozygous for the wild-type allele [11]. In November 2004, the FDA Advisory Committee for Pharmaceutical Science – Clinical Pharmacology Subcommittee (CPSC) discussed these findings [19]. Based on their recommendation, the label of irinotecan was updated to include *UGT1A1* genetic information and the recommendation that patients who are homozygous for *UGT1A1\*28* alleles start irinotecan therapy with a reduced dose because of an increased risk of neutropenia [11].

Additional *UGT1A* polymorphisms have been evaluated, and Cecchin *et al.* [20] suggested that *UGT1A1* variants in addition to *UGT1A1\*28* or haplotypes of *UGT1A1, UGT1A7,* and *UGT1A9* may describe better the SN-38 glucuronidation and thus contribute to the individual variations of the clinical

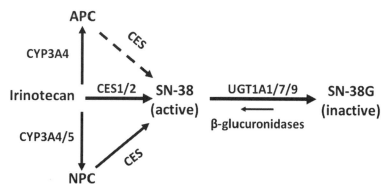

**FIGURE 17.3** Metabolism of irinotecan. Irinotecan is metabolized into its active metabolite SN-38 (7-ethyl-10-hydroxycamptothecin) via carboxylesterases (CES). SN-38 is then inactivated into its glucuronide conjugate, SN-38G, by one of the following uridine diphosphate glucuronosyltransferases (UGTs), listed from most to least significant: UGT1A1, 1A7, and 1A9. Hepatobiliary excretion occurs, then SN-38G is reconverted into active SN-38 by β-glucuronidases from intestinal bacteria. A second irinotecan detoxification pathway is the CYP3A (cytochrome P450 isoforms 3A4 and 3A5)-mediated oxidation of irinotecan in APC (7-ethyl-10-[4-*N*-(5-aminopentanoic acid)-1-piperidino]-carbonyloxy-camptothecin) and NPC (7-ethyl-10-[4-amino-1-piperidino]-carbonyloxy-camptothecin). CES facilitates conversion of NPC, and possibly APC, into SN-38 [121–123].

effects of irinotecan. Another recent study has explored the association of a haplotype of ABCC2, which encodes MRP2 (an efflux transporter), with irinotecan-related diarrhea, and suggested that the reduced diarrhea observed in patients with this haplotype may be a consequence of their reduced hepatobiliary secretion of irinotecan [21]. The significance of this association in modifying patient treatment awaits further evaluation.

## Transporter- Mediated Pharmacogenomic Mechanisms of Drug Toxicity

Genes associated with exposure-related drug toxicity also include drug transporters, which play a role in both influx and efflux into all cells in the body [22, 23]. Polymorphisms in transporter genes may enhance drug accumulation into target tissues for toxicity directly or indirectly through pharmacokinetic mechanisms, thereby enhancing susceptibility to ADRs. For example, a polymorphism in a hepatic transporter may result in reduced hepatic uptake and metabolism of a drug, and therefore higher systemic drug levels (Figure 17.4) [23, 24]. The resulting higher systemic levels may in turn cause toxicity in various body organs. Other mechanisms by which transporter polymorphisms may be associated with drug toxicity include modulation of the accumulation of endogenous substrates. For example, polymorphisms in bile

acid transporters such as multidrug resistance protein (MRP) 2 (or ABCC2) and bile salt export pump (BSEP) (ABCB11) may be associated with drug-induced cholestasis through changes in bile salt transport [22, 25]. Mechanisms by which variants may alter transport activity include changes in the expression levels of transporters or alteration in their interaction with drugs, which can be either substrates or inhibitors.

### The Organic Anion Transporter 1B1 (OATP1B1) and Statin-Induced Myopathy

OATP1B1 is a genetically polymorphic influx transporter that is encoded by SLCO1B1 and is expressed on the sinusoidal membrane of human hepatocytes (Figure 17.4). OATP1B1 mediates the hepatic uptake of many endogenous compounds and xenobiotics, including many clinically important drugs [26, 27]. The clinical significance of SLCO1B1 genetic polymorphisms is best exemplified by statin-induced myopathy. In general, statin-induced myopathy is mild and reversible, but at times a more severe myopathy may result after treatment with statins [28, 29]. Symptoms of statin-induced myopathy include fatigue, muscle pain, tenderness, weakness, and cramping, which can occur with or without an increase in blood creatine kinase concentration. The clinical spectrum of statin-induced myopathy ranges

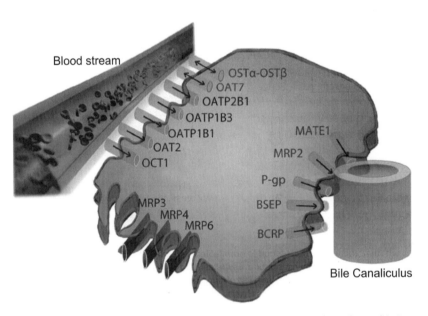

**FIGURE 17.4** Selected transporters for endogenous compounds and xenobiotics, expressed on the sinusoidal and canalicular membranes of human hepatocytes [58, 116]. BSEP, bile salt export pump; MATE1, multidrug and toxin extrusion protein 1; MRP, Multiple drug resistance protein; OAT, organic anion transporter; OCT, organic cation transporter; OSTα-OSTβ, heteromeric organic solute transporter.

from a mild and relatively common myalgia (5–10% of statin users/year) to a life-threatening and rare rhabdomyolysis (0.001–0.005% of statin users/year) [30, 31]. Known risk factors for statin-induced myopathy and rhabdomyolysis include a high statin dose, drug–drug interactions (especially those that raise statin plasma concentrations), old age, existence of multiple concomitant diseases, hypothyroidism, and certain inherited muscle disorders [30, 31]. The mechanism by which statins cause myopathy remains unknown, but appears to be related to statin concentrations in blood and muscle [32]. Polymorphisms in SLCO1B1 have been associated with altered hepatic uptake of pravastatin [33, 34], and a genetic variant of SLCO1B1 was reported in a patient with pravastatin-induced myopathy [35]. Additional data indicate that genetic variations in SLCO1B1 also might affect outcomes in patients treated with simvastatin (Figure 17.5). These studies and others have led some to speculate that

SLCO1B variants are associated with increased susceptibility to statin-induced myopathy.

The Study of the Effectiveness of Additional Reductions in Cholesterol and Homocysteine (SEARCH) Collaborative Group [36] conducted a genome-wide association study (GWAS) and identified a common single-nucleotide variation (c.521T>C, rs4149056) in the SLCO1B1 gene (OATP1B1) that was associated with simvastatin-induced myopathy (Figure 17.5B). This variant had been previously shown to cause reduced function of OATP1B1, resulting in markedly increased plasma concentrations of several statins, including simvastatin and pravastatin [37, 38]. The variant was associated with an enhanced risk of statin-induced myopathy and a lower therapeutic index of simvastatin. The study used two groups of patients and controls from large trials involving approximately 12,000 participants (6000 received 80 mg, 6000 received 20 mg in the initial GWAS study) and 20,000 participants (10,000 received

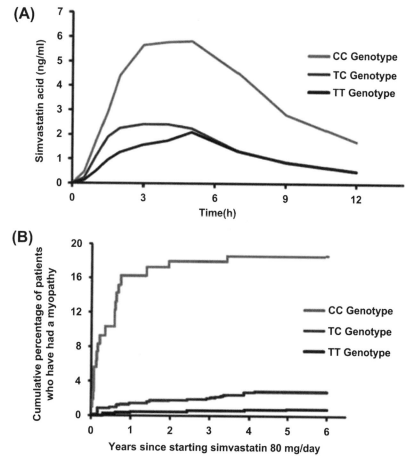

**FIGURE 17.5** Effects of the *SLCO1B1* c.521T>C variant (A) on the plasma concentrations of active simvastatin acid after a single 40-mg dose of simvastatin in healthy volunteers, and (B) on the cumulative incidence of myopathy during treatment with 80 mg/day simvastatin. Panel A modified from Pasanen *et al.* Pharmacogenet Genomics 2006;16:873–9 [124]; Panel B modified from SEARCH Collaborative Group *et al.* N Engl J Med 2008;359:789–99 [36].

40 mg and 10,000 received placebo). DNA samples from 85 patients with myopathy on high-dose (80 mg/day) simvastatin and 90 matched control subjects who had been enrolled as a part of the 12,000-patient SEARCH Collaborative Group were analyzed by GWAS [36]. This study revealed that a non-coding SNP in the SLCO1B1 gene, which is in strong linkage disequilibrium with the c.521T>C SNP ($r^2 = 0.97$), was associated with simvastatin-induced myopathy (Figure 17.5). The odds ratio for myopathy was 4.5 per allele of the c.521C allele and as high as 16.9 in CC homozygotes compared with TT homozygotes. More than 60% of the myopathy cases were attributed to the C allele. Of the patients with the CC genotype, 18.2% developed myopathy during the first 5 years of high-dose simvastatin therapy, with most cases occurring during the first year, compared with an overall risk of 2.83% in TC heterozygotes and 0.63% in TT homozygotes [36]. The association was replicated in 10,000 patients on 40 mg/day simvastatin in the Heart Protection Study, yielding a relative risk of 2.6 per copy of the C allele [36]. The SLCO1B1 c.521T>C SNP has also been associated with milder forms of simvastatin-, atorvastatin-, and pravastatin-induced adverse reactions, even with use of low statin doses [39].

The molecular mechanism by which the SLCO1B1 c.521T>C SNP reduces transport has been investigated in functional genomic studies. In particular, a systematic investigation of SLCO1B1 variants identified 14 non-synonymous single-nucleotide polymorphisms (SNPs) in 15 haplotypes, many of which (c.217T>C, c.245T>C, c.467A>G, c.521T>C, c.1058T>C, c.1294A>G, c.1463G>C, c.1964A>G) conferred reduced transporter activity of OATP1B1 [40]. The SLCO1B1 c.521T>C SNP in exon 5 resulted in a decreased membrane expression of OATP1B1 and decreased transport activity of estrone-3-sulfate and estradiol-17β-D-glucuronide. Consistent with its decreased membrane expression, the c.521T>C SNP affected mainly the maximum transport velocity [40]. Many non-synonymous transporter variants have been shown to reduce membrane expression levels of transporters, presumably by altering protein stability or trafficking [41, 42].

The degree of myopathy in patients in the GWAS study was mild, in stark contrast to statin-induced rhabdomyolysis – a potentially fatal ADR that involves severe muscle damage accompanied by toxic effects in other organs such as the kidney [31]. There is a need to test for SLCO1B1 variants in patients with statin-induced rhabdomyolysis. However, this ADR is rare with a reported incidence as low as 0.000044 event per person per year [24, 31]. The potential of concomitant medications that interact with certain statins, such as amiodarone or gemfibrozil [43–45], to enhance the susceptibility to statin-induced myopathy also should be evaluated, particularly in patients carrying the c.521T>C SNP. Other genetic factors, such as the *ABCG2* c.421G>A SNP, which was recently found to significantly raise the plasma concentrations of rosuvastatin, atorvastatin, and fluvastatin [46, 47], might have an additive effect with the SLCO1B1 c.521T>C SNP or interacting drugs.

Though further studies are clearly needed, the pharmacogenomic findings by the SEARCH Collaborative Group have important clinical implications for treatment with simvastatin. Because the SLCO1B1 c.521T>C SNP markedly reduces the uptake of simvastatin acid into hepatocytes and increases its plasma concentrations, it thereby enhances the risk of myopathy, particularly during high-dose simvastatin therapy. Thus, high-dose simvastatin should be avoided in carriers of this SNP. Genotyping SLCO1B1 polymorphisms may be useful in the future for both tailoring the statin dose and safety monitoring, especially when statins are used in combination with certain other drugs and during the first year of treatment, when the absolute risk of myopathy is greatest. Since approximately 60% of the cases of simvastatin-induced myopathy were attributed to variant SLCO1B1, avoiding the administration of high-dose simvastatin to those who are homozygous or heterozygous for the variant allele could reduce the incidence of myopathy by nearly 60%. Alternatively, one could reduce the incidence of myopathy by choosing to avoid prescribing simvastatin to those who are homozygous for the risk allele and by prescribing relatively low dose of the drug to patients who are heterozygous for this allele, but further investigation is needed to identify the optimal therapeutic approach [24]. The US FDA has recently restricted the use of 80 mg of simvastatin to patients who have been taking simvasatin 80 mg chronically (e.g., for 12 months or more) without evidence of muscle toxicity [48].

These pharmacogenetic findings may apply to some other statins because myopathy is a class effect, and SLCO1B1 polymorphisms affect the blood levels of several statins. However, the SLCO1B1 c.521T>C SNP does not appear to significantly affect the pharmacokinetics of fluvastatin, so it is possible that the variant does not confer an increased risk of fluvastatin-induced myopathy [49]. Thus, fluvastatin may represent an alternative therapy for individuals who carry the c.521T>C SNP. Finally, variants in SLCO1B1 are relevant to toxicities associated with other classes of drugs transported by OATP1B1 and, for example, are associated with increased risk of gastrointestinal toxicity in children with acute lymphoblastic leukemia treated with methotrexate [49].

### Transporters and Tenofovir Renal Toxicity

Tenofovir disoproxil fumarate (TDF) is an orally bioavailable prodrug of tenofovir (TFV), an acyclic nucleotide analog reverse transcriptase inhibitor that can cause a proximal tubulopathy [50]. TDF is among the most popular antiretroviral agents for treating HIV-infected patients due to its high efficacy, low toxicity, and once-daily dosing schedule [51]. However, cases of renal failure and kidney tubular dysfunction, including development of Fanconi syndrome, have been reported, and concerns exist regarding long-term TDF use [52]. In fact, TFV currently is the drug most associated with this syndrome [53], which leads to bone demineralization and osteomalacia [54]. The proximal tubular cell is the main target of tenofovir toxicity, in large part due to its large complement of cell membrane transporters that favor tenofovir intracellular accumulation (Figure 17.6). Though controversial, recent studies suggest that mitochondria are the target organelles of tenofovir cytotoxicity that is possibly mediated through inhibition of mitochondrial DNA polymerase $\gamma$ and decreased mitochondrial DNA (mtDNA) replication [55–57]. This results in structural mitochondrial abnormalities that include mitochondrial depletion and wide changes in mitochondria size and shape, with clumping, loss, and disorientation of cristae, which may lead to apoptosis of tubular cells [58]. The main clinical symptoms of tenofovir nephrotoxicity are either proximal tubular dysfunction with preserved renal function, or proximal tubular dysfunction associated with decreased renal function. Two studies have demonstrated tubular dysfunction with tenofovir in 17–22% of tenofovir-treated patients (vs 6% and 12% of HAART-treated or -naïve HIV patients, respectively) [59, 60]. Compared to controls, the risk difference for developing acute kidney injury with renal failure in tenofovir treated patients was estimated to be 0.7% (95% CI 0.2–1.2%) in a recent meta-analysis [52].

Owing to the high interindividual variability in the presentation of kidney function abnormalities, researchers have recently focused on host genetic factors predisposing to TFV-associated renal dysfunction [61]. Transporter proteins involved in the renal elimination of TFV, such as organic anion transporters (OATs) or MRP 2, 4 or 10, have been the focus of these studies (Figure 17.6). Notably, several genetic polymorphisms in these transporters have been associated with an increased risk of kidney tubulopathy in

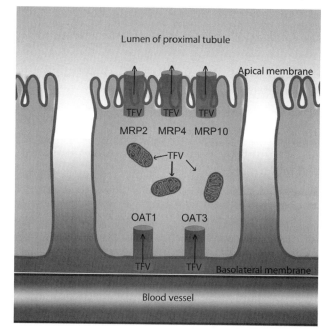

**FIGURE 17.6** Transporter proteins involved in TFV elimination through proximal tubular cells. Tenofovir secretion by proximal tubular cells: 20–30% of tenofovir is excreted unchanged in the urine through active secretion by proximal tubular cells. OAT1 is the main transporter taking tenofovir into the proximal tubular cell, although OAT3 also contributes. Once in the proximal tubular cells, tenofovir must be extruded into the tubular lumen by MRP2 and MRP4. Recently, MRP10 has also been implicated in TFV transport (not shown in figure). Proximal tubular cells are uniquely susceptible to tenofovir toxicity because they express the transporters that increase intracellular concentrations of the drug, and they are rich in mitochondria [58]. MRP, multidrug resistant protein; OAT, organic anion transporter protein; TFV, tenofovir.

patients treated with TDF [49, 61–63]. Relevant pharmacogenetic factors that may play a role in the risk of renal toxicity associated with the use of tenofovir are summarized in Table 17.2.

MRP2, encoded by the *ABCC2* gene, is localized apically in cellular membranes. Associations between polymorphisms in this gene and TFV-associated tubulopathy have been reported in two studies. The first reported an association between the "CATC" haplotype, defined as the combination of the polymorphisms at positions g.-24C>T, c.1249G>A, c.3563T>A, and c.3972C>T (the number is relative to the translational start site) within the *ABCC2* gene, and a greater risk of proximal tubulopathy in patients receiving TFV [61]. The study examined DNA from 13 human immunodeficiency virus type 1 (HIV-1)-infected patients (cases) presenting with TDF-induced renal proximal tubulopathy and 17 unrelated HIV-1-infected patients who had received TDF therapy and who did not have renal proximal tubulopathy (controls) in a case–control analysis, to assess the

**TABLE 17.2**   Polymorphisms In the Transporters and Their Association With Renal Damage

| Gene (protein) | rs number | SNPs/haplotypes | Amino acid change | Functional alteration | Association with renal damage |
|---|---|---|---|---|---|
| ABCC2 (MRP2) | rs717620 | −24C>T | 5′-UTR | No clear influence on DNA-protein binding and the mRNA stability did not differ significantly. In transfected HEK293T/17 cells; significantly lower protein expression [125] | The carriers of the -24 T allele excreted 19% more TFV than carriers of the common allele; CC genotype is more frequent in patients with tubular damage [60, 62] |
| ABCC2 (MRP2) | rs7080681 | 1058G>A | Arg353His | N.A. | No association with renal damage |
| ABCC2 (MRP2) | rs2273697 | 1249G>A | Val417Ile | Vmax ↓; Km ↓ (for certain substrates in sf9 cell [126]; significantly increased protein expression (HEK293T/17 cell) [125] | AA genotype is more frequent in patients with proximal tubular damage; no association with renal damage [60, 61] |
| | rs8187694 | 3563T>A | Val1188Glu | N.A. | TT genotype is more frequent in patients with proximal tubular damage; no association with renal damage [60, 61] |
| | rs3740066 | 3972C>T | Ile1324Ile | Significantly increased protein expression (HEK293T/17 cell) [125] | No association with renal damage [60, 61] |
| | rs8187710 | 4544G>A | Cys1515Tyr | N.A. | A allele is not present in patients with proximal tubular damage; no association with renal damage [60, 61] |
| ABCC2 (MRP2) | – | Haplotype CATC | – | Significantly increased protein expression (HEK293T/17 cell) [125] | Risk of proximal tubular damage [61] |
| ABCC4 (MRP4) | rs11568685 | 559G>T | Gly187Trp | Reduced function and Decreased expression (HEK 293T) [42] | No association with renal damage [61] |
| | rs899494 | 669C>T | Ile223Ile | N.A. | |

| Gene | rs number | Nucleotide | Amino acid | Functional effect | Clinical association |
|---|---|---|---|---|---|
| | rs2274407 | 912G>T | Lys304Asn | No functional alternation (HEK 293T) [42] | T allele is more frequent in patients with proximal tubular damage; no association with renal damage [60, 61] |
| | rs2274406 | 951G>A | Arg317Arg | N.A. | No association with renal damage [61] |
| | rs2274405 | 969G>A | Ser323Ser | N.A. | |
| | rs1557070 | 1497C>T | Tyr499Tyr | N.A. | |
| | rs11568655 | 3310T>C | Leu1104Leu | N.A. | |
| | rs1751034 | 3348A>G | Lys1116Lys | N.A. | |
| | rs11568695 | 3609G>A | Ala1203Ala | N.A. | |
| ABCC4 (MRP4) | rs3742106 | 4135T>G | 3'UTR | N.A. | No association with TFV clearance and no association with renal damage [60, 62] |
| ABCC10 (MRP7) | rs9349256 | 2137G>A | Intron | N.A. | Significantly associated with kidney tubular dysfunction (KTD); urine phosphorus wasting and $\beta2$ microglobulinuria [63] |
| ABCC10 (MRP7) | rs2125739 | 2843T>C | Ile948Thr | N.A. | |
| ABCC10 (MRP7) | – | HaplotypeGGC | – | N.A. | |
| ABCC10 (MRP7)–ABCC1 (MRP2) | – | HaplotypeGGC-CGTC | – | N.A. | Significantly higher in the KTD group than in the controls [63] |
| ABCB1 (P-gp) | rs1128503 | 1236 C>T | Gly412Gly | N.A. | No association with renal damage [60, 61] |
| | rs2032582 | 2677 G>A/T | Ala893Ser / Thr | Enhanced efflux of digoxin [127] | |
| | rs1045642 | 3435 C>T | Ile1145Ile | N.A. | |
| SLC22A6 (OAT1) | rs11568634 | 1361 G>A | Arg454Gln | Non-functional with respect to adenovir assayed in X. laevis oocytes [128] | No difference in renal clearance and secretory clearance of adefovir in family-based studies [60, 62] |
| SLC22A11 (OAT4) | rs11231809 | g.64302950 T>A | – | N.A. | No association with renal damage [60] |

N.A., not available.

influence of single-nucleotide polymorphisms (SNPs) identified in ABCC2 and ABCC4. A complete linkage between the CATC haplotype and *ABCC2* c.1249G>A was found, suggesting that the CATC haplotype might impair TFV secretion by tubular cells. These authors also identified a protective CGAC haplotype that might confer a phenotype with higher TFV secretion. However, their results could not be replicated in a second study, which also included polymorphisms in *ABCC4* (MRP4), *SCL22A6* (OAT1), and *ABCB1*(P-glycoprotein), and identified another SNP in the ABCC2 gene (−24C) as a risk allele for TFV toxicity [60]. The authors of this study suggested that TFV was excreted less efficiently by tubular cells in the individuals who were *ABCC2-24C* variants, and that increased TFV concentrations within renal tubular cells were deleterious. However, in cellular assays, −24C>T, in the MRP2 5′UTR, demonstrated no effect of this variant on mRNA expression or downstream open reading frame translation, and various ABCC2 haplotypes have been shown to lower expression levels of MRP2 by posttranscriptional modification of protein expression rather than by a direct effect on transporter function [64].

Whereas the role of MRP2 in TFV renal excretion is questionable, MRP4, coded by the *ABCC4* gene, appears to play an important role in TFV tubular secretion. In one study, the polymorphism *ABCC4* 669C>T was found in a higher proportion of TFV-treated individuals who were developing renal tubular damage [61]. However, this finding was not confirmed by others [60]. Since then, other SNPs have been examined, including *ABCC4* 559G>T, 912G>T, 951G>A, 969G>A, 1497C>T, 3310T>C, and 3348A>G. None of them has definitively been proven to be associated with a greater risk of TFV-associated kidney damage [60, 61]. Although the *ABCC4* 4131T>G allele has previously been associated with higher intracellular levels of lamivudine in patients harboring the 4131GG genotype (20% higher lamivudine-triphosphate concentrations than carriers of the common allele), this polymorphism did not show any association with TFV intracellular levels [65]. Collectively, the role of MRP4 genetic variants in modulating TFV kidney toxicity has not been confirmed.

A recent study of ABCC10 (MRP10), which is functionally similar to ABCC4 and is highly expressed in the kidney, established that TFV is a substrate for this transporter [63]. Because genetic variability within the ABCC10 gene may influence TFV renal tubular transport and contribute to the development of kidney tubule toxicity, a case–control association study was undertaken to investigate common variants in ABCC10 in HIV-positive patients in TFV-containing regimens [63]. Two SNPs and their haplotypes were significantly associated with kidney tubule damage: rs9349256 located in intron 4, and rs2125739 (a non-synonymous SNP) in exon 12, resulting in an amino acid change (p.I920T) [63]. The functional effects of the ABCC10 polymorphisms identified in this study are not known. A bioinformatics approach using FastSNP software [66] found rs2125739 to be located in a putative splice site that may cause the splicing apparatus to use nearby cryptic splice sites or skip exons, leading to an altered protein. ABCC10 rs9349256, was associated with urine phosphorus wasting and β2-microglobulinuria. Urine phosphorus wasting is among the three criteria defining Fanconi syndrome, and the ABCC10–ABCC2 combination haplotype was more prevalent in patients with abnormal urine phosphorus excretion. However, the above results need to be replicated in other cohorts.

Polymorphisms in ABCB1 and OAT1, which is the main transporter taking tenofovir into the proximal tubular cell, although *OAT3* also contributes, have also been associated with renal toxicity due to TFV; however, the overall results suggest that polymorphisms in these two genes have no effect on TFV-associated renal dysfunction [60, 61]. In addition to genetic factors, non-genetic factors such as age, body weight, and gender have to some extent been related to the incidence of renal dysfunction in TFV-treated patients. For example, it has been reported that renal toxicity occurs more frequently in males than females [62, 67]. Other variables that may increase risk of renal toxicity from TFV include pre-existing renal impairment and the concomitant use of nephrotoxic drugs didanosine (DDI) or protease inhibitors, and in particular ritonavir [68].

## GENETIC MECHANISMS FOR DRUG-INDUCED HYPERSENSITIVITY REACTIONS

As discussed in Chapter 16, ADRs are generally classified into two major subtypes: A and B. Type A reactions are mechanism-based, dose-dependent, and generally predictable, whereas type B reactions are not predictable. Among type B reactions, hypersensitivity reactions have been the most thoroughly studied and are responsible for substantial morbidity and mortality. Drug allergies are a class of hypersensitivity reactions that can range in symptoms from mild skin rashes to more severe, less common syndromes. In particular, toxic epidermal necrolysis (TEN) and Stevens-Johnson syndrome (SJS) are two life-threatening hypersensitivity reactions in which drugs or their metabolites are implicated. Particular drugs and classes of drugs that are associated with drug hypersensitivity reactions such as SJS and TEN include non-steroidal anti-inflammatory drugs (NSAIDS), sulfonamides, antiretroviral drugs, antibiotics, corticosteroids, anti-epileptic agents, methotrexate, and allopurinol.

For years, hypersensitivity reactions have been known to vary in prevalence among human populations. For example, East Asians are particularly sensitivity to carbamazepine-induced hypersensitivity reactions. More recently, genetic polymorphisms in the human leukocyte antigen (HLA) system, the major histocompatibility complex (MHC), have been implicated in drug-induced hypersensitivity reactions. Though the mechanisms by which HLA polymorphisms may lead to risk for drug hypersensitivity reactions are not well understood, recent studies have

shed some light on the genetic mechanisms of abacavir-induced hypersensitivity reactions.

## Haptens Interact with HLA Molecules in a Polymorphic-Specific Manner

To produce a robust T-cell or immunologic response, the neoself peptides, formed by the drug reacting with proteins and the proteins being digested into smaller peptides, must bind to the HLA molecule (Figure 17.7). HLA-B polymorphisms have been associated with a variety of drug-induced hypersensitivity reactions. HLA genes are found on chromosome 6 in the region of the MHC. MHC class 1, including HLA-A, HLA-B and HLA-C, are primarily involved in the presentation of peptides on the cell surface, which, if foreign, will attract CD8-positive T-cells. The HLA-B gene, located on chromosome

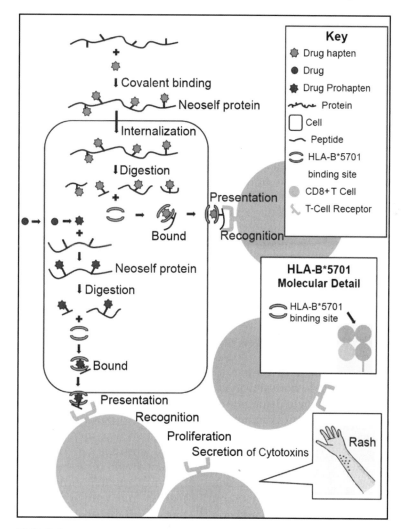

**FIGURE 17.7** Mechanisms by which HLA-B*5701 mediates hypersensitivity reactions of drugs including abacavir. The key describes the symbols, and the details of the mechanisms are described in the text.

6 p21.3, is involved in hypersensitivity reactions to various drugs, including allopurinol, carbamazepine, and abacavir [69–71], and in flucloxacillin hepatotoxicity [72]. Hundreds of HLA-B polymorphisms have been described. These are numbered, and many have been associated with human disease, including infectious disease such as AIDS and reactive arthritis [73–75]. Though the exact drug-modified peptide for abacavir sensitivity has not been discovered, the reaction appears to be dependent on key residues in HLA-B*5701, which are not present in other HLA-B polymorphisms. This mechanism, which will be described in more detail below, explains how an HLA polymorphism may lead to a drug-induced hypersensitivity reaction.

Though patients with particular HLA-B polymorphisms are at increased risk for SJS and TEN, most do not get these hypersensitivity reactions when exposed to the drugs that have the potential to cause these ADRs. Thus, HLA-B polymorphisms seem to be necessary, but not sufficient, to elicit these drug-hypersensitivity reactions. The mechanisms for this phenomenon are not clear. However, it is possible that patients with certain T-cell receptor polymorphisms may be at risk for drug-induced hypersensitivity reactions [76]. Additional studies are clearly needed to explain why many individuals with polymorphic HLA-B risk alleles do not get these hypersensitivity reactions. Further, in addition to hapten-specific binding to HLA-B polymorphisms, other mechanisms should be studied which may lead to HLA-B polymorphism-specific drug-hypersensitivity reactions [76].

### Abacavir-Induced Hypersensitivity Reactions

Abacavir hypersensitivity reactions have been associated in many studies with the HLA polymorphism HLA-B*5701 [70, 77]. These reactions are known to vary in frequency among ethnic groups, paralleling the allele frequencies of HLA-B*5701 in these populations [78]. Abacavir is a prodrug that is activated to carbovir triphosphate, a reactive drug which may be responsible for the formation of immunogenic peptides in the body. The mechanism of the HLA-B*5701-dependent abacavir hypersensitivity reaction was recently studied by Chessman and coworkers [79], who conducted *in vitro* experiments suggesting that abacavir-induced hypersensitivity reactions are mediated by the activation of cytotoxic CD8$^+$ T cells, which corresponded to the known increased abundance of CD8$^+$ T cells in the skin of patients with abacavir hypersensitivity reactions (Figure 17.7). Abacavir stimulation of CD8$^+$ T cells *in*

*vitro* occurred with lymphoblastoid cell lines expressing HLA-B*5701, but not HLA-B*5702 or HLA-B*5801. By comparing the amino acid substitutions in the antigen binding pocket among the three HLA-B polymorphisms, the investigators speculated that HLA-B*5702 and *5801 may not bind abacavir neoself peptide(s) (which was not identified) because of differences in the antigen binding cleft (Figure 17.8). Alternatively, they speculated that these HLA-B polymorphisms may bind abacavir neoself peptides, but present them in an altered configuration that is not recognized by CD8$^+$ T-cells. Further site-directed mutagenesis studies demonstrated that the amino acid substitution of a polar serine at position 116 of HLA-B*5701 to a tyrosine residue of HLA-B*5702 resulted in lack of recognition by abacavir-specific CD8$^+$ T cells. Though residue 116 is clearly critical in the hypersensitivity reaction of abacavir, the study did not identify the abacavir hapten. Collectively, the data suggest that a unique ligand(s) or neoself peptide(s) is created with abacavir and an endogenous protein(s). Importantly, there is selective binding and presentation of the abacavir neoself peptide(s) by cells expressing the HLA-B*5701, due to amino acid differences in the antigen binding cleft (Figure 17.8).

### Granulysin Produced by CD8$^+$ T-Cells is a Key Determinant of Disseminated Keratinocyte Death in Patients with SJS and TEN

Because the number of inflammatory cells that infiltrate the skin are too few to explain the toxic skin reactions that occur in SJS and TEN, Chung *et al.* [69] measured the cytotoxic molecules in blister cells from patients with allergies to amoxicillin, phenytoin and carbamazepine. Granulysin was the predominant cytotoxic molecule in the blister cells. When directly injected into mouse skin, granulysin produced extensive lesions, characterized by inflammation and necrosis, that were consistent with it being a key factor involved in drug-induced hypersensitivity reactions. In addition, depleting granulysin from blister cells attenuated the cytotoxicity.

### Drug-Induced Liver Injury (DILI) Mediated by the HLA System

Studies of polymorphisms in the HLA system and ADRs have primarily centered on drug-induced skin rashes, SJS, and TEN. However, recently it has become increasingly clear that hypersensitivity reactions may lead to other adverse drug reactions, in particular in

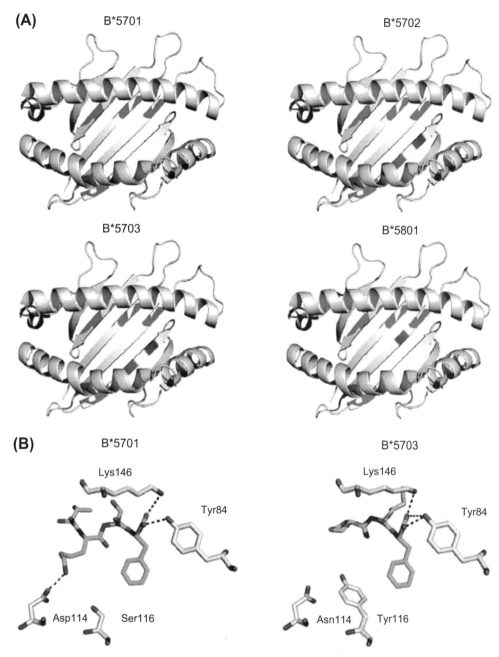

**FIGURE 17.8** Binding pocket of HLA-B*5701 compared with other HLA-B polymorphisms. (A) Abacavir-specific CD8 cells are raised *in vitro* from HLA-B*5701 donors, but not from HLA-B*5702, HLA-B*5703 or HLA-B*5801 donors. Differences in the binding pocket of the HLA polymorphisms are shown, and include variants in several amino acid residues in HLA-B*5701: Asp114 and Ser116. These are mutated to Asp114 and Tyr116 in B*5702 and B*5703. In addition, B*5702 has a polymorphism at position 156, Leu157Arg. B*5801 has distinct differences in other residues (compared with B*5701): Met45Thr, Ala46Glu, Val97Arg, Val103Leu. Selected variations are indicated as dark bands. (B) Interaction between a neoself peptide and the Asp114 is shown for HLA-B*5701, but not with the Asn114 in HLA-B*5703.

the liver [80]. Notably, Daly *et al.* [72] conducted a GWAS that showed a strong association with DILI caused by treatment with flucloxacillin. In 51 cases of flucloxacillin DILI and 282 controls, a highly significant association ($P < 8.7 \times 10^{-33}$) was identified with a genetic polymorphism (rs2395029) in complete linkage disequilibrium with HLA-B*5701 (Figure 17.9). The association of this rare adverse drug reaction was replicated in a second, smaller cohort in which HLA-B*5701 was present in 64% of the cases of

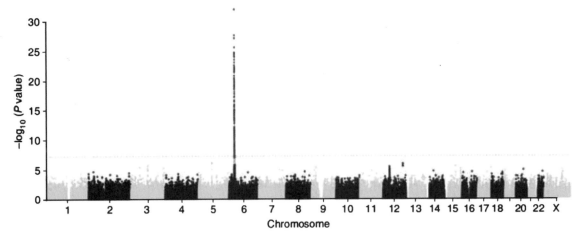

**FIGURE 17.9**  Flucloxacillin DILI GWAS result. Each dot represents a SNP. The *x*-axis represents the position of the SNP on chromosomes. The *y*-axis represents the −log10 of Cochran-Armitage trend P value of the SNP in the case–control association study. We included 51 DILI cases and 282 population controls in the study. The strong signal in chromosome 6 lies in the MHC region. Reproduced with permission from Daly, Donaldson PT, Bhatnagar P *et al.* Nat Genet 2009;41:816–9 [72].

flucloxacillin DILI. This striking association raised awareness in the field of pharmacogenomics that HLA polymorphisms may also contribute to DILI in addition to TEN and SJS.

DILI due to ximelagatran, an anticoagulant, has also been associated with an HLA polymorphism, in particular, HLA-DRB1*0701 [81]. HLA polymorphisms have been found to be associated with DILI due to administration of several drugs used in the treatment of tuberculosis, including isoniazid, rifampin, and ethambutol [82]. Since most of these reports have been published only recently, the mechanisms responsible for their polymorphism-based risk for DILI have not been elucidated, but this is likely to be the subject of considerable research in the future.

## FDA LABELING OF DRUGS FOR PHARMACOGENOMIC INFORMATION

After the draft of the human genome was published a decade ago [83, 84], there was high hope that this information could be utilized to develop personalized medicines. The past decade has seen exponential growth in research exploring the utility of this genomic information, and there has been rapid advancement in understanding the mechanisms that underlie interindividual differences in drug response, resulting in greater appreciation of the role that genetic factors play in such response. One result has been that many drugs have been relabeled to describe these new findings when they have critical implications for patient treatment. The timing of relabeling varies depending on the availability of new information, and

may occur within a few years after the drugs have been on the market, as shown for abacavir in Figure 17.10, or decades after their initial approvals, as with warfarin and codeine, which have been relabeled (Table 17.1) to include critical pharmacogenomic information 50 and 60 years, respectively, after their initial approvals.

Considerable controversy exists about the clinical utility of genomic tests and how to translate pharmacogenomic findings to useful tools in clinical practice [85–87]. Although randomized clinical trials (RCTs) have been considered as the gold standard, providing evidential basis for many interventions of medicine, there are other complementary sources of evidence (mechanistic, pharmacological, and observational studies) that can all contribute to establishing clinical utility [88, 89]. For example, the recommendation and high utility of a test for patients' HLA genotype prior to treatment with abacavir [90, 91] were based on a prospective RCT that showed associations between hypersensitivity and HLA-B*5701 [92]. On the other hand, case–control or cohort studies have identified the genetic basis of other ADRs, including in patients taking carbamazepine [93].

To transition from the discovery of a diagnostic test, such as the genetic tests related to ADRs discussed in this chapter, to their routine clinical use, key questions related to their clinical utility must be addressed, and can include the following [88]:

1. Is there an informative marker that correlates with a clinical state?
2. Does the test measure the biomarker reliably?
3. Does the test predict the clinical state?

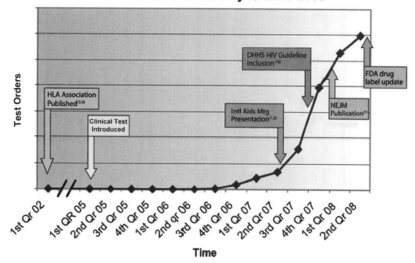

**FIGURE 17.10** HLA-B*5701 test orders received by quarter at a US-based National Reference Laboratory showing rapid adoption of the HLA-B*5701 genetic test. Adapted with permission from Lai-Goldman M, Faruki H. Genet Med 2008;10:874–8 [91].

4. Does the test provide reliable information?
5. Is the test worth doing?
6. Does the test predict the desired clinical response?
7. Is the test worth paying for?
8. Is the test worth doing in the real world, as compared with other options?

Some of the above questions have been addressed via RCTs, others via case–control, cohort studies, or clinical studies in naturalistic settings [94].

A drug's labeling may be changed after an association has been established between a gene and a drug response. This often follows intensive review of the available association data and their clinical implication at various FDA internal interdisciplinary team meetings, open public meetings such as the FDA advisory committee meetings, other public scientific debates and publications, and FDA meetings with the NDA/BLA holders of the affected drug products and with other regulatory agencies such as EMA.

After the drug labeling has been revised, many factors affect the clinical uptake and implementation of the genetic tests. These may include the knowledge of the healthcare providers, the test's availability when the drug is initially prescribed, the peer-reviewed guidelines, and the availability of alternate dosages or drugs for patients with high-risk genotypes [95]. For example, the management of hypersensitivity reactions, via the requirement of the HLA-B*5701 genotyping prior to prescription of abacavir was adopted by the HIV community as soon as strong clinical association data became available

[91], even before the FDA labeling change to include a blackbox warning about this association (Figure 17.10). On the other hand, widespread implementation of the warfarin genetic test has not occurred, and reimbursement for this test remains uncertain or restricted [96, 97] even after FDA relabeling to describe how patients' CYP2C9 and VKORC1 genotypes can affect warfarin dosing requirements. As discussed in Chapter 18, the FDA has published both procedural guidance on biomarker qualifications and recommendations related to the evaluation of pharmacogenomic associations prior to marketing approval [98, 99]. The European Medicinal Agent has also provided guidelines in these areas [100].

## THE ROLE OF SIMULATION IN ELUCIDATING PHARMACOGENOMIC ADR MECHANISMS

As most ADRs cannot be attributed to a single patient factor, it is important to understand the risks associated with multiple factors – both genetic and non-genetic. Mathematical simulations using population-based, physiological models (e.g., physiologically-based pharmacokinetic (PBPK) models) that simultaneously integrate various patient intrinsic and extrinsic factors can provide an understanding of the potential complex changes in exposure–response relationships in patients in whom multiple covariates are present. Some applications of these physiologically-based models include the design of clinical trials

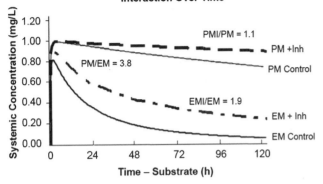

**Mean Systemic Concentration in Plasma of *S*-Warfarin With and Without Interaction Over Time**

**FIGURE 17.11** Highest ranked gene/drug pairs, based on a survey of American Society for Clinical Pharmacology and Therapeutics Members in 2010. Data related to the percentages of respondents who ranked the gene/drug pairs as 1 or 2 (on a scale of 1–5) are plotted along the *y*-axis.

to evaluate the effects of drug-metabolizing enzyme polymorphisms on pharmacokinetics and pharmacodynamics are described in Chapter 32 and have been summarized in a recent review [101]. For example,

simulations have been used to evaluate the impact of drug interactions on patients with CYP2C9 polymorphisms. Simulations indicated that co-administration of a CYP2C9 inhibitor to warfarin-treated patients who are extensive metabolizers of CYP2C9 substrates could result in a two-fold increase in the plasma levels of *S*-warfarin, the active isomer of warfarin (Figure 17.11) [102]. On the other hand, if a patient has two copies of variant alleles of CYP2C9 *3 and has been on a stable warfarin dosing regimen, co-administration of drugs that are strong inhibitors of CYP2C9 is not expected to lead to any significant increase in plasma *S*–warfarin levels.

In addition, PBPK models can be developed to simulate tissue levels at the sites of drug action, both beneficial and adverse, and evaluate their relationships (or lack thereof) with systemic exposure levels [103]. Simulations can also be used to provide hypotheses on observed clinical effects not predicted by systemic drug levels, or to provide optimal study designs to address further questions. Finally, PBPK modeling and simulation can play an important role in regulatory review, and their utility and limitations

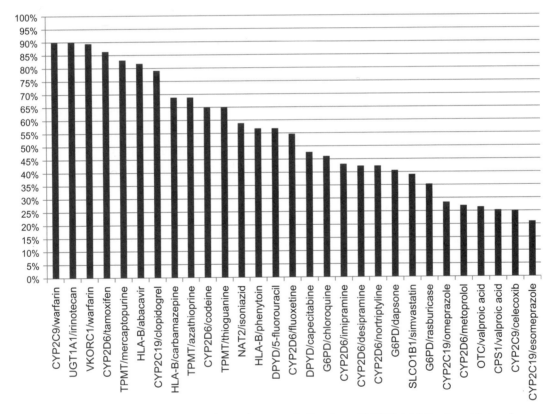

**FIGURE 17.12** Simulated inhibition of *S*-warfarin metabolism by a CYP2C9 inhibitor in subjects who are extensive vs poor metabolizers of CYP2C9 (simulation, simcyp v8.20; PM, poor metabolizer of CYP2C9; EM, extensive metabolizer of CYP2C9; male/female ratio = 1; age 20–40 years. *S*-warfarin single dose, 10 mg on Day 1, sulfaphenzole (CYP2C9 inhibitor) once a day 2000 mg for 5 days). The intrinsic clearance values for 7-hydroxy warfarin (μL/min/pmol of CYP) were assigned to be 0.034 and 0.005, for EM (*1/*1) and PM (*3/*3) of CYP2C9 respectively.

have been discussed in both FDA publications [104, 105] and in guidance documents [106].

## THE ROLE OF CONSORTIA IN ELUCIDATING PHARMACOGENOMIC ADR MECHANISMS

Various consortia have been established to address many of the priority areas related to drug safety [107]. For example, a Serious Adverse Events Consortium (SAEC) [108] is focused on understanding the genetic basis of serious ADRs such as drug-induced liver injury (DILI) and serious skin reactions. Recent studies, based on either candidate gene approaches or GWAS using DNA samples from patients taking ticlopidine, flucloxacillin, amoxicillin-clavulanate, lumiracoxib and ximelagatran, have resulted in the discovery of various HLA genotypes that can predispose individuals to DILI, and exemplify these efforts [109]. Other consortia have a general focus on drugs, such as the NIH Pharmacogenomics Research Network (PGRN) [110]; focus on specific drugs, such as the International Warfarin Pharmacogenetic Consortium [111] and the International Tamoxifen Pharmacogenetic Consortium [112]; or focus on a class of proteins, such as the International Transporter Consortium. These consortia have all demonstrated the critical need and fruitfulness of these collaborations [113, 114].

The establishment of various consortia to conduct pre-competitive research has been instrumental in identifying key pharmacogenomic mechanisms of various serious ADRs [107–109, 111, 112, 115] and in providing important guidance about the particular transporters that may need to be evaluated during drug development [88, 113, 116]. Recently, implementation consortia, such as the clinical pharmacogenetic implementation consortium, have been formed to provide peer-reviewed guidelines for gene/drug pairs [95]. Figure 17.12 shows the results of a recent survey of members of the American Society for Clinical Pharmacology and Therapeutics who were asked to rank gene/drug pairs based on their perceived importance. Many of the 29 gene/drug pairs surveyed and deemed important are related to systemic exposure changes due to genetic variations in metabolizing enzymes. Other consortia, such as the Taiwan SJS Consortium [117], provide data assessing the impact of prospective screening using pharmacogenetic tests on the occurrence of serious ADRs.

The recent implementation of active surveillance programs (e.g., the Mini-Sentinel program) [118], in addition to continual collaborations among various stakeholders (industry, academia, government agencies, health benefit management and/or consumer groups), will leverage public and private health care databases and contribute to identification of risk factors, including genomics, in specific patient groups predisposed to experiencing adverse drug reactions.

## ACKNOWLEDGEMENT

The authors would like to acknowledge support from GM61390, a grant from the National Institutes of Health.

## REFERENCES

[1] Giacomini KM, Krauss RM, Roden DM, Eichelbaum M, Hayden MR, Nakamura Y. When good drugs go bad. Nature 2007;446:975–7.

[2] Friedman MA, Woodcock J, Lumpkin MM, Shuren JE, Hass AE, Thompson LJ. The safety of newly approved medicines: Do recent market removals mean there is a problem? JAMA 1999;281:1728–34.

[3] Berndt ER, Gottschalk AH, Philipson TJ, Strobeck MW. Industry funding of the FDA: Effects of PDUFA on approval times and withdrawal rates. Nat Rev Drug Discov 2005;4(7):545–54.

[4] CDER, CBER. Safety labeling changes – implementation of section 505(o)(4) of the Federal Food, Drug, and Cosmetic Act. Guidance for Industry. Rockville, MD: FDA (Internet at, www.fda.gov/downloads/Drugs/GuidanceCompliance RegulatoryInformation/Guid, 1988. cited April 15, 2011.).

[5] CDER, CBER, CDRH. Clinical pharmacogenomics: Premarketing evaluation in early phase clinical studies. Guidance for Industry. Rockville, MD: FDA (Internet at, http://www.fda.gov/downloads/Drugs/GuidanceComplianceRegulatoryInformation/Guidances/UCM243702.pdf, 2011. cited April 7, 2011.).

[6] Amur S, Frueh FW, Lesko LJ, Huang SM. Integration and use of biomarkers in drug development, regulation and clinical practice: A US regulatory perspective. Biomark Med 2008;2(3):305–11.

[7] Woodcock J, Lesko LJ. Pharmacogenetics – tailoring treatment for the outliers. N Engl J Med 2009;360(8):811–3.

[8] Xenazine® (Tetrabenazine) [package insert issued 5/2008]. Washington, DC: Prestwick Pharmaceuticals, Inc. (Internet at, www.accessdata.fda.gov/drugsatfda_docs/label/2008/021894lbl.pdf.)

[9] Huang SM, Temple R. Is this the drug or dose for you? Impact and consideration of ethnic factors in global drug development, regulatory review, and clinical practice. Clin Pharmacol Ther 2008;84(3):287–94.

[10] Yasuda SU, Zhang L, Huang SM. The role of ethnicity in variability in response to drugs: Focus on clinical pharmacology studies. Clin Pharmacol Ther 2008;84(3):417–23.

[11] Drugs@FDA. Internet at, www.accessdata.fda.gov/scripts/cder/drugsatfda.

[12] Zaza G, Cheok M, Krynetskaia N, Thorn C, Stocco G, Hebert JM, et al. Thiopurine pathway. Pharmacogenet Genomics 2010;20(9):573–4.

[13] Otterness D, Szumlanski C, Lennard L, Klemetsdal B, Aarbakke J, Park-Hah JO, et al. Human thiopurine methyltransferase pharmacogenetics: Gene sequence polymorphisms. Clin Pharmacol Ther 1997;62(1):60–73.

[14] McLeod HL, Krynetski EY, Relling MV, Evans WE. Genetic polymorphism of thiopurine methyltransferase and its

clinical relevance for childhood acute lymphoblastic leukemia. Leukemia 2000;14(4):567–72.

[15] CDER. Pediatric Subcommittee of the Oncology Drug Advisory Committee meeting transcript. Rockville, MD: FDA (Internet at, www.fda.gov/OHRMS/DOCKETS/AC/03/transcripts/3971T1.pdf. 2003.).

[16] van den Akker-van Marle ME, Gurwitz D, Detmar SB, Enzing CM, Hopkins MM, Gutierrez de Mesa E, et al. Cost-effectiveness of pharmacogenomics in clinical practice: A case study of thiopurine methyltransferase genotyping in acute lymphoblastic leukemia in Europe. Pharmacogenomics 2006;7(5):783–92.

[17] Hanioka N, Ozawa S, Jinno H, Ando M, Saito Y, Sawada J. Human liver UDP-glucuronosyltransferase isoforms involved in the glucuronidation of 7-ethyl-10-hydroxycamptothecin. Xenobiotica 2001;31(10):687–99.

[18] Innocenti F, Undevia SD, Iyer L, Chen PX, Das S, Kocherginsky M, et al. Genetic variants in the UDP-glucuronosyltransferase 1A1 gene predict the risk of severe neutropenia of irinotecan. J Clin Oncol 2004;22(8):1382–8.

[19] CDER. Clinical Pharmacology Subcommittee of the Advisory Committee for Pharmaceutical Science. Briefing information. Gaithersburg, MD: FDA (Internet at, www.fda.gov/ohrms/dockets/ac/04/briefing/2004-4079b1.htm. 2004.).

[20] Cecchin E, Innocenti F, D'Andrea M, Corona G, De Mattia E, Biason P, et al. Predictive role of the UGT1A1, UGT1A7, and UGT1A9 genetic variants and their haplotypes on the outcome of metastatic colorectal cancer patients treated with fluorouracil, leucovorin, and irinotecan. J Clin Oncol 2009;27(15):2457–65.

[21] de Jong FA, Scott-Horton TJ, Kroetz DL, McLeod HL, Friberg LE, Mathijssen RH, et al. Irinotecan-induced diarrhea: Functional significance of the polymorphic ABCC2 transporter protein. Clin Pharmacol Ther 2007;81(1):42–9.

[22] Ho RH, Leake BF, Kilkenny DM, Meyer Zu Schwabedissen HE, Glaeser H, Kroetz DL, et al. Polymorphic variants in the human bile salt export pump (BSEP; ABCB11): Functional characterization and interindividual variability. Pharmacogenet Genomics 2010;20(1):45–57.

[23] Wilke RA, Lin DW, Roden DM, Watkins PB, Flockhart D, Zineh I, et al. Identifying genetic risk factors for serious adverse drug reactions: Current progress and challenges. Nat Rev Drug Discov 2007;6(11):904–16.

[24] Nakamura Y. Pharmacogenomics and drug toxicity. N Engl J Med 2008;359(8):856–8.

[25] Choi JH, Ahn BM, Yi J, Lee JH, Lee JH, Nam SW, et al. MRP2 haplotypes confer differential susceptibility to toxic liver injury. Pharmacogenet Genomics 2007;17(6):403–15.

[26] Neuvonen PJ, Niemi M, Backman JT. Drug interactions with lipid-lowering drugs: Mechanisms and clinical relevance. Clin Pharmacol Ther 2006;80(6):565–81.

[27] Kalliokoski A, Niemi M. Impact of OATP transporters on pharmacokinetics. Br J Pharmacol 2009;158(3):693–705.

[28] Niemi M, Pasanen MK, Neuvonen PJ. SLCO1B1 polymorphism and sex affect the pharmacokinetics of pravastatin but not fluvastatin. Clin Pharmacol Ther 2006; 80(4):356–66.

[29] Ghatak A, Faheem O, Thompson PD. The genetics of statin-induced myopathy. Atherosclerosis 2010;210(2):337–43.

[30] Staffa JA, Chang J, Green L. Cerivastatin and reports of fatal rhabdomyolysis. N Engl J Med 2002;346(7):539–40.

[31] Graham DJ, Staffa JA, Shatin D, Andrade SE, Schech SD, La Grenade L, et al. Incidence of hospitalized rhabdomyolysis in patients treated with lipid-lowering drugs. JAMA 2004;292(21):2585–90.

[32] Thompson PD, Clarkson P, Karas RH. Statin-associated myopathy. JAMA 2003;289(13):1681–90.

[33] Nishizato Y, Ieiri I, Suzuki H, Kimura M, Kawabata K, Hirota T, et al. Polymorphisms of OATP-C (SLC21A6) and OAT3 (SLC22A8) genes: Consequences for pravastatin pharmacokinetics. Clin Pharmacol Ther 2003;73(6):554–65.

[34] Mwinyi J, Johne A, Bauer S, Roots I, Gerloff T. Evidence for inverse effects of OATP-C (SLC21A6) 5 and 1b haplotypes on pravastatin kinetics. Clin Pharmacol Ther 2004; 75(5):415–21.

[35] Morimoto K, Oishi T, Ueda S, Ueda M, Hosokawa M, Chiba K. A novel variant allele of OATP-C (SLCO1B1) found in a japanese patient with pravastatin-induced myopathy. Drug Metab Pharmacokinet 2004;19(6):453–5.

[36] SEARCH Collaborative Group, Link E, Parish S, Armitage J, Bowman L, Heath S, et al. SLCO1B1 variants and statin-induced myopathy – a genomewide study. N Engl J Med 2008;359(8):789–99.

[37] Niemi M, Schaeffeler E, Lang T, Fromm MF, Neuvonen M, Kyrklund C, et al. High plasma pravastatin concentrations are associated with single nucleotide polymorphisms and haplotypes of organic anion transporting polypeptide-C (OATP-C, SLCO1B1). Pharmacogenetics 2004;14(7):429–40.

[38] Niemi M. Transporter pharmacogenetics and statin toxicity. Clin Pharmacol Ther 2010;87(1):130–3.

[39] Voora D, Shah SH, Spasojevic I, Ali S, Reed CR, Salisbury BA, et al. The SLCO1B1*5 genetic variant is associated with statin-induced side effects. J Am Coll Cardiol 2009;54(17):1609–16.

[40] Tirona RG, Leake BF, Merino G, Kim RB. Polymorphisms in OATP-C: Identification of multiple allelic variants associated with altered transport activity among European- and African-Americans. J Biol Chem 2001;276(38):35669–75.

[41] Shu Y, Leabman MK, Feng B, Mangravite LM, Huang CC, Stryke D, et al. Evolutionary conservation predicts function of variants of the human organic cation transporter, OCT1. Proc Natl Acad Sci USA 2003;100(10):5902–7.

[42] Abla N, Chinn LW, Nakamura T, Liu L, Huang CC, Johns SJ, et al. The human multidrug resistance protein 4 (MRP4, ABCC4): Functional analysis of a highly polymorphic gene. J Pharmacol Exp Ther 2008;325(3):859–68.

[43] Backman JT, Luurila H, Neuvonen M, Neuvonen PJ. Rifampin markedly decreases and gemfibrozil increases the plasma concentrations of atorvastatin and its metabolites. Clin Pharmacol Ther 2005;78(2):154–67.

[44] Neuvonen PJ. Drug interactions with HMG-CoA reductase inhibitors (statins): The importance of CYP enzymes, transporters and pharmacogenetics. Curr Opin Investig Drugs 2010;11(3):323–32.

[45] Becquemont L, Neuvonen M, Verstuyft C, Jaillon P, Letierce A, Neuvonen PJ, et al. Amiodarone interacts with simvastatin but not with pravastatin disposition kinetics. Clin Pharmacol Ther 2007;81(5):679–84.

[46] Keskitalo JE, Pasanen MK, Neuvonen PJ, Niemi M. Different effects of the ABCG2 c.421C>A SNP on the pharmacokinetics of fluvastatin, pravastatin and simvastatin. Pharmacogenomics 2009;10(10):1617–24.

[47] Keskitalo JE, Zolk O, Fromm MF, Kurkinen KJ, Neuvonen PJ, Niemi M. ABCG2 polymorphism markedly affects the pharmacokinetics of atorvastatin and rosuvastatin. Clin Pharmacol Ther 2009;86(2):197–203.

[48] Zocor, Simvastatin [package insert issued 6/2011]. Cramlington, UK: Merck Sharp & Dohme. (Internet at, www.accessdata.fda.gov/drugsatfda_docs/label/2011/019766s077s082lbl.pdf.)

[49] Neuvonen PJ, Backman JT, Niemi M. Pharmacokinetic comparison of the potential over-the-counter statins simvastatin, lovastatin, fluvastatin and pravastatin. Clin Pharmacokinet 2008;47(7):463–74.

[50] Fernandez-Fernandez B, Montoya-Ferrer A, Sanz AB, Sanchez-Nino MD, Izquierdo MC, Poveda J, et al. Tenofovir nephrotoxicity: 2011 update. AIDS Res Treat 2011;2011:354908.

[51] Rodriguez-Novoa S, Labarga P, Soriano V. Pharmacogenetics of tenofovir treatment. Pharmacogenomics 2009; 10(10):1675–85.

[52] Cooper RD, Wiebe N, Smith N, Keiser P, Naicker S, Tonelli M. Systematic review and meta-analysis: Renal safety of

tenofovir disoproxil fumarate in HIV-infected patients. Clin Infect Dis 2010;51(5):496–505.

[53] Izzedine H, Isnard-Bagnis C, Hulot JS, Vittecoq D, Cheng A, Jais CK, et al. Renal safety of tenofovir in HIV treatment-experienced patients. AIDS 2004;18(7):1074–6.

[54] Earle KE, Seneviratne T, Shaker J, Shoback D. Fanconi's syndrome in HIV+ adults: Report of three cases and literature review. J Bone Miner Res 2004;19(5):714–21.

[55] Birkus G, Hitchcock MJ, Cihlar T. Assessment of mitochondrial toxicity in human cells treated with tenofovir: Comparison with other nucleoside reverse transcriptase inhibitors. Antimicrob Agents Chemother 2002;46(3):716–23.

[56] Martin JL, Brown CE, Matthews-Davis N, Reardon JE. Effects of antiviral nucleoside analogs on human DNA polymerases and mitochondrial DNA synthesis. Antimicrob Agents Chemother 1994;38(12):2743–9.

[57] Gayet-Ageron A, Ananworanich J, Jupimai T, Chetchotisakd P, Prasithsirikul W, Ubolyam S, et al. No change in calculated creatinine clearance after tenofovir initiation among Thai patients. J Antimicrob Chemother 2007;59(5):1034–7.

[58] Klaassen CD, Aleksunes LM. Xenobiotic, bile acid, and cholesterol transporters: Function and regulation. Pharmacol Rev 2010;62(1):1–96.

[59] Labarga P, Barreiro P, Martin-Carbonero L, Rodriguez-Novoa S, Solera C, Medrano J, et al. Kidney tubular abnormalities in the absence of impaired glomerular function in HIV patients treated with tenofovir. AIDS 2009;23(6):689–96.

[60] Rodriguez-Novoa S, Labarga P, Soriano V, Egan D, Albalater M, Morello J, et al. Predictors of kidney tubular dysfunction in HIV-infected patients treated with tenofovir: A pharmacogenetic study. Clin Infect Dis 2009;48(11):e108–16.

[61] Izzedine H, Hulot JS, Villard E, Goyenvalle C, Dominguez S, Ghosn J, et al. Association between ABCC2 gene haplotypes and tenofovir-induced proximal tubulopathy. J Infect Dis 2006;194(11):1481–91.

[62] Kiser JJ, Carten ML, Aquilante CL, Anderson PL, Wolfe P, King TM, et al. The effect of lopinavir/ritonavir on the renal clearance of tenofovir in HIV-infected patients. Clin Pharmacol Ther 2008;83(2):265–72.

[63] Pushpakom SP, Liptrott NJ, Rodriguez-Novoa S, Labarga P, Soriano V, Albalater M, et al. Genetic variants of ABCC10, a novel tenofovir transporter, are associated with kidney tubular dysfunction. J Infect Dis 2011;204(1):145–53.

[64] Kiser JJ, Aquilante CL, Anderson PL, King TM, Carten ML, Fletcher CV. Clinical and genetic determinants of intracellular tenofovir diphosphate concentrations in HIV-infected patients. J Acquir Immune Defic Syndr 2008;47(3):298–303.

[65] Anderson PL, Lamba J, Aquilante CL, Schuetz E, Fletcher CV. Pharmacogenetic characteristics of indinavir, zidovudine, and lamivudine therapy in HIV-infected adults: A pilot study. J Acquir Immune Defic Syndr 2006;42(4):441–9.

[66] Yuan HY, Chiou JJ, Tseng WH, Liu CH, Liu CK, Lin YJ, et al. FASTSNP: An always up-to-date and extendable service for SNP function analysis and prioritization. Nucleic Acids Res 2006;34(Web Server issue):W635–41.

[67] Madeddu G, Bonfanti P, De Socio GV, Carradori S, Grosso C, Marconi P, et al. Tenofovir renal safety in HIV-infected patients: Results from the SCOLTA project. Biomed Pharmacother 2008;62(1):6–11.

[68] Zimmermann AE, Pizzoferrato T, Bedford J, Morris A, Hoffman R, Braden G. Tenofovir-associated acute and chronic kidney disease: A case of multiple drug interactions. Clin Infect Dis 2006;42(2):283–90.

[69] Chung WH, Hung SI, Hong HS, Hsih MS, Yang LC, Ho HC, et al. Medical genetics: A marker for Stevens-Johnson syndrome. Nature 2004;428:486.

[70] Hetherington S, Hughes AR, Mosteller M, Shortino D, Baker KL, Spreen W, et al. Genetic variations in HLA-B region and hypersensitivity reactions to abacavir. Lancet 2002;359(9312):1121–2.

[71] Tassaneeyakul W, Tiamkao S, Jantararoungtong T, Chen P, Lin SY, Chen WH, et al. Association between HLA-B*1502 and carbamazepine-induced severe cutaneous adverse drug reactions in a Thai population. Epilepsia 2010;51(5):926–30.

[72] Daly AK, Donaldson PT, Bhatnagar P, Shen Y, Pe'er I, Floratos A, et al. HLA-B*5701 genotype is a major determinant of drug-induced liver injury due to flucloxacillin. Nat Genet 2009;41:816–9.

[73] Brown MA, Crane AM, Wordsworth BP. Genetic aspects of susceptibility, severity, and clinical expression in ankylosing spondylitis. Curr Opin Rheumatol 2002;14(4):354–60.

[74] Colmegna I, Cuchacovich R, Espinoza LR. HLA-B27-associated reactive arthritis: Pathogenetic and clinical considerations. Clin Microbiol Rev 2004;17(2):348–69.

[75] Carrington M, O'Brien SJ. The influence of HLA genotype on AIDS. Annu Rev Med 2003;54:535–51.

[76] Pichler WJ, Naisbitt DJ, Park BK. Immune pathomechanism of drug hypersensitivity reactions. J Allergy Clin Immunol 2011;127(Suppl 3.):S74–81.

[77] Martin AM, Nolan D, Gaudieri S, Almeida CA, Nolan R, James I, et al. Predisposition to abacavir hypersensitivity conferred by HLA-B*5701 and a haplotypic Hsp70-hom variant. Proc Natl Acad Sci USA 2004;101:4180–5.

[78] Hughes AR, Mosteller M, Bansal AT, Davies K, Haneline SA, Lai EH, et al. Association of genetic variations in HLA-B region with hypersensitivity to abacavir in some, but not all, populations. Pharmacogenomics 2004;5(2):203–11.

[79] Chessman D, Kostenko L, Lethborg T, Purcell AW, Williamson NA, Chen Z, et al. Human leukocyte antigen class I-restricted activation of CD8$^+$ T Cells provides the immunogenetic basis of a systemic drug hypersensitivity. Immunity 2008;28:822–32.

[80] Posadas SJ, Pichler WJ. Delayed drug hypersensitivity reactions – new concepts. Clin Exp Allergy 2007;37:989–99.

[81] Kindmark A, Jawaid A, Harbron CG, Barratt BJ, Bengtsson OF, Andersson TB, et al. Genome-wide pharmacogenetic investigation of a hepatic adverse event without clinical signs of immunopathology suggests an underlying immune pathogenesis. Pharmacogenomics J 2008;8:186–95.

[82] Sharma SK, Balamurugan A, Saha PK, Pandey RM, Mehra NK. Evaluation of clinical and immunogenetic risk factors for the development of hepatotoxicity during antituberculosis treatment. Am J Respir Crit Care Med 2002;166:916–9.

[83] Venter JC, Adams MD, Myers EW, Li PW, Mural RJ, Sutton GG, et al. The sequence of the human genome. Science 2001;291(5507):1304–51.

[84] Lander ES, Linton LM, Birren B, Nusbaum C, Zody MC, Baldwin J, et al. Initial sequencing and analysis of the human genome. Nature 2001;409(6822):860–921.

[85] Lesko LJ, Zineh I, Huang SM. What is clinical utility and why should we care? Clin Pharmacol Ther 2010;88(6):729–33.

[86] O'Kane D. An outsider's viewpoint: The FDA should regulate clinical pharmacogenetic/genomic tests, but... Clin Pharmacol Ther 2010;88(6):746–8.

[87] Epstein RS. Pharmacy benefit managers: Evaluating clinical utility in the real world. Clin Pharmacol Ther 2010;88(6):880–2.

[88] Woodcock J. Assessing the clinical utility of diagnostics used in drug therapy. Clin Pharmacol Ther 2010;88(6):765–73.

[89] Temple R. Enrichment of clinical study populations. Clin Pharmacol Ther 2010;88(6):774–8.

[90] ZIAGEN®, Abacavir sulfate [package insert, issued 2008]. Research Triangle Park, NC: GlaxoSmithKline. (Internet at, www.accessdata.fda.gov/drugsatfda_docs/label/2008/020977s019, 020978s022lbl.pdf, accessed April 15, 2011.)

[91] Lai-Goldman M, Faruki H. Abacavir hypersensitivity: A model system for pharmacogenetic test adoption. Genet Med 2008;10(12):874–8.

[92] Mallal S, Nolan D, Witt C, Masel G, Martin AM, Moore C, et al. Association between presence of HLA-B*5701, HLA-DR7, and HLA-DQ3 and hypersensitivity to HIV-1 reverse-transcriptase inhibitor abacavir. Lancet 2002;359:727–32.

[93] Hung S, Chung W, Chen Y. HLA-B genotyping to detect carbamazepine-induced Stevens-Johnson syndrome: Implications for personalizing medicine. Pers Med 2005;2(3):225–37.

[94] Epstein RS, Moyer TP, Aubert RE, O, Kane DJ, Xia F, et al. Warfarin genotyping reduces hospitalization rates results from the MM-WES (Medco-Mayo Warfarin Effectiveness Study). J Am Coll Cardiol 2010;55(25):2804–12.

[95] Relling MV, Klein TE. CPIC: Clinical pharmacogenetics implementation consortium of the pharmacogenomics research network. Clin Pharmacol Ther 2011;89(3):464–7.

[96] CMS. Pharmacogenomic testing for warfarin response. Medicare Learning Network Matters (Internet at, www.cms.gov/MLNMattersArticles/downloads/MM6715.pdf, 2010. accessed April 15, 2011.).

[97] Ansell J, Hirsh J, Hylek E, Jacobson A, Crowther M, Palareti G, et al. Pharmacology and management of the vitamin K antagonists: American College of Chest Physicians evidence-based clinical practice guidelines (8th edition). Chest 2008;133(Suppl 6.):160S–98S.

[98] CDER. Qualification process for drug development tools. Guidance for Industry. Rockville, MD: FDA (Internet at, www.fda.gov/downloads/Drugs/GuidanceCompliance RegulatoryInformation/Guidances/UCM230597.pdf. 2010.).

[99] CDER, CBER, CDRH. Clinical Pharmacogenomics: Premarketing evaluation in early phase clinical studies. Guidance for Industry. Rockville, MD: FDA (Internet at, www.fda.gov/downloads/Drugs/GuidanceComplianceRegulatory Information/Guidances/UCM243702.pdf, 2011. cited April 15, 2011.).

[100] European Medicines Agency (EMA). Guideline on the use of pharmacogenetic methodologies in the pharmacokinetic evaluation of medicinal products. London: EMA (Internet at, www.ema.europa.eu/docs/en_GB/document_library/Scientific_guideline/2010/05/WC500090323.pdf. 2010.).

[101] Rowland M, Peck C, Tucker G. Physiologically-based pharmacokinetics in drug development and regulatory science. Annu Rev Pharmacol Toxicol 2011;51:45–73.

[102] Zhao P, Zhang L, Lesko L, Huang SM. Evaluating complex drug–drug interactions using modeling and simulations: Application and challenges in regulatory review. Presentation at the Land o' Lakes Conference on Drug Metabolism/Applied Pharmacokinetics, Merrimac, WI: September 17, 2009.

[103] Watanabe T, Kusuhara H, Maeda K, Shitara Y, Sugiyama Y. Physiologically based pharmacokinetic modeling to predict transporter-mediated clearance and distribution of pravastatin in humans. J Pharmacol Exp Ther 2009;328(2):652–62.

[104] Zhao P, Zhang L, Grillo JA, Liu Q, Bullock JM, Moon YJ, et al. Applications of physiologically based pharmacokinetic (PBPK) modeling and simulation during regulatory review. Clin Pharmacol Ther 2011;89(2):259–67.

[105] Huang S, Rowland M. The role of physiologically-based pharmacokinetic modeling in regulatory review. Clin Pharmacol Ther 2012 (in press).

[106] CDER, CBER. Study design, data analysis, and implications for dosing and labeling. Draft Guidance. Rockville, MD: FDA (Internet at, www.fda.gov/downloads/Drugs/GuidanceComplianceRegulatoryInformation/Guidances/ucm072101.pdf, 2006. cited April 7, 2011.).

[107] Buckman S, Huang SM, Murphy S. Medical product development and regulatory science for the 21st century: The critical path vision and its impact on health care. Clin Pharmacol Ther 2007;81(2):141–4.

[108] The International Serious Adverse Event Consortium (Internet at, www.saeconsortium.org/2011.).

[109] Aithal GP, Daly AK. Preempting and preventing drug-induced liver injury. Nat Genet 2010;42(8):650–1.

[110] Giacomini KM, Brett CM, Altman RB, Benowitz NL, Dolan ME, Flockhart DA, et al. The pharmacogenetics research network: From SNP discovery to clinical drug response. Clin Pharmacol Ther 2007;81(3):328–45.

[111] International Warfarin Pharmacogenetics Consortium, Klein TE, Altman RB, Eriksson N, Gage BF, Kimmel SE, et al. Estimation of the warfarin dose with clinical and pharmacogenetic data. N Engl J Med 2009;360(8):753–64.

[112] The International Tamoxifen Pharmacogenomics Consortium (Internet at, www.pharmgkb.org/contributors/consortia/itpc_profile.jsp. 2011.).

[113] Huang SM, Zhang L, Giacomini KM. The International Transporter Consortium: A collaborative group of scientists from academia, industry, and the FDA. Clin Pharmacol Ther 2010;87(1):32–6.

[114] Huang SM, Woodcock J. Transporters in drug development: Advancing on the critical path. Nat Rev Drug Discov 2010;9(3):175–6.

[115] Dieterle F, Sistare F, Goodsaid F, Papaluca M, Ozer JS, Webb CP, et al. Renal biomarker qualification submission: A dialog between the FDA-EMEA and Predictive Safety Testing Consortium. Nat Biotechnol 2010;28(5):455–62.

[116] International Transporter Consortium, Giacomini KM, Huang SM, Tweedie DJ, Benet LZ, Brouwer KL, et al. Membrane transporters in drug development. Nat Rev Drug Discov 2010;9(3):215–36.

[117] Chen P, Lin JJ, Lu CS, Ong CT, Hsieh PF, Yang CC, et al. Carbamazepine-induced toxic effects and HLA-B*1502 screening in taiwan. N Engl J Med 2011;364(12):1126–33.

[118] Behrman RE, Benner JS, Brown JS, McClellan M, Woodcock J, Platt R. Developing the sentinel system – a national resource for evidence development. N Engl J Med 2011;364(6):498–9.

[119] Roberts RL, Gearry RB, Barclay ML, Kennedy MA. IMPDH1 promoter mutations in a patient exhibiting azathioprine resistance. Pharmacogenomics J 2007;7(5):312–7.

[120] Dubinsky MC, Feldman EJ, Abreu MT, Targan SR, Vasiliauskas EA. Thioguanine: A potential alternate thiopurine for IBD patients allergic to 6-mercaptopurine or azathioprine. Am J Gastroenterol 2003;98(5):1058–63.

[121] Klein TE, Chang JT, Cho MK, Easton KL, Fergerson R, Hewett M, et al. Integrating genotype and phenotype information: An overview of the PharmGKB project. Pharmacogenomics J 2001;1:167–70.

[122] de Jong FA, van der Bol JM, Mathijssen RH, van Gelder T, Wiemer EA, Sparreboom A, et al. Renal function as a predictor of irinotecan-induced neutropenia. Clin Pharmacol Ther 2008;84(2):254–62.

[123] van der Bol JM, Mathijssen RH, Loos WJ, Friberg LE, van Schaik RH, de Jonge MJ, et al. Cigarette smoking and irinotecan treatment: Pharmacokinetic interaction and effects on neutropenia. J Clin Oncol 2007;25(19):2719–26.

[124] Pasanen MK, Neuvonen M, Neuvonen PJ, Niemi M. SLCO1B1 polymorphism markedly affects the pharmacokinetics of simvastatin acid. Pharmacogenet Genomics 2006;16(12):873–9.

[125] Laechelt S, Turrini E, Ruehmkorf A, Siegmund W, Cascorbi I, Haenisch S. Impact of ABCC2 haplotypes on transcriptional and posttranscriptional gene regulation and function. Pharmacogenomics J 2011;11(1):25–34.

[126] Megaraj V, Zhao T, Paumi CM, Gerk PM, Kim RB, Vore M. Functional analysis of nonsynonymous single nucleotide polymorphisms of multidrug resistance-associated protein 2 (ABCC2). Pharmacogenet Genomics 2011;21(8):506–15.

[127] Kim RB, Leake BF, Choo EF, Dresser GK, Kubba SV, Schwarz UI, et al. Identification of functionally variant MDR1 alleles among European Americans and African Americans. Clin Pharmacol Ther 2001;70(2):189–99.

[128] Fujita T, Brown C, Carlson EJ, Taylor T, de la Cruz M, Johns SJ, et al. Functional analysis of polymorphisms in the organic anion transporter, SLC22A6 (OAT1). Pharmacogenet Genomics 2005;15(4):201–9.

# ASSESSMENT OF DRUG EFFECTS

# 18

# Physiological and Laboratory Markers of Drug Effect

Janet Woodcock[1], Arthur J. Atkinson, Jr.[2] and Paul Rolan[3]

[1]Center for Drug Evaluation and Research, US Food and Drug Administration, Silver Spring, MD 20903
[2]Department of Molecular Pharmacology & Biochemistry, Feinberg School of Medicine, Northwestern University, Chicago, IL 60611
[3]Discipline of Pharmacology, School of Medical Sciences, University of Adelaide, Adelaide, Australia 5005

## CONCEPTUAL FRAMEWORK

The selection and measurement of relevant drug effects is an important part of clinical pharmacology. *Clinical endpoints*, defined as characteristics that directly measure how a patient feels, functions, or survives, have been traditionally used to evaluate the impact of drug therapy [1]. Clinical endpoints are quantifiable outcomes, such as survival, myocardial infarction, stroke, bone fracture, jaundice, anuria, or recurrence of cancer. However, these endpoints have obvious disadvantages when used to monitor patient response to drug therapy. As a result, these endpoints are routinely supplemented by more accessible and informative laboratory and physiological *biomarkers*. The term *biomarker* has been formally defined as "a characteristic that is objectively measured and evaluated as an indicator of normal biologic processes, pathogenic processes, or pharmacologic responses to a therapeutic intervention" [1]. A biomarker could be an analyte in blood or some other body fluid, an image, or the result of some other test (EEG, ECG, etc.); however, in all cases, it must be quantifiable. Biomarkers do not directly measure how patients feel, function, or survive, but are expected to have a mechanistic relationship to such outcomes.

Biomarkers are used widely in clinical medicine. Diagnostic biomarkers are frequently used to detect or confirm the presence of disease. Prognostic biomarkers can categorize various risk strata within a particular disease. Drug-response biomarkers (also known as *classifiers*) can be used to identify people with a higher probability of positive or negative response to a drug. Biomarkers are also frequently used to monitor response to treatment. A single biomarker can be used in many ways. For example, blood pressure is a biomarker that often is used in clinical practice to diagnose hypertension, assess the risk of stroke and other hypertension-related cardiovascular complications, evaluate the response to antihypertensive drugs, and assess hypotension in patients with shock or who are receiving a variety of drugs that may lower blood pressure (e.g. intravenous morphine for pain). Thus, this single biomarker (blood pressure), depending on the context, can provide many different types of information.

Because biomarkers can be assessed more easily and rapidly than many clinical endpoints and because they are often more informative about pharmacologic processes, they are playing an increasingly central role in pharmaceutical development [2]. During early clinical development, biomarkers are often used to define specific patient subsets for inclusion or exclusion in trials and to assess whether a candidate drug has the anticipated receptor binding or pharmacodynamic effects (so-called proof of mechanism). They are also widely used to assess drug safety. During later development, biomarkers are often used to provide a preliminary assessment of drug efficacy and to monitor for organ toxicity. In a few cases, biomarkers may be accepted as *surrogate endpoints* (i.e., as substitutes for clinical effect) for regulatory approval.

A great deal of attention has been paid to using biomarkers as surrogate endpoints. Nevertheless, in future drug development it is likely that biomarkers will be used much more commonly for patient selection, proof of concept and of mechanism, pharmacodynamic assessment, and safety monitoring than as surrogate endpoints. Unfortunately, the controversy surrounding the use of surrogate endpoints has obscured the need to develop evidence to support the use of biomarkers in these settings. More recently, it has become clear that the utility of a biomarker (whether as a surrogate endpoint or other use) must be evaluated in relation to its intended use and demonstrated to be *fit for purpose* before regulatory adoption. Thus, the appropriate use of a biomarker or a surrogate endpoint is context-dependent – contingent on the extent to which the biomarker has been validated and qualified for its intended use [3, 4]. *Validation*, in this context, refers to the process of demonstrating that a biomarker can be reliably measured with sufficient reliability for its intended use, and includes the characterization of measurement performance in terms of sensitivity, specificity, and reproducibility. *Qualification* encompasses the evidentiary process of linking a biomarker with biological processes and clinical endpoints (Table 18.1). *Clinical utility* is a final evidentiary standard for evaluating biomarkers that are intended for use with a specific drug in patient care [5]. Examples of some commonly used biomarkers and surrogate endpoints are listed, along with clinical endpoints for several therapeutic drug classes, in Table 18.2.

**TABLE 18.1  Definition of Biomarker and Endpoint Terms[a]**

| | |
|---|---|
| Clinical endpoint | A characteristic or variable that reflects how a patient feels, functions, or survives. |
| Biological marker (**biomarker**) | A characteristic that is objectively measured and evaluated as an indicator of normal biologic processes, pathogenic processes, or pharmacologic responses to an intervention. |
| Surrogate endpoint | A biomarker intended to substitute for a clinically meaningful endpoint. A surrogate endpoint is expected to predict clinical benefit (or harm, or lack of benefit) based on epidemiologic, therapeutic, pathophysiologic, or other scientific evidence. |
| Analytical validation | Assessing an assay and its measurement performance characteristics, determining the range of conditions under which the assay will give reproducible and accurate data. |
| Qualification | The evidentiary process of linking a biomarker with biological processes and clinical endpoints. |
| Utilization | Contextual analysis based on proposed use and applicability of available evidence, including analytical validation and qualification, to support this use. |

[a]The term *surrogate marker* is not included in this table and its use is discouraged because it can cause confusion by suggesting that the substitution is for a marker rather than for a clinical endpoint. See Biomarkers Definitions Working Group. Clin Pharmacol Ther 2001;69:89–95 [1].

## IDENTIFICATION AND EVALUATION OF BIOMARKERS

Most of the traditional biomarkers listed in Table 18.2 were identified in studies of pathophysiology and epidemiology that demonstrated an association between the marker and the presence or prognosis of the underlying clinical condition. Often, these markers were studied for decades prior to regulatory adoption.

**TABLE 18.2  Examples of Biomarkers and Surrogate Endpoints**

| | Therapeutic class | Biomarker/surrogate | Clinical endpoint |
|---|---|---|---|
| **Physiologic Markers** | Antihypertensive drugs | ↓ Blood pressure | ↓ Stroke |
| | Drugs for glaucoma | ↓ Intraocular pressure | Preservation of vision |
| | Drugs for osteoporosis | ↑ Bone density | ↓ Fracture rate |
| | antiarrhythmic drugs | ↓ Arrhythmias | ↑ Survival |
| **Laboratory Markers** | Antibiotics | Negative culture | Clinical cure |
| | Antiretroviral drugs | ↑ CD4 count, ↓ Viral RNA | ↑ Survival |
| | Antidiabetic drugs | ↓ Blood glucose | ↓ Morbidity |
| | Lipid-lowering drugs | ↓ Cholesterol | ↓ Coronary artery disease |
| | Drugs for prostate cancer | ↓ Prostate-specific antigen | Tumor response |

More recently developed biomarkers are likely to have originated with the identification of a serum protein, gene sequence, gene expression profile, or imaging technique that was linked to a particular physiologic state, disease, or condition.

Newly discovered candidate biomarkers typically follow a similar life cycle [5]. After their discovery in academic laboratories and introduction to the biomedical community through scientific publications, they are initially used in research laboratories. Confirmation of the initial findings through additional academic studies subsequently leads to their increasing use, first by medical specialists, then in more general medical practice after their provision by commercial laboratories as laboratory developed tests. These commercial laboratories usually conduct analytical validation of the marker and may participate in academic studies of its performance. However, formal demonstration of clinical utility is seldom undertaken, and reliance is placed on the haphazard evidence that accumulates through clinical use. As a result, the appropriate clinical use of many biomarkers remains controversial, despite their long-standing widespread incorporation into clinical practice. Such biomarkers have not been adopted for regulatory use because they lack the objective evidence that is needed for this purpose. In fact, the standards for biomarker adoption for various purposes have not been well established. The Institute of Medicine (IOM) has outlined an evaluation framework, shown schematically in Figure 18.1, by which candidate biomarkers can be evaluated with respect to the critical components of analytical validity, qualification, and intended use [6]. However, the evidentiary threshold for use in regulatory or clinical decision-making remains controversial.

## Biomarker Discovery

Fields as disparate as physics and genomics are providing candidate biomarkers that are unprecedented in their power and specificity [5]. In some cases, biomarkers are developed on the basis of drug-metabolizing enzyme polymorphisms, known as Mendelian disorders or virus sequences, that have previously been well characterized. As a result, the association of the biomarker with a clinical state has already been established and assay development can be relatively straightforward and rapid. In most cases, the discovery process entails developing diagnostic and assessment methods that are not simply building on known biological relationships. In these instances, substantial scientific work is needed to establish correlations between the candidate marker and

a particular clinical event or disease state. Given the complexity of genotype–phenotype interactions in health and disease, it is likely that systems biology approaches will play an increasing role in the mechanistic evaluation of candidate biomarkers, as well as in identifying targets for new therapies [7].

## Analytical Validation

*Analytical validation* is defined as an assessment of assays and their measurement performance [6]. The validation process includes characterizing the accuracy, precision, bias, and inter-operator variability of the candidate biomarker assay, as well as its performance under a range of conditions that may affect its ability to give reliable and reproducible results. The wide array of biomarker formats presents a corresponding diversity of qualification challenges. Analytical validation is relatively straightforward in the case of the drug concentration measurements in biological fluids that are a widely used substitute for clinical endpoints in the regulatory evaluation of generic drug products. The FDA has provided guidance on bioanalytical methods for developing both assays that use the established chromatographic and mass spectrometric methods described in Chapter 12,

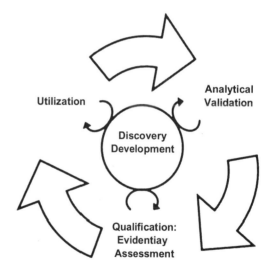

**FIGURE 18.1** Proposed framework for evaluating biomarkers. The individual steps in the evaluation process are interdependent. For example, while analytical validation is required before qualification and utilization can be completed, biomarker uses may impose new analytical requirements, and biomarker use may indicate the need to evaluate more evidence. The circle in the center indicates ongoing processes that should continually inform each evaluation step. Reproduced with permission from Institute of Medicine Committee on Qualification of Biomarkers and Surrogate Endpoints in Chronic Disease, Michael CM, Ball JR, editors. Evaluation of biomarkers and surrogate endpoints in chronic disease. Washington, DC: The National Academies Press; 2010 [6].

as well as for those that are based on immunological and microbiological procedures [8]. Nevertheless, many recently developed biomarkers typically have more complex validation pathways. For example, the AIDS Clinical Trials Group has implemented rigorous programs for standardization and quality control of biomarker measurements in patients with HIV-1 infection [9]. A more recent example is the testing for HER2 status, which is now recommended for all patients with breast cancer since overexpression of this protein is a prerequisite for patients to be treated with trastuzumab (Herceptin™). Out of the multiplicity of tests initially developed by research laboratories, measurement of HER2 protein by immunohisto-chemistry (IHC) and HER2 gene amplification by fluorescence *in-situ* hybridization (FISH) emerged as the preferred analytical procedures [10]. There has been considerable debate about the choice and conduct of these procedures – even about whether to perform testing when breast cancer is first diagnosed, or only after metastases have occurred. Early attempts to improve the quality of HER2 testing included identifying the need for a standard reference material to be developed for proficiency testing and standard-ization of results [11]. Even as recently as 2007, it was estimated that about 20% of HER2 testing was inac-curate, and an expert panel was convened to recom-mend detailed guidelines for both the conduct of IHC and FISH testing and the interpretation of testing results [12].

The validation of imaging biomarkers for evalu-ating tumor response involves even greater complexity. Although validation is particularly chal-lenging for newly introduced imaging modalities, such as diffusion-weighted magnetic resonance imaging, where an anatomical truth standard often cannot be used for comparison [13], it also remains a challenge for more established imaging techniques, like computed tomography, magnetic resonance imaging, and flurodeoxyglucose positron emission tomography [14]. Consequently, the approach to formulating recommendations and guidelines for validating these imaging biomarkers has been based on the consensus developed by panels of experts.

## Qualification

Biomarker qualification requires some level of consensus [15]. The traditional qualification of biomarkers has been haphazard, in that no structured pathway has been followed to accumulate the evidence needed to link biomarkers with biological processes and clinical endpoints. In many instances, epidemio-logic studies initially established the prognostic utility

of candidate biomarkers and provided a measure of mechanistic plausibility. Subsequent statistical analysis of therapeutic interventions in clinical trials then generated further consensus around the appropriate role of candidate biomarkers.

The important role that biomarkers currently play in drug development has generated increasing interest in qualifying new biomarkers, creating the need for a formal, evidence-based regulatory path for advancing candidate biomarkers from their initial exploratory introduction to context-dependent clinical qualification [16]. In response to this need, the FDA has issued draft guidance for the qualification of biomarkers and patient-reported outcomes that outlines a new two-stage regulatory process that is independent of the development of specific drugs [16]. In the initial stage, the FDA encourages sponsors to consult with the agency about the data that will be needed for qualification. The sponsor is asked to describe the biomarker, its context of use, available data supporting this use, and the proposed additional studies to support qualification in the given context. The second stage involves submission and regulatory review of the results from the agreed-upon studies, which would be followed by a letter of qualification from the FDA if the data were found sufficient. This process is intended to support the qualification of global, rather than product-specific, fitness for use, and is best suited for sponsors who represent a consortium of interested parties and who can integrate pre-existing data and fill gaps in the infor-mation that is initially available [5, 17]. Qualification will allow the biomarker to be used in regulatory submissions, in the qualified setting, without addi-tional data submission. The FDA is working closely with the European Medicines Agency (EMA), which has also established a qualification process. The first biomarkers qualified through this process were urinary protein biomarkers for early identification of glomerular and tubular nephrotoxicity in rat studies. The biomarkers were submitted by the Critical Path Institute's Predictive Safety Testing Consortium [18]. Further studies should enable these biomarkers to be qualified for additional uses, such as for determining whether a drug is safe for human use, for monitoring drug toxicity during clinical use, or even as the basis for approving less nephrotoxic drugs.

## Surrogate Endpoints

A particularly high level of evidentiary stringency and consensus is required when a biomarker response is substituted for a clinical outcome and is used as the basis for regulatory approval of an application to market a new drug. For this reason, very few biomarkers have been qualified to serve as surrogate endpoints. Blood pressure and serum cholesterol level are the only surrogate endpoints currently being used as a basis for new drug approvals (i.e., cardiovascular drugs) [19]. Perhaps the most widely used surrogate endpoint is the substitution of drug concentration measurements for clinical endpoints in the registration of new formulations and generic drug products [20]. Acceptance of this surrogate is based on very strong evidence about the relationship between drug concentration and drug effect for systemically acting drugs. This surrogate is also used for evaluating the effect of manufacturing changes for innovator drugs.

Enthusiasm about using surrogate endpoints for demonstrating efficacy for regulatory approval has waxed and waned over the decades. In a number of clinical trials, initial conclusions based on the response of a candidate surrogate endpoint were not borne out by the subsequent clinical response. These unexpected results have fueled concerns that many proposed surrogate endpoints may not accurately predict meaningful clinical outcomes [21–23]. The Cardiac Arrhythmia Suppression Trial (CAST) offers the most notable example of this concern. In this trial, a dichotomy was found between suppression of ventricular ectopy and increased mortality in patients who received long-term therapy with antiarrhythmic drugs [24]. The impetus for the trial was the fact that patients who have sustained a myocardial infarction, and subsequently have ventricular ectopy with more than 10 premature ventricular depolarizations per hour, have a four-fold increase in mortality rate. A total of 1498 patients were entered in the trial and were randomized to receive encainide, flecainide, or placebo. After a mean treatment period of 10 months, the safety monitoring board stopped the trial because 63 patients died while receiving these antiarrhythmic drugs whereas only 26 placebo-treated patients had died ($P = 0.0001$). Although complete understanding of the mechanisms underlying the excess mortality is lacking, it is presumed that the adverse pro-arrhythmic effects of drug therapy outweighed the benefit provided by the intended suppression of arrhythmias resulting from underlying cardiac disease (Figure 18.2). Supporting this interpretation is the finding that patients receiving antiarrhythmic drugs had an increased incidence of fatal arrhythmias and of shock after recurrent myocardial infarction.

Statistical approaches have played an important role in assessing the predictive utility of surrogate endpoints (*criterion validity*). Prentice [25] initially proposed that the ideal substitute for a clinical endpoint should completely capture the relationship between the treatment and the true endpoint. However, this expectation is unrealistic given the multidimensionality of pathogenic factors underlying patient outcomes, as illustrated by the relationship between hypertension, antihypertensive therapy, and the incidence of coronary heart disease (Figure 18.3). To address this complexity, Shatzkin *et al.* [26] proposed a means for calculating the extent to which response measured by the clinical endpoint can be attributed to a biomarker. Their formula for calculating this *attributable proportion (AP)* is:

$$AP = S\left(1 - \frac{1}{R}\right)$$

where $S$ is the sensitivity of the biomarker – the proportion of patients with the clinical endpoint who are biomarker positive; and $R$ is the relative risk – the incidence of the clinical endpoint in patients who are biomarker positive divided by the incidence in those who are biomarker negative. More elaborate analyses have been proposed for estimating the proportion of treatment effect explained by a biomarker [27, 28]. These and other statistical approaches for evaluating the correlation between candidate surrogate endpoints and clinical endpoints in clinical trials were reviewed

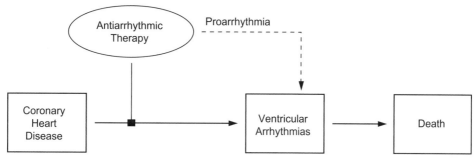

**FIGURE 18.2** Path diagram illustrating the potential of adverse proarrhythmic effects of anti-arrhythmic drug therapy (*broken line and arrow*) to outweigh the potential benefit of suppressing ventricular arrhythmias in patients with coronary heart disease.

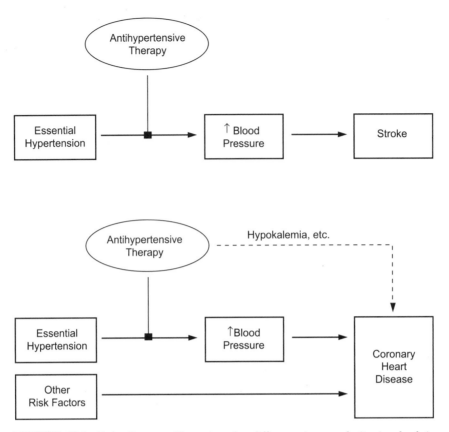

**FIGURE 18.3** Path diagrams illustrating the difference in complexity involved in demonstrating the efficacy of antihypertensive therapy in reducing the incidence of stroke and coronary heart disease. The anticipated benefit in reducing the incidence of coronary heart disease is offset by the deleterious effects of some antihypertensive drug regimens. In addition, hypertension is just one of many factors that contribute to the risk of developing coronary heart disease.

and discussed at a workshop sponsored by the National Institutes of Health [29].

Despite the important role that statistical criteria have played in establishing the linkage between biomarkers and clinical endpoints, it is always hazardous to equate causation with statistical association. For that reason, the *biological plausibility*, or *construct validity*, of candidate biomarkers also needs to be considered. Evidence supporting the biological plausibility of a biomarker rests on an understanding of both pharmacologic action and disease mechanism and is often summarized in path diagrams, such as those shown in Figure 18.3. In this figure, a disease mechanism biomarker is shown as a reduction in the elevated blood pressure that accounts for disease progression. A more proximal pharmacologic biomarker might represent the interaction of an antihypertensive drug with its receptor. The latter type of biomarker is easier to evaluate and may play an important role early in the process of drug development, but lacks the capacity for generalization and overall clinical utility of biomarkers that are based on

an understanding of disease mechanism. On the other hand, even biomarkers based on a thorough understanding of disease mechanism often fail to encompass all facets of a therapeutic intervention, and their utility is often confounded by off-target effects, such as the hypokalemia that occurs when excessive doses of some diuretics are prescribed to control hypertension [21].

The regulatory decision to classify a biomarker as a surrogate endpoint is a matter of scientific judgment. Temple [21] has laid out evidentiary standards for plausibility that include documented success in clinical trials and public health and risk–benefit considerations, such as the availability of alternative effective therapy, the safety database of the drug in question, and the difficulty of obtaining clinical endpoint data. Status as a surrogate endpoint may be granted only to drugs in a particular class, as is the case for inhibitors of 3-hydroxy-3-methylglutaryl coenzyme A (HMG-CoA) reductase inhibitors, or more generally when the surrogate has predictive validity for several classes of drugs, such as antihypertensive agents.

Since full regulatory reliance on a surrogate endpoint requires a significant evidence base, a *provisional acceptance* is needed for cases involving a serious or life-threatening disease when more uncertainty about the true effect can be tolerated. In the 1990s, the urgent need for effective therapy against human immunodeficiency virus (HIV) infections prompted the use of biomarkers both in clinical practice and in the development and regulatory approval of antiretroviral drugs. In 1992, the FDA published the accelerated approval regulations, which stipulate, in part, that:

> FDA may grant marketing approval for a new drug product on the basis of adequate and well-controlled trials establishing that the drug product has an effect on a surrogate endpoint that is reasonably likely, based on epidemiologic, therapeutic, pathophysiologic, or other evidence, to predict clinical benefit or on the basis of an effect on a clinical endpoint other than survival or irreversible morbidity.
>
> Title 21, Section 314.50, Subpart H of the Code of Federal Regulations [30]

These regulations state further that such approvals are subject to the requirement that the sponsor complete additional studies intended to verify and describe the clinical benefit of the drug. The first approvals under these new regulations were for antiretroviral drugs using CD4 lymphocyte counts and subsequently HIV RNA levels as surrogate endpoints. There have been additional approvals in cancer and other serious diseases using a variety of surrogate endpoints.

In 2000, a collaborative group reported a meta-analysis of 16 clinical trials of nucleoside analog antiretroviral drugs that supported the use of both CD lymphocyte counts in blood and plasma HIV RNA levels as prognostic and therapeutic response biomarkers and as surrogate endpoints [31]. However, short-term changes in these biomarkers were found to be imperfect surrogate endpoints because treatments that showed similar changes in these markers were not always accompanied by similar clinical outcomes, measured as survival or time to progression of acquired immunodeficiency disease. Despite this drawback, the use of these biomarkers facilitated the rapid development of a variety of antiretroviral drugs, and in 2002 the FDA issued guidance on the development and use of plasma HIV RNA measurements for both accelerated and traditional approval pathways for these drugs [32]. This example illustrates that regulatory decisions based on surrogate endpoints entail an explicit trade-off between faster drug access and certainty about drug effectiveness [5, 33]. For this reason, when a drug is granted accelerated approval, continued marketing of the drug is conditional on the conduct of further studies to establish clinical benefit.

On the other hand, a biomarker need not achieve surrogate endpoint status to play an important role in advancing our understanding of disease mechanism and natural history, in facilitating the process of drug development, or in guiding clinical practice [20].

## USES OF BIOMARKERS

All of the biomarkers listed in Table 18.2 have some degree of clinical utility, even though they differ with respect to their ability to substitute as a clinical endpoint. The process of determining biomarker utility is not only linked to biomarker qualification (Figure 18.1), it is similar to it in that the process is highly situational and depends on the circumstances surrounding the intended use of the biomarker [5]. Thus, the standards for determining utility of a test used for population screening or prenatal diagnosis might differ from the standards for tests used to assess the risk of a rare, serious adverse event. In many cases, the clinical utility of a biomarker has been based on epidemiologic studies and established only after a period of years. However, in the future the development of many drugs, such as those listed at the top of Table 18.3 [72] as already requiring testing for a pharmacogenetic marker, will most likely proceed in tandem with the development of a *companion diagnostic* test on which its safe and effective use depends. A number of these tests are now required for patient selection, and a draft FDA guidance provides recommendations for conjoint development of both a drug and an appropriately validated and qualified patient-selection biomarker [34]. In such cases, much of the evidence about clinical utility of the biomarker (and performance of the specific assay) will derive from the clinical trials conducted to assess the investigational drug under development. It is also likely that new drugs will be developed in parallel with assays for biomarkers that are intended to identify patients who are ***not*** candidates for therapy, because of either lower response probability or higher likelihood of an adverse effect. All the above are enrichment strategies that are expected to become increasingly common in drug development as biological knowledge accrues. The following examples illustrate the wide utility of biomarkers in drug development.

### Application of Blood Pressure in Hypertension

Blood pressure is a biomarker that is relied on in clinical practice to diagnose hypertension, to estimate its severity, and to monitor response to antihypertensive therapy. The term *essential hypertension* initially

**TABLE 18.3  Currently Required and Recommended Pharmacogenetic and Pharmacogenomic Tests**

|  | Pharmacogenetic marker | Therapeutic indication | Drug(s) |
|---|---|---|---|
| Required Test | HER overexpression | Breast cancer | Trastuzumab |
|  | BCR-ABL fusion gene | Acute lymphoblastic leukemia | Dasatinib |
|  | CCR-5 receptor tropic HIV-1 virus | HIV infection | Maraviroc |
|  | EGFR expression + wild-type KRAS | Colon cancer | Cetuximab and Panitumumab |
|  | Anaplastic lymphoma kinase (ALK) positive (FISH) | NSC lung cancer | Crizotinib |
|  | BRAF v600E mutation | Melanoma | Vemurafenib |
| Recommended Test | G6PD deficiency | Hyperuricemia | Rasburicase |
|  | Thiopurine methyltransferase variants | Acute lymphocytic leukemia | 6-MP, Azathioprine, Thioguanine |
|  | UGT1A1 variants | Colorectal cancer | Irinotecan |
|  | CYP2C9 and VKORC1 variants | Anticoagulation | Warfarin |
|  | HLA-B*1502 | Seizure disorders, neuralgia | Carbamazepine |
|  | HLA-B*5701 | HIV infection | Abacavir |

Modified from Ikediobi ON, Shin J, Nussbaum RL *et al.* Clin Pharmacol Ther 2009;86:28–31 [72].

was coined in the belief that an elevated blood pressure was required to provide adequate organ perfusion in patients with sclerotic arteries [35]. This concept was accepted by some clinicians well into the 1970s and, aside from the therapeutic imperative presented by malignant hypertension, accounted for their continued reluctance to treat patients with asymptomatic elevations in blood pressure. However, epidemiologic data developed during the Framingham Study convincingly demonstrated the impact of hypertension on the full clinical spectrum of cardiovascular disease [36]. This epidemiologic data, accumulated over several decades, finally dispelled the notion of benign essential hypertension, introduced the concept of cardiovascular disease as the outcome of multiple risk factors, and provided evidence for treating elevations in systolic as well as diastolic blood pressure. During the same period, research studies in humans and in animal models contributed an important dimension of biological plausibility by elucidating the pathophysiologic basis for the linkage between hypertension and cerebral hemorrhage and infarction [37]. However, owing to the multifactorial nature of its pathogenesis, experimental evidence for the impact of hypertension on the outcome of coronary heart disease was more difficult to establish (Figure 18.3).

As these epidemiological and experimental findings emerged, the pharmaceutical industry began to develop a wide variety of antihypertensive drugs, conducting clinical studies to demonstrate their efficacy in reducing adverse cardiovascular events. Subsequently, the power of these individual studies was amplified and focused through the use of meta-analysis. For example, a recent meta-analysis of 147

clinical trials of antihypertensive agents demonstrated that, except for β–adrenergic blocking drugs that have additional myocardial protective effects in patients with a prior myocardial infarction and high-dose diuretic therapy that resulted in an increased incidence of sudden cardiac death, all classes of antihypertensive drugs provide equivalent benefits that are dependent only on the extent of blood-pressure lowering [38]. The authors of this meta-analysis found that the proportional reduction in stroke and coronary heart disease events varied according to patient age. However, the proportional reduction in these events for a given reduction in blood pressure was the same within each age group, irrespective of pretreatment blood pressures down to diastolic pressure levels of at least 70 mm Hg. On the basis of this observation, the authors recommended instituting antihypertensive therapy in all patients over a certain age. This recommendation is certainly at variance with current clinical practice and is in opposition to the view that excessive lowering of diastolic blood pressure may be detrimental in some patients, particularly in those who have underlying coronary artery disease [35]. It appears, then, that not only has the clinical use of blood pressure as a biomarker evolved slowly, but also certain aspects of its use continue to generate controversy.

Blood pressure may also be used as a marker of drug safety or adverse effect. A number of drugs and drug classes raise blood pressure as a pharmacologic effect. Although the effect of lowering BP on stroke and cardiovascular disease has been well documented, the effects of small, acute, or chronic pharmacologically driven increases in BP are not well understood.

This issue continues to be of importance in drug development and postmarket drug safety. These effects can be seen in trials when such drugs are compared in placebo-treated or matched control subjects. It is notable that the FDA, in 2000, took steps to remove phenylpropanolamine from the market after an epidemiologic study using matched control subjects revealed an increased rate of hemorrhagic stroke that was particularly marked in women who were using this drug as an appetite suppressant [39, 40]. More recently, the weight-loss drug sibutramine was withdrawn from the worldwide market after the SCOUT study showed an excess of non-fatal MI and stroke in obese patients with cardiovascular risk factors taking the drug, compared to placebo [41]. Although BP decreased in both groups, the systolic and diastolic BPs were slightly higher in individuals taking sibutramine. It is not known if the BP differences had any relationship to the observed adverse outcomes.

## Use of Biomarkers in Contemporary Drug Development

As summarized in Figure 18.4, biomarkers play in important role in all phases of contemporary drug development [42]. Many of the biomarkers were developed under time constraints that preclude the accumulation of supporting data from epidemiological studies, or involve novel technology for which traditional evaluation approaches are unsuitable. For example, the clinical diagnosis of Alzheimer's disease is currently based on psychological tests which detect cognitive impairment that occurs only at an advanced stage of the disease, when therapeutic interventions can be anticipated to have little disease-modifying effect [43]. As a result, identification and development of effective therapeutic interventions for patients with Alzheimer's disease is critically dependent on the availability of biomarkers that reflect the early pathophysiological changes that occur before the onset of cognitive loss. Amyloid β and the microtubule protein tau are the main components of the plaques and neurofibrillary tangles that are hallmarks of Alzheimer's disease and are thought to be primarily responsible for neuronal degeneration and cognitive loss. Positron emission tomography, using amyloid tracers (amyloid PET), shows particular promise in being able to diagnose Alzheimer's disease patients before the clinical onset of dementia, and in differentiating this disease from frontotemporal lobar degeneration and other forms of cognitive deterioration in elderly patients [44]. Concentration measurements of amyloid β and P-tau in cerebrospinal fluid (CSF) have been used as proximal biomarkers to reflect brain amyloid and tangle pathophysiology and, together with amyloid PET, have potential use in identifying the mechanism of action of candidate drugs [43]. Other markers, such as CSF concentrations of T–tau and magnetic resonance imaging measurements of brain

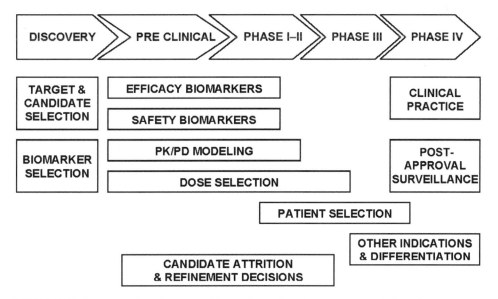

**FIGURE 18.4** Potential applications of biomarkers along the continuum of drug discovery and development to utilization in clinical practice. In general, biomarkers used for internal decision-making early in the development process need lesser degrees of qualification than those used later in the continuum. Modified from Lee JW, Hall M. J Chromatogr B Analyt Technol Biomed Life Sci 2009;877:1259–71 [42].

atrophy, have potential use for monitoring the rate of neuronal degeneration. Despite the apparent utility of these biomarkers in facilitating the transition from preclinical investigations in animal models of Alzheimer's disease to initial clinical studies, their further evaluation will need to progress within the context of future clinical trials of candidate drugs. As part of its Critical Path Initiative, the FDA has proposed guidance intended to facilitate the development of biomarkers within this context of use [16].

PET imaging also has been used to provide *proof of mechanism* by providing *in vivo* demonstration that a drug binds to its targeted receptor or ion channel. For example, PET imaging was used in an innovative dose-ranging study to demonstrate that a 0.48-mg/kg dose of a reversible monamine oxidase type B (MAO-B) inhibitor was needed to achieve more than 90% blockade of irreversible L-[$^{11}$C]deprenyl binding to central nervous system MAO-B [45]. Here, blockade of irreversible L-[$^{11}$C]deprenyl binding was used as the biomarker, and it was estimated that a 1-year Phase II study in patients with Parkinson's disease would have been required had conventional clinical endpoints been used for dose-ranging studies.

In preclinical and early clinical development, biomarkers can provide evidence of *in vivo* pharmacologic activity and can provide a rational basis for the selection of lead compounds. By substituting for clinical endpoints they can define the dose or range of plasma concentrations that is likely to be effective in subsequent studies, and can shorten development time and expense by facilitating early decision-making. In later phases of clinical development, disease biomarkers can be used to guide patient selection and stratification, thereby reducing the number of patients that need to be enrolled to demonstrate statistically significant therapeutic responses. In some cases it is advantageous to co-develop a drug along with a biomarker that will be used in clinical practice for patient selection, as was the case for traztuzumab and tests for HER2 overexpression [5]. Even after marketing approval, drugs that show lower than hoped for efficacy and unexpected toxicity sometimes can be *rescued* by using patient selection biomarkers, and pharmacogenetic and pharmacogenomic biomarkers are particularly likely to be useful for this purpose, as described in Chapter 13 for cetuximab [5]. However, only a few well-qualified biomarkers will be judged suitable to provide the basis for initial marketing approval by serving as surrogate endpoints, and this will be of primary utility for drugs being developed to treat chronic diseases [5].

Although most attention has been focused on biomarkers that are intended to substitute for measures of clinical efficacy, recent emphasis has shifted to include biomarkers that can be used primarily to monitor drug safety in either the preclinical or clinical phases of drug development and use [46]. The most credible of these biomarkers will be linked directly to the pathogenic mechanism of a given toxic reaction. Because serum creatinine and blood urea nitrogen concentrations are measures of renal function that are insensitive indicators of renal injury, efforts are underway to develop more sensitive biomarkers of acute nephrotoxicity [18]. Pharmacogenetic biomarkers are likely to play an increasingly important role in identifying patients who have an increased susceptibility to serious adverse reactions. For example, patients with one or two non-functional TPMT alleles have a high risk of hematopoietic toxicity when treated with standard doses of 6-mercaptopurine (6-MP) and other thiopurine drugs [47]. Consequently, measurement of TPMT activity has become an accepted biomarker for identifying patients at high risk of thiopurine drug toxicity [47]. As discussed in previous chapters, the finding that Han Chinese patients homozygous for the *HLA-B\*1502* allele are at increased risk of developing Stevens-Johnson syndrome and toxic epidermal necrolysis also illustrates the important role that pharmacogenetic biomarkers factors may play in identifying patients who are particularly likely to experience adverse reactions [48].

The potential lethality of drug-induced ventricular arrhythmias has drawn attention to this adverse event, and has resulted in published guidance for evaluating drug-induced QT-interval prolongation that may precipitate these arrhythmias [49]. Since QT-interval prolongation is integral to the mechanism of action of many antiarrhythmic drugs, emphasis is placed in this guidance on drugs that are intended for other uses than arrhythmia control. Further refinements in assessing proarrhythmic risk have been proposed that include a covariate analysis of T-wave morphology along with measurements of QTc prolongation [50]. Particularly intriguing in the context of future biomarker development and use has been the application of systems biology approaches in a multi-scale model that provided a useful *in silico* assessment of the arrhythmogenic potential of a few drugs [51].

## CASE STUDY: DEVELOPMENT AND USE OF SERUM CHOLESTEROL AS A BIOMARKER AND SURROGATE ENDPOINT

Although serum cholesterol measurements are a currently accepted surrogate endpoint for lipid-

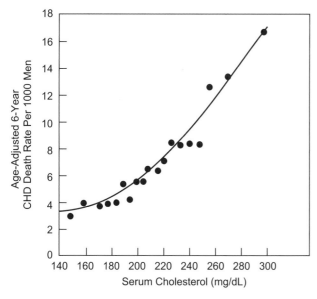

**FIGURE 18.5** Relation of serum cholesterol to coronary heart disease death in a population of 361,662 men aged 35–57. The average duration of follow-up was 6 years. Reproduced with permission from LaRosa JC, Hunninghake D, Criqui MH *et al.* Circulation 1990;81:1721–33 [53].

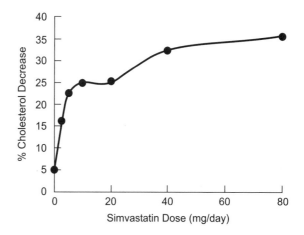

**FIGURE 18.6** Results of a study which established the dose–response relationship between simvastatin dose and percent reduction in serum cholesterol levels in patients with heterozygous familial hypercholesterolemia. Data from Mol MJTM, Erkelens DW, Gevers Leuven JA *et al.* Lancet 1986;ii:936–9 [55].

lowering therapy, there is a long history of controversy regarding the value of this therapy in preventing coronary heart disease [52]. Epidemiologic studies provided initial evidence that increasing serum cholesterol concentrations were associated with an increased risk of death from coronary heart disease (Figure 18.5) [53]. This relationship was confirmed by studies conducted in a number of animal models [54]. Taken together, this evidence provided strong support for the hypothesis that reducing cholesterol levels would lower morbidity and mortality from coronary heart disease. Accordingly, serum cholesterol has played an important role as a biomarker in the clinical development of HMG-CoA reductase inhibitors and other lipid-lowering agents. This experience illustrates both some important uses of biomarkers and some of the continuing limitations surrounding their use as surrogate endpoints.

## Role of Serum Cholesterol in the Simvastatin Development Program

Measurements of serum cholesterol were used in a Phase II dose-ranging study in which simvastatin doses, ranging from 2.5 to 40 mg once daily to 1.25 to 40 mg twice daily, were administered to 43 patients with heterozygous familial hypercholesterolemia [55]. The study duration was just 6 weeks, and only four study centers were needed for patient recruitment.

Based on the results shown in Figure 18.6, it was concluded that simvastatin had suitable efficacy whether given once or twice daily, and that 20 mg/day represented an appropriate starting point for dosing in subsequent studies. These results were then incorporated in a definitive randomized, placebo-controlled Phase III trial in which 4444 patients with coronary heart disease were followed in 94 centers for a median of 5.4 years [56]. Patients receiving simvastatin were initially treated with a daily dose of 20 mg that subsequently was adjusted as needed to lower serum cholesterol concentrations to the range of 117–200 mg/dL. The study demonstrated that simvastatin therapy reduced total cholesterol by a mean of 25% during the study (average LDL cholesterol reduction was 34%), and was associated with a 34% reduction in the incidence of major coronary events. Total mortality was 30% less for patients who were treated with simvastatin than for those who received placebo.

The inclusion of clinical endpoints in this larger Phase III study provided the first definite evidence that lipid-lowering therapy could reduce total mortality in patients with coronary heart disease. Subgroup analysis subsequently indicated that the relationship between lowering LDL cholesterol and reducing major clinical events was curvilinear, in that decreases in cholesterol level resulted in continuing, but progressively smaller, reductions in major coronary events [57]. This is consistent with the epidemiologic findings shown in Figure 18.5, and supports clinical practice guidelines that recommend lowering LDL cholesterol levels to 100 mg/dL or below for patients who have established coronary heart disease or a greater than 20% 10-year risk of myocardial infarction or coronary heart disease death, and to less than 130 mg/dL for high-risk patients with a 10–20% risk of these events [58]. An even more aggressive LDL cholesterol goal of less than 70 mg/dL that may be of additional benefit for high-risk patients is currently optional and is under further evaluation [58].

## Unanticipated Therapeutic Benefit from HMG-CoA Reductase Inhibitors

Several findings suggest that HMG-CoA reductase inhibitors have therapeutic effects that extend beyond lipid lowering. This is suggested by the fact that HMG-CoA reductase inhibitors have demonstrated in most studies a more rapid onset of therapeutic benefit than would be expected just from their lipid-lowering properties [59]. Of particular interest are the results of the West of Scotland Coronary Prevention Study, in which the relationship between the observed incidence of coronary heart disease events was compared with that predicted from an equation that incorporates cholesterol levels, smoking history, diabetes, blood pressure, and other risk factors that were known at the time [60]. These results, shown in Figure 18.7, indicate that the predicted and observed event rates in patients who received placebo were similar. On the other hand, coronary event rates in pravastatin-treated patients were consistently lower than those predicted. Statistical evidence has subsequently further qualified elevated high-sensitivity C-reactive protein (CRP) levels as a biomarker that is independent of serum lipid levels in assessing coronary heart disease risk [61, 62]. Nevertheless, studies have not yet shown that therapy specifically designed to lower CRP levels

affects patient outcome, and several other mechanisms have been proposed to account for the non-lipid-lowering beneficial effects of HMG-CoA reductase inhibitors [63].

## Cholesterol-Lowering Disappointments

It is relatively uncommon for the clinical benefit of therapeutic interventions to exceed predictions based on biomarker response. Far more often, unanticipated adverse effects diminish or nullify the clinical benefits expected from drug effects on a biomarker. This is illustrated by the example of probucol, a drug structurally unrelated to HMG-CoA reductase inhibitors that exerted pronounced lipid-lowering effects and received marketing approval in the 1970s, even though long-term survival studies were not conducted. Probucol also was known to prolong the electrocardiographic QT interval. In a scenario reminiscent of that encountered with antiarrhythmic drugs (Figure 18.2), subsequent investigations indicated that this drug was proarrhythmic and that it caused *torsades de pointes* ventricular tachycardia in some patients [64]. It is thus hazardous to assume *a priori* that any drug that lowers cholesterol will also improve patient survival.

More recently, the guideline-driven widespread adoption of HMG-CoA reductase inhibitors has been followed by efforts to assess the further impact of adjunctive lipid-lowering measures. Given the expense and duration of large clinical outcome trials, these interventions generally have been evaluated using biomarkers [65]. The trial Ezetimibe and Simvastatin in Hypercholesterolemia Enhances Atherosclerosis Regression (ENHANCE), in which ezetimibe,

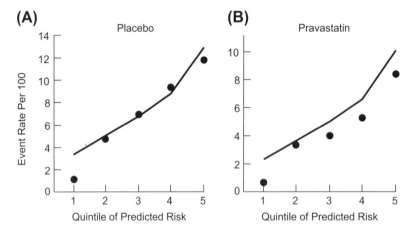

**FIGURE 18.7** Comparison of observed risk of a coronary heart disease event (*circles*) and predicted risk (*lines*) for patients receiving either placebo or pravastatin over the 4.4-year duration of the West of Scotland Coronary Prevention Study. Reproduced with permission from West of Scotland Coronary Prevention Group. Circulation 1998;97:1440–5 [60].

a marketed inhibitor of intestinal cholesterol absorption, was combined with simvastatin, has been particularly problematic in that contradictory results were obtained with two different biomarkers [66]. A total of 642 patients with primary hypercholesterolemia completed the 2-year study in which a difference in changes of carotid artery intimal-medial thickness (CIMT) was chosen as the primary endpoint. Whereas combined therapy yielded the expected lowering of serum low-density lipoprotein (LDL) cholesterol concentrations and also reduced CRP levels, there was no significant difference in the progression of atherosclerosis as assessed by ultrasound CIMT measurement. This paradox is particularly troubling, because single-measurement CIMT has been shown to be a strong predictor of myocardial infarction and other vascular events [67]. Partly because variability in estimates of CIMT progression is much larger than that of single-measurement CIMT, more evidence is needed to support reliance on CIMT progression as a surrogate for vascular risk in clinical trials [68]. Additional explanations of these discordant results have included criticisms of the small sample size and short duration of the ENHANCE study, and the fact that, before study entry, approximately 80% of the study subjects were being treated with HMG-CoA reductase inhibitors which might have caused baseline CIMT measurements to be lower than they otherwise would have been [65]. Although serum cholesterol lowering has been accepted as a surrogate endpoint for HMG-CoA reductase inhibitors, these examples raise additional questions about the extent of its applicability to other drug classes or even to its use in studies designed to evaluate combinations of cholesterol lowering drugs that by themselves have been deemed effective.

## FUTURE DEVELOPMENT OF BIOMARKERS

So far, we have considered biomarkers the use of which has been either somewhat established or discredited by their application in clinical practice or in clinical trials. However, the utility of biomarkers in aiding drug development and the diagnosis and management of patients is stimulating the introduction of many new biomarkers, many of which are based on the development of new imaging and genetics-based technologies and are less well characterized. Innovative but incompletely evaluated biomarkers are particularly likely to play an important role in exploratory studies of new drug candidates, but are increasingly being deployed as well in later-phase clinical trials and in clinical practice. Unfortunately, the degree of innovation represented by a biomarker is likely to vary inversely with the extent of its qualification [69]. This is because prior use in clinical trials is an important component of the biomarker qualification process.

One scheme for categorizing the multitude of established and candidate biomarkers is presented in Figure 18.8. Type 1 biomarkers reflect a drug's initial pharmacologic action. As such, they confirm primary pharmacology, but may not be correlated with downstream events or clinical effects. Because Type 1 biomarkers reflect fundamental mechanisms, they are likely to emerge from a *bottom–up* elucidation of disease mechanism and drug action. These biomarkers generally find utility in *in vitro* studies to confirm that a drug binds to a certain receptor or ion channel, or elicits an *in vivo* response that is easily measured but separate from an effect on disease mechanism. Positron emission tomography is example of an

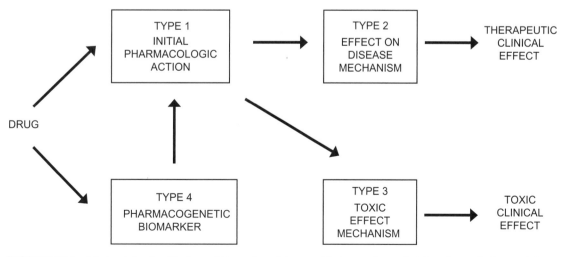

**FIGURE 18.8** Mechanistic classification of biomarkers interposed between drug administration and observed therapeutic or toxic clinical effects. Further explanation is provided in text.

imaging technology that has been useful in assessing receptor binding even in early-phase clinical studies. The development and application of Type 1 biomarkers is most likely to be undertaken by the pharmaceutical industry.

Type 2 biomarkers reflect drug effects on the targeted disease mechanism and, like blood pressure, serum cholesterol, and CRP, are more likely to be predictive of beneficial clinical response to a therapeutic intervention. Because they are properties of biological systems, Type 2 biomarkers are more likely to be qualified by academic investigators.

There has been increasing interest in developing Type 3 biomarkers, which could provide an early warning of possible drug toxicity [70]. Many of the biomarkers in this category, such as biomarkers of early nephrotoxicity, can be considered *pre-competitive* and amenable to being developed by consortia of industry, academia, and regulatory scientists.

Recent advances in pharmacogenetics have led to the development of Type 4 biomarkers, which could reflect interindividual differences in genes that encode for transporters, enzymes, receptors, and other proteins involved in drug action or in the processes of drug absorption and disposition [71].

It is likely that advances in pharmacogenetics and pharmacogenomics will expand the current repertoire of biomarkers. Pharmacogenomics already has played an important role in the mechanism-driven development of trastuzumab and several other oncology drugs, and Table 18.3 lists a number of pharmacogenetic and pharmacogenomic biomarkers that are either required companion diagnostic tests or recommended in drug labels to be used as an integral part of clinical practice [72]. Nevertheless, the pathophysiology of most common diseases is multifactorial, so it is likely that most disease states will be characterized by a typical pattern in the expression of several genes in one or more tissues of relevance. For this reason, studies of the expression pattern of multiple genes should lead to a better understanding of the complex genetic basis for these diseases and to the identification of promising molecular targets for new drug development [73]. After appropriate validation and qualification, these expression patterns could be used as a *genomic signature* to confirm diagnosis, establish prognosis, choose the most appropriate therapy for an individual patient, and monitor patient response.

Accordingly, the future development of pharmacogenomic biomarkers is likely to extend beyond the use of single-gene markers to include the analysis of the differential expression of as many as 10,000 genes in a single experiment [74, 75]. The promising potential of this approach in matching patients with appropriate therapy is illustrated by a retrospective investigation of the expression of 2453 genes in breast-cancer tissue from patients who were treated with docetaxel [76]. Tumor samples from 44 patients were analyzed with a high-throughput reverse polymerase chain reaction technique. An 85-gene signature was identified that predicted the docetaxel response of 26 additional patients with 80% accuracy. Moreover, the signature of non-responders was characterized by overexpression of genes controlling the cellular redox environment, thus providing insight into an important mechanism underlying docetaxel resistance.

Expression proteomics also has considerable potential to aid in characterizing multifactorial diseases. Proteomics can provide valuable data beyond what is available from genomic studies, because the proteome varies between time points and is affected by environmental conditions that may also be relevant to the causation of multifactorial diseases [77]. The analytical approaches that have been used for proteomic studies are usually based either on the use of two-dimensional gel electrophoresis or immunological methods to analyze a limited number of critical markers, or on mass spectrometry combined with different interfaces, such as matrix-assisted laser desorption and ionization (MALDI) or surface-enhanced laser desorption and ionization (SELDI), to identify a disease-specific protein fragment ion pattern that can serve as a biomarker. Although most women with ovarian cancer are only diagnosed when the disease is advanced and prognosis is poor, several proteomic approaches are being investigated that may be able to identify biomarker signatures which in the future could be suitable for patient screening and permit early diagnosis of this disease [78, 79]. The best currently available single biomarker used for detecting ovarian cancer is CA-125; it is the only biomarker approved for monitoring ovarian cancer progression and treatment response; however, by itself, CA-125 lacks the sensitivity and specificity needed for a screening tool. In response to this unmet need, Petricoin *et al.* [80] used mass spectrometry to demonstrate that differential expression of low molecular weight serum proteins had the potential to identify patients with diagnosed ovarian cancer with near 100% sensitivity and specificity. Nevertheless, questions arose about the reproducibility and reliability of these results [81], and the inability to identify the specific proteins involved precluded subsequent validation with immunologic methods [82]. To circumvent the problems encountered in validating and qualifying mass spectrometry assays, an immunoassay using a multiplex bead array was subsequently developed that incorporates CA-125 and five other molecularly defined biomarkers [83]. A signature based on the expression level of these six proteins was found to detect ovarian cancer with a sensitivity of 95.3% and a specificity of 99.4%. This signature is being commercially developed for patient screening.

The use of gene expression array and differential protein expression technologies poses a bioinformatics challenge, but substantial progress has been made in developing relational database management systems that can store, process, and analyze the data that are generated by high-throughput methods [84–86]. Currently available bioinformatics packages and heuristic cluster algorithms have the potential to provide panels of relevant biomarkers that can transform drug development and patient therapy, and supersede reliance on single biomarkers, at least in patients with cancer and other multifactorial diseases.

## REFERENCES

[1] Biomarkers Definitions Working Group. Biomarkers and surrogate endpoints: Preferred definitions and conceptual framework. Clin Pharmacol Ther 2001;69:89–95.

[2] Frank R, Hargreaves R. Clinical biomarkers in drug discovery and development. Nat Rev Drug Discov 2003;2:566–80.

[3] Wagner JA. Overview of biomarkers and surrogate endpoints in drug development. Dis Markers 2002;18:41–6.

[4] Wagner JA. Strategic approach to fit-for-purpose biomarkers in drug development. Ann Rev Pharmacol Toxicol 2008;48:631–51.

[5] Woodcock J. Assessing the clinical utility of diagnostics used in drug therapy. Clin Pharmacol Ther 2010;88:765–73.

[6] Institute of Medicine Committee on Qualification of Biomarkers and Surrogate Endpoints in Chronic Disease. In: Michael CM, Ball JR, editors. Evaluation of biomarkers and surrogate endpoints in chronic disease. Washington, DC: The National Academies Press; 2010.

[7] Kohl P, Crampin EJ, Quinn TA, Noble D. Systems biology: An approach. Clin Pharmacol Ther 2010;88:25–33.

[8] CDER, CVM. Bioanalytical method validation. Guidance for Industry. Rockville, MD: FDA (Internet at, www.fda.gov/downloads/Drugs/GuidanceComplianceRegulatoryInformation/Guidances/ucm070107.pdf; 2001).

[9] Mildvan D, Landay A, De Gruttola V, Machado SG, Kagan J. An approach to the validation of markers for use in AIDS clinical trials. Clin Infect Dis 1997;24:764–74.

[10] Di Leo A, Dowsett M, Horten B, Penault-Liorca F. Current status of HER2 testing. Oncology 2002;63(Suppl. 1):25–32.

[11] Elizabeth M, Hammond H, Barker P, Taube S, Gutman S. Standard reference material for HER2 testing: Report of a National Institute of Standards and Technology-sponsored Consensus Workshop. Appl Immunohistochem Mol Morphol 2003;11:103–6.

[12] Wolff AC, Elizabeth M, Hammond H, Schwartz JN, Hagerty KL, Aldred DC, et al. American Society of Clinical Oncology/College of American Pathologists guideline recommendations for human epidermal growth factor receptor 2 testing in breast cancer. J Clin Oncol 2007;25:118–45.

[13] Padhani AR, Liu G, Mu-Koh D, Chenevert TL, Thoeny HC, Takahara T, et al. Diffusion-weighted magnetic resonance imaging as a cancer biomarker: Consensus and recommendations. Neoplasia 2009;11:1102–25.

[14] Shanbhogue AKP, Karnand AB, Prasad SR. Tumor response evaluation in oncology: Current update. J Comput Assist Tomogr 2010;34:479–84.

[15] Goodsaid FM, Frueh FW. Mattes. Strategic paths for biomarker qualification. Toxicology 2008;245:219–23.

[16] CDER. Qualification process for drug development tools. Draft Guidance for Industry. Silver Spring, MD: FDA (Internet at, www.fda.gov/downloads/Drugs/ Guidance Compliance RegulatoryInformation/Guidances/UCM230597.pdf; 2010).

[17] Goodsaid FM, Mendrick DL. Translational medicine and the value of biomarker qualification. Sci Transl Med 2010;2:47.ps44.

[18] Goodsaid FM, Blank M, Dieterle F, Harlow P, Hausner E, Sistare F, et al. Novel biomarkers of acute kidney toxicity. Clin Pharmacol Ther 2009;86:490–6.

[19] Temple R. Are surrogate markers adequate to assess cardiovascular disease drugs? JAMA 1999;282:790–5.

[20] Lesko LJ, Atkinson AJ Jr. Use of biomarkers and surrogate endpoints in drug development and regulatory decision making. Ann Rev Pharmacol 2001;41:347–66.

[21] Temple RJ. A regulatory authority's opinion about surrogate endpoints. In: Nimmo WS, Tucker GT, editors. Clinical measurement in drug evaluation. New York, NY: J Wiley; 1995.

[22] Fleming TR, DeMets DL. Surrogate endpoints in clinical trials: Are we being misled? Ann Intern Med 1996;125:605–13.

[23] Temple R. Are surrogate markers adequate to assess cardiovascular disease drugs? JAMA 1999;282:790–5.

[24] Echt DS, Liebson PR, Mitchell B, Peters RW, Obias-Manno D, Barker AH, et al. CAST Investigators. Mortality and morbidity of patients receiving encainide, flecainide or placebo: The Cardiac Arrhythmia Suppression Trial. N Engl J Med 1991;324:781–8.

[25] Prentice RL. Surrogate endpoints in clinical trials: Definition and operational criteria. Stat Med 1989;8:431–40.

[26] Shatzkin A, Freedman LS, Schiffman MH, Dawsey SM. Validation of intermediate endpoints in cancer research. J Natl Cancer Inst 1990;82:1746–52.

[27] Freedman LS, Graubard BI. Statistical validation of intermediate endpoints for chronic diseases. Stat Med 1992;11:167–78.

[28] Lin DY, Fleming TR, De Gruttola V. Estimating the proportion of treatment effect explained by a surrogate marker. Stat Med 1997;16:1515–27.

[29] De Gruttola VG, Clax P, DeMets DL, Downing GJ, Ellenberg SS, Friedman L, et al. Considerations in the evaluation of surrogate endpoints in clinical trials: Summary of a National Institutes of Health workshop. Control Clin Trials 2001;22:485–502.

[30] Code of Federal Regulations, Title 21, Vol. 5, Parts 300–499. Washington, DC: US Government Printing Office; April 1, 1997.

[31] HIV Surrogate Marker Collaborative Group. Human immunodeficiency virus type 1 RNA level and CD4 count as prognostic markers and surrogate endpoints: A meta-analysis. AISA Res Hum Retroviruses 2000;16:1123–32.

[32] CDER. Antiretroviral drugs using plasma HIV RNA measurements – clinical considerations for accelerated and traditional approval. Guidance for Industry. Rockville, MD: FDA (Internet at, www.fda.gov/downloads/Drugs/GuidanceComplianceRegulatoryInformation/Guidances/ucm070968.pdf; 2002).

[33] Lathia CD, Amakye D, Girman C, Madani S, Mayne J, MacCarthy P, et al. The value, qualification and regulatory use of surrogate endpoints in drug development. Clin Pharmacol Ther 2009;86:32–43.

[34] CDRH, CBER CDER. In vitro companion diagnostic devices. Draft Guidance for Industry, Rockville, MD: FDA (Internet at, www.fda.gov/downloads/MedicalDevices/DeviceRegulationandGuidance/GuidanceDocuments/UCM262327.pdf; 2011).

[35] Messerli FH, Panjrath GS. The J-curve between blood pressure and coronary artery disease or essential hypertension. J Am Coll Cardiol 2009;54:1827–34.

[36] Kannel WB. Hypertension: Reflections on risks and prognostication. Med Clin North Am 2009;93:541–56.

[37] Russell RWR. How does blood-pressure cause stroke? Lancet 1975;ii:1283–5.

[38] Law MR, Morris JK, Wald NJ. Use of blood pressure lowering drugs in the prevention of cardiovascular disease: Meta-analysis of 147 randomised trials in the context of expectations from prospective epidemiological studies. BMJ 2009;32:729–41.

[39] Kernan WN, Viscoli CM, Brass LM, Broderick JP, Brott T, Feldmann E, et al. Phenylpropanolamine and the risk of hemorrhagic stroke. N Engl J Med 2000;343:1826–32.

[40] Fleming GA. The FDA, regulation, and the risk of stroke. N Engl J Med 2000;343:1886.

[41] Philip W, James T, Caterson ID, Coutinho W, Finer N, Van Gaal LF, et al., for the SCOUT Investigators. Effect of sibutramine on cardiovascular outcomes in overweight and obese subjects. N Engl J Med 2010;363:905–17.

[42] Lee JW, Hall M. Method validation of protein biomarkers in support of drug development or clinical diagnosis/prognosis. J Chromatogr B Analyt Technol Biomed Life Sci 2009;877:1259–71.

[43] Blennow K. Biomarkers in Alzheimer's disease drug development. Nat Med 2010;16:1218–22.

[44] Rowe CC, Ackerman U, Browne W, Mulligan R, Pike KL, O'Keefe G, et al. Imaging of amyloid β in Alzheimer's disease with 18F-BAY94-9172, a novel PET tracer: Proof of mechanism. Lancet Neurol 2008;7:129–35.

[45] Bench CJ, Price GW, Lammertsma AA, Cremer JC, Luthra SK, Turton D, et al. Measurement of human cerebral monamine oxidase type B (MAO-B) activity with positron emission tomography (PET): A dose ranging study with the reversible inhibitor Ro 19-6327. Eur J Clin Pharmacol 1991;40:169–73.

[46] Rolan P, Danhof M, Stanski D, Peck C. Current issues relating to drug safety especially with regard to the use of biomarkers: A meeting report and progress update. Eur J Pharm Sci 2007;30:107–13.

[47] Krynetski E, Evans WE. Drug methylation in cancer therapy: Lessons from the TPMT polymorphism. Oncogene 2003;22:7403–13.

[48] Chung W-H, Hung S-I, Hong H-S, Hsih M-S, Yang L-C, Ho H-C, et al. A marker for Stevens-Johnson syndrome. Nature 2004;428:486.

[49] CDER, CBER. E14 clinical evaluation of QT/QTc interval prolongation and proarrhythmic potential for non-antiarrhythmic drugs. Guidance for Industry. Rockville, MD: FDA (Internet at, www.fda.go/downloads/Drugs/GuidanceComplianceRegulatoryInformation/Guidances/ucm073153.pdf; 2005 ).

[50] Graff C, Struijk JJ, Matz J, Kanters JK, Andersen MP, Nielsen J, et al. Covariate analysis of QTc and T-wave morphology: New possibilities in the evaluation of drugs that affect cardiac repolarization. Clin Pharmacol Ther 2010;88:88–94.

[51] Rodriguez B, Burrage K, Gavaghan D, Grau V, Kohl P, Noble D. The systems biology approach to drug development: Application to toxicity assessment of cardiac drugs. Clin Pharmacol Ther 2010;88:130–4.

[52] Davey Smith G, Pekkanen J. Should there be a moratorium on the use of cholesterol lowering drugs? BMJ 1992;304:431–4.

[53] LaRosa JC, Hunninghake D, Criqui MH, Getz GS, Gotto AM. Jr, Grundy SM, et al. The cholesterol facts: A summary of the evidence relating dietary fats, serum cholesterol, and coronary heart disease: A joint statement by the American Heart Association and the National Heart, Lung, and Blood Institute. Circulation 1990;81:1721–33.

[54] Wissler RW, Vesselinovitch D. Can atherosclerotic plaques regress? Anatomic and biochemical evidence from nonhuman animal models. Am J Cardiol 1990;65:33F–40F.

[55] Mol MJTM, Erkelens DW. Gevers Leuven JA, Schouten JA, Stalenhoef AFH. Effects of synvinolin (MK-733) on plasma lipids in familial hypercholesterolaemia. Lancet 1986;ii:936–9.

[56] Scandinavian Simvastatin Survival Study Group. Randomised trial of cholesterol lowering in 4444 patients with coronary heart disease: The Scandinavian Simvastatin Survival Study (4S). Lancet 1994;344:1383–9.

[57] Pedersen TR, Olsson AG, Færgeman O, Kjekshus J, Wedel H, Berg K, et al., for the Scandinavian Simvastatin Survival Study Group. Lipoprotein changes and reduction in the incidence of major coronary heart disease events in the Scandinavian Simvastatin Survival Study. Circulation 1998;97:1453–60.

[58] Grundy SM, Cleeman JI, Merz CN, Brewer HB. Jr, Clark LT, Hunninghake DB, et al. Coordinating Committee of the National Cholesterol Education Program. Implications of recent clinical trials for the National Cholesterol Education Program Adult Treatment Panel III Guidelines. J Am Coll Cardiol 2004;44:720–32.

[59] Vaughan CJ, Murphy MB, Buckley BM. Statins do more than just lower cholesterol. Lancet 1996;348:1079–82.

[60] West of Scotland Coronary Prevention Study Group. Influence of pravastatin and plasma lipids on clinical events in the West of Scotland Coronary Prevention Study (WOSCOPS). Circulation 1998;97:1440–5.

[61] Buckley DL, Fu R, Freeman M, Rogers K, Helfand M. C-reactive protein as a risk factor for coronary heart disease: A systematic review and meta-analysis for the US Preventive Services Task Force. Ann Intern Med 2009;151:483–96.

[62] Corrado E, Rizzo M, Coppola G, Fattouch K, Novo G, Marturana I, et al. An update on the role of markers of inflammation in atherosclerosis. J Atheroscler Thromb 2010;17:1–11.

[63] Blum A, Shamburek R. The pleiotropic effects of statins on endothelial function, vascular inflammation, immunomodulation and thrombogenesis. Atherosclerosis 2009;203:325–30.

[64] Reinoehl J, Frankovich D, Machado C, Kawasaki R, Baga JJ, Pires LA, et al. Probucol-associated tachyarrhythmic events and QT prolongation: Importance of gender. Am Heart J 1996;131:1184–91.

[65] Silverman MG, Blaha MJ, Blumenthal RS. Adjunctive lipid lowering therapy in the era of surrogate endpoints. Cardiol Rev 2011;19:17–22.

[66] Kastelein JJP, Akdim F, Stroes ESG, Zwinderman AH, Bots ML, Stalenhoef AFH, et al. ENHANCE Investigators. Simvastatin with or without ezetimibe in familial hypercholesterolemia. N Engl J Med 2008;358:1431–43.

[67] Lorenz MW, Markus HS, Bots ML, Rosvall M, Sitzer M. Prediction of cardiovascular events with carotid intima–media thickness – a systemic review and meta-analysis. Circulation 2007;115:459–67.

[68] Lorenz MW, Bickel H, Bots ML, Breteler MMB, Catapano AL, Desvarieux M, et al. PROG-IMT Study Group. Individual progression of carotid intima media thickness as a surrogate for vascular risk (PROG-IMT): Rationale and design of a meta-analysis project. Am Heart J 2010;159:730–6.

[69] Rolan P. The contribution of clinical pharmacology surrogates and models to drug development – a critical appraisal. Br J Clin Pharmacol 1997;44:219–25.

[70] Abernethy DR, Woodcock J, Lesko LJ. Pharmacological mechanism-based drug safety assessment and prediction. Clin Pharm Ther 2011;89:793–7.

[71] Lesko LJ, Woodcock J. Translation of pharmacogenomics and pharmacogenetics: A regulatory perspective. Nat Rev Drug Discov 2004;3:763–9.

[72] Ikediobi ON, Shin J, Nussbaum RL, Phillips KA. UCSF Center for Translational and Policy Research on Personalized Medicine, Walsh JM, Ladabaum U, Marshall D. Addressing the challenges of the clinical application of pharmacogenetic testing. Clin Pharmacol Ther 2009;86(1):28–31.

[73] Kim K, Zakharkin SO, Allison DB. Expectations, validity, and reality in gene expression profiling. J Clin Epidemiol 2010;63:950–9.

[74] Debouck C, Goodfellow PN. DNA microarrays in drug discovery and development. Nat Genet 1999;21:48–50.

[75] Hiltunen MO, Niemi M, Ylä-Herttuala S. Functional genomics and DNA array techniques in atherosclerosis research. Curr Opin Lipidol 1999;10:515–9.

[76] Iwao-Koizumi K, Matoba R, Ueno N, Kim SJ, Ando A, Miyoshi Y, et al. Prediction of docetaxel response in human breast cancer by gene expression profiling. J Clin Oncol 2005; 23:422–31.

[77] Street JM, Dear JW. The application of mass-spectrometry-based protein biomarker discovery to theragnostics. Br J Clin Pharmacol 2009;69:367–78.

[78] Kim G, Minig L, Kohn EC. Proteomic profiling in ovarian cancer. Intl J Gynecol Cancer 2009;19:S2–6.

[79] Husseinzadeh N. Status of tumor markers in epithelial ovarian cancer: Has there been any progress? A review. Gynecol Oncol 2011;120:152–7.

[80] Petricoin EF. III, Ardekani AM, Hitt BA, Leviine PJ, Fusaro VA, Steinberg SM, et al. Use of proteomic patterns in serum to identify ovarian cancer. Lancet 2002;359:572–7.

[81] Ransohoff DF. Lessons from controversy: Ovarian cancer screening and proteomics. J Natl Cancer Inst 2005; 97:315–9.

[82] Meani F, Pecorelli S, Liotta L, Petricoin EF. Clinical application of proteomics in ovarian cancer prevention and treatment. Mol Diag Ther 2009;13:297–311.

[83] Kim K, Vishintin I, Alvero AB, Mor G. Development and validation of a protein based signature for the detection of ovarian cancer. Clin Lab Med 2009;29:47–55.

[84] Braxton S, Bedilion T. The integration of microarray information in the drug development process. Curr Opin Biotechnol 1998;9:643–9.

[85] Carlisle AJ, Prabhu VV, Elkahloun A, Hudson J, Trent JM, Linehan WM, et al. Development of a prostate cDNA microarray and statistical gene expression analysis package. Mol Carcinogen 2000;28:12–22.

[86] Jacob RJ. Bioinformatics for LC-MS/MS-based proteomics. Methods Mol Biol 2010;658:61–91.

# Imaging in Drug Development

Richard J. Hargreaves[1] and Michael Klimas[2]

[1]*Discovery Neuroscience Merck Research Laboratories, West Point, PA 19486*
[2]*Imaging, Merck Research Laboratories, West Point, PA 19486*

## INTRODUCTION

Novel drug discovery is becoming progressively more difficult. Many diseases are today well served by existing agents, making the hurdle increasingly high for the differentiation of novel therapeutics that clearly demonstrate increased therapeutic benefits. Additionally, diseases with the greatest impact on quality of life and health economics are both chronic, developing over years to decades, and multifactorial in contributing factors including diet and exercise. Examples include Alzheimer's disease, diabetes, and heart failure. There is still, however, room for improvement in the treatment of many disorders. Increased scientific understanding has recognized that what appeared as one disease can in fact be deconstructed into constellations of disease subtypes and "symptom clusters" that are only partly treated by current therapeutics, giving opportunity for new therapies to improve patient care.

New drug candidates need to differentiate from currently available drugs, and novel unprecedented mechanisms are often the means to reach this goal. Novel mechanisms carry greater inherent risk of failure, as they generally lack clinical validation. Strategies for early decision-making are therefore critical to cost-effective drug development, as deferring proof of concept on poorly validated targets to late clinical trials is financially unsustainable if we are to obtain a satisfactory return on investment. Paul Matthews, the head of imaging at GlaxoSmithKline, recently commented that a fundamentally optimistic future scenario for the drug industry is to make drug discovery more successful by being smarter in our early Go/No Go decision with the disciplined use of biomarkers [1].

Development of drugs for novel targets requires good lab to clinic translational markers to guide dosing in early proof of biology experimental medicine and clinical proof-of-concept tests to drive early decision-making. The use of a biomarker strategy can pose different degrees of development risk, dependent on when biomarkers are used for decision-making. As discussed earlier in this volume, pre-investment is required to make biomarkers available at the right time, with the right fit-for-purpose level of analytical validation, and clinical qualification. Biomarkers that come too late have no impact on decisions and waste resources.

New, more efficient drug discovery paradigms could fundamentally allow evaluation of a greater number of targets, many of which today have only preclinical face validity, and prevent late-stage testing and extensive human exposure to molecules that have no chance of clinical success. Stopping work on targets and mechanisms that show little early evidence of significant biological benefit allows clinical development resources and energy to be focused on the best candidates and the best-validated hypotheses. Thus, the use of biomarkers has the promise to reinvigorate the drug discovery process through improved success rates that help bring useful medicines to patients sooner [2].

This chapter will discuss the promise and challenges of using imaging biomarkers in drug development, with examples from oncology, cardiovascular disease, respiratory disease, bone biology,

**327**

and central nervous system disorders. Additional information and "live updates" on molecular imaging can be found through the professional imaging societies (Society of Nuclear Medicine: Molecular Imaging Center of Excellence, www.snm.org/mi; World Molecular Imaging Society, www.wmis.org; International Society for Magnetic Resonance in Medicine, www.ismrm.org; and Radiological Society of North America, www.rsna.org/).

## THE CASE FOR MOLECULAR IMAGING

### Enabling Clinical Proof of Concept Testing

Advances in molecular imaging science, coupled with evolution of the imaging toolbox (Table 19.1), are playing an increasingly important role in our ability to use imaging as a translational endpoint in the assessment of molecules, mechanisms, and therapeutic hypotheses [3, 4]. In the laboratory setting, molecular imaging can help validate drug targets in models of disease and symptomatology and focus research on those drug candidates that achieve the highest target engagement with the lowest exposure, thereby maximizing the therapeutic index. Linking the degree of target engagement and the time-on-target to preclinical measures of efficacy is critical to molecule selection and hypothesis generation. In

early clinical development, molecular imaging can be used to link target engagement to drug-induced biological changes that are expected to produce clinical benefit – so-called proof-of-mechanism or activity testing. Proof of concept can be declared when target engagement can be linked to a change in a clinically meaningful imaging endpoint. If a drug has adequate target engagement but does not produce the expected biological or clinical effects, the therapeutic concept is flawed and development can be stopped.

### Accelerating Drug Development

Molecular imaging can be used to speed cycle times in drug development. To be optimally effective, simultaneous parallel discovery efforts in medicinal chemistry and radiochemistry are required to ensure radiotracers reach the clinic at the same time as drug candidates. The link between drug and tracer discovery efforts is important, as unique radiotracers are required for each new protein target. Phase I protocols can then be devised to weave together first-in-human single- or multiple-dose safety and tolerability testing with positron emission tomography (PET) imaging assessment of target engagement by central nervous system (CNS) drugs. This allows early assessment of the relationship between safety/tolerability and target engagement at peak levels,

TABLE 19.1   The Molecular Imaging Toolbox

| Modality | Parameter | Probe dosing characteristics | Spatial Resolution | Molecular Sensitivity | Applications |
|---|---|---|---|---|---|
| CT | X-rays | High mass contrast | ~ 20–50 μm | * | Tissue anatomy/density<br>Tumors<br>Bone |
| MRI/MRS | Radiowaves | High mass contrast (nanoparticles) | ~100 μm | ** | Tissue anatomy /blood flow/ content<br>Tumors<br>Atherosclerotic plaque<br>Vascular edema<br>Brain structure, function, and biochemistry |
| US | High-frequency acoustic | High mass microbubbles (targeted) | ~100 μm | *** | Anatomy/blood flow/tissue structure<br>Atherosclerotic plaque |
| SPECT/PET | Low-/high-energy gamma radiation | Low mass high specific activity (targeted) | PET: 1~2 mm | **** | Blood flow/ metabolism receptor density/molecular markers of health and disease<br>Brain receptors/pathology<br>Tumor physiology |
| Optical | Fluorescence Bioluminescence Near-IR | Gene reporters and activatable probes | μm to mm | ***** | Enzyme activity/metabolism/ receptors/genes<br>Tumors<br>Atherosclerosis |

accelerating Go/No Go decisions and enabling dose selection for later Phase II clinical trials. Vertically integrated research strategies that encompass animal imaging models which are aligned with early experimental imaging paradigms in humans, and in turn guide subsequent clinical studies in patients, are becoming core translational research approaches today.

## Improving the Efficiency of Drug Development

There is a growing interest in patient-specific, disease-specific, and outcome-specific imaging biomarkers that are independent of specific therapeutic mechanisms and molecules. Molecular imaging approaches that can be used to stratify patients for clinical trials will enable enrichment of clinical proof-of-concept studies, potentially leading to shorter, smaller, and more definitive clinical trials. Stratification using molecular imaging may not only improve the drug development process but ultimately could also drive personalized medicine approaches to therapy, delivering the right drug at the right dose to the right patient. There is additionally increasing interest in disease- and outcome-specific imaging biomarkers that can be used to study disease progression and remission, potentially serving as surrogate endpoints that could support and speed marketing approval of new disease modifying drug therapies.

## CHALLENGES TO USING IMAGING IN DRUG DEVELOPMENT

Perhaps the biggest challenge for the use of imaging in clinical drug development is making the shift from its qualitative use to detect disease to a quantitative discipline that provides objective numerical measurements of tissue characteristics suitable for incorporation into hypothesis-testing clinical trial designs [5, 6]. In routine clinical practice, images are subject to qualitative radiographic interpretation and are used to identify lesions or disease, thereby facilitating diagnosis and monitoring response to treatment. However, rigorous quantification and reproducibility are most important for drug development applications. The development of novel imaging biomarkers alongside drug candidates requires resource expenditure, so can add time and expense to early-stage drug development programs. But the elimination of potential failures early in development holds the promise of focusing resources and subsequent clinical research on higher quality molecules that have demonstrated

adequate target engagement and proven biology for further hypothesis testing in therapeutic clinical trials.

As with all biomarkers, imaging markers undergo the fit-for-purpose scientific validation and clinical qualification process that is described elsewhere in this volume [3, 7]. However, there are diverse practical challenges that are specific to using imaging markers to characterize patients, identify responders, monitor drug actions, and define therapeutic outcomes. Imaging requires specialized equipment and trained individuals, but its successful routine use most importantly depends on assay validation through assessment of the true magnitude of effect and purposeful harmonization of data acquisition techniques, together with the development of "turn-key" applications using standardized tools for data collection and analysis. These requirements add complexity, especially in multicenter clinical imaging trials in as much as detailed imaging manuals, standardized acquisition protocols (across different instruments from different manufacturers), data transfer, image reconstruction and data-processing algorithms (to annotate images with patient-specific information to permit confidential independent data review) are also required. Clinical qualification is a graded evidentiary process linking the biomarker to biology and clinical endpoints, and is dependent upon the intended use of the biomarker (Figure 19.1). The intended use may be for internal, regulatory, or clinical trial design and decision-making. But qualifying imaging biomarkers for use in regulatory approval processes is especially difficult, even when a biomarker is scientifically validated and well defined, ultimately requiring assessment in the context of clinical care or through integration into trials with proven active agents. This is clearly an issue when novel mechanisms and novel markers are developed together. Indeed, most biomarkers continue to be used at risk for decision-making during drug discovery and development, and few ever reach the level of surrogacy where they can substitute for a clinical outcome.

Proprietary molecular imaging biomarkers rarely have applicability across different targets even within the same disease area, and the cost of developing them has to be justified and accounted for in the context of specific drug discovery programs. In contrast, disease imaging biomarkers can generally be considered platform technologies that can characterize patient populations, disease state, and therapeutic response, so they have a potentially broad cross-target utility with value to diverse therapeutic approaches within a common disease area. In this case, the barrier is that there is little incentive for any one company to bear the

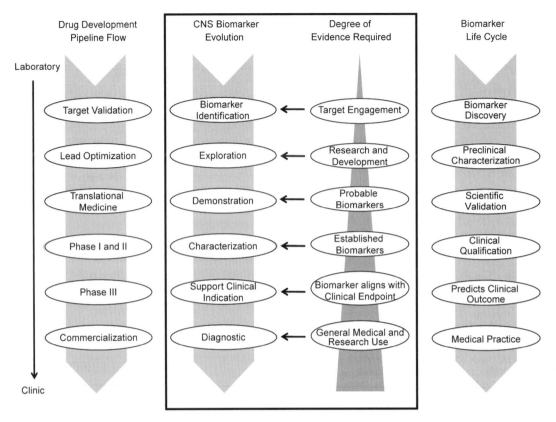

**FIGURE 19.1** Biomarker development. The *left-hand panel* shows the classic drug development pipeline flow from initial discovery in the laboratory to its clinical use. The *middle panel* shows CNS biomarker evolution from initial identification of the potential biomarker through processes that include exploration, demonstration, classification, and its clinical qualification before it becomes a diagnostic in general medical and research use. Note that as progress toward a diagnostic use becomes more defined, increasing levels of evidence for the biomarker are required. The *right-hand panel* shows the biomarker life cycle from initial definition to adoption. An initial observation suggesting a potential CNS biomarker may be observed in a small study which then needs to be evaluated in a larger clinical trial that contributes to validation. Validation, demonstrating specificity and sensitivity of the biomarker assay, is followed by qualification (with demonstration of robust reproducibility) of the biomarker and then regulatory adoption. Once adopted, the process of continued biomarker evaluation defines its status and includes potential refinements as technologies and larger clinical data sets become available. Adapted from Hargreaves RJ, Borsook D, Becerra L. Expert Opin Drug Discov 2011;6:597–617 [7].

considerable cost of clinical qualifying of the biomarker, so a different shared solution is required, in some cases entailing creation of public–private consortia.

## MOLECULAR IMAGING TECHNOLOGIES

Molecular imaging uses a variety of imaging technologies and specialized imaging agents to visualize, characterize, and quantify anatomical structures and biological processes at the cellular and subcellular levels in a physiologically relevant tissue context with high spatial and biochemical resolution [8]. Each technology generates images in different ways, and each has its strengths and weaknesses in terms of

spatial resolution, sensitivity, and imaging probe characteristics (Table 19.1). X-ray computed tomography (CT) is a mainstay for anatomical (structural) and perfusion imaging. Magnetic resonance imaging (MRI), on the other hand, yields rich information on structure, metabolites, and functional physiology. Molecular imaging modalities enable the spatial, temporal, and *in vivo* characterization of biological processes at the molecular level by employing various types of exogenously applied imaging probes. Molecular imaging and the generation of molecular imaging agents requires coordination and integration of many disciplines, including medicine, biology, chemistry, pharmacology, medical imaging physics, applied computer sciences and mathematics, and bioinformatics.

The most commonly used molecular imaging technique is nuclear imaging, which visualizes radio-labeled probes or radiotracers interacting with protein targets within or on the surface of cells. The two key radionuclide imaging modalities are PET, which uses tracers labeled with positron-emitting radioisotopes ($^{11}C$ and $^{18}F$), and single photon emission computed tomography (SPECT), which detects tracers labeled with gamma-emitting radioactive isotopes (e.g., $^{123}I$). Both can be used to track small molecule and biologic therapeutics. Radiotracers are versatile and sensitive, and can be designed to track the drug itself, image the drug target, or monitor key biochemical and physiological processes. Novel molecular tracer probes are the only way to quantitatively measure receptor populations and pharmacology at picomolar to nanomolar concentrations *in vivo* in both animals and humans. The use of structural imaging modalities such as CT and MRI in combination with PET or SPECT enables precise spatial and anatomical localization of molecular activity. Advances in the development of small animal tomographic cameras (microPET or microSPECT with CT) have facilitated translational bridging between preclinical and clinical research. Radionuclide imaging modalities, especially PET, have become powerful tools for drug discovery and development, particularly in oncology, where [$^{18}F$] FDG PET imaging of glucose metabolism is part of routine clinical care, and in the neurosciences, due to the inaccessibility of the brain and the paucity of specific CNS-specific markers to drive accurate drug dosing.

## IMAGING BIOMARKER EXAMPLES

### Selecting and Monitoring the Right Patients

The development of disease-modifying agents for Alzheimer's disease provides an example where a range of imaging biomarkers are being used to select patients and to monitor treatment response in clinical trials designed to test the amyloid-deposition hypothesis. PET imaging with radiotracers that visualize amyloid is being used to select patients with high amyloid burden, structural MRI to detect early brain atrophy in the entorhinal cortex and hippocampus – regions markedly affected during the progression of the disease- and functional imaging with fMRI or FDG PET to provide objective measurements of responses to cognitive tasks and brain metabolic function. These imaging metrics can of course also be used to monitor treatment response by providing objective measures of the preservation, slowing, or reversal of pathological, anatomical or

fluid-based biomarkers and brain function that could be used to support subjective cognition testing outcomes and claims of therapeutic disease modification. Future efforts will be aimed towards the development of molecular tracers for other hallmark pathologies in Alzheimer's disease. For example, tau diagnostics directed towards tau neurofibrillary tangles could support development of anti-tau therapeutics (Figure 19.2).

The validation and qualification of disease-based platform biomarkers that are independent of drug target and mechanism is now increasingly being addressed through formation of public–private consortia that share the risk and considerable cost of these long-term studies. Large consortia are developing and standardizing CNS imaging biomarker measurements in Alzheimer's disease (ADNI: Alzheimer's Disease Neuroimaging Initiative; www.nia.nih.gov/ Alzheimers/ResearchInformation/ClinicalTrials/ADNI. htm) and Parkinson's disease (www.michaeljfox. org/ living_PPMI.cfm Parkinson's Progression Markers Initiative) that characterize disease progression in patient populations to provide robust baselines for therapeutic trials. Data collected from these initiatives could therefore lead to the development of objective standard assessment tools to define the most appropriate patients to treat, and to monitor the effects of drugs in clinical trials, and so could become an important part of personalized medicine and the drug application, review, and approval process. In the US, the foundation for the National Institutes of Health (fNIH) set up the Biomarker Consortium (www.fnih. org) as a direct response to the FDA Critical Path Initiative that called for a greater emphasis on biomarkers to speed drug discovery and development. Other groups, such as the Innovative Medicines Initiative (IMI: www.imi.europa.eu/ a partnership between the EU and pharmaceutical companies) and the European Medicines Agency (www.ema.europa. eu), have also championed these approaches.

### Target Engagement Imaging

The goal of any early development program is always to test the mechanism and not the molecule in order to support additional research investments in late-phase clinical trials. Confirmation that drugs reach their targets using imaging markers of engagement and pharmacodynamics is therefore central to successful clinical proof-of-concept testing, particularly in CNS drug development. All too often, suboptimal molecules that fail to test hypotheses have been advanced to the clinic and so confuse and complicate paths for future development of new drug

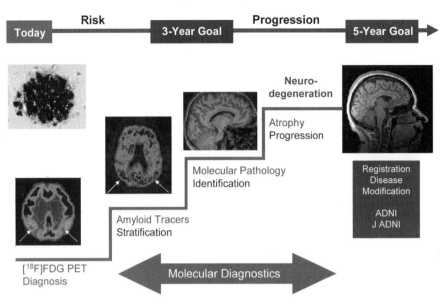

**FIGURE 19.2**   Imaging roadmap for Alzheimer's disease in which steps of increasing value are shown as we move from today's imaging with [$^{18}$F] FDG positive emission tomography (PET) to the development and registration of PET tracers that detect amyloid deposits in the brain for patient identification and clinical trial stratification, to imaging markers of molecular pathology such as tau-containing neurofibrillary tangles, to coordinated imaging consortia initiatives to characterize progression of Alzheimer's disease under conditions of today's standards of care. These consortia efforts will characterize patient populations and stages of disease to set the baseline metrics for clinical trials evaluating disease-modifying therapeutic approaches. Adapted from Hargreaves RJ. Clin Pharmacol Ther 2007;83:349–53 [4], with thanks to Drs WE Klunk, CA Mathis, P Shughrue and M Weiner for the use of the images.

entities, especially in neuropsychiatric disease. Indeed, the lack of an appropriate imaging "biomarker tool box" probably explains why so many neuroscience targets from the 1990s are still being pursued and have not yet been shown to work. It is a sobering thought that many different companies may keep failing on the same targets because they continue to lack the CNS biomarkers needed to guide Go/No Go decision-making and dose selection in clinical development.

In nuclear medicine, medicinal chemists together with radiochemists now play an increasingly important role in developing PET tracers to establish brain penetration and target engagement of candidate drugs that can guide interpretation of preclinical experiments and help select doses for clinical trial. Accordingly, an important feature of most CNS drug discovery programs is now the design, in parallel with drug candidate synthesis, of precursor molecules suitable for rapid labeling at high specific activity with $^{11}$C and $^{18}$F radionuclides to produce imaging radioligands that have high receptor affinity, target selectivity, fast brain penetration, and physicochemical properties that minimize non-specific binding to maximize signal-to-noise sensitivity.

The goal of the Neuroscience group in Merck Research Laboratories (MRL) is to supply a PET tracer alongside a drug candidate for all our CNS targets. We developed a PET tracer to assess the ability of a putative anti-obesity drug candidate to engage NPY5 receptors in the brain, which were believed to be critical components of a pathway that stimulates food intake and decreases energy expenditure. However, despite full engagement of the therapeutic target, the degree of weight-loss induced using the drug candidate alone was relatively modest and therefore not clinically useful. Since these results suggested that further development of this drug candidate would not produce therapeutic value, the program was terminated [9].

Subsequently, [$^{18}$F] MK-9470, an $^{18}$F-labeled inverse agonist of the cannabinoid-1 receptor (CB1R), was used to characterize CB1R distribution in the human brain and measure receptor occupancy of potential therapeutic anti-obesity CB1R agonists [10]. Despite having marked clinical efficacy, this program was also terminated since even at low receptor occupancies there was no therapeutic window between weight loss and adverse psychiatric effects [11]. However, as the cannabinoid system is thought to be involved in neuromodulation of a variety of CNS functions, $[^{18}F]$ MK-9470 has continued to be used as a research tool to study CB1R biology and pharmacology in CNS disorders [12].

Recently, we have described an $H_3$ receptor PET tracer $[^{11}C]$ MK-8278 [13] and have used it to evaluate the clinical experimental pharmacology and therapeutic index of $H_3$-receptor inverse agonist drugs which have an ability to promote wakefulness and prevent excessive daytime sleepiness (EDS) but also the potential side effect of disrupting sleep [14, 15]. Pharmacodynamic effects on quantitative electroencephalography (qEEG) were apparent at receptor occupancies of ~70% and higher. In a stimulant-referenced sleep deprivation model (SRSDM), the $H_3$-receptor inverse agonist MK-0249 had alerting activity that was statistically superior to placebo at doses associated with ~90% receptor occupancy. Consistent with this finding, using the Leeds Sleep Evaluation Questionnaire (LSEQ), subjects reported difficulty getting to sleep when receptor occupancy was ~70% after dosing MK-0249 at 10 pm,, and sleep was disrupted when occupancy was estimated to be between ~77% and 84% over the entire sleep period. In addition, polysomnography (PSG) during the recovery sleep period after sleep deprivation showed some evidence for sleep disturbance 19–31 hours after dosing, corresponding to brain $H_3$-receptor occupancy levels between ~78% and 69% [16]. These studies indicated that although clinically significant alerting efficacy could clearly be attributed to the $H_3$ inverse agonist mechanism, the pharmacodynamic profile of MK-0249 did not allow the wanted alerting and unwanted sleep disrupting effects to be separated. Nevertheless, these imaging studies have been useful in guiding the future goals of the $H_3$ inverse agonist program by showing that the profile of the optimal EDS molecule would need to rapidly achieve high levels of receptor occupancy but have a shorter half-life than MK-0249 so that drug would be cleared from the brain when it came to time to sleep.

We have also used PET imaging to facilitate Go/No Go decisions on MRK-409 an $\alpha_3$-subunit-preferring $GABA_A$ agonist [17]. MRK-409 produced anxiolytic-like activity in rodent and primate unconditioned and conditioned models of anxiety with minimum effective doses corresponding to $GABA_A$ receptor occupancies ranging from ~35% to 65%, depending on the particular model used. However, animals showed minimal overt signs of sedation at occupancies > 90%. Nonetheless, safety and tolerability studies in humans showed that there was pronounced sedation at a dose of 2 mg that was predicted from animal occupancy data to have low levels of occupancy. This set the maximum clinically tolerated single dose of MRK-409 at 1 mg, but PET studies showed that $[^{11}C]$flumazenil uptake following this dose was comparable to that after placebo administration, indicating that occupancy of $GABA_A$ receptor benzodiazepine binding sites by MRK-409 was below the limits of detection (i.e., < 10%). Thus, the preclinical non-sedating anxiolytic profile of MRK-409 did not translate into humans, and further development of this class of compound was halted. Similarly, PET was used to help interpret Phase I safety and tolerability data for a $\alpha_5$- selective inverse agonist of the $GABA_A$ receptor which, unlike non-selective inverse agonists at $GABA_A$ receptors such as FG7142, was shown to be devoid of anxiogenic effects at receptor occupancies that enhanced cognitive performance in preclinical species [18].

Dose-ranging using molecular imaging data can facilitate the registration of new therapies. For example, PET imaging (see Figure 19.3) was used to support final dose selection for aprepitant (EMEND®), a selective neurokinin-1-(NK1) receptor antagonist [19] that prevents acute and delayed chemotherapy-induced nausea and vomiting (19). In this application, PET studies were used to pick the lowest doses that demonstrated full CNS target engagement, thereby maximizing efficacy while optimizing the therapeutic window [2, 20]. This was especially important as aprepitant is used in conjunction with complex oncology drug therapy regimes where the potential for drug interactions is high. More recently, NK-1R PET imaging was used in a novel study to show receptor occupancy over 5 days of dosing with a single IV dose of 150 mg fosaprepitant (the water-soluble phosphate prodrug of aprepitant) that was equivalent to that provided by a single oral dose of 165 mg aprepitant given orally [21]. This study provided critical support for registration of new single-dose options for the drug. Finally, imaging was also used to select doses of aprepitant or the investigational NK-1R antagonist L-759,274 needed to block central NK1 receptors "around the clock" in a series of unsuccessful Phase II/III trials of this mechanism in patients with depression [22] and anxiety [23].

## IMAGING BIOLOGY AND PREDICTING RESPONSE

Molecular imaging has great potential to aid the development of oncology therapeutics since it fits into the existing framework of medical care, where PET/CT is a mainstay of diagnostic evaluation and

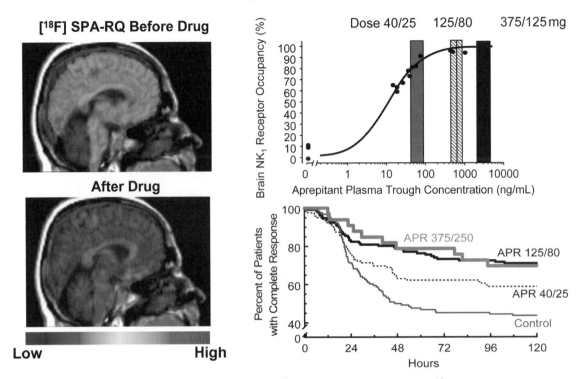

**FIGURE 19.3** Substance P NK1-receptor imaging with [$^{18}$F] SPA-RQ. The *left panels* show [$^{18}$F] SPA-RQ imaging of NK1 receptors in the brain (*top*) in the absence of aprepitant (EMEND®) and (*bottom*) after a fully blocking dose of aprepitant. The *right lower panel* shows dose–response curves for aprepitant in preventing emesis caused by a highly emetogenic chemotherapy such as cisplatin. Note that the response is submaximal at 40/25 mg and then is complete at doses of 125/80 mg, with no further effect at the higher dose of 375/250 mg. The *right upper panel* shows that this is the case because receptor occupancy is ~75% at the lowest dose and then > 90% saturated at the higher doses. The 125/80-mg dose was chosen for registration because it optimized the therapeutic window for aprepitant.

response monitoring [24, 25]. PET radiotracers are being developed as early-response markers to assess the impact of novel therapeutics on various universal molecular characteristics of tumor physiology (Figure 19.4). The most widely used molecular imaging marker in oncology is [$^{18}$F]-fluorodeoxyglucose ([$^{18}$F] FDG), which is used routinely as a diagnostic to monitor glucose uptake and metabolism by glycolysis and thereby can identify and track tumors and metastases that have increased glucose demands. Decreases in [$^{18}$F] FDG uptake, resulting from downregulation of glucose transporters, decreased glucose metabolism by cells, or fewer cells, have been proposed as an early signal that an experimental treatment may show promise in affecting tumor physiology [26, 27].

An important feature of the clinical evaluation of cancer therapeutics is the assessment of changes in tumor burden, and tumor shrinkage (objective response) and disease progression are useful endpoints in clinical trials. Guidelines for these evaluations, called RECIST (Response Evaluation Criteria in Solid Tumors), were published in 2000 and revised in 2009, and have been widely used for assessment of treatment outcomes. These guidelines cover imaging recommendations on the optimal anatomical assessment of lesions, which and how many lesions to measure, and clear definitions of progression. Interestingly, detection of new lesions, including the interpretation of [$^{18}$F] FDG scan assessment, is now a consideration [28].

One of the most contentious issues for RECIST has been the use of an anatomic unidimensional assessment (single longest dimension) of tumor burden and whether it is now time, given the improvement in imaging instrumentation and computing image reconstruction power, to move to volumetric anatomical assessment or to functional assessment with PET or MRI. Whether [$^{18}$F] FDG PET imaging can be used as an adjunct to anatomical imaging to determine progression and provide a potential endpoint for drug registration is currently being assessed. The fNIH launched consortia to look at [$^{18}$F] FDG PET in the context of treatments for lung cancer and non-Hodgkin's lymphoma (www.biomarkersconsortium.org/index.php?option=com_content&task=view&id=93&Itemid=143), but

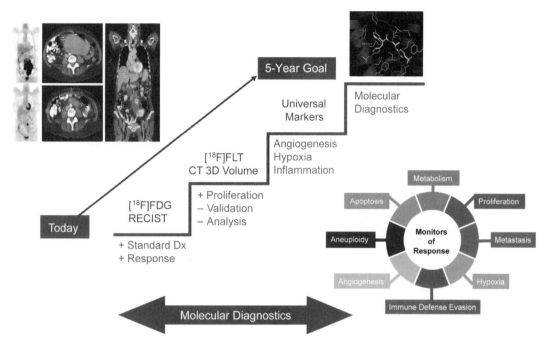

**FIGURE 19.4**   An oncology imaging roadmap in which steps of increasing value are shown as we move from today's imaging metrics to the development of universal markers of tumor physiology and molecular diagnostics for cancer pathways. Adapted from Hargreaves RJ. Clin Pharmacol Ther 2007;83:349-53 [4], with thanks to Dr S Stroobants for use of the PET/CT images.

these appear to be making only slow progress. A particular challenge is that these new three-dimensional volumetric methodologies and functional imaging modalities need to be standardized before current RECIST guidelines can be abandoned.

In comparison to [$^{18}$F] FDG PET, other applications of nuclear tracer imaging for oncologic drug development are more nascent but growing fast. The most mature effort is in the validation of tracers that can monitor cell proliferation ([$^{18}$F] FLT and [$^{18}$F] FMAU), but novel tracers for angiogenesis (integrin $\alpha v \beta 3$ directed tracers), hypoxia ([$^{18}$F] MISO and [$^{64}$Cu] ATSM), and apoptosis (Annexin-V based tracers and caspase-3 and -9 directed tracers) are following rapidly [29]. In the future it is also likely that optical and MR-based tracers will monitor cell physiology in cancer [30, 31].

Finally, MRI techniques also play an important role in anatomical and molecular imaging. One technique of particular note is dynamic contrast-enhanced magnetic resonance imaging (T$_1$-weighted DCE-MRI), which is now frequently used to assess dose-dependent biological responses in early clinical trial assessment of many anti-angiogenic drug candidates [32]. Whether DCE-MRI changes are predictive of drug efficacy or could be used as a tumor progression marker are still subjects of debate. As with many imaging modalities, critical issues for the future development and

application of DCE-MRI are standardization of data acquisition, analysis, and modeling.

## IMAGING THERAPEUTIC DRUG EFFECTS

### Respiratory Imaging

Chronic obstructive pulmonary disease (COPD) and asthma are heterogeneous diseases that have many different clinical presentations, prognosis, and therapeutic responses to medications. With the advent of novel imaging modalities (Figure 19.5), it is now possible to evaluate COPD and asthma phenotypes in clinical studies using non-invasive or minimally invasive imaging methods such as CT and MRI to complement traditional physiological measurements such as forced expiratory volumes (FEV$_1$) [33, 34]. Over the past few years CT has become the imaging modality of choice for the lung, enabling the extent of emphysema to be estimated objectively in patients with COPD. The advent of multidetector CT scanners (MDCT) has made it possible to obtain high-resolution images of the lung with less than a 10-second breath-hold. The volume of the lung and its individual lobes can be measured and lung mass, tissue volume, and airspace volumes can be calculated by using the apparent X-ray attenuation values of the lung to estimate lung density.

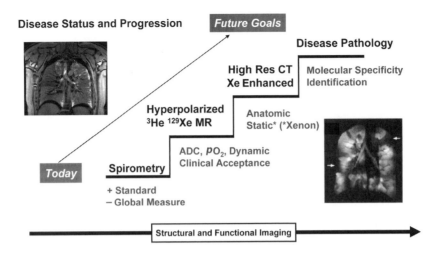

**FIGURE 19.5**   A respiratory imaging roadmap in which steps of increasing value are shown as we move from today's respiratory physiology measurements to imaging lung structure and function with a goal of discovering molecular diagnostics for respiratory disease pathology. Lung images kindly provided by Dr G Parraga.

At Merck, we sponsored experimental clinical MR imaging studies to explore the potential of lung imaging with the hyperpolarized noble gases $^{129}$Xe and $^{3}$He to help in developing drugs for respiratory diseases such as asthma and COPD. Inhalation of $^{3}$He gas provides the strongest MR signal, but $^{3}$He is expensive and its availability is limited, so $^{129}$Xe has become more widely used. These imaging agents provide excellent MRI contrast and, within a single breath-hold, enable quantitative images of the airways and airspaces of the entire lung to be captured that distinguish areas involved in ventilation from those that are impaired by disease. Diffusion-weighted MR methods are used to detect signals that reflect the random Brownian motion of the hyperpolarized gas. During inhalation, gas diffusion is restricted by the dimension of the airways and airspaces, so the average displacement of the gas is similar to alveolar diameters (a few hundred micrometers) and thus reflects alveolar integrity. An apparent diffusion coefficient (ADC) can be derived from the MRI and mapped quantitatively to examine lung integrity in pulmonary disease. In healthy young adults the ADC signal is homogeneous, whereas "focal" defects are observed in COPD and, as shown in Figure 19.6, the ADC can be used to map disease progress and severity [35]. More recently, fluorine-based MRI imaging of sulfur hexafluoride (SF6) has been investigated, eliminating the need for hyperpolarization and its associated technical challenges [36].

## Cardiovascular Imaging

Cardiovascular medicine is another area in which imaging has become a routine part of medical practice.

The chronic and progressive nature of atherosclerosis requires the registration of new therapies for this condition to be based on long-term clinical outcome trials. As with any disease-modifying therapy, there is a critical need to select and prioritize drug targets and to personalize therapy by identifying plaque subtypes (e.g., high-risk vulnerable plaques) that can be linked to the most appropriate therapeutic interventions (www.hrpinitiative.com/hrpinit). Molecular imaging agents directed against plaque-specific targets could be used to highlight patients for clinical trials in drug development and in the future could form the basis of diagnostic molecular imaging alongside conventional CT- and MRI-based structural and intravascular imaging approaches [37, 38]. However, despite considerable efforts using genetic and proteomic analysis of atherosclerotic plaque to identify targets, no molecular imaging agents have yet progressed into routine experimental use or been incorporated into clinical trials.

Recent studies have attempted to use [$^{18}$F] FDG to highlight active plaque by imaging increased glucose metabolic rates due to macrophage infiltration [39], and these have had varying degrees of success [40]. In the field of vascular imaging, important advances have been made in three-dimensional carotid ultrasound techniques to quantitatively capture plaque volumes. Developments in optical coherence tomography (OCT) may advance intravascular coronary imaging beyond the intravascular ultrasound (IVUS) techniques used today by enabling imaging of the vessel wall at the ultrastructural (macrophage) level [41], and all the intravascular techniques are now combining

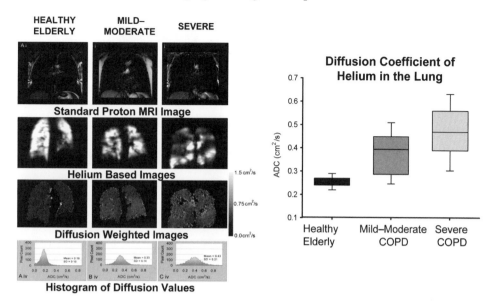

**FIGURE 19.6** Imaging studies in patients with chronic obstructive pulmonary disease (COPD) in which the *left panels* show representative standard proton MRI images, ³He images, and calculated diffusion weighted images for healthy elderly, mild–moderate and severe COPD patients. The histograms of diffusion values show the increasing spread with disease indicative of loss of alveolar integrity and increased diffusional characteristics (ADC) of the hyperpolarized gas. The *right panel* shows the mean data for each group, and indicates that ADC derived from ³He MR imaging could be a sensitive marker for disease progression and therapeutic outcome. Preliminary data from studies with Drs G Santyr, G Parraga, and R Fogel.

measurements (ultrasound, OCT, near IR spectroscopy) into single catheters [42].

## Bone Imaging

The field of bone imaging biomarkers has advanced quickly [43]. This has been spurred by the development of effective drug therapies such as the bisphosphonates, new drug registrations such as the RANK ligand denosumab [44], and investigational drugs such as the cathepsin K inhibitor odanacatib [45]. Biomarkers have advanced from fluid markers of bone formation and resorption to include dual energy X-ray imaging (DEXA) of bone density (allowing bone to be distinguished from soft tissue due to differential absorption at the two energies) and, most recently, high-resolution CT and MR imaging of bone architecture (Figure 19.7). These high-resolution structural measurements can be combined with *ex vivo* biomechanical testing of bone to form the basis for computational algorithms, such as finite element analysis (FEA), that can estimate bone strength and thereby complement bone density estimates and potentially differentiate between treatment effects [46]. It is hoped that these estimates of bone strength ultimately could displace the current need to use bone fracture development as a metric in clinical drug development trials (Figure 19.8).

## Functional CNS Imaging

Brain function is manifest by behaviors, and behavior is the integrated output of neuronal circuits and systems. Until the recent advent of non-invasive functional imaging, it has been impossible to observe the brain in action in health and disease and to monitor its response to therapy [47, 48]. The broad potential of using functional imaging for drug discovery in CNS disorders has been covered in a number of recent publications, including a recent review of the usefulness and current limitations of applying functional, morphological, and chemical imaging techniques in CNS drug development [49–51].

fMRI techniques now allow us to "look into functional aspects of living brain" and correlate these observations with our understanding of brain neurobiology and the effects of drugs on brain systems, in order to add to our understanding of where and how drugs may act to produce their therapeutic effects and perhaps also give insight into the etiology of the CNS disease itself [52]. The neuroimaging readouts available for CNS biomarker discovery include molecular, functional, morphometric/anatomical, and chemical measures (Figure 19.9).

Pain and analgesia have been a focus of many fMRI studies because they provide objective measures that can complement subjective pain reporting in drug

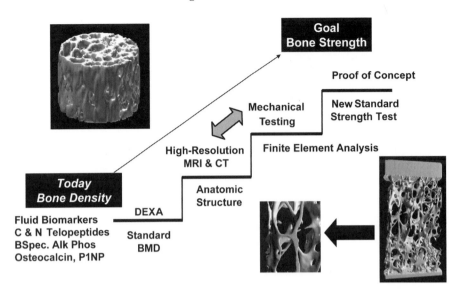

**FIGURE 19.7** A bone imaging roadmap in which steps of increasing value are shown as we move from today's fluid biomarkers of bone formation and resorption, to measurements of bone density (DEXA), to imaging of bone architecture accompanied by functional analysis of bone strength through mechanical testing and finite element analysis.

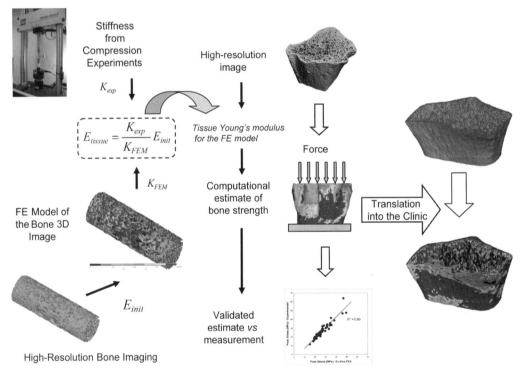

**FIGURE 19.8** Steps in the finite element analysis calculation of bone strength, starting with the acquisition of the *in vivo* bone trabecular images, leading to a mathematical model derived from mechanical testing of bone samples that allows virtual testing and calculation of an index of bone strength from the images. Images kindly provided by Drs D Williams and A Cabal.

development studies [53]. The sensorimotor neuro-anatomy of *acute* pain is relatively well characterized, and acute experimental pain paradigms lend themselves well to fMRI studies in both healthy volunteers

and pain patients. However, the structural anatomy and neurophysiology of chronic, persistent, or neuropathic pain and its modulation by physiological, psychological, and cognitive factors is much less well

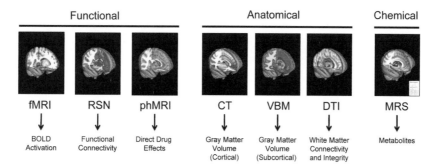

**FIGURE 19.9**  Functional, structural, and chemical approaches to measuring brain function. Reading from the left, functional imaging methods for blood oxygen level dependent (BOLD) fMRI, resting state network (RSN), and pharmacological MRI (phMRI). Morphological or anatomical structural methods that measure changes in gray matter volume include cortical thickness (CT) and voxel-based morphometry (VBM) of subcortical regions. Diffusion tensor imaging (DTI) measures white matter connectivity and integrity and magnetic resonance spectroscopy (MRS) can be used to measure chemical or metabolite changes in the brain that result from the action of drugs on transmitter systems or neurodegenerative disease. Reproduced with permission from Hargreaves RJ, Borsook D, Becerra L. Expert Opin Drug Discov 2011;6:597–617 [7].

understood, and so is currently an important area of imaging research [54–56]. The successful identification and qualification of functional brain "signatures" for both drug action (analgesia) and disease state (neuropathic pain) could provide objective biomarkers to guide drug development and clinical practice [57, 58]. Recent fMRI studies have begun to track the activation of brain systems during arthritis pain and to link these to preclinical fMRI experiments in murine arthritis pain models in which genetic molecular signatures have fingerprinted the brain circuits that were activated by pain and deactivated by analgesic treatment with TNF-α [59]. Clinical imaging studies clearly show the usefulness of fMRI to rapidly evaluate the effects of drugs with (fentanyl [60], buprenorphine [61]) and without (substance P NK1 receptor antagonists) clinical analgesic efficacy [62] by examining responses across the matrix of circuits activated by pain. In the future, combination PET/fMRI imaging together with the administration of highly selective CNS drugs has the marvelous potential to dissect the neurochemical basis of brain function and unravel the interactive systems–neuroscience basis of complex CNS-mediated behaviors in health and disease.

## CONCLUSION

Imaging has the potential to play an important role in the clinical evaluation and development of new molecules and mechanisms across diverse therapeutic areas. The value proposition in drug discovery is to use imaging biomarkers to focus research activities on

the patients and molecules most likely to test therapeutic hypotheses and achieve beneficial clinical outcomes. The hope is that the use of imaging biomarkers in early discovery and development, despite adding cost to early trials, will increase return on research investments by leading to fewer expensive late-stage failures by quickly eliminating the approaches that are most likely to fail. Perhaps most valuable are imaging biomarkers that could be used to drive new medical practice paradigms for patients in the latent phase of progressive disorders that will enable prediction, prevention, and tracking of disease in a paradigm shift from today's approaches that have to see overt disease before treating it.

## REFERENCES

[1] Matthews PM. Preface. In: Borsook D, Becerra L, Bullmore E, Hargreaves R, editors. Imaging in CNS drug discovery and development. New York, NY: Springer; 2009. pp. v–vii.

[2] Frank R, Hargreaves R. Clinical biomarkers in drug discovery and development. Nat Rev Drug Discov 2003;2: 566–80.

[3] Hargreaves R, Wagner J. Imaging as a biomarker for decision making in drug development. In: Beckmann N, editor. *In vivo* MR techniques in drug discovery and development. New York, NY: Taylor & Francis; 2006. p. 31–46.

[4] Hargreaves RJ. The role of molecular imaging in drug discovery and development. Clin Pharmacol Ther 2007;83:349–53.

[5] Schwarz A, Becerra L, Upadyhay J, Anderson J, Baumgartner R, Coimbra A, et al. A procedural framework for good imaging practice in pharmacological fMRI studies applied to drug development #1: Processes and requirements. Drug Discov Today 2011;16:583–93.

[6] Schwarz A, Becerra L, Upadyhay J, Anderson J, Baumgartner R, Coimbra A, et al. A procedural framework

for good imaging practice in pharmacological fMRI studies applied to drug development #2: Protocol optimization and best practices. Drug Discov Today 2011;16:671–82.

[7] Hargreaves RJ, Borsook D, Becerra L. Can functional magnetic resonance imaging improve success rates in central nervous system drug discovery? Expert Opin Drug Discov 2011;6:597–617.

[8] Rudin M, Weissleder R. Molecular imaging in drug discovery and development. Nat Rev Drug Discov 2003;2:123–31.

[9] Erondu N, Gantz I, Musser B, Suryawanshi S, Mallick M, Addy C, et al. Neuropeptide Y5 receptor antagonism does not induce clinically meaningful weight loss in overweight and obese adults. Cell Metab 2006;4:275–82.

[10] Burns HD, van Laere K, Sanabria-Bohorquez S, Hamill T, Bormans G, Eng W, et al. [18F] MK-9470, a positron emission tomography tracer (PET) for in vivo human PET brain imaging of the cannabinioid-1 receptor. Proc Nat Acad Sci USA 2007;104:9800–5.

[11] Addy C, Wright DH, Van Laere K, Gantz I, Erondu NE, Musser BJ, et al. The acyclic CB1R inverse agonist taranabant mediates weight loss by increasing energy expenditure and decreasing caloric intake. Cell Metab 2008;7:68–78.

[12] Van Laere K, Casteels C, Dhollander I, Goffin K, Grachev I, Bormans G, et al. Widespread decrease of type 1 cannabinoid receptor availability in Huntington disease in vivo. J Nucl Med 2012;51:1413–7.

[13] Hamill T, Sato N, Jitsuoka M, Tokita S, Sanabria S, Eng W, et al. Inverse agonist histamine H3 receptor PET tracers labeled with carbon -11 or fluorine-18. Synapse 2009; 2009(63):1122–32.

[14] Iannone R, Palcza JS, Renger JJ, Calder NA, Cerchio KA, Gottesdiener KM, et al. Acute alertness promoting effects of a novel histamine subtype-3 receptor inverse agonist in healthy sleep-deprived male volunteers. Clin Pharmacol Ther 2010;88:831–9.

[15] Iannone R, Renger J, Potter W, Dijk D, Boyle J, Palcza J, et al. The relationship between brain receptor occupancy and alerting effects in humans support MK-0249 and MK-3134 as inverse agonists at the histamine subtype-3 pre-synaptic receptor. (Poster). American College of Neuropsychopharmacology (ANCP) 48th Annual Conference. Hollywood: Florida; December, 2009.

[16] James LM, Iannone R, Palcza J, Renger JJ, Calder N, Cerchio K, et al. Effect of a novel histamine subtype-3 receptor inverse agonist and modafinil on EEG power spectra during sleep deprivation and recovery sleep in male volunteers. Psychopharmacology 2011;215:643–63.

[17] Atack JR, Wafford KA, Street LJ, Dawson GR, Tye S, Van Laere K, et al. MRK–409 (MK-0343), a GABA$_A$ receptor subtype-selective agonist, is a non-sedating anxiolytic in preclinical species but causes sedation in humans. J Psychopharmacol 2011;25:314–28.

[18] Eng W, Atack JR, Bergström M, Sanabria S, Appel L, Dawson GR, et al. Occupancy of human brain GABA$_A$ receptors by the novel α5 subtype-selective benzodiazepine site inverse agonist α5IA as measured using [$^{11}$C]flumazenil PET imaging. Neuropharmacology 2010;59:635–9.

[19] Hargreaves RJ, Arjona Ferreira JC, Brands J, Hale JJ, Hughes DL, Mattson B, et al. Development of aprepitant, the first neurokinin-1 receptor antagonist for the prevention of chemotherapy-induced nausea and vomiting. Ann NY Acad Sci 2011;1222:40–8.

[20] Bergström M, Hargreaves RJ, Burns HD, Goldberg MR, Sciberras D, Reines SA, et al. Human positron emission tomography studies of brain neurokinin 1 receptor occupancy by aprepitant. Biol Psychiatry 2004;55:1007–12.

[21] Van Laere K, de Hoon J, Bormans G, Koole M, Derdelinckx I, De Lepeleire I, et al. Equivalent dynamic human brain NK1-receptor occupancy following single-dose IV fosaprepitant versus oral aprepitant as assessed by PET imaging. Clin Pharmacol Ther 2012 (in press).

[22] Keller M, Montgomery S, Ball W, Morrison M, Snavely D, Liu G, et al. Lack of efficacy of the substance P (neurokinin$_1$ receptor) antagonist aprepitant in the treatment of major depressive disorder. Biol Psychiatry 2006;59:216–23.

[23] Michelson D, Hargreaves RJ, Alexander RC, Ceesay TP, Hietala J, Lines CR, et al. Lack of efficacy of L-759274, a novel neurokinin1 (substance P) receptor antagonist, for the treatment of generalized anxiety disorder. Intl J Neuropsychopharmacol 2012 (in press).

[24] Shields AF. Positron emission tomography measurement of tumor metabolism and growth: Its expanding role in oncology. Mol Imaging Biol 2006;8:141–50.

[25] Weissleder R. Molecular imaging in cancer. Science 2006;312:1168–71.

[26] Stroobants S, Goeminne J, Seegers M, Dimitrijevic S, Dupont P, Nuyts J, et al. $^{18}$FDG-Positron emission tomography for the early prediction of response in advanced soft tissue sarcoma treated with imatinib mesylate (Glivec®). Eur J Cancer 2003;39:2012–20.

[27] MacManus MP, Seymour JF, Hicks RJ. Overview of early response assessment in lymphoma with FDG-PET. Cancer Imaging 2007;7:10–8.

[28] Eisenhauer EA, Therasse P, Bogaerts J, Schwartz LH, Sargent D, Ford R, et al. New response evaluation criteria in solid tunours: Revised RECIST guideline (version1.1). Eur J Cancer 2009;45:228–47.

[29] Shields AF, Grierson JR, Dohmen BM, Machulla HJ, Stayanoff JC, Lawhorn-Crews JM, et al. Imaging proliferation in vivo with [F-18]FLT and positron emission tomography. Nat Med 1998;4:1334–6.

[30] Weissleder R, Pittet MJ. Imaging in the era of molecular oncology. Nature 2008;452:580–9.

[31] Pysz MA, Gambhir SS, Willmann JK. Molecular imaging: Current status and emerging strategies. Clin Radiol 2010;65:500–16.

[32] O'Conner JPB, Jackson A, Parker GJM, Jayson GC. DCE-MRI biomarkers in the clinical evaluation of antiangiogenic and vascular disrupting agents. Br J Cancer 2007; 96:189–95.

[33] Schuster DP. The opportunities and challenges of developing imaging biomarkers to study lung function and disease. Am J Respir Crit Care Med 2007;176:224–30.

[34] Coxson HO, Mayo J, Lam S, Santyr G, Parraga G, Sin DD. New and current clinical imaging techniques to study chronic obstructive pulmonary disease. Am J Respir Crit Care Med 2009;180:588–97.

[35] Kirby M, Mathew L, Heydarian M, Etemad-Rezai R, McCormack DG, Parraga G. Chronic obstructive pulmonary disease: Quantification of bronchodilator effects by using hyperpolarized $^3$He MR imaging. Radiology 2011; 261:283–92.

[36] Ruiz-Cabello J, Barnett BP, Bottomley PA, Bulte JW. Fluorine ($^{19}$F) MRS and MRI in biomedicine. NMR Biomed 2011;24:114–29.

[37] Jaffer FA, Libby P, Weissleder R. Molecular imaging of cardiovascular disease. Circulation 2007;116:1052–61.

[38] Sanz J, Fayad ZA. Imaging of atherosclerotic cardiovascular disease. Nature 2008;451:953–7.

[39] Rudd JH, Myers KS, Bansilal S, Machac J, Pinto CA, Tong C, et al. Atherosclerosis inflammation imaging with $^{18}$F-FDG PET: Carotid, iliac, and femoral uptake reproducibility, quantification methods, and recommendations. J Nucl Med 2008;49:871–8. 2008.

[40] Myers KS, Rudd JH, Hailman EP, Bolognese JA, Burke JP, Pinto CA, et al. Correlations among arterial FDG uptake and biomarkers in peripheral artery disease. JACC Cardiovasc Imaging 2012;5:38–45.

[41] Liu L, Gardecki JA, Nadkarni SK, Toussaint JD, Yagi Y, Bouma BB, et al. Imaging the subcellular structure of human coronary atherosclerosis using micro-optical coherence tomography. Nat Med 2011;17:1010–4.

[42] Yoo H, Kim JW, Shishkov M, Namati E, Morse T, Shubochkin R, et al. Intra-arterial catheter for simultaneous microstructural and molecular imaging *in vivo*. Nat Med 2011;17:1680–4.

[43] Guglielmi G, Muscarella S, Bazzocchi A. Integrated imaging approach to osteoporosis: State of the art review and update. Radiographics 2011;31:1343–64.

[44] Kendler DL, Roux C, Benhamou CL, Brown JP, Lillestol M, Siddhanti S, et al. Effects of denosumab on bone mineral density and bone turnover in post-menopausal women transitioning from alendronate therapy. J Bone Miner Res 2010;25:72–81.

[45] Eisman JA, Bone HG, Hosking DJ, McClung MR, Reid IR, Rizzoli R, et al. Odancatib in the treatment of postmenopausal women with low bone mineral density: Three-year continued therapy and resolution of effects. J Bone Miner Res 2011;26:242–51.

[46] Jayakar R, Cabal A, Szumiloski J, Sardesai S, Phillips EA, Laib A, et al. Evaluation of high resolution peripheral quantitative computer tomography, finite element analysis and biomechanical testing in a pre-clinical model of osteoporosis: A study with odanacatib treatment in the ovariectomized adult rhesus monkey. Bone 2012 (in press).

[47] Borsook D, Becerra L, Hargreaves RJ. A role for fMRI in CNS drug development. Nat Rev Drug Discov 2006;5:411–24.

[48] Wise RG, Tracey I. The role of fMRI in drug discovery. J Magn Reson Imaging 2006;23:862–76.

[49] Borsook D, Bleakman D, Hargreaves RJ, Upadhyay J, Schmidt KF, Becerra L. A "BOLD" experiment in defining the utility of fMRI in drug development. Neuroimage 2008;42:461–6.

[50] Borsook D, Becerra L, Bullmore E, Hargreaves R. The challenges and opportunities. In: Borsook D, Becerra L, Bullmore E, Hargreaves R, editors. Imaging in CNS drug discovery and development. New York, NY: Springer; 2009. p. 3–9.

[51] Borsook D, Becerra L, Bullmore E, Hargreaves R. Reasons to believe: The potential of imaging in CNS drug development. In: Borsook D, Becerra L, Bullmore E, Hargreaves R, editors. Imaging in CNS drug discovery and development. New York, NY: Springer; 2009. p. 381–5.

[52] Hargreaves RJ, Becerra L, Borsook D. Imaging as a CNS biomarker. In: Braddock M, editor. The chemistry of labels, probes and contrast agents. Cambridge: The Royal Society of Chemistry; 2011. p. 411–40.

[53] Tracey I. Imaging pain. Br J Anaesth 2008;101:32–9.

[54] Wartolowska K, Hough MG, Jenkinson M, Andersson J, Wordsworth BP, Tracey I. Structural changes of the brain in rheumatoid arthritis. Arthritis Rheum 2012;64:371–9.

[55] May A. Structural brain imaging: A window into chronic pain. Neurosceintist 2011;17:209–20.

[56] Howard MA, Krause K, Khawaja N, Massat N, Zelaya F, Schumann G, et al. Beyond patient reported pain: Perfusion magnetic resonance imaging demonstrates reproducible cerebral representation of ongoing post-surgical pain. PLoS One 2011;6:e17096.

[57] Borsook D, Becerra L, Hargreaves RJ. Biomarkers for chronic pain and analgesia. Part 1: The need, reality, challenges, and solutions. Discov Med 2011;11:197–207.

[58] Borsook D, Becerra L, Hargreaves RJ. Biomarkers for chronic pain and analgesia. Part 2: How, where, and what to look for using functional imaging. Discov Med 2011;11:209–19.

[59] Hess A, Axmann R, Rech J, Finzel S, Heindl C, Kreitz S, et al. Blockade of TNF–$\alpha$ rapidly inhibits pain responses in the central nervous system. Proc Natl Acad Sci USA 2011;108:3731–6.

[60] Zelaya FO, Zois E, Muller-Pollard C, Lythgoe DJ, Lee S, Andrews C et al. The response to rapid infusion of fentanyl in the human brain measured using pulsed arterial spin labeling. MAGMA. (Internet at, DOI 10.1007/s10334-011-0293-4, published Nov 24, 2011).

[61] Upadhyay J, Anderson J, Baumgartner R, Coimbra A, Schwarz A, Nutile L, et al. Modulation of CNS pain circuitry by intravenous and sublingual doses of buprenorphine. Neuroimage 2012;59:3762–73.

[62] Upadhyay J, Anderson J, Schwarz A, Coimbra A, Baumgartner R, Pendse G, et al. Imaging drugs with and without clinical analgesic efficacy. Neuropsychopharmacology 2011;36:2659–73.

# 20

# Dose–Effect and Concentration–Effect Analysis

Elizabeth S. Lowe[1] and Juan J.L. Lertora[2]

[1]Clinical Development, AstraZeneca Pharmaceuticals, Wilmington, DE 19803
[2]Clinical Pharmacology Program, Clinical Center, National Institutes of Health, Bethesda, MD 20892

## BACKGROUND

The intensity and duration of a drug's pharmacological effect are proportional to the dose of the drug administered and the concentration of the drug at its site of action. This simple fundamental principle of pharmacology has a pervasive influence on our approach to the study and use of drugs, from the basic research laboratory to the management of patients receiving drug therapy in the clinic. *Pharmacodynamics* is the discipline that quantifies the relationship between drug concentration at the site of drug action and the drug's pharmacological effect. A drug's pharmacological effect can be monitored and quantified at several levels, including at a molecular or cellular level *in vitro*, in a tissue or organ *in vitro* or *in vivo*, or in the whole organism (Table 20.1). The endpoint that is used to measure effect may differ at each level even for the same drug, and at the organism level the overall pharmacological effect may be the sum of multiple drug effects and the physiologic response of the organism to these drug effects.

Figure 20.1 is an example of a dose–effect study with a molecular endpoint. Patients who were scheduled for resection of their brain tumor received a dose of $O^6$-benzylguanine ($O^6$-BG) intravenously 10 to 27 hours prior to surgery [1]. $O^6$-BG irreversibly inactivates the DNA repair protein $O^6$-alkylguanine-DNA alkyltransferase (AGT), which mediates resistance to some alkylating-agent therapy in brain tumors. To determine the dose of $O^6$-BG that most effectively inhibits AGT activity, a sample of tumor tissue was snap-frozen and tumor AGT levels were measured

and related to the dose. The dose–effect curve shows an inverse relationship between the $O^6$-BG dose and the amount of remaining tumor AGT activity (fmol/mg protein), with higher doses resulting in lower tumor AGT activity. The optimal biological dose was defined as the dose achieving AGT levels < 10 fmol/mg protein in at least 11 of 13 patients treated at that dose level. As shown in Figure 20.1, all 11 patients at the 100-mg/m$^2$ dose level had tumor AGT levels < 10 fmol/mg protein. There was no $O^6$-BG-related toxicity from this dose [1].

When the drug-effect endpoint, such as change in blood pressure, is measured on a continuous scale the dose–effect relationship is termed *graded*, whereas an all-or-none endpoint, such as alive or dead, results in a dose–effect relationship that is *quantal*. Graded dose–effect relationships can be measured in a single biological unit that is exposed to a range of doses, and dose or drug concentration is related to the *intensity* of the effect. Quantal dose–effect relationships are measured in a population of subjects that are treated with a range of doses, and the dose is related to the *frequency* of the all-or-none effect at each dose level.

Figure 20.2 illustrates a graded dose–effect relationship for recombinant human erythropoietin (rhEPO) in patients with end-stage renal disease [2]. Erythropoietin, which is produced by the kidney in response to hypoxia, is a naturally occurring hematopoietic growth factor that stimulates bone-marrow production of red blood cells. Patients with end-stage renal disease are deficient in erythropoietin, and, as a result, they are usually severely anemic and transfusion dependent. In this dose-finding study, 18

*PRINCIPLES OF CLINICAL PHARMACOLOGY, THIRD EDITION*
DOI: http://dx.doi.org/10.1016/B978-0-12-385471-1.00020-9

**TABLE 20.1  Endpoints for Measuring Drug Effect at Different Levels for the New Class of Molecularly-Targeted Anticancer Drugs that Inhibit Farnesyl Protein Transferase**

| Level | Endpoint |
|---|---|
| Molecular | Inhibition of farnesyl protein transferase, farnesylation of target substrate proteins such as HDJ2 |
| Cellular | Inhibition of cellular proliferation *in vitro* <br> Induction of apoptosis |
| Tissue | Change in the size of measurable tumors |
| Organism | Prolonged survival <br> Reduction in tumor-related symptoms <br> Enhanced quality of life |

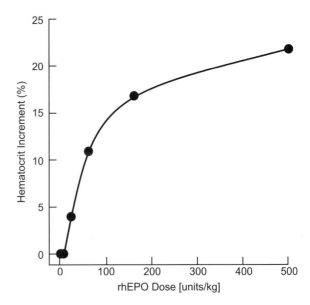

FIGURE 20.2  Dose–effect curve for recombinant human erythropoietin in patients with end-stage renal disease. Each point represents the mean absolute increase in hematocrit in a cohort of three to five patients. Adapted from data published by Eschbach JW, Egrie JC, Downing MR *et al.* N Eng J Med 1987;316:73–8 [2].

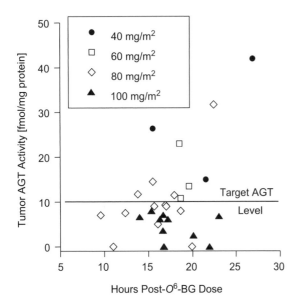

FIGURE 20.1  Activity level of the DNA repair protein, $O^6$-alkylguanine-DNA-alkyltransferase (AGT) in brain tumor surgical specimens from patients treated with escalating doses of the irreversible AGT inhibitor, $O^6$-benzylguanine ($O^6$-BG,) prior to surgery. All 11 patients treated at the 100-mg/m$^2$ dose level had undetectable levels of the target enzyme in tumor specimens. Adapted from data published by Friedman HS, Kokkinakis DM, Pluda J *et al.* J Clin Oncol 1998;16:3570–5 [1].

asymptotically approaches a maximum effect. This means that there is a "diminishing return" at higher doses because the incremental increase in hematocrit is smaller with each incremental increase in rhEPO dose.

## DRUG–RECEPTOR INTERACTIONS

The pharmacological effects of rhEPO and most drugs result from their non-covalent interaction with *receptors* (Figure 20.3). A receptor can be any cellular macromolecule to which a drug selectively binds to initiate its pharmacological effect. Cellular proteins are the most important class of drug receptors, especially cellular proteins that are receptors for endogenous regulatory ligands, such as hormones, growth factors, and neurotransmitters. The drug's chemical structure is the primary determinant of the class of receptors with which the drug will interact. Receptors on the cell surface have two functional domains – a *ligand-binding domain*, which is the drug-binding site, and an *effector domain*, which propagates a signal and results in an effect (Figure 20.3). The interaction of a drug and its receptor is reversible and conforms to the *law of mass action*:

$$C + R \underset{k_2}{\overset{k_1}{\rightleftharpoons}} C - R$$

patients with end-stage renal disease and baseline hematocrit < 20% were treated with rhEPO at doses ranging from 1.5–500 units/kg in cohorts of three to five patients per dose level. The effect of the rhEPO is measured as the peak absolute increment in the hematocrit. At the lowest dose levels (1.5 and 5 units/kg) there was no effect on hematocrit, but starting at a dose of 15 units/kg the hematocrit increased by 4–22% as the rhEPO dose increased. The shape of the dose–effect curve is a rectangular hyperbola, which

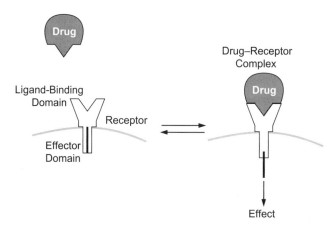

**FIGURE 20.3**  Drug–receptor interaction. A drug molecule binds reversibly to the ligand-binding domain of a receptor on the cell surface and the receptor propagates the signal into the cell via its effector domain, resulting in a pharmacological effect.

where $C$ is the free drug concentration at the site of action, $R$ is the concentration of unoccupied receptor in tissue, $C - R$ is the concentration of receptors occupied by drug, and $k_1$ and $k_2$ are the proportionality constants for the formation and dissociation of the drug–receptor complex.

## Receptor Occupation Theory

The receptor *occupation theory* of drug action equates drug effect to receptor occupancy. The intensity of drug effect is proportional to the number of receptors that are occupied by drug and the maximum effect occurs when all receptors are occupied by drug. The relationship between drug effect and the concentration of free drug at the site of action ($C$) can be described at equilibrium by the following equation:

$$\text{Effect} = \frac{\text{Maximum Effect} \cdot C}{K_D + C}$$

where Maximum Effect is the intensity of the pharmacological effect that occurs when all of the receptors are occupied, and $K_D$, which equals $k_2/k_1$, is the equilibrium dissociation constant of the drug–receptor complex. The dissociation constant ($K_D$) is also a measure of the affinity of a drug for its receptor, analogous to the Michaelis-Menten constant ($K_m$), which is a measure of the affinity of a substrate for its enzyme. The expression $C/K_D + C$ in this equation represents the fraction of receptors that are occupied with drug. When $C \gg K_D$, the expression equals 1 (i.e., all of the receptors are occupied with drug), and the Effect = Maximum Effect.

The equation relating a drug's pharmacological effect to its concentration describes a hyperbolic function that is shown graphically in Figure 20.4A. As free drug concentration increases, the drug effect asymptotically approaches the maximum effect. When the free drug concentration on the $x$-axis is transformed to a logarithmic scale, the dose–effect curve becomes sigmoidal, with a central segment that is nearly log-linear (Figure 20.4B). Semilogarithmic dose–effect curves allow for a better assessment of the dose–effect relationship at low doses and of a wide range of doses on the same plot. The $EC_{50}$ is the dose at which 50% of the maximum effect is produced or the concentration of drug at which the drug is half-maximally effective. On a semilogarithmic plot, the $EC_{50}$ is located at the midpoint or inflection point of the curve. When the relationship between receptor occupancy and effect is linear, $K_D = EC_{50}$. If there is amplification between receptor occupancy and effect, such as if the receptor has catalytic activity when the receptor ligand is bound, then the $EC_{50}$ lies to the left of the $K_D$.

## Receptor-Mediated Effects

Figure 20.5A shows dose–effect curves for the types of pharmacological effects that can be elicited when a drug interacts with its receptor. Drugs that interact with a receptor and elicit the same stimulatory effect as the receptor's endogenous ligand are called *agonists*. An agonist that produces less than the maximum effect at doses or concentrations that saturate the receptor is a *partial agonist*. An *antagonist* binds to a receptor but produces no effect. Antagonists produce their pharmacological effects by inhibiting the action of an agonist that binds to the same receptor.

Dose–effect curves are also useful for studying pharmacodynamic drug interactions (Figure 20.5B). A *competitive antagonist* binds to the same binding site as does the agonist, and the competitive antagonist can be displaced from the binding site by an excess of the agonist. Therefore, the maximum effect of an agonist can still be achieved in the presence of a competitive antagonist, if a sufficient dose or concentration of the agonist is used. The competitive antagonist lowers the potency of the agonist, but does not alter its efficacy. A *non-competitive antagonist* binds irreversibly to the same binding site as does the agonist, or it interacts with other components of the receptor to diminish or eliminate the effect of the drug binding to the receptor. A non-competitive antagonist prevents the agonist, at any concentration, from producing its maximum effect. Typically, a dose–effect curve with this type of interaction will reveal a reduced apparent efficacy, but the potency of the drug is unchanged.

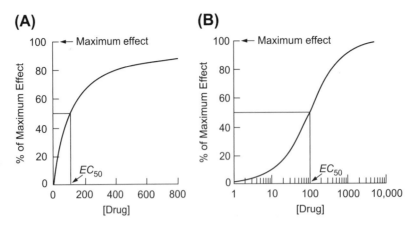

**FIGURE 20.4**   Dose–effect curves plotted using a (A) linear or (B) logarithmic scale for drug dose/concentration on the *x*-axis. The function relating effect to dose/concentration is based on the receptor occupation theory, described in the text. The relationship is non-linear, and with each increment in dose/concentration there is diminishing increment in effect. $EC_{50}$ is the dose/concentration producing half of the maximum effect.

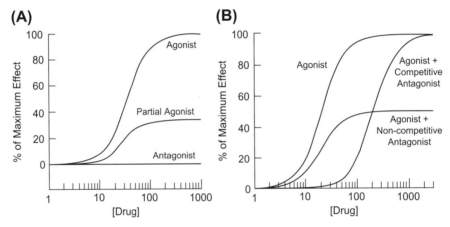

**FIGURE 20.5**   (A) Dose–effect curves describing the types of pharmacological effects produced when a drug interacts with its receptor. An *agonist* produces the maximum stimulatory effect, a *partial agonist* produces less than the maximum stimulatory effect, and an *antagonist* elicits no effect, but inhibits the effect of an agonist. (B) Dose–effect curves for the combination of an agonist and antagonist. A competitive antagonist reduces the potency of the agonist, but not the maximum effect. A non-competitive antagonist reduces the efficacy (maximum effect), but does not alter the potency of the agonist.

## THE GRADED DOSE–EFFECT RELATIONSHIP

The drug–receptor concept of drug action and the receptor occupation theory describe a graded dose–effect relationship in which the responding system is capable of showing progressively increasing effect with increasing dose or drug concentration. Graded dose–effect relationships are measured by exposing a single subject or a specific organ or tissue to increasing amounts of drug, and quantifying the resulting effect on a continuous scale. Although the

dose–effect curve can take on a variety of shapes, the classical graded dose–effect curve is the rectangular hyperbola that was described previously (Figure 20.4).

Figure 20.6 demonstrates a graded concentration-effect study of an intravenous infusion of lidocaine at a rate of 8.35 mg/min in patients with neuropathic pain [3]. The severity of pain was measured at 10-minute intervals using a visual analog pain scale (0 to 10), and blood levels of lidocaine were also measured at 10-minute intervals. Patients had a median pain score of 7 prior to the initiation of

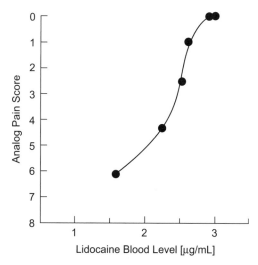

**FIGURE 20.6** Graded concentration–effect curve for intravenous lidocaine in patients with neuropathic pain. Pain was scored from 0 to 10 with an analog pain scale. The median pretreatment pain score was 7 and a score of 0 meant no pain. Blood levels of lidocaine were measured every 10 minutes, and pain was scored at the same time points. The graph relates the blood level of lidocaine to the severity of pain. Adapted from data published by Ferrante FM, Paggioli J, Cherukuri S, Arthur GR. Anesth Analg 1996;82:91–7 [3].

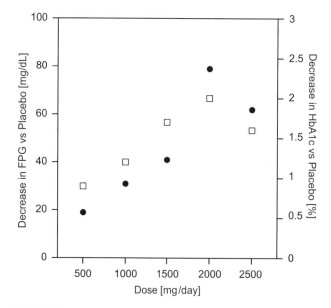

**FIGURE 20.7** Graded dose–effect curves for the oral anti-hyperglycemic agent, metformin, relative to a placebo in patients with a fasting plasma glucose (FPG) exceeding 180 mg/dL. Reductions in FPG (●) and HbA$_{1c}$ (□) occurred in a dose-dependent manner. Adapted from data published by Garber AJ, Duncan TG, Goodman AM. Am J Med 1997;102;491–7 [4].

therapy, and the maximal effect, no pain, had a score of 0. The concentration–effect curve for lidocaine is very steep. The pain decreased over a concentration range of 0.62 μg/mL. This steep concentration–effect curve indicates that the response to intravenous lidocaine is characterized by a precipitous break in pain over a narrow range in lidocaine concentrations.

Figure 20.7 demonstrates a typical example of a graded dose–effect curve from a study that evaluated the dose–effect relationship for the antihyperglycemic agent metformin. Metformin lowers blood glucose concentrations by increasing insulin sensitivity in peripheral tissues and inhibiting hepatic glucose production. Patients with a fasting plasma glucose (FPG) exceeding 180 mg/dL were randomized to receive either a placebo or metformin at one of five escalating doses ranging from 500 to 2500 mg/day [4]. The monitored endpoints of the study included FPG and levels of glycosylated hemoglobin (HbA$_{1c}$), a biomarker for chronic hyperglycemia. At the end of the study, FPG had declined by 19–84 mg/dL and HbA$_{1c}$ had declined by 0.6–2.0% in patients receiving metformin compared to placebo. Predictably, the decreases in FPG and HbA$_{1c}$ were disproportionate due to the slow turnover of hemoglobin. Metformin reduced both FPG and HbA$_{1c}$ in a dose-related fashion, with the maximum effect on both endpoints occurring at the upper limits of the dose range (2000 mg). The minimum effective dose was found to be 500 mg/day rather than 1500 mg/day, as was previously thought,

allowing, in subsequent clinical practice, an upward titration of metformin doses above this minimum if needed to achieve the target effect.

## Dose–Effect Parameters

*Potency* and *efficacy* are parameters that are derived from graded dose–effect curves and that can be used to compare drugs that elicit the same pharmacological effect. Potency, which is a measure of the sensitivity of a target organ or tissue to a drug, is a relative term that relates the amount of one drug required to produce a desired level of effect to the amount of a different drug required to produce the same effect. On the semilogarithmic graded dose–effect plot, the curve of the more potent agent is to the left, and the $EC_{50}$ is lower. A drug's potency is influenced by its affinity for its receptor. In Figure 20.8, Drug A is more potent than Drug B.

Figure 20.9 shows the *in vitro* dose–effect curves for two thiopurine analogs, thioguanine (TG) and mercaptopurine (MP). The thiopurines are antimetabolites that are used in the treatment of acute leukemia. Both drugs have multiple sites of action, but their primary mechanism of action is felt to be the result of their incorporation into DNA strands. Effect is measured *in vitro* as the percentage of leukemic cells killed in the presence of drug compared to untreated controls for three different leukemic cell lines [5].

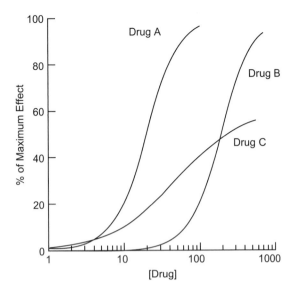

**FIGURE 20.8** Evaluation of the relative potency and efficacy of drugs that produce the same pharmacological effect. Drug A is more potent than Drug B, and Drugs A and B are more efficacious than Drug C.

The dose–effect curves show that TG is approximately 10-fold more potent than MP, despite the fact that they have very similar chemical structures and are converted to the same active intracellular metabolite (deoxy-thioguanosine triphosphate) prior to their incorporation into DNA. The two drugs appear to have similar efficacy in this *in vitro* study. Considerable

weight is placed on these *in vitro* concentration–effect studies for anticancer drugs because it has not been possible to define therapeutic concentrations *in vivo* in either animal models or patients.

*Efficacy* is the drug property that allows the receptor-bound drug to produce its pharmacological effect. The relative efficacy of two drugs that elicit the same effect can be measured by comparing the maximum effects of the drugs. In Figure 20.8, Drugs A and B are more efficacious than is Drug C. *Intrinsic activity* ($\alpha$), which is a proportionality factor that relates drug effect in a specific tissue to receptor occupancy, has become a standard parameter for quantifying the ability of a drug to produce a response:

$$\text{Effect} = \left(\frac{\text{Maximum Effect} \cdot \text{Dose}}{K_D + \text{Dose}}\right)$$

The value for intrinsic activity ranges from 1 for a full agonist to 0 for an antagonist, and the fractional values between these extremes represent partial agonists. Intrinsic activity is a property of both the drug and the tissue in which drug effect is measured.

Comparing the dose–effect curves of drugs that produce the same pharmacological effect can also provide information about the site of action of the drugs. Drugs A and B in Figure 20.8 have parallel dose–effect curves with identical shapes and the same level of maximal response. This suggests, but does not prove, that these two drugs act through the same receptor. Conversely, Drugs A and C have non-parallel dose–response curves, suggesting that they have different sites of action.

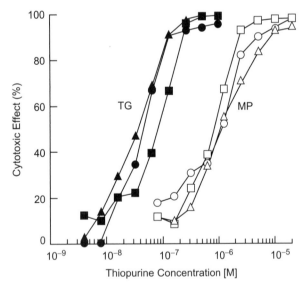

**FIGURE 20.9** Concentration–effect curves for the thiopurine analogs, mercaptopurine (MP, *open symbols*) and thioguanine (TG, *closed symbols*). Effect is the percentage of cells killed *in vitro* relative to an untreated control in MOLT 4 (*squares*), CCRF-CEM (*triangles*), and Wilson (*circles*) leukemia cell lines. TG is 10-fold more potent than is MP. Reproduced with permission from Adamson PC, Poplack DG, Balis FM. Leukemia Res 1994;18:805–10 [5].

## Dose Effect and Site of Drug Action

Graded concentration–effect studies may be useful for establishing the mechanism of action of a drug at a molecular or biochemical level by assessing the drug–receptor interaction. The xanthine analog, theophylline, which is a potent relaxant of bronchial smooth muscle, is used for the treatment of asthma. However, theophylline has a narrow therapeutic range, and at concentrations above this therapeutic range patients can experience vomiting, tremor, seizures, and cardiac arrhythmias. Theophylline interacts with multiple receptors that could account for its anti-asthmatic effect and its toxicity. Theophylline is an adenosine receptor antagonist and it inhibits phosphodiesterase (PDE). These two mechanisms have been proposed as the basis for the anti-asthmatic effects of theophylline and other xanthines.

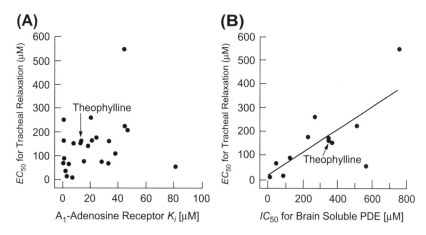

**FIGURE 20.10** Correlation between concentration–effect at the tissue level measured by $EC_{50}$ for relaxation of guinea pig trachea and concentration–effect at the receptor level for (A) antagonism of the $A_1$-adenosine receptor and (B) inhibition of phosphodiesterase for a series of xanthine analogs, including theophylline. The correlation between $EC_{50}$ for tracheal relaxation and $IC_{50}$ for phosphodiesterase inhibition suggests that phosphodiesterase inhibition is the primary site of action for the anti-asthmatic effects of these drugs. Reproduced with permission from Brackett LE, Shamim MT, Daly JW. Biochem Pharmacol 1990;39:1897–904 [6].

In Figure 20.10, the drug concentration that is required to elicit *in vitro* relaxation of tracheal smooth muscle in isolated guinea pig tracheal segments for a series of xanthine analogs, including theophylline, is related to the drug concentration required to antagonize the $A_1$-adenosine receptor (Figure 20.10A) or to inhibit brain-soluble PDE (Figure 20.10B) [6]. The relative potency of these xanthine analogs as adenosine receptor antagonists does not correlate with their potencies as tracheal relaxants. However, there is an association between PDE inhibition and tracheal relaxant activity, suggesting that PDE inhibition is the primary site of drug action. This type of graded concentration–effect analysis can lead to the development of more selective agents. In this case, xanthine analogs that are more potent PDE inhibitors and weaker adenosine-receptor antagonists may be more effective and less toxic anti-asthmatics.

## Biphasic Dose–Response Relationships (Hormesis)

*Hormesis* refers to a biphasic dose–response relationship characterized by stimulation at low doses and inhibition at high doses [7]. Numerous endogenous compounds and their synthetic agonists, including dopamine, display hormetic-like biphasic dose–response relationships in various models of pain assessment and modulation [8]. Dopamine is involved in learning and memory formation, which are processes that depend on synaptic modifications like long-term potentiation and long-term depression. Although the effect of dopamine on neuroplasticity is not well understood, it has been proposed that the specific dopaminergic impact on neuroplasticity depends on the concentration of dopamine to which the receptor is exposed, the specificity of the dopamine subreceptor involved in the interaction, and the type of cortical plasticity that is affected. It has been found that cognitive function is impaired when dopamine concentrations at D1 receptors are either insufficient or excessive, with a concentration–response curve that is biphasic and has the shape of an inverted U.

Similarly, D2-like receptor activation results in a dose-dependent inverted U-shaped impact on neuroplasticity [9]. To determine the dose-dependent effects of D2-like receptor activation on non-focal and focal neuroplasticity in the human cortex, 12 healthy volunteers participated in two experiments to assess the effects of D2-like activity on (a) focal plasticity, induced by paired associative stimulation (PAS; ISI of 10 or 25 ms) and (b) non-focal plasticity, induced by anodal or cathodal transcranial direct current stimulation (tDCS). Ropinirole is a non-ergoline synthetic D2/D3-specific dopamine agonist that is used either alone or in combination with other drugs to treat patients with Parkinson's disease, and was used in this study to activate D2-like receptors. Low (0.125 and 0.25 mg in the tDCS experiments; 0.125 mg in the PAS experiments), medium (0.5 mg), or high (1.0 mg) doses of ropinirole or an equivalent placebo were taken by subjects 1 hour prior to the start of plasticity-inducing cortical stimulation. Transcranial magnetic stimulation-elicited motor-evoked potentials (TMS-elicited MEPs) were recorded to measure excitability changes of the representational motor cortical area of the right abductor digiti minimi muscle (ADM). As shown in Figure 20.11, modulation of the D2-like receptor by ropinirol exerted a dose-dependent non-linear effect on neuroplasticity in the human motor cortex which differed for the type of plasticity induced. Both too little and too much D2-like activation impaired non-focal plasticity induced by tDCS and focal plasticity generated by excitatory PAS (ePAS). These results suggest that there is a limited range of D2-like receptor activity that is needed for optimal brain function, possibly resulting from presynaptic activation at lower doses and post-synaptic stimulation at higher doses.

## THE QUANTAL DOSE–EFFECT RELATIONSHIP

Whereas a graded dose–effect relationship relates drug dose and concentration to the intensity of a drug's effect measured on a continuous scale in a single biological unit, the *quantal* dose–effect relationship relates dose to the frequency of the all-or-none effect in a population of individuals. The minimally effective dose, or *threshold dose*, of the drug that evokes the all-or-none effect is identified by gradually increasing the dose in each subject. When displayed graphically as a frequency distribution histogram with threshold dose levels as the independent variable ($x$–axis) and the number of subjects who respond at each threshold dose level on the $y$-axis, the quantal dose–effect curve assumes a normal frequency distribution or bell-shaped curve (Figure 20.12A). The threshold dose level at which the effect occurs with maximum frequency is in the middle portion of the dose range. For most drugs, a wide range of threshold doses is required to produce the all-or-none effect in a population of individuals. This variability results from differences in pharmacokinetics and in end-organ or tissue sensitivity to the drug (pharmacodynamics) within the population.

A quantal dose–effect relationship can also be graphically displayed as a cumulative dose–effect curve, in which the cumulative percentage of individuals experiencing an effect is plotted as a function of the threshold dose. The normal frequency distribution in Figure 20.12A takes on a sigmoidal shape when the same data are plotted as a cumulative dose–effect curve (Figure 20.12B). The median effective

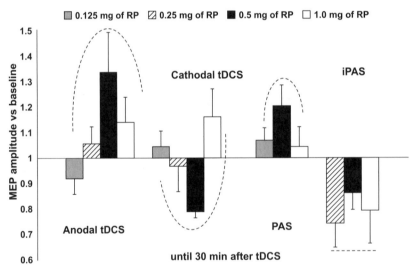

**FIGURE 20.11** Dose-dependent effect of D2-like receptor activation on non-focal and focal plasticity, indicated by changes in motor-evoked potentials (MEP) induced by transcranial direct stimulation (tDCS) and paired associative stimulation (PAS). D2-like receptor activation by ropinirole (RP) has an inverted U-shaped effect on neuroplasticity induced by tDCS and excitatory PAS (ePAS), with high or low D2-like agonist dosage resulting in impaired plasticity. No dose-dependent alterations were observed in after-effects induced by inhibitory PAS (iPAS). Each bar represents the mean of baseline-standardized MEP amplitudes ± SEM until 30 minutes after stimulation. Reproduced with permission from Monte-Silva K, Kuo M-F, Thirugnanasambandam N *et al.* J Neurosci 2009; 29:6121–34 [9].

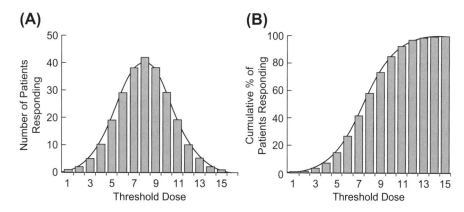

**FIGURE 20.12** Population-based, quantal dose-effect curves plotted in (A) as a frequency distribution histogram relating the threshold dose that is required to produce an all-or-none effect to the number of patients responding at each threshold dose; and in (B) as a cumulative distribution, in which the cumulative fraction of patients responding at each dose is plotted as a function of the dose.

dose ($ED_{50}$) for the quantal dose–effect relationship is the dose at which 50% of the population on the cumulative dose–effect curve responds to the drug. The cumulative dose–effect curve reflects the manner in which most quantal dose–effect studies are performed in a population of individuals. It is usually not practical in human or animal trials to define the threshold dose for each subject by gradually increasing the dose in each individual. Therefore, in most studies, groups of individuals are treated at each different dose level, and the fraction of individuals who respond at each dose level represents the cumulative proportion of those whose threshold dose is at or below the administered dose. This is equivalent to the cumulative distribution.

When administered to an organism, a drug that produces a desired therapeutic effect is also likely to produce at least one toxic effect. As a result, a single dose–effect curve does not adequately characterize the full spectrum of effects from the drug. The toxic effects of a drug can also be described by separate quantal dose–effect curves, and the safety of a drug depends on the degree of separation between the dose that produces the therapeutic effect and the dose that produces unacceptable toxic effects.

Cardiotoxicity, which can lead to congestive heart failure and death, is a toxic effect of the anticancer drug, doxorubicin. A cumulative dose–effect analysis demonstrated that doxorubicin cardiotoxicity is related to the lifetime dose of the drug (Figure 20.13) and provided the basis for the definition of safe lifetime dose levels [10]. The lifetime dose of doxorubicin is now limited to less than 400–450 mg/m², which is associated with a < 5% risk of developing congestive heart failure.

## Therapeutic Indices

*Therapeutic indices* quantify the relative safety of a drug, and can be estimated from the cumulative quantal dose–effect curves of a drug's therapeutic and toxic effects. Figure 20.14 shows the doses that are used in the calculation of these indices.

The *therapeutic ratio* is a ratio [$TD_{50}/ED_{50}$] of the dose at which 50% of subjects experience the toxic effect to the dose at which 50% of patients experience the therapeutic effect. A therapeutic ratio of 2.5 means that approximately 2.5 times as much drug is required to cause toxicity in half of the patients than is needed to produce a therapeutic effect in the same proportion of patients. However, this ratio of toxic to therapeutic

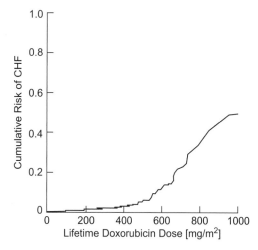

**FIGURE 20.13** Cumulative risk of developing congestive heart failure (CHF) as a function of the lifetime dose of doxorubicin. Reproduced with permission from Von Hoff DD, Layard MW, Basa P *et al.* Ann Intern Med 1979;91:710–7 [10].

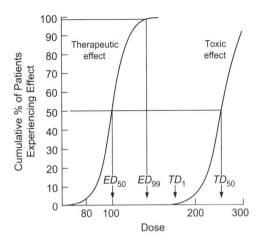

**FIGURE 20.14** Cumulative quantal dose–effect curves for a drug's therapeutic and toxic effects. The $ED_{50}$ and $ED_{99}$ are the doses required to produce the drug's therapeutic effect in 50% and 99% of the population, respectively. The $TD_1$ and $TD_{50}$ are the doses that cause the toxic effect in 1% and 50% of the population, respectively.

dose may not be consistent across the entire dose range if the dose–effect curves for the therapeutic and toxic effects are not parallel.

The goal of drug therapy is to achieve the desired therapeutic effect in all patients without producing toxic effects in any patients. Therefore, an index that uses the lowest toxic and highest therapeutic doses is more consistent with this goal than the therapeutic ratio. The *certainty safety factor* (CSF) is the ratio of $[TD_1/ED_{99}]$. A CSF $> 1$ indicates that the dose effective in 99% of the population is less than the dose that would be toxic in 1% of the population. If the CSF $< 1$, there is overlap between the maximally effective ($ED_{99}$) and minimally toxic ($TD_1$) doses. Unlike the therapeutic ratio, this measure is independent of the shapes of the cumulative quantal dose–effect curves for the therapeutic and toxic effects. The *standard safety margin* $\{[(TD_1 - ED_{99})/ED_{99}] \times 100\}$ also uses $TD_1$ and $ED_{99}$, but is expressed as the percentage by which the $ED_{99}$ must be increased before the $TD_1$ is reached.

## Dose–Effect and Defining Optimal Dose

Characterization of the dose–effect relationship is an important component of clinical trials performed during the initial stages of clinical drug development. These early trials frequently follow a dose-escalation design, in which increasing dose levels of drug are administered to cohorts of patients until the maximal effect is achieved or dose-limiting toxicity is encountered. The optimal dose is identified from these dose–effect relationships for the therapeutic and toxic effects.

Johnston [11] reviewed the dose-finding studies of a variety of antihypertensive agents and compared the initial recommended dosage range from these dose-finding studies with the lowest effective dose identified in subsequent randomized clinical trials and the currently recommended dose (Table 20.2). Based on this dose–effect meta-analysis, he concluded that many antihypertensive agents were introduced into clinical practice at excessively high doses. He attributed this to reliance on a dose-escalation trial design in which the dose was escalated too rapidly, resulting in a failure to define the lower part of the dose–effect relationship. In many of the cases the initial dose produced the maximum therapeutic effect, but the dose continued to be escalated without any clear evidence of increased efficacy. The initial recommended doses often appeared to be on the plateau of the dose–effect curve, considerably higher than the range of doses adequate to achieve the desired therapeutic response. At these higher doses, there is very little added benefit but a significantly greater risk for toxicity. A current trend is to avoid this pitfall by identifying the minimum dose required for satisfactory effect (MDSE) [12].

For anticancer drugs, tumor response is often related to *dose intensity*, and this dose–effect relationship is the basis for treating cancer patients with the maximum tolerated dose of these drugs, administered at the shortest possible dosing interval. Dose intensity, or dose rate, is the amount of drug administered

**TABLE 20.2** Comparison of Recommended Doses for Antihypertensive Agents Based on Initial Dose-Finding Clinical Trials and Subsequent Experience in Randomized Clinical Trials and Clinical Practice

| | Dose Range (mg) | | Lowest Effective Dose (mg) |
|---|---|---|---|
| Drug | Early Studies | Present Dose | |
| Propranolol | 160–5000 | 160–320 | 80 |
| Atenolol | 100–2000 | 50–100 | 25 |
| Hydrochlorothiazide | 50–400 | 25–50 | 12.5 |
| Captropril | 75–1000 | 50–150 | 37.5 |
| Methyldopa | 500–6000 | 500–3000 | 750 |

Data from Johnston GD. Pharmacol Ther 1992;55:53–93 [11].

within a defined period of time (e.g., mg/week). The strong relationship between doxorubicin dose intensity and the percentage of patients with osteogenic sarcoma who achieved greater than 90% tumor necrosis is shown in Figure 20.15 [13]. A dose-intensity analysis such as this one is useful in defining the optimal dose of an anticancer drug if a relationship between dose and therapeutic effect is observed.

The maximal effect achieved by a drug can be measured not only as a biomarker but also as a behavior or patient-reported outcome. Tobacco smoking is the most prevalent modifiable risk factor for morbidity and mortality associated with cancer, cardiovascular disease, and respiratory disease. Varenicline is a drug approved in many countries throughout the world as an effective treatment for smoking cessation. Varenicline targets the $\alpha 4\beta 2$ nicotinic acetylcholine receptor associated with nicotine-induced behaviors. In humans, varenicline is predominantly excreted unchanged via the kidney, and its pharmacokinetic profile is linear over the recommended dosing range. Population PK/PD analyses of varenicline were carried out on three groups of cigarette smokers [$n = 1099$ (51% women); $n = 1892$ (47% women); $n = 2238$ (47% women)] pooled from five randomized, placebo-controlled, multicenter clinical trials in order to determine the continuous abstinence rate (CAR) for weeks 9–12 after 12 weeks of continuous

treatment with varenicline, based on the subject's oral self-report of smoking and use of any nicotine-containing products since the last study visit [14]. In these clinical trials, an exhaled carbon monoxide measurement of $\leq 10$ ppm was used as a biomarker to confirm the CAR behavior outcome. Figure 20.16 demonstrates the exposure–response relationships for CAR at weeks 9–12 of varenicline in adult smokers. In the reference population [white, male, 45 years of age, and time to first cigarette upon waking (6–30 min)], the quit probability at 9–12 weeks (95% CI) increased from 22% (19–26%) in subjects receiving placebo to 38% (34–42%) in subjects receiving varenicline 0.5 mg BID and to 56% (51–61%) in subjects receiving varenicline 1 mg BID. The effects of patient population characteristics as covariates (time to first cigarette in the morning, age, gender, and race) could then be estimated relative to the baseline population (data not shown). These population PK/PD analyses provided an understanding of dose, exposure, response, and relevant patient covariates as they relate to the efficacy of varenicline for smoking cessation.

## FDA Guidance on Exposure–Response Relationships

In 2003, the United States Food and Drug Administration (FDA) produced a document with non-binding recommendations for sponsors of investigational new drugs (INDs) and applicants submitting new drug applications (NDAs) or biologics license applications (BLAs) on the use of exposure–response information in the development of drugs, including therapeutic biologics [15]. This guidance document recognizes that exposure–response information lies at the heart of the determination of the safety and effectiveness of drugs. However, like all FDA guidance documents, it does not establish legally enforceable responsibilities but describes the FDA's current thinking on a topic, and so represents only recommendations.

## PHARMACODYNAMIC MODELS

Pharmacodynamic models mathematically relate a drug's pharmacological effect to its concentration at the effect site. Examples of the types of pharmacodynamic models that have been employed include the fixed-effect model, maximum-effect models ($E_{max}$ and sigmoid $E_{max}$), and linear and log-linear models [16]. Unlike pharmacokinetic models, pharmacodynamic models are time independent. However, these models can be linked to pharmacokinetic models as discussed in Chapter 21.

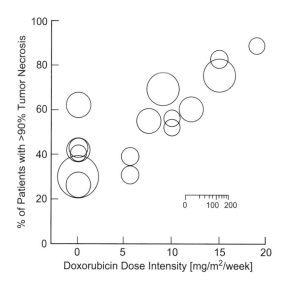

**FIGURE 20.15** Dose intensity meta-analysis for doxorubicin in patients with osteosarcoma. Each bubble represents a separate clinical trial, and the size of the bubble is proportional to the number of patients treated during the trial. Doxorubicin was administered prior to definitive surgical resection and effect is > 90% necrosis of tumor in the resected specimen. Dose intensity or dose rate is measured in mg/m²/week. Reproduced with permission from Smith MA, Ungerleider RS, Horowitz ME, Simon R. J Natl Cancer Inst 1991;83:1460–70 [13].

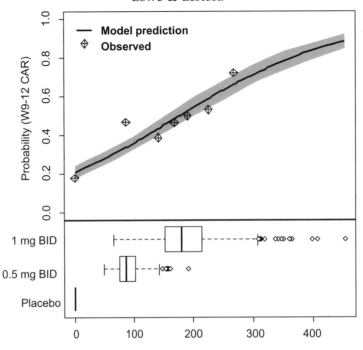

**FIGURE 20.16** Exposure–response relationships for the efficacy of varenicline in adult smokers. Varenicline population exposure–response relationships for continuous abstinence rate (CAR) at weeks 9–12 in adult smokers. The solid line and shaded area represent respectively the predicted probability and bootstrap 95% prediction interval of smoking cessation. The diamond symbols are the observed probabilities for each of six exposure ranges, as assessed by varenicline $AUC(0–24)ss$, with exposure set to zero for the placebo group. The box-and-whiskers plots at the bottom describe the distribution of the exposure data. The box itself indicates the difference between the first and third quartiles of the data, showing the spread of the data. The solid line in the middle of the box is the median value, and the whiskers indicate the range of the data or $1.5\times$ the interquartile distance, whichever is less. Open circles plotted outside the whiskers exceed these limits and may be considered outliers. Reproduced with permission from Ravva P, Gastonguay MR, French JL *et al*. Clin Pharm Ther 2010;87:336–44 [14].

## Fixed-Effect Model

The fixed-effect pharmacodynamic model is a simple model that relates drug concentration to a pharmacological effect that is either present or absent, such as sleep, or is a defined cutoff for a continuous effect, such as diastolic blood pressure < 90 mm Hg in a patient with hypertension. The specific pharmacological effect is present when the drug concentration is greater than a threshold level required to produce the effect, and the effect is absent when the drug concentration is below the threshold. This threshold concentration varies among individuals, and the fixed-effect model quantifies the likelihood or probability that a given concentration will produce an all-or-none effect based on the population distribution of threshold concentrations. This model is used primarily in the clinical setting. For example, based on a study correlating digoxin levels with toxicity, the probability of toxicity is 50% at a digoxin level of 3 ng/mL [17].

## Maximum-Effect ($E_{max}$ and Sigmoid $E_{max}$) Models

Although the maximum-effect pharmacodynamic models are empirically based, they do incorporate the concept of a maximum effect predicted by the drug–receptor interactions described earlier. The Hill equation, which takes the same form as the equation describing drug effect as a function of receptor occupancy, relates a continuous drug effect to the drug concentration at the effect site as shown:

$$\text{Effect} = \frac{E_{max} \cdot C^n}{EC_{50}^n + C^n}$$

where $E_{max}$ is the maximum effect, $EC_{50}$ is the drug concentration producing 50% of $E_{max}$, $C$ is the drug concentration, and the exponential constant, $n$ (the *Hill constant*), controls the slope of the resulting sigmoid-shaped curve, as shown in Figure 20.17 [18].

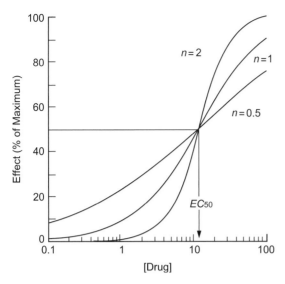

**FIGURE 20.17** Sigmoid $E_{max}$ pharmacodynamic model relating drug effect to the drug concentration at the effect site. The three curves show the effect of the exponential Hill constant ($n$) on the slope of the sigmoid curves.

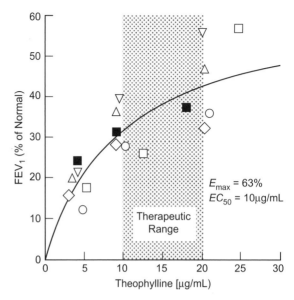

**FIGURE 20.18** Theophylline pharmacodynamics in patients with asthma. Effect, which was measured as improvement in forced expiratory volume in 1 second ($FEV_1$), is related to the serum drug level in six patients, who were studied after placebo and three incremental doses of theophylline. An $E_{max}$ model is fit to the concentration–effect data. Based on this analysis, a therapeutic range of 10–20 μg/mL was proposed (*shaded area*). Adapted from data published by Mitenko PA, Ogilvie RI. N Engl J Med 1973;289:600–3 [19].

If there is a baseline effect in the absence of drug, the effect term on the left-hand side of the equation can be expressed as the absolute or percentage change from baseline. Maximum-effect models describe a hyperbolic relationship between drug concentration and effect such that there is no effect in the absence of drug, there is a maximum effect ($E_{max}$) when concentrations approach infinity, and there is a diminishing increment in effect as the concentration rises above the $EC_{50}$.

The $E_{max}$ model is a simpler form of the sigmoid $E_{max}$ model, with a slope factor $n = 1$, so that:

$$\text{Effect} = \frac{E_{max} \cdot C}{EC_{50} + C}$$

In Figure 20.18, the $E_{max}$ model is used to quantify the relationship between theophylline serum level and improvement in pulmonary function as measured by the increase in forced expiratory volume in 1 second ($FEV_1$) in six patients who were treated with placebo and three incremental doses of theophylline [19].

## Linear and Log-Linear Model

In the linear model, concentration–effect relationships are described by the equation:

$$\text{Effect} = E_0 + \beta \cdot C$$

where $E_0$ is the baseline effect prior to treatment, $\beta$ is the slope of the line, and $C$ is the drug concentration. Although the linear model will predict no effect when drug concentrations are zero, it cannot predict a maximum effect. Therefore, for many effects, this model is only applicable over a narrow concentration range. At low drug concentrations ($<< EC_{50}$), the slope will approach the value of $E_{max}/EC_{50}$.

When the maximum-effect models are plotted on a semilogarithmic scale, the sigmoidal curves are log-linear within the range of 20–80% of the maximum effect, and can be described by the *log-linear model* (Effect $= \beta \cdot \log C + I$, where $I$ is the intercept). The disadvantages of this approach are that the pharmacologic effect cannot be predicted when the drug concentration is zero because of the logarithmic function, and the maximum effect cannot be predicted at very high concentrations. For example, the data shown in Figure 20.18 were linearized in the original article by plotting them with a logarithmic abscissa [19]. This linearized version of the plot unfortunately obscured the fact that theophylline levels above 15 μg/mL result in relatively little gain in therapeutic efficacy. Thus, maximum-effect models, which do not have these limitations, may be preferable to the linear models over a broad drug concentration range. Although simpler linear models are necessary when effects are linear over narrow concentration ranges, semilogarithmic plots should not be used to linearize curvilinear dose–effect relationships.

## CONCLUSION

The dose– or concentration–effect relationship is a central tenet of pharmacology. Dose–effect studies contribute to our understanding of the site of action of a drug, the selection of a dose and dosing schedule, the determination of an agent's potency and efficacy, and the elucidation of drug interactions. An essential aspect of the preclinical and clinical evaluation of any new drug is the careful delineation of the dose–effect relationship over the anticipated dosing range for the drug's therapeutic and toxic effects. More rational individualized dosing regimens that incorporate adaptive dosing, therapeutic drug monitoring, and the determination of risk/benefit from therapeutic indices have evolved from the integration of our knowledge of pharmacokinetics and pharmacodynamics.

## REFERENCES

[1] Friedman HS, Kokkinakis DM, Pluda J, Friedman AH, Cokgor I, Haglund MM, et al. Phase I trial of O$^6$-benzylguanine for patients undergoing surgery for malignant glioma. J Clin Oncol 1998;16:3570–5.

[2] Eschbach JW, Egrie JC, Downing MR, Browne JK, Adamson JW. Correction of the anemia of end-stage renal disease with recombinant human erythropoietin: Results of a combined phase I and II clinical trial. N Engl J Med 1987;102:491–7.

[3] Ferrante FM, Paggioli J, Cherukuri S, Arthur GR. The analgesic response to intravenous lidocaine in the treatment of neuropathic pain. Anesthes Analges 1996;82:91–7.

[4] Garber AJ, Duncan TG, Goodman AM, Mills DJ, Rohlf JL. Efficacy of metformin in type II diabetes: Results of a double-blind, placebo-controlled, dose–response trial. Am J Med 1997;102:491–7.

[5] Adamson PC, Poplack DG, Balis FM. The cytotoxicity of thioguanine vs mercaptopurine in acute lymphoblastic leukemia. Leukemia Res 1994;18:805–10.

[6] Brackett LE, Shamim MT, Daley JW. Activities of caffeine, theophylline, and enprofylline analogs as tracheal relaxants. Biochem Pharmacol 1990;39:1897–904.

[7] Calabrese EJ, Baldwin LA. Hormesis: The dose–response revolution. Annu Rev Pharmacol Toxicol 2003;43:175–97.

[8] Calabrese EJ. Pain and U-shaped dose responses: Occurrence, mechanisms, and clinical implications. Crit Rev Toxicol 2008;38:579–90.

[9] Monte-Silva K, Kuo M-F, Thirugnanasambandam N, Liebetanz D, Paulus W, Nitsche MA. Dose-dependent inverted U-shaped effect of dopamine (D$_2$-like) receptor activation on focal and nonfocal plasticity in humans. J Neurosci 2009;29:6124–31.

[10] Von Hoff DD, Layard MW, Basa P, Davis HL, Von Hoff AL, Rozencweig M, et al. Risk factors for doxorubicin-induced congestive heart failure. Ann Intern Med 1979;91:710–7.

[11] Johnston GD. Dose–response relationships with antihypertensive drugs. Pharmacol Ther 1992;55:53–93.

[12] Rolan P. The contribution of clinical pharmacology surrogates and models to drug development – a critical appraisal. Br J Clin Pharmacol 1997;44:219–25.

[13] Smith MA, Ungerleider RS, Horowitz ME, Simon R. Influence of doxorubicin dose intensity on response and outcome for patients with osteogenic sarcoma and Ewing's sarcoma. J Natl Cancer Inst 1991;83:1460–70.

[14] Ravva P, Gastonguay MR, French JL, Tensfeldt G, Faessel HM. Quantitative assessment of exposure–response relationships for the efficacy and tolerability of varenicline for smoking cessation. Clin Pharm Ther 2010;87:336–44.

[15] CDER, CBER. Exposure–response relationships – study design, data analysis, and regulatory applications. Guidance for Industry. Rockville, MD: FDA (Internet at, www.fda.gov/downloads/Drugs/GuidanceComplianceRegulatory Information/Guidances/UCM072109.pdf; 2003).

[16] Holford NHG, Scheiner LB. Understanding the dose–effect relationship: Clinical applications of pharmacokinetic–pharmacodynamic models. Clin Pharmacokinet 1981; 6:429–53.

[17] Piergies AA, Worwag EM, Atkinson AJ Jr. A concurrent audit of high digoxin plasma levels. Clin Pharmacol Ther 1994; 55:353–8.

[18] Wagner JG. Kinetics of pharmacologic response. J Theor Biol 1968;20:173–201.

[19] Mitenko PA, Ogilvie RI. Rational intravenous doses of theophylline. N Engl J Med 1973;289:600–3.

# Time Course of Drug Response

**Nicholas H.G. Holford[1] and Arthur J. Atkinson, Jr.[2]**

[1]*Department of Pharmacology and Clinical Pharmacology, University of Auckland, Auckland, New Zealand 1142*
[2]*Department of Molecular Pharmacology & Biochemistry, Feinberg School of Medicine,
Northwestern University, Chicago, IL 60611*

Therapeutic drug responses are a consequence of drug exposure. Exposure describes the intensity and time course of drug treatment. Most clinicians and patients behave as if they believe drug exposure is defined by the drug dose. However, a central dogma of clinical pharmacology is that drug actions are determined by drug concentration. Events leading up to such concentrations include the therapeutic consultation between patient and prescriber, the patient's decision to obtain and take the medication, and the time course of delivery and loss of drug from the site of action. The act of taking a drug dose is only one step in this chain of events, and provides only part of the information needed to predict the time course of response.

Pharmacokinetics provides a rational framework for understanding how the time course of observable drug concentration (usually in plasma) is related to the dose. The principles of pharmacodynamics described in Chapter 20 provide a companion framework for understanding the relationship between concentration and response. However, pharmacokinetics and pharmacodynamics are not enough by themselves to describe the time course of drug response for two main reasons:

1. Plasma is not the site of action of most drugs, so responses will be delayed in relation to pharmacokinetic predictions of plasma concentrations. The only exceptions are a limited number of drugs (e.g., heparin) whose action directly affects physical components of plasma.

2. The action of a drug is not the same as the drug response. In many cases, a network of events links receptor activation to physiological changes. These in turn are linked via complex pathophysiological mechanisms, often including homeostatic feedback, before the appearance of either therapeutic or adverse pharmacologic responses.

Recognizing these processes, it is useful to distinguish between the pharmacologic *action* (e.g., stimulation of a receptor, inhibition of an enzyme), the physiologic *effect* (e.g., bronchodilatation, lowering of cholesterol), and the clinical *outcome* (e.g., relief of an asthma attack, reduction of risk of a cardiovascular event).

These two reasons give rise to two basic conceptual approaches for describing the delay between plasma concentrations and changes in physiological effect [1]. In the first approach, the effect is considered to be an immediate consequence of drug action and the delay is thought to reflect the time required for the drug to reach its site of pharmacologic action, or *biophase*. In the second approach, the drug is thought to alter the turnover (synthesis or degradation) of some factor, usually an endogenous compound, that mediates the physiological effect. With each approach, the basic relationships between drug concentration and intensity of effect that were described in Chapter 20 can be applied to the analysis of drug response. The relationship between drug-induced effects on pathophysiology and clinical outcome is often too complex to describe in detailed mechanistic terms, and usually involves the pragmatic application of pharmacodynamic models linking observable biomarkers of drug effect to outcome as if the biomarkers, rather than drug concentrations, were themselves the driving force of drug response.

## PHARMACOKINETICS AND DELAYED PHARMACOLOGIC EFFECTS

In some cases, it is biologically plausible to identify the site of drug action as one of the compartments used to characterize the kinetics of drug distribution. As described in Chapter 3, Sherwin *et al.* [2] noted that the time course of insulin-stimulated glucose utilization parallels expected insulin concentrations in the slowly equilibrating compartment of a three-compartment model of insulin distribution (Figure 3.4). Since the kinetics of drug in this compartment may correspond to insulin concentrations in skeletal muscle interstitial fluid [3], it is reasonable to use this pharmacokinetic compartment to predict the time course of this particular insulin effect. In a study of digoxin pharmacokinetics and inotropic effects, Kramer *et al.* [4] observed that there is a close relationship between the time course of these effects and estimated digoxin concentrations in the slowly equilibrating peripheral compartment of a three-compartment pharmacokinetic model (Figure 21.1). Although the heart comprises only a small fraction of total body muscle mass, there is some

physiological justification for identifying myocardium as a component of this compartment. The authors noted that the time course of inotropic response could also reflect a delay due to the time required for the chain of digoxin-initiated intracellular events to result in increased myocardial contractile force. However, it has been shown that neither the distribution of digoxin from plasma to the myocardium nor the intracellular consequences of $Na^+$, $K^+$-ATPase inhibition are the key determinants of the slow onset of digoxin action. It is the slow dissociation of digoxin from $Na^+$, $K^+$-ATPase that best explains the slow equilibration between plasma digoxin and intensity of enzyme inhibition [5]. In this regard, models in which the effects of lysergic acid diethylamide on arithmetic performance are related to concentrations in a peripheral compartment of a pharmacokinetic model also appear to represent just a coincidence and do not have an obvious physiological rationale [6].

### The Biophase Compartment

Because only a small fraction of an administered drug dose actually binds to receptors or in other ways produces an observed effect, it is reasonable to suppose that the biophase may have kinetic properties that are distinct from those of the splanchnic and somatic tissues that, as discussed in Chapter 3, are involved in the distribution of most of an administered drug dose. This was first appreciated by Segre [7], who introduced the concept of a separate biophase compartment to explain the fact that the pressor effects of norepinephrine lagged appreciably behind its concentration profile in blood. Hull *et al.* [8] and Sheiner *et al.* [9] independently incorporated a biophase compartment in their pharmacokinetic–pharmacodynamic models linking plasma concentrations of neuromuscular blocking drugs to their skeletal muscle paralyzing effects.

Figure 21.2 is a schematic diagram of a pharmacokinetic–pharmacodynamic model in which a biophase compartment links drug concentrations in plasma to observed effects. The mathematical characteristics of this biophase compartment have been described in detail by Sheiner *et al.* [9] and by Holford and Sheiner [10]. In Figure 21.2, the pharmacokinetics of drug distribution and elimination are characterized by a single compartment ($V_1$). Since no drug actually passes from $V_1$ to $V_B$, the amount of drug X in compartment $V_1$ merely serves as a forcing function with respect to the biophase, and the differential equation for drug in $V_1$ can be written as:

$$dX/dt = -k_{01}X$$

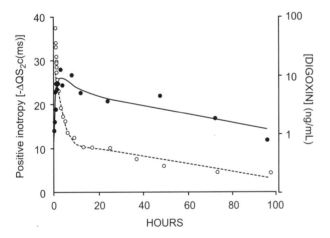

**FIGURE 21.1** An experiment in which a bolus injection of digoxin was administered and a model describing the slow binding of this drug to its receptor was used to fit the solid and dotted lines to average measurements of plasma digoxin concentration (○) and inotropic effect assessed from the heart-rate-corrected change in the $QS_2$ interval (●). Reproduced with permission from Weiss M, Kang W. Pharm Res 2004; 21:231–6 [5], who based this analysis on plasma concentration and effect data taken from Kramer WG, Kolibash AJ, Lewis RP *et al.* J Pharmacokinet Biopharm 1979;7:47–61 [4].

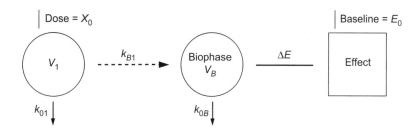

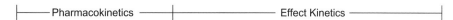

**FIGURE 21.2** A delayed pharmacodynamic model in which the kinetics of drug distribution and elimination are modeled with a single compartment ($V_1$), which receives a bolus input dose ($X_0$) and has an elimination rate constant $k_{01}$. Plasma concentrations are linked to a biophase compartment ($V_B$), and $\Delta E$ transduces drug concentrations in the biophase compartment into changes in the observed effect ($E$). The baseline value for the effect is given by $S_0$ so that $E = S_0 + \Delta E$. The time course of the observed effects is governed by the rate constant $k_{0B}$. The arrow linking $V_1$ and $V_B$ is dotted to indicate that no mass transfer occurs between these compartments and that $k_{B1}$ is not an independent parameter of the system (see text).

The differential equation for drug in the biophase compartment, B, is:

$$dB/dt = k_{B1}X - k_{0B}B \qquad (21.1)$$

Expressing these in Laplace notation (see Appendix I) gives the following two simultaneous equations (Equations 21.2 and 21.4):

$$s\,X(s) - X_0 = -k_{01}X(s) \qquad (21.2)$$

or:

$$X(s) = \frac{X_0}{s + k_{01}} \qquad (21.3)$$

and:

$$s\,B(s) = k_{B1}X(s) - k_{0B}\,B(s) \qquad (21.4)$$

or:

$$B(s) = \frac{k_{B1}X(s)}{s + k_{0B}} \qquad (21.5)$$

Substituting $X(s)$ as defined by Equation 21.3 into Equation 21.5 yields:

$$B(s) = \frac{X_0\,k_{B1}}{(s + k_{01})(s + k_{0B})}$$

Taking the inverse Laplace transform of this expression for the general case when $k_{01} \neq k_{0B}$:

$$B = \frac{X_0\,k_{B1}}{(k_{0B} - k_{01})}(e^{-k_{01}t} - e^{-k_{0B}t}) \qquad (21.6)$$

From Equation 21.1, we see that at steady state:

$$k_{B1}\,X_{SS} = k_{0B}\,B_{SS}$$

where $X_{SS}$ and $B_{SS}$ are the respective steady-state values for $X$ and $B$. To interpret biophase concentration-related effects in terms of their equivalent steady-state plasma concentrations, we equate their steady-state concentrations by letting $B_{SS} = X_{SS}$ and $V_B = V_1$. Therefore, $k_{B1} = k_{0B}$, and Equation 21.6 can be rewritten to describe biophase concentrations as:

$$[B] = \frac{X_0\,k_{0B}}{V_1(k_{0B} - k_{01})}(e^{-k_{01}t} - e^{-k_{0B}t}) \qquad (21.7)$$

$k_{0B}$ is the only additional parameter required to characterize the biophase compartment that is not obtained from the conventional kinetic analysis of drug distribution and elimination.

If we make the assumptions that drug distribution to and from the site of action is first order (i.e., no active transport is involved) and that drug actions are directly determined by the unbound, unionized drug concentration in water at the site of action, then at steady state the drug concentration in plasma water will be directly proportional to its concentration at the site of action. From a practical viewpoint, the parameters estimated from biophase concentrations (such as the $EC_{50}$) to predict the drug effects will correspond to the concentrations (e.g., plasma) used for the pharmacokinetic forcing function.

A characteristic feature of delayed response is the existence of a hysteresis loop when plasma concentrations are plotted against effects occurring at the same time. This is shown in Figure 21.3, in which

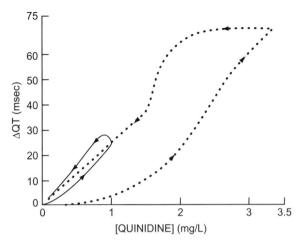

**FIGURE 21.3** Predicted changes in QT interval after administration of intravenous (*dotted line*) and oral (*solid line*) single doses of quinidine to healthy subjects [12]. The delay in effect with respect to plasma concentration causes *hysteresis* loops. The slope of the biophase concentration–effect relationship is greater after oral doses due to active metabolites formed during quinidine absorption. Reproduced with permission from Holford NHG, Coates PE, Guentert TW *et al.* Br J Clin Pharmacol 1981;11:187–95 [12].

plasma concentrations of quinidine have been related to changes in electocardiographic QT intervals. When the effect of the drug increases with concentration then the loop has a counterclockwise direction, but if the effect decreases with concentration then the loop goes clockwise (e.g., if potassium channel conductance had been used to describe the effect of quinidine). In both cases, the loop is described as showing hysteresis.

## Incorporation of Pharmacodynamic Models

The models described in Chapter 20 that are used to relate steady-state plasma concentrations of drug to observed effects can also be applied to the time course of drug effects.

### Linear Response Models

If the relationship between change in effect ($\Delta E$) and biophase concentration is linear, biophase concentrations can be related to $\Delta E$ by a constant ($\beta$) such that:

$$\Delta E = \beta [B] \qquad (21.8)$$

Biophase concentrations then are related to observations made on the effect variable ($E$) as follows:

$$E = S_0 + \beta [B] \qquad (21.9)$$

where $S_0$ is the baseline observed effect, termed *baseline state* in Chapter 22. The arithmetic sign of the value

of $\beta$ determines if the change in effect is either added to or subtracted from the baseline value.

A linear model was used to show that the blood-pressure lowering effects and blockade of transmission across sympathetic ganglia caused by *N*-acetylprocainamide (NAPA) followed a similar time course in dogs [11]. This pharmacokinetic–pharmacodynamic analysis was used to provide supporting evidence for the conclusion that the observed hypotensive effect of the drug was mediated by its ganglionic blocking action. This detailed analysis in dogs then was extended to demonstrate that the hypotensive effects of NAPA in a human subject were similar in intensity and time course.

A linear model was used also to relate biophase quinidine concentrations to the time course of electrocardiographic QT interval changes after intravenous and oral dosing [12]. As shown in Figure 21.3, the slope was greater after oral than after intravenous doses. This phenomenon was attributed to the formation of active metabolites of quinidine during first-pass metabolism of the oral dose [13].

### $E_{max}$ Models

The apparent linear relationship between biophase concentration and pharmacologic effect usually indicates that effects have been analyzed over only a limited concentration range [14]. In many cases, an $E_{max}$ model is required to analyze more pronounced effects, such as the blood pressure response of cats to norepinephrine. This was the concentration–effect relationship initially analyzed by Segre [7] when he proposed a model for the time course of biophase concentrations. For the $E_{max}$ model, $\Delta E$ in Equation 21.8 is described by:

$$\Delta E = \frac{E_{max}}{EC_{50} + [B]} \qquad (21.10)$$

where $E_{max}$ is a presumed maximal effect that is predicted from the observed non-linearity of response and $EC_{50}$ is the biophase concentration at which effects are half maximal. The linear-effect model defines this relationship adequately as long as biophase drug concentrations, $[B]$, are substantially less than the $EC_{50}$. However, the decision to use an $E_{max}$ rather than a linear model is usually determined by the available data rather than by theoretical considerations. For example, in one study of QT interval prolongation by an antiarrhythmic drug, a linear effect model was satisfactory for analyzing the response of four patients but an $E_{max}$ model was required to analyze the more pronounced effect seen in a fifth patient [15].

Although the mathematical form of the $E_{max}$ model is pharmacologically realistic [7], no physiological significance has been assigned to $E_{max}$ and $EC_{50}$ estimates in most applications of this model. Nonetheless, $E_{max}$ values in some cases may provide an indication of the maximal degree to which a particular intervention can affect enzyme or receptor activity. It also may be possible to find similarities between $EC_{50}$ values and drug binding affinity. For example, $\varepsilon$-aminocaproic acid is a lysine analog that has clot-stabilizing antifibrinolytic effects because it binds to lysine binding sites on plasminogen, preventing its attachment to fibrin. A study of $\varepsilon$-aminocaproic acid kinetics and antifibrinolytic effects in human subjects provided an estimate of half-maximal inhibitory biophase concentration ($IC_{50}$) of 63.0 μg/mL, which was similar to the *in vitro* estimate of 0.55 mM or 72 μg/mL for the $\varepsilon$-aminocaproic acid-plasminogen dissociation constant [16]. In fact these *in vivo* and *in vitro* results both represent an oversimplification of physiological reality, since plasminogen has one high-affinity and four low-affinity sites that bind $\varepsilon$-amino-caproic acid, rather than a single binding site [17].

### Sigmoid $E_{max}$ Models

In some cases, Equation 21.10 will need to be modified to account for the fact that the biophase concentration–effect relationship is sigmoid rather than hyperbolic. This modification was necessary in analyzing the pharmacokinetics and effects of d-tubocurarine [9]. In this case, the following equation was used to relate estimated biophase concentrations of d-tubocurarine to the degree of skeletal muscle paralysis ($\Delta E$), ranging from normal function to complete paralysis ($E_{max} = 1$) caused by this drug:

$$\Delta E = \frac{E_{max}}{EC_{50}^n + [B]^n}[B]^n \qquad (21.11)$$

Equation 29.11 was developed initially by Hill [18] to analyze the oxygen-binding affinity of hemoglobin. For normal human hemoglobins and those of most other mammalian species, $n$ has values ranging from 2.8 to 3.0 [19]. This reflects cooperative subunit interactions between the four heme elements of the hemoglobin tetramer. Proteins such as myoglobin that have a single heme subunit, and tetrameric hemoglobins such as hemoglobin H that lack subunit cooperativity, have $n$ values of 1.0. On the other hand, if oxygenation of one hemoglobin subunit caused an infinite increase in the oxygen binding affinity of the other subunits, $n$ would equal 4. Therefore, the $n$ values for normal hemoglobins indicate that there is strong but not infinite cooperativity in oxygen binding by the four heme subunits.

Wagner [20] first proposed using the Hill equation to analyze the relationship between drug concentration and pharmacologic response. However, the physiologic significance of $n$ values estimated in pharmacokinetic–pharmacodynamic studies is far less well understood than it is in the case of oxygen binding to hemoglobin. Accordingly, $n$ is currently regarded in these studies as simply an empirical parameter that confers sigmoidicity and steepness to the relationship between biophase concentrations and pharmacologic effect. This is illustrated by Figure 21.4, in which Equation 21.11 was used to analyze the relationship between tocainide plasma concentration and antiarrhythmic response [21]. It can be seen from this figure that the shape of the concentration–response curves approximates that of a step function as $n$ values increase. In fact, pharmacokinetic–pharmacodynamic models can be developed for *quantal responses* simply by fixing $n$ at an arbitrary large value, such as 20 [14]. In that case, the $EC_{50}$ parameter will indicate the threshold concentration of drug needed to provide the quantal response.

Sigmoid $E_{max}$ models have been particularly useful in the pharmacokinetic–pharmacodynamic analysis of anesthetic drugs [22]. Waveform analyses of electroencephalographic (EEG) morphology have served as biomarkers for anesthetic effects, and show characteristic changes that are different for barbiturates, benzodiazepines, and opiates. Since it often is impossible to conduct clinical studies of these agents at steady state, pharmacokinetic–pharmacodynamic investigations have been performed under conditions in which drug concentrations in plasma and effects are constantly changing. The time delay between changes in drug concentration and effect has been analyzed using a biophase compartment, such as that shown in Figure 21.2.

Of practical clinical importance is the role that pharmacokinetic–pharmacodynamic analysis played in optimizing dosing guidelines for using midazolam as an intravenous anesthetic agent [22]. Drug approval was based on results of traditional studies from which it was estimated that midazolam was no more than twice as potent as diazepam, the benzodiazepine with which clinicians had the greatest familiarity [23]. However, after considerable patient morbidity and mortality was encountered in routine clinical practice, pharmacokinetic–pharmacodynamic studies provided a significantly greater estimate of midazolam relative potency [24]. The EEG effect chosen in comparing midazolam with diazepam was total voltage from 0 to 30 Hz, as obtained from aperiodic waveform analysis.

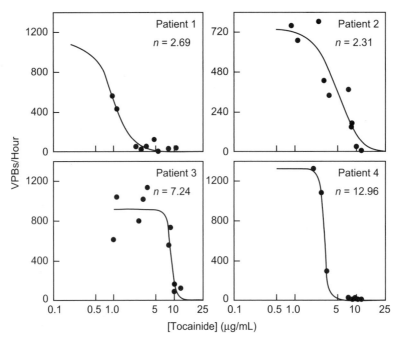

**FIGURE 21.4** Relationship between plasma concentrations of tocainide and suppression of ventricular premature beats (VPBs) for four representative patients. The relationship between VPB frequency and tocainide concentrations shown by the solid curves was obtained from a non-linear least-squares regression analysis of the data using Equation 21.11. The estimate of $n$ for each patient can be compared with the shape of the tocainide concentration–antiarrhythmic response curve. Reproduced with permission from Meffin PJ, Winkle RA, Blaschke TF *et al.* Clin Pharmacol Ther 1977;22:42–57 [21].

The results summarized in Table 21.1 show that the two agents have similar $E_{max}$ values, indicating similar efficacy, but that the $EC_{50}$ of midazolam is 5.5 times that of diazepam, demonstrating that midazolam is much more potent than diazepam. In addition, the equilibration half-life between plasma and the biophase compartment, calculated as:

$$t_{1/2(k_{0B})} = \frac{0.693}{k_{0B}}$$

is three times longer for midazolam (5.6 min) than for diazepam (1.9 min). This means that a longer time is needed after rapid injection for the effects of midazolam to become apparent [22]. No physiological significance has been attached to the values of the Hill

coefficient, $n$, that were obtained in these studies. However, investigations in rats have demonstrated a correlation between the $EC_{50}$ of EEG effects and estimates of $K_i$ obtained from *in vitro* studies of the ability of a series of benzodiazepines to displace [³H]flumazenil from benzodiazepine receptors (Figure 21.5) [25].

## PHYSIOKINETICS – THE TIME COURSE OF EFFECTS DUE TO PHYSIOLOGICAL TURNOVER PROCESSES

In almost all cases effects are mediated by an endogenous substance, and drugs modulate these effects indirectly by affecting either the production or elimination of this effect mediator (Figure 21.6). In addition to delays in drug effect due to pharmacokinetic distribution to the site of action, there are delays determined by the turnover of these effect mediators. The time course of the physiological mediator can be described as *physiokinetics*. Delays of a few minutes, or perhaps an hour or so, might plausibly be explained by distribution of a drug to its site of action, but the rate-limiting step for longer delays is likely to be physiokinetic rather than pharmacokinetic.

**TABLE 21.1** Comparison of Parameters Describing Midazolam and Diazepam Effect Kinetics

|            | $t_{1/2(k_{0B})}$ (min) | $E_{max}$ (µV) | $EC_{50}$ (ng/mL) | $n$ |
|------------|-------------------------|----------------|-------------------|-----|
| Midazolam  | 5.6                     | 141            | 171               | 1.8 |
| Diazepam   | 1.9                     | 137            | 946               | 1.7 |

Parametric analysis results from Bührer M, Maitre PO, Crevoisier C, Stanski DR. Clin Pharmacol Ther 1990;48:555–67 [24].

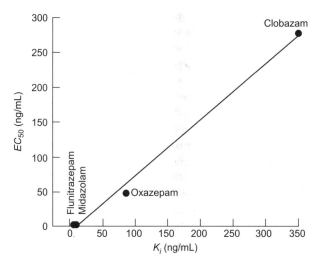

**FIGURE 21.5** Relationship in rats between the $EC_{50}$ of EEG effects (averaged amplitude in the 11.5- to 30-Hz frequency band) and estimates of $K_i$ obtained from *in vitro* studies of the ability of four benzodiazepines to displace [$^3$H]flumazenil from benzodiazepine receptors on brain tissue homogenates. Estimates of $EC_{50}$ were based on free benzodiazepine concentrations not bound to plasma proteins. Data from Mandema JW, Sansom LN, Dios-Vièitez MC *et al.* J Pharmacol Exp Ther 1991;257:472–8 [25].

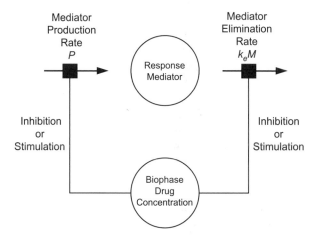

**FIGURE 21.6** Basic concept of physiological turnover or *physiokinetic* models. Observed effects are mediated by an endogenous substance (*effect mediator*). Drugs modulate these effects by either inhibiting or stimulating the production or elimination of this mediator. This accounts for the fact that the development of these drug effects is delayed beyond the time required for the drug to reach its pharmacologic site of action (*biophase*).

If the production rate ($P$) of the mediator ($M$) is regarded as a zero-order process and the elimination rate of the mediator is regarded as first order, the following equation describes the mass balance of the mediator:

$$dM/dt = P - k_e M \qquad (21.12)$$

where $k_e$ is the first-order elimination rate constant. Drugs can be modeled as exerting their effects by altering either $P$ or $k_e$ from their initial values. Implicit in Equation 21.12 is the fact that the rate of onset of effect is governed by the elimination rate of the mediator.

Warfarin is a classic example of a delayed action drug that exerts its anticoagulant effects by blocking synthesis of vitamin K-dependent clotting factors (factors II, VII, IX, and X). This effect can be analyzed by adding to Equation 21.12 a forcing function ($f_c$) to relate the degree of inhibition of clotting factor production ($P$) to the plasma concentration of warfarin:

$$dM/dt = P \cdot f_c - k_e M \qquad (21.13)$$

Nagashima *et al.* [26] developed a model in which the forcing function was modeled as proportional to the logarithm of the warfarin concentration in plasma. However, Pitsiu *et al.* [27] subsequently found that a sigmoid $E_{max}$ model (Equation 21.11) is more suitable for modeling the relationship between plasma concentrations of *S*-warfarin, the active isomer of warfarin, and inhibition of coagulation factor production.

Any of the pharmacodynamic models that we have described for other pharmacologic effects can serve as forcing functions in Equation 21.13, and model choice is guided best by an understanding of the mechanism of drug action and by the information content of the available data. For example, Sharma and Jusko [1] have selected the following modification of the $E_{max}$ model to illustrate the general use of a forcing function to model inhibition of either mediator production or elimination:

$$f_c = 1 - \frac{I_{max}[B]}{IC_{50} + [B]}$$

where $I_{max}$ is the maximal fractional degree of inhibition provided by any drug concentration $[B]$ and $IC_{50}$ is the concentration required for half-maximal inhibitory effect. The corresponding forcing function for stimulatory drug effects would be given by:

$$f_c = 1 + \frac{E_{max}[B]}{EC_{50} + [B]}$$

In addition to warfarin, Sharma and Jusko [1] have listed a large number of other drugs with delays attributable to changes in mediator turnover. These range from $H_2$-receptor antagonists, diuretics, and bronchodilators to corticosteroids, non-steroidal anti-inflammatory drugs, and interferon.

## Time-Varying Changes in the Relationship between Concentration and Drug Effect

So far, we have considered examples in which the relationship between drug concentration at the site of action and the effect is time invariant. This is not the case for drugs that exhibit *pharmacologic tolerance*, in which the intensity of an effect after initial drug exposure subsequently declines despite maintenance of similar biophase drug concentrations. Pharmacologic tolerance is characteristically revealed by plotting plasma concentration against effect and observing a *proteresis* loop. If the drug causes an increase in effect the loop will have a clockwise direction, while an inhibitory drug effect will have a loop with a counterclockwise direction.

There is now general agreement that tolerance develops rapidly to the cardiovascular and euphoric effects of cocaine [28, 29]. This phenomenon has been characterized by studies in which a bolus injection of cocaine was followed by an exponentially tapering infusion, so that relatively constant plasma concentrations were maintained while pharmacologic effects were observed [30]. Both the cardiovascular and euphoric effects of cocaine were analyzed with a biophase effect compartment and linear pharmacodynamic model. Function generators were used to characterize the acute development of tolerance by reducing over time the effect intensity, $\beta$ in Equation 21.8. The increase in heart rate that followed cocaine administration decreased with a 31-minute average half-life from its peak to a plateau that averaged 33% of peak values. Changes in blood pressure paralleled the increase and subsequent decline in heart rate [28]. However, subjective evaluation of cocaine-induced euphoria declined to baseline with an average half-life of 66 minutes. The slower development of tolerance to the euphoric response might reflect other phenomena such as a placebo response based on subjective expectations or a different physiological feedback system. Alternative models for tolerance have been evaluated by Gårdmark *et al.* [31]. Among the mechanisms proposed are the formation of a drug metabolite that acts as an antagonist, and the depletion of a precursor substance when conversion to an active mediator is stimulated by the drug.

*Sensitization* refers to an increase in pharmacologic response despite maintenance of constant biophase concentrations of drug. Adverse clinical consequences of sensitization are commonly observed following abrupt withdrawal of β-adrenergic blocking drug therapy in patients with coronary heart disease, and include ventricular arrhythmias, worsening of angina, and myocardial infarction [32].

Although several mechanisms have been proposed, these adverse events primarily reflect the fact that chronic therapy with β-adrenergic receptor-blocking drugs causes an increase in the number of available β-adrenergic receptors, a phenomenon termed *up-regulation* [32, 33]. When therapy with β-adrenergic receptor blocking drugs is stopped abruptly, the decline in up-regulated receptors lags behind the elimination of the receptor-blocking drug, resulting in a period of exaggerated responses to normal circulating catecholamine levels.

Using data describing the time course of receptor up-regulation in lymphocytes, Lima *et al.* [34] have developed a kinetic model of the fractional increase in β-adrenergic receptors that occurs with the institution of β-adrenergic receptor-blocking drug therapy, and of its subsequent decline when this therapy is stopped. A modification of Equation 21.10 was used to characterize the initial intensity of β-adrenergic receptor agonist-induced chronotropic response in the presence of a β-adrenergic receptor antagonist. Supersensitivity was then modeled by simply multiplying this estimate of initial intensity by the expected increase in β-adrenergic receptor density.

## THERAPEUTIC RESPONSE, CUMULATIVE DRUG EFFECTS, AND SCHEDULE DEPENDENCE

So far, we have focused our attention on the time course of drug effect. While the study of these effects can be helpful in understanding the mechanism of drug action and factors affecting drug effectiveness and potency, it usually does not provide information on how drug exposure influences clinical outcome.

Clinical outcome can be defined as the effect of drug treatment on the clinical endpoint of how the patient feels, functions, or survives. Some clinical outcomes can be described by composite scales that are commonly used in drug development for regulatory approval [e.g., the Unified Parkinson's Disease Scale (UPDRS) and the Alzheimer's Disease Assessment Scale (ADAS)]. These scales can be treated as if they were continuous measures of drug response and, as discussed in Chapter 22, are amenable to pharmacokinetic–pharmacodynamic modeling involving delayed effects even if no concentrations are available [35]. This seemingly broad definition of clinical outcome nevertheless excludes almost all of the drug effects we have discussed so far. For example, some outcomes are related to the cumulative effects of previous drug doses.

The acute treatment of congestive heart failure commonly involves the use of a diuretic to get rid of excess fluid that has accumulated as edema of the lungs and lower extremities. As shown in Figure 21.7, a high-efficacy diuretic like furosemide has a steep concentration–effect relationship, with a clearly defined maximum effect on sodium excretion. After an oral furosemide dose of 120 mg that causes almost maximal sodium excretion, the time course of drug concentrations reaches a peak of about 6 mg/L, which is well above the $EC_{50}$ of 1.5 mg/L (Figure 21.8). A lower dose of 40 mg produces concentrations which are one-third of the 120-mg dose, but the natriuretic effects are not decreased in proportion to the dose. When three 40-mg doses are given over 12 hours, the cumulative effect measured by total sodium excretion is 50% greater than that seen after a single 120-mg dose. Despite the same total dose and the same cumulative area under the concentration vs time curve from the two patterns of dosing, the clinical outcome would be less with the single 120-mg dose. This is an example of the phenomenon of *schedule dependence*.

Schedule dependence occurs when the drug effect is reversible, the concentrations exceed the $EC_{50}$ so that effects approach $E_{max}$ with proportionately less drug effect at high concentrations, and the clinical outcome is related to the cumulative drug effect. The phenomenon is expected to be quite common but is not often recognized clinically because of wide variability in response and other confounding factors such as disease progression.

The reduction of pain and other symptoms due to peptic ulceration may be quite closely linked to the current effect of a drug on acid secretion, but the rate of healing and eventual disappearance of an ulcer is a slow process determined in part by the extent and

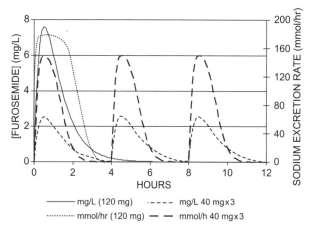

**FIGURE 21.8** The time course of furosemide concentration and natriuretic effect after three doses of 40 mg compared with those after a single 120-mg dose. Note that the concentrations after 120 mg are exactly three times higher than after 40 mg, but the peak effect after 40 mg is quite close to the peak after 120 mg because response to the 120-mg dose is limited by effects approaching $E_{max}$. The cumulative sodium loss after 120 mg is 400 mmol, while the three 40-mg doses produce a 600-mmol loss.

duration of gastric acid secretion suppression over several weeks. The clinical outcome of ulcer healing is therefore a consequence of the cumulative degree of acid inhibition. Proton pump inhibitors such as omeprazole bind irreversibly to the proton pump to suppress gastric acid secretion. The extent of inhibition is close to 100%, and outcomes are related to cumulative effects, but the irreversible nature of the drug action means that schedule dependence is not observed.

Many clinical outcomes are described in terms of *events*. An event might be death, a stroke, a myocardial infarction, an epileptic seizure, admission to hospital, need for supplementary treatment, and so on. The occurrence of an event or the time to an event can be modeled using a survivor function. The word *survival* relates most obviously to a death event, but the term is commonly used in a much broader context to describe the probability that the event under study will not occur.

The hazard function approach allows complex pharmacokinetic–pharmacodynamic influences to affect the occurrence of an event. The hazard [$h(t)$, sometimes called instantaneous risk] of an event at time $t$ is shown as:

$$h(t) = f(\mathbf{B}, X) \qquad (21.14)$$

where $\mathbf{B}$ is a set of parameters describing the hazard as a function of $X$ (time, dose, etc). The hazard is exactly equivalent to the elimination rate constant in a pharmacokinetic model. Indeed, the time course of drug concentration can be described by thinking of each

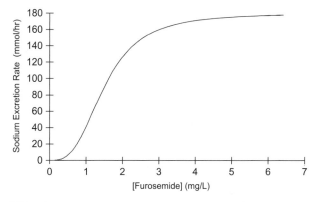

**FIGURE 21.7** The diuretic effect of furosemide is to increase the excretion rate of sodium. The pharmacodynamics of furosemide show a steep concentration–effect relationship with a clear maximum effect (180 mmol/h of $Na^+$). The $EC_{50}$ is 1.5 mg/L and the Hill coefficient ($n$) is 3.

molecule as having a risk of "dying" when it is eliminated. It is the survival of the molecules that have yet to be eliminated that determines the drug concentration. Potential time-varying covariates for the hazard are cholesterol concentrations (heart attack event), blood pressure (stroke event), or concentration of an anticonvulsant drug (seizure event). The chances of an event are related both to the size of the hazard and to the time that the patient is exposed to the hazard. The cumulative hazard $[H(t)]$ from 0 to $t$ can be related to the probability of an event, as illustrated by Equation 21.15 for the case of a constant hazard.

$$
\begin{aligned}
H(t) &= \int_0^t h(t) \\
&= \int_0^t \beta_0 \qquad (21.15) \\
&= \beta_0 \cdot t
\end{aligned}
$$

In this equation, $\beta_0$ is the instantaneous risk of an event when the hazard is constant.

A constant hazard is not typically realistic for biological events, and time-varying hazards are more commonly needed to describe clinical outcome events. The probability of surviving from time 0 to time $t$ is known as the survivor function, $S(t)$, and is shown in Equation 21.16.

$$ S(t) = \exp(-H(t)) \qquad (21.16) $$

Note the exact similarity between Equation 21.16 and the equation describing the time course of drug concentration being eliminated from a one-compartment system. Cox et al. [36, 37] describe the use of the hazard and the survivor function for modeling the likelihood of an event $(L)$ whose time is known, $L(t)$:

$$ L(t) = S(t) \cdot h(t) \qquad (21.19) $$

More often, an event is known to have occurred in an interval of time but the exact time is not known. The likelihood of an event in the interval $t[j-1]$ to $t[j]$ is given by:

$$ L(t[j] - t[j-1]) = S(t[j-1]) - S(t[j]) \qquad (21.20) $$

Hu and Sale [38] give interesting examples of applying this idea to simulating clinical trials with dropout events that may be determined by the underlying disease progress.

The use of a hazard function to describe time-varying risk of an event is a flexible method for bringing together pharmacokinetics, changes in drug effects on biomarkers, and other risk factors such as concomitant changes in disease severity. It has been applied to understand the need for additional pain medication in clinical trials of analgesics [39] and the suppression of vomiting events caused by chemotherapy [37]. The hazard function idea can be extended to describe clinical outcomes that are described in terms of frequency (e.g., epileptic seizures per month) and categorical scales of severity (e.g., heartburn pain) [40]. Study of long-term drug effects requires incorporation of a disease progression model into the analysis, and this will be the subject of the next chapter.

## REFERENCES

[1] Sharma A, Jusko WJ. Characteristics of indirect pharmacodynamic models and applications to clinical drug responses. Br J Clin Pharmacol 1998;45:229–39.

[2] Sherwin RS, Kramer KJ, Tobin JD, Insel PA, Liljenquist JE, Berman M, Andres R. A model of the kinetics of insulin in man. J Clin Invest 1974;53:1481–92.

[3] Steil GM, Meador MA, Bergman RN. Thoracic duct lymph. Relative contribution from splanchnic and muscle tissue. Diabetes 1993;42:720–31.

[4] Kramer WG, Kolibash AJ, Lewis RP, Bathala MS, Visconti JA, Reuning RH. Pharmacokinetics of digoxin: Relationship between response intensity and predicted compartmental drug levels in man. J Pharmacokinet Biopharm 1979;7:47–61.

[5] Weiss M, Kang W. Inotropic effect of digoxin in humans: Mechanistic pharmacokinetic/pharmacodynamic model based on slow receptor binding. Pharm Res 2004;21:231–6.

[6] Wagner JG, Aghajanian GK, Bing OHL. Correlation of performance test scores with "tissue concentration" of lysergic acid diethylamide in human subjects. Clin Pharmacol Ther 1968;9:635–8.

[7] Segre G. Kinetics of interaction between drugs and biological systems. Farmaco Sci 1968;23:907–18.

[8] Hull CJ, Van Beem HBH, McLeod K, Sibbald A, Watson MJ. A pharmacodynamic model for pancuronium. Br J Anaesth 1978;50:1113–23.

[9] Sheiner LB, Stanski DR, Vozeh S, Miller RD, Ham J. Simultaneous modeling of pharmacokinetics and pharmacodynamics: Application to d-tubocurarine. Clin Pharmacol Ther 1979;25:358–71.

[10] Holford NHG, Sheiner LB. Understanding the dose–effect relationship: Clinical application of pharmacokinetic–pharmacodynamic models. Clin Pharmacokinet 1981;6:429–53.

[11] Eudeikis JR, Henthorn TK, Lertora JJL, Atkinson AJ Jr, Chao GC, Kushner W. Kinetic analysis of the vasodilator and ganglionic blocking actions of N-acetylprocainamide. J Cardiovasc Pharmacol 1982;4:303–9.

[12] Holford NHG, Coates PE, Guentert TW, Riegelman S, Sheiner LB. The effect of quinidine and its metabolites on the electrocardiogram and systolic time intervals: Concentration–effect relationships. Br J Clin Pharmacol 1981;11:187–95.

[13] Vozeh S, Bindschedler M, Ha HR, Kaufmann G, Guentert TW, Follath F. Pharmacodynamics of 3-hydroxyquinidine alone and in combination with quinidine in healthy persons. Am J Cardiol 1987;59:681–4.

[14] Holford NHG, Sheiner LB. Pharmacokinetic and pharmacodynamic modeling in vivo. CRC Crit Rev Bioengineer 1981;5:273–322.

[15] Piergies AA, Ruo TI, Jansyn EM, Belknap SM, Atkinson AJ Jr. Effect kinetics of *N*-acetylprocainamide-induced QT interval prolongation. Clin Pharmacol Ther 1987;42:107–12.

[16] Frederiksen MC, Bowsher DJ, Ruo TI, Henthorn TK, Ts'ao C-H, Green D, Atkinson AJ Jr. Kinetics of epsilon-aminocaproic acid distribution, elimination, and antifibrinolytic effects in normal subjects. Clin Pharmacol Ther 1984;35:387–93.

[17] Markus G, DePasquale JL, Wissler FC. Quantitative determination of the binding of ε-aminocaproic acid to native plasminogen. J Biol Chem 1978;253:727–32.

[18] Hill AV. The possible effects of the aggregation of the molecules of hemoglobin on its dissociation curves. J Physiol 1910;40:iv–vii.

[19] Bunn HF, Forget BG, Ranney HM. Human hemoglobins. Philadelphia, PA: WB Saunders; 1977.

[20] Wagner JG. Kinetics of pharmacologic response: I. Proposed relationships between response and drug concentration in the intact animal and man. J Theor Biol 1968;20:173–201.

[21] Meffin PJ, Winkle RA, Blaschke TF, Fitzgerald J, Harrison DC. Response optimization of drug dosage: Antiarrhythmic studies with tocainide. Clin Pharmacol Ther 1977;22:42–57.

[22] Stanski DR. Pharmacodynamic modeling of anesthetic EEG drug effects. Annu Rev Pharmacol Toxicol 1992;32:423–47.

[23] Magni VC, Frost RA, Leung JWC, Cotton PB. A randomized comparison of midazolam and diazepam for sedation in upper gastrointestinal endoscopy. Br J Anaesth 1983;55:1095–101.

[24] Bührer M, Maitre PO, Crevoisier C, Stanski DR. Electroencephalographic effects of benzodiazepines. II. Pharmacodynamic modeling of the electroencephalographic effects of midazolam and diazepam. Clin Pharmacol Ther 1990;48:555–67.

[25] Mandema JW, Sansom LN, Dios-Vièitez MC, Hollander-Jansen M, Danhof M. Pharmacokinetic–pharmacodynamic modeling of the electroencephalographic effects of benzodiazepines. Correlation with receptor binding and anticonvulsant activity. J Pharmacol Exp Ther 1991;257:472–8.

[26] Nagashima R, O'Reilly RA, Levy G. Kinetics of pharmacologic effects in man: The anticoagulant action of warfarin. Clin Pharmacol Ther 1969;10:22–35.

[27] Pitsiu M, Parker EM, Aarons L, Rowland M. Population pharmacokinetics and pharmacodynamics of warfarin in healthy young adults. Eur J Pharm Sci 1993;1:151–7.

[28] Ambre JJ. Acute tolerance to pressor effects of cocaine in humans. Ther Drug Monit 1993;15:537–40.

[29] Foltin RW, Fischman MW, Levin FR. Cardiovascular effects of cocaine in humans: Laboratory studies. Drug Alcohol Depend 1995;37:193–210.

[30] Ambre JJ, Belknap SM, Nelson J, Ruo TI, Shin S-G, Atkinson AJ Jr. Acute tolerance to cocaine in humans. Clin Pharmacol Ther 1988;44:1–8.

[31] Gårdmark M, Brynne L, Hammarlund-Udenaes M, Karlsson MO. Interchangeability and predictive performance of empirical tolerance models. Clin Pharmacokinet 1999;36:145–67.

[32] Nattel S, Rangno RE, Van Loon G. Mechanism of propranolol withdrawal phenomenon. Circulation 1979;59:1158–64.

[33] Houston MC, Hodge R. Beta-adrenergic blocker withdrawal syndromes in hypertension and other cardiovascular diseases. Am Heart J 1988;116:515–23.

[34] Lima JJ, Krukenmyer JJ, Boudoulas H. Drug- or hormone-induced adaptation: Model of adrenergic hypersensitivity. J Pharamacokinet Biopharm 1989;17:347–64.

[35] Holford NHG, Peace KE. Results and validation of a population pharmacodynamic model for cognitive effects in Alzheimer patients treated with tacrine. Proc Natl Acad Sci USA 1992;89:11471–5.

[36] Cox EH, Sheiner LB. Repeated measures time to event with time-varying concentration and hazard (Internet at, ftp://ftp.globomaxnm.com/Public/nonmem/non-continuous; 2001).

[37] Cox EH, Veyrat-Follet C, Beal SL, Fuseau E, Kenkare S, Sheiner LB. A population pharmacokinetic–pharmacodynamic analysis of repeated measures time-to-event pharmacodynamic responses: The antiemetic effect of ondansetron. J Pharmacokinet Biopharm 1999;27:625–44.

[38] Hu C, Sale ME. A joint model for nonlinear longitudinal data with informative dropout. J Pharmacokinet Pharmacodyn 2003;30:83–103.

[39] Sheiner LB. A new approach to the analysis of analgesic drug trials, illustrated with bromfenac data. Clin Pharmacol Ther 1994;56:309–22.

[40] Plan EL, Karlsson KE, Karlsson MO. Approaches to simultaneous analysis of frequency and severity of symptoms. Clin Pharmacol Ther 2010;88:255–9.

# Disease Progress Models

**Nicholas H.G. Holford[1], Diane R. Mould[2] and Carl C. Peck[3]**

[1]*Department of Pharmacology and Clinical Pharmacology, University of Auckland, Auckland, New Zealand 1142*
[2]*Projections Research Inc, Phoenixville, PA 19460*
[3]*Center for Drug Development Science, University of California at San Francisco,*
*University of California Washington Center, Washington, DC 20036*

## CLINICAL PHARMACOLOGY AND DISEASE PROGRESS

Clinical pharmacology, like many disciplines, can be viewed from several perspectives. In the context of a clinical trial of a therapeutic agent, clinical pharmacology provides a conceptual framework for relating drug treatment to responses and differentiating possible mechanisms of action. Disease progression refers to the evolution of a disease over time. It typically implies worsening of the disease, but also may include spontaneous recovery. Disease progress, in a broader sense, is a description of the disease and its response to treatment. In the context of simulation and modeling, it is useful to think of clinical pharmacology itself as a model that combines disease progression with drug action:

$$\text{Clinical pharmacology} = \text{Disease progression} + \text{Drug action} \quad (22.1)$$

Thus, the study of clinical pharmacology is the study of disease progress. Disease progress models may be used to describe the time course of a biomarker or clinical outcome reflecting the status of a disease and the effects of drug treatment. The disease status in a clinical trial may also be modified by participation in the trial (called the placebo response), which can occasionally be distinguished from the natural history of disease progression. Disease status is a reflection of the state of the disease at a point in time. The disease status may improve or worsen over time, or may be a cyclical phenomenon – for example, malarial quartan fever or seasonal affective disorder. Therefore, a model of disease progress is a quantitative expression that describes the expected changes in disease status over time.

Drug action refers to all the pharmacokinetic and pharmacodynamic processes involved in producing a drug effect on the disease. The effect of the drug is assumed to influence the disease status. Pharmacokinetic and pharmacodynamic drug properties are the major attributes determining drug action and its effect on the time course of progression of the disease. Disease progress models can be extended to include terms that account for the changes in disease progression that are affected by drug treatment. We call such a combined model the "clinical pharmacology model" for the drug (Equation 22.1).

## DISEASE PROGRESS MODELS

In this chapter, we describe the basic elements of clinical pharmacology models for use in describing the time course of disease progression and the changes in progress in response to treatment. These models have two basic components; the first describes the disease progression without therapeutic intervention, and the second defines the change in progress as a result of treatment.

## "No Progress" Model

The simplest model of disease progress assumes there is no change in disease status during the period of observation. Previously this has been reflected in simple pharmacodynamic models, such as those described in Chapter 21, by the constant "baseline effect" parameter, often symbolized by $E_0$ [1]. The symbol $E_0$ is misleading because the "$E$" implies a drug effect, but by definition the drug effect is zero at baseline before the drug has been administered. A constant baseline is a common assumption made in the design and analysis of clinical trials. Such an analysis ignores the progress of disease during the course of the trial by comparing the effect of drug treatment groups at similar points in time. This is a reflection of a "minimalist" approach to clinical trial design and analysis that seeks only to reject the null hypothesis and which is a lost opportunity to learn by employing an informative description of the observed phenomena [2, 3]. The assumption that there is no change in disease status over time does not allow learning about the effect of the drug on the rate of disease progress.

## Linear Progression Model

The linear disease progression model (Equation 22.2) assumes a constant rate of change of a biomarker or clinical outcome that reflects the disease status ($S$) at any time, $t$, from the initial observation of the patient – for example, at the time of entry into a clinical trial. It can be defined in terms of a baseline disease status ($S_0$) and a slope ($\alpha$), which reflects the change from baseline status with time:

$$S(t) = S_0 + \alpha \cdot t \qquad (22.2)$$

$S_0$ is a preferable to $E_0$ because it refers to the disease status before drug is given. Using this model as a basis to describe the effect of drug on the time course of disease progression, there are three drug-effect patterns possible. Treatment can influence the patient's disease status without affecting the rate of progress (offset pattern), it can alter the rate of progression of the disease (slope pattern), or it can do both (combined slope and offset pattern).

### Offset Pattern

We define a drug-induced shift upwards or downwards without a change in slope of the disease status line as the offset pattern. The effect of the drug is a function of concentration ($C_{e,A}$) at the effect site,

constant $E_{OFF}$, and can be thought of as modifying the baseline parameter $S_0$ as shown in Equation 22.3:

$$S(t) = S_0 + E_{OFF}(C_{e,A}) + \alpha \cdot t \qquad (22.3)$$

This model can be used to describe a transient drug effect (sometimes termed "symptomatic") – for example, lowering of blood pressure by an antihypertensive agent that persists during periods of exposure to the drug but with a return to pretreatment status on cessation of therapy. The onset of drug effect may be delayed by adding an effect compartment to the drug action part of the model, which incorporates more realism by making active drug concentrations at the effect site delayed in relation to plasma drug concentrations [4].

### Slope Pattern

We define a drug-induced increase or decrease in the rate of progression of disease status as the slope pattern. The effect of the drug, $E_{SLOPE}$, can be thought of as modifying the slope parameter $\alpha$ as shown in Equation 22.4:

$$S(t) = S_0 + [E_{SLOPE}(C_{e,A}) + \alpha] \cdot t \qquad (22.4)$$

Compared to the offset pattern, this model can be used to describe a more permanent drug effect, such as slowing the progression of a disease such as rheumatoid arthritis. This kind of change in the rate of change of disease progression is called a "disease-modifying" effect. In this case, the cessation of therapy would not be expected to result in a return to pretreatment status. In general we might expect some delay in the onset of effect (predicted by $C_{e,A}$), but an instantaneous effect model to describe the drug effect on the slope parameter may be sufficient because changes in status tend to develop slowly when the slope changes.

### Combined Offset and Slope Pattern

Both an offset effect and a slope effect may be combined to describe the changes in disease status (Equation 22.5 ):

$$S(t) = S_0 + E_{OFF}(C_{e,A}) + [E_{SLOPE}(C_{e,A}) + \alpha] \cdot t \qquad (22.5)$$

Figure 22.1 illustrates the offset and slope models and the combination of both types of effect. The offset pattern of drug effect provides an explicit definition of a temporary or symptomatic effect of a drug. In contrast, the slope pattern of drug effect defines a drug with a disease-modifying effect. The pattern of disease progress in the absence of drug is usually referred to as the natural history of the disease.

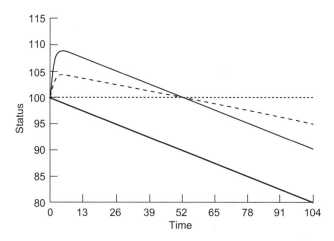

**FIGURE 22.1** The *thick line* depicts the natural course ("natural history") of disease progress without therapeutic intervention (Equation 22.2). The *thin line* describes an offset pattern ("symptomatic") as a consequence of treatment (Equation 22.3). The *dotted line* reflects a slope pattern with a change in the rate of progress of the disease ("disease modifying") (Equation 22.4). The *dashed line* shows the combination of both offset and slope patterns (Equation 22.5).

A study by Griggs *et al.* [5] reporting temporary increases in muscle strength of muscular dystrophy patients treated with prednisone illustrates an application of the offset drug effect pattern (Figure 22.2). Figure 22.3 shows a similar offset pattern of the effect of zidovudine in CD4 cell measurements in HIV patients [6]. However, in this case the model of disease progress is comprised of functions that are not simply straight lines (polynomial; Equation 22.6) and

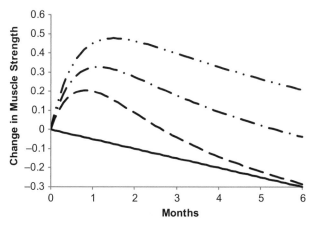

**FIGURE 22.2** Example of linear disease progress and offset drug effect pattern when prednisone is used to treat muscular dystrophy. The *heavy solid line* is the expected natural history of progressive loss of muscle strength. The *dashed line* shows the transient improvement due to the placebo response. The two upper lines demonstrate the delayed offset pattern of drug effect at two doses of prednisone. Based on Griggs RC, Moxley RT III, Mendell JR *et al.* Arch Neurol 1991;48:383–8 [5].

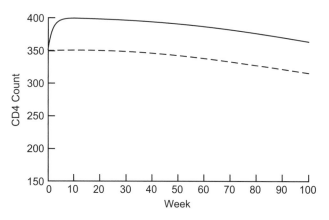

**FIGURE 22.3** Time course of CD4 count in placebo- (*dashed line*) and zidovudine- (*solid line*) treated patients. Reproduced with permission from Sale M, Sheiner LB, Volberding P *et al.* Clin Pharmacol Ther 1993;54:556–66 [6].

zidovudine treatment (combined polynomial and exponential; Equation 22.7):

$$\text{No Treatment }(t) = \text{CD4}_0 - k_1 \cdot t - k_2 \cdot t^2 \quad (22.6)$$

$$\text{Treatment }(t) = \left[ B + (k_5 \cdot \text{CD4}_0) + \left( k_6 \cdot \text{CD4}_0^2 \right) \right]$$
$$\cdot \left( e^{-k_3 \cdot t} - e^{-k_4 \cdot t} \right)$$
$$(22.7)$$

The parameters $B$ and $k_1$ through $k_6$ are used to describe how *CD4* can be predicted from baseline $\text{CD4}_0$ and time. The model for the placebo group that did not receive treatment ("*No Treatment*") most likely reflects the natural history of HIV progression as observed in a clinical trial, but it is not possible to distinguish a placebo response component in this case.

Models for multiple periods of treatment with placebo and active drug (with different doses) in a clinical trial have been used with a disease progress model to describe the response to tacrine in Alzheimer's disease. By assuming the disease progression model is linear, it was possible to identify a placebo response time course that was independent of the natural history of progression. Figure 22.4 shows the placebo and active treatment components, as well as the disease progression [7]. The predicted time course of response in patients with Alzheimer's disease in a complex clinical trial design combining disease progress, placebo and tacrine effects is shown in Figure 22.5 [8]. In this figure, the upper curve reflects the expected patient disease status, which would reflect a combination of disease progress and the effect of placebo on the time course of disease progress. In the lower curve, the sequential effects of varying treatments including doses of placebo (P) and 40 mg/day and 80 mg/day of tacrine were

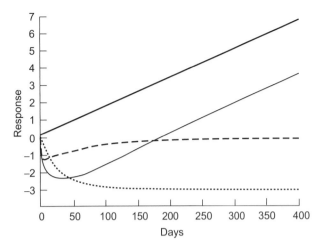

**FIGURE 22.4**  Models of Alzheimer's disease progress (*thick line*), placebo effect (*dotted line*) and drug effect (*dashed line*) in absence of disease progress, and combined (drug plus placebo) response to active drug in the presence of disease progress (*thin line*). Drug effect is assessed by subtracting placebo response and disease progress from the combined response that is observed with drug therapy. Reproduced with permission from Holford NHG. Population models for Alzheimer's and Parkinson's disease. In: Aarons L, Balant LP, editors. The population approach: measuring and managing variability in response, concentration and dose. Brussels: COST B1 European Commission; 1997. pp. 97–104 [7].

simulated. The difference between the control and active groups increases notably over the duration of the trial. This underscores the need to incorporate appropriate models of disease progress as well as to account for placebo effect, if possible, in descriptions of clinical trials.

Finally, a disease progress model can reflect more complex drug action phenomena such as a drug

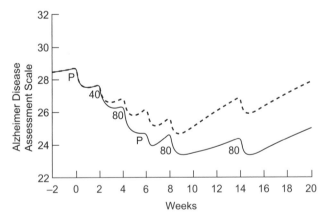

**FIGURE 22.5**  The *upper curve* shows the time course of predicted responses in a patient receiving placebo treatments as part of the three-part trial design used to evaluate tacrine in Alzheimer's disease. The *lower curve* shows the simulated response in a patient receiving a particular sequence of placebo (P) followed by tacrine (40 or 80 mg/day). Reproduced with permission from Holford NH, Peace KE. Proc Natl Acad Sci USA 1992;89:11466–70 [8].

concentration–effect delay, and tolerance and rebound to both placebo and active treatments For instance, a delay to onset can be accounted for by the addition of an effect site compartment, and tolerance and rebound effects can be described by the addition of a precursor pool compartment, which would limit the effect of drug activity.

The offset and slope models account for open-ended monotonic disease progression in time, suitable for describing disease progression during a clinical trial that comprises a brief time of observation relative to the duration of disease. The following asymptotic models provide for disease stabilization or return to a non-disease state, applicable to a clinical trial that encompasses disease progression to an eventual unchanging state.

## Asymptotic Progress Model

### Zero Asymptote

A common pattern of disease progress provides for the patient's return to health or recovery. For example, the time course of postoperative pain can be expected to start at a baseline state, which involves intense levels of pain. However, over a few days the level of pain experienced by the patient usually decreases until eventually pain is no longer perceived. This recovery can be approximated by an exponential model with an asymptote of zero, indicating the absence of pain. As shown in Figure 22.8, the parameters of this model are the baseline pain status $S_0$ and the half-life of progression, $T_{prog}$:

$$S(t) = S_0 \cdot e^{-\ln 2/T_{prog} \cdot t} \qquad (22.8)$$

The asymptote model is particularly useful for illustrating one of the primary potential drawbacks of not accounting for disease progress. Because patients are expected to improve over time, a simple minimalist approach to the comparison of different drug effects would be expected to be dependent on the time of comparative assessment. If the comparison were made at a point in time where recovery has largely occurred, the difference between treatments would probably be un-detectable.

As with the linear model of disease progress, the consequences of therapeutic intervention on the asymptotic model of disease progress can be described by including terms to account for the expected action of a drug. Drugs may exert an immediate and transient symptomatic effect, or they may act to alter the progress of the disease, such as shortening the time to recovery, or they may do both.

### Zero Asymptote Offset Model Pattern

As shown in Figure 22.9, drug action models based on the zero asymptote model can be extended to include an offset term $[E_{OFF}(C_{e,A})]$ in the model of progress describing symptomatic benefit, such as the relief of pain from a simple analgesic:

$$S(t) = E_{OFF}(C_{e,A}) + S_0 \cdot e^{-\ln 2/T_{prog} \cdot t} \qquad (22.9)$$

As with the offset model for the linear disease progress model, the effect of drug would be expected to disappear on cessation of therapy in this offset model. Again, a delay to the onset of drug effect can be incorporated with the use of an effect site compartment component.

### Zero Asymptote Slope Pattern

In addition, an exponentially progressing pattern of disease progress (parameterized by a half-life of progression) can reflect a disease-modifying benefit of drug treatment, if the therapeutic intervention accelerates the return to the normal state or shortens the half-life of the recovery process. Equation 22.10 describes the disease-modifying benefit:

$$S(t) = S_0 \cdot e^{-\ln 2/[E_{TP}(C_{e,A}) + T_{prog}] \cdot t} \qquad (22.10)$$

### Combined Offset and Slope Pattern

The effects of a therapeutic agent $(E_{TP})$ on the progress of a disease may include both an immediate palliative effect and a reduction in the overall recovery time. Equation 22.11 describes the combination of these actions on the zero-asymptote disease progress model:

$$S(t) = E_{OFF}(C_{e,A}) + S_0 \cdot e^{-\ln 2/[E_{TP}(C_{e,A}) + T_{prog}] \cdot t} \qquad (22.11)$$

Figure 22.6 illustrates the expected changes in the progress of a disease, which can be described using the zero-asymptote model.

## Non-Zero Asymptote

Another pattern of disease progress encompasses reaching a "burned out" state $(S_{SS})$. This state is thought to happen when diseases such as rheumatoid arthritis reach a point when disease processes damage tissue beyond repair by any therapeutic means. This irreversibly damaged state can be described by another exponential model. The model can be expressed as follows, where $t$ is time after the start of observing the disease from a baseline state $(S_0)$ and the half-life of progression is $T_{prog}$:

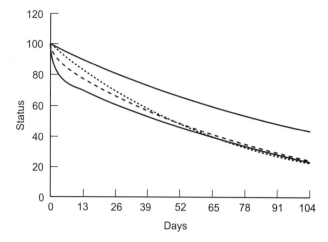

**FIGURE 22.6** Patterns of drug effect with the zero-asymptote progress model. The *thick line* describes the normal expected time course of recovery without therapeutic intervention. The *thin line* shows the change when a drug that affects symptoms is administered. The *dotted line* illustrates the expected time course of disease when an agent is given which hastens recovery (disease modifying) and the *dashed line* describes the expected results from administering an agent that exhibits both an immediate symptomatic effect and a disease-modifying effect on the time course of disease progress.

$$S_0 \cdot e^{-\ln 2/T_{prog} \cdot t} + S_{SS} \cdot \left(1 - e^{-\ln 2/T_{prog} \cdot t}\right) \qquad (22.12)$$

### Offset Pattern

Therapeutic treatment can affect disease status without altering the time to reach a burned out steady-state status, $S_{SS}$. This improvement in status would be expected to be transient, and dependent on continual drug exposure. Equation 22.13 describes the effect of adding a drug that has a symptomatic effect $[E_{OFF}(C_{e,A})]$ on patient disease status:

$$S(t) = E_{OFF}(C_{e,A}) + S_0 \cdot e^{-\ln 2/T_{prog} \cdot t}$$
$$+ S_{SS} \cdot \left(1 - e^{-\ln 2/T_{prog} \cdot t}\right) \qquad (22.13)$$

### Slope Pattern

Additional models for drug effects on the non-zero asymptote model include two patterns of disease-modifying drug effects. These assume a drug effect either changing the burned out state, $S_{SS}$,

$$S_0 \cdot e^{-\ln 2/T_{prog} \cdot t} + [E_{OFF}(C_{e,A}) + S_{SS}] \cdot \left(1 - e^{-\ln 2/T_{prog} \cdot t}\right)$$
$$(22.14)$$

or affecting the half-life of progression, $T_{prog}$,

$$S(t) = S_0 \cdot e^{-\ln2/[E(C_{e,A})+T_{prog}] \cdot t}$$
$$+ S_{SS} \cdot \left(1 - e^{-\ln2/[E(C_{e,A})+T_{prog}] \cdot t}\right) \quad (22.15)$$

### Offset and Slope Patterns

Figure 22.7 illustrates the non-zero asymptote model with all three patterns of disease progress influenced by drug effect. Drug exposure starts at 1.0 time units and is stopped at 8.0 time units. In Equation 22.16, the effects of symptomatic improvement and the two functions describing the action of drug on both the burned out state and on the time to reach this state have been included.

$$S(t) = E_{OFF}(C_{e,A}) + S_0 \cdot e^{-\ln2/[E_{TP}(C_{e,A})+T_{prog}] \cdot t}$$
$$+ [E_{SS}(C_{e,A}) + S_{SS}] \cdot \left(1 - e^{-\ln2/[E_{TP}(C_{e,A})]+T_{prog} \cdot t}\right)$$
$$(22.16)$$

The above models are descriptive and are not based on underlying biological mechanisms or pathophysiology. The following models employ physiological concepts and may be considered to be semi-empirical models.

## Physiological Turnover Models

The time course of drug effect can often be understood in terms of drug-induced changes in physiological turnover processes controlling synthesis rate ($R_{syn}$) or elimination of a physiological mediator [9, 10]. These models can be readily extended to

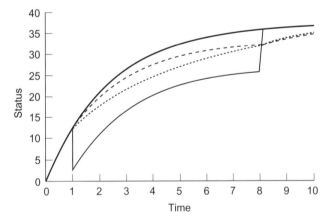

**FIGURE 22.7** Non-zero asymptote model with natural history (*thick line*) offset pattern (*thin line*) and two types of disease-modifying drug effects: effect on steady-state burned out state ($S_{ss}$) (*dashed line*), and effect on half-life of disease progress ($T_{prog}$) (*dotted line*).

describe disease progress by incorporating a time-varying inhibitory effect of the drug (Pharmaco Dynamic Inhibition, *PDI*) on either synthesis or elimination of the physiological mediator. For example, if the rate constant ($k_{loss}$) describing loss of a physiological mediator starts from a baseline state, $k_{loss0}$, and decreases with a half-life of $T_{50_{loss}}$, then the time course of the disease state can be described by solving the differential equation given in Equation 22.17:

$$\frac{ds}{dt} = R_{syn} - k_{loss} \cdot PDI \cdot S \quad (22.17)$$

where

$$k_{loss} = k_{loss0} \cdot \left[1 + (Maxprog - 1) \cdot \left(1 - e^{\ln2/T_{50_{loss}} \cdot t}\right)\right]$$
$$(22.18)$$

*MaxProg* is a parameter that determines the fractional change in $k_{loss0}$ at infinite time. The effect of a drug might be to inhibit loss, in which case *PDI* would be modeled by Equation 22.19, where $C_{e,A}$ is the effect site concentration and $C_{50}$ is the value of $C_{e,A}$ causing a 50% inhibition of loss:

$$PDI = \frac{c_{e,A}}{c_{50} + c_{e,A}} \quad (22.19)$$

Figure 22.8 illustrates the four basic drug-effect patterns when the input or output parameter changes with an exponential time course. This type of mechanism for disease progression has subsequently been described as a model in which time-varying changes in the disease state model parameters comprise a disease progress model [11].

As an example of this type of disease progression model, consider postmenopausal osteoporosis reflected by the net loss of bone mass that may be due to decreased formation or increased resorption of bone. Figure 22.9 illustrates the time course of bone mass change due to increased bone loss and the effect of administering a drug to reduce that loss. For example, raloxifene has been shown to be beneficial in women with postmenopausal osteoporosis [12]. The pattern of increase in bone mineral density observed after treatment with raloxifene or placebo resembles the curves shown in Figure 22.10. However, the treatment duration in this dataset was too short to identify the actual mechanism of raloxifene effect on disease progress.

## Growth and Decay Models

Another semi-empirical approach to modeling the course of disease progression is to use models

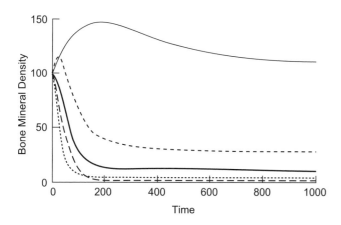

**FIGURE 22.8** Disease progression due to a time varying increase in the rate of loss of a physiological mediator of the response. The *thick line* shows the time course of response in the untreated state with an increase in the loss of physiological mediator. If the response was "change in bone mass from a baseline of 100 at time 0" then the rate of bone loss would be increased by a factor of 10, reaching a new steady state after 200 time units. The time to steady state is determined both by the time course of change in rate of bone loss and the turnover time of bone. The other four lines show the patterns expected from four different kinds of drug effect. Potentially therapeutic effects are inhibition of bone loss (*thin line*) and stimulation of bone synthesis (*upper dashed line*). Deleterious drug effects are inhibition of synthesis (*lower dashed line*) and stimulation of bone loss (*dotted line*).

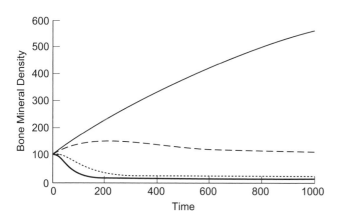

**FIGURE 22.9** The pattern and time course of response to treatment is crucially dependent on the dose. This shows the same model as that illustrated in Figure 22.8 without treatment (*thick line*) and with three different dose rates of a drug which reduces the rate of loss of physiological substance (*dotted line* = dose rate of 10, *broken line* = dose rate of 100, *thin line* = dose rate of 1000).

originally developed to describe growth. The growth function might be used to describe something such as tumor growth or bacterial cell increase, where growth is dependent on the number of actively dividing cells. A simple function that can be used to describe the growth of a response $R$ is given in Equation 22.20 [13, 14]:

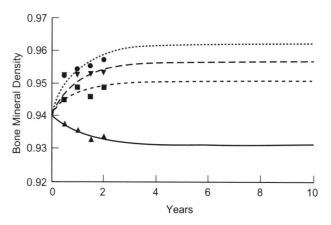

**FIGURE 22.10** Bone mineral density change with placebo and three doses of raloxifene. Symbols indicate observed responses to placebo (▲) and daily doses of 30 mg (■), 60 mg (▼) and 150 mg (●). Curves show predictions assuming disease progress is due to increased loss and raloxifene reduces loss. The model is the same as that shown in Figure 22.8 and Figure 22.9. Curves fit to lumbar spine data from Delmas PD, Bjarnason NH, Mitlak BH *et al.* N Engl J Med 1997;337:1641–7 [12].

$$\frac{dR}{dt} = k_{growth} \cdot R - k_{death} \cdot R \qquad (22.20)$$

The solution to this equation describes an exponential increase in cell count with time.

As with the other physiological models, the effect of drug treatment may be realized by slowing the growth rate ($k_{growth}$) or increasing the cell death rate ($k_{death}$). In the latter case, this effect can be incorporated by including a term for the effect of drug concentration ($C_{e,A}$) on the rate constant for cell decrease, as shown in Equation 22.21:

$$\frac{dR}{dt} = k_{growth} \cdot R - k_{death} \cdot R \cdot C_{e,A} \qquad (22.21)$$

A more realistic refinement of the simple cell growth model would describe cells that, through mutation or other processes, may become resistant to drug treatment. The change of cell characteristic from a responsive to an unresponsive state can be either reversible or irreversible. Equations 22.22 and 22.23 describe the reversible case, which may be reflective of cells moving between sensitive phases ($R_S$) and phases that are not sensitive to therapeutic intervention ($R_R$) [15]:

$$\frac{dR_S}{dt} = k_{growth} \cdot R_S - k_{SR} \cdot R_S + K_{RS} \cdot R_R - k_{death} \cdot R_S$$

$$(22.22)$$

and

$$\frac{dR_R}{dt} = k_{SR} \cdot R_S - k_{RS} \cdot R_R \qquad (22.23)$$

where the rates of transformation to and from the resistant state are indicated by $k_{SR}$ and $k_{RS}$, respectively.

Another series of functions frequently used to describe growth kinetics is the Gompertz functions [16]. These functions are useful because they describe a rapid initial rapid rate of growth ($\beta$), followed by a slower phase of growth until a finite limit ($\beta_{max}$) is reached. This behavior makes the Gompertz functions particularly appropriate for describing disease progress where there is a maximum level of impairment associated with the disease (e.g., a burned out state). Consequently, Gompertz functions have been used to describe the pharmacodynamics of antibacterial agents [17], as well as an empirical description of disease progression in Parkinson's disease [18]. Equations 22.24 and 22.25 describe a Gompertz function of cell growth in which the cells oscillate between a therapeutically sensitive state ($R_S$) and a resistant state ($R_R$). The effect of drug concentration ($C_{e,A}$) is described using an $E_{max}$ equation that acts to reduce the number of responsive cells in the system by increasing loss ($k_{SO}$) independently of transformation to or from the resistant state:

$$\frac{dR_S}{dt} = k_{RS} \cdot R_R + \beta \cdot R_S \cdot (\beta_{max} - R_S)$$

$$- \left[ k_{SR} + \left( 1 + \frac{E_{max} \cdot C_{e,A}}{EC50 + C_{e,A}} \right) \cdot k_{SO} \right] \cdot R_S \tag{22.24}$$

$$\frac{dR_{SR}}{dt} = k_{SR} \cdot R_S - k_{RS} \cdot R_R \tag{22.25}$$

Figure 22.11 shows the expected pattern of cell growth in three different treatment groups. In the low-dose treatment group cell regrowth is expected to be rapid, and there is some evidence of regrowth near the 20-day time point even in the high-dose group.

Weibull functions are used in another class of semi-empirical models to describe disease progression. Pennypacker *et al.* [19] first proposed using the Weibull function to describe the progression of plant diseases such as fungal infections and black rot.

Although commonly employed in epidemiology and in models of plant disease, Weibull functions have not been used widely to describe the time course of human disease. Freeman *et al.* [20] used this function to describe the progression from Hepatitis C to cirrhosis. Similarly, Foucher *et al.* [21] implemented the Weibull function with a Markov chain to describe the progression of HIV through various states as life without disease, appearance of symptoms, disease progression, and eventual death.

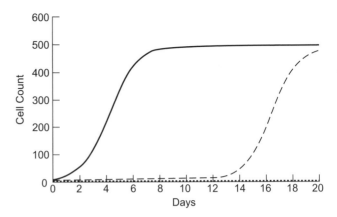

**FIGURE 22.11**  Growth curves for responsive cells exposed to three different treatment regimens: untreated (*solid line*), inadequately treated with a low drug dose (*broken line*), and adequately treated with a higher drug dose (*dashed line*). The curves show that cell regrowth following inadequate treatment is rapid.

The function was evaluated for numerical stability by Thal *et al.* [22] The authors reported that the Weibull function was generally robust, and allowed for a variety of inflection points that made this function suitable for describing a variety of disease progression scenarios. The authors, however, also pointed out that if the parameters exhibited high correlation, simplification of the Weibull function would provide more reasonable confidence intervals for the parameters. In order to maintain numerical plausibility, a modified Weibull function (Equation 22.26) may be implemented. This function can take on several characteristics depending on the value of the shape function WE3 (Figure 22.12). When all parameters are constrained to be positive and the parameter WE3 is at or below 1, the function mimics an exponential model, which describes a rapid fall-off from a baseline value to a new lower plateau in the time course of response. However, as WE3 increases to values greater than 1, the function approximates a Weibull model, which allows for a delay in the onset of change before the function falls to a plateau. The rate of change of the score between baseline and plateau is controlled by the parameter WE2, and WE1 describes the maximum decrease from the baseline value. $S_i(t)$ is the Weibull function value at a given time "$t$".

$$S_i(t) = \text{WE1} \cdot \left( 1 - e^{-(\text{WE2}/t)^{\text{WE3}}} \right) \tag{22.26}$$

Depending on the Weibull parameter values, the function can either describe a decay over time, as shown in Figure 22.11, or describe an increase in disease score over time to a new higher plateau. The application of a logit transform can be used to constrain the modified Weibull function to fall

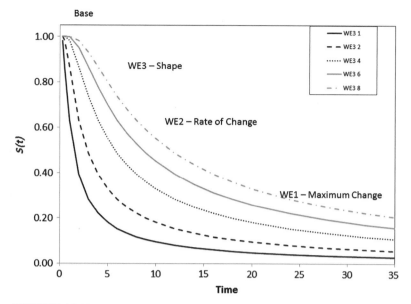

**FIGURE 22.12** Weibull decay curves for a variety of values of WE3 or shape parameter values. When the value of WE3 is low ($\leq 1$) the function mimics an exponential decay, with a rapid fall-off from its BASE level to a new lower plateau level. When the value of WE3 increases, there is a delay prior to the fall-off and the rate of decline is slower. Although not shown here, ultimately all values for WE3 would eventually stabilize at the same new lower plateau value.

within the upper and lower bounds of a disease assessment score, thus ensuring that the disease progression model will not simulate inappropriate values.

$$LGT = S_i(t)$$

$$UB = 100$$

$$LB = 0$$

$$Score_i(t) = (UB - LB) \cdot \frac{e^{LGT}}{\left(1 + e^{LGT}\right)} + LB \qquad (22.27)$$

In this equation, LGT is the Weibull function shown in Equation 22.7, $UB$ is the upper bound of the clinical disease assessment score, and $LB$ is the lower bound of the disease score. Then $Score_i(t)$ is the disease score at any time "$t$".

## DESIGN OF TRIALS TO STUDY DISEASE PROGRESS

The study of disease progress requires trial designs that can identify the time course of disease status. It is not sufficient just to measure a response at baseline and at the end of a period of treatment in order to describe the effect of a drug on disease progression. For example, the ELLODOPA study was intended to determine if levodopa affected the rate of progression of Parkinson's disease [23]. This study used a washout design which involved withdrawal of treatment and seeing if the disease status was the same in the placebo and levodopa-treated groups after 2 weeks without levodopa. However, the results of the study were inconclusive because the 2-week study period was not long enough to be sure that all the effects of prior therapy had been washed out and the primary analysis was based only on change from baseline. A prediction of the ELLDOPA results based on earlier studies [18, 24] accurately described the observed differences and also confirmed a disease-modifying effect of levodopa.

Another trial design, the delayed start design, has been proposed for identifying disease-modifying effects. The basic idea is that if two groups of patients are observed in a trial in which treatment is delayed for one group, then if there is a disease-modifying effect, the disease status will show greater improvement (less progress) in the early start group. This trial design, like the washout design, requires an assumption about the time required for the effects of prior therapy to decline to asymptotic values. If this assumption is made *a priori* and is not borne out by the data, the prespecified analysis is invalidated. This is what happened with the ADAGIO trial, which aimed to identify disease-modifying effects of rasagiline on Parkinson's disease [25]. A model-based analysis that uses the observed data to describe the time course of the symptomatic effect does not suffer from this limitation [26].

The importance of trial design for identifying disease-modifying effects may be studied by clinical trial simulation. For example, a simulation study has shown that a washout design is more powerful than a delayed start design for identifying symptomatic vs disease-modifying drug effects in patients with Parkinson's disease [27]. The use of clinical trial simulation also is an important tool for understanding complex diseases and trial designs which try to distinguish the effects of treatments from natural disease progression [28]. In addition, the inclusion of quantitative models for disease progress in the regulatory and drug development process has been advocated as a means of sharing knowledge and improving trial design [29].

## CONCLUSION

The use of models to describe disease progress is an important tool that allows the clinical pharmacologist and clinical trialist to evaluate the effects of drug treatment on the time course of disease. In the "learning vs confirming" paradigm of drug development strategy [3], inclusion of models for disease progress can focus attention more clearly on the objectives of a clinical trial. In early, "learning phase" studies, the model of disease progress can be developed and the mechanism of drug action elucidated. Subsequently, clinical trials can be designed to account for variability in the natural history of disease, which increases the statistical power to distinguish effects of different treatments and thus "confirm" the effectiveness of the drug. Once the disease progress model has been defined and an effect of the drug on progress has been accepted, study designs can be defined that optimize dosage regimens to achieve clinical benefit.

In this chapter, we have described some examples of models that can be used to illustrate the natural history of disease. We have also suggested modifications to these models that can be used to account for the effect of drug treatment. The development of an appropriate model for disease progress is ideally a team-based approach. It requires the input of clinical experts as to the validity of the status measure used to describe the progress of the disease, statisticians to advise on the inferences that can be drawn from clinical trial observations, and pharmacometricians to determine the appropriateness and utility of the clinical pharmacology model for predicting the response to treatment and to provide guidance to the patient and prescriber on how to use the drug safely and effectively.

## REFERENCES

[1] Holford NHG, Sheiner LB. Understanding the dose–effect relationship: Clinical application of pharmacokinetic–pharmacodynamic models. Clin Pharmacokinet 1981;6:429–53.

[2] Sheiner LB. Clinical pharmacology and the choice between theory and empiricism. Clin Pharmacol Ther 1989;46:605–15.

[3] Sheiner LB. Learning versus confirming in clinical drug development. Clin Pharmacol Ther 1997;61:275–91.

[4] Holford NHG, Sheiner LB. Kinetics of pharmacologic response. Pharmacol Ther 1982;16:143–66.

[5] Griggs RC, Moxley III RT, Mendell JR, Fenichel GM, Brooke MH, Pestronik A, et al. Prednisone in Duchenne dystrophy: A randomized, controlled trial defining the time course and dose response. Arch Neurol 1991;48:383–8.

[6] Sale M, Sheiner LB, Volberding P, Blaschke TF. Zidovudine response relationships in early human immunodeficiency virus infection. Clin Pharmacol Ther 1993;54:556–66.

[7] Holford NHG. Population models for Alzheimer's and Parkinson's disease. In: Aarons L, Balant LP, editors. The population approach: Measuring and managing variability in response, concentration and dose. Brussels: COST B1 European Commission; 1997. p. 97–104.

[8] Holford NHG, Peace KE. Methodologic aspects of a population pharmacodynamic model for cognitive effects in Alzheimer patients treated with tacrine. Proc Natl Acad Sci USA 1992;89:11466–70.

[9] Holford NHG. Physiological alternatives to the effect compartment model. In: D'Argenio DZ, editor. Advanced methods of pharmacokinetic and pharmacodynamic systems analysis. New York, NY: Plenum Press; 1991. p. 55–68.

[10] Dayneka NL, Garg V, Jusko WJ. Comparison of four basic models of indirect pharmacodynamic responses. J Pharmacokinet Biopharm 1993;21:457–78.

[11] Post TM, Freijer JI, DeJongh J, Danhof M. Disease system analysis: Basic disease progression models in degenerative disease. Pharm Res 2005;22:1038–49.

[12] Delmas PD, Bjarnason NH, Mitlak BH, Ravoux A-C, Shah AS, Huster WJ, et al. Effects of raloxifene on bone mineral density, serum cholesterol concentrations, and uterine endometrium in postmenopausal women. N Engl J Med 1997;337:1641–7.

[13] Jusko W. Pharmacodynamics of chemotherapeutic effects: Dose–time–response relationships for phase-nonspecific agents. J Pharm Sci 1971;60:892–5.

[14] Zhi J, Nightingale C, Quintiliani R. A pharmacodynamic model for the activity of antibiotics against microorganisms under non saturable conditions. J Pharm Sci 1986;25:1063–7.

[15] Jusko W. A pharmacodynamic model for cell cycle-specific chemotherapeutic agents. J Pharmacokinet Biopharm 1973;1:175–200.

[16] Prior JC, Vigna YM, Schulzer M, Hall.E Bonen A. Determination of luteal phase length by quantitative basal temperature methods: Validation against the midcycle LH peak. Clin Invest Med 1990;13:123–31.

[17] Yano Y, Oguma T, Nagata H, Sasaki S. Application of a logistic growth model to pharmacodynamic analysis of *in vitro* bacteriocidal kinetics. J Pharmacokinet Biopharm 1998;87:1177–83.

[18] Holford NH, Chan PL, Nutt JG, Kieburtz K, Shoulson I. Disease progression and pharmacodynamics in Parkinson disease – evidence for functional protection with levodopa and other treatments. J Pharmacokinet Pharmacodyn 2006;33:281–311.

[19] Pennypacker SP, Knoble HD, Antle CE, Madden. V. A flexible model for studying plant disease progression. Phytopathology 1980;70:232–5.

[20] Freeman AJ, Law MG, Kaldor JM, Dore GJ. Predicting progression to cirrhosis in chronic hepatitis C virus infection. J Viral Hepatol 2003;10:285–93.

[21] Foucher Y, Mathieu E, Saint-Pierre P, Durand JF, Daures JP. A semi-Markov model based on generalized Weibull distribution with an illustration for HIV disease. Biom J 2005;47:825–33.

[22] Thal WM, Campbell CL, Madden LV. Sensitivity of Weibull model parameter estimates to variation in simulated disease progression data. Phytopathology 1984;74:1425–30.

[23] The Parkinson Study Group. Levodopa and the progression of Parkinson's disease. N Engl J Med 2004;351:2498–508.

[24] Hauser RA, Holford NH. Quantitative description of loss of clinical benefit following withdrawal of levodopa-carbidopa and bromocriptine in early Parkinson's disease. Mov Disord 2002;17:961–8.

[25] Olanow CW, Rascol O, Hauser R, Feigin PD, Jankovic J, Lang A, et al. A double-blind, delayed-start trial of rasagiline in Parkinson's disease. N Engl J Med 2009;361:1268–78.

[26] Holford NHG, Nutt J. Interpreting the results of Parkinson's disease clinical trials: Time for a change. Mov Disord 2011;26:569–77.

[27] Ploeger BA, Holford NH. Washout and delayed start designs for identifying disease modifying effects in slowly progressive diseases using disease progression analysis. Pharm Stat 2009;8:225–38.

[28] Holford N, Ma SC, Ploeger BA. Clinical trial simulation: A review. Clin Pharmacol Ther 2010;88:166–82.

[29] Gobburu JVS, Lesko LJ. Quantitative disease, drug and trial models. Annu Rev Pharmacol Toxicol 2009;49:291–301.

# OPTIMIZING AND EVALUATING PATIENT THERAPY

# 23

# Pharmacological Differences between Men and Women

Ameeta Parekh

*Office of Translational Sciences, Center for Drug Evaluation and Research, US Food and Drug Administration, Silver Spring, MD 20993*

## INTRODUCTION

The 1980s era of drug development was accompanied by renewed attention to response differences in population subgroups determined by age, race, and sex, and led to studies of intrinsic and extrinsic factors and their impact on pharmacokinetics (PK), pharmacodynamics (PD), and overall treatment response. As a result, the safety and efficacy of drug products in representative patient populations and the biological bases for interindividual differences in treatment response are now routinely studied prior to their marketing approval. This approach can optimize risks and benefits of therapeutic products by helping to base drug, dose, and regimen selection on individual patient needs. Guidances and regulations have also been developed by the US Food and Drug Administration (FDA) in order to provide drug developers and regulatory reviewers with a better understanding and appreciation of interindividual differences in treatments and outcomes [1]. In accordance with currently accepted usage, those differences reflecting differences between men and women that are biological or chromosomal based are referred to as *sex differences*, whereas cultural, social, and societal differences are referred to as *gender differences* [2]. This chapter focuses primarily on differences and similarities between men and women, as it relates to sex-based pharmacological response to therapy.

In the 1960s and 1970s, the fetal malformations that resulted from the exposure of pregnant women to thalidomide led to the 1977 recommendation by FDA that women of child-bearing potential be excluded from the earliest dose-ranging studies, although they could be included in further studies once satisfactory safety information was generated from animal fertility and teratology studies and after adequate information on efficacy and safety was amassed from early clinical trials [3]. This cautionary guidance from the FDA contributed to an unfortunate under-representation or exclusion of women from clinical trials. However, the burgeoning AIDS epidemic in the 1980s rapidly became a major cause of death in women and fueled the concern that women's access to breakthrough antiviral and anticancer treatments might be hampered if this pattern continued [4, 5]. This concern also focused attention on the potential for response differences between patients and the importance of understanding sex differences in treatment outcomes. Important milestones were reached in 1993 with the passage of the NIH Revitalization Act, directing NIH to include women and minorities in NIH-sponsored clinical research, and the development of the FDA's guidance on *Study and Evaluation of Gender Differences in the Clinical Evaluation of Drugs* [6, 7]. These measures facilitated accrual of clinical information in both sexes and served to reverse the practice of excluding women of child-bearing potential from clinical research that had been fostered by the previous 1977 guidelines.

Sex differences in response to drug therapy can manifest as differences in safety and/or efficacy outcomes. In some cases the observed sex differences can be attributed to differences in plasma concentrations of the active drug and/or its metabolites, and can be monitored in population subgroups who receive the drug. The magnitude of response differences based on dose alone may display far greater variability than when response assessments are based on drug and metabolite concentrations in the systemic circulation. This discordance reflects interindividual and intraindividual differences in the processes of drug absorption, distribution, metabolism, and excretion that determine the time course of systemic drug and/or metabolite concentrations after administration of a drug dose. These PK differences between subjects may be due to intrinsic (e.g., genetic predisposition, renal function, body weight) and extrinsic (e.g., smoking, concomitant drug and dietary intake and their interactions) factors. In addition to PK differences, sex-related PD differences, hormonal influence, extent of medication use (e.g., prescription medicine, over-the-counter drugs, alternative medicines, dietary supplements), healthcare utilization, and reporting bias may further contribute to the differences that are reported for men and women [8].

## PHARMACOKINETICS

The first medication to be analyzed for sex-based PK differences was antipyrine, in 1971 [9]. This drug is eliminated entirely by hepatic metabolism, and its half-life was reported to be shorter in women than in men. A subsequent study concluded that the clearance of antipyrine was the same for women and men only on day 5 of the menstrual cycle [10]. Sex-based differences for acetaminophen were studied in the 1970s and 1980s, and the clearance of this drug was reported to be faster in men than in women [11]. Benzodiazepines were examined in the 1980s for sex-specific differences in pharmacokinetics, and several of these studies concluded that women had higher clearances for this class of drugs than men [12]. In the ensuing years there has been a heightened interest in understanding sex differences and, as a result, reports of studies investigating PK and PD differences for new drugs in both sexes have grown. A recent survey of new chemical entity drugs and biologics approved by the FDA from September 2007 to August 2010 reported that most medications are now evaluated for sex differences in PK and the findings are reported in the regulatory reviews and product labels [13].

Currently, more than 95% of the systemically absorbed products that are used in both men and women have been studied with respect to sex-specific

PK differences [13]. These PK studies are typically conducted in 12–24 healthy volunteers in the early phases of drug development when clinical pharmacology and early dose-ranging studies are conducted. Women's participation in late-phase clinical trials has also increased over the years, and these studies are being analyzed for sex-based differences in both safety and efficacy [14]. Additionally, post-approval monitoring of a drug's clinical performance has furthered and will continue to further the understanding of response differences in subgroup populations [15]. This growing interest in understanding sex differences in drug exposure and response is contributing to better information on the underlying mechanisms contributing to response differences between individuals.

## Drug Transport

Drug transport has been discussed in Chapter 14, and transporter proteins play an important role both in the absorption and in the hepatobiliary and urinary excretion of xenobiotics. The two major classes of drug transporters are the uptake and efflux transporters. Uptake carriers, such as $H^+$/ditripeptide transporter, organic anion transporting polypeptide (OATPs), and other unidentified proteins, mediate greater uptake of drugs into cells and facilitate drug absorption [16]. Sex differences in hepatic OATP have been described for both human and animal models and have been related to differences in mRNA protein expression and the presence of gonadal hormones [17]. Sex differences have also been identified in efflux transporters. A study of P-glycoprotein (P-gp) expression in normal liver biopsies has shown an approximately 2.4-fold higher P-gp expression in men compared with women [18]. There is also higher hepatic expression of BCRP/Bcrp1 in men compared to women, and this may contribute to sex-specific variability seen in the transport of BCRP substrates [19].

## Absorption

Most drugs are developed for oral administration, and factors potentially influencing sex differences in oral absorption include gastric pH, gastrointestinal motility, enzymatic activity, and the intestinal expression of transporter proteins. It has been shown that gastric emptying of solids is slower in women than in men, and this could delay drug absorption from distal gastrointestinal sites [20]. The mechanism is unknown, but it may be related to sex differences in steroid hormone levels that may modify gastric acid secretion, gastric pH, and gastric emptying time [21]. Gastric pH is reported to be lower in men than in women [22]. In one study of aspirin bioavailability in men and women, it was found that aspirin was absorbed more rapidly in women, but that there was no sex difference in the extent of aspirin absorption [23]. However, another study reported that women had increased aspirin exposure compared to men who received the same aspirin doses [24]. In this study, the higher aspirin plasma concentrations in women were attributed to intrinsically lower blood concentrations of aspirin esterase in women, rather than to sex differences in aspirin absorption.

Other gastrointestinal enzymes may account for important differences between men and women in first-pass metabolism and bioavailability. For example, women have less alcohol dehydrogenase in the gut than men, and this partly explains women's higher blood alcohol levels after consuming the same amount of ethyl alcohol as men [25]. Higher oral bioavailability in women compared to men was also shown for midazolam, a probe for intestinal CYP3A [26]. The extent of drug absorption is also determined by first-pass metabolism in the liver as well as in the intestine, and sex differences in hepatic CYP3A4 activity have been documented [27]. However, the extent of CYP3A4 expression in the gut and liver can differ, so it is possible that sex differences noted after intravenous administration of CYP3A4 substrates may not be the same as those after oral administration.

Intestinal expression of proteins that modulate intestinal transport of drugs may also result in sex-based differences in plasma drug concentrations. For example, as discussed in Chapter 4, P-gp is expressed at the luminal surface of enterocytes, where it facilitates back-transport of cellularly absorbed drugs. The co-expression of P-gp and CYP3A4 in the intestinal mucosa plays an important role in determining the overall systemic availability of drugs. Although hepatic P-gp expression was shown to be higher in men than in women [18], a duodenal biopsy study showed high variability and no sex differences in P-gp expression [28]. Because of the interplay between CYP3A4 and P-gp in the intestinal lumen and liver, differentiating the role of each pathway in absorption of drugs that are co-substrates is a challenging yet important consideration. Finally, life stages need to be considered in evaluating the absorption of a chemical entity. For example, gastrointestinal absorption of calcium is decreased in menopause, but this decrease can be reversed with estrogen hormone replacement therapy [29, 30].

Unfortunately, there are only a few examples in the literature that document sex differences in drug absorption from routes other than the gastrointestinal tract, such as muscle, subcutaneous fat, and lung. It was shown in one study that women absorbed the lysine salt of aspirin at a slower rate than men after intramuscular injection [23]. Although minor sex differences in regional blood flow have been reported, and might have contributed to this observation, the authors considered that the more likely cause of this difference was drug injection into subcutaneous fat of the women, rather than the gluteus muscle.

## Distribution

The rate and extent of drug distribution are determined by multiple factors such as body mass index (BMI), body composition in terms of muscle and fat content, plasma volume, organ blood flow, and the extent of tissue and plasma protein binding of the drug. Compared to men, women have a higher body fat content, a lower average BMI, a smaller average plasma volume, and a lower average organ blood flow [31]. These differences may contribute to sex differences in the rate and extent of drug distribution, and should be considered in calculating loading or bolus doses in order to avoid unnecessary adverse reactions in women. Thus, a study on the action of anesthetics concluded that sex-modified dosing should be considered for anesthetics when rapid onset or short duration of action is important [32].

Total body fat is estimated at about 13.5 kg in an adult male and at 16.5 kg in an adult female [33]. Owing to this disparity, lipophilic drugs may exhibit a relatively greater volume of distribution in women than in men when normalized on the basis of body weight. For example, lipophilic drugs such as diazepam, nitrazepam, and chlordiazepoxide have larger L/kg distribution volumes in women than in men [34–36]. Conversely, total body water constitutes a lower proportion of body mass in women than in men, so the distribution volume of hydrophilic drugs is generally lower in women than in men on a L/kg basis. Thus, the distribution volume of ethanol is smaller in women than in men and contributes to its higher peak plasma concentrations and greater initial effects in women [37]. Some other hydrophilic drugs that exhibit a smaller distribution volume in women are metronidazole, prednisolone, and the water-soluble fluoroquinolones [31].

The main drug-binding proteins in plasma are albumin, $\alpha_1$-acid-glycoprotein (AAG) and globulins. Drug binding to albumin is not greatly influenced by sex [38]. Estrogens have been shown to decrease plasma levels of AAG by inducing its hepatic glycosylation, presumably accounting for less binding to this protein in women than in men [39]. Exogenous estrogens increase the levels of some other proteins, such as sex hormone binding globulin, corticosteroid binding globulin and thyroxine binding globulin, that may contribute to observed sex differences in drug binding to plasma proteins [40].

## Drug Metabolism

The large body of literature on drug metabolic clearance suggests that the high variability associated with drug metabolism is due to the influence of both intrinsic factors, such as age, race, sex, body composition, disease states, genetic makeup, hormonal status, and extrinsic factors, such as smoking, drinking, diet, dietary supplements, administration of multiple medications, and other environmental exposures. Of relevance to this chapter are the sex differences that have been reported for both the Phase I and Phase II metabolic pathways described previously in Chapter 11.

### Phase I Metabolic Pathways

Phase I metabolic reactions (e.g., oxidation, reduction, and hydrolysis) are primarily catalyzed by the cytochrome P450 (CYP) multigene superfamily of enzymes. The major CYP families (CYP1, CYP2, CYP3) have specific isoenzymes that are involved in drug metabolism, and the most extensively studied are CYP1A2, CYP2C9, CYP2C19, CYP2D6, CYP2E1, and CYP3A4 [31]. Because sex differences affect the activity of some of these enzymes, it is recommended that these differences be studied and that their clinical implications be evaluated during drug development.

**CYP3A4**: Greater than 50% of drugs are metabolized by CYP3A4 and its activity in the liver is higher in women than in men [41], as indicated by the observation that metabolic ratio of 6β-hydroxycortisol to cortisol, the endogenous marker for CYP3A activity, is higher in women than in men [42]. A retrospective analysis concluded that women have about a 20–30% higher clearance of drugs that are CYP3A4 substrates than men [43]. Midazolam, erythromycin, verapamil, cyclosporine, methylprednisolone, diazepam, and tirilazad are some of the CYP3A4 substrate drugs that have a higher clearance in women than in men [44].

The unsuccessful attempt to develop tirilazad to treat patients with aneurismal subarachnoid hemorrhage provides a cautionary example of the importance of designing clinical trials in which dosage is adjusted to account for sex differences in drug metabolism. In two large clinical trials intended to demonstrate the efficacy of this drug in these patients, men and women were both treated with the same tirilazad dose but only men appeared to have a therapeutic response [45, 46]. PK studies indicated that young women had 40–60% higher clearance than men, although middle-aged premenopausal women's clearance was about 10% lower than in younger women, and postmenopausal women's clearance was similar to that in men [47, 48]. Unfortunately in these and in subsequent failed clinical trials, plasma-level monitoring was not used to adjust dosage in order to minimize the impact on tirilazad clearance of either sex differences or CYP3A4 induction by drugs, such as phenobarbital, that were concurrently administered to the patients [49].

Many compounds are co-substrates of both the CYP 3A4 and the efflux drug transporter P-gp, so it is challenging to evaluate the specific role played by each of these mechanisms in altering drug clearance. It has been suggested that membrane-bound P-gp may lower the intracellular drug concentrations that would be available for CYP3A4 metabolism. Because men have higher levels of hepatic P-gp than women, this could result in their having lower intracellular drug levels available for metabolism and might account for the observation that women have a higher clearance of CYP3A4 substrates than men [50, 51].

**CYP2D6**: The CYP2D6 isoenzyme metabolizes several drugs in current use, including antidepressants, antiarrhythmics, analgesics, and beta blockers. Several drugs metabolized partially or exclusively by CYP2D6 have shown higher activity in men than in women, and the combined data suggest higher activity of CYP2D6 in men than in women. For example, studies in extensive CYP2D6 metabolizers have shown faster clearance for dextromethorphan and metoprolol in men than in women [52]. Mirtazapine is primarily metabolized by CYP2D6 and CYP3A, and a higher clearance has been reported for men than in women [53]. Sex differences in propranolol clearance also have been reported, with a higher clearance found in men than in women [54].

**CYP2C19**: The CYP2C19 isoenzyme is responsible for metabolizing drugs such as the proton pump inhibitors, citalopram, and diazepam. Sex differences have been reported for drugs metabolized by the CYP2C19 pathway; however, these findings may have been confounded by other factors. Using S-mephenytoin as a probe, CYP2C19 activity was shown to be about 60% lower in women receiving oral contraceptives as compared to women not receiving these drugs. Sex differences for drugs metabolized by CYP2C19 were reported to be ethnic-population specific. However, since oral contraceptive use was not reported in these studies it is likely that its use was not controlled for, and thus the results of these studies may have been confounded by oral contraceptive use [55].

**CYP2C9**: CYP2C9 metabolizes drugs such as *S*-warfarin, phenytoin, toldutamide, and ketoprofen. No sex differences have been reported with these drugs [55].

**CYP1A2**: Caffeine is a common probe for CYP1A2, and this isoenzyme also oxidizes drugs such as theophylline, clozapine, olanzapine, tacrine, and ondansetron. Studies have consistently shown a higher activity of CYP1A2 in males as compared to females. Smoking also induces the activity of CYP1A2 to a greater extent in males than in females [55–57].

**CYP2E1**: Limited information for CYP2E1 suggests an approximately 30% lower metabolic activity in women as compared to men in studies with chlorzoxazone. CYP2E1 is an alcohol-inducible enzyme, and sex differences were not observed under conditions of alcohol-induced CYP2E1 induction [58, 59].

### Phase II Metabolic Pathways

Phase II metabolic pathways include glucuronidation, sulfation, acetylation, or methylation of either a parent drug or its Phase I metabolite to form polar conjugates that are more readily excreted by the kidneys. Sex differences have been identified in some of these drug conjugation reactions.

**Glucuronidation**: Glucuronide conjugates are formed by UDP-glucuronosyltransferases (UGT). UGT conjugation of oxazepam and temazepam has been reported to be slower in women than in men, and the clearance of these drugs is faster in men [60, 61]. The clearance of acetaminophen, which undergoes both glucuronidation and sulfate conjugation, is also 22% higher in men than in women [62]. However, sex differences in glucuronidation are not universally seen, and no sex differences in clearance were reported for clofibric acid and ibuprofen [63, 64]. Oral contraceptives increase the glucuronidation rates in women, and it is possible that their co-administration may have confounded the observation of sex differences in UGT activity that were observed in some studies [62, 65].

**Acetylation**: There are no sex differences reported for *N*-acetyltransferase activity as assessed with isoniazid, caffeine, and sulfamethazine [66].

**Methylation**: Human liver biopsies have shown higher thiopurine methyl transferase (TPMT) activity in men compared to women. Azathioprine and 6-mercaptopurine undergo TPMT metabolism, and patients with low TPMT activity are at higher risk for bone marrow toxicity from these drugs. It is also reported that higher doses of 6-mercaptopurine are needed for equivalent therapeutic efficacy in boys compared with girls with leukemia. Concentrations of catechol-*O*-methyltransferase (COMT) are reported to be higher in men compared to women. Although COMT is responsible for the metabolism of norepinephrine, epinephrine, and dopamine, this sex difference does not appear to have clinically significant consequences [66].

**Sulfation**: Limited and conflicting evidence exists for sex differences in sulfotransferase activity. Environmental and genetic factors have been suggested as possibly contributing to these inconsistent findings [67, 68].

### Multiple Metabolic Pathways

Although a number of drugs have been associated with a specific metabolic pathway, the metabolism of many drugs actually involves multiple pathways operating either in series or in parallel. As described previously, many drugs are first oxidized in a Phase I reaction that is followed by Phase II conjugation. It is also common for several isoenzymes to participate in the Phase I metabolism of a drug. For example, propranolol undergoes ring oxidation, side-chain cleavage, and glucuronidation, involving several isoenzymes in both Phase I and Phase II pathways. Therefore, sex differences in these multiple pathways may contribute to the observation that propranolol clearance is lower in women than in men [54].

## Renal Excretion

Glomerular filtration rate (GFR), tubular secretion, and tubular reabsorption need to be considered in evaluating the renal excretion of drugs. In general, women have a lower renal clearance for drugs that are predominantly eliminated unchanged in urine (e.g., vancomycin, ceftazidime, cefepime, fleroxacin) [55]. This partly reflects the fact that, after correcting for body size, GFR is about 10% lower in women than in men [69]. There are limited data regarding sex differences in renal tubular secretion. Men have been shown to have approximately 50% higher renal clearance for amantadine than women. Amantadine is actively secreted in the kidneys by the organic cationic transporter 2 (OCT2) and, mechanistically, testosterone has been shown to upregulate renal OCT2 in animals [55]. Digoxin is predominantly eliminated by the kidneys, is a substrate for the P-gp efflux transporter, and its oral clearance is about 12–14% lower in women than in men [55]. These differences may account for the fact that about 3.4% of women but only about 2.3% of men were reported in one study to have digoxin concentrations higher than 2 ng/ml.

## Effects of Menstrual Cycle and Menopause on Pharmacokinetics

The follicular, ovulatory, and luteal phases of the menstrual cycle are accompanied by substantial hormonal changes, and these may result in PK differences for drugs administered during various phases of the menstrual cycle. There have been a few studies that have encompassed all different phases of the menstrual cycle and the results of these studies have been conflicting, with the result that clinically relevant changes have not been consistently identified in the processes of drug absorption, distribution, metabolism, and excretion. For instance, although highest peak alcohol concentrations were reported in premenstrual women and the rate of absorption varied during the menstrual cycle, these results were not replicated in subsequent studies [70]. No absorption differences were reported for sodium salicylate solution during the menstrual cycle phases [71]. Studies with antipyrine, nitrazepam, and phenytoin also have shown no significant differences in distribution volume across the menstrual cycle phases [70, 72–74]. Protein-binding changes were not seen during the menstrual cycle phases for nitrazepam, phenytoin, phenobarbital, carbamazepine, or sodium salicylate [70–73, 75]. However, some studies have shown that the clearance of some drugs is higher during the ovulation phase and lower during the luteal phase of the menstrual cycle. For example, a two-fold increase in methaqualone clearance was reported during the ovulation phase [70, 76]. The clearance rates of acetaminophen, caffeine and theophylline also were decreased during the luteal phase, but these changes were not considered clinically important [70]. On the other hand, the menstrual cycle has not been found to affect the PK of some other drugs, including propranolol, ethylmorphine, dextromethorphan, alprazolam, nitrazepam, carbamazepine, midazolam, and methylprednisolone, and studies with antipyrine, phenytoin, and alcohol have yielded conflicting results [70].

American women spend one-third of their life in menopause, a time when plasma levels of estrogen and progesterone are greatly reduced, and these changes also affect PK. The renal clearance of many drugs also decreases with age in parallel with a gradual decline in renal function. In addition, the metabolic clearance of a number of drugs has been shown to decline in postmenopausal women, whereas decreases were not found in men of corresponding age. Studies have shown a 20% decrease in the intestinal CYP3A4 content in biopsy samples from postmenopausal women as compared to premenopausal women [77]. In another study of women ranging in age from 25 to 79 years, alfentanil clearance was shown to decrease with advancing age but a similar trend was not seen in men [78]. A lower clearance in postmenopausal women as compared to premenopausal women was also shown for tirilazad and for intravenous midazolam, administered concomitantly as a CYP3A4 probe [79]. However, other studies with midazolam have shown conflicting findings, and erythromycin studies showed no difference in clearance between pre- and postmenopausal women [31]. As mentioned before, calcium absorption is decreased in menopause, and this may explain changes in the absorption of drugs that have absorptive profiles which are similar to that of this mineral.

## PHARMACODYNAMICS

There has been increased awareness of sex-related differences in drug exposure and response since the 1980s. Analysis of sex differences in PD as well as combined PK and PD has also generated research interest, although published reports have focused on certain therapeutic areas more than others. Currently, the most information has been provided on the cardiovascular effects of drugs, followed by pharmacodynamic studies of analgesics, immunosuppressants, and antidepressants.

### Cardiovascular Effects

Emerging clinical evidence is suggestive of sexually dimorphic profiles in both drug safety and efficacy. Perhaps the most prominent and widely discussed example of sex differences in pharmacologic response is that of the life-threatening ventricular arrhythmia called *torsades de pointes* (TdP) [80–82]. Women have a risk of developing drug-induced TdP that is at least twice as high as that of men [82–85]. As discussed in Chapter 1, the demonstration that TdP is an important side effect of terfenadine first attracted widespread attention to the severity of this problem and led to the withdrawal of this non-sedating antihistamine from the market in 1998. The 2001 GAO report entitled *Drug Safety: Most Drugs Withdrawn in Recent Years Had Greater Risks for Women* has drawn further attention to women's susceptibility to drug-induced QTc interval prolongation. This report lists the drugs withdrawn from the market during 1997–2000; of the 10 drugs listed, 4 had TdP potential (cisapride, astemizole, grepafloxacin, and terfenadine) [86].

Terfenadine and presumably other drugs that cause TdP block the delayed rectifier potassium current, which initially lengthens the electrocardographic QT interval [87]. However, TdP does not occur in every patient who is treated with these drugs, and other factors that may predispose patients to this arrhythmia include hypokalemia, hypomagnesemia, and hypothyroidism [82, 88, 89]. Women appear to be at an increased risk of TdP because the heart rate-corrected QT interval in women is longer than it is in men [84]. Several attempts have been made to elucidate the underlying mechanism for women's higher sensitivity to QTc interval prolongation and TdP. Baseline QTc assessments through puberty and the changes during the menstrual cycle have revealed that pre-pubertal baseline QTc is similar for both the sexes [90, 91]. At puberty, testosterone exerts a protective effect in men through shortening of the baseline QTc intervals, with women's QTc remaining unchanged. Manifestation of this longer QTc interval for women at baseline is explained as one of the causes of physiological divergence in men and women leading to higher arrhythmia and TdP propensity in women [92].

An example that illustrates the importance of including women in clinical trials is given by probucol, a cholesterol-lowering drug that was withdrawn from the market after its initial approval. The safety database cited as evidence of probucol's long-term safety leading to its approval was based on studies that were confined to men, and it was only when probucol was studied in women that its propensity to cause TdP was recognized [93]. Quinidine is a drug that for many years has been recognized to cause of TdP, with a reported prevalence of this arrhythmia in females of 60% as compared with 43% in males [82, 94]. Although there is no PK difference between men and women, there is a PD difference in that QT interval prolongation is more likely to occur in women than in men who are treated with quinidine [95]. Similarly, women have three times the risk of developing TdP while receiving sotalol and dofetilide [81, 96, 97].

Propranolol is an example of a drug with sex differences in both PK and PD. In the Beta-Blocker Heart Attack Trial, both sexes received equal doses of propranolol but women were found to have higher plasma concentrations of this drug than men [54, 98]. However, when an isoproterenol challenge infusion was used to assess the actual degree of β-adrenoreceptor blockade, it was found that women had a reduced sensitivity to propranolol that compensated for their higher plasma concentration [99, 100]. These offsetting PK and PD effects obviated the need to reduce propranolol doses in women – an action which could reduce the overall effectiveness of the drug in this sex.

Sex differences in patient response also were noted in a trial that was designed to assess the efficacy of aspirin and dipyridamole in preventing recurrence of stroke [101]. It was found that this regimen reduced the frequency of strokes and reduced mortality in males, but was much less effective in females. *In vitro* studies have shown that when the same amounts of aspirin were added to the blood of males and females, platelet aggregation decreased more in men than in women [102]. Further investigation indicated that when aspirin was added to blood from orchiectomized subjects there was only a modest change in platelet aggregation. However, when testosterone also was added to these blood samples, platelet aggregation was similar to that seen with blood from nonorchiectomized males, so it is possible that testosterone may be contributing to the clinical findings of sex differences in aspirin-mediated inhibition of platelet aggregation.

## Pain

Studies in the area of pain perception and response to analgesics have shown that women have an overall lower pain threshold and are less tolerant to experimental pain than men [103, 104]. A higher level of pain intensity and prevalence has also been reported for women [105–107]. However, various factors complicate the reporting and interpretation of sex differences in pain response. Social behavior, genetic factors, PK and PD differences, pain models utilized, and hormonal contributions have been discussed as contributing to these observed sex differences. In addition, women in the periovulatory, luteal, and premenstrual phases of the menstrual cycle were reported to have a lower pain threshold than women in the follicular phase [103]. These various contributing factors, combined with the inconsistencies in observed pain response, pose challenges for the future research that is needed to elucidate the clinical significance and underlying cause of sex differences in the response to and treatment of pain. However, some studies have already indicated that there can be substantial sex differences in the analgesic response to both opioid and non-steroidal anti-inflammatory drugs.

Using a clinical pain model in which the μ-agonist morphine was administered to men and women emerging from general anesthesia after surgical procedures, it was found that, compared to men, women had more intense pain and required about 30% more morphine to achieve a similar degree of analgesia despite the lack of a PK sex difference and after adjusting for type of surgery, age, and body weight [108]. In a study using an electric pain model, it was found that morphine provided greater μ-opioid analgesic potency but a slower onset and offset of analgesic effect in women than in men [109]. A recent systematic review and meta-analysis indicated higher efficacy of morphine in women in patient-controlled analgesia studies. The data on non-morphine μ-opioids and mixed μ-/κ-opioids are less certain and require further research [110]. The opioid side effects of respiratory depression, nausea, and vomiting have also been reported to be more pronounced in women than in men [109–112].

Sex differences were noted with the κ-agonist–antagonist drugs pentazocine, butorphanol, and nalbuphine in the setting of postoperative dental pain [113]. In this study, a greater degree of analgesia was reported in women after the third-molar extraction as compared to men. It is suggested that this sex difference is a general characteristic of the κ-agonist–antagonist drug class and may be partly responsible for the lower usage of these drugs as compared to the μ-opioid drug class. The relevance of genotypic characteristics in pain response to κ-agonist–antagonist analgesic drugs has also been discussed in a study in which pain was induced using thermal and ischemic pain stimuli [114]. It was found that women with two variant *MC1R* alleles exhibited a higher analgesic response to pentazocine as compared to men or to women with either 1 or no variant *MC1R* alleles. However, no sex differences were found between men and women without the two variant *MC1R* alleles. On the other hand, standard doses of ibuprofen appeared to be more effective in men than in women when they were challenged with different degrees of ear lobe pain, even though there was no sex difference in PK profile [115].

## Immunology and Immunosuppression

Although women are more susceptible than men to autoimmune diseases, there are few sex-analyzed studies of immunosuppressant therapy in patients with these disorders. Heart transplantation is followed by a higher incidence of organ rejection in women than in men which suggests that there may be sex differences in the PK and PD of immunosuppressant drugs, although others factors may also be involved [116]. Cyclosporine, prednisolone, and methylprednisolone frequently are administered to these patients as immunosuppressants and these

drugs are metabolized by CYP3A4, which is known to be more active in women than in men. In addition, it was observed that duration of survival after heart transplantation was inversely correlated with the length of time required to withdraw patients from maintenance corticosteroid therapy [117]. Although the basis for this difference is unclear, it may reflect the clinical observation that it is more difficult to withdraw steroid therapy from women than from men. Further complexity emerges from a study of methylprednisolone PK and PD in healthy volunteers [118]. It was found in this study that even though women cleared the drug faster than men, they were more sensitive than men to suppression of endogenous cortisol production and had an $IC_{50}$ value for cortisol suppression that was 17 times lower than in men. However, these PK and PD sex differences were offsetting, so the observed clinical response to a given dose of methylprednisolone was similar in both men and women.

## EFFECTS OF EXTRANEOUS FACTORS

Extraneous factors contributing to apparent sex differences include differences between men and women in the use of prescription medicines, over-the-counter drugs, herbal medicines, dietary supplements, and smoking. In the United States, nearly one in five women is a smoker [119]. Smoking increases CYP1A2 activity and therefore increases the clearance of caffeine and theophylline. However, sex differences in the extent of this increase were not consistently observed, as the effect on caffeine clearance is greater in men than in women [120] but the opposite is true for theophylline [121]. Olanzapine dosing presents an interesting case of dosing in women who smoke [122]. It also is metabolized by CYP1A2, and its clearance in nonsmokers is lower in women than in men and also lower in the elderly ($\geq 65$ years) than in subjects less than 65 years old. However, olanzapine metabolism is induced by cigarette smoking and as a result its clearance is about 40% higher in smokers than in nonsmokers. Although each of these factors may not independently justify olanzapine dosing adjustment, the combined effects of age, smoking status, and patient's sex could lead to substantial PK differences in certain populations and increase the likelihood of adverse effects from higher exposures. Although specific recommendations are not made for women or smokers, the labeling for olanzapine recommends a lower starting dose for patients who exhibit a combination of certain factors (e.g., non-smoking female patients $\geq 65$ years of age) [122].

Women use medications, including herbal products and dietary supplements, more frequently than men [123]. As more and more patients are combining these alternative therapies with conventional pharmaceuticals, drug–herb and drug–nutrient interactions are becoming increasingly important [124]. St John's wort, for instance, contains numerous compounds, some of which have documented biological activity [125]. It has been reported that St John's wort induces CYP1A2, which could lower plasma concentrations of drugs metabolized by this isoenzyme (e.g., theophylline and olanzapine) [126, 127]. Studies have shown that St John's wort also induces hepatic and intestinal CYP3A4 and the P-gp efflux transporter, and may cause clinically important drug interactions through its effect on these pathways [128, 129]. St John's wort increases clearance of indinavir, a protease inhibitor that is metabolized by CYP3A4, and its concurrent use may compromise therapeutic response to this drug [129]. Concurrent use of St John's wort has also been shown to decrease blood concentrations of cyclosporine, a CYP3A4 and P-gp substrate. There have been reports of graft rejection in organ transplant patients, and lower cyclosporine levels due to interaction with St John's wort have been implicated [129]. Since sex steroids are metabolized by CYP3A4, one would expect plasma concentrations of oral contraceptives also to decrease in patients taking St John's wort. Breakthrough bleeding among women taking both St John's wort and oral contraceptives have been reported [129]. Based on such findings, information regarding concomitant use of oral contraceptives and St John's wort is included in the FDA-approved labels for these drugs, and patients are cautioned about the potential for lower efficacy and advised to consider using other birth control methods [130]. Exposure to digoxin, a P-gp substrate, is also influenced by concomitant use of St John's wort, likely reflecting induction of this efflux transporter by St John's wort [129].

## SUMMARY

Historically, sex differences in response to treatment have often been attributed to differences in body weight or, alternatively, a higher propensity to report adverse events by women. Most PK and PD differences discussed in this chapter discount these variables as the only source of the reported differences. The heightened interest in the underlying causes of variable inter- and intraindividual patient outcomes, combined with increasingly supportive NIH and FDA policies and practices, has provided the impetus to study and understand sex differences through clinical research. Continued attention to the influence of intrinsic and extrinsic factors on the physiological changes throughout a woman's life cycle, a mechanistic understanding of PK and/or PD changes brought about by these factors, and their relationship to therapeutic response differences will further our existing understanding of the sex-specific treatment needs of men and women.

## ACKNOWLEDGEMENT

Portions of the chapter were retained from previous editions

## REFERENCES

[1] CDER. Guidances (Drugs) (Internet at, www.fda.gov/Drugs/GuidanceCompliance RegulatoryInformation/Guidances/default.htm.)

[2] Kim JS, Nafziger AN. Is it sex or is it gender? Clin Pharmacol Ther 2000;68:1–3.

[3] CDER. General considerations for the clinical evaluation of drugs. Guidance for industry. Rockville, MD: FDA (Internet at, www.fda.gov/downloads/Drugs/Guidance Compliance RegulatoryInformation/Guidances/ucm071682.pdf. last accessed February 15, 2012).

[4] Merkatz RB. Women in clinical trials: An introduction. Food Drug Law J 1993;48:161–6.

[5] McCarthy C. Historical background of clinical trials involving women and minorities. Acad Med 1994;69:695–8.

[6] CDER Guideline for the study and evaluation of gender differences in the clinical evaluation of drugs. Guidance for Industry. Rockville, MD: FDA; February 1997, initially published as a Guideline in the Federal Register on July 22, 1993. (Internet at, http://www.fda.gov/downloads/Drugs/GuidanceComplianceRegulatoryInformation/Guidances/UCM072044.pdf.)

[7] United States General Accounting Office. GAO Report to Congressional Requesters. Women's health. NIH has increased its efforts to include women in research. Washington, DC: Publication No GAO/HEHS–00–96; May 2000.

[8] Tran C, Knowles SR, Liu BA, Shear NH. Gender differences in adverse drug reactions. J Clin Pharmacol 1998;38:1003–9.

[9] Berg MJ. Drugs, vitamins and gender. J Gend-Specif Med 1999;2:18–20.

[10] Nayak VK, Kshirsagar NA, Desai NK, Satoskar RS. Influence of menstrual cycle on antipyrine pharmacokinetics in healthy Indian female volunteers. Br J Clin Pharmacol 1988;26:604–6.

[11] Miners JO, Attwood J, Birkett DJ. Influence of sex and oral contraceptive steroids on paracetamol metabolism. Br J Clin Pharmacol 1983;16:503–9.

[12] Cotreau MM, von Molke LL, Greenblatt DJ. The influence of age and sex on the clearance of cytochrome P450 3A substrates. Clin Pharmacokinetics 2005;44:33–60.

[13] Copeland V, Parekh A. FDA approved drug labels 2007–10: Dose adjustments for women based on exposure. Drug Information Association 2011 47th Annual Meeting, June 19–23, 2011, Chicago, IL. Poster Presentation. (Internet at, www.fda.gov/Science Research/SpecialTopics/WomensHealthResearch/ucm201358.htm.)

[14] Poon R, Khanijow K, Umarjee S, Zhang L, Fadiran E, Yu M, et al. Tracking women's participation and sex analyses in late-phase clinical trials of new molecular entity (NME) drugs and biologics approved by FDA between 2007–2009. Drug

Information Association 2011 47th Annual Meeting, June 19–23, 2011, Chicago, IL. Poster Presentation. (Internet at, www.fda.gov/ScienceResearch/SpecialTopics/WomenshealthResearch/ucm201358.htm.)

[15] FDA's Sentinel Initiative. Transforming how we monitor the safety of FDA-regulated products. (Internet at, www.fda.gov/Safety/FDAsSentinelInitiative/default.htm.; May 2008).

[16] Tamai I, Saheki A, Saitoh R, Sai Y, Yamada I, Tsuji A. Nonlinear intestinal absorption of 5-hydroxytryptamine receptor antagonist caused by absorptive and secretory transporters. J Pharmacol Exp Ther 1997;283:108–15.

[17] Morris ME, Lee HJ, Predko LM. Gender differences in the membrane transport of endogenous and exogenous compounds. Pharmacol Rev 2003;55:229–40.

[18] Shuetz EG, Furuya KN, Shuetz JD. Interindividual variation in expression of P-gp in normal human liver and secondary hepatic neoplasm. J Pharmacol Exp Ther 1995;275:1011–8.

[19] Merino G, van Herwaarden AE, Wagenaar E, Jonker JW, Schinkel AH. Sex dependent expression and activity of the ATP-binding cassette transporter breast cancer resistance protein (BCRP/ABCG2) in liver. Mol Pharmacol 2005;67:1765–71.

[20] Datz FL, Christian PE, Moore J. Gender-related differences in gastric emptying. Nucl Med 1987;28:1204–7.

[21] Carrasco-Portugal M, Flores-Murrieta F. Gender Differences in the pharmacokinetics of oral drugs. Pharmacol Pharm 2011;2:31–41.

[22] Soldin OP, Mattison DR. Sex differences in pharmacokinetics and pharmacodynamics. Clin Pharmacokinet 2009;48:143–57.

[23] Aarons L, Hopkins K, Rowland M, Brossel S, Thiercelin J-F. Route of administration and sex differences in the pharmacokinetics of aspirin, administered as its lysine salt. Pharm Res 1989;6:660–6.

[24] Ho PC, Triggs EJ, Bourne DW, Heazlewood VJ. The effects of age and sex on the disposition of acetylsalicylic acid and its metabolites. Br J Clin Pharmacol 1985;19:675–84.

[25] Seitz H, Egerer G, Srianowsk U, Waldherr R, Eckey R, Agarwal D, et al. Human gastric alcohol dehydragenase activity: Effect of age, sex and alcoholism. Gut 1993;34:1433–7.

[26] Gorski JC, Jones DR, Haehner-Daniels BD, Hamman MA, O'Mara EM, Hall SD. The contribution of intestinal and hepatic CYP3A to the interaction between midazolam and clarithromycin. Clin Pharmacol Ther 1998;64:133–43.

[27] Nicolas JM, Espie P, Molimard M. Gender and interindividual variability in pharmacokinetics. Drug Metab Rev 2001;41:408–21.

[28] Paine MF, Ludington SS, Chen ML, Stewart PW, Huang SM, Watkins PB. Do men and women differ in proximal small intestinal CYP3A or P-glycoprotein expression? Drug Metab Dispos 2005;33:426–33.

[29] Arjmandi BH, Salih MA, Herbert DC, Sims SH, Kalu DN. Evidence for estrogen receptor-linked calcium transport in the intestine. Bone Miner 1993;21:63–74.

[30] Gennari C, Agnussdei D, Nardi P, Civitelli R. Estrogen preserves a normal intestinal responsiveness to 1,25-dihydroxyvitamin D$_3$ in oophorectomized women. J Clin Endocrinol Metab 1990;71:1288–93.

[31] Gandhi M, Aweeka F, Greenblatt RM, Blaschke TF. Sex differences in pharmacokinetics and pharmacodynamics. Annu Rev Pharmacol Toxicol 2001;44:499–523.

[32] Ueno K. Gender differences in pharmacokinetics of anesthetics. Masui 2009;58:51–8.

[33] Soldin OP, Chung SH, Mattison DR. Sex differences in drug disposition. J Biomed Biotech 2011;2011:187103. Epub.

[34] Ochs HR, Greenblatt DJ, Divoll M, Abernethy DR, Feyerabend H, Dengler HJ. Diazepam kinetics in relation to age and sex. Pharmacology 1981;23:24–30.

[35] Greenblatt DJ, Abernethy DR, Lochniskai A, Ochs HR, Harmatz JS, Shader RI. Age, sex and nitrazepam kinetics: Relation to antipyrene disposition. Clin Pharmacol Ther 1985;38:697–703.

[36] Roberts RK, Desmond PV, Wilkinson GR, Schenker S. Disposition of chlordiazepoxide: Sex differences and effects of oral contraceptives. Clin Pharmacol Ther 1979;25:826–31.

[37] Wedel M, Pieters JE, Pikaar NA, Ockhuizen T. Application of a three-compartment model to a study of the effects of sex, alcohol dose and concentration, exercise and food consumption on the pharmacokinetics of ethanol in healthy volunteers. Alcohol Alcohol 1991;26:329–36.

[38] Verbeeck RK, Cardinal JA, Wallace SM. Effect of age and sex on the plasma binding of acidic and basic drugs. Eur J Clin Pharmacol 1984;27:91–7.

[39] Succari M, Foglietti MJ, Percheron F. Microheterogeneity of alpha1-acid glycoprotein: Variation during the menstrual cycle. Clin Chim Acta 1990;187:35–41.

[40] Wiegratz I, Kutschera E, Lee JH, Moore C, Mellinger U, Winkler UH. Effect of four different oral contraceptives on various sex hormones and serum-binding globulins. Contraception 2003;67:25–32.

[41] Wolbold R, Klein K, Burk O, Nüssler AK, Neuhaus P, Eichelbaum M, et al. Sex is a major determinant of CYP3A4 expression in human liver. Hepatology 2001;38:978–88.

[42] Lutz U, Bittner N, Ufer M, Lutz WK. Quantification of cortisol and 6 beta-hydroxycortisol in human urine by LC-MS/MS, and gender-specific evaluation of the metabolic ratio as biomarker of CYP3A activity. J Chromatogr B Analyt Technol Biomed Life Sci 2010;878:97–101.

[43] Greenblatt DJ, von Moltke LL. Gender has a small but statistically significant effect on clearance of CYP3A substrate drugs. J Clin Pharmacol 2008;48:1350–5.

[44] Sakuma T, Kawasaki Y, Jarukamjorn K, Nemoto N. Sex differences of drug-metabolizing enzymes: Female predominant expression of human and mouse cytochrome P450 3A isoforms. J Health Sci 2009;55:325–37.

[45] Kassell NF, Haley Jr EC, Apperson-Hansen C, Alves WM. Randomized, double-blind, vehicle-controlled trial of tirilazad mesylate in patients with aneurysmal subarachnoid hemorrhage: A cooperative study in Europe, Australia, and New Zealand. J Neurosurg 1996;84:221–8.

[46] Haley Jr EC, Kassel NF, Apperson-Hansen C, Maile MH, Alves WM. A randomized, double-blind, vehicle-controlled trial of tirilazad mesylate in patients with aneurysmal subarachnoid hemorrhage: A cooperative study in North America. J Neurosurg 1997;86:467–74.

[47] Fleishaker JC, Hulst-Pearson LK, Peters GR. Effect of gender and menopausal status on the pharmacokinetics of tirilazad mesylate in healthy subjects. Am J Ther 1995;2:553–60.

[48] Hulst LK, Fleishaker JC, Peters GR, Harry JD, Wright DM, Ward P. Pharmacokinetics and drug disposition: Effect of age and gender on tirilazad pharmacokinetics in humans. Clin Pharmacol Ther 1994;55:378–84.

[49] Lanzino G, Kassell NF, Dorsch NW, Pasqualin A, Brandt L, Schmiedek P, et al. Double-blind, randomized, vehicle-controlled study of high-dose tirilazad mesylate in women with aneurismal subarachnoid hemorrhage. Part I. A cooperative study in Europe, Australia, New Zealand, and South Africa. J Neurosurg 1999;90:1011–7.

[50] Benet LZ, Cummins C, Wu CY. Unmasking the dynamic interplay between efflux transporters and metabolic enzymes. Intl J Pharm 2004;277:3–9.

[51] Benet LZ. The drug transporter–metabolism alliance: Uncovering and defining the interplay. Mol Pharm 2009;6:1631–43.

[52] Labbé L, Sirois C, Pilote S, Arseneault M, Robitaille NM, Turgeon J, et al. Effect of gender, sex hormones, time variables and physiological urinary pH on apparent CYP2D6 activity as assessed by metabolic ratios of marker substrates. Pharmacogenetics 2000;10:425–38.

[53] Timmer CJ, Sitsen JM, Delbressine LP. Clinical pharmacokinetics of mirtazapine. Clin Pharmacokin 2000;38:461–74.

[54] Walle T, Walle UK, Cowart TD, Conradi EC. Pathway-selective sex differences in metabolic clearance of propranolol in human subjects. Clin Pharmcol Ther 1989;46:257–63.

[55] Anderson GD. Sex and racial differences in pharmacological response: Where is the evidence? Pharmacogenetics, pharmacokinetics, and pharmacodynamics. J Womens Health (Larchmt) 2005;14:19–29.

[56] Ereshefsky L, Saklad SR, Watanabe MD, Davis CM, Jann MN. Thiothixene pharmacokinetic interactions: A study of hepatic enzyme inducers, clearance inhibitors, and demographic variables. J Clin Psychopharmacol 1991;11:296–301.

[57] Bruno R, Vivier N, Montay G, Le Liboux A, Powe LK, Delumeau JC, et al. Population pharmacokinetics of riluzole in patients with amyotrophic lateral sclerosis. Clin Pharmacol Ther 1997;62:518–26.

[58] Lucas D, Ménez C, Girre C, Berthou F, Bodenez P, Joannet I, et al. Cytochrome P450 2E1 genotype and chlorzoxazone metabolism in healthy and alcoholic Caucasian subjects. Pharmacogenetics 1995;5:298–304.

[59] Kim RB, O'Shea D. Interindividual variability of chlorzoxazone 6-hydroxylation in men and women and its relationship to CYP2E1 genetic polymorphisms. Clin Pharmacol Ther 1995;57:645–55.

[60] Divoll M, Greenblatt DJ, Harmatz JS, Shader RJ. Effect of age and gender on disposition of temazepam. J Pharm Sci 1981;70:1104–7.

[61] Greenblatt DJ, Divoll M, Harmatz JS, Shader RJ. Oxazepam kinetics: Effects of age and sex. J Pharmacol Exp Ther 1980;215:86–91.

[62] Bock KW, Schrenk D, Forster A, Griese EU, Mörike K, Brockmeier D, et al. The influence of environmental and genetic factors on CYP2D6, CYP1A2 and UDP-glucuronosyltransferases in man using sparteine, caffeine, and paracetamol as probes. Pharmacogenetics 1994;4: 209–18.

[63] Miners JO, Robson RA, Birkett DJ. Gender and oral contraceptive steroids as determinants of drug glucuronidation: Effects on clofibric acid elimination. Br J Clin Pharmacol 1984;18:240–3.

[64] Greenblatt DJ, Abernethy DR, Matlis R, Harmatz JS, Shader RI. Absorption and disposition of ibuprofen in the elderly. Arthritis Rheum 1984;27:1066–9.

[65] Macdonald JI, Herman RJ, Verbeeck RK. Sex-difference and the effects of smoking and oral contraceptive steroids on the kinetics of diflunisal. Eur J Clin Pharmacol 1990;38:175–9.

[66] Schwartz JB. The influence of sex on pharmacokinetics. Clin Pharmacokinet 2003;42:107–21.

[67] Meibohm B, Beierle I, Derendorf H. How important are gender differences in pharmacokinetics? Clin Pharmacokinet 2002;41:329–42.

[68] Song WC, Qian Y, Li AP. Estrogen sulfotransferase expression in the human liver: Marked interindividual variation and lack of gender specificity. J Pharmacol Exp Ther 1998;284:1197–202.

[69] Gross JL, Friedman R, Azevedo MJ, Silveiro SP, Pecis M. Effect of age and sex on glomerular filtration rate measured by 51Cr-EDTA. Braz J Med Biol Res 1992;25:129–34.

[70] Kashuba AD, Nafziger AN. Physiological changes during the menstrual cycle and their effects on the pharmacokinetics and pharmacodynamics of drugs. Clin Pharmacokinet 1998; 34:203–18.

[71] Miaskiewicz SL, Shively CA, Vesell ES. Sex differences in absorption kinetics of sodium salicylate. Clin Pharmacol Ther 1982;31:30–7.

[72] Jochemsen R, van der Graaff M, Boeijinga JK, Breimer DD. Influence of sex, menstrual cycle and oral contraception on the disposition of nitrazepam. Br J Clin Pharmacol 1982;13:319–24.

[73] Shavit G, Lerman P, Korczyn AD, Kivity S, Bechar M, Gitter S. Phenytoin pharmacokinetics in catamenial epilepsy. Neurology 1984;34:959–61.

[74] Riester EF, Pantuck EJ, Pantuck CB, Passananti GT, Vesell ES, Conney AH. Antipyrine metabolism during the menstrual cycle. J Pharmacol Ther 1980;28:384–91.

[75] Bäckström T, Jorpes P. Serum phenytoin, phenobarbital, carbamazepine, albumin and plasma estradiol progesterone concentrations during the menstrual cycle in women with epilepsy. Acta Neurol Scand 1979;58:63–71.

[76] Wilson K, Oram M, Horth CE, Burnett D. The influence of the menstrual cycle on the metabolism and clearance of methaqualone. Br J Clin Pharmacol 1982;14:333–9.

[77] Nicolas JM, Espie P, Molimard M. Gender and interindividual variability in pharmacokinetics. Drug Metab Rev 2009;41:408–21.

[78] Lemmens HJ, Burm AG, Hennis PJ, Gladines MP, Bovill JG. Influence of age on the pharmacokinetics of alfentanil. Gender dependence. Clin Pharmacokinet 1990;19:416–22.

[79] Fleishaker JC, Pearson LK, Pearson PG, Wienkers LC, Hopkins NK, Peters GR. Hormonal effects on tirilazad clearance in women: Assessment of the role of CYP3A. J Clin Pharmacol 1999;39:260–7.

[80] Nicolson TJ, Mellor HR, Roberts RR. Gender differences in drug toxicity. Trends Pharmacol Sci 2010;31:108–14.

[81] Parekh A, Fadiran EO, Uhl K, Throckmorton DC. Adverse effects in women: Implications for drug development and regulatory policies. Exp Rev Clin Pharmacol 2011;4:453–66.

[82] Ebert SN, Liu XK, Woosley RL. Female gender as a risk factor for drug-induced cardiac arrhythmias: Evaluation of clinical and experimental evidence. J Women's Health 1998;7:547–57.

[83] Woosley RL. Drugs that prolong the Q-T interval and/or induce *torsades de points*. Tucson, AZ: University of Arizona (Internet at. www.atforum.com/SiteRoot/pages/addiction_resources/QTDrugs%209-03-02.pdf.; 2002).

[84] Makkar RR, Fromm BS, Steinman RT, Meissner MD, Lehmann MH. Female gender as a risk factor for *torsades de points* associated with cardiovascular drugs. JAMA 1993;270:2590–7.

[85] Drici MD, Knollmann BC, Wang WX, Woosley RL. Cardiac actions of erythromycin: Influence of female sex. JAMA 1998;280:1774–6.

[86] US General Accounting Report. Drug safety: Most drugs withdrawn in recent years had greater health risks for women. GAO-01-286R Drugs Withdrawn From Market (Internet at, www.gao.gov/new.items/d01286r.pdf).

[87] Woosley RL, Chen Y, Freiman JP, Gillis RA. Mechanism of the cardiotoxic actions of terfenadine. JAMA 1993;269:1532–6.

[88] Kumar A, Bhandari AK, Rahimtoola SH. *Torsades de points* and marked QT prolongation in association with hypothyroidism. Ann Intern Med 1987;106:712–3.

[89] Bagchi N, Brown TR, Parish RF. Thyroid dysfunction in adults over age 55 years. A study in an urban US community. Arch Intern Med 1990;150:785–7.

[90] Drici MB, Clément N. Is gender a risk factor for adverse drug reactions? The example of drug-induced long QT syndrome. Drug Saf 2001;24:575–85.

[91] Rodriguez I, Kilborn JM, Liu XK, Pezzullo JC, Woosley RL. Drug-induced QT prolongation in women during the menstrual cycle. JAMA 2001;285:1322–6.

[92] Rautaharju PM, Zhou SH, Wong S, Calhoun HP, Berenson GS, Prineas R, et al. Sex differences in the evolution of electrocardiographic QT Interval with age. Can J Card 1992;8:690–5.

[93] Reinoehl J, Frankovich D, Machado C, Kawasaki R, Baga JJ, Pires LA, et al. Probucol-associated tachyarrhythmic events and QT prolongation: Importance of gender. Am Heart J 1996;131:184–91.

[94] Benton RE, Sale M, Flockhart DA, Woosley RL. Greater quinidine-induced QTc interval prolongation in women. Clin Pharmacol Ther 2000;67:413–8.

[95] Roden DM, Woosley RL, Primm RK. Incidence and clinical features of the quinidine-associated long QT syndrome: Implications for patient care. Am Heart J 1986;111:1088–93.

[96] Lehmann MH, Hardy S, Archibald D, Quart B, MacNeil DJ. Sex difference in risk of *torsades de points* with d, l-sotalol. Circulation 1996;94:2535–41.

[97] Tikosyn (dofetilide) US FDA Drug Pruduct Labeling (Internet at, http://dailymed.nlm.nih.gov/dailymed/search.cfm? startswith=tikosyn).

[98] Walle T, Byington RP, Furberg CD, McIntyre KM, Vokanas PS. Biologic determinants of propranolol disposition: Results from 1308 patients in the Beta-Blocker Heart Attack Trial. Clin Pharmacol Ther 1985;38:509–18.

[99] Flockhart DA, Drici MD, Samuel C, Abernethy DR, Woosley RL. Effects of gender on propranolol pharmacokinetics and pharmacodynamics [Abstract]. FASEB J 1996; 10:A429.

[100] Berg MJ. Pharmacokinetics and pharmacodynamics of cardiovascular drugs. J Gender-Specif Med 1999;2:22–4.

[101] Sivenius J, Laakso M, Penttilä I, Smets P, Lowenthal A, Riekkinen PJ. The European Stroke Prevention Study: Results according to sex. Neurology 1991;41:1189–92.

[102] Spranger M, Aspey BS, Harrison MJ. Sex differences in antithrombotic effect of aspirin. Stroke 1989;20:34–7.

[103] Riley III JL, Robison ME, Wise EA, Price DD. A meta-analytic review of pain perception across the menstrual cycle. Pain 1999;81:225–35.

[104] Kest B, Sarton E, Dahan A. Gender differences in opioid-mediated analgesia: Animal and human studies. Anesthesiology 2000;93:539–47.

[105] Cepeda MS, Africano JM, Manrique AM, Fragoso W, Carr DB. The combination of low dose of naloxone and morphine in PCA does not decrease opioid requirements in the postoperative period. Pain 2002;96:73–9.

[106] Unruh AM. Gender variations in clinical pain experience. Pain 1996;65:123–67.

[107] Barsky AJ, Peekna HM, Borus JF. Somatic symptom reporting in women and men. J Gen Intern Med 2001;16:266–75.

[108] Cepeda MS, Carr DB. Women experience more pain and require more morphine than men to achieve a similar degree of analgesia. Anesth Analg 2003;97:1464–8.

[109] Sarton E, Olofsen E, Romberg R, den Hartigh J, Kest B, Nieuwenhuijs D, et al. Sex differences in morphine analgesia: An experimental study in healthy volunteers. Anesthesiology 2000;93:1245–54.

[110] Niesters M, Dahan A, Kest B, Zacny J, Stijnen T, Aarts L, et al. Do sex differences exist in opioid analgesia? A systematic review and meta-analysis of human experimental and clinical studies. Pain 2010;151:61–8.

[111] Dahan A, Sarton E, Teppema L, Olivier C. Sex-related differences in the influence of morphine on ventilatory control in humans. Anesthesiology 1998;88:903–13.

[112] Sarton E, Teppema L, Dahan A. Sex differences in morphine-induced ventilatory depression reside within the peripheral chemoreflex loop. Anesthesiology 1999;90:1329–38.

[113] Gear RW, Miaskowski C, Gordon NC, Paul SM, Heller PH, Levine JD. Kappa-opioids produce significantly greater analgesia in women than in men. Nat Med 1996;2:1248–50.

[114] Mogil JS, Wilson SG, Chesler EJ, Ramkin AL, Nemmani KVS, Lariviere WR, et al. The melanocortin-1 receptor gene mediates female specific mechanisms of analgesia in mice and humans. Proc Natl Acad Sci USA 2003; 100:4867–72.

[115] Walker JS, Carmody JJ. Experimental pain in healthy human subjects: Gender differences in nociception and a response to ibuprofen. Anesth Analg 1998;86:1257–62.

[116] Esmore D, Keogh A, Spratt P, Jones B, Chang V. Heart transplantation in females. J Heart Lung Transplant 1991;10: 335–41.

[117] Taylor DO, Bristow MR, O'Connell JB, Price GD, Hammond EH, Doty DB. Improved long-term survival after heart transplantation predicted by successful early withdrawal from maintenance corticosteroid therapy. J Heart Lung Transplant 1996;15:1039–46.

[118] Lew K, Ludwig E, Milad M, Donovan K, et al. Gender-based effects on methylprednisolone pharmacokinetics and pharmacodynamics. Clin Pharmacol Ther 1993;54:402–14.

[119] Women and smoking. Legacy for longer healthier lives. Washington, DC: December 2010. (Internet at, www.legacyforhealth. org/PDFPublications/Women_and_Smoking.pdf).

[120] Carrillo JA, Benitez J. CYPIA2 activity, gender and smoking as variables influencing the toxicity of caffeine. Br J Clin Pharmacol 1996;41:605–8.

[121] Jennings TS, Nafziger AN, Davidson L, Bertino Jr JS. Gender differences in hepatic induction and inhibition of theophylline pharmacokinetics and metabolism. J Lab Clin Med 1993;122:208–16.

[122] Olanzepine Label (Internet at, http://pi.lilly.com/us/ zyprexa-pi.pdf.)

[123] Barnes PM, Powell-Griner E, McFann K, Nahin RL. Complementary and alternative medicine use among adults: United States, 2002. Adv Data May 27, 2004;3431–19.

[124] Fugh-Berman A. Herb–drug interactions. Lancet 2000;355:134–8.

[125] Butterweck V. St John's wort: Quality issues and active compounds. In: Cooper R, Kronenberg F, editors. Botanical medicine: From bench to bedside. New Rochelle, NY: Mary Ann Liebert, Inc.; 2009. Chapter 4.

[126] Wenk M, Todesco L, Krähenbühl S. Effect of St John's wort on the activities of CYP1A2, CYP3A4, CYP2D6, *N*-acetyltransferase 2, and xanthine oxidase in healthy males and females. Br J Clin Pharmacol 2004;57:495–9.

[127] Nebel A, Schneider BJ, Baker RV, Kroll DJ. Potential metabolic interaction between St John's wort and theophylline. Ann Pharmacother 1999;33:502.

[128] Zhou S, Chan E, Pan SQ, Huang M, Lee EJ. Pharmacokinetic interactions of drugs with St John's wort. J Psychopharmacol 2004;18:262–76.

[129] Henderson L, Yue QY, Bergquist C, Gerden B, Arlett P. St John's wort (*Hypericum perforatum*): Drug interactions and clinical outcomes. Br J Clin Pharmacol 2002;54:349–56.

[130] CDER. Labeling for combined oral contraceptives. Draft guidance for industry. Rockville, MD: FDA (Internet at, www.fda. gov/downloads/Drugs/GuidanceComplianceRegulatory Information/Guidances/UCM075075.pdf; March 2004. last accessed February 15, 2012).

# Drug Therapy in Pregnant and Nursing Women

Catherine S. Stika and Marilynn C. Frederiksen

*Department of Obstetrics and Gynecology, Feinberg School of Medicine, Northwestern University, Chicago, IL 60611*

The pregnant woman is perhaps the last true therapeutic orphan. Because of the ethical, medicolegal, and fetal safety concerns regarding pregnant women, few pharmacokinetic, pharmacodynamic, or clinical trials are conducted during pregnancy. The majority of drugs that are marketed in the United States therefore carry statements such as the following [1] in their labeling:

> There are, however, no adequate and well-controlled studies in pregnant women. Because animal reproductive studies are not always predictive of human response, this drug should be used during pregnancy only if clearly needed.
>
> [Zinacef (cefuroxime) labeling; PDR; 2005. p. 1678]

This places the burden squarely on the practitioner to assess the risks and benefits of a particular agent in a given clinical situation. The risk most often considered is the fetal risk of teratogenesis, or drug-induced malformation, irrespective of the gestational age during the pregnancy when therapy is initiated. Pregnant women are more often than not left untreated in an attempt to avoid any perceived fetal risk related to use of a pharmacologic agent, and the effect of untreated maternal disease on either the pregnancy outcome or the offspring is not a usual consideration. On those occasions when pharmacotherapy is initiated, issues of appropriate dosage and frequency of administration are often not evaluated, so that the usual adult dose is prescribed without thought to any changes dictated by physiologic differences between non-pregnant and pregnant women.

There are two compelling reasons for studying drugs and drug therapy during pregnancy. The first relates to the changing age of reproduction. Pregnancy once was mainly undertaken by healthy, younger women, but the age of reproduction now includes women ranging from 10 to approximately 50 years, and, with *in vitro* fertilization and egg donation, even older women undertake pregnancy. Moreover, the age of a woman's first pregnancy has been steadily rising in the United States, with an increasing number of first pregnancies occurring after age 30 [2]. The expansion of the reproductive age range, coupled with the occurrence of pregnancy later in life, increases the number of women who may require drug therapy for diseases present prior to pregnancy and who may need to continue therapy during pregnancy. Knowledge of drug therapy during pregnancy is needed if these women with underlying diseases are to be optimally treated.

The second reason supporting the need to study drugs during pregnancy relates to the physiologic changes that occur with gestation. To accommodate fetal growth and development, and perhaps provide a measure of safety for the woman, pregnancy alters a woman's underlying physiology. This altered physiology can affect the pharmacokinetics of drugs. These physiologic changes may affect drug absorption, decrease drug binding to plasma proteins, increase drug distribution volume, and cause variations in either renal and/or hepatic drug clearance. Mere extrapolation of pharmacokinetic data from drug studies largely conducted in non-pregnant subjects to pregnant women fails to account for the impact of these multiple physiologic changes that

*PRINCIPLES OF CLINICAL PHARMACOLOGY, THIRD EDITION*
DOI: http://dx.doi.org/10.1016/B978-0-12-385471-1.00024-6

occur during pregnancy. This disregard for the changes in maternal physiology may affect drug efficacy and ultimately impact the overall pregnancy outcome.

These issues were addressed by the US Food and Drug Administration in a lengthy process which has led to a re-vamping of the sections of the drug label that address pregnancy, labor and delivery, and nursing mothers. To provide more human data on the use of drugs during pregnancy, the FDA is requiring the establishment of a pregnancy registry after initial marketing of a drug. In August 2002, an FDA guidance for industry was published regarding pregnancy registries and the incorporation of the data from registries into drug labels [3]. Subsequently, a guidance for industry on the design and conduct of pharmacokinetic studies in pregnant women was published in November 2004 [4], and a guidance regarding clinical lactation studies was published in February 2005 [5]. These new labeling requirements were published for comment in the Federal Register in May 2008 [6]. As detailed in Table 24.1, the proposed new labels will be divided to include the following sections: general information, which will include pregnancy registry information; a fetal risk summary;

clinical considerations, which will include inadvertent exposure, and dosage adjustments, during pregnancy; and a summary of the data available. However, a time-line for adopting these new labeling requirements has not been established at this time.

## PREGNANCY PHYSIOLOGY AND ITS EFFECTS ON PHARMACOKINETICS

Rather than present a list of the many changes in maternal physiology that occur during pregnancy, the focus here is to select those changes which have the greatest potential to alter the absorption, distribution, and elimination of drugs in pregnant women.

### Gastrointestinal Changes

The effect of progesterone on smooth muscle activity has long been thought to prolong gastric emptying and gastrointestinal transit time during all of pregnancy. In addition, pregnant women have been found to have a decrease in gastric acid secretion that results in a correspondingly higher gastric pH [7], which theoretically could also affect absorption.

---

**TABLE 24.1    Pregnancy Information Proposed for Inclusion in Drug Labels**

**General Information**

Contact information if pregnancy registry available

General statement about background risk

**Fetal Risk Summary**

Based on all available data, this section characterizes the likelihood that the drug increases the risk of developmental abnormalities in humans and other relevant risks

More than one risk conclusion may be needed

For drugs that are not systemically absorbed, there is a standard statement that states that maternal use is not expected to result in fetal exposure

For drugs that are systemically absorbed, include:
   When there are human data, a statement about the likelihood of increased risk based on this data
   This statement is followed by a description of findings
   A standard statement about likelihood of increased risk based upon animal data

**Clinical Considerations**

This section provides information of the following topics:

Inadvertent exposure: known predicted risk to the fetus from inadvertent exposure to drug early in pregnancy

Prescribing decisions for pregnant women: describe any known risk to the pregnant woman and fetus from the disease or condition the drug is intended to treat — information about dosing adjustments during pregnancy, maternal adverse reactions unique to pregnancy or increased in pregnancy, effects of dose, timing, and duration of exposure to drug during pregnancy, potential neonatal complications and needed interventions

**Data**

Human and animal data are presented separately, with human data presented first

Describe study type, exposure information (dose, duration, timing), and identified fetal developmental abnormality or other adverse effects

For human data, include positive and negative experiences, number of subjects, and duration of study

For animal data, include species studied and describe doses in terms of human dose equivalents (provide basis for calculation)

However, most of the early studies of gastrointestinal function were done in women during labor [8, 9]. More recent studies of acetaminophen absorption in non-laboring women using real-time ultrasonography have shown no differences in gastric emptying during the first and third trimesters of pregnancy, as compared with the postpartum period [10, 11]. Only in the third trimester are orocecal transit times prolonged. This effect is due to the lower level of plasma pancreatic polypeptide that occurs in the third trimester of pregnancy and results in reduced gastrointestinal motility [10].

Only a few studies have been conducted in pregnant woment to evaluate the effects of these pregnancy-related gastrointestinal changes on the actual rate and extent of drug absorption. In all these studies, women received both intravenous and oral drug doses while they were pregnant as well as after pregnancy, thus serving as their own controls. Sotalol, a beta-adrenergic receptor antagonist, showed no significant difference in bioavailability between the two time periods [12] The antibiotics cephazolin, ampicillin, and cephradine also were studied during pregnancy and in the postpartum period [13, 14]. Peak drug levels were found to be lower during pregnancy, but pregnancy did not appear to change the extent of drug absorption or the time to peak drug concentration ($t_{max}$).

## Cardiovascular Effects

The cardiovascular effects which occur during pregnancy include plasma volume expansion, an increase in cardiac output, and changes in regional blood flow. By the sixth to eighth week of pregnancy, plasma volume has expanded, and continues to increase until approximately 32–34 weeks of pregnancy [15]. For a singleton gestation, this increase in plasma volume is 1200–1300 mL, or approximately 40% higher than the plasma volume of non-pregnant women. Plasma volume expansion is even greater for multiple gestations [16]. There are also significant increases in extracellular fluid space and total body water that vary somewhat with patient weight. These changes in body fluid spaces are summarized in Table 24.2 [17, 18].

The increase in plasma volume is accompanied by a gradual increase in cardiac output that begins in the first trimester of pregnancy. By 8 weeks' gestation, cardiac output can be as much as 50% greater, and by the third trimester it is at least 30–50% greater, than in the non-pregnant state [19]. Early in pregnancy, an increase in stroke volume accounts for the increased cardiac output. In later pregnancy, the

**TABLE 24.2   Body Fluid Spaces in Pregnant and Non-Pregnant Women**

| | Weight (kg) | Plasma volume (mL/kg) | ECF space (L/kg) | TBW (L/kg) | Ref. |
|---|---|---|---|---|---|
| Non-pregnant | | 49 | | | [9] |
| | < 0 | | 0.189 | 0.516 | [11] |
| | 70−80 | | 0.156 | 0.415 | [11] |
| | > 80 | | 0.151 | 0.389 | [11] |
| Pregnant | | 67 | | | [9] |
| | < 70 | | 0.257 | 0.572 | [12] |
| | 70−80 | | 0.255 | 0.514 | [12] |
| | > 80 | | 0.240 | 0.454 | [12] |

Modified from Frederiksen MC, Ruo TI, Chow MJ, Atkinson AJ Jr. Clin Pharmacol Ther 1986;40:321–8 [26].

increase in cardiac output is the result of both elevated maternal heart rate and a continued increase in stroke volume [20].

Regional blood flow changes also occur in pregnant women and can affect drug distribution and elimination. Blood flow increases to the uterus, kidneys, skin, and mammary glands, with a compensatory decrease in skeletal muscle blood flow. At full term, blood flow to the uterus represents about 20–25% of cardiac output and renal blood flow is 20% of cardiac output [21]. There is increased blood flow to the skin to dissipate the additional heat produced by the fetus [22]. Blood flow to the mammary glands is increased during pregnancy in preparation for lactation postpartum [23]. As shown in Figure 24.1, arterial hepatic blood flow is maintained relatively unchanged during pregnancy but constitutes a lower percentage of cardiac output than in the non-pregnant condition because of the increased proportion of blood flow to the uterus and kidneys [24]. Portal venous blood flow has been shown by Doppler ultrasonography to increase beginning at 28 weeks of pregnancy, and has been measured to be 150–160% over the non-pregnant portal blood flow [25]. As a result of these hemodynamic changes, there is a decreased proportion of cardiac output available to skeletal muscle and other vascular beds.

These multiple physiological changes in pregnant women may affect drug distribution. In some cases, it is possible to correlate pregnancy-associated changes in distribution volume ($V_d$) with changes in extracellular fluid space (ECF), total body water (TBW), and drug binding to plasma proteins using the following equation, which was developed in Chapter 3:

$$V_d = \text{ECF} + f_U(\text{TBW} - \text{ECF}) \qquad (24.1)$$

where $f_U$ is the fraction of unbound drug.

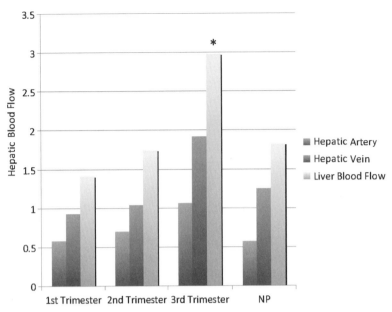

**FIGURE 24.1** Hepatic blood flow as measured by Doppler ultrasound. Portal venous blood flow is shown to be markedly increased in the third trimester of pregnancy as compared with hepatic blood flow in non-pregnant (NP) women ($* = P < 0.5$). Data from Nakai A, Seklya I, Oya A et al. Arch Gynecol Obstet 2002;266:25–9 [25].

## Blood Composition Changes

Plasma albumin concentration decreases during pregnancy [26, 27]. The fall in albumin concentration from 4.2 g/dL in the non-pregnant woman to 3.6 g/dL in the midtrimester of pregnancy (Figure 24.2) has long been erroneously attributed to a "dilutional effect" caused by plasma volume expansion. However, it follows from pharmacokinetic principles that this decrease in plasma albumin concentration represents either a reduction in the rate of albumin synthesis or an increase in the rate of albumin clearance (see Chapter 1, Equation 1.2). Additional support for this explanation is provided by the fact that the plasma concentrations of total protein [27] and $\alpha_1$-acid glycoprotein [28], which binds many basic drugs, are relatively unchanged during pregnancy.

The reduction in albumin concentration potentially can alter the binding of drugs commonly bound to serum albumin. In a study of theophylline pharmacokinetics during the second and third trimesters of pregnancy, theophylline protein binding to plasma proteins was reduced to only 11% and 13% of total plasma concentrations, respectively, compared with 28% 6 months postpartum [26]. Although the decrease in the serum concentration of albumin may be thought to account for these differences, a subsequent study showed that the albumin binding sites for theophylline were actually increased during pregnancy, but the

binding affinity constant was significantly lower during pregnancy than in the non-pregnant state [29].

Pregnancy is also associated with a partially compensated respiratory alkalosis that may affect the protein binding of some drugs. Respiratory changes in pregnancy include a decrease in arterial partial pressure of carbon dioxide to 30.9 mm Hg, most likely due to the effect of progesterone [30, 31]. In compensation,

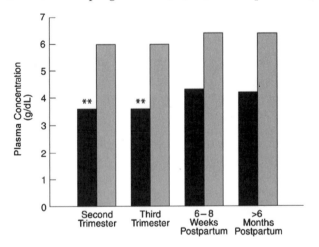

**FIGURE 24.2** Albumin (*black bars*) and total protein (*gray bars*) concentrations during the second and third trimesters of pregnancy and in the postpartum period. Albumin concentrations are reduced significantly during pregnancy when compared to > 6 months postpartum values ($** = P < 0.01$). Data from Frederiksen MC, Ruo TI, Chow MJ, Atkinson AJ Jr. Clin Pharmacol Ther 1986;40:321–8 [26].

serum bicarbonate decreases and maternal serum pH increases slightly to 7.44 [30].

## Renal Changes

Accompanying the increased blood flow to the kidneys is an increase in glomerular filtration rate (GFR). This increase begins by the sixth week of gestation, gradually rises in the early portion of the third trimester [32], and plateaus or falls slightly until delivery. This increase in GFR is reflected in an increase in inulin and creatinine clearance during pregnancy. Tubular reabsorption processes, however, do not appear to be changed during pregnancy [33].

For drugs predominantly cleared by the kidney, the increase in GFR will increase drug clearance during pregnancy. Cefuroxime, a cephalosporin predominantly eliminated by the kidneys, has a significantly greater clearance in the midtrimester of pregnancy than during either delivery or the postpartum period [34]. Tobramycin clearance mirrors the GFR changes in pregnancy, with the highest clearance and shortest half-life found in the midtrimester, with a fall in clearance and corresponding longer half-life in the third trimester [35].

Even for a drug primarily eliminated by hepatic metabolism in non-pregnant women, the increase in GFR can significantly affect total drug clearance during pregnancy. For example, the renal clearance of theophylline, a drug largely eliminated by CYP1A2 metabolism which is reduced during pregnancy, was found to increase during pregnancy so that its total elimination clearance was not significantly reduced but was maintained at 86% of its value 6 months postpartum [26].

## Hepatic Drug Metabolizing Changes

The activity of hepatic drug-metabolizing enzymes also changes during pregnancy and can affect drug elimination clearance. Pregnancy is an estrogenic state with 100-fold increases in estradiol levels over a woman's non-pregnant baseline [36, 37]. Progesterone, the hormone responsible for sustaining gestation, also rises dramatically during pregnancy from luteal levels of 30–40 ng/mL to levels of 100–200 ng/mL [38–40]. These changes in estrogen and progesterone, as well as in other placental hormones, are probably responsible for the alteration in hepatic enzymatic activity.

Recent studies during the second and third trimesters of pregnancy and again postpartum, using caffeine metabolism as a marker of CYP1A2 activity, dextromethorphan O-demethylation as a marker of CYP2D6 activity, and dextromethorphan N-demethylation as a marker of CYP3A activity, have led to a better characterization of the changes in the drug-metabolizing enzymes activity during pregnancy [41]. CYP1A2 activity decreases, with a 22% reduction in activity in the early second trimester gradually progressing to a 65% reduction in the late third trimester. CYP2D6 activity increases, with a 25% increase in activity in the early second trimester gradually progressing to a 48% increase in the late third trimester. CYP3A activity, however, is consistently increased by some 35–38% during the second and third trimesters of pregnancy.

### CYP3A4 Substrates

The clearances of drugs metabolized by CYP3A4 have been shown to be consistently increased in multiple studies of pregnant women. Because midazolam is exclusively eliminated by CYP3A4 metabolism [42, 43], midazolam clearance and the 1′-hydroxymidazolam to midazolam serum concentration ratio are recognized markers of CYP3A4 activity [44, 45]. In pregnant women at term, the clearance of midazolam has been shown to be 2.9-fold greater than in non-pregnant women [46]. The metabolic ratio of cortisol, a non-specific probe of CYP3A4 activity, was increased in pregnant women near term when compared to the same women 1 week and 3 months postpartum [47]. Betamethasone, used antenatally to decrease the incidence of respiratory distress syndrome in neonates born prematurely, is metabolized by CYP3A4 [48, 49]. Its clearance was found to be 1.2- to 1.6-fold higher in the third trimester of pregnancy as compared with non-pregnant women [50–52]. The clearance of nifedipine was increased four-fold in women during the third trimester of pregnancy in comparison to historical controls [53]. Methadone, a drug used to treat heroin addiction during pregnancy, also is a CYP3A4 substrate. In a study of methadone pharmacokinetics during pregnancy, methadone clearance doubled in the midtrimester but fell somewhat in the third trimester [54]. This change was both statistically and clinically significant, because the lower methadone plasma levels will result in symptoms of methadone withdrawal unless methadone dosage is increased during pregnancy. In a study of the extended release formulation of metronidazole, which is primarily metabolized by CYP3A4, the total oral clearance in pregnant women during the second and early third trimesters was 27% greater than in non-pregnant women [55]. The mean maximum concentration of metronidazole was approximately 25% lower in pregnancy, and the difference in areas under the plasma-concentration vs time curves (AUCs) in pregnant vs non-pregnant women approached significance.

The critical stimulus for CYP3A4 induction in pregnancy has not been identified. However, both estradiol and estrone, as well as the natural progestins, including progesterone, pregnenolone, 17-hydroxyprogesterone, and 5β-3-20-pregnanedione, have been shown to activate the human orphan nuclear pregnane X receptor (PXR). As described in Chapter 11 (see Figure 11.3), PXR forms a heterodimer complex with the 9-cis-retinoic acid receptor (RXR). This hPXR/RXR complex then binds to the promotor region of the CYP3A4 gene, also called the rifampicn/dexamethasone response element, and serves as a key transcriptional regulator [56, 57].

## CYP1A2 Substrates

The elimination clearance of caffeine, a marker of CYP1A2 enzymatic activity, was shown to decrease by a factor of two by midgestation and by a factor of three by the third trimester compared to the postpartum period [58]. Although the intrinsic hepatic clearance of theophylline was reduced during pregnancy, there was substantially less change in its hepatic clearance because of the pregnancy-associated decrease in theophylline binding to plasma proteins [26]. As a result of the off-setting changes in renal and hepatic clearance referred to previously, the total elimination clearance of theophylline was unchanged in the third trimester of pregnancy.

## CYP2D6 Substrates

Although, as detailed in Chapter 13, CYP2D6 activity is known to show considerable pharmacogenetic variation, this enzyme is not inducible by other xenobiotics. Hogstedt et al. [59, 60] reported that the CYP2D6 substrate metoprolol had a four- to five-fold increase in clearance during pregnancy. Wadelius et al. [61] used dextromethophan to characterize CYP2D6 activity in the late third trimester of pregnancy. He found that CYP2D6 activity increased during pregnancy in individuals who were homozygous and heterozygous extensive metabolizers but decreased in homozygous poor metabolizers. However, a more extensive characterization subsequently showed that CYP2D6 activity increased by 25% in the early portion of the second trimester and gradually increased further throughout pregnancy to as much as 48% by the late third trimester [41].

## CYP2C9 Substrates

The hepatic clearance of phenytoin, a restrictively eliminated drug that is predominantly a CYP2C9 substrate, increases during pregnancy, resulting in correspondingly lower total plasma concentrations [62]. This is in large part a reflection of the decrease in protein binding that is well documented for phenytoin, as free plasma concentrations of this drug have been shown to remain relatively constant until late in pregnancy, when the intrinsic clearance of this drug does increase [63, 64].

Glyburide has been shown in non-pregnant patients to be primarily metabolized by CYP2C9 [65], and its clearance was found to be two-fold higher in pregnant women [66]. While effective twice-daily doses generally range from 1.25 to 10.0 mg in non-pregnant women, simulations predicted that doses would have to be increased to as much as 23.75 mg twice daily for optimal glucose control during pregnancy. However, the safety of glyburide for the fetus is open to question, since steady state glyburide concentrations in serum from cord blood are approximately 70% of maternal serum concentrations.

## CYP2C19 Substrates

The metabolism of proguanil, an antimalarial drug, to its active metabolite cycloguanil is dependent on CYP2C19 activity. The metabolic ratio of proguanil to cycloguanil has been shown to increase by approximately 60% during pregnancy [67]. In a population-based study, CYP2C19 dependent clearance decreased by 50% [68].

## NAT2 Substrates

Using caffeine to examine the changes in hepatic enzymatic activity during pregnancy, Bologna et al. [69] studied both pregnant and non-pregnant epileptic women and showed that the activity of N-acetyltransferase was decreased during pregnancy. Tsutsumi et al. [70] also used caffeine to show that the activity of N-acetyltransferase-2 was decreased in normal healthy women during pregnancy.

## Glucuronidation

The anticonvulsant and mood-stabilizing drug lamotrigine is metabolized primarily by glucuronidation via uridine 5'-diphosphate glucuronosyltransferase 1A4 (UGT1A4). Estradiol, with the assistance of the transcription factor, specificity protein-1 (Sp1), and the estrogen receptor α (ERα), upregulates UGT1A4 expression [71]. Studies in pregnant women have shown a dramatic increase in lamotrigine clearance that begins as early as 6 weeks' gestation and continues to progressively increase into the third trimester [72–75]. By the second month of gestation lamotrigine levels decrease by 27% [76], and this enhanced clearance continues to rise and, in the third trimester, peaks at 248–330% over baseline [74, 77]. Serial dose increases are necessary to maintain stable therapeutic antiseizure lamotrigine levels during pregnancy, and dose-to-plasma-concentration (D/C) ratios by the third trimester are typically 250–295% greater than at baseline [72, 78]. By late pregnancy this ratio of the metabolite, 2-*N*-lamotrigine glucuronide, to the parent drug increases approximately by 150% over baseline [72, 79]. Because this increase occurs despite little change in the blood concentration of 2-*N*-GLUC, this finding supports increased glucuronidation as the primary mechanism responsible for the increased clearance of lamotrigine during pregnancy. After delivery, clearance of lamotrigine falls rapidly and returns to non-pregnant levels by 3 weeks postpartum. For this reason, dose reductions need to be started promptly within the first week after delivery in order to prevent possible lamotrigine toxicity [73, 74].

Several studies have investigated the pharmacokinetics of lamotrigine in pregnancy when administered with other anticonvulsant drugs [78, 80, 81]. Co-administration with oxcarbazepine, which is also glucuronidated by unknown isoforms, does not affect the pregnancy-induced increase in lamotrigine clearance [81]. On the other hand, valproic acid, a known inhibitor of UGT1A4, partially blocks the pregnancy-associated increase in lamotrigine clearance, with the result that women receiving both lamotrigine and valproic acid during the third trimester have a lamotrigine D/C ratio that is only 60% greater than baseline [78].

## Peripartum Changes

The physiologic changes which begin early in gestation are most pronounced in the third trimester of pregnancy. Further physiologic changes occur during labor and delivery, when there is an even further increase in cardiac output, blood flow to muscle mass decreases, and there is a cessation of gastrointestinal activity [82]. The onset of uterine contractions decreases placental blood flow and drug distribution to the fetus. During the intrapartum period there also may be a change in the pharmacodynamics of drugs, but this is largely unstudied.

Drugs are very commonly studied during the intrapartum period, probably for no other reason than that the amount of drug distributed to the fetus can be estimated from cord blood obtained at delivery. However, the pharmacokinetics of drugs given during this period has been shown to be different from their pharmacokinetics during the antepartum period. An intrapartum study of cefuroxime showed that clearance was lower than during pregnancy but higher than in the remote postpartum period [34]. Morphine clearance has been shown to be markedly increased during labor, resulting in a shortening of its elimination half-life that reduces the dosing interval required for adequate pain relief during labor [83].

## Postpartum Changes

In the early postpartum period, maternal pregnancy physiologic changes are sustained with an elevated cardiac output, decreased plasma albumin concentration, and increased GFR [84, 85]. The cardiovascular changes of pregnancy are sustained as long as 12 weeks after delivery [86]. However, maternal hepatic enzymatic activity may either rapidly reverse within 24 hours of delivery or gradually return to normal during the first months after delivery [73, 87].

The physiology of the postpartum period seems to have great interindividual variability, since pharmacokinetic studies during this period show greater between-subject variability than studies conducted in women who have not recently been pregnant. As shown in Figure 24.3, a study of clindamycin pharmacokinetics in five postpartum women demonstrated that there was a 15-fold variation in peak drug concentrations and that $t_{max}$ varied from 1 to 6 hours after oral administration of this drug [88]. Similarly, a study of gentamicin in the postpartum period showed distribution volume estimates that varied from 0.1 to 0.5 L/kg, as compared with distribution volume estimates from studies in non-pregnant volunteers that only ranged from 0.2 to 0.3 L/kg [89].

## PHARMACOKINETIC STUDIES DURING PREGNANCY

### Results of Selected Pharmacokinetic Studies in Pregnant Women

Although an exhaustive survey of pharmacokinetic studies is not possible, the purpose here is to present illustrative studies that best demonstrate the effects of maternal physiologic changes on pharmacokinetics and potentially on drug dosing requirements and efficacy.

### *Ampicillin/Amoxicillin*

The pharmacokinetics of both intravenously and orally administered ampicillin were studied serially in 26 women who served as their own controls [13].

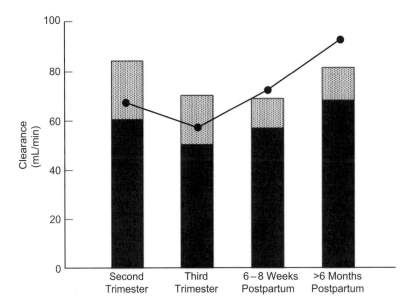

**FIGURE 24.3** Theophylline clearance measured during the second and third trimesters of pregnancy and in the postpartum period. During pregnancy, the substantial drop in the intrinsic hepatic clearance (●) of this CYP1A2 substrate is attenuated by decreased theophylline binding to plasma proteins and increased glomerular filtration rate so that overall elimination clearance, consisting of the sum of hepatic clearance (*solid bars*) and renal clearance (*stippled bars*), is relatively unaffected. Data from Frederiksen MC, Ruo TI, Chow MJ, Atkinson AJ Jr. Clin Pharmacol Ther 1986;40:321–8 [26].

Perhaps because both intravenous and oral doses need to be administered, ampicillin is one of the few medications for which absolute bioavailability has been examined during pregnancy. No difference in the extent of ampicillin absorption or in time to peak drug concentrations was seen between pregnant and non-pregnant women, but peak levels were lower than in non-pregnant women. Although this study demonstrated an absolute increase in the distribution volume of ampicillin, it did not include an analysis of the effect of the change in maternal weight on the volume of distribution. Both renal and total elimination clearance of ampicillin increased by approximately 50% during pregnancy and resulted in correspondingly lower plasma concentrations. Unfortunately, the study combined data from women whose pregnancies ranged from 13 to 33 weeks' gestation, which blurred assessment of the effects of the progression of changes in maternal physiology that is known to occur during the second and third trimesters of pregnancy. Another study of ampicillin pharmacokinetics in the third trimester of pregnancy showed an increase in the steady-state volume of distribution on a L/kg basis, but used results in male controls as an historic reference population [90].

The pharmacokinetics of a similar antibiotic, amoxicillin, was studied in 17 pregnant women during the second and third trimesters of pregnancy and again postpartum [91]. This was a single oral-dose study to evaluate whether the drug would be an appropriate drug for treating anthrax infections during pregnancy. Both the *AUC*s and peak concentrations were lower and the elimination half-life was shorter during the second and third trimesters of pregnancy as compared with the postpartum period because of increased amoxicillin renal clearance. This increase in renal clearance consisted of an increase in renal filtration of amoxicillin and either a 50% increase in amoxicillin renal secretory transport or a similar decrease in its renal reabsorption. The authors concluded that amoxicillin would need to be dosed every 4 hours to achieve adequate serum concentrations.

### Caffeine

The pharmacokinetics of caffeine was also studied serially during and after pregnancy [58]. Although only oral doses were administered, $V_d/F$ showed no change when calculated on a L/kg basis to take into account the change in weight during and after pregnancy. On the other hand, $CL/F$ was decreased by a factor of two by midgestation and by a factor of three in the third trimester compared to the postpartum period [58].

## Theophylline

The pharmacokinetics of intravenously administered theophylline has been studied serially in women during and after pregnancy [26]. As described previously, theophylline binding to plasma proteins was reduced during the second and third trimesters of pregnancy to 11% and 13% of total plasma concentrations, respectively, compared with 28% 6 months postpartum. This appears to reflect the fact that the albumin binding affinity constant for theophylline is significantly lower during pregnancy than in the non-pregnant state, even though there is an increased number of albumin binding sites [29]. The steady-state distribution volume of theophylline was increased during the second and third trimesters of pregnancy. As shown in Table 24.3, the increases were similar to what was predicted from Equation 24.1 (see also Chapter 3, Figure 3.1) using measured values for protein binding and the estimates of extracellular fluid volume and total body water shown in Table 24.2.

Renal clearance of theophylline paralleled the pregnancy-associated increase in creatinine clearance and accounted for 30% and 28% of total theophylline elimination in the second and third trimesters, respectively, compared to only 16% at 6 months postpartum. As shown in Figure 24.4, the intrinsic clearance of theophylline was reduced substantially during pregnancy. Hepatic clearance showed substantially less change because of the pregnancy-associated decrease in theophylline binding to plasma proteins. As a result of the offsetting changes in renal and hepatic clearance, total elimination clearance of theophylline in the third trimester of pregnancy averaged 86% of its value 6 months postpartum. Although this reduction in elimination clearance was not statistically significant, it combined with the increase in theophylline distribution volume to significantly increase theophylline elimination half-life

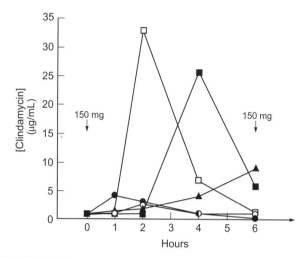

**FIGURE 24.4** Plasma concentrations of clindamycin measured in five postpartum women over a 6-hour period after oral administration of a 150-mg dose. Reproduced with permission from Steen B, Rane A. Br J Clin Pharmacol 1982;13:661–4 [88].

from an average of 4.4 hours in the non-pregnant state (assessed 6 months postpartum) to 6.5 hours in the third trimester of pregnancy.

## Cefuroxime

The pharmacokinetics of intravenously administered cefuroxime was studied serially in seven women during pregnancy, at delivery, and in the remote postpartum period [34]. Distribution volume ($V_{d(extrap)}$) during pregnancy and at delivery approximated the expected ECF volumes shown in Table 24.2. However, the difference in these volumes and the postpartum value was not statistically significant and there was no change in the weight-normalized distribution volumes. On the other hand, cefuroxime is largely eliminated by renal excretion, and renal clearance was significantly greater during pregnancy than that measured either at delivery or in non-pregnant women. As a result, plasma cefuroxime concentrations resulting from a 750-mg dose were significantly lower during pregnancy.

## Methadone

The pharmacokinetics of orally administered methadone was studied serially in nine women at 20–24 weeks and 35–40 weeks of pregnancy, and at 1–4 weeks and 8–9 weeks postpartum [54]. There was no significant change in methadone binding to plasma proteins during pregnancy. Renal methadone clearance during pregnancy was approximately twice its value in the postpartum periods. However, renal clearance

**TABLE 24.3** Comparison of Expected with Measured Values of Theophylline Distribution Volume

| | $V_{d(ss)}$ [a] | |
|---|---|---|
| | Expected (L) | Measured (L) |
| Pregnant | | |
|   24–26 Weeks | 32.0 ± 2.0 | 30.3 ± 6.6 |
|   36–38 Weeks | 37.9 ± 1.9 | 36.8 ± 4.2 |
| Postpartum | | |
|   6–8 Weeks | 28.0 ± 1.1 | 28.4 ± 3.0 |
|   > 6 Months | 26.9 ± 2.3 | 30.7 ± 4.4 |

[a]Mean values for five women ± SD

Data from Frederiksen MC, Ruo TI, Chow MJ, Atkinson AJ Jr. Clin Pharmacol Ther 1986;40:321–8 [26].

contributed only minimally to total methadone clearance, and this change did not reach statistical significance. On the other hand, estimates of *CL/F* during pregnancy were also doubled and this change was both statistically and clinically significant, resulting in a corresponding lowering of methadone plasma levels and symptoms of methadone withdrawal in some women near the end of gestation. Because the clearance of other CYP3A4 substrates is increased during pregnancy, the authors concluded that increased metabolic clearance rather than decreased bioavailability was responsible for the decrease in *CL/F*.

### Anticonvulsants

The total plasma concentrations of most anticonvulsant drugs have been shown to decrease during pregnancy. This is in large part a reflection of the decrease in protein binding that is well documented for phenytoin [62, 63], carbamazepine [63], and phenobarbital [64]. However, these drugs are restrictively eliminated and unbound concentrations of carbamazepine [63, 92] and phenobarbital [64] remain unchanged during pregnancy, reflecting the fact that their intrinsic clearance is unchanged. As is the case for patients with impaired renal function (see Chapter 5), dosage of phenytoin and these other anticonvulsants should not be increased in pregnant women based solely on decreases in total plasma concentration. On the other hand, Tomson *et al.* [63] monitored phenytoin plasma levels serially in 36 women during pregnancy and in the non-pregnant state. Intrinsic clearance was increased only during the third trimester of pregnancy, resulting in unbound plasma concentrations that averaged 16% lower than in the non-pregnant woman (Figure 24.5), and this may warrant increasing phenytoin doses for some women late in pregnancy.

### Other Drugs

The clearance of a number of other drugs that are eliminated primarily by renal excretion has also been shown to increase during pregnancy. For example, the pharmacokinetics of subcutaneously administered enoxaprin, a low molecular weight heparin, was studied serially in 13 women at 12–15 weeks' and 30–33 weeks' gestation and 6–8 weeks postpartum [93]. Compared to postpartum values, elimination clearance was increased by approximately 50% in the first gestational study period but was not significantly increased in the later period. In another study, the clearance of tobramycin was shown to peak in the mid-trimester and fall during the third trimester [35].

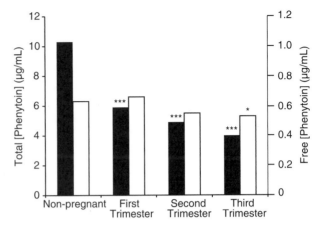

**FIGURE 24.5** Total (*solid bars*) and free (*open bars*) plasma concentrations of phenytoin in non-pregnant and pregnant women ($* = P < 0.05$, $***P = 0.001$). Data from Tomson T, Lindbom U, Ekqvist B, Sundqvist A. Epilepsia 1994;35:122–30 [62].

Metformin is an orally effective hypoglycemic agent used to treat women with polycystic ovarian disease and women with gestational, as well as pre-existing, diabetes during pregnancy. Metformin is a small molecule not bound to plasma proteins [94] and is a substrate for organic cation transporters (OCT) [95–97]. It is primarily eliminated by renal clearance, correlating with creatinine clearance, but exceeding glomerular filtration rate, thus indicating net renal tubular secretion [98, 99]. Pharmacokinetic studies in pregnant women have shown that metformin clearance is increased by 49% during the second trimester and by 29% during the third trimester of pregnancy. The increase in clearance was found to be the result of a combination of the increased GFR known to occur during pregnancy, and also to an increase in the tubular secretion of the drug which increased by 45% in the second trimester and by 38% during the third trimester. In fact, the renal clearance of metformin was better correlated with tubular secretion ($r = 0.97$) than with creatinine clearance ($r = 0.80$). This increased clearance was thought to be due to an increase in renal plasma flow during pregnancy, but a change in the expression and/or function of the OCT during pregnancy could also be possible [100].

Plasma concentrations of orally administered nifedipine, another CYP3A4 substrate, have been reported to be decreased in 15 women with pregnancy-induced hypertension who were studied during the third trimester of pregnancy but not subsequently postpartum [53]. Estimates of *CL/F* averaged 2.0 L/h per kg, compared to a value of 0.49 L/h per kg that was reported in a study of non-pregnant subjects. Another study of nifedipine pharmacokinetics in eight patients with pre-eclampsia indicated that *CL/F* remains elevated in the immediate postpartum period, averaging 3.3 L/h per kg in this clinical setting [101].

First-pass conversion of a prodrug to an active drug has been studied in pregnancy with the drug valacyclovir [102]. Orally administered valacyclovir produced three times higher plasma levels of acyclovir than when acyclovir was administered orally. However, the levels achieved with valacyclovir are somewhat lower than that reported in normal volunteers. On the other hand, acyclovir pharmacokinetics were, overall, similar to what have been reported in non-pregnant women.

## Guidelines for the Conduct of Drug Studies in Pregnant Women

Although abstinence from the use of pharmacologic agents is held forth as the ideal during pregnancy, studies have shown that most pregnant women use either prescribed or over-the-counter drugs during pregnancy and this creates the need for careful pharmacokinetic studies to be conducted in this subset of patients [103, 104]. Studying drugs in pregnancy requires special considerations, and guiding principles for these studies were formally published in October 2004 by the Pharmacokinetics in Pregnancy Working Group of the Pregnancy Labeling Task Force in the Guidance for Industry – Pharmacokinetics in Pregnancy – Study Design, Data Analysis, and Impact on Dosing and Labeling [4]. Ethically, drug studies in pregnancy cannot be done in normal pregnant "volunteers", but only in women who require a drug for a clinical reason. For this reason, study design for these trials must include the ethical justification that the woman would be using the particular agent during pregnancy to treat a medical condition. FDA approval of drugs specific to pregnancy, such as tocolytic agents, oxytocic agents, and a drug to treat pre-eclampsia, requires that studies be done during pregnancy. However, drugs commonly used by women of childbearing potential, such as antidepressants, asthma medications, antihypertensive agents, and antihistamines also can be justifiably studied during pregnancy. Drugs can be studied not only when given for maternal indications (e.g., hypertension or asthma) but also when given for fetal indications (e.g., fetal supraventricular tachycardia).

Some subpopulations of pregnant women, however, often have disease-related alterations in physiology that may affect pharmacokinetics. Therefore, pharmacokinetic studies in these women should be designed so that maximal information is obtained that separates the effects of their pathophysiology from those resulting from more general pregnancy-related changes. As a

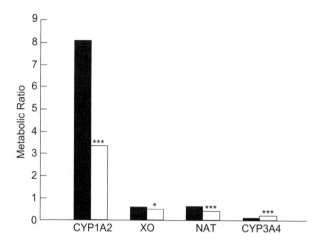

**FIGURE 24.6**   Paired comparisons of measured ratios of caffeine metabolites to parent drug in non-pregnant (*solid bars*) and pregnant (*open bars*) women. Comparisons were made of the metabolic activities of CYP 1A2, xanthine oxidase (XO), *N*-acetyltransferase (NAT), and CYP3A4 (* = $P < 0.05$, *** = $P < 0.005$). Data from Bologa M, Tang B, Klein J, Tesoro A, Koren G. J Pharmacol Exp Ther 1991;257:735–40 [69].

first step, population pharmacokinetic techniques can serve as a screening tool to establish the need for further intensive pharmacokinetic studies. For drugs that are chronically administered, these intensive studies should be conducted serially during the second and third trimesters of pregnancy and in the postpartum period, so that each woman serves as her own control. Ideally, both an early and a remote postpartum evaluation should be included. However, drugs used only during the peripartum period need only be studied at that time. Studies should incorporate *in vitro* measurements of drug binding to plasma proteins, and use established tracer substances or concurrent non-invasive measures of physiology as reference markers. For bioavailability evaluations, the stable isotope method described in Chapter 4 would decrease the number of studies necessary and decrease the biologic variation between studies. As shown in Figure 24.6, caffeine has been used as a probe to assess the effects of pregnancy on a number of drug metabolic pathways [69]. This has the advantage over the "cocktail" approaches described in Chapter 7 in that only a single drug is needed to simultaneously assess a number of metabolic pathways. However, a multiprobe study designed to assess the effects of pregnancy has also been conducted [41].

## PLACENTAL TRANSFER OF DRUGS

The placenta was long thought to be a barrier that protected the fetus from drugs and chemicals administered to the mother. However, the thalidomide tragedy, reported independently by McBride [105] and Lenz [106], showed that the placenta was capable of transferring drugs ingested by the mother to the fetus, with the potential for great harm. On the other hand, placental transfer of drugs administered to the mother has been used to treat fetal arrhythmias, congestive heart failure, and other conditions [107].

The placenta develops from a portion of the zygote, and thus has the same genetic endowment as the developing fetus [108]. The embryonic/fetal component consists of trophoblastic-derived chorionic villi, which invade the maternal endometrium and are exposed directly to maternal blood in lake-like structures called lacunae. These villi create the large surface area necessary for maternal–fetal transfer in what becomes the intervillous space of the placenta. Here, the maternal blood pressure supplies pulsatile blood flow in jet-like streams from the spiral arteries of the endometrium to bathe the chorionic villi and allow for transfer of gases, nutrients, and metabolic products. Biologically, the human placenta is classified as a hemochorial placenta because maternal blood is in direct contact with the fetal chorionic membrane. It is this membrane that determines what is transferred to the fetus.

For the most part, drugs and other substances given to the mother will be transferred to the fetus. Drugs cross the placenta largely by simple diffusion. Factors affecting drug transfer are similar to those affecting transfer across other biological membranes, and include the molecular weight, lipid solubility, protein binding, and degree of ionization of the compound.

Generally, drugs and chemicals with a molecular weight of less than 600 Da traverse the placenta readily, while drugs with a molecular weight larger than 1000 Da transfer less readily, if at all. Compounds that are uncharged and more lipid soluble are also more readily transferred.

There are factors which affect the transfer of drugs and chemicals that are unique to the placenta. The placenta has a pore system which allows for bulk water flow across the placenta and can be responsible for small drugs and chemicals crossing the membrane by solvent drag. Within the placenta there is also a process of endocytosis that is capable of transferring large immunoglobulins to the fetus. Placental tissue has a full complement of cytochrome enzymes capable of metabolizing drugs and chemicals, and some of these metabolites may then transfer more readily to the fetus than the parent drugs. The permeability and diffusion properties of the placenta may increase as the placenta matures due to a decrease in thickness of

the trophoblastic epithelium forming the chorionic membrane from more than 50 μm in the first trimester to less than 5 μm at term [109, 110].

One of the factors affecting drug transfer to the fetus is the amount of drug delivered to the intervillous space by utero-placental blood flow. Blood flow to the uterus and placenta increases during pregnancy from 50 mL/min at 10 weeks' gestation to 500–600 mL/min at term [108]. Maternal blood flow to the uterus is also influenced by posture, diseases affecting maternal vasculature (such as hypertension and diabetes), placental size, and uterine contractions. For example, maternal cardiac output and utero-placental blood flow are reduced in the supine position and placental perfusion virtually ceases during a contraction. Placentas that are small for gestational age, or those with diffuse calcifications, are less efficient at transferring any maternal compounds to the fetus. Diseases, such as diabetes, which can thicken the chorionic membrane may also potentially affect diffusion of drugs into the fetal circulation.

In addition to passive and facilitated diffusion, the placenta contains a rich complement of numerous drug transporters that actively move compounds against their concentration gradient into and out of the fetus. Transporters are found on both surfaces of the syncytiotrophoblast – on the apical brush border facing maternal blood (ATP-binding cassette transporters: multidrug resistance protein MDR-1/P-glycoprotein, breast cancer resistance protein BCRP/ABCG2, and the multidrug resistance-associated proteins MRP-2 and MRP-3; plus serotonin transporter SERT, organic anion-transporter polypeptide OATP-E, and organic cation transporter OATN2) and on the basolateral membrane adjacent to fetal capillaries (multidrug resistance protein MDR-3, multidrug resistance-associated proteins MRP-1 and MRP-5, organic anion transporter polypeptide OATP-2B1, OATP-B, organic cation transporter OCT-3, and noradrenalin transporter NET). Additional transporters have been identified on fetal capillary endothelium (multidrug resistance-associated proteins MRP-1, MRP-3, MRP-5, and BRCP) [111]. Because these membranes express different transporters, polarized movement of compounds can occur, sometimes with efflux and uptake transporters in different locations working synergistically [111–116].

Of the placental transporters, the most extensively studied is P-glycoprotein (P-gp), which has been shown to play a critical role in transporting a large number of maternally administered drugs back into maternal circulation and away from the fetus. As described in Chapter 14, P-gp is a large 140- to 170-kDa transmembrane phospho-glycoprotein whose role as an energy-dependent efflux transporter was first elucidated in the investigation of cellular multidrug resistance. Coded for by the *MDR1* gene, P-gp belongs to a superfamily of ATP binding cassette transporters which are present in all organisms from bacteria to humans [117–119]. Actively excreting absorbed molecules from the cytoplasm, the evolutionary job of P-gp has been to reduce exposure to xenobiotics, or foreign, natural toxins [120, 121]. Numerous seemingly structurally unrelated drugs are substrates for this transporter.

In humans, although P-gp is expressed on trophoblastic cells throughout pregnancy, it undergoes a two-fold decline in expression between late first trimester and term [122–125]. It has been located in the vesicles of the apical brush-border membrane of the syncytiotrophoblast that directly faces human maternal blood, but not within maternal vascular endothelium [111, 123, 126]. Actively transporting molecules in a basolateral-to-apical direction, the role of P-gp within the placenta is similar to its function at other sites: it extrudes drugs from the placenta back into maternal circulation, thereby protecting the developing fetus from potential toxic factors within the maternal circulation [126].

In genetically altered *mdr1a/b(−/−)* knockout mice without P-gp, both transplacental transport of P-gp substrates and the incidence of fetal malformations increase [127]. Transplacental transport of the P-gp substrates digoxin, saquinavir, and paclitaxel was increased 2.4-, 7-, and 16-fold, respectively, in the knockout mice compared to transport in the wild-type animals. In another murine study, *mdr1a/b(−/−)* fetuses were susceptible to cleft palate malformation induced by prenatal exposure to a photoisomer of avermectin B1a, whereas their wild-type littermates were protected from this teratogen [114].

An active transport mechanism has long been suspected to account for the placental barrier that causes maternal and fetal concentrations for many drugs to differ [110, 128]. Studies of maternal–fetal transport of medications used during pregnancy in HIV positive women have shown variable penetration into the fetus [129, 130]. Whereas the maternal–fetal drug ratios for zidovudine, lamivudine, and nevirapine (approximately 0.85, 1.0, and 0.9, respectively) demonstrate good fetal penetration, most protease inhibitors, including nelfinavir, ritonavir, saquinivir, lopinavir, and indinavir, are known P-gp substrates and do not cross the placenta in detectable levels [130–132].

Several studies have examined the interaction between selective serotonin reuptake inhibitors (SSRIs) and P-gp and have shown that not all members of this class of drugs are P-gp substrates. Concentrations of paroxetine and venlafaxine, but not fluoxetine, were significantly increased in the brains of *mdr1a/b−/−* knockout mice compared to concentrations in the wild-type mice [133]. In cell culture studies, sertraline, its metabolite, desmethylsertraline, and paroxetine were shown to be potent inhibitors of Pgp; however, citalopram and venlafaxine were only weak inhibitors [134, 135]. P-glycoprotein polymorphisms may also alter drug transport across the placenta and influence fetal exposure. Whereas the P-gp SNP C3435T allele has no effect on saquinavir placental transport [136], its presence is associated with significantly increased maternal to fetal transfer of quetiapine [137]. Both C3435T and G2677T alleles have also been associated with lower levels of placental P-gp expression [138, 139].

Another ATP-binding cassette transporter located on the apical brush border of the syncytiotrophoblast and the chorionic villi fetal vessels is breast cancer resistance protein (BCRP, also referred to as ABCG2). BCRP has also been shown to play a critical role in limiting fetal drug exposure [140–143]. BCRP mRNA expression is higher in the human placenta than any other organ [144], its expression may increase with advancing gestation [141], and the expression of BCRP transcripts in the human term placenta is 10-fold higher than is P-gp expression [143]. Using pregnant mice and a specific inhibitor of Bcrp1 (the murine homolog of human BCRP), Jonker *et al.* [145] demonstrated that Bcrp1 limited fetal exposure to topotecan and both reduced maternal to fetal passage of cimetidine and actively removed existing drug from the fetal circulation [146]. Other studies with Bcrp1 knockout mice have shown that this transporter reduces fetal exposure to phytoestrogens [147] and nitrofurantoin [148, 149]. Fetal exposure to the oral hypoglycemic glyburide has been shown to be limited by BCRP efflux transport in human [150, 151] and rat [152] placental perfusion models, in human placental tissue [153], in pregnant mice [154], and in fetal umbilical cord samples [66]. Maternal to fetal transport of bupropion is also restricted by BCRP, but its primary active metabolite, OH-bupropion, freely passes across the placenta [155].

The precise function and significance of additional transporters is currently under active study [111, 115]. Similarly not yet well understood is the influence of the chemical environment, including steroid hormones, growth factors, and inflammation and infection on the expression and activity of these transporters which can then alter placental drug disposition and fetal exposure [156–159].

## TERATOGENESIS

During the 38 weeks that comprise human gestation the human conceptus develops from a one-cell zygote to a fully developed newborn infant. This complicated process has a high degree of wastage, with approximately 65% of conceptions lost prior to implantation, 20% lost from spontaneous abortion, and 15% born prematurely. Major congenital abnormalities that are recognized at birth occur in approximately 2–3 infants per 100. Minor anomalies occur in another 7–14 infants per 100. Major birth defects cause 20% of infant mortality and are responsible for the majority of childhood hospitalizations.

From the patient's perspective, a birth defect may be any abnormality of the infant found at birth. This may include birth injuries, such as a cephalohematoma or a brachial plexus injury. However, birth defects are usually considered to be structural defects of the newborn. Structural defects have been broken down into four major categories: a *malformation*, which is a structural defect caused by an intrinsic problem in embryologic differentiation and/or development; a *disruption*, which is an alteration in shape or structure of a normally differentiated part, such as a limb amputation from an amniotic band or a vascular event; a *deformation*, which is an alteration in the shape or structure of a normally differentiated part, such as a Potter's facies or metatarsus adductus, which is often due to a mechanical constraint; and a *dysplasia*, which is a primary defect in cellular organization into tissues [160]. A *teratogen* is a chemical substance which can induce a malformation during development. An expansion of the definition includes an adverse effect on the developing fetus either in causing a structural abnormality or in altering organ function. This should be distinguished from a *mutagen*, which causes a genetic mutation whose effects cannot be seen for at least a generation.

Underlying causes of birth defects are shown in Table 24.4. It should be appreciated that approximately 90% of birth defects have a genetic component. Birth defects caused by drugs represent the one group of anomalies that can potentially be prevented. However, there is only a small list of drugs that have been proven to cause human anomalies (Table 24.5). Potential effects of drugs on the developing fetus include altered structural development during the first trimester, producing a dysmorphic infant; altered fetal growth during the second and third trimesters of pregnancy; and altered function of organ systems.

### Principles of Teratology

The principles of teratology have been articulated by Wilson [161]. The first principle is that teratogens act with specificity. A teratogen produces a specific abnormality or constellation of abnormalities. For example, thalidomide produces phocomelia, and valproic acid produces neural tube defects. This specificity also applies to species, because drug effects may be seen in one species and not another. The best example is cortisol, which produces cleft palate in mice but not in humans.

The next principle is that teratogens demonstrate a dose–effect relationship. Given to the mother at a specific time during gestation, low doses can produce no effect, intermediate doses can produce the characteristic pattern of malformation, and higher doses will be lethal to the embryo. Dose–effect curves for most teratogens are steep, changing from minimal to maximal effect by dose-doubling. Increasing the dose beyond that found to be lethal to the embryo will eventually lead to maternal death. This is used as an endpoint in animal teratogenicity studies.

The third principle is that teratogens must reach the developing conceptus in sufficient amounts to cause their effects. The extent of fetal exposure to drugs and other xenobiotics is determined not only by maternal dose, route of elimination, and placental transfer, but also by fetal elimination mechanisms. Because the fetal liver is interposed between the umbilical vein and systemic circulation, drugs transferred across the placenta are subject to fetal first-pass metabolism [107]. This protective mechanism is compromised by ductus venosus shunting, which enables 30–70% of umbilical venous blood flow to bypass the liver. After drugs reach the fetal systemic circulation, hepatic metabolism constitutes the primary elimination mechanism and renal excretion is relatively ineffective, because the fetal kidney is immature and fetal urine passing into the amniotic fluid is swallowed by the fetus. CYP3A7 is a fetal-specific enzyme that accounts for about one-third of fetal hepatic cytochrome P450. CYP1A1, CYP2C8, CYP2D6, and

---

TABLE 24.4   Human Reproductive Risk

| Causes of anomalies | Percent of total anomalies |
|---|---|
| Chromosomal | 5 |
| Single gene | 20 |
| Polygenic/multifactorial | 65 |
| Environmental | 10 |
|    Irradiation | < 1 |
|    Maternal disease | 1–2 |
|    Infection | 2–3 |
|    Drugs and chemicals | 4–5 |

**TABLE 24.5    Known Human Teratogens**

| Agent | Teratogenic effect |
| --- | --- |
| Carbamazepine | Facial dysmorphogenesis, neural tube defect |
| Phenytoin | Facial dysmorphogenesis, mental retardation, growth retardation, distal digital hypoplasia |
| Valproate | Lumbosacral spina bifida, facial dysmorphogenesis |
| Trimethadione | Facial dysmorphogenesis, intrauterine growth retardation, intrauterine fetal demise, neonatal demise |
| Coumadin | Nasal hypoplasia, epiphyseal stippling, optic atrophy |
| Alcohol | Facial dysmorphogenesis, growth retardation, mental retardation |
| Diethylstilbesterol | Vaginal adenosis, uterine anomalies, vaginal carcinogenesis |
| Androgens | Masculinization of the female genitalia |
| Methyl mercury | Growth retardation, severe mental retardation |
| ACE inhibitors | Oligohydramnios, potential lung hypoplasia, postnatal renal failure |
| Folic acid antagonists (aminopterin, methotrexate) | Abortion, intrauterine growth retardation, microcephaly, hypoplasia of frontal bones |
| Thalidomide | Phocomelia |
| Isotretinoin | CNS anomalies, including optic nerve abnormalities; craniofacial anomalies; cardiovascular malformations, thymic abnormalies |
| Inorganic iodides | Fetal goiter |
| Tetracycline | Bone deposits, teeth discoloration |
| Lithium | Ebstein's anomaly |

CYP3A3/4 have also been identified in fetal liver. These enzymes are not only protective, but, as described in Chapter 16, their presence in fetal tissues other than liver is also capable of converting drugs into chemically reactive teratogenic intermediates such as phenytoin epoxide (see Chapter 11, Scheme 11.7) or phenytoin free radicals (see Chapter 16, Figure 16.15).

The fourth principle is that the effect that a teratogenic agent has on a developing fetus depends upon the stage during development when the fetus is exposed. From conception to implantation there is an all-or-nothing effect, in that the embryo, if exposed to a teratogen, either survives unharmed or dies. This concept developed from Brent's studies of the effects of radiation on the developing embryo, and may or may not apply to fetal exposure to chemicals [162]. After implantation, during the process of differentiation and embryogenesis, the embryo is very susceptible to teratogens. However, since teratogens are capable of affecting many organ systems, the pattern of anomalies produced depends on which organ systems are differentiating at the time of teratogenic exposure. A difference of 1 or 2 days can result in a slightly different pattern of anomalies. After organogenesis, a teratogen can affect the embryo by producing growth retardation, or by changing the size or function of a specific organ. Giving a teratogen after the fetus has developed normally has no effect on the development of organs already formed. For example,

beginning lithium after cardiac development, or valproic acid after the closure of the neural tube, will not produce either drug's characteristic anomalies. However, of particular interest is the effect of psychoactive agents, such as cocaine, crack, or antidepressants, on the developing central nervous system during the second and third trimesters of pregnancy, as these drugs can potentially affect the function and behavior of the infant after delivery.

The fifth principle is that susceptibility to teratogens is influenced by the genotype of the mother and fetus. Animal studies have shown that certain animal strains are more susceptible to the production of malformations when exposed to a teratogen compared to other animal strains. In humans, the fetus homozygous for the recessive allele associated with decreased epoxide hydrolase activity has an increased risk of developing the full fetal hydantoin syndrome [163]. Maternal smoking increases the risk for the development of cleft lip and palate in a fetus carrying the atypical allele for tranforming growth factor α [164]. Single mutant genes or polygenic inheritance may explain why certain fetuses are unusually susceptible to teratogens.

Mechanisms of teratogenesis include genetic interference, gene mutation, chromosomal breakage, interference with cellular function, enzyme inhibition, and altered membrane characteristics. The response of the developing embryo to these insults is failure of cell–cell interaction crucial for development, interference with cell migration, or mechanical cellular disruption. The common endpoint is cell death–teratogenesis causing fewer cells. Most mechanisms of teratogenesis are theoretical, not well understood, and imply a genetic component. One exception is the mechanism of thalidomide teratogenesis. In susceptible species, thalidomide causes oxidative DNA damage and one active metabolite, CPS49, directly prevents blood vessel formation or angiogenesis in the limbs [165]. Pretreatment with PBN, a free radical trapping agent, reduces the occurrence of thalidomide embryopathy, suggesting that the mechanism is free radical-mediated oxidative DNA damage [166].

## Measures to Minimize Teratogenic Risk

All new drug applications filed with the FDA include data from developmental and reproductive toxicology (DART) studies. These studies examine the effects of the particular agent on all aspects of reproduction, including oogenesis, spermatogenesis, fertility, and fecundity, as well as effects on litter size, spontaneous resorption, fetal malformation, fetal size, and newborn pup function. Most studies are conducted in mice, rats, and rabbits. All studies are designed with dose escalations and with maternal death as the endpoint. Information from these teratologic experiments is included in the drug labeling. Some, but not all, human teratogenic reactions of new drugs have been predicted from animal studies, in large part because most animals have a shorter gestational clock than humans. In addition, species vary in their susceptibility to teratogens, with some animal models being either more or less susceptible to teratogenesis than humans. Thus, if an agent does not produce an anomaly in animal studies, it does not necessarily prove that it is safe for humans.

Safety of a drug for use in human pregnancy is demonstrated by observational studies conducted after the drug is marketed. Better studies are conducted prospectively with an exposed and unexposed control population found before pregnancy outcome is known. Although population-based large cohort studies begun prior to pregnancy are considered the best type, they are expensive to conduct and limited to those agents used at the time of the study. Epidemiologic clues to teratogenesis are often found in case reports of abnormal infants, but these are biased in that an abnormal infant is more likely reported than a normal infant, and the background rate of malformations is high. Proof of teratogenicity in humans is supported by the following criteria: a recognizable pattern of anomalies; a higher prevalence of the particular anomaly or anomalies in patients exposed to an agent than in a control population; presence of the agent during the stage of organogenesis of the organ system affected; increased incidence of the anomaly after introduction of the agent; and production of the anomaly in experimental animals by administration of the agent during the appropriate stage of organogenesis.

A general approach to reduce the risk of human teratogenesis includes planning for pregnancy. Prior to conception, women with medical problems should be counseled about the medications they chronically use, which ones can safely be continued throughout pregnancy, and which ones should be discontinued. Medications should be evaluated and changed if necessary to decrease teratogenic risk. Plasma level monitoring of unbound concentrations of antiepileptic drugs may be helpful in optimizing seizure control, decreasing the need for multiple drug therapy, and minimizing dosage and fetal risk. Since more than 50% of pregnancies in the United States are unplanned, all women of childbearing potential should be treated as antenatal patients and counseled regarding use of any new drug in a potential pregnancy. Therefore, when a woman of childbearing potential develops a new medical problem, counseling for pregnancy should be included in management. In general, the use of agents that are already widely used during pregnancy is preferred to use of newer agents. Just stopping pharmacologic therapy or leaving the issue up to the woman does not help her and may place both the mother and fetus at risk for adverse pregnancy outcome or an uncontrolled medical condition during pregnancy.

When using a known human teratogen, particular attention should be given to preventing pregnancy. This includes counseling the patient on the fetal effects of the drug being used and on the use of one or more effective forms of contraception. Therapy should be begun with a normal menstrual period, or no more than 2 weeks from a negative pregnancy test. Pregnancy tests bear repeating every 2–4 weeks, depending upon the form of contraception being used and the woman's menstrual history. When renewing prescriptions for these drugs, it is necessary to repeat a pregnancy test to verify that the patient is not pregnant.

To allow thalidomide, a known teratogen on the market, the FDA required the development of a program called System for Thalidomide Education and Prescribing Safety (STEPS) which ensures that pregnant women will not be exposed to the drug [167]. All patients, physicians, and pharmacists involved in thalidomide usage must be registered with the program. Women who can become pregnant must have a negative pregnancy test within 24 hours before therapy is begun. Pregnancy tests are then required once per week for the first 4 weeks of therapy and every 2–4 weeks while on therapy. Two forms of acceptable contraception must be used for 4 weeks prior to use, during use, and for 4 weeks after use.

## DRUG THERAPY OF NURSING MOTHERS

Transfer of drugs into breast milk is generally bidirectional, reflecting passive diffusion of unbound drug between plasma and blood rather than active secretion. Factors that affect the milk concentration include binding to maternal plasma proteins, protein binding in milk, lipid content of milk, and physiochemical factors of the drug [168]. As shown for theophylline in Figure 24.7, drug concentrations in breast milk are usually less than plasma concentrations, and there usually is a fixed ratio between milk and plasma concentrations [169]. In the usual case, drug concentrations measured in plasma and breast milk can be used to calculate a milk:plasma ratio (M/P), from which the daily drug dose to the infant is estimated as follows:

$$\text{Infant Dose/Day} = C_{maternal} \times M/P \times V_{milk} \quad (24.2)$$

where $C_{maternal}$ is the average maternal plasma concentration of drug during nursing and $V_{milk}$ is the volume of maternal milk ingested each day, usually estimated as 150 ml/kg [168]. This estimate of infant

dose is often reported as a percentage of administered maternal dose. However, concentration-dependent saturation of the plasma protein binding precludes calculation of a fixed milk:plasma ratio for a few drugs (Figure 24.8) [170]. In addition, there are drugs that, because of physiochemical properties or their active transport into milk, can give a higher dose to the infant than would otherwise be expected. For example, cimetidine has been shown to be actively transported into human breast milk, giving an M/P of 5.5 – far higher than expected on the basis of passive diffusion, milk-protein binding, ion trapping, or lipid solubility [171]. Despite this high M/P, the estimated infant dose is still low and no infant toxicity has been reported. Dapsone, used in the therapy of dermatitis herpetiformis, is a weak base with a pKb of 13, is highly protein bound at physiologic pH, and has a half-life of 20 hours that ensures significant serum concentrations during the entire 24-hour dosing period. These physiochemical properties result in infants receiving dapsone doses that are higher than expected, and use of this drug with breast-feeding has been reported to cause hemolytic anemia in infants [172].

The prodrug codeine and its active metabolite morphine have been shown to pass into breast milk in generally insignificant amounts, and short-term use of codeine for postpartum pain relief has been considered safe for mothers breast-feeding their infants

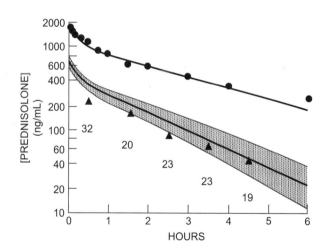

**FIGURE 24.8** Kinetic analysis of prednisolone plasma (●) concentrations after intravenous administration of a 50-mg prednisolone dose. The solid lines represent the least-squares fit of the measured plasma concentrations. Measured milk concentrations (▲) are plotted along with the range (*shaded area*) of unbound prednisolone plasma concentrations expected if serum transcortin binding capacity is allowed to vary ± 1 SD from its reported mean. The volume (in milliliters) of each breast-milk sample is shown by the numbers below the milk concentrations. Reproduced with permission from Greenberger PA, Odeh YK, Frederiksen MC, Atkinson AJ Jr. Clin Pharmacol Ther 1993;53:324–8 [170].

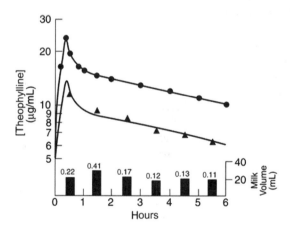

**FIGURE 24.7** Kinetic analysis of theophylline plasma (●) and milk (▲) concentrations after intravenous administration of a 3.2- to 5.3-mg/kg aminophylline dose. The solid lines represent the least-squares fit of the measured concentrations. The interval and volume of each milk collection are shown by the solid bars. The milligram recovery of theophylline in each breast-milk collection is shown by the numbers above the bars. Reproduced with permission from Stec GP Greenberger P, Ruo TI *et al.* Clin Pharmacol Ther 1980;28:404–8 [169].

[173, 174]. However, a report of an infant death secondary to maternal codeine use prompted a reappraisal of the use of codeine in breast-feeding mothers [175]. In this case, the mother was found to be heterozygous for a CYP2D6*2 A allele with CYP2D6*2×2 gene duplication, and was thus an ultrarapid metabolizer who converted codeine to morphine at an increased rate. As discussed in Chapter 13, the incidence of ultra-rapid CYP2D6 metabolizers ranges from 1% in the Scandinavian population to as high as 29% in the Ethiopian population. In addition, although morphine is metabolized through glucuronidation mainly to the inactive metabolite morphine-3-glucuronide, it also is metabolized to a lesser extent by uridyl glucuronsyltransferase 2B7 (UGT2B7) to morphine-6-glucuronide (M6G), which is equipotent to morphine [176]. A UGT2B7*2 variant has been reported that increases the proportion of morphine that is metabolized to M6G [177]. So an infant whose mother is an ultra-rapid CYP2D6 metabolizer and also carries the UGT2B7*2 variant would be at a particularly high risk of life-threatening CNS depression from maternal codeine usage [178].

Although some drugs are specifically contra-indicated during lactation, including antineoplastics, immune suppressants, ergot alkaloids, gold, iodine, lithium carbonate, radiopharmaceuticals, social drugs of abuse, and certain antibiotics, drugs considered safe for pregnancy are usually safe during the lactation period. In some cases, it may be advisable to monitor infant blood levels to ensure that they are less than those required for pharmacologic effects. Finally, an important clinical point is that infant exposure can be minimized by breast-feeding just prior to drug administration, when drug concentrations in milk are lowest [169].

## REFERENCES

[1] Zinacef (cefuroxime) Labeling. In: Physicians' Desk Reference. 54th ed. Montvale, NJ: Medical Economics; 2005. p. 1678.

[2] CDC. Births: Preliminary data for 1999. National Vital Statistics Reports 48(14). Atlanta, GA: Centers for Disease Control; 2000.

[3] CDER, CBER. Establishing pregnancy exposure registries. Guidance for industry. Rockville, MD: FDA (Internet at, www.fda.gov/downloads/Drugs/GuidanceComplianceRegulatoryInformation/Guidances/UCM071639.pdf.; August 2002).

[4] CDER. Pharmacokinetics in pregnancy – study design, data analysis, and impact on dosing and labeling. Draft guidance for industry. Rockville, MD: FDA (Internet at, www.fda.gov/downloads/Drugs/GuidanceComplianceRegulatoryInformation/Guidances/UCM072133.pdf.; October 2004).

[5] CDER, CBER. Clinical lactation studies-study design, data analysis, and recommendations for labeling. Draft guidance for industry. Rockville, MD: FDA (Internet at, http://www.fda.gov/downloads/RegulatoryInformation/Guidances/ucm127505.pdf; February 2005).

[6] Content and format of labeling for human prescription drug and biological products; requirements for pregnancy and lactation labeling. Proposed Rule in the US Code of Federal Regulations: 21 CFR Part (Internet at, http://www.regulations.gov/#!docketDetail;rpp=10;po=0;s=Proposed%252Brule; D=FDA-2006-N-0515. May 29, 2008;201).

[7] Gryboski WA, Spiro HM. The effect of pregnancy on gastric secretion. N Engl J Med 1956;255:1131–4.

[8] Hunt JN, Murray FA. Gastric function in pregnancy. J Obstet Gynaecol Br Emp 1958;65:78–83.

[9] Parry E, Shields R, Turnbull AC. Transit time in the small intestine in pregnancy. J Obstet Gynaecol Br Commonw 1970;77:900–1.

[10] Chiloiro M, Darconza G, Piccioli E, De Carne M, Clemente C, Riezzo G. Gastric emptying and orocecal transit time in pregnancy. J Gastroenterol 2001;36:538–43.

[11] Wong CA, Loffredi M, Ganchiff JN, Zhao J, Wang Z, Avram MJ. Gastric emptying of water in term pregnancy. Anesthesiology 2002;96:1395–400.

[12] O'Hare MF, Leahey W, Mumaghan GA. McDevitt. Pharmacokinetics of sotalol during pregnancy. Eur J Clin Pharmacol 1983;24:521–4.

[13] Philipson A. Pharmacokinetics of ampicillin during pregnancy. J Infect Dis 1977;136:370–6.

[14] Philipson A, Stiernstedt G, Ehrenbo M. Comparison of the pharmacokinetics of cephradine and cefazolin in pregnant and non-pregnant women. Clin Pharmacokinet 1987;12:136–44.

[15] Lund CV, Donovan JC. Blood volume during pregnancy: Significance of plasma and red cell volumes. Am J Obstet Gynecol 1967;98:394–403.

[16] Hytten F. Blood volume changes in normal pregnancy. Clin Haematol 1985;14:601–12.

[17] Petersen VP. Body composition and fluid compartments in normal, obese and underweight human subjects. Acta Med Scand 1957;108:103–11.

[18] Plentl AA, Gray MJ. Total body water, sodium space and total exchangeable sodium in normal and toxemic pregnant women. Am J Obstet Gynecol 1959;78:472–8.

[19] Lees MM, Taylor SH, Scott DM, Kerr MR. A study of cardiac output at rest throughout pregnancy. J Obstet Gynaecol Br Commonw 1967;74:319–28.

[20] Robson SC, Hunter S, Boys RJ, Dunlop W. Serial study of factors influencing changes in cardiac output during human pregnancy. Am J Physiol 1989;256:H1060–5.

[21] Metcalfe J, Romney SL, Ramsey LH, Burwell CS. Estimation of uterine blood flow in women at term. J Clin Invest 1955;34:1632–8.

[22] Ginsburg J, Duncan SL. Peripheral blood flow in normal pregnancy. Cardiovasc Res 1967;1:132–7.

[23] Thoresen M, Wesch J. Doppler measurements of changes in human mammary and uterine blood flow during pregnancy and lactation. Acta Obstet Gynecol Scand 1988;67:741–5.

[24] Robson SC, Mutch E, Boy RJ, Woodhouse KH. Apparent liver blood flow during pregnancy: A serial study using indocyanine green clearance. Br J Obstet Gynaecol 1990;97:720–4.

[25] Nakai A, Seklya I, Oya A, Koshino T, Araki T. Assessment of hepatic arterial and portal venous blood flows during pregnancy with Doppler ultrasonography. Arch Gynecol Obstet 2002;266:25–9.

[26] Frederiksen MC, Ruo TI, Chow MJ, Atkinson AJ Jr. Theophylline pharmacokinetics in pregnancy. Clin Pharmacol Ther 1986;40:321–8.

[27] Mendenhall HW. Serum protein concentrations in pregnancy: I. Concentrations in maternal serum. Am J Obstet Gynecol 1970;106:388–99.

[28] Wood M, Wood AJJ. Changes in plasma drug binding and $\alpha_1$-acid glycoprotein in mother and newborn infant. Clin Pharmacol Ther 1981;29:522–6.

[29] Connelly RJ, Ruo TI, Frederiksen MC, Atkinson AJ Jr. Characterization of theophylline binding to serum proteins in nonpregnant and pregnant women. Clin Pharmacol Ther 1990;47:68–72.

[30] Lucius H, Gahlenbeck H, Kleine HO, Fabel H, Bartels H. Respiratory functions, buffer system and electrolyte concentrations of blood during human pregnancy. Respir Physiol 1970;9:311–7.

[31] Lyons HA, Antonio R. The sensitivity of the respiratory center in pregnancy and after the administration of progesterone. Trans Assoc Am Physicians 1959;72:173–80.

[32] Davison JM, Hytten FE. Glomerular filtration during and after pregnancy. J Obstet Gynaecol Br Commonw 1974;81:588–95.

[33] Davison JM, Hytten FE. The effect of pregnancy on the renal handling of glucose. J Obstet Gynaecol Br Commonw 1975;82:374–81.

[34] Philipson A, Stiernstedt G. Pharmacokinetics of cefuroxime in pregnancy. Am J Obstet Gynecol 1982;142:823–8.

[35] Bourget P, Fernandez H, Delouis C, Taburet AM. Pharmacokinetics of tobramycin in pregnant women, safety and efficacy of a once-daily dose regimen. J Clin Pharm Ther 1991;16:167–76.

[36] Buster JE, Abraham GE. The applications of steroid hormone radioimmunoassys to clinical obstetrics. Obstet Gynecol 1975;46:489–99.

[37] Devroey P, Camus M, Palermo G, Smitz J, Van Waesberghe L, Wsanto A, et al. Placental production of estradiol and progesterone after oocyte donation in patients with primary ovarian failure. Am J Obstet Gynecol 1990;162:66–70.

[38] Schneider MA, Davies MC, Honour JW. The timing of placental competence in pregnancy after oocyte donation. Fertil Steril 1993;59:1059–64.

[39] Mishell DR, Thorneycroft IH, Nagata Y, Murata T, Nakamura RM. Serum gonadotropin and steroid patterns in early human gestation. Am J Obstet Gynecol 1971;117:631–42.

[40] Tulchinsky D, Hobel CJ. Plasma human and chorionic gonadotropin, estrone, estradiol, estriol, progesterone and 17α-hydroxyprogesterone in human pregnancy. 3. Early normal pregnancy. Am J Obstet Gynecol 1973;117:884–93.

[41] Tracy TS, Venkataramanan R, Glover DD, Caritis SN. National Institute for Child Health and Human Development Network of Maternal–Fetal Medicine Units. Temporal changes in drug metabolism (CYP1A2, CYP2D6 and CYP3A4 activity) during pregnancy. Am J Obstet Gynecol 2005;192:633–9.

[42] Kronbach T, Mathys D, Umeno M, Gonzalez FJ, Meyer UA. Oxidation of midazolam and triazolam by human liver cytochrome P450IIIA4. Mol Pharmacol 1989;36:89–96.

[43] Gorski JC, Hall SD, Jones DR, VandenBranden M, Wrighten SA. Regioselective biotransformation of midazolam by members of the human cytochrome P450 3A (CYP 3A) subfamily. Biochem Pharmacol 1994;47:1643–53.

[44] Thummel KE, Shen DD, Podoll TD, Kunze KL, Trager WF, Hartwell PS, et al. Use of midazolam as a human cytochrome P450 3A probe: I. *In vitro–in vivo* correlations in liver transplant patients. J Pharmacol Exper Ther 1994;271:549–56.

[45] Thummel KE, Shen DD, Podoll TD, Kunze KL, Trager WF, Bacchi CE, et al. Use of midazolam as a human cytochrome P450 3A probe: II. Characterization of inter- and intra-individual hepatic CYP3A variability after liver transplantation. J Pharmacol Exp Ther 1994;271:557–66.

[46] Kanto J, Sjövall S, Erkkola R, Himberg J-J, Kangas L. Placental transfer and maternal midazolam kinetics. Clin Pharmacol Ther 1983;33:786–91.

[47] Ohkita C, Goto M. Increased 6-hydroxycortisol excretion in pregnant women: Implication of drug-metabolizing enzyme induction. DICP 1990;24:814–6.

[48] Varis T, Kivistö KT, Backman JT, Neuvonen PJ. The cytochrome P450 3A4 inhibitor itraconazole markedly increases the plasma concentrations of dexamethasone and enhances

its adrenal-suppressant effect. Clin Pharmacol Ther 2000;68:487–94.

[49] Gentile DM, Tomlinson ES, Maggs JL, Park BK, Back DJ. Dexamethasone metabolism by human liver *in vitro*. Metabolite identification and inhibition of 6-hydroxylation. J Pharmacol Exp Ther 1996;277:105–12.

[50] Della Torre M, Hibbard JU, Jeong H, Fischer JH. Betamethasone in pregnancy: Influence of maternal body weight and multiple gestation on pharmacokinetics. Am J Obstet Gynecol 2010;203:254.e1–12.

[51] Petersen MC, Collier CB, Ashley JJ, McBride WG, Nation RL. Disposition of betamethasone in parturient women after intravenous administration. Eur J Clin Pharmacol 1983;25:803–10.

[52] Petersen MC, Nation RL, McBride WG, Ashley JJ, Moore RG. Pharmacokinetics of betamethasone in healthy adults after intravenous administration. Eur J Clin Pharmacol 1983;25:643–50.

[53] Prevost RR, Aki SA, Whybrew WD, Sibai BM. Oral nifedipine pharmacokinetics in pregnancy-induced hypertension. Pharmacother 1992;12:174–7.

[54] Pond SM, Kreek MJ, Tong TG, Raghunath J, Benowitz NL. Altered methadone pharmacokinetics in methadone-maintained pregnancy women. J Pharmacol Exp Ther 1985;233:1–6.

[55] Stika CS, Andrews W, Frederiksen MC, Mercer B, Sabai B, Antal E. Steady state pharmacokinetic study of Flagyl® ER in pregnant patients during the second to third trimester of pregnancy [Abstract]. Clin Pharmacol Ther 2004;75:24.

[56] Lehmann JM, McKee DD, Watson MA, Willson TM, Moore JT, Kliewer SA. The human orphan nuclear receptor PXR is activated by compounds that regulate CYP3A4 gene expression and cause drug interactions. J Clin Invest 1998;102:1016–23.

[57] Goodwin B, Hodgson E, Liddle C. The orphan human pregnane X receptor mediates the transcription activation of CYP3A4 by rifampicin through a distal enhancer module. Mol Pharmacol 1999;56:1329–39.

[58] Aldridge A, Bailey J, Neims AH. The disposition of caffeine during and after pregnancy. Semin Perinatol 1981;5:310–4.

[59] Högstedt S, Lindberg B, Peng DR, Regårdh CG, Rane A. Pregnancy-induced increase in metoprolol metabolism. Clin Pharmacol Ther 1985;37:688–92.

[60] Högstedt S, Lindberg B, Rane A. Increased oral clearance of metoprolol in pregnancy. Eur J Clin Pharmacol 1983;24:217–20.

[61] Wadelius M, Darj E, Freene G, Rane A. Induction of CYP2D6 in pregnancy. Clin Pharmacol Ther 1997;62:400–7.

[62] Tomson T, Lindbom U, Ekqvist B, Sundqvist A. Epilepsy in pregnancy: A prospective study of seizure control in relation to free and total plasma concentrations of cabamazepine and phenytoin. Epilepsia 1994;35:122–30.

[63] Tomson T, Lindbom U, Ekqvist B, Sundqvist A. Disposition of cabamazepine and phenytoin in pregnancy. Epilepsia 1994;35:131–5.

[64] Chen SS, Perucca E, Lee JN, Richens A. Serum protein binding and free concentration of phenytoin and phenobarbitone in pregnancy. Br J Clin Pharmacol 1982;3:547–52.

[65] Niemi M, Cascorbi I, Timm R, Kroemer HK, Neuvonen PJ, Kvistö KT. Glyburide and glimepride pharmacokinetics in subjects with different CYP2C9 genotypes. Clin Pharmacol Ther 2002;73:326–32.

[66] Hebert MF, Ma X, Naraharisettti SB, Krudys KM, Umans JG, Hankins GD, et al. Are we optimizing gestational diabetes treatment with glyburide? The pharmacologic basis for better clinical practice. Clin Pharmacol Ther 2009;85:607–14.

[67] McGready R, Stepniewska K, Seaton E, Cho D, Cho A, Ginsberg MD. Pregnancy and use of oral contraceptives reduces the biotransformation of proguanil to cycloguanil. Eur J Clin Pharmacol 2003;59:553–7.

[68] McGready R, Stepniewska K, Edstein MD, Cho T, Gilveray G, Looareesuwan S, et al. The pharmacokinetics of atovaquone

and proguanil in pregnant women with acute falciparum malaria. Eur J Clin Pharmacol 2003;59:545–52.

[69] Bologa M, Tang B, Klein J, Tesoro A, Koren G. Pregnancy-induced changes in drug metabolism in epileptic women. J Pharmacol Exp Ther 1991;257:735–40.

[70] Tsutsumi K, Kotegawa T, Matsuki S, Tanaka Y, Ishii Y, Kodama Y, et al. The effect of pregnancy on cytochrome P4501A2, xanthine oxidase, and N-acetyltransferase activities in humans. Clin Pharmacol Ther 2001;70:121–5.

[71] Chen H, Yang K, Choi S, Fischer JH, Jeong H. Up-regulation of UDP-glycuronosyltransferase (UGT) 1A4 by 17beta-estradiol: A potential mechanism of increased lamotrigine elimination in pregnancy. Drug Metab Dispos 2009;37:1841–7.

[72] Ohman I, Beck O, Vitols S, Tomson T. Plasma concentrations of lamotrigine and its 2-N-glucuronide metabolite during pregnancy in women with epilepsy. Epilepsia 2008;49:1075–80.

[73] Ohman I, Vitois S, Tomson T. Lamotrigine in pregnancy: Pharmacokinetics during delivery, in the neonate, and during lactation. Epilepsia 2000;41:709–13.

[74] Pennell PB, Newport DJ, Stowe ZN, Helmers SL, Montgomery JQ, Henry TR. The impact of pregnancy and childbirth on the metabolism of lamotrigine. Neurology 2004;62:292–5.

[75] Tomson T, Ohman I, Vitols S. Lamotrigine in pregnancy and lactation: A case report. Epilepsia 1997;38:1039–41.

[76] Reimers A, Heilde G, Bråthen G, Brodtkorb E. Lamotrigine and its N2-glucuronide during pregnancy: The significance of renal clearance and estradiol. Epilepsy Res 2011 (Epub ahead of print).

[77] Fotopoulou C, Kretz R, Bauer S, Schefold JC, Schmitz B, Dudenhausen JW, et al. Prospectively assessed changes in lamotrigine-concentration in women with epilepsy during pregnancy, lactation and the neonatal period. Epilepsy Res 2009;85:60–4.

[78] Tomson T, Luef G, Sabers A, Pittschieler S, Ohman I. Valproate effects on kinetics of lamotrigine in pregnancy and treatment with oral contraceptives. Neurology 2006;67: 1297–9.

[79] Ohman I, Luef G, Tomson T. Effects of pregnancy and contraception on lamotrigine disposition: New insights through analysis of lamotrigine metabolites. Seizure 2008;17:199–202.

[80] Reimers A, Skogvoll E, Sund JK, Spigset O. Drug interactions between lamotrigine and psychoactive drugs: Evidence from a therapeutic drug monitoring service. J Clin Psychopharmacol 2005;25:342–8.

[81] Wegner I, Edelbroek P, de Haan GJ, Lindhout D, Sander JW. Drug monitoring of lamotrigine and oxcarbazepine combination during pregnancy. Epilepsia 2010;51:2500–2.

[82] Lees MM, Scott DH, Kerr MG. Haemodynamic changes associated with labour. J Obstet Gynaecol Br Commonw 1970;77:29–36.

[83] Gerdin E, Salmonson T, Lindberg B, Rane A. Maternal kinetics of morphine during labour. J Perinat Med 1990;18:479–87.

[84] Ueland K, Metcalfe J. Circulatory changes in pregnancy. Clin Obstet Gynecol 1975;18:41–50.

[85] Sims EAH, Krantz KE. Serial studies of renal function during pregnancy and the puerperium in normal women. J Clin Invest 1958;37:1764–74.

[86] Capeless EL, Clapp JF. When do cardiovascular parameters return to their preconception values? Am J Obstet Gynecol 1991;165:883–6.

[87] Dam M, Christiansen J, Munck O, Mygind KI. Antiepileptic drugs: Metabolism in pregnancy. Clin Pharmacokin 1979;4:53–62.

[88] Steen B, Rane A. Clindamycin passage into human milk. Br J Clin Pharmacol 1982;13:661–4.

[89] Del Priore G, Jackson-Stone M, Shim EK, Garfinkel J, Eichmann MA, Frederiksen MC. A comparison of once-daily and eight hour gentamicin dosing in the treatment of postpartum endometritis. Obstet Gynecol 1996;87:994–1000.

[90] Kubacka RT, Johnstone HE, Tan HSI, Reeme PD, Myre SA. Intravenous ampicillin pharmacokinetics in the third trimester of pregnancy. Ther Drug Monit 1983;5:55–60.

[91] Andrew MA, Easterling TR, Carr DB, Shen D, Buchanan ML, Rutherford T, et al. Amoxicillin pharmacokinetics in pregnant women: Modeling and simulations of dosage strategies. Clin Pharmacol Ther 2007;81:547–56.

[92] Yerby MS, Friel PN, Miller DQ. Carbamazepine protein binding and disposition in pregnancy. Ther Drug Monit 1985;7:269–73.

[93] Casele HL, Laifer SA, Woelders DA, Venkataramanan R. Changes in the pharmacokinetics of the low-molecular-weight heparin enoxaparin sodium during pregnancy. Am J Obstet Gynecol 1999;181:1113–7.

[94] Scheen AJ. Clinical pharmacokinetics of metformin. Clin Pharmacokinet 1996;30:359–71.

[95] Wang DS, Jonker JW, Kato Y, Kusuhara H, Schinkel AH, Sugiyama Y. Involvement of organic cation transporter 1 in hepatic and intestinal distribution of metformin. J Pharmacol Exp Ther 2002;302:510–5.

[96] Kimura N, Okuda M, Inui K. Metformin transport by renal basolateral organic cation transporter hOCT2. Pharm Res 2005;22:255–9.

[97] Zhou M, Xia L, Wang J. Metformin transport by a newly cloned proton-stimulated organic cation transporter (plasma membrane monoamine transporter) expressed in human intestine. Drug Metab Dispos 2007;35:1956–62.

[98] Pentikainen PJ, Neuvonen PJ, Penttila A. Pharmacokinetics of metformin after intravenous and oral administration to man. Eur J Clin Pharmacol 1979;16:195–202.

[99] Tucker GT, Casey C, Phillips PJ, Connor H, Ward JD, Woods HF. Metformin kinetics in healthy subjects and in patients with diabetes mellitus. Br J Clin Pharmacol 1981;12:235–46.

[100] Eyal S, Easterling TR, Carr D, Umans JG, Miodovnik M, Hankins GD, et al. Pharmacokinetics of metformin during pregnancy. Drug Metab Dispos 2010;38:833–40.

[101] Barton JR, Prevost RR, Wilson DA, Whybrew WD, Sibai BM. Nifedipine pharmacokinetics and pharmacodynamics during the immediate postpartum period in patients with preeclampsia. Am J Obstet Gynecol 1991;165:951–4.

[102] Kimberlin DF, Weller S, Whitley RJ, Andrews WW, Hauth JC, Lakeman F, et al. Pharmacokinetics of oral valacyclovir and acyclovir in late pregnancy. Am J Obstet Gynecol 1998;179:846–51.

[103] Nelson MM, Forfar JO. Association between drugs administered during pregnancy and congenital abnormalities of the fetus. Br Med J 1971;1:523–7.

[104] Bonati M, Bortolus R, Marchetti F, Romero M, Tognoni G. Drug use in pregnancy: An overview of epidemiological (drug utilization) studies. Eur J Clin Pharmacol 1990;38:325–8.

[105] McBride WG. Thalidomide and congenital abnormalities [Letter]. Lancet 1961:ii1358.

[106] Lenz W. Kindliche missbildungen nach medikament während der gravidität. Deutsch Med Wschr 1961;86:2555–6.

[107] Morgan DJ. Drug disposition in mother and foetus. Clin Exp Pharmacol Physiol 1997;24:869–73.

[108] Martin CB. The anatomy and circulation of the placenta. In: Barnes AC, editor. Intra-uterine development. Philadelphia, PA: Lea & Febiger; 1968. p. 35–67.

[109] Castellucci M, Kaufmann P. Basic structure of the villous trees. In: Benirschke K, Kaufmann P, Baergen R, editors. Pathology of the human placenta. New York, NY: Springer; 2006. p. 50–120.

[110] van der Aa EM, Peereboom-Stegeman JH, Noordhoek J, Gribnau FW, Russel FG. Mechanisms of drug transfer across the human placenta. Pharm World Sci 1998;20:139–48.

[111] Vahakangas K, Myllynen P. Drug transporters in the human blood–placental barrier. Br J Pharmacol 2009; 158:665–78.

[112] Evseenko D, Paxton JW, Keelan JA. Active transport across the human placenta: Impact on drug efficacy and toxicity. Expert Opin Drug Metab Toxicol 2006;2:51–69.

[113] Grube M, Reuther S, Meyer Zu Schwabedissen H, Köch K, Draber K, Ritter CA, et al. Organic anion transporting polypeptide 2B1 and breast cancer resistance protein interact in the transepithelial transport of steroid sulfates in human placenta. Drug Metab Dispos 2007;35:30–5.

[114] Lankas GR, Wise LD, Cartwright ME, Pippert T, Umbenhauer DR. Placental P-glycoprotein deficiency enhances susceptibility to chemically induced birth defects in mice. Reprod Toxicol 1998;12:457–63.

[115] Prouillac C, Lecoeur S. The role of the placenta in fetal exposure to xenobiotics: Importance of membrane transporters and human models for transfer studies. Drug Metab Dispos 2010;38:1623–35.

[116] Syme MR, Paxton JW, Keelan JA. Drug transfer and metabolism by the human placenta. Clin Pharmacokinet 2004;43:487–514.

[117] Gottesman MM, Pastan I, Ambudkar SV. P-glycoprotein and multidrug resistance. Curr Opin Immunol 1996;6:610–7.

[118] Higgins CF. ABC transporters: From microorganisms to man. Annu Rev Cell Biol 1992;8:67–113.

[119] Schinkel AH, Wagenaar E, Mol CAAM, van Deemter L. P-glycoprotein in the blood–brain barrier of mice influences the brain penetration and pharmacological activity of many drugs. J Clin Invest 1996;97:2517–24.

[120] Mylona P, Glazier JD, Greenwood SL, Slides MK, Sibley CP. Expression of the cystic fibrosis (CF) and multidrug resistance (MDR1) genes during development and differentiation in the human placenta. Mol Hum Reprod 1996;2:693–8.

[121] Nakamura Y, Ikeda S, Furukawa T, Sumizawa T, Tani A, Akiyama S, et al. Function of P-glycoprotein expressed in placenta and mole. Biochem Biophys Res Commun 1997;235:849–53.

[122] Gil S, Saura R, Rorestier F, Farinotti R. P-glycoprotein expression of the human placenta during pregnancy. Placenta 2005;26:268–70.

[123] MacFarland A, Abramovich DR, Ewen SW, Pearson CK. Stage-specific distribution of P-glycoprotein in first-trimester and full-term human placenta. Histochem J 1994;26:417–23.

[124] Mathias AA, Hitti J, Unadkat JD. P-glycoprotein and breast cancer resistance protein expression in human placentae of various gestational ages. Am J Physiol Regul Integr Comp Physiol 2005;289:R963–9.

[125] Sun M, Kingdom J, Baczyk D, Lye SJ, Matthews SG, Gibb W. Expression of the multidrug resistance P-glycoprotein, (ABCB1 glycoprotein) in the human placenta decreases with advancing gestation. Placenta 2006;27:602–9.

[126] Ushigome F, Takanaga H, Matsuo H, Yanai S, Tsukimori K, Nakano H, et al. Human placental transport of vinblastine, vincristine, digoxin and progesterone: Contribution of P-glycoprotein. Eur J Pharmacol 2000;408:1–10.

[127] Smit JW, Huisman MT, van Tellingen O, Wiltshire HR, Schinkel AH. Absence or pharmacological blocking of placental P-glycoprotein profoundly increases fetal drug exposure. J Clin Invest 1999;104:1441–7.

[128] Pacifici GM, Nottoli R. Placental transfer of drugs administered to the mother. Clin Pharmacokinet 1995;28:235–69.

[129] Casey BM, Bawdon RE. Placental transfer of ritonavir with zidovudine in the ex vivo placental perfusion model. Am J Obstet Gynecol 1998;179:758–61.

[130] Marzolini C, Rudin C, Decosterd LA, Telenti A, Schreyer A, Biollaz J, et al. Transplacental passage of protease inhibitors at delivery. AIDS 2002;16:889–93.

[131] Sudhakaran S, Ghabriel M, Nation RL, Kong DC, Gude NM, Angus PW, et al. Differential bidirectional transfer of indinavir in the isolated perfused human placenta. Antimicrob Agents Chemother 2005;49:1023–8.

[132] Marzolini C, Kim RB. Placental transfer of antiretroviral drugs. Clin Pharmacol Ther 2005;78:118–22.

[133] Uhr M, Steckler T, Yassouridis A, Holsboer F. Penetration of amitriptyline, but not of fluoxetine, into brain is enhanced in mice with blood–brain barrier deficiency due to mdr1a P-glycoprotein gene disruption. Neuropsychopharmacology 2000;22:380–7.

[134] Weiss J, Dorrman S-MG, Martin-Facklam M, Kerpen CJ, Ketabi-Kiyanvash N, Haefell WE. Inhibition of P-glycoprotein by newer antidepressants. J Pharmacol Exp Ther 2003;305:197–204.

[135] Weiss J, Kerpen CJ, Lindenmaier H, Dormann S-MG, Haefelll WE. Interaction of antiepileptic drugs with human P-glycoprotein in vitro. J Pharmacol Exp Ther 2003;307:262–7.

[136] Rahi M, Heikkinen T, Hakkola J, Hakala K, Wallerman O, Wadelius M, et al. Influence of adenosine triphosphate and ABCB1 (MDR1) genotype on the P-glycoprotein-dependent transfer of saquinavir in the dually perfused human placenta. Hum Exp Toxicol 2008;27:65–71.

[137] Rahi M, Heikkinen T, Härtter S, Hakkola J, Hakala K, Wallerman O, et al. Placental transfer of quetiapine in relation to P-glycoprotein activity. J Psychopharmacol 2007;21:751–6.

[138] Hitzl M, Schaeffeler E, Hocher B, Slowinski T, Halle H, Eichelbaum M, et al. Variable expression of P-glycoprotein in the human placenta and its association with mutations of the multidrug resistance 1 gene (MDR1, ABCB1). Pharmacogenetics 2004;14:309–18.

[139] Tanabe M, Ieiri I, Nagata N, Inoue K, Ito S, Kanamori Y, et al. Expression of P-glycoprotein in human placenta: Relation to genetic polymorphism of the multidrug resistance (MDR)-1 gene. J Pharmacol Exp Ther 2001;297:1137–43.

[140] Evseenko DA, Paxton JW, Keelan JA. ABC drug transporter expression and functional activity in trophoblast-like cell lines and differentiating primary trophoblast. Am J Physiol Regul Integr Comp Physiol 2006;290:R1357–65.

[141] Yeboah D, Sun M, Kingdom J, Baczyk D, Lye SJ, Matthews SG, et al. Expression of breast cancer resistance protein (BCRP/ABCG2) in human placenta throughout gestation and at term before and after labor. Can J Physiol Pharmacol 2006;84:1251–8.

[142] Maliepaard M, Scheffer GL, Faneyte IF, van Gastelen MA, Pijnenborg AC, Schinkel AH. Subcellular localization and distribution of the breast cancer resistance protein transporter in normal human tissues. Cancer Res 2001;61:3458–64.

[143] Ceckova M, Libra A, Pavek P, Nachtigal P, Brabec M, Fuchs R, et al. Expression and functional activity of breast cancer resistance protein (BCRP, ABCG2) transporter in the human choriocarcinoma cell line BeWo. Clin Exp Pharmacol Physiol 2006;33:58–65.

[144] Allikmets R, Schriml LM, Hutchinson A, Romano-Spica V, Dean M. A human placenta-specific ATP-binding cassette gene (ABCP) on chromosome 4q22 that is involved in multidrug resistance. Cancer Res 1998;58:5337–9.

[145] Jonker JW, Smit JW, Brinkhuis RF, Maliepaard M, Beijnen JH, Schellens JH, et al. Role of breast cancer resistance protein in the bioavailability and fetal penetration of topotecan. J Natl Cancer Inst 2000;92:1651–6.

[146] Staud F, Vackova Z, Pospechova K, Pavek P, Ceckova M, Libra A, et al. Expression and transport activity of breast cancer resistance protein (Bcrp/Abcg2) in dually perfused rat placenta and HRP-1 cell line. J Pharmacol Exp Ther 2006;319:53–62.

[147] Enokizono J, Kusuhara H, Sugiyama Y. Effect of breast cancer resistance protein (Bcrp/Abcg2) on the disposition of phytoestrogens. Mol Pharmacol 2007;72:967–75.

[148] Zhang Y, Wang H, Unadkat JD, Mao Q. Breast cancer resistance protein 1 limits fetal distribution of nitrofurantoin in the pregnant mouse. Drug Metab Dispos 2007;35:2154–8.

[149] Merino G, Jonker JW, Wagenaar E, van Herwaarden AE, Schinkel AH. The breast cancer resistance protein (BCRP/ABCG2) affects pharmacokinetics, hepatobiliary excretion, and milk secretion of the antibiotic nitrofurantoin. Mol Pharmacol 2005;67:1758–64.

[150] Pollex E, Lubetsky A, Koren G. The role of placental breast cancer resistance protein in the efflux of glyburide across the human placenta. Placenta 2008;29:743–7.

[151] Elliott BD, Langer O, Schenker S, Johnson RF. Insignificant transfer of glyburide occurs across the human placenta. Am J Obstet Gynecol 1991;165:807–12.

[152] Cygalova LH, Hofman J, Ceckova M, Staud F. Transplacental pharmacokinetics of glyburide, rhodamine 123, and BODIPY FL prazosin: Effect of drug efflux transporters and lipid solubility. J Pharmacol Exp Ther 2009;331:1118–25.

[153] Gedeon C, Anger G, Piquette-Miller M, Koren G. Breast cancer resistance protein: Mediating the trans-placental transfer of glyburide across the human placenta. Placenta 2008;29:39–43.

[154] Zhou L, Naraharisetti SB, Wang H, Unadkat JD, Hebert MF, Mao Q. The breast cancer resistance protein (Bcrp1/Abcg2) limits fetal distribution of glyburide in the pregnant mouse: An Obstetric–Fetal Pharmacology Research Unit Network and University of Washington Specialized Center of Research Study. Mol Pharmacol 2008;73:949–59.

[155] Hemauer SJ, Patrikeeva SL, Wang X, Abdelrahman DR, Hankins GD, Ahmed MS, et al. Role of transporter-mediated efflux in the placental biodisposition of bupropion and its metabolite, OH-bupropion. Biochem Pharmacol 2010;80:1080–6.

[156] Evseenko DA, Paxton JW, Keelan JA. Independent regulation of apical and basolateral drug transporter expression and function in placental trophoblasts by cytokines, steroids, and growth factors. Drug Metab Dispos 2007;35: 595–601.

[157] Morgan ET, Goralski KB, Piquette-Miller M, Renton KW, Robertson GR, Chaluvadi MR, et al. Regulation of drug-metabolizing enzymes and transporters in infection, inflammation, and cancer. Drug Metab Dispos 2008;36:205–16.

[158] Wang H, Lee EW, Zhou L, Leung PC, Ross DD, Unadkat JD, et al. Progesterone receptor (PR) isoforms PRA and PRB differentially regulate expression of the breast cancer resistance protein in human placental choriocarcinoma BeWo cells. Mol Pharmacol 2008;73:845–54.

[159] Wang H, Unadkat JD, Mao Q. Hormonal regulation of BCRP expression in human placental BeWo cells. Pharm Res 2008;25:444–52.

[160] Jones KL. Smith's recognizable patterns of human malformation. 5th ed. Philadelphia, PA: WB Saunders; 1997.

[161] Wilson JG. Current status of teratology – general principles and mechanisms derived from animal studies. In: Wilson JG, Fraser FC, editors. Handbook of teratology. Vol. I: General principles and etiology. New York, NY: Plenum Press; 1977. p. 47–74.

[162] Brent RL. Radiation teratogenesis. Teratology 1980;21:281–98.

[163] Buehler BA, Delimont D, van Waes M, Finnell RH. Prenatal prediction of risk of the fetal hydantoin syndrome. N Engl J Med 1990;31:1567–72.

[164] Shaw GM, Wasserman CR, Lammer EJ, O'Malley CD, Murray JC, Basart AM, et al. Orofacial clefts, parental cigarette smoking, and transforming growth factor-alpha gene variants. Am J Hum Genet 1996;58:551–61.

[165] Therapontos C, Erskine L, Gardner ER, Figg WD, Vargesson N. Thalidomide induces limb defects by preventing angiogenic outgrowth during early limb formation. Proc Natl Acad Sci USA 2009;106:8573–8.

[166] Parman T, Wiley MJ, Wells PG. Free radical-mediated oxidative DNA damage in the mechanism of thalidomide teratogenicity. Nat Med 1999;5:582–5.

[167] Thalidomide product information. Summit NJ: Celgene Corporation. Internet at, www.thalomid.com/pdf/Thalomid%20PI%2072991-10.pdf.

[168] Begg EJ, Atkinson HC, Duffull SB. Prospective evaluation of a model for the prediction of milk : plasma drug concentrations from physicochemical characteristics. Br J Clin Pharmacol 1992;33:501–5.

[169] Stec GP, Greenberger P, Ruo TI, Henthorn T, Morita Y, Atkinson AJ Jr, et al. Kinetics of theophylline transfer to breast milk. Clin Pharmacol Ther 1980;28:404–8.

[170] Greenberger PA, Odeh YK, Frederiksen MC, Atkinson AJ Jr. Pharmacokinetics of prednisolone transfer to breast milk. Clin Pharmacol Ther 1993;53:324–8.

[171] Oo CY, Kuhn RJ, Desai N, McNamara PJ. Active transport of cimetidine into human milk. Clin Pharmacol Ther 1995;58:548–55.

[172] Sanders SW, Zone JJ, Foltz RL, Tolman KG, Rollins DE. Hemolytic anemia induced by dapsone transmitted through breast milk. Ann Intern Med 1982;96:465–6.

[173] Kwit NT, Hatcher RA. Excretion of drugs in milk. Am J Dis Child 1935;49:900–4.

[174] Meny RG, Naumburg EG, Alger LS, Brill-Miller JL, Brown S. Codeine and the breastfed neonate. J Hum Lact 1993;9:237–40.

[175] Koren G, Cairns J, Chitayat D, Gaedigk A, Leeder SJ. Pharmacogenetics of morphine poisoning in a breastfed neonate of a codeine-prescribed mother. Lancet 2006;368:704.

[176] Coffman BL, Rios GR, King CD, Tephly TR. Human UGT2B7 catalyzes morphine glucuronidation. Drug Metab Dispos 1997;25:1–4.

[177] Sawyer MB, Innocenti F, Das S, Cheng C, Ramirez J, Pantle-Fisher FH, et al. A pharmacogenetic study of uridine diphosphate-glucuronosyltransferase 2B7 in patients receiving morphine. Clin Pharmacol Ther 2003;73:566–74.

[178] Madadi P, Ross CJ, Hayden MR, Carleton BC, Gaedigk A, Leeder JS, et al. Pharmacogenetics of neonatal opioid toxicity following maternal use of codeine during breastfeeding: A case–control study. Clin Pharmacol Ther 2009;85:31–5.

# 25

# Pediatric Clinical Pharmacology and Therapeutics

Bridgette L. Jones[1,2], John N. Van Den Anker[3] and Gregory L. Kearns[1,4]

[1]Department of Pediatrics, and Divisions of Pediatric Clinical Pharmacology and Medical Toxicology,
University of Missouri–Kansas City School of Medicine, Kansas City, MO 64109
[2]Department of Medical Research, The Children's Mercy Hospital, Kansas City, MO 64108
[3]Departments of Pediatrics, Integrative Systems Biology, Pharmacology & Physiology, and Division of Pediatric Clinical Pharmacology,
The George Washington University School of Medicine and Health Sciences/Children's
National Medical Center, Washington, DC 20010
[4]Department of Pediatrics, University of Kansas School of Medicine, Kansas City, KS 66160

## INTRODUCTION

Children younger than 15 years old account for 28% of the population worldwide and about one quarter of the US population. As one must undergo the developmental trajectory of childhood to reach adulthood, any discussion of clinical pharmacology would be incomplete without inclusion of how development, the most dynamic period of human life, influences drug disposition and action and creates unique therapeutic scenarios that are not seen in adults.

Development, despite being a continuum of physiologic events that culminates in maturity, is often arbitrarily divided into the stages of infancy, childhood, adolescence, and even early adulthood. Across this period of time organ size and function change, as do body composition, protein expression, and cellular function. Some cellular components are active during early development and subsequently lose function with age, and *vice versa*. Some tissues may be more sensitive to pharmacologic effects early in life, whereas function may decline later in life. As these developmental changes in function and form occur, their implications must be considered, with respect both to the clinical pharmacology of drugs and to their appropriate place in pediatric pharmacotherapy.

## History of Pediatric Clinical Pharmacology

The practice of pediatrics developed out of the realization that illness affects children differently from adults. The same realization regarding the need to "individualize" drug therapy for infants and children fostered the birth of pediatric clinical pharmacology. In 1968, Dr Harry Shirkey wrote that "By an odd and unfortunate twist of fate, infants and children are becoming therapeutic or pharmaceutical orphans" [1]. Many of the laws regulating drug manufacturing, testing, and distribution, which were often the result of therapeutic tragedies in children, had the unfortunate result that relatively few drugs were being labeled for use in children. One specific pediatric tragedy was the death from renal failure of nearly 100 children who had ingested an elixir of sulfanilamide preparation made with diethylene glycol. As discussed in Chapter 36, this precipitated the US Food, Drug and Cosmetic Act of 1938 and the birth of the US Food and Drug Administration (FDA). In 1962 the Kefauver-Harris Amendment was enacted following another tragic event in which more than 10,000 children in 46 countries were born with limb deformities as a consequence of thalidomide exposure *in utero*, the drug being taken by pregnant mothers for nausea. The German pediatrician Widukind Lenz suspected a link between birth defects and the drug, which he subsequently proved in 1961. Prior to this knowledge, Dr Frances Oldham Kelsey, a clinical pharmacologist serving as a medical officer at the FDA, became an at-the-time unknown hero (she was later awarded the medal for Distinguished Federal Civilian Service by President John F. Kennedy) by denying approval (and subsequent marketing) of thalidomide in the United States due to a lack safety data. Dr Kelsey's apprehension regarding the drug was partly spurred by her previous research in which she found that pregnant rabbits and embryonic rabbits metabolized quinine differently than non-pregnant mature rabbits. She also had suspicions that thalidomide might be toxic in developing fetuses after hearing reports that the drug was a possible cause of nerve damage in adults [2]. Thus, it was her understanding of developmental and clinical pharmacology that led Dr Kelsey to a decision that prevented this pediatric drug tragedy from reaching the US.

The bitter irony of these early laws and regulatory decisions is that they put forward the practice of therapeutic restriction as the primary means to maximize drug safety in pediatric patients. Thus, these laws did not actually benefit children as much as they could have because pediatric patients were excluded from the study of therapeutic drugs, many of which even were intended for pediatric use. In fact, the laws actually led to drug labeling that included warnings for most new drugs, stating that they were not recommended for use in children because inadequate (or non-existent) data had been obtained in these patients. This led Dr Shirkey to describe children as "therapeutic orphans", and to issue a call to academia, industry, and government to actively take responsibility for prudently including children in the development programs of drugs intended for pediatric use [1]. Despite this profound unmet need, little progress in making safe and effective drugs for children was made for almost three decades after this call to action was issued.

However, government mandates were initiated in the mid-1990s that provided provisions to ensure future progress in pediatric drug development. In 1994, the FDA issued a Pediatric Rule stating that if the course of the disease and/or the response to a given drug was similar in children and adults, labeling of drugs for pediatric use would be allowed based on extrapolation of efficacy in adults and additional pharmacokinetic (PK), pharmacodynamic (PD), and safety studies in pediatric populations. Unfortunately, this rule prompted the conduct of only a small number of well-designed and well-executed pediatric studies. For this reason the FDA Modernization Act (FDAMA) was passed in 1997, which granted sponsors 6 months of extended market exclusivity for new drugs in exchange for pediatric studies that were completed in accordance with a written request from the FDA. This Act also mandated that a list be compiled of already approved drugs for which additional information was needed for pediatric labeling, and again provided additional market exclusivity if pediatric studies were performed for these drugs [3]. In 2002 the Best Pharmaceuticals for Children Act was signed, which provided mechanisms for studying on- and off-patent drugs in children. This act extended the 6 months' exclusivity provided in 1997 under the FDAMA to include pediatric studies of drugs currently under patent in addition to non-patent drugs in which studies are initiated via an FDA Written Request. In 2003 the Pediatric Research Equity Act (PREA) was passed into US law, and mandated the conduct of pediatric clinical trials for drugs under development that had the potential for significant pediatric use. The Act also expanded labeling of approved drugs that were used extensively in infants and children but did not have adequate pediatric labeling. Finally, the BPCA and PREA provisions were renewed in the 2007 Food and Drug Administration Amendments Act (FDAAA) and sections were added pertaining to the study of pediatric devices, requiring the FDA to actively monitor the safety of all the drugs studied under the provisions of this legislation.

Collectively, these initiatives have brought about a marked increase in the number of pediatric clinical trials that characterize the clinical pharmacology of both the old and new drugs that are used in pediatric patients, and have led to improvements in pediatric dosing and labeling. As of 2012, 426 drugs had a new pediatric label which included new dosing, dosing changes, or PK information, new safety data, lack-of-efficacy data, new formulations, and dosing instructions that extend the age limits for use in children [4]. These initiatives also have had global impact in creating the framework for similar European regulations which require that children be included in clinical trials of drugs intended to be used in their treatment. Despite the improvements in pediatric therapeutics that have been driven by these regulations, a significant number of drugs, particularly many that have been used for years in pediatric practice, have both insufficient pediatric labeling and incomplete knowledge regarding their pharmacologic properties. Thus, many information gaps exist which pose serious safety concerns as drugs continue to be used in pediatric patients in the absence of complete knowledge of their clinical pharmacology.

## Developmental Clinical Pharmacology

Normal human development represents a dynamic continuum with aspects that are overtly evident (e.g., acquisition of speech, mobility, linear growth, accretion of body weight, pubertal onset) and others that are not (e.g., maturation of renal and hepatic function, neuronal development). Throughout development, the impact of ontogeny on PK and PD is, to a great degree, predictable and follows definable physiologic "patterns". Examples are illustrated in Figure 25.1 [5] and described in greater detail in the sections that follow.

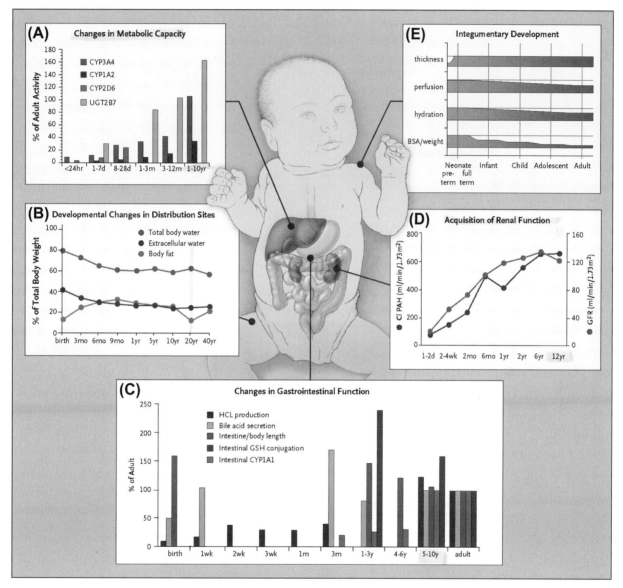

**FIGURE 25.1** Developmental changes in physiologic in multiple organs and organ systems during development are responsible for age-related differences in drug disposition. *Panel A* shows that the activity of many cytochrome P450 (CYP) isoforms and a single glucuronosyltransferase (UGT) isoform is markedly diminished during the first 2 months of life. The acquisition of adult activity over time also is enzyme- and isoform-specific. *Panel B* shows age-dependent changes in body composition, which influence the apparent distribution volume for drugs. Infants in the first 6 months of life have larger TBW and ECF relative to total body weight than older infants and adults. *Panel C* shows the age-dependent changes in gastrointestinal tract structure and function. As with hepatic drug-metabolizing enzymes, the activity of CYP1A1 in the intestine is low during early life. *Panel D* summarizes the effect of postnatal development on the GFR and active tubular secretion, both of which approximate adult activity by 6–12 months of age. *Panel E* shows age dependence in the thickness, extent of perfusion, and extent of hydration of the skin and the relative size of the skin surface area, which are reflected in the ratio of body surface area to body weight). Modified from Kearns GL, Abdel-Rahman SM, Alander SW *et al.* N Engl J Med 2003;349:1157–67 [5].

# ONTOGENY OF PHARMACOKINETICS IN CHILDREN

## Oral Absorption

As in adults, most medications administered to infants and children are given via the peroral route, and development can influence both the rate and extent of drug absorption. During the first few years of life, there are significant changes in gastric pH related to the density and function of parietal cells which are present early in fetal life in the antrum and body of the stomach. However, at term only about 20% of neonates possess the proportion of parietal cells in the antrum that is observed in adults [6]. The highest gastric pH levels (6–8) occur in the neonate immediately after birth and within hours drop to 2–3. With parietal cell maturation, gastric pH gradually decreases over the next few years, reaching adult levels by 3–7 years of age (Figure 25.1C). In the case of drugs that are weak organic acids with a narrow therapeutic index (e.g., phenytoin), this developmental difference may result in the need for more frequent dose adjustments to achieve the desired therapeutic level in younger children. During the neonatal period and infancy, the oral bioavailability of acid labile drugs (e.g., beta-lactam antibiotics) may be increased because higher gastric pH results in their reduced degradation. Similar considerations should also be made for sick preterm infants in whom gastric pH is lower than in healthy preterm infants [7]. In addition, one must consider the impact of feeding on gastric pH and its effects on drug absorption, because feedings with infant formula increase gastric pH, buffering it to levels > 4 for up to 90 minutes after a feed. Finally, human breast milk contains large amounts of epidermal growth factor, a peptide that also inhibits gastric acid secretion.

Gastric emptying rates also exhibit significant developmental differences that may alter the rate of drug absorption. In the fetus, between 26 weeks gestational age and term (38 weeks) the liquid gastric emptying time is approximately 45 minutes, compared with a normal adult emptying time of about 20 minutes [6]. Prolonged gastric emptying times in infancy can delay delivery of orally administered drugs to the small intestine, where the majority of absorption takes place. By 6–8 months of age, gastric emptying times are faster and usually comparable to rates observed in adults. For drugs with limited water solubility (e.g., carbamazepine, phenytoin), gastric emptying rate may significantly influence both the rate and extent of bioavailability by reducing their residence time in the small intestine.

Finally, intestinal drug-metabolizing enzymes (e.g., CYP3A4/5, CYP1A, *N*-acetyltransferase, xanthine oxidase, glutathione-*S*-transferase) and transporters (e.g., P-glycoprotein, organic anion and cation transporters) whose activity likely varies with developmental stage may also alter the bioavailability of drugs [8]. In humans, the expression of these proteins appears to reach adult levels between 6 and 12 months of age. Glutathione-*S*-transferase activity and bile acid secretion also exhibit developmental differences that may affect drug exposure (Figure 25.1C). Other factors, such as differences in intestinal microbial flora, have also been proposed to affect intestinal drug absorption in infants.

## Extravascular Absorption

Development can also alter the systemic exposure to drugs given by extravascular routes of administration (e.g., dermal, subcutaneous, buccal, intramuscular, rectal, intraosseous, intrapulmonary). For example, the perfusion and hydration status of the stratum corneum is altered in young infants (Figure 25.1E) and this can facilitate transdermal absorption of specific drugs, thereby predisposing neonates and young infants to potential systemic toxicity as has been reported for corticosteroid- and diphenhydramine-containing drug products [9]. Such toxicity can be further exacerbated by conditions (e.g., eczema) that disrupt the integumentary barrier.

The rate of absorption of intramuscularly administered drugs in neonates can be reduced (i.e., slower absorption rate relative to older children and adults) consequent to their reduced skeletal muscle blood flow and inefficient muscular contractions, which together work to disperse drug within large muscles. However, the density of skeletal muscle capillaries is higher in infants than in older children and adults, and appears to lead to a more efficient intramuscular absorption of specific agents (e.g., amikacin and cephalothin) in this age group.

Absorption of rectally administered agents may be reduced in infants because they have a greater number of high-amplitude pulsatile contractions in the rectum than adults and are prone to premature expulsion of solid rectal drug formulations (e.g., suppositories). In contrast, rectal solutions of drugs such as diazepam (which is commonly prescribed for outpatient emergency treatment of seizures) are readily and rapidly absorbed in children, achieving therapeutic plasma concentrations within 4 minutes of administration [10]. On the other hand, the bioavailability of some rectally administered drugs is greater in neonates and young infants than in older infants (i.e., > 6–12 months) and children because of the reduced activity of many of their hepatic drug metabolizing enzymes (Figure 25.1A).

Inhaled medications are often used to treat conditions that commonly occur in the pediatric population, such as bronchiolitis, croup, cystic fibrosis, chronic lung disease of prematurity, and asthma. Developmental differences in airway surface area, chest wall compliance, functional residual capacity, and hypoxic drive have the potential to influence both the local and systemic exposure to drugs that are administered via inhalation. For example, impactor studies, which measure amounts of deposited drug on body surface areas after inhalation, have shown that a larger proportion of inhaled drug is deposited in the oropharyngeal area (greater than five-fold for some agents) relative to adults because infants have smaller upper airway dimensions [11]. In addition, lung deposition increases and oropharyngeal deposition decreases with increasing age (lung deposition from the same inhaler/spacer combination 1–2% in infants, 4–6% in 2- to 6-year-old children, and 12% in a 10-year-old child). The efficacy of medications administered by inhalation may also be affected by psychomotor development (e.g., manual dexterity, coordination of actuation with inhalation) which can limit their effective delivery to the lung.

## Distribution

Changes in drug distribution during development are largely associated with changes in body composition and the quantity and nature of plasma proteins capable of drug binding. As reflected in Figure 25.1B, significant age-dependent changes in body composition occur. When expressed as a percentage of total body mass, neonates and young infants have significantly higher extracellular fluid (ECF) and total body water (TBW) volumes (e.g., TBW = 80% in infants vs 65% in adults). In contrast, the percentage of intracellular water (ICW) as a function of body mass remains stable from the first months of life through adulthood (Figure 25.1B). Age-dependent changes in body composition can alter the apparent volume of distribution ($V_d$) for both hydrophilic and lipophilic drugs. For example, as described in Chapter 3, aminoglycoside antibiotics distribute in a central compartment that corresponds to ECF, so the corresponding $V_d$ for these drugs is increased in neonates (0.4–0.7 L/kg) relative to adults (usually ~0.2 L/kg). While higher relative body fat is observed in infants and children (Figure 25.1B), this does not appear to markedly alter L/kg estimates of $V_d$ for most therapeutic drugs, although it must be considered under certain circumstances (e.g., obesity) and for extremely lipophilic agents (see Chapter 3). Although neonates tend to have a lower percentage of total body fat than older infants, lipid content in the developing central nervous system (CNS) is high and this situation has implications for the distribution of lipophilic drugs and their CNS effects (e.g., propranolol) in neonates. Special consideration must also be made for overweight and obese children, as prevalence of obese children has been reported to have doubled between 1970 and 1990 [12]. Studies have found that obese children have significantly higher body volume, lean mass, fat mass, and TBW than non-obese children [13]. Drug dose adjustments, especially for agents with a narrow therapeutic index (e.g., aminoglycosides, cancer chemotherapeutic agents), must therefore be made in obese children so as to prevent either under- or over-dosing and thus provide the optimal systemic exposure for the desired drug effects [14].

Circulating plasma protein concentrations, albumin and $\alpha_1$-acid glycoprotein, are influenced by disease state, nutrition, and age. The proteins are present in relatively low concentrations (~80% of adult) in the young infant and neonate, but adult levels are usually reached by 1 year of age. Similar patterns are also observed for $\alpha_1$-acid glycoprotein, where neonatal plasma concentrations are approximately three times lower than in maternal plasma and attain adult values by approximately 1 year of age. These proteins are not only quantitatively diminished in young children but are also immature and, compared to adults, their drug-binding ability is reduced because fetal albumin present in neonates has a lower binding capacity for weak acids. For example, phenytoin is more extensively (~94% to 98%) bound to albumin in adults than in neonates (80–85%), and, as described in Chapter 5 for adults with impaired renal function, the resultant six- to eight-fold difference in the free fraction can in neonates result in CNS adverse effects when total plasma phenytoin concentrations are within the generally accepted "therapeutic range" of 10–20 mg/L. Endogenous substances in the neonate, such as bilirubin and free fatty acids, may also displace drugs from their albumin binding sites and *vice versa*. For example, sulfonamides have an albumin binding affinity that exceeds that of bilirubin, and their administration to neonates can lead to excess free bilirubin concentrations that have the potential to produce CNS injury (e.g., kernicterus).

## Drug Transport

Drug transporters, such as P-glycoprotein (P-gp), multidrug resistance protein 1 (MRP1), and breast cancer resistance protein (BCRP), may influence both drug distribution and elimination. Limited data in humans suggest that both P-gp and MRP1 expression follow a developmental pattern [15]. P-gp is expressed in the human CNS as early as 27 weeks' gestation, with expression intensity becoming highest at 33 weeks' gestation. There is also differential expression within various regions of the brain in relation to age [15]. P-gp in the liver also follows a developmental pattern of expression in which activity increases during the first few months of life and adult levels are reached by 2 years of age [16].

## Drug Metabolism

Drug metabolism exhibits marked developmental dependence, especially during fetal and early postnatal life. The liver undergoes significant development during fetal and early childhood after its origin in the fourth week of gestation as a duodenal diverticulum. By the sixth week of fetal life hepatic lobules are present, and the liver represents 10% of fetal weight by the ninth week of gestation [17]. As the architecture of the liver develops, so do the families of enzymes responsible for the biosynthesis and metabolism of both endogenous and exogenous substrates.

### Cytochrome P450 Enzymes

The cytochrome P450 family of enzymes (CYPs) is responsible for the biotransformation of numerous endogenous substrates (e.g., adrenal steroids) and therapeutic agents, and there are considerable changes in the expression and activity of these enzymes during development. At birth the total hepatic CYP concentration is approximately 30% that of adults, and there are variable rates of both quantitative and functional maturation [18, 19]. As illustrated by Figure 25.1A, CYP1A2 activity begins to rise at 8–28 days of postnatal life and reaches adult activity by 1 year of age [20]. Diet has also been shown to affect the ontogeny of CYP1A2 activity, and formula-fed infants acquire function more rapidly than do breast-fed infants [21].

The CYP3A subfamily is the most abundant of the hepatic CYPs and is responsible for the biotransformation of approximately 50% of the therapeutic drugs that are administered to pediatric patients (e.g., salmeterol, cyclosporine, tacrolimus, midazolam, fentanyl, macrolide antibiotics), with CYP3A4, CYP3A5, and CYP3A7 being the enzymes that are most relevant for pediatric pharmacotherapy. CYP3A7 was found to be the most abundant CYP3A isoform in fetal liver samples obtained from 76 days to 32 weeks of gestation, and continues to be the predominant CYP

enzyme during the first 1–2 months of life [22]. However, a "switch" from CYP3A7 to CYP3A4 predominance begins to occur at birth, with the activity of the former progressively declining toward adult levels during the first year of life to a level that is approximately 7% of fetal levels [23]. The high activity of this enzyme early in fetal life is associated with its function in forming a precursor for estriol biosynthesis, a hormone that is important in fetal growth and timing of parturition. In contrast, the activity of CYP3A4 is minimal in the fetus and only 10% of adult levels at birth, but rises steadily during the neonatal period and early childhood, probably reaching adult levels in early adolescence (Figure 25.1A) [23, 24]. CY3A4 and CY3A5 have overlapping substrate specificities and in the case of the latter, polymorphic expression with racial differences in the genotype–phenotype relationship exist that can have significant effects on the biotransformation of drugs that are substrates for this isoform [25, 26]. While the presence of CYP3A5 has been demonstrated across the developmental continuum, a clear developmental pattern for its expression has not yet been fully elucidated.

As discussed in Chapter 13, CYP2D6 is a polymorphically expressed enzyme in humans and is responsible for the biotransformation of approximately 12% of drugs used in pediatric practice (e.g. β-receptor antagonists, antiarrhythmics, antidepressants, morphine derivatives, antipsychotics, dextromethorphan, diphenhydramine, atomoxetine, metoclopramide). CYP2D6 has not been consistently detected in the fetal period, and its activity remains low (approximately 5–10% of adult activity) during the first few weeks of life. Interestingly, expression of this enzyme appears to be independent of gestational age in newborns, which suggests that there is a birth-dependent process that activates its expression. After birth there is a steady increase in CYP2D6 activity, with levels approximating 30% and 70% of adult activity at 1 month and 1–5 years of life, respectively [27]. However, *in vivo* longitudinal phenotyping studies have revealed that genotype–phenotype relationships are present as early as 2 weeks postnatal age and that genotype contributes more importantly than ontogeny to the interindividual variability of CYP2D6 enzyme activity [28].

CYP2C9 is a polymorphically expressed enzyme that catalyzes the biotransformation of several important drugs used in pediatrics (e.g., phenytoin, ibuprofen, indomethacin). CYP2C9 has been detected at very low levels (1% of adult levels) in early gestation (earliest at 8 weeks). At term, activity increases to approximately 10% of that observed in adults, and is approximately 25% of adult levels by 5–6 months of age. A similar pattern of developmental expression is demonstrated for CYP2C19, an enzyme that is also polymorphically expressed and is largely responsible for the biotransformation of proton pump inhibitors (e.g., lansoprazole, omeprazole, pantoprazole, esomeprazole, rabeprazole) – a drug class used extensively in neonates and infants with gastroesophageal reflux. As illustrated in Figure 25.2, CYP2C19 activity increases quickly after birth and reaches adult levels at approximately 6 months postnatally [29]. As is the case for CYP2C9, genotype–phenotype concordance is expected at this point and predictive relationships appear between the *CYP2C19* genotype and the activity of the enzyme [29]. In examining the ontogeny of both CYP2C9 and CYP2C19, as is the case with most of the cytochrome P450 isoforms, significant intersubject variability occurs across the developmental continuum (Figure 25.2). Also, when constitutive activity of the enzyme is normally low shortly after birth, genotype–phenotype discordance can lead to erroneous classification of metabolizer status.

Of the CYP isoforms quantitatively important for drug metabolism in humans, all studied to date appear to have a developmental pattern with respect to the attainment of activity. Although it is beyond the scope of this chapter to provide a detailed description for each enzyme, this has been accomplished in a recent review [30], and an overview is summarized in Table 25.1 [31].

### Phase II Biotransformations

A historical catastrophe in pediatric clinical pharmacology, the chloramphenical-associated "Grey Baby Syndrome", was a sentinel event that demonstrated the impact of development on the activity of a Phase II drug-metabolizing enzyme (UDP glucuronosyltransferase, or UGT). More importantly, this event illustrated how failure to recognize these differences and account for them in determining age-appropriate drug doses can lead to unnecessary morbidity and mortality. As with chloramphenicol, morphine, acetaminophen and zidovudine are also UGT substrates that require dose regimen alterations to compensate for reduced enzyme activity in the first weeks and months of life. In premature infants (gestational age 24–37 weeks), the plasma clearance of morphine, a predominant UGT2B7 and UGT1A1 substrate, is five-fold lower relative to older children and generally reaches adult levels between 2 and 6 months of life, although considerable variability exists [32]. Acetaminophen glucuronidation, mediated by UGT1A6 and UGT1A9, is present in the fetus and newborn at very low levels (1–10% of adults). Following birth, activity steadily increases, with levels approaching ~50% of adult levels by 6 months of age and with full maturation by puberty. A similar maturation pattern is seen for zidovudine, a substrate for UGT2B7. Zidovudine clearance is significantly reduced in children < 2 years of age relative to older children, with the result that they have a higher risk of hematologic toxicity (anemia) from this drug [33]. Similar to what is seen for the UGT isoforms, ontogenic profiles also exist for glutathione-S-transferase (GST), *N*-acetyltransferase (NAT), epoxide hydroxylase, and the sulfotransferases (SULT). These profiles are summarized in Table 25.2 [34], and are discussed in a previously published authoritative review [30].

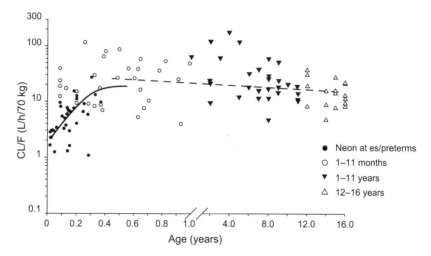

**FIGURE 25.2** *In vivo* assessment of drug-metabolizing activity as a function of age, using oral clearance of pantoprazole as a marker for CYP2C19 activity. The activity of this enzyme is considerably reduced in neonates and preterm infants relative to older age groups. Reproduced from Kearns GL, Leeder JS, Gaedigk A. Drug Metab Dispos 2010;38:894–7 [29].

**TABLE 25.1** Developmental Patterns for the Ontogeny of Phase I Drug- Metabolizing Enzymes in Humans[a]

| Enzymes | Known developmental pattern |
|---|---|
| CYP2D6 | Low to absent in fetal liver but present at 1 week of age. Poor activity (i.e., 20% of adult) by 1 month. Adult competence by 3—5 years of age. |
| Substrates | SSRIs (fluoxetine, paroxetine, sertraline), risperidone, atomoxetine, promethazine, dextromethorphan, diphenhydramine, chlorpheneramine. |
| CYP2C19 | Apparently absent in fetal liver. Low activity in first 2—4 weeks of life, with adult activity reached by approximately 6 months. Activity may exceed adult levels during childhood and declines to adult levels after conclusion of puberty. |
| Substrates | Proton pump inhibitors (omeprazole, pantoprazole, lansoprazole), propranolol. |
| CYP2C9 | Detected at very low levels (1% of adult levels) in early gestation (earliest at 8 weeks). At term, activity increases to approximately 10% of that observed in adults; by 5—6 months of age, activity is approximately 25% of adult levels. |
| Substrates | Warfarin, phenytoin, ibuprofen, indomethacin. |
| CYP1A2 | Not present in appreciable levels in human fetal liver. Adult levels reached by approximately 4 months and exceeded in children at 1—2 years of age. Adult activity reached after puberty. |
| Substrates | Clozapine, clomipramine, caffeine, haloperidol, ondansetron, theophylline. |
| CYP3A7 | Fetal form of CYP3A which is functionally active (and inducible) during gestation. Virtually disappears by 1—4 weeks postnatal, when CYP3A4 activity predominates, but remains present in approximately 5% of individuals. |
| CYP3A4 | Extremely low activity at birth reaching approximately 30—40% of adult activity by 1 month and full adult activity by 6 months. May exceed adult activity between 1 and 4 years of age, decreasing to adult levels after puberty |
| Substrates (3A7 & 3A4) | Cyclosporine, erythromycin, lidocaine, midazolam, nifedipine, tacrolimus, verapamil, zolpidem. |
| CYP2E1 | Undetectable expression in the fetal liver. In newborn livers, levels are 10% those in adults. Steady increase of expression with age. Adult levels are reached in children between 1 and 10 years of age. There is a strong association between protein levels and activity along the developmental spectrum. |
| Substrates | Anesthetics (halothane, isoflurane, enflurane), acetaminophen. |
| CYP2B6 | Variable detection in fetal liver and at low levels relative to adults (median levels approximately 15% of adult). There is an approximate two-fold increase in median expression after the neonatal period (birth to 30 days postnatal) with considerable variability. Expression is less variable in infants and children, with median levels reported at approximately 40% of adults. |

Abbreviations: CYP, cytochrome P450; SSRIs, serotonin selective reuptake inhibitors.
Adapted from Leeder JS, Kearns GL. Pediatr Clin North Am 1997;44:55—57 [31].

## Drug Elimination

Drug elimination in pediatric patients can occur via multiple routes, including exhalation, biliary secretion, and renal clearance. Of these, the kidney is the primary organ responsible for the excretion of drugs and their metabolites. The development of renal function begins during early fetal development, and is complete by early childhood (Figure 25.1D). From a developmental perspective, renal function is highly dependent on gestational age and postnatal adaptations. Renal function begins to mature early during fetal organogenesis and is complete by early childhood. Increases in glomerular filtration rate (GFR) result from both nephrogenesis, a process that is completed by 34 weeks of gestation, and changes in renal and intrarenal blood flow [35]. GFR varies widely among different postconceptional ages and ranges from approximately $2-4 \, \text{ml}/\text{min}/1.73 \, \text{m}^2$ in term neonates to a low of $0.6-0.8 \, \text{ml}/\text{min}/1.73 \, \text{m}^2$ in preterm neonates. GFR increases rapidly during the first 2 weeks of life, then more slowly until adult values are reached by 8–12 months of postnatal age [36–38] (Table 25.3). Development impacts not only GFR but also tubular secretion, which is immature at birth and reaches adult capacity during the first year of life (Figure 25.1D).

Developmental changes in renal function are better characterized than for any other organ system. For drugs that have substantial renal clearance, kidney function serves as a major determinant of age-specific drug dosing regimens. Failure to account for the ontogeny of renal function and adjust dosing regimens accordingly can result in a degree of systemic exposure that increases the risk of drug-associated adverse events. For example, digoxin is predominantly eliminated by the kidneys and its plasma clearance is markedly reduced in neonates and young infants,

**TABLE 25.2 Ontogeny of Phase II Drug Metabolizing Enzymes in the Neonate**

| Enzyme | Prenatal trimester | | | Neonate | 1 month to 1 year |
|---|---|---|---|---|---|
| | 1 | 2 | 3 | | |
| GSTA1/A2 | + | + | + | + | + |
| GSTM | + | + | + | + | + |
| GSTP1 | + | + | + | + | 0 |
| NAT2 | + | + | + | + | + |
| UGT1A1 | 0 | 0 | 0 | + | + |
| UGT1A3 | ? | + | + | + | + |
| UGT1A6 | 0 | 0 | 0 | + | + |
| UGTB7 | ? | + | + | + | + |
| UGTB17 | ? | + | + | + | + |
| EPHX1 | + | + | + | + | + |
| EPHX2 | ? | + | + | + | + |
| SULT1A1 | ? | + | + | + | + |
| SULT1A3 | ? | + | + | + | + |
| SULT2A1 | 0 | 0 | + | + | + |

+, Activity or protein detectable; 0, activity or protein not detectable; ?, undetermined.

Abbreviations: GST, glutathione *S*-transferase; NAT, *N*-acetyltransferase; UGT, uridine 5'-diphospho-glucuronosyltransferase; EPHX, epoxide hydrolase; SULT, sulfotransferase

Adapted from Blake MJ, Castro L, Leeder JS, Kearns GL. Semin Fetal Neonatal Med 2005;10:123-38 [34].

**TABLE 25.3 Glomerular Filtration Rate According to Age**

| Age (sex) | Mean GFR ± SD (mL/min/1.73 m²) |
|---|---|
| 1 week (males and females) | 40.6 ± 14.8 |
| 2–8 weeks (males and females) | 65.8 ± 24.8 |
| > 8 weeks (males and females) | 95.7 ± 21.7 |
| 2–12 years (males and females) | 133.0 ± 27.0 |
| 13–21 years (males) | 140.0 ± 30.0 |
| 13–21 years (females) | 126.0 ± 22.0 |

Reproduced with permission from National Kidney Foundation. Clinical practice guidelines (Internet at, http://www.kidney.org/professionals/kdoqi/ guidelines_ckd/Gif_File/kck_t24.gif [38]).

approaching adult values only when both GFR and active tubular secretory capacity mature (Figure 25.1D) [39]. Failure to adjust the dose and dosing interval for digoxin to compensate for developmentally associated differences in its plasma clearance can produce significant toxicity, especially given the low therapeutic index for this drug [40]. Another example is provided by gentamicin, for which a starting dosage interval of 12 hours in infants of any gestational age, or a starting dosage interval of

24 hours for infants of less than 30 weeks gestational age, has been shown to lead to serum gentamicin trough levels in the toxic range [41]. It is also important to note that use of some medications concomitantly (i.e., betamethasone and indomethacin) may alter the normal progress of renal maturation in the neonate [42]. Therefore, both maturation and concomitant treatment can affect renal function and are important to consider when designing appropriate drug dose regimens in neonates and infants.

As denoted above, development produces profound differences in processes that collectively, can influence all facets of drug disposition (i.e., absorption, distribution, metabolism, and excretion). Knowledge of the impact of ontogeny on the physiologic determinants of drug disposition enables prediction of how development can impact PK, and also enables prescribers to use this information to design age-appropriate pediatric drug regimens. A recent review by Rakhmanina and van den Anker describes the implications of developmental PK on pediatric therapeutics, and the information presented is summarized in Table 25.4 [43].

## DEVELOPMENTAL PHARMACODYNAMICS

As with drug disposition, drug action appears in many instances to have a profound dependence upon development. Developmental PD has been described as the study of age-related maturation of the structure and function of biologic systems and how this affects drug response. Relative to PK data, there is paucity of information regarding developmental PD. However, studies in animals and the few studies that have been conducted in children provide important insight into some of the potential differences that must be considered in the pediatric age group.

### Drug Receptors

There is evidence that differences in receptor number, density, distribution, function, and ligand-binding affinity differ among children of differing ages and adults. Much of the data demonstrating these differences is acquired from studies of the CNS and peripheral nervous systems. Specifically, receptors for γ-aminobutyric acid (GABA), the most prevalent inhibitory neurotransmitter, have been found in animals to be reduced early in infancy [44]. A recent study in humans found that the GABA$_A$ receptor, which binds benzodiazepines and barbiturates, has significantly higher CNS expression levels in children at the age of 2 years as compared to older children and

**TABLE 25.4    Summary of Developmentally Dependent Changes in Drug Disposition**

| Physiologic system | Age-related trends | Pharmacokinetic implications | Clinical implications |
|---|---|---|---|
| Gastrointestinal tract | Neonates and young infants: reduced and irregular peristalsis with prolonged gastric emptying time. Neonates: greater intragastric pH ($> 4$) relative to infants. Infants: enhanced lower GI motility. | Slower rate of drug absorption (e.g., increased $T_{max}$) without compensatory compromise in the extent of bioavailability. Reduced retention of suppository formulations. | Potential delay in the onset of drug action following oral administration. Potential for reduced extent of bioavailability from rectally administered drugs. |
| Integument | Neonates and young infants: thinner stratum corneum (neonates only), greater cutaneous perfusion, enhanced hydration and greater ratio of total BSA to body mass. | Enhanced rate and extent of percutaneous drug absorption. Greater relative exposure of topically applied drugs as compared to adults. | Enhanced percutaneous bioavailability and potential for toxicity. Need to reduce amount of drugs applied to skin. |
| Body compartments | Neonates and infants: decreased fat, decreased muscle mass, increased extracellular and total body water spaces. | Increased apparent volume of distribution for drugs distributed to body water spaces and reduced apparent volume of distribution for drugs that bind to muscle and/or fat. | Requirement of higher weight normalized (i.e., mg/kg) drug doses to achieve therapeutic plasma drug concentrations. |
| Plasma protein binding | Neonates: decreased concentrations of albumin and $\alpha_1$-acid glycoprotein with reduced binding affinity for albumin-bound weak acids. | Increased unbound concentrations for highly protein-bound drugs with increased apparent volume of distribution and potential for toxicity if the amount of free drug increases in the body. | For highly bound (i.e., $> 70\%$) drugs, need to adjust dose to maintain plasma levels near the low end of the recommended "therapeutic range". |
| Drug-metabolizing enzyme (DME) activity | Neonates and young infants: immature isoforms of cytochrome P450 and phase II enzymes with discordant patterns of developmental expression. Children 1–6 years: apparent increased activity for selected DMEs over adult normal values. Adolescents: attainment of adult activity after puberty. | Neonates and young infants: decreased plasma drug clearance early in life with an increase in apparent elimination half life. Children 1–6 years: increased plasma drug clearance (i.e., reduced elimination half-life) for specific pharmacologic substrates of DMEs. | Neonates and young infants: increased drug dosing intervals and/or reduced maintenance doses. Children 1–6 years: for selected drugs, need to increase dose and/or shorten dose interval in comparison to usual adult dose. |
| Renal drug excretion | Neonates and young infants: decreased glomerular flitration rates (first 6 months) and active tubular secretion (first 12 months) with adult values attained by 24 months. | Neonates and young infants: accumulation of renally excreted drugs and/or active metabolites with reduced plasma clearance and increased elimination half-life, greatest during first 3 months of life. | Neonates and young infants: increased drug dosing intervals and/or reduced maintenance doses during the first 3 months of life. |

Reproduced with permission from Rakhmanina NY, van den Anker JN. Adv Drug Deliv Rev 2006;58:4–14 [43].

adults. These data suggest that the expression of GABA receptors increases rapidly early in infancy, then subsequently declines with age. In addition, there is evidence in animal models that GABA actually has excitatory functions early in development because neurons have relatively high chloride concentrations when GABA opens chloride channels, and this leads to neuronal depolarization and excitation. With maturation, intracellular chloride concentrations decrease when GABA opens these chloride channels, causing neuronal hyperpolarization and inhibition of excitation. These changes may explain why infants require relatively larger doses of anti-epileptic medications (e.g., midazolam) to control seizures and furthermore explain why some infants experience seizures when treated with benzodiazepines. In animal studies, neonatal exposure to GABAergic agents (anticonvulsants, IV and inhaled anesthetics) during synaptogenesis accelerates apoptotic cell death in the CNS [45]. On the other hand, GABA has a trophic role early in brain development, so interference with this neurotransmitter early in life may affect neurodevelopment and lead to cognitive deficits, such as reported in children who were exposed to phenobarbital *in utero* [46].

Another example receptor development in the CNS is the μ-opioid receptor, the numbers of which are markedly reduced (i.e., > 50%) in newborn as compared to adult rats [47, 48]. Regional opioid receptor distribution in the brain also exhibits developmental differences. In neonates, receptor density is lower in the areas of the brain responsible for analgesic effect (e.g., cortex, thalamus, hippocampus) as compared to those areas of the brain responsible for autonomic side effects (e.g., pons, medulla, hypothalamus), where receptor density approximates that observed in adults [47, 49]. These findings suggest that efficacy in the neonate is limited by its side-effect profile because the higher relative doses required for desired effect may not be tolerated. Finally, CNS developmental changes have been suggested for the glutamate and acetylcholine receptors, and for the serotonin and adrenergic neurotransmitter systems (Figure 25.3), which have potential implications for the pharmacodynamics of drugs whose action involves their modulation [46].

## Immune Function

The ontogenic pathway by which the human immune system acquires full immunocompetence has been well described. As might be expected, age-dependent differences in the action of immunomodulatory drugs have also been reported. For example, cyclosporine, a calcineurin-inhibitor, has an $EC_{50}$ (measured using an *in vitro* monocyte proliferation assay and IL-2 expression) in infants less than 1 year of

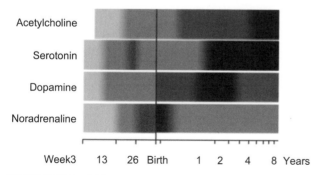

**FIGURE 25.3** Differences in expression of central nervous system neurotransmitters in humans along the developmental spectrum. Lighter shading indicates decreased expression and darker shading indicates increased expression. Reproduced from Herlenius E, Lagercrantz H. Exp Neurol 2004;190 (Suppl 1):S8–21 [46].

age which is approximately 50% of that in older children and adults (Figure 25.4) [50]. Furthermore, T-lymphocyte sensitivity to dexamethasone has been found to be greater in preterm infants and term infants relative to adults. Specifically, concentrations of dexamethasone needed to suppress T-lymphocyte proliferation in newborns are significantly lower in preterm newborns (0.29 n*M*) compared to adults (1.90 n*M*) [50]. Consequently, young children exposed to immunomodulatory medications may be at a greater risk of side effects than older children and adults.

## Pharmacodynamic Biomarkers

A recent editorial stressed the importance of expanding pediatric pharmacology studies beyond descriptions of age-dependence in PK to include data on PD [51]. A hindrance in accomplishing this goal in pediatric patients relative to adults resides in the greater difficulty of defining and validating pharmacodynamic endpoints that can be applied to pediatric patients (e.g., the use of repeated upper gastrointestinal endoscopy to validate the effect of acid-modifying drugs). To address this disparity, there is a need to develop pharmacodynamic "biomarkers" that are sufficiently non-invasive and robust that they can be used to assess the relationship of drug exposure and response across the developmental continuum [52]. Creative and selective use of non-invasive biomarkers that are appropriately qualified for their intended use, as described in Chapter 18, can add to the current body of knowledge pertaining to the ontogeny of pharmacodynamic response. This is essential to facilitate and expedite expansion of pediatric drug development when exposure–response relationships are used to determine age-appropriate drug doses and therapeutic regimens.

Specific examples of biomarkers currently used for pharmacodynamic assessments in the pediatric population include gastric pH monitoring and stable isotope breath tests ($^{13}C$ acetate and $^{13}C$ octonoate) which are used to assess acid modifying and prokinetic agents, respectively. Other examples are the histamine skin-prick test, used to determine the pharmacodynamic properties of antihistamines, and spirometry, used to determine the effect of drugs on pulmonary function in children with asthma and other chronic lung diseases. Hemoglobin $A_{1c}$ plasma concentrations are often used to determine efficacy of hypoglycemic agents. Drug minimal inhibitory (MIC) and minimal bactericidal concentrations (MBC) are used as hybrid PK/PD parameters (e.g., MIC/AUC and % time above MIC) to comparatively assess antibiotic and antimycobacterial drug regimens.

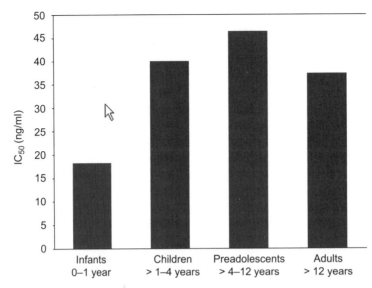

**FIGURE 25.4** Differences in IC$_{50}$ of cyclosporine across the developmental spectrum. Based on data from Marshall JD, Kearns GL. Clin Pharmacol Ther 1999;66:66–75 [50].

Several biomarkers also have been used in pediatric studies to assess drug disposition or effect. For example, urinary excretion of 6-β hydroxycortisol has been used to assess induction of CYP3A4. Finally, genotypes of drug receptors and metabolizing enzymes are used to predict the PK (e.g., CYP2C19 and proton pump inhibitors) or PD (e.g., leukotriene synthase and drugs that inhibit the enzyme) profile of some drugs.

## THERAPEUTIC CONSIDERATIONS

### Formulation

In addition to inadequate labeling of medications in children, there is also a significant lack of drug formulations that are suitable for use in all pediatric patients. As in adults, oral drug administration represents the most common route of administration. However, data obtained in 2008 from the US Pharmacopeia identified over 70 drug products which lacked an appropriate formulation for use in children, and the FDA also has compiled a priority list of medications which lack an appropriate pediatric formulation (Table 25.5) [53, 54]. Many times it is impractical and not feasible to use conventional solid oral dosage forms in children because of the need to administer weight-based doses, or a child's inability or refusal to swallow tablets or capsules. When compared to other routes of administration used in infants and children (e.g., transdermal, rectal,

inhalation), age-appropriate oral formulations (e.g., solutions, suspensions, chewable tablets, rapidly disintegrating oral tablets) offer the greatest flexibility and accuracy in dosing.

Even a formulation that is elegant from the standpoint of its physicochemical characteristics (e.g., stability, disintegration/dissolution properties) may not provide successful treatment for children unless it is palatable and has a flavor that is not objectionable. As reviewed at a recent workshop sponsored by the Eunice Kennedy Shriver National Institute for Child

**TABLE 25.5  Drugs that Lack a Suitable Formulation for Use in Children**

| | |
|---|---|
| Isoniazid | Methotrexate |
| Benznidazole | Prednisone |
| Nifurtimox | Isotretinoin |
| Albendazole | Baclofen |
| Mefloquine | *l*-Thyroxine |
| Sulfadoxine | Zinc Sulfate |
| Pyrimethamine | Sildenafil |
| Dapsone | Famciclovir |
| Hydroxyurea | Saquinavir |
| 6-Mercaptopurine | Lisinopril |

Adapted from NICHD, NIH. Priority list of needs in pediatric therapyeutics for 2008-2009 as of September 2, 2009 (Internet at, http://bpca. nichd.nih.gov/about/ process/upload/2009-Summary-091509-1-rev.pdf [53]).

Health and Human Development, flavor results from an interaction between the five basic tastes (i.e., bitter, sweet, salty, sour, umami) and odor or smell [55]. Umami is a savory taste sensation experienced with the ingestion of specific foods such as mushrooms, aged cheeses, and even breast milk. Flavor is linked to an oral medication via a basic taste (e.g., sweet) combined with an odor (e.g., cherry) which is transmitted retro-nasally from the back of the oral cavity to the nasal pharynx and subsequently to the olfactory receptors. A large number of receptors on the tongue, oral cavity, pharynx, and esophagus transmit a bitter taste that is believed to be associated with potentially toxic or harmful substances found in nature. This taste can be effectively masked by preparing bitter-tasting drugs in an oral solid formulation (e.g., tablet, granule, microcapsules). Because these are of limited utility in infants and younger children, amelioration of bitter tastes in pediatric formulations has mainly focused on two methods: blocking, through pharmacologic antagonism of bitter pathways, and psychological masking to interfere with bitter perception. Sodium salts are one method of reducing bitter taste, and studies have shown that children prefer salty tastes more than adults [56]. Salty tastes also enhance the flavor of sweet in liquid formulations, presumably by blocking bitter perception.

Taste and olfactory preferences are also influenced by the developmental stage of the child. Rejection of bitter tastes and preference for sweet and umami tastes is present hours after birth. Preference for salty tastes is not acquired until around 4 months of age. Children in general have a much stronger preference than adults for tastes that are sweet, salty, and even sour [56, 57]. Sweet-tasting solutions have even been found to produce an analgesic affect in both infants and children. Preference for sweets declines during childhood and appears near adult preference levels during adolescence [58]. The olfactory system is well-developed at birth, and there is evidence that an infant's preference for certain odors/flavors is influenced by flavors experienced *in utero* and with breast-feeding, as well as by culture and dietary experience [59]. For example, children in the United States prefer medications that are cherry- or bubblegum-flavored, while those in other parts of the world prefer different flavors (e.g., lemon in England and Australia, licorice in The Netherlands).

Given the complexity and cost of preparing pediatric drug formulations and the relatively small market offered by the pediatric population, age-specific drug formulations are still often prepared extemporaneously by pharmacists. In a few instances (e.g., captopril, benazepril hydrochloride, clonazepam, lisinopril, losartan potassium, rifampin) the approved product labeling contains specific instructions on how to prepare an oral liquid formulation of the drug from the marketed tablets [54]. There also are established compendia (e.g., the European Paediatric Formulations Initiative, the American Society of Health-Systems Pharmacists guidance on extemporaneous formulations) and primary medical literature which describe methods to prepare extemporaneous formulations of many drugs. When these are used, the practitioner should determine that appropriate data on stability, purity/sterility, and storage conditions have been provided for the extemporaneous formulation. Unfortunately, the most common practice is to prepare an extemporaneous formulation at the time of dosing by mixing the powdered content of a tablet or capsule (either through emptying a capsule or pulverization of a solid dosage form) with a liquid or foodstuff that is known to be generally palatable to patients of similar age (e.g., formula or breast milk for infants; cherry syrup, apple sauce or puddings for children). In these situations, stability of the drug with the vehicle is an important consideration, as is accuracy of preparation/dosing and the potential adverse effects associated with excipients in tableted drug formulations. Other limitations associated with this "point of administration" approach to extemporaneous drug formulation include the inaccuracy in dose delivery associated with dividing a solid formulation (i.e., tablet, capsule or suppository), insuring equal dispersion of the solid phase into the liquid phase of the vehicle, and the accuracy of the device chosen for drug administration (e.g., oral dosing syringe vs kitchen teaspoon). Finally, it is important to note that, in most instances, extemporaneous formulations have not been evaluated in controlled trials for efficacy or safety. Consequently, monitoring children who are given these medications for efficacy and adverse effects is important.

## Adherence (Compliance)

Adherence is currently the medically preferred term to describe a patient's willingness to take medications as prescribed. However, the term compliance (defined as to conform, submit, or adapt) may actually be more appropriate in pediatrics, as most children are dependent upon the actions and directions of caregivers who are responsible for the oversight of their medical treatment. Until children reach the age at which they can self-administer a drug in an accurate, proficient fashion, and can mentally assume responsibility for doing this (generally from 7 to 14 years of age), adherence to a drug regimen is the responsibility of an adult who is able to ensure that age-appropriate doses and dosing regimens are followed. Developmental challenges to adherence are observed in school-aged children (e.g., ensuring adequate access to treatment that may be too complicated to execute in a normal school environment) and during puberty, especially in the face of chronic medical conditions where the adolescent must increasingly assume responsibility for his or her treatment in order for it to be effective (e.g., asthma, type 1 diabetes, cystic fibrosis).

Difficulties with adherence in the adolescent patient can be the result of normal psychological development whereby children seek to gain independence, question values of parents/institutions, may participate in risk-taking and/or acting out, and have strong concerns about views of peers [60]. Average adherence rates in children with chronic diseases are approximately 50%, and are similar to rates observed in adults. However, rates decrease with increasing age as children enter into adolescence, presumably due to less parental supervision [61]. Several strategies for improving adherence have been evaluated in the pediatric population, and strategies that provide families with individualized and group education have met with some success. Involvement of schools and other social supports is also valuable in facilitating adherence in children. New technologies, such as text messaging and automated audiovisual alerts via cell phone and electronic device applications, may also be used in older children and adolescents to foster good adherence practices, and have great promise to "personalize" therapeutics given that they enable real-time monitoring and intervention by physicians, health professionals, and caregivers.

## Adverse Drug Reactions in Children

Due to the paucity of controlled clinical trials in children, clinical trial data regarding adverse drug reactions (ADRs) are generally lacking in this population. Spontaneous ADR reporting is also much less than for adult patients for various reasons, which include: (1) greater off-label use of drugs in pediatric patients; (2) an under-appreciation for ADRs that appear to have a predilection for infants and children (e.g., hepatotoxicity associated with valproic acid, weight gain from the use of psychoactive medications, paradoxical CNS responses to commonly used drugs) and cannot always be reliably predicted from adult ADR profiles; (3) the relative inability of young children (especially those that are non-verbal) to report symptoms that may be associated with an ADR; and (4) the fact that available reporting systems are largely designed to capture ADRs in adults. Incidence of ADRs in children has been reported to be between 14% and 17%, and ADRs are reported to be responsible for 2–4% of all pediatric hospitalizations. Moreover, 12.3% of pediatric ADRs have been reported to be classified as severe [62, 63]. So despite a lack of systematic data, it is well known that ADRs in children represent a significant public health concern.

The incidence of ADRs is particularly likely to be significantly increased in special populations, such as the sick newborn, children with chronic disease, and/ or in children with multiorgan dysfunction, as these children often have simultaneous exposure to multiple medications. Infants and children are also at an increased risk of ADRs during the maturation of the organs and biological processes that collectively are responsible for drug disposition, consequent to either inappropriate systemic exposure (i.e., associated with improper individualization of dose) or, potentially, developmentally-based pharmacodynamic differences. Furthermore, ADRs occurring early in development may have lifelong consequences. Some examples include aminoglycoside-associated hearing loss in neonates, developmental delay in infants treated for seizures with phenobarbital, and linear growth retardation associated with corticosteroid use for lung disease. Other adverse events appear to be relatively specific to children, such as aspirin-associated Reye's syndrome, serum sickness-like reactions produced by cefaclor, and behavioral adverse events (increased activity, impulsivity, disinhibition and insomnia) associated with serotonin selective reuptake inhibitor (SSRI) exposure. In most instances, the specific mechanisms which underlie these "pediatric-specific" ADRs are not known (e.g., the "neonatal SSRI syndrome" produced by *in utero* exposure). Enhanced reporting is needed to establish the true incidence of pediatric ADRs, as is the use of current technology (e.g., pharmacogenomics, metabolomics) to understand the biological basis of their genesis and, eventually, to enable their prediction and avoidance.

## Special Therapeutic Considerations in the Neonate

In addition to growth and development, there are several other major variables that will influence the PK and PD of drugs used in the neonatal nursery. These include inborn or acquired diseases, pharmacogenomic variants, patent ductus arteriosus (PDA), extracorporeal membrane oxidation (ECMO), and environmental influences such as therapeutic hypothermia. While a complete description of these variables is outside the scope of this chapter, several of the more predominant therapeutic considerations in this special population can be highlighted.

### Patent Ductus Arteriosus

The ductus arteriosus is a normal fetal vascular connection between the left pulmonary artery and the descending aorta. *In utero*, the ductus serves to allow the majority of blood flow leaving the right ventricle to circumvent the high resistance pulmonary circulation and flow directly into the descending aorta. This directs oxygen-deprived blood to the placenta, the fetal source for reoxygenation. After birth, the elimination of the low-resistance placenta results in an increase in systemic vascular resistance, and the exchange of air for fluid in the lungs creates decreased pulmonary resistance. Constriction of the ductus arteriosus and functional closure generally are spontaneous after birth so that blood flow is redirected to the lungs. Factors crucial to the closure of the ductus arteriosus are oxygen tension, concentration of circulating prostenoids, and available muscle mass in the ductus. In preterm infants, higher circulating concentrations of prostaglandins, an immature ductus, or an immature respiratory system contribute to continued patency of the ductus [64].

The primary physiological consequences of a patent ductus arteriosus (PDA) result from hypoxia, hypoperfusion, fluid overload, and acidosis. As a consequence, the apparent $V_d$ of drugs may be altered in neonates with a PDA [64, 65]. Thus, drugs that distribute primarily into body water may demonstrate an increased $V_d$ as the result of fluid overload. The presence of acidosis may decrease protein binding of some drugs and thereby increase their apparent $V_d$ [66]. Acidosis may also reduce the ionization of agents with a $pK_a$ close to 7.4, permitting an increased concentration of unionized molecules that are available to cross biological membranes and distribute into tissues [67]. PK studies in neonates with PDA have shown that the $V_d$ of several drugs is increased [68–70]. In addition to changes in $V_d$, a PDA decreases renal and hepatic blood flow, and this may reduce drug elimination capacity [65]. However, the interpretation of drug clearance in neonates with a PDA is often confounded by the effects of pharmacological (e.g., indomethacin, ibuprofen) or surgical treatment of the PDA, which both significantly alter blood flow to the liver and kidneys [68–72]. Therefore, the increase in digoxin, gentamicin, amikacin, and vancomycin levels that occurs with concurrent use of indomethacin appears to be the consequence of the dual effects of decreasing renal elimination secondary to indomethacin and, only on a temporary basis, a decreased $V_d$ once the PDA closes. As either or both interactions may play a role, drug concentrations should be monitored closely, both when indomethacin or ibuprofen therapy is initiated and after it has been completed.

### Extracorporeal Membrane Oxygenation

Extracorporeal membrane oxygenation (ECMO) is used in a variety of conditions, and is another example in neonatal therapeutics where physiological intervention can alter drug disposition. Neonatal indications include congenital diaphragmatic hernia, meconium aspiration syndrome, persistent pulmonary hypertension of the newborn, congenital heart defects, and sepsis. ECMO provides gas exchange and circulatory support by pumping blood from the patient through an extracorporeal circuit that includes a pump, a heater, and an oxygenator to oxygenate the blood and extract carbon dioxide. Blood is drawn from a venous access site, preferably the right atrium, and returned either into the right atrium via a double lumen catheter (venovenous ECMO) for respiratory support, or via the carotid artery (venoarterial ECMO) for cardiopulmonary support. Alternatively, access can be achieved via the femoral vein or artery.

On average, neonates on ECMO generally receive more than 10 different drugs per day. All patients on ECMO must be heparinized to prevent clotting of the ECMO circuit, and often receive sedatives and analgesics to alleviate pain and discomfort, diuretics to manage fluid overload, and antibiotics or antiviral medication to treat infections [73]. As only sparse PK and PD are available for neonates treated with ECMO, drug therapy must be individualized using a combination of existing knowledge of the drug (e.g., expected "normal" PK data in neonates and knowledge of how renal and/or hepatic compromise would impact drug disposition), the physical properties of the ECMO circuit (e.g., composition of tubing and oxygenator membrane and their capability to adsorb drugs to their surfaces, the volume and type of fluids used to prime the ECMO circuit), and therapeutic drug monitoring data. For example, circuit material, size, and priming fluid composition could affect the increase in $V_d$ that occurs with cannulation and attachment to the extracorporeal circuit [74–78]. Silicone membranes have a higher capacity for drug adsorption compared to the newer microporous membranes, presenting a potential problem for highly lipophilic drugs. While the extent of drug adsorption to ECMO circuit components can be predicted based upon *in vitro* data, its significance with regard to a drug's *in vivo* PK profile can only be discerned by measuring drug concentrations simultaneously from both the patient and the ECMO circuit. The volume of an ECMO circuit also increases the total circulating volume of a patient by between 5% and 100%, which in turn influences not only $V_d$ but also blood composition, coagulation, and circulation, as well as organ perfusion and function. These ECMO effects can compound the innate alterations in function that are expected in critically ill patients treated with this modality. When all these factors are considered in the context of how ontogeny influences drug disposition, it is easy to understand many of the reasons for altered PK in neonates and young infants treated with ECMO [5, 79–82]. The few studies that have been published report that ECMO alters PK for a variety of drugs, including antibiotics (gentamicin, vancomycin), sedative agents, and opiate analgesics [83–90]. Most of these studies have demonstrated changes in $V_d$ as well as in total plasma clearance [73].

## Therapeutic Hypothermia

Therapeutic hypothermia is being used in some centers to treat acute perinatal asphyxia. The exact mechanism of neuroprotection produced by hypothermia is unknown, but is believed to occur by reducing apoptosis and thus interrupting early cell necrosis. In asphyxiated neonates, hypothermia reduces metabolic rate and decreases the release of nitric oxide and endogenous excitotoxins, thereby reducing the likelihood they will develop neonatal encephalopathy. The effects of hypothermia on neonatal PK and PD in neonates are incompletely understood because there are only limited pediatric clinical data and most research has been done in animals and in adults [91]. Some of these studies were done under conditions of severe hypothermia (28°C), rather than the moderate hypothermia (33–34°C) that is used to treat neonatal asphyxia.

Therapeutic hypothermia causes a redistribution of regional blood flow that may significantly alter drug distribution and clearance [92]. Thus, hypothermia increases the $V_d$ of phenobarbital and midazolam and reduces the $V_d$ of gentamicin, fentanyl, morphine, and pancuronium. Since most enzymatic processes exhibit temperature dependency, alterations in the activity of drug-metabolizing enzymes also is expected [93]. This likely explains why the clearance of morphine in asphyxiated neonates treated with hypothermia is prolonged when compared to normothermic controls [94]. Diminished renal blood flow may also decrease

drug clearance. However, a recent study in neonates showed that the effects of asphyxia on renal function overwhelm any hypothermia-related changes in gentamicin clearance [95].

## Pediatric Dose and Regimen Selection

Historically, pediatric dose selection was driven by scaling, in that the dose for a child was determined from their weight relative to that of an adult. Thus, if the dose of a drug for a 100-kg adult was 500 mg, the pediatric dose for a child weighing 20 kg would be 100 mg. However, this approach does not consider known developmental differences in drug disposition, and has, in almost all cases, been demonstrated to be ineffective in producing a degree of systemic drug exposure for a pediatric patient which would approximate that in an adult. Unfortunately, incomplete developmental profiles for hepatic and extrahepatic drug metabolizing enzymes and drug transporters that may influence drug clearance and/or bioavailability also prevent the use of allometric scaling or other simple formulas for consistently effective pediatric dose prediction. While these approaches may have some potential clinical utility in older children (i.e., > 8 years of age) and adolescents whose organ function and body composition approximates that of young adults, their utility is severely limited in neonates, infants, and young children, where ontogeny produces dramatic differences in drug disposition. This is especially problematic for drugs whose doses cannot be easily individualized using patient-specific PK data obtained from therapeutic drug monitoring. In the absence of such data and/or established pediatric dosing guidelines, alternate methods must often be employed.

To date, more than 20 different approaches for initial selection of a drug dose for pediatric patients have been described. The majority of these utilize either total body weight (BW) or body surface area (BSA) as surrogates that reflect the developmental changes in either body composition or the function of those organs that collectively determine drug disposition. Selection based on BW or BSA will generally produce similar relationships between drug dose and resultant plasma concentration, except for those drugs whose apparent $V_d$ approximates ECF (i.e., $V_d$ ~0.3 L/kg), in which case a BSA-based approach is preferable (e.g. warfarin, heparin). In contrast, for drugs whose apparent $V_d$ exceeds ECF (i.e., $V_d$ > 0.3 L/kg), a BW-based approach for dose selection is preferable and this method is most frequently used in pediatrics. When the pediatric dose for a given drug is not known, these principles can be used to best approximate a proper dose for beginning treatment, as is illustrated by the following equations:

$$\text{Child dose (if } V_d < 0.3 \text{ L/kg)}$$
$$= (\text{child BSA in m}^2/1.73 \text{ m}^2)$$
$$\times \text{ adult dose} \qquad (25.1)$$

$$\text{Infant dose (if } V_d \geq 0.3 \text{ L/kg)}$$
$$= (\text{infant BW in kg/70 kg})$$
$$\times \text{ adult dose} \qquad (25.2)$$

It should be noted that this approach assumes that the child's weight, height, and body composition are age appropriate and normal, and that the "reference" normal adult has a BW and BSA of 70 kg and 1.73 m$^2$, respectively.

Additional factors need to be considered in order to estimate an appropriate dosing interval. For example, in neonates and young infants with developmental immaturity in either glomerular filtration and/or active tubular secretion, it is often necessary to adjust the dosing interval normally used for older infants and children who have attained more developed renal function for drugs with significant (i.e., > 50%) renal elimination, so as to prevent excessive drug accumulation (and possible associated toxicity) when multiple doses are administered. To accomplish this therapeutic goal, it is necessary to estimate the apparent elimination half-life of the drug and to use these data, along with age-appropriate estimates of the apparent $V_d$, to project a dosing regimen for a given patient.

## APPLICATION OF PEDIATRIC PHARMACOLOGY TO CLINICAL STUDY DESIGN

The accumulated knowledge of how ontogeny influences both PK and PD should be used together with available pharmacogenetic information to guide the design of ethical and rational clinical drug trials in neonates, infants, children, and adolescents. The application of these clinical pharmacology principles to the study of drugs in pediatrics is, in most respects, similar to what must be done in adults. What is different are the approaches and, in some instances, the restrictions that are imposed by facets of normal human development.

Increasingly, *in silico* approaches are used to design pediatric clinical trials and, specifically, to predict dose–exposure relationships. This is particularly useful for drugs for which effective plasma concentration ranges and/or systemic exposure (i.e., area under the curve) are known from adult data and can be plausibly extrapolated to produce similar PD effects in pediatric patients. Approaches to accomplish these objectives range from using simple allometric models (see Chapter 32) to the use of known and/or approximated PK parameter estimates, obtained by applying known profiles for maturation of specific drug-metabolizing enzymes, transporters, renal function ontogeny, and body composition. These PK parameter estimates are particularly helpful in that they can support modeling and simulation that incorporates the impact of ontogeny on the PK–PD interface. One such approach is that afforded by the application of physiologically-based PK (PBPK) modeling. As described in Chapter 32, these models draw together the physiological and biochemical information that determines drug disposition and then link it in a physiologically-based systems model which incorporates additional information on developmental physiology and relevant biochemistry. The value of PBPK models in pediatric drug development resides in their ability to refine initial dose projections, and thereby improve safety, by an adaptive approach to control systemic exposure. PBPK models also can be used to explore mechanistic reasons underlying altered PK during development, to explore the potential impact of development on important drug–drug interactions, and to improve the efficiency of pediatric clinical trials by reducing the number of subjects needed to characterize the impact of development and disease on drug disposition and action [96, 97].

## REFERENCES

[1] Shirkey H. Therapeutic orphans. J Pediatr 1968;72:119–20.
[2] Bren L. Frances Oldham Kelsey. FDA medical reviewer leaves her mark on history. FDA Consum 2001;35:24–9.
[3] Food and Drug Cost of Administration Modernization Act of 1997. Public Law 105–115. In the US Code of Federal Regulations 21 CFR 355a.111 Stat 2296, Nov 21, 1997. (Internet at, www.fda.gov/cber/fdama.htm.)
[4] FDA. Pediatric labeling changes table. (Internet at, www.fda.gov/downloads/Science Research/SpecialTopics/Pediatric Therapeutics Research/UCM163159.pdf.)
[5] Kearns GL, Abdel-Rahman SM, Alander SW, Blowey DL, Leeder JS, Kauffman RE. Developmental pharmacology – drug disposition, action, and therapy in infants and children. N Engl J Med 2003;349:1157–67.
[6] Kelly EJ, Newell SJ. Gastric ontogeny: Clinical implications. Arch Dis Child 1994;71:F136–41.
[7] Sankaran K, Hayton S, Duff E, Waygood B. Time-wise sequential analysis of gastric aspirate for occult blood and pH in sick preterm infants. Clin Invest Med 1984;7:115–8.
[8] Fakhoury M, Litalien C, Medard Y, et al. Localization and mRNA expression of CYP3A and P-glycoprotein in human

duodenum as a function of age. Drug Metab Dispos 2005;33:1603–7.

[9] Turner JW. Death of a child from topical diphenhydramine. Am J Forensic Med Pathol 2009;30:380–1.

[10] Choonara IA. Giving drugs per rectum for systemic effect. Arch Dis Child 1987;62:771–2.

[11] Pedersen S, Dubus JC, Crompton GK. ADMIT Working Group. The ADMIT series – issues in inhalation therapy. 5) Inhaler selection in children with asthma. Prim Care Respir J 2010;19:209–16.

[12] Wang Y, Lobstein T. Worldwide trends in childhood overweight and obesity. Intl J Pediatr Obes 2006;1:11–25.

[13] Wells JC, Fewtrell MS, Williams JE, Haroun D, Lawson MS, Cole TJ. Body composition in normal weight, overweight and obese children: Matched case–control analyses of total and regional tissue masses, and body composition trends in relation to relative weight. Intl J Obes (Lond) 2006;30:1506–13.

[14] Kendrick JG, Carr RR, Ensom MHH. Pharmacokinetics and drug dosing in obese children. J Pediatr Pharmacol Ther 2010;15:94–108.

[15] Daood M, Tsai C, Ahdab-Barmada M, Watchko JF. ABC transporter (P-gp/ABCB1, MRP1/ABCC1, BCRP/ABCG2) expression in the developing human CNS. Neuropediatrics 2008;39:211–8.

[16] Johnson TN, Thomson M. Intestinal metabolism and transport of drugs in children: The effects of age and disease. J Pediatr Gastroenterol Nutr 2008;47:3–10.

[17] G.Miethke A, Balistreri WF. Morphogenesis of the liver and biliary system. In: Kliegman RM, Stanton BF, Schor NF, III JWSG, Behram RE, editors. Nelson textbook of pediatrics. Philadelphia, PA: Elsevier; 2011.

[18] Treluyer JM, Cheron G, Sonnier M, Cresteil T. Cytochrome P-450 expression in sudden infant death syndrome. Biochem Pharmacol 1996;52:497–504.

[19] Treluyer JM, Gueret G, Cheron G, Sonnier M, Cresteil T. Developmental expression of CYP2C and CYP2C-dependent activities in the human liver: *In-vivo/in-vitro* correlation and inducibility. Pharmacogenetics 1997;7:441–52.

[20] Sonnier M, Cresteil T. Delayed ontogenesis of CYP1A2 in the human liver. Eur J Biochem 1998;251:893–8.

[21] Blake MJ, Abdel-Rahman SM, Pearce RE, Leeder JS, Kearns GL. Effect of diet on the development of drug metabolism by cytochrome P-450 enzymes in healthy infants. Pediatr Res 2006;60:717–23.

[22] Leeder JS, Gaedigk R, Marcucci KA, et al. Variability of CYP3A7 expression in human fetal liver. J Pharmacol Exp Ther 2005;314:626–35.

[23] Lacroix D, Sonnier M, Moncion A, Cheron G, Cresteil T. Expression of CYP3A in the human liver – evidence that the shift between CYP3A7 and CYP3A4 occurs immediately after birth. Eur J Biochem 1997;247:625–34.

[24] Stevens JC, Hines RN, Gu C, Koukouritaki SB, Manro JR, Tandler PJ, et al. Developmental expression of the major human hepatic CYP3A enzymes. J Pharmacol Exp Ther 2003;307:573–82.

[25] Min DI, Ellingrod VL, Marsh S, McLeod H. CYP3A5 polymorphism and the ethnic differences in cyclosporine pharmacokinetics in healthy subjects. Ther Drug Monit 2004;26:524–8.

[26] Kuehl P, Zhang J, Lin Y, Lamba J, Assem M, Schuetz J, et al. Sequence diversity in CYP3A promoters and characterization of the genetic basis of polymorphic CYP3A5 expression. Nat Genet 2001;27:383–91.

[27] Treluyer JM, Jacqz-Aigrain E, Alvarez F, Cresteil T. Expression of CYP2D6 in developing human liver. Eur J Biochem 1991;202:583–8.

[28] Blake MJ, Gaedigk A, Pearce RE, Bomgaars LR, Christensen ML, Stowe C, et al. Ontogeny of dextromethorphan O- and N-demethylation in the first year of life. Clin Pharmacol Ther 2007;81:510–6.

[29] Kearns GL, Leeder JS, Gaedigk A. Impact of the CYP2C19*17 allele on the pharmacokinetics of omeprazole and pantoprazole in children: Evidence for a differential effect. Drug Metab Dispos 2010;38:894–7.

[30] Hines RN. The ontogeny of drug metabolism enzymes and implications for adverse drug events. Pharmacol Ther 2008;118:250–67.

[31] Leeder JS, Kearns GL. Pharmacogenetics in pediatrics. Implications for practice. Pediatr Clin North Am 1997;44:55–77.

[32] Choonara IA, McKay P, Hain R, Rane A. Morphine metabolism in children. Br J Clin Pharmacol 1989;28:599–604.

[33] Capparelli EV, Englund JA, Connor JD, Spector SA, McKinney RE, Palumbo P, et al. Population pharmacokinetics and pharmacodynamics of zidovudine in HIV-infected infants and children. J Clin Pharmacol 2003;43:133–40.

[34] Blake MJ, Castro L, Leeder JS, Kearns GL. Ontogeny of drug metabolizing enzymes in the neonate. Semin Fetal Neonatal Med 2005;10:123–38.

[35] Robillard JE, Petershack JA. Renal function during fetal life. In: Barratt T, Avner E, Harmon W, editors. Pediatric nephrology. 4th ed. Baltimore, MD: Lippincott Williams & Wilkins; 1999. p. 21–37.

[36] Arant Jr BS. Developmental patterns of renal functional maturation compared in the human neonate. J Pediatr 1978; 92:705–12.

[37] van den Anker JN, Schoemaker RC, Hop WC, van der Heijden BJ, Weber A, Sauer PJ, et al. Ceftazidime pharmacokinetics in preterm infants: Effects of renal function and gestational age. Clin Pharmacol Ther 1995;58:650–9.

[38] National Kidney Foundation. Clinical practice guidelines: Table 24. Normal GFR in children and young adults. (Internet at, www.kidney.org/professionals/kdoqi/ guidelines_ckd/ Gif_File/kck_t24.gif.)

[39] Steinberg C, Notterman DA. Pharmacokinetics of cardiovascular drugs in children. Inotropes and vasopressors. Clin Pharmacokinet 1994;27:345–67.

[40] Wells TG, Young RA, Kearns GL. Age-related differences in digoxin toxicity and its treatment. Drug Saf 1992;7:135–51.

[41] Davies MW, Cartwright DW. Gentamicin dosage intervals in neonates: Longer dosage interval – less toxicity. J Paediatr Child Health 1998;34:577–80.

[42] van den Anker JN, Hop WC, de Groot R, van der Heijden BJ, Broerse HM, Lindemans J, et al. Effects of prenatal exposure to betamethasone and indomethacin on the glomerular filtration rate in the preterm infant. Pediatr Res 1994;36:578–81.

[43] Rakhmanina NY, van den Anker JN. Pharmacological research in pediatrics: From neonates to adolescents. Adv Drug Deliv Rev 2006;58:4–14.

[44] Brooksbank BW, Atkinson DJ, Balazs R. Biochemical development of the human brain. III. Benzodiazepine receptors, free gamma-aminobutyrate (GABA) and other amino acids. J Neurosci Res 1982;8:581–94.

[45] Henschel O, Gipson KE, Bordey A. GABAA receptors, anesthetics and anticonvulsants in brain development. CNS Neurol Disord Drug Targets 2008;7:211–24.

[46] Herlenius E, Lagercrantz H. Development of neurotransmitter systems during critical periods. Exp Neurol 2004; 190(Suppl. 1):S8–21.

[47] Kretz FJ, Reimann B. Ontogeny of receptors relevant to anesthesiology. Curr Opin Anaesthesiol 2003;16:281–4.

[48] Georges F, Normand E, Bloch B, Le Moine C. Opioid receptor gene expression in the rat brain during ontogeny, with special reference to the mesostriatal system: An *in situ* hybridization study. Brain Res Dev Brain Res 1998; 109:187–99.

[49] Freye E. Development of sensory information processing – the ontogenesis of opioid binding sites in nociceptive afferents and their significance in the clinical setting. Acta Anaesthesiol Scand Suppl 1996;109:98–101.

[50] Marshall JD, Kearns GL. Developmental pharmacodynamics of cyclosporine. Clin Pharmacol Ther 1999;66:66–75.

[51] Holford N. Dosing in children. Clin Pharmacol Ther 2010;87:367–70.

[52] Kearns GL. Beyond biomarkers: An opportunity to address the "pharmacodynamic gap" in pediatric drug development. Biomark Med 2010;4:783–6.

[53] NICHD, NIH. Priority list of needs in pediatric theapeutics for 2008–2009 as of September 1, 2009. (Internet at, http://bpca.nichd.nih.gov/about/process/upload/2009-Summary-091509-1-rev.pdf.)

[54] Nahata MC, Allen Jr LV. Extemporaneous drug formulations. Clin Ther 2008;30:2112–9.

[55] Mennella JA, Beauchamp GK. Optimizing oral medications for children. Clin Ther 2008;30:2120–32.

[56] Beauchamp GK, Cowart BJ. Preferences for high salt concentrations among children. Dev Psychol 1990;26:539–45.

[57] Segovia C, Hutchinson I, Laing DG, Jinks AL. A quantitative study of fungiform papillae and taste pore density in adults and children. Brain Res Dev Brain Res 2002;138:135–46.

[58] Desor JA, Beauchamp GK. Longitudinal changes in sweet preferences in humans. Physiol Behav 1987;39:639–41.

[59] Mennella JA, Jagnow CP, Beauchamp GK. Prenatal and postnatal flavor learning by human infants. Pediatrics 2001;107:E88.

[60] Hazen E, Scholzman S, Beresin E. Adolescent psychological development: A review. Pediatr Rev 2008;29:161–8.

[61] Bender B, Wamboldt FS, O'Connor SL, Rand C, Szefler S, Milgrom H, et al. Measurement of children's asthma medication adherence by self report, mother report, canister weight, and doser CT. Ann Allergy Asthma Immunol 2000;85:416–21.

[62] Martinez-Mir I, Garcia-Lopez M, Palop V, Ferrer JM, Rubio E, Morales-Olivas FJ. A prospective study of adverse drug reactions in hospitalized children. Br J Clin Pharmacol 1999;47:681–8.

[63] Gonzalez-Martin G, Caroca CM, Paris E. Adverse drug reactions (ADRs) in hospitalized pediatric patients. A prospective study. Intl J Clin Pharmacol Ther 1998;36:530–3.

[64] Bhatt V, Nahata MC. Pharmacologic management of patent ductus arteriosus. Clin Pharm 1989;8:17–33.

[65] Huhta JC. Patent ductus aretiosus in the preterm neonate. In: Long WA, editor. Fetal and neonatal cardiology. Philadelphia, PA: WB Sanders; 1990. p. 389–400.

[66] Vallner JJ, Speir Jr WA, Kolbeck RC, Harrison GN, Bransome Jr ED. Effect of pH on the binding of theophylline to serum proteins. Am Rev Respir Dis 1979;120:83–6.

[67] Waddell WJ, Butler TC. The distribution and excretion of phenobarbital. J Clin Invest 1957;36:1217–26.

[68] Collins C, Koren G, Crean P, Klein J, Roy WL, MacLeod SM. Fentanyl pharmacokinetics and hemodynamic effects in preterm infants during ligation of patent ductus arteriosus. Anesth Analg 1985;64:1078–80.

[69] Watterberg KL, Kelly HW, Johnson JD, Aldrich M, Angelus P. Effect of patent ductus arteriosus on gentamicin pharmacokinetics in very low birth weight (less than 1,500 g) babies. Dev Pharmacol Ther 1987;10:107–17.

[70] Gal P, Ransom JL, Weaver RL, et al. Indomethacin pharmacokinetics in neonates: The value of volume of distribution as a marker of permanent patent ductus arteriosus closure. Ther Drug Monit 1991;13:42–5.

[71] van den Anker JN, Hop WC, Schoemaker RC, van der Heijden BJ, Neijens HJ, de Groot R. Ceftazidime pharmacokinetics in preterm infants: Effect of postnatal age and postnatal exposure to indomethacin. Br J Clin Pharmacol 1995;40:439–43.

[72] Van Overmeire B, Touw D, Schepens PJ, Kearns GL, van den Anker JN. Ibuprofen pharmacokinetics in preterm infants with patent ductus arteriosus. Clin Pharmacol Ther 2001;70:336–43.

[73] Buck ML. Pharmacokinetic changes during extracorporeal membrane oxygenation: Implications for drug therapy of neonates. Clin Pharmacokinet 2003;42:403–17.

[74] Buylaert WA, Herregods LL, Mortier EP, Bogaert MG. Cardiopulmonary bypass and the pharmacokinetics of drugs. An update. Clin Pharmacokinet 1989;17:10–26.

[75] D'Arcy PF. Drug interactions with medicinal plastics. Adverse Drug React Toxicol Rev 1996;15:207–19.

[76] Mulla H, Lawson G, von Anrep C, Burke MD, Upton DU, Firmin RK. In vitro evaluation of sedative drug losses during extracorporeal membrane oxygenation. Perfusion 2000;15:21–6.

[77] Rosen DA, Rosen KR, Silvasi DL. In vitro variability in fentanyl absorption by different membrane oxygenators. J Cardiothorac Anesth 1990;4:332–5.

[78] Yahya AM, McElnay JC, D'Arcy PF. Drug sorption to glass and plastics. Drug Metabol Drug Interact 1988;6:1–45.

[79] de Wildt SN. Profound changes in drug metabolism enzymes and possible effects on drug therapy in neonates and children. Expert Opin Drug Metab Toxicol 2011;7:935–48.

[80] Lopez SA, Mulla H, Durward A, Tibby SM. Extended-interval gentamicin: Population pharmacokinetics in pediatric critical illness. Pediatr Crit Care Med 2010;11:267–74.

[81] Peeters MY, Bras LJ, DeJongh J, Wesselink RM, Aarts LP, Danhof M, et al. Disease severity is a major determinant for the pharmacodynamics of propofol in critically ill patients. Clin Pharmacol Ther 2008;83:443–51.

[82] Vet NJ, de Hoog M, Tibboel D, de Wildt SN. The effect of critical illness and inflammation on midazolam therapy in children. Pediatr Crit Care Med 2012;13:e48–50.

[83] Bhatt-Mehta V, Johnson CE, Schumacher RE. Gentamicin pharmacokinetics in term neonates receiving extracorporeal membrane oxygenation. Pharmacotherapy 1992;12:28–32.

[84] Buck ML. Vancomycin pharmacokinetics in neonates receiving extracorporeal membrane oxygenation. Pharmacotherapy 1998;18:1082–6.

[85] Mulla H, Lawson G, Peek GJ, Firmin RK, Upton DR. Plasma concentrations of midazolam in neonates receiving extracorporeal membrane oxygenation. ASAIO J 2003;49:41–7.

[86] Mulla H, McCormack P, Lawson G, Firmin RK, Upton DR. Pharmacokinetics of midazolam in neonates undergoing extracorporeal membrane oxygenation. Anesthesiology 2003;99:275–82.

[87] Peters JW, Anderson BJ, Simons SH, Uges DR, Tibboel D. Morphine pharmacokinetics during venoarterial extracorporeal membrane oxygenation in neonates. Intensive Care Med 2005;31:257–63.

[88] Peters JW, Anderson BJ, Simons SH, Uges DR, Tibboel D. Morphine metabolite pharmacokinetics during venoarterial extra corporeal membrane oxygenation in neonates. Clin Pharmacokinet 2006;45:705–14.

[89] Wells TG, Fasules JW, Taylor BJ, Kearns GL. Pharmacokinetics and pharmacodynamics of bumetanide in neonates treated with extracorporeal membrane oxygenation. J Pediatr 1992;121:974–80.

[90] Wells TG, Heulitt MJ, Taylor BJ, Fasules JW, Kearns GL. Pharmacokinetics and pharmacodynamics of ranitidine in neonates treated with extracorporeal membrane oxygenation. J Clin Pharmacol 1998;38:402–7.

[91] Zanelli S, Buck M, Fairchild K. Physiologic and pharmacologic considerations for hypothermia therapy in neonates. J Perinatol 2011;31:377–86.

[92] van den Broek MP, Groenendaal F, Egberts AC, Rademaker CM. Effects of hypothermia on pharmacokinetics and pharmacodynamics: A systematic review of preclinical and clinical studies. Clin Pharmacokinet 2010;49:277–94.

[93] Tortorici MA, Kochanek PM, Poloyac SM. Effects of hypothermia on drug disposition, metabolism, and response: A focus of hypothermia-mediated alterations on the

cytochrome P450 enzyme system. Crit Care Med 2007;35: 2196–204.

[94] Roka A, Melinda KT, Vasarhelyi B, Machay T, Azzopardi D, Szabo M. Elevated morphine concentrations in neonates treated with morphine and prolonged hypothermia for hypoxic ischemic encephalopathy. Pediatrics 2008; 121:e844–9.

[95] Liu X, Borooah M, Stone J, Chakkarapani E, Thoresen M. Serum gentamicin concentrations in encephalopathic infants are not affected by therapeutic hypothermia. Pediatrics 2009; 124:310–5.

[96] Edginton AN. Knowledge-driven approaches for the guidance of first-in-children dosing. Paediatr Anaesth 2011;21:206–13.

[97] Johnson TN, Rostami-Hodjegan A. Resurgence in the use of physiologically based pharmacokinetic models in pediatric clinical pharmacology: Parallel shift in incorporating the knowledge of biological elements and increased applicability to drug development and clinical practice. Paediatr Anaesth 2011;21:291–301.

# 26

# Drug Therapy in the Elderly

**S.W. Johnny Lau and Darrell R. Abernethy**

*Office of Clinical Pharmacology, Center for Drug Evaluation and Research,*
*US Food and Drug Administration, Silver Spring, MD 20993*

## INTRODUCTION

A hallmark of aging in humans is the development of multiple, coexisting physiological and pathophysiological changes which may benefit from drug therapy. It is not uncommon for the older individual to have 5 to 10 diagnoses, each of which has one or more proved beneficial therapies (Table 26.1) [1–4]. Examples abound: hypertension, coronary artery disease, osteoarthritis, osteoporosis, type 2 diabetes mellitus, and treated prostate or breast cancer often coexist in an individual patient. In addition, treatable insomnia, depression, and anxiety may be present, either independently or associated with these medical illnesses. As the number of individuals who are greater than 85 years old dramatically increases, the prevalence of Alzheimer's disease and other forms of cognitive impairment for which somewhat effective treatment is available will increase as well (Figure 26.1) [5]. This results in increased medication exposure and the potential for drug interactions (see Chapter 15) even more [6]. With the availability of medications that are in many instances dramatically effective, it is imperative to understand the impact of multiple current medications (high drug burden) on the older individual.

A number of studies over the past three decades have demonstrated that the likelihood of adverse drug effect increases with the number of drugs prescribed [7, 8]. There is a disproportionate increase in both total and severe adverse drug reactions when more than five drugs are co-administered [9]. Adverse drug effects also are more likely in older patients when certain drugs such as warfarin, theophylline, or digoxin are among the drugs prescribed. However, the absolute number of drugs the patient concurrently receives is probably the best predictor of an adverse drug event (Figure 26.2) [8, 10].

Further complicating this issue is the fact that the relative therapeutic benefit of treatments such as thrombolytic therapy, hypocholesterolemic therapy, post-myocardial infarction β-blocker treatment, and angiotensin-converting enzyme inhibitor treatment in congestive heart failure in patients over the age of 75 is similar to that seen in younger patients. Disease-specific clinical practice guidelines have reflected this by including specific recommendations for treatment. However these practice guidelines do not adequately recognize the presence of multiple comorbid diseases in older patients, with the result that if all pertinent guidelines are followed for a given patient, contradictory medication regimens and excessive polypharmacy results [11, 12]. This has led to a call in the geriatric medicine community for patient-centered, not disease-centered, treatment guidelines that make adequate provision for older patients with multiple comorbid conditions. Unfortunately, this creates a dilemma in that dramatic therapeutic advances have been made for many illnesses that afflict the elderly, yet administration of multiple medications increases the likelihood of adverse drug events.

## PATHOPHYSIOLOGY OF AGING

It is useful to think of the aging process in physiological, not chronological, terms. That being said,

**TABLE 26.1   Age-Related Chronic Medical Conditions**

|  | Frequency per 1000 persons in USA | | |
|---|---|---|---|
|  | Age < 45 years | Age 46–64 years | Age > 65 years |
| Arthritis | 30 | 241 | 481 |
| Hypertension | 129 | 244 | 372 |
| Hearing impairment | 37 | 141 | 321 |
| Heart disease | 31 | 134 | 295 |
| Diabetes | 9 | 57 | 99 |
| Visual impairment | 19 | 48 | 79 |
| Cerebrovascular disease | 1 | 16 | 63 |
| Constipation | 11 | 19 | 60 |

Reproduced from Zisook S, Downs NS. J Clin Psych 1998;59 (Suppl 4):80–91 [3]; data from Dorgan CA, editor. Statistical record of health and medicine. New York, NY: International Thompson Publishing Co; 1995 [4].

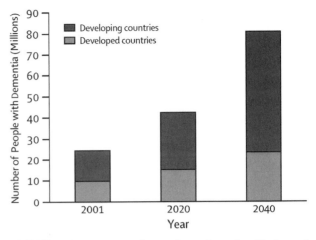

**FIGURE 26.1**   Projections for numbers of people with dementia in developing and developed countries. Reproduced with permission from Ferri CP, Prince M, Brayne C *et al.* Lancet 2005;366:211–27 [5].

a chronological definition is often used to stratify the aging population into three groups: *young old*, age 65–75; *old*, age 75–85 years; and *old old*, age $\geq 85$ years. Nearly all of the research which describes pharmacokinetics and pharmacodynamics in older individuals has been obtained from study of the young old – that is, individuals $\leq 75$ years. Therefore, the validity of extrapolating these findings to the older age groups may be questioned. In contrast, the data describing adverse drug events in older as compared to younger patients are obtained from patient populations and databases that include the full age-spectrum of the elderly. The general physiological changes that occur with aging can be characterized as a decrease in maximum performance capacity and loss of homeostatic reserve [13]. Although these changes occur to different degrees for each organ system or function, they are present in individuals who are in good health and are accentuated during illness.

Placed in the context of response to drugs, it is most useful to discuss age-related physiological changes that occur in integrated functions. Systemic drug responses are the result of the complex interaction of specific and non-specific drug effects, and the direct and indirect physiological or pathological responses to these drug effects. The sum of these effects is the pharmacodynamic response that is observed, whether therapeutic or toxic. Therefore, the age-related changes that occur in physiological or psychological function prior to drug exposure are helpful in predicting and describing a particular drug response.

The observed pharmacodynamic response is the result of extent of drug exposure, determined by drug pharmacokinetics (Table 26.2), and sensitivity to a given drug exposure, determined by the state of function of the effectors of drug response such as receptor-cellular transduction processes (Figure 26.3). We will discuss the age-related changes that have been described for renal drug elimination and hepatic and extrahepatic drug biotransformations, and then briefly review the age-related changes that have been described for central nervous system function, autonomic nervous system function, cardiovascular function, and renal function. These functions are selected as each has been rather comprehensively evaluated in the healthy elderly, and a great diversity of drugs can have adverse as well as beneficial effects on these functions. We will describe and/or predict the effect of these changes on drug pharmacodynamics at a given drug exposure for drug groups commonly used in older patients. Due to the high incidence and prevalence of cancer in older patients, we will review the information available to guide cancer chemotherapy in this patient group. Similarly, osteoporosis is prevalent in older individuals, and we will discuss therapeutic alternatives. Finally, we will discuss drug groups for which increased age confers greater risk for drug toxicity, along with the mechanism, when known.

## AGE-RELATED CHANGES IN PHARMACOKINETICS

### Age-Related Changes in Drug Distribution

With aging, body fat increases as a proportion of total body weight and lean body mass and total body

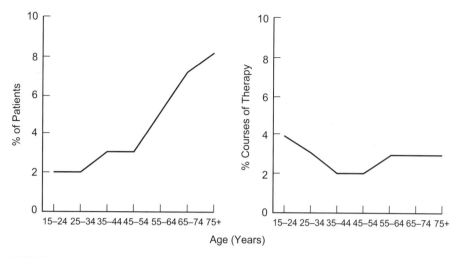

**FIGURE 26.2** The relationship of increasing age and likelihood of adverse drug events (*left panel*), and the relationship of increasing age and adverse drug reactions when corrected for number of drugs per patient (*right panel*). Reproduced with permission from Gurwitz JH, Avorn J. Ann Intern Med 1991;114:956–66 [10].

**TABLE 26.2 Pharmacokinetic Changes in the Elderly**

| Process | Change with age[a] |
| --- | --- |
| *Gastrointestinal absorption* | — |
| *Drug distribution* | |
| Central compartment volume | — or ↓ |
| Peripheral compartment volume | |
| Lipophilic drugs | ↑↑ |
| Hydrophilic drugs | ↓↓ |
| Plasma protein binding | |
| Binding to albumin | ↓ |
| Binding to α₁-acid glycoprotein | — or ↑ |
| *Drug elimination* | |
| Renal elimination | ↓↓ |
| Hepatic metabolism | |
| Phase I reactions | |
| CYP3A | ↓ |
| CYP1A2 | — or ↓ |
| CYP2D6 | — or ↓ |
| CYP2C9 | — or ↓ |
| CYP2C19 | — or ↓ |
| CYP2E1 | — or ↓ |
| Phase II reactions | |
| Glucuronidation | — |
| Sulfation | — |
| Acetylation | — |

[a]—, no change.

water decreases [14]. Accordingly, the volume of distribution per unit total body weight decreases for polar drugs such as digoxin, theophylline, and aminoglycosides, and increases for lipophilic drugs such as diazepam [15]. Assuming that the therapeutic goal is to achieve average plasma concentrations in the elderly that are similar to those in younger patients, the changes in drug volume of distribution will generally be relevant only for drugs which are administered as single doses or for the determination of loading dose for drugs in which use of a loading dose is appropriate. However, as discussed in Chapter 2, distribution volume changes will also affect the observed elimination-phase half-life, as well as the peak and trough drug concentrations that are achieved during a dosing interval, and the changes described above may, for example, adversely affect the response of elderly patients to therapy with sedative-hypnotic drugs (see Figure 2.7).

Serum albumin concentrations may slightly decrease or be unchanged, whereas α₁-acid glycoprotein tends to increase with age. These changes in plasma proteins are generally not attributed to age *per se*, but to pathophysiological changes or disease states that may occur more frequently in older patients. Again, these changes affect unbound drug exposure only for drugs administered as a single dose or with a loading dose [16], but are also of importance when therapeutic drug monitoring is limited to measurement of just total drug concentrations (see Chapter 5 and Figure 5.3).

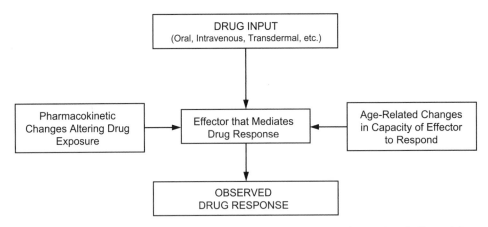

**FIGURE 26.3** Observed drug responses in elderly patients represent the combined effects of drug input and age-related pharmacokinetic and pharmacodynamic changes.

## Age-Related Changes in Renal Clearance

The most consistent and predictable age-related change in pharmacokinetics is that of renal drug clearance. Renal function, including renal blood flow, glomerular filtration rate (GFR), and active renal tubular secretory processes, all decline with increasing age [17]. Measured GFR is the best overall index of renal function, but it is cumbersome to collect urine over extended periods of time and this procedure is prone to measurement error. For this reason, the following two formulae are commonly used to estimate GFR based on serum creatinine.

The Cockcroft-Gault (CG) equation, described in Chapter 1 and discussed as a guide to drug dosing in Chapter 5, has traditionally been used to estimate creatinine clearance as a surrogate for measured GFR [18]. For men, creatinine clearance is estimated as follows:

$$CL_{CR}(\text{mL/min}) = \frac{(140 - \text{age})(\text{weight in kg})}{72(\text{serum creatinine in mg/dL})}$$

For women, this estimate should be reduced by 15%.

As discussed in Chapter 1, the Modification of Diet in Renal Disease (MDRD) equation for estimating GFR has also been proposed as a guide for adjusting drug dosage [19]. In the current iteration of this equation, GFR is estimated as:

$$\text{GFR}(\text{mL/min/1.73 m}^2)$$

$$= 175 \times (\text{serum creatinine})^{-1.154} \times (\text{age})^{-0.203}$$

$$\times (0.742 \text{ if female})$$

$$\times (1.210 \text{ if African American})$$

Although the CG equation-estimated creatinine clearance predicts a linear decrease with age that is steeper than the non-linear decline predicted via the MDRD equation, either of these equations gives a reasonable estimate that is sufficiently accurate to determine drug dose for drugs that have predominant renal clearance. The relative merits of these estimates of creatinine clearance have been extensively discussed, with no clear resolution [20]. The disadvantage of the MDRD equation is that only limited information is available on its use to guide drug dosage adjustments, as most published age-adjusted recommendations are based on the CG equation. Perhaps the greatest limitation for both of these equations is that they were not derived from significant numbers of people over the age of 70 years [21].

Drugs that are eliminated primarily by glomerular filtration, including aminoglycoside antibiotics, lithium, and digoxin, have an elimination clearance that decreases with age in parallel with the decline in measured or calculated creatinine clearance [22–24]. The renal clearance of drugs undergoing active renal tubular secretion also decreases with aging (Table 26.3). For example, the decrease in renal tubular secretion of cimetidine has been shown to parallel the decrease in creatinine clearance in older patients [25]. On the other hand, the renal clearance/creatinine clearance *ratio* of both procainamide and N-acetylprocainamide decreases in the elderly, indicating that with aging the renal tubular secretion of these drugs declines more rapidly than creatinine clearance does [26].

## Age-Related Changes in Hepatic and Extrahepatic Drug Biotransformations

Drug biotransformations occur in quantitatively important amounts in the liver, gastrointestinal tract,

**TABLE 26.3** Some Drugs with Decreased Clearance in the Elderly

| Route of clearance | Representative drugs |
|---|---|
| Renal | All aminoglycosides |
|  | Vancomycin |
|  | Digoxin |
|  | Procainamide |
|  | Lithium |
|  | Sotalol |
|  | Atenolol |
|  | Dofetilide |
|  | Cimetidine |
| Single Phase I metabolic pathway |  |
| CYP3A | Alprazolam |
|  | Midazolam |
|  | Triazolam |
|  | Verapamil |
|  | Diltiazem |
|  | Dihydropyridine calcium channel blockers |
|  | Lidocaine |
| CYP2C | Diazepam |
|  | Phenytoin |
| CYP1A2 | Celecoxib |
|  | Theophylline |
| Multiple Phase I metabolic pathways | Imipramine |
|  | Desipramine |
|  | Trazodone |
|  | Hexobarbital |
|  | Flurazepam |

kidneys, lung, and skin. However, nearly all organs have some metabolic activity. As described in Chapter 11, *in vivo* drug biotransformations are commonly separated into Phase I and Phase II biotransformations. Phase I biotransformations are catalyzed by membrane-bound enzymes found in the endoplasmic reticulum and Phase II biotransformations occur predominantly in the cytosol, with the exception of the UDP-glucuronosyltransferases that are membrane-bound to the endoplasmic reticulum. Phase I biotransformations are primarily catalyzed by enzymes of the cytochrome P450 monoxygenase system (CYP450), with the important members of this enzyme family for drug biotransformations being CYP3A, CYP2D6, CYP2C9, CYP2C19, CYP1A2, CYP2B6, and CYP2E1. No general approach has been developed to estimate age-related changes in hepatic and extrahepatic drug biotransformation, perhaps in part because hepatic and extrahepatic biotransformation processes are influenced by complex and heterogenous factors that include both genetic and environmental influences [15]. In any case it is not needed, as it will be seen from the following that age-related changes in drug exposure are at most modest.

Data from *in vitro* studies using human liver tissue indicate that the content and activities of various CYP isozymes from liver microsomal preparations have high intersubject variability and do not significantly change with advancing age over the range of 10–85 years (Figure 26.4) [27]. *In vivo* hepatic drug clearance via CYP metabolism has been studied for a number of drugs in older individuals and was found to be either

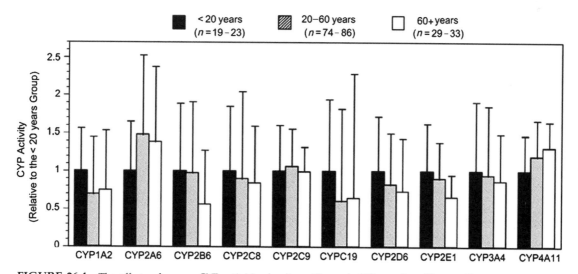

**FIGURE 26.4** The effects of age on CYP activities *in vitro* with nearly 150 samples of human liver microsomes are shown. The subjects represent three age groups, namely < 20 years, 20–60 years, and 60+ years. The liver microsomal CYP activity is highly variable and not significantly different in the CYP activities between the age group of 20–60 years and the age group over 60 years. Reproduced with permission from Parkinson A, Mudra DR, Johnson C *et al.* Toxicol Appl Pharmacol 2004;199:193–209 [27].

unchanged or modestly decreased, with clearance reductions reported to be in the range of 10–40% for young-old and old subjects who were generally in good health [28, 29]. The clearance of two CYP3A substrates, amlodipine and erythromycin, was evaluated in old and old-old frail as well as nursing home patients, and was not changed compared to younger individuals [30, 31]. At present it is not clear how to interpret these findings in relation to other studies in which drugs such as midazolam and triazolam, both CYP3A substrates, were found to have decreased clearance in young-old and old individuals [28, 29]. There is limited information on the pharmacodynamic consequences of such clearance changes. However, when altered drug effects have been reported in older individuals, they most likely result from a combination of age-related pharmacokinetic and physiologic changes [32].

Phase II biotransformations are little changed with aging, based on studies of glucuronidation, sulfation, and acetylation. Prototype substrates studied for glucuronidation have been lorazepam, oxazepam, and acetaminophen; for sulfation, acetaminophen; and for acetylation, isoniazid and procainamide.

## AGE-RELATED CHANGES IN EFFECTOR SYSTEM FUNCTION

### Central Nervous System

It is important to separate age-related and disease-related changes in central nervous system (CNS) function. A number of changes have been noted in the absence of dementing illness, Parkinson's disease, and primary psychiatric disease. Brain aging proceeds in a relatively selective fashion, with the prefrontal cortex and the subcortical monoaminergic nuclei most affected. In the case of the prefrontal cortex, progressive loss of volume with aging is consistently shown. Age-related slowing in mental-processing function is a consistent finding, but the mechanism is uncertain. Aging has been associated with changes in brain activation during encoding and retrieval processes of memory function. Older individuals have more widespread task-related brain activation to conduct the same tasks as compared to younger individuals. One postulate has been that older individuals need to recruit greater brain resources to conduct the same memory function [33]. Even in the absence of Parkinsonism, the dopaminergic systems are diminished as a function of age. The dopaminergic impairment has been most clearly defined for processes related to dopamine D2 receptors [34].

An important pharmacodynamic principle is that older individuals have increased sensitivity to a given exposure of some CNS depressant drugs. After accounting for age-related pharmacokinetic changes that may cause greater drug exposure at a given dose, the aged individual is more sensitive to the opiate anesthetic induction agents propofol, fentanyl, and alfentanil [35–37]. In the case of propofol, the concentration needed to induce anesthesia in a 75-year-old healthy individual was approximately one-half that required for a 25-year-old individual [35, 36]. A similar increase in pharmacodynamic sensitivity to fentanyl and alfentanil has been described, with, again, a 50% decrease in the dose required to induce the same degree of drug effect in older individuals (up to 89 years) as compared to younger individuals [37]. The mechanism for the increased pharmacodynamic sensitivity to these opiates is unknown.

These findings for opiates are in contrast to findings with the barbiturate thiopental and the benzodiazepines midazolam and triazolam [30, 38, 39]. Although a substantially lower dose of these drugs is needed to induce anesthesia or the same degree of sedation in older than younger individuals, this is the result of the pharmacokinetic changes of aging. When drug effect is normalized to arterial drug concentration, the concentration–effect relationship is similar in the young and the elderly. For ambulatory elderly patients, the clinical consequences of increased exposure to benzodiazepines due to decreased Phase I metabolic clearance can be devastating, with an increased incidence of hip fracture noted in older patients taking long half-life benzodiazepines [40]. These drugs (e.g., flurazepam and diazepam) undergo Phase I biotransformation, and the decreased clearance seen in the elderly results in markedly greater drug accumulation, even when taken once daily as a sedative-hypnotic [41, 42].

There are fewer data on adverse drug effects caused by neuroleptic and antidepressant drugs in older patients. However, as shown in Figure 26.5, it is now clear that older patients have three- to five-fold higher incidence of tardive dyskinesia than younger patients when "typical" neuroleptics (e.g., phenothiazines and haloperidol) are administered [43–46]. Across studies, 10–20% of younger patients develop tardive dyskinesia after 3 years or more of neuroleptic treatment, while 40–60% of older patients are affected within the same treatment period [45]. It is unknown if this is related to age-dependent pharmacokinetic or pharmacodynamic changes. The newer neuroleptics, such as risperidol and olanzapine, have a much lower incidence of tardive dyskinesia in all patient groups studied, and may be of considerable clinical utility for this reason [47]. However, it should be noted that all

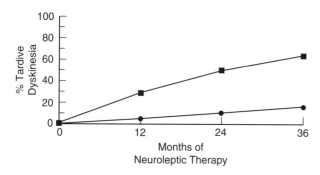

**FIGURE 26.5** Cumulative incidence of neuroleptic-induced tardive dyskinesia in old (■) and young (●) adults. Reproduced with permission from Jeste DV. J Clin Psychiatry 2000;61(Suppl 4):27–32 [46].

neuroleptics are associated with increased mortality in older patients [48, 49], and, although they are often prescribed for behavioral and psychological symptoms in dementia, there is no evidence for their efficacy for this indication [50].

There has been less comprehensive analysis of other classes of CNS active drugs, but the general clinical impression is that older patients are more sensitive to side effects and require a lower dose of drug to achieve similar therapeutic benefit. Pharmacokinetic studies for lithium, which undergoes renal elimination, and tricyclic antidepressants, which undergo Phase I biotransformation, show decreased clearance on the basis of age-related decrease in renal function and age-related decrease in Phase I drug-metabolizing capacity, respectively [23, 51]. In addition, drugs in a wide range of therapeutic classes, such as antihypertensives, antiarrhythmics, antihistamines, antidepressants, and neuroleptics, have "off-target" anticholinergic and sedative drug effects, and sensitivity to these drug effects is also greater in older patients. This is at least in part due to increased central nervous system depressant effects when such drugs are administered to older patients. The need for tools and methods to evaluate anticholinergic and sedative drug effects on physical function in older individuals has prompted development of a *Drug Burden Index* that links extent of anticholinergic and sedative drug exposure to physical functional status [52, 53]. Although not conclusively established, this tool also may have some capacity to predict future decreased functional status in the context of anticholinergic and/or sedative drug exposure [54, 55].

## Autonomic Nervous System

The age-related changes in autonomic nervous system (ANS) function are very diverse, and are likely to be associated with many of the age-related changes observed in drug response and toxicity across many therapeutic classes of drugs. Cardiovagal function is diminished, as indicated by age-related decreases in resting heart rate and beat-to-beat heart rate variability. Older individuals have lower vagal tone, as indicated by less increase in heart rate with atropine administration. Other findings consistent with this conclusion are that older individuals have decreased heart rate variation with deep breathing and reduced increases in heart rate in response to standing. Baroreflex function is also impaired in the healthy elderly, and this is accentuated in the presence of illness common in older patients, such as hypertension and diabetes mellitus [56]. Cardiac sympathetic function is also altered, as demonstrated by decreased tachycardic response to isoproterenol and increased circulating plasma norepinephrine concentrations [57, 58]. An integrated response that reflects many of these age-related changes is that of orthostatic hypotension, which is substantially increased in older individuals [59]. The degree of orthostatic decrease in blood pressure in older patients may be particularly evident in the postprandial state, and may be exacerbated when older patients are treated with diuretics [60, 61]. Thermoregulatory homeostasis is also impaired in the elderly, who have a higher thermoreceptor threshold and decreased sweating when perspiration is initiated [56].

Data that conclusively establish that altered drug effects result from impaired ANS function are sparse, perhaps due to the difficulty in ascribing a particular drug effect to a particular ANS function. However, increased orthostatic hypotension seen at baseline, in addition to drugs that cause sympathetic blockade, such as typical neuroleptics and tricyclic antidepressants, is likely to be a contributing factor to the increased incidence of hip fracture noted in patients receiving these drugs [62]. Similarly, the anticholinergic effects of many drugs, including antihistamines and neuroleptics, may not only accentuate orthostatic blood pressure changes but also be associated with greater cognitive impairment in older individuals. Impaired thermoregulation under baseline conditions may also be accentuated by administration of these drugs because they have potent anticholinergic effects that further disable thermoregulatory responses. It is unclear at this time how age-related ANS changes may relate to the cardiac proarrhythmic effects of drugs that prolong the electrocardiographic QT interval. However, there is a clear association of increasing age with the proarrhythmic effects of neuroleptic drugs [63]. It is clear that these ANS changes markedly alter systemic cardiovascular responses to a drug such as the α- and β–adrenergic blocking drug labetalol, which, as shown in Figure 26.6, lowers blood pressure to a greater extent in older than in younger hypertensive patients while decreasing heart rate to a much lesser extent [64].

## Cardiovascular Function

The age-related changes in cardiovascular function that relate to drug responses are usefully separated into changes in cardiac and changes in peripheral vascular function. However, this separation must be made with the understanding that the pharmacodynamic responses seen are generally an integrated function of ANS, cardiac, and peripheral vascular function.

Cardiac output at rest is not substantially changed with age in the absence of superimposed cardiac disease. However, components of the cardiac cycle are indeed changed. Heart rate is decreased, reflecting the decrease in parasympathetic withdrawal noted previously, and perhaps impaired β-adrenergic and sinoatrial function. Left ventricular mass and left ventricular stroke volume are increased, which allows cardiac output to be maintained in the face of decreased heart rate. However, diastolic relaxation is slowed, making the late left ventricular filling that is associated with atrial contraction a more important determinant of stroke volume in the elderly. Chronotropic response to β-adrenergic stimulation is impaired, but it is uncertain if this is the cause or the result of increased circulating norepinephrine levels [65]. Cellular and molecular mechanisms for these changes have been studied in some detail in animal models, and may offer some insight into drug responses. The prolonged left ventricular contraction period and slowed diastolic relaxation may be associated with decreased uptake of calcium by the sarcoplasmic reticulum [66]. Many potential mechanisms for the impairment in β-adrenoceptor function have been suggested, but this remains controversial.

The pharmacodynamic consequences of these age-related changes can be substantial. Impaired β₁-adrenergic responsiveness results in a decreased tachycardic response to both direct pharmacologic stimulation by drugs, such as isoproterenol [57], and indirect reflex sympathetic stimulation induced by vasodilating drugs, such as the calcium antagonist nisoldipine [67]. Conversely, the decrease in heart rate caused by β₁-adrenoceptor blockade is reduced in elderly patients [64]. Although diastolic relaxation is slowed as a usual consequence of aging, this slowing progresses in many older patients to the extent that symptoms of congestive heart failure occur. As many as 40% of elderly patients with clinical congestive heart failure have normal left ventricular function when it is defined as left ventricular ejection fraction ≥ 40% [68, 69]. When these patients with diastolic dysfunction are treated with loop diuretics, they are particularly susceptible to intravascular volume depletion that is manifest clinically as increased orthostatic hypotension [70]. If the volume depletion is sufficient to decrease vital organ perfusion, other symptoms may occur, such as central nervous system depression and decreased renal function [71].

Vascular stiffness increases with age, even in the absence of disease. This may be due to both structural and functional changes, with increased deposition of collagen and other ground substance evident on microscopic or molecular examination [72]. In addition, advanced age by itself decreases endothelial-mediated relaxation, even in the absence of concurrent diseases, such as hypertension and hypercholesterolemia, and environmental exposures,

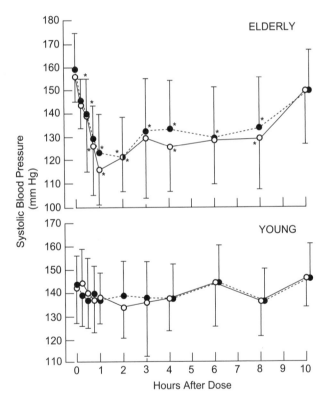

**FIGURE 26.6** Comparison of changes in erect (O——O) and sitting (●- -●) systolic blood pressures between elderly (*upper panel*) and young (*lower panel*) hypertensive patients treated with a daily oral labetalol dose of 200 mg. Bars represent the standard deviation from the mean, and asterisks indicate values that are significantly different (*P* < 0.05) from the baseline in that posture for the respective group. No differences were noted between sitting and standing blood pressure for either group. Reproduced with permission from Abernethy DR, Schwartz JB, Plachetka JR *et al*. Am J Cardiol 1987;60:697–702 [64].

such as cigarette smoking, that are associated with impaired vascular endothelial relaxation [73]. Not only is β–adrenergic function impaired, but β2-adrenergic-mediated peripheral vasodilatation is impaired as well, due to decreased β-adrenergic vascular relaxation [74]. The clinical result of these changes is an increase in pulse pressure, with systolic blood pressure disproportionately increased relative to diastolic blood pressure.

The pharmacodynamic consequences of these age-related cardiovascular changes are quite diverse. With initial administration of a non-selective β-adrenoceptor blocking drug, the decrease in heart rate is diminished. However, one would predict as well that the β2–adrenoceptor blockade-mediated increase in peripheral vascular resistance would be diminished simultaneously. Clinical data indicate that β-blocker therapy for hypertension may indeed be somewhat less effective in older hypertensive patients. However, the limited data available indicate that β-blocker therapy is as efficacious in older as in younger patients after myocardial infarction and for the treatment of congestive heart failure. Administration of an α-adrenergic blocking drug (e.g., terazosin for the treatment of urinary retention due to prostate hypertrophy) results in greater hypotensive response in the older individual due to lack of reflex β-adrenergic stimulation [75].

The response of older individuals to calcium channel antagonists is a combination of changes in direct drug effects and age-related alterations in reflex responses to drug effect. Hypotensive responses are maintained because direct arterial vasodilatation remains intact, even though there is the previously noted age-related impairment in reflex sympathetic stimulation [76]. For verapamil and diltiazem, atrioventricular nodal conduction delay is less in older than in younger individuals, while sinoatrial suppression is greater in the elderly [77, 78]. Mechanisms for these changes are unclear, but are thought to entail a complex summation of changes in direct drug effects and age-related ANS and cardiac function changes.

Angiotensin-converting enzyme inhibitors may be less effective in treating hypertension in older than in younger patients [79]. The mechanism for this is probably related to the low-renin state and resulting decreased role of the circulating renin–angiotensin–aldosterone axis in maintaining blood pressure in older hypertensive patients [80, 81]. Conversely, available data indicate that angiotensin-converting enzyme inhibitors are an extremely effective treatment for congestive heart failure in older as well as younger patients [82].

## Renal Function

Kidney morphology and renal function change markedly with aging. These changes have been associated with pharmacokinetic changes (decreased renal drug clearance) and also changes in pharmacodynamics for three drug classes important for the elderly – non-steroidal anti-inflammatory drugs, angiotensin-converting enzyme inhibitors, and diuretics – and each may have responses altered by renal aging.

The anatomic changes associated with aging include a decrease in kidney weight that, from the fourth to the ninth decade of life, may fall by as much as one-third. This loss of renal mass occurs primarily from the renal cortex, and results in decreased numbers and size of glomeruli. The remaining renal blood vessels may then produce shunts between afferent and efferent arterioles. The functional result is a decline in GFR that averages 0.75 mL/min/year, but is quite variable. Perhaps as many as one-third of individuals have no decrease in GFR while others have more rapid decreases. Renal plasma flow, measured by para-aminohippurate clearance, decreases more with age than GFR as measured by inulin clearance, and may be decreased as much as 50% in individuals in the ninth decade as compared to the fourth decade of life. The result is that filtration fraction (GFR/renal plasma flow) increases in the elderly [13, 83]. These findings also may be related to intrarenal impairment in vascular endothelial vasodilating function as demonstrated by an attenuated vasodilatory response to acetylcholine. Consistent with findings in other vascular beds, intrarenal vasoconstrictive responses to angiotensin II are maintained in the elderly. Circulating atrial natriuretic hormone is increased in older individuals, and this may be responsible for suppressing renal renin secretion. This suppression leads to decreased basal activation of the renin–angiotensin–aldosterone axis [84]. As mentioned previously, the age-associated decrease renal tubular secretion parallels the decrease in GFR for some drugs [23], but occurs more rapidly for others [24]. The decrease in renal tubular reabsorption, at least as measured by glucose reabsorption, appears to parallel the decline in GFR. A final impairment in renal tubular function that occurs with aging is manifest as a decreased capacity to concentrate or dilute urine that results in an impaired ability to excrete a free-water load and to excrete sodium during states of volume depletion [85].

Altered or accentuated responses to nonsteroidal anti-inflammatory drugs in elderly patients include azotemia, decreased GFR, sodium retention, and hyperkalemia [86, 87]. A common basis for these effects is likely to rest in part on the increased dependence of the aging kidney on vasodilating prostaglandins that results from the age-related decrease in renal plasma flow. Furthermore, selective inhibition of cyclooxygenase-2 in older patients may decrease GFR to the same extent as occurs with non-selective cyclooxygenase inhibitors [88, 89]. The increased likelihood of sodium retention in older patients may also be associated with the loss of action of vasodilating prostaglandins, decreased glomerular filtration, and decreased renal tubular capacity to concentrate sodium in the decreased urine volume. The increased likelihood of hyperkalemia may reflect a pre-existing state of relative hyporeninemic hypo-aldosteronism in older individuals, exacerbated either by loss of prostaglandin effect on renin secretion or by increased effective intravascular volume due to drug-induced sodium retention [84–89].

Treatment with angiotensin-converting enzyme inhibitors is also more likely to be associated with hyperkalemia in older individuals [90]. Impaired angiotensin II formation limits this potent stimulus for aldosterone secretion, and this is superimposed on the already age-related decrease in activity of the renin–angiotensin–aldosterone axis. The same drug-induced hyporeninemic hypoaldosteronism is predicted for the angiotensin receptor blockers. However, to date this has not been documented clinically.

Thiazide diuretic-induced hyponatremia is much more common in older than in younger patients, probably due to thiazide-mediated impairment in renal diluting capacity superimposed on the already present age-related decrease in capacity to dilute urine. Older studies indicated this was an extremely common cause of moderate to severe hyponatremia. However, this may occur less frequently now that lower doses of thiazide diuretics are used to treat hypertension [91–93].

## Hematopoietic System and the Treatment of Cancer

Available data suggest that the antitumor thera-peutic response of older patients is optimal when exposure to appropriate chemotherapy is the same as for younger patients. For example, the treatment of non-Hodgkin's lymphoma with cyclophosphamide, doxorubicin, vincristine, and prednisone (CHOP) or etoposide, mitoxantrone and prednimustine (VMP) is less effective in older patients when dose reductions are made [94, 95]. Similarly, treatment of metastatic breast cancer in younger and older patients with the same dose intensity of doxorubicin-based chemotherapy results in similar outcomes as measured by time to progression of disease and overall survival [96].

However, these findings must be coupled with the known increased risk of hematopoietic toxicity in older patients undergoing cancer chemotherapy. The risk of myelosuppression is increased in patients over the age of 70 [97], leading to the recommendation that these patients receive hematopoietic growth factor treatment during cancer chemotherapy [97, 98]. Such treatment also has been associated with a decrease in febrile neutropenia and sepsis-related mortality [97, 99, 100]. Anemia, defined as a hemoglobin concentration of less than 13 g/dL in men and 12 g/dL in women, is common in older adults [101], and its presence is an independent risk factor for myelotoxicity associated with anthracycline, epi-podophyllotoxin, and camptothecin chemotherapy [102]. This is at least in part due to changes in the tissue distribution of these drugs that are highly bound to red blood cells. These findings have led to a recom-mendation that hemoglobin levels should be main-tained at 12 g/dL in older patients undergoing chemotherapy [103]. Irrespective of the age of cancer patients, comorbid conditions (e.g., heart disease, renal dysfunction, and hepatobiliary disease) and functional status are the most important predictors of survival [104, 105]. Identification of comorbid condi-tions by clinical and laboratory assessment and of functional status using comprehensive geriatric assessment has been proposed as the most effective way to target therapeutic interventions in older cancer patients [106].

With respect to the pharmacokinetics and pharma-codynamics of specific cancer chemotherapy drugs in older patients, the goal is to achieve a desired tissue exposure to the drug(s) in the context of the age-related changes in drug disposition described in other sections of this chapter. Specific for anticancer agents is the role of erythrocyte and platelet binding of these drugs. Chemotherapy itself may cause anemia and/or thrombocytopenia in older patients. In the case of anemia, a diminished response to chemotherapy has been described that perhaps is due to decreased tissue delivery of drugs [107]. A summary of reported age-associated pharmacokinetic and pharmacodynamic changes for specific drugs is shown in Table 26.4 [108–115]. However, for many anticancer drugs and tumors similar information is not available to guide therapy, despite the demonstration that such information can be used to treat older patients more effectively.

## Musculoskeletal System and the Treatment of Osteoporosis

Osteoporosis is a highly prevalent disease in older individuals, affecting as many as 75% of women and

TABLE 26.4   Summary of Age-Related Changes in Disposition and Effect of Chemotherapeutic Agents

| Drug | Pharmacokinetic change in older patients[a] | Pharmacodynamic change in older patients | Ref(s) |
|---|---|---|---|
| Cyclophosphamide | — | ↑ Myelosuppression | [108] |
| Ifosfamide | ↑ $V_d$, ↓ CL, ↑ $t_{1/2}$ (Dose reduction for decreased renal function)[b] | ? | [109] |
| Melphalan | Dose reduction for decreased renal function[b] | ? | [109] |
| Chlorambucil | — | —? | [108] |
| Dacarbazine | Dose reduction for decreased renal function[b] | —? | [109] |
| Temozolomide | — | ↑ Hematotoxicity | [108] |
| Busulfan | — | ? | [108] |
| Carmustine | ? ↑ $V_d$, Dose reduction for decreased renal function[b] | ? | [109] |
| Cisplatin | Dose reduction for decreased renal function[b] | ↑ Hematotoxicity, ↑ Nausea | [108, 109] |
| Carboplatin | Dose reduction for decreased renal function[b] | ? | [108] |
| Oxaliplatin | ? | ? | [108, 109] |
| Vincristine | ? | ? | [108] |
| Vinblastine | ? | ? | [108] |
| Vinorelbine | — | — | [108] |
| Paclitaxel | — | — | [110] |
| Docetaxel | ↓ CL (CYP3A4) | ? | [108] |
| Etoposide | ↓ CL, Dose reduction for decreased renal function[b] | ? | [108] |
| Teniposide | ? | ? | [108] |
| Irinotecan | ↑ AUC | ? | [111] |
| Topotecan | ↓ CL, Dose reduction for decreased renal function[b] | — ? | [108, 112] |
| Methotrexate | ↓ CL, ↑ $t_{1/2}$, Dose reduction for decreased renal function[b] | — | [108, 113] |
| 5-Fluorouracil | — | ? — | [108] |
| Capecitabine | ? — | — | [108] |
| Cytarabine | ↓ CL, Dose adjustment for decreased renal function[b] | — | [108] |
| Gemicitabine | ↓ CL, ↑ $t_{1/2}$ | — | [114] |
| Fludarabine | Dose adjustment for decreased renal function[b] | — | [108] |
| Hydroxyurea | Dose adjustment for decreased renal function[b] | — | [108] |
| Doxorubicin | — | ↑ cardiotoxicity | [108] |
| Daunorubicin | — | ? | [108] |
| Idarubicin | Dose adjustment for decreased renal function[b] | ? | [108] |
| Epirubicin | — | ? | [108] |
| Mitoxantrone | — | ? ↑ hematotoxicity | [108] |
| Bleomycin | — | — | [108, 109] |
| Mitomycin C | ? ↑ AUC | ? ↑ myelosuppression | [115] |

[a]— Indicates no change, often based on steady-state plasma concentration rather than full pharmacokinetic analysis.

[b]Dose adjustment for renal function is in some cases recommended based on clinical experience rather than documented pharmacokinetic changes.

50% of men over the age of 80 years in the United States [116]. In addition, it is present as a comorbid condition in a number of other diseases that occur commonly in the elderly, including renal impairment, cardiovascular disease, and stroke [117]. Bone homeostasis is the result of a balance between osteoblastic bone formation and osteoclastic bone resorption. Mesenchymal stem cells differentiate either into osteoblasts or adipocytes in the bone, while osteoclasts are of hematopoietic origin. Age-related increases in PPAR-γ2 may decrease the differentiation of mesenchymal stem cells to osteoblasts and increase the formation of bone adipocytes [118]. Other local regulatory factors, including IGF-1, are positively correlated with bone mass, and age-related decreases in IGF-1 have been associated with age-related bone loss [119]. Also important is local "cross-talk" between osteoblasts and osteoclasts that involves ephrinB2 on osteoclasts and EphB4, its receptor, on osteoblasts [120]; receptor activator of NF-κB ligand (RANKL); and macrophage colony stimulating factor (M-CSF) [121]. A number of these modulators of osteoblast and osteoclast function have been therapeutic targets for treating patients with osteoporosis in order to prevent bone fractures.

The primary treatment for osteoporosis is physical activity combined with calcium and vitamin D supplementation. There is evidence that older individuals require a higher daily intake of vitamin D and calcium than do younger individuals, so the Institute of Medicine's Recommended Dietary Allowance (IOM-RDA) for vitamin D is 600 IU/day for individuals younger than 70 years of age and 800 IU/day for individuals older than 70 years of age [122]. Measures to avoid vitamin D deficiency are also recommended to include intake of 800–1000 IU of vitamin $D_3$ day$^{-1}$ for individuals older than 50 years, as they contain a decreased amount of 7–dehydrocholesterol in their skin [123]. The IOM-RDA for calcium intake is 1000 mg/day for men between 51 and 70 years of age, but is increased to 1200 mg/day for women between 51 and 70 years of age and for anyone older than 70 years of age [122].

Pharmacological therapies for the treatment of postmenopausal osteoporosis in the United States include bisphosphonates, a selective estrogen receptor modulator, estrogen, calcitonin, denosumab, and teriparatide. An effort to review comparative effectiveness among the various agents concluded that although these agents individually have been demonstrated to decrease bone fracture incidence, there are insufficient data to compare the effectiveness of specific agents [124]. Bisphosphonates (alendronate, risedronate, ibandronate, and zoledronic acid) have become the mainstay for the treatment of osteoporosis. Though as a group they clearly decrease incidence of bone fracture, there are limitations to their use in older patients because they are renally eliminated and should not be used in patients with marked renal impairment (creatinine clearance < 35 mL/min). In addition nephrotoxicity occurs with excessive bisphosphonate exposure, so renal function needs to be monitored during bisphosphonate treatment [125].

The selective estrogen receptor modulator, raloxifene, increases spine bone mineral density slightly and decreases the risk of vertebral fracture by 40% in osteoporotic women, but it has no effect on the risk of non-vertebral fracture [126]. Raloxifene may be most appropriate for patients at high risk for vertebral

fractures but who cannot tolerate bisphosphonate therapy, but a primary concern is that it is associated with an increased risk of deep vein thrombosis and pulmonary embolism. Older patients with additional comorbidities that result in low mobility may be at a particularly high risk of developing deep vein thrombosis during raloxifene therapy [125]. Estrogens (estradiol and conjugated estrogens), which act by blocking cytokine signaling to osteoclasts, have also been used to slow bone resorption in elderly patients [127, 128]. Although estrogens continue to be used to prevent postmenopausal osteoporosis, and the Women's Health Initiative study confirmed that they increased both hip and vertebral bone mineral density, this study also documented that they increased the incidence of breast cancer and thromboemboli to the extent that these risks are generally considered to outweigh the therapeutic benefit [129]. These risks may increase with increasing age, as older women tend to have higher breast cancer and thromboembolic event rates while receiving postmenopausal hormone replacement therapy [130].

Several other therapeutic options are available but are not as widely used as other treatments. Calcitonin (salmon calcitonin) has been shown in a single randomized trial to reduce the incidence of vertebral (but not non-vertebral) fracture [131]. The fully humanized monoclonal antibody against receptor activator of nuclear factor-kappa B ligand (RANKL) (denosumab) is an inhibitor of osteoclastic bone resorption [132]. It is the newest class of antiresorptive drug, but its place in therapy is not yet fully established. Teriparatide is the N-terminal chain 34-amino acid fragment of parathyroid hormone. It requires intermittent administration to result in anabolic effects [133, 134]. The usual adverse effect is mild hypercalcemia, which occurs in 1–3% of patients and is usually corrected by reducing calcium or vitamin D supplementation

## DRUG GROUPS FOR WHICH AGE CONFERS INCREASED RISK FOR TOXICITY

In addition to the adverse pharmacodynamic consequences described, for which there is at least a potential mechanistic understanding, it is more difficult to formulate a mechanistic explanation for a number of drug toxicities that are more frequent in older than younger patients.

Theophylline neurotoxicity and cardiotoxicity are increased in older patients. Although it is unclear whether decreased theophylline clearance and increased exposure in older patients fully explain this apparent sensitivity, clinical reports are uniform in identifying age as a major contributing risk factor for theophylline toxicity [135, 136]. This has resulted in much less use of theophylline in older patients.

Isoniazid-induced hepatotoxicity is more likely to occur in individuals who are more than 35 years old [137]. Attempts to establish a pharmacokinetic or pharmacogenetic explanation have been unsatisfactory. Nevertheless, this clinical finding led to the subsequent recommendation that isoniazid be withheld from individuals with a positive tuberculin skin test ($\geq 15$ mm) but no other risk factors [138]. Because approximately 5–10 % of patients with a positive tuberculin test will develop active tuberculosis and elderly individuals are at highest risk, there currently is concern that appropriate chemoprophylaxis is not being made available to individuals who are $\geq 50$ years of age [139]. In view of the fact that routine clinical monitoring has reduced the risk of severe heptatotoxicity in recent years, current guidelines do not put an age limit on the use of isoniazid to treat latent tuberculosis but simply discourage tuberculin testing in low-risk individuals [140].

Neuroleptic-induced tardive dyskinesia has been discussed. However, the mechanism for tardive dyskinesia is not well established. It is clear that increased patient age contributes significantly to the risk of developing tardive dyskinesia with the "typical" neuroleptics [44–47].

Non-steroidal anti-inflammatory drugs are probably more likely to induce gastric ulceration in older than in younger patients [141]. This may be the result of decreases in gastric mucosal prostaglandins in the elderly [142], with drug-induced inhibition of gastric prostaglandins being superimposed on this age-related decrease.

Oral anticoagulation therapy with vitamin K antagonists is more likely to be associated with bleeding, and, particularly with intracranial hemorrhage, in older as compared to younger patients. This may be in part related to impaired drug clearance [143]. Although the potential therapeutic benefit of oral anticoagulation for the treatment of venous thromboembolism or atrial fibrillation is maintained in older patients, their risk from these adverse events is higher, even when the extent of their anticoagulation is controlled by maintaining the INR in the therapeutic range of 2–3 [144, 145]. Due to these risks and the difficulty in treating older patients with vitamin K antagonists, there has been considerable interest in the thrombin and factor Xa inhibitors that have recently become available. However, there is no information available at this time about the relative risk and benefit of these alternative anticoagulants in older patients.

## CONCLUSIONS

Older patients frequently have multiple coexisting diseases that are often very effectively treated with medications. There is little doubt that the risk of a specific drug therapy, such as angiotensin-converting enzyme inhibitor treatment of patients with congestive heart failure, is in most instances far outweighed by the benefit of therapy. However, the concurrent presence of multiple diseases in older patients results in their being treated with multiple medications, which itself is a risk factor for adverse drug events. Therefore, it is an appropriate generalization to assume that the risk/benefit ratio, or the therapeutic index, of any given therapy is narrowed for older patients. Understanding age-related pathophysiology can in some instances allow for prediction of age-related changes in drug disposition and effect. However, drug therapy continues to be a significant contributor to morbidity and mortality in the elderly.

## REFERENCES

[1] Weiss CO, Boyd CM, Yu Q, Wolff JL, Leff B. Patterns of prevalent major chronic disease among older adults in the United States. JAMA 2007;298:1160–2.

[2] Boyd CM, Leff B, Wolff JL, Yu Q, Zhou J, Rand C, et al. Informing clinical practice guideline development and implementation: Prevalence of coexisting conditions among adults with coronary heart disease. J Am Geriatr Soc 2011;59:797–805.

[3] Zisook S, Downs NS. Diagnosis and treatment of depression in late life. J Clin Psych 1998;59(Suppl. 4):80–91.

[4] Dorgan CA, editor. Statistical record of health and medicine. New York, NY: International Thompson Publishing Co; 1995.

[5] Ferri CP, Prince M, Brayne C, Brodaty H, Fratiglioni L, Ganguli M, et al. Global prevalence of dementia: A Delphi consensus study. Lancet 2005;366:2112–7.

[6] Kaufman DW, Kelly JP, Rosenberg L, Anderson TE, Mitchell AA. Recent patterns of medication use in the ambulatory adult population of the United States. The Slone Survey. JAMA 2002;287:337–44.

[7] Smith JW, Seidl LG, Cluff LE. Studies on the epidemiology of adverse drug reactions. V. Clinical factors influencing susceptibility. Ann Intern Med 1966;65:629–40.

[8] Hutchinson TA, Flegel KM, Kramer MS, Leduc DG, Kong HH. Frequency, severity and risk factors for adverse drug reactions in adult outpatients. J Chronic Dis 1986;39:533–42.

[9] Gurwitz JH, Field TS, Avorn J, McCormick D, Jain S, Eckler M, et al. Incidence and preventability of adverse drug events in the nursing home setting. Am J Med 2000;109:87–94.

[10] Gurwitz JH, Avorn J. The ambiguous relation between aging and adverse drug reactions. Ann Intern Med 1991;114:956–66.

[11] Tinetti ME, Bogardus ST, Agostini JV. Potential pitfalls of disease-specific guidelines for patients with multiple conditions. N Engl J Med 2004;351:2870–4.

[12] Boyd CM, Darer J, Boult C, Fried LP, Boult L, Wu AW. Clinical practice guidelines and quality of care for older patients with multiple comorbid diseases. JAMA 2005;295:716–24.

[13] Hall DA. The biomedical basis of gerontology. Littleton, MA: John Wright PSG, Inc; 1984.

[14] Borkan GA, Hults DE, Gerzof SG, Robbins AH, Silbert CK. Age changes in body composition revealed by computed tomography. J Gerontol 1983;38:673–7.

[15] Klotz U. Pharmacokinetics and drug metabolism in the elderly. Drug Metab Rev 2009;41:67–76.

[16] Benet LZ, Hoener B-A. Changes in plasma protein binding have little clinical significance. Clin Pharmacol Ther 2002;71:115–21.

[17] Davies DF, Shock NW. Age changes in glomerular filtration rate, effective renal plasma flow, and tubular excretory capacity in adult males. J Clin Invest 1950;29:496–507.

[18] Cockcroft DW, Gault MH. Prediction of creatinine clearance from serum creatinine. Nephron 1976;16:31–41.

[19] Levey AS, Bosch JP, Lewis JB, Greene T, Rogers N, Roth D. A more accurate method to estimate glomerular filtration rate from serum creatinine: A new prediction equation. Modification of Diet in Renal Disease Study Group. Ann Intern Med 1999;130:461–70.

[20] Nyman HA, Dowling TC, Hudson JQ, St. Peter WL, Joy MS, Nolin TD. Comparative evaluation of the Cockcroft-Gault equation and the modification of diet in renal disease (MDRD) study equation for drug dosing: An opinion of the Nephrology Practice and Research Network of the American College of Clinical Pharmacy. Pharmacotherapy 2011;31:1130–44.

[21] Schwartz JB, Abernethy DR. Aging and medications: Past, present, future. Clin Pharmacol Ther 2009;85:3–10.

[22] Bauer LA, Blouin RA. Age and phenytoin kinetics in adult epileptics. Clin Pharmacol Ther 1982;31:301–4.

[23] Sproule BA, Hardy BG, Shulman KI. Differential pharmacokinetics of lithium in elderly patients. Drugs Aging 2000;16:165–77.

[24] Cusack B, Kelly J, O'Malley K, Noel J, Lavan J, Horgan J. Digoxin in the elderly: Pharmacokinetic consequences of old age. Clin Pharmacol Ther 1979;25:772–6.

[25] Drayer DE, Romankiewicz J, Lorenzo B, Reidenberg MM. Age and renal clearance of cimetidine. Clin Pharmacol Ther 1982;31:45–60.

[26] Reidenberg MM, Camacho M, Kluger J, Drayer DE. Aging and renal clearance of procainamide and acetylprocainamide. Clin Pharmacol Ther 1980;28:732–5.

[27] Parkinson A, Mudra DR, Johnson C, Dwyer A, Carroll KM. The effects of gender, age, ethnicity, and liver cirrhosis on cytochrome P450 enzyme activity in human liver microsomes and inducibility in cultured human hepatocytes. Toxicol Appl Pharmacol 2004;199:193–209.

[28] Greenblatt DJ, Abernethy DR, Locniskar A, Harmatz JS, Limjuco RA, Shader RI. Effect of age, gender, and obesity on midazolam kinetics. Anesthesiology 1984;61:27–35.

[29] Greenblatt DJ, Divoll M, Abernethy DR, Moschitto LJ, Smith RB, Shader R. Reduced clearance of triazolam in old age: Relation to antipyrine oxidizing capacity. Br J Clin Pharmacol 1983;15:303–9.

[30] Kang D, Verotta D, Schwartz JB. Population analyses of amlodipine in patients living in the community and patients living in nursing homes. Clin Pharmacol Ther 2006;79:114–24.

[31] Schwartz JB. Erythromycin breath test results in elderly, very elderly, and frail elderly persons. Clin Pharmacol Ther 2006;79:440–8.

[32] Greenblatt DJ, Harmatz JS, Shapiro L, Engelhardt N, Gouthro TA, Shader RI. Sensitivity to triazolam in the elderly. N Engl J Med 1991;324:1691–8.

[33] Raz N. Aging of the brain and its impact on cognitive performance: Integration of structural and functional findings. In: Craik FIM, Salthouse TA, editors. The handbook of aging and cognition. 2nd ed. Mahwah, NJ: Lawrence Erlbaum Associates; 2000. p. 1–90.

[34] Volkow ND, Gur RC, Wang G-J, Fowler JS, Moberg PJ, Ding Y-S, et al. Association between decline in brain dopamine activity with age and cognitive and motor impairment in healthy individuals. Am J Psychiatry 1998;155:344–9.

[35] Schnider TW, Minto CF, Shafer SL, Gambus PL, Andresen C, Goodale DB, et al. The influence of age on propofol pharmacodynamics. Anesthesiology 1999;90:1502–16.

[36] Olmos M, Ballester JA, Vidarte A, Elizalde JL, Escobar A. The combined effect of age and premedication on the propofol requirements for induction by target controlled infusion. Anesth Analg 2000;90:1157–61.

[37] Scott JC, Stanski DR. Decreased fentanyl and alfentanil dose requirements with age. A simultaneous pharmacokinetic and pharmacodynamic evaluation. J Pharmacol Exp Ther 1987;240:159–66.

[38] Stanski DR, Maitre PO. Population pharmacokinetics and pharmacodynamics of thiopental: The effect of age revisited. Anesthesiology 1990;72:412–22.

[39] Jacobs JR, Reves JG, Marty J, White WD, Bai SA, Smith LR. Aging increases pharmacodynamic sensitivity to the hypnotic effects of midazolam. Anesth Analg 1995;80:143–8.

[40] Ray WA, Griffin MR, Downey W. Benzodiazepines of long and short elimination half-life and the risk of hip fracture. JAMA 1989;262:3303–7.

[41] Greenblatt DJ, Shader RI, Abernethy DR. Drug therapy. Current status of benzodiazepines. N Engl J Med 1983;309:354–8, 410–6.

[42] Greenblatt DJ, Allen MD, Shader RI. Toxicity of high-dose flurazepam in the elderly. Clin Pharmacol Ther 1977;21:355–61.

[43] Saltz BL, Woerner MG, Kane JM, Lieberman JA, Alvir JMJ, Bergmann KJ, et al. Prospective study of tardive dyskinesia incidence in the elderly. JAMA 1991;266:2402–6.

[44] Jeste DV, Caligiuri MP, Paulsen JS, Heaton RK, Lacro JP, Harris J, et al. Risk of tardive dyskinesia in older patients: A prospective longitudinal study of 266 outpatients. Arch Gen Psychiatry 1995;52:756–65.

[45] Woerner MG, Alvir JMJ, Saltz BL, Lieberman JA, Kane JM. Prospective study of tardive dyskinesia in the elderly: Rates and risk factors. Am J Psychiatry 1998;155:1521–8.

[46] Jeste DV. Tardive dyskinesia in older patients. J Clin Psychiatry 2000;61(Suppl. 4):27–32.

[47] Jeste DV, Lacro JP, Bailey A, Rockwell E, Harris MJ, Caligiuri MP. Lower incidence of tardive dyskinesia with risperidone compared with haloperidol in older patients. J Am Geriatr Soc 1999;47:716–9.

[48] Ballard C, Creese B, Corbett A, Aarsland D. Atypical antipsychotics for the treatment of behavioral and psychological symptoms in dementia, with a particular focus on longer term outcomes and mortality. Expert Opin Drug Saf 2011;10:35–43.

[49] Rochon PA, Normand S-L, Gomes T, Gill SS, Anderson GM, Melo M, et al. Antipsychotic therapy and short-term serious events in older adults with dementia. Arch Intern Med 2008;168:1090–6.

[50] Schneider LS, Tariot PN, Dagerman KS, Davis SM, Hsaio JK, Ismail S, et al. for the CATIE-AD Study Group. Effectiveness of atypical antipsychotic drugs in patients with Alzheimer's disease. N Engl J Med 2006;355:1525–38.

[51] Abernethy DR, Greenblatt DJ, Shader RI. Imipramine and desipramine disposition in the elderly. J Pharmacol Exp Ther 1985;232:183–8.

[52] Hilmer SN, Mager DE, Simonsick EM, Cao Y, Ling SM, Windham BG, et al. A drug burden index to define the functional burden of medications in older people. Arch Intern Med 2007;167:781–7.

[53] Cao Y-J, Mager DE, Simonsick EM, Hilmer SN, Ling SM, Windham BG, et al. Physical and cognitive performance and burden of anticholinergics, sedatives, and ACE inhibitors. Clin Pharmacol Ther 2008;83:422–9.

[54] Hilmer SN, Mager DE, Simonsick EM, Ling SM, Windham BG, Harris TB, et al, for the Health ABC Study. Drug burden index and functional decline in older people. Am J Med 2009;122:1142–9.

[55] Gnjidic D, Le Couteur DG, Abernethy DR, Hilmer SN. A pilot randomized clinical trial utilizing the drug burden index to reduce exposure to anticholinergic and sedative medications in older people. Ann Pharmacother 2010;44:1725–32.

[56] Low PA. The effect of aging on the autonomic nervous system. In: Low PA, editor. Clinical autonomic disorders. 2nd ed. Philadelphia, PA: Lippincott-Raven; 1977. p. 161–75.

[57] Vestal RE, Wood AJJ, Shand DG. Reduced beta-adrenoceptor sensitivity in the elderly. Clin Pharmacol Ther 1979;26:181–6.

[58] Ziegler MG, Lake CR, Kopin IJ. Plasma noradrenaline increases with age. Nature 1976;261:333–5.

[59] Rodstein M, Zeman FD. Postural blood pressure changes in the elderly. J Chronic Dis 1957;6:581–8.

[60] Lipsitz LA, Nyquist RP, Wei JY, Rowe JW. Postprandial reduction in blood pressure in the elderly. N Engl J Med 1983;309:81–3.

[61] van Kraaij DJW, Jansen RWMM, Gribnau FWJ, Hoefnagels WHL. Diuretic therapy in elderly heart failure patients with and without left ventricular systolic dysfunction. Drugs Aging 2000;16:289–300.

[62] Ray WA, Griffin MR, Schaffner W, Baugh DK, Melton LJ. Psychotropic drug use and the risk of hip fracture. N Engl J Med 1987;316:363–9.

[63] Reilly JG, Ayis SA, Ferrier IN, Jones SJ, Thomas SHL. QT$_c$-interval abnormalities and psychotropic drug therapy in psychiatric patients. Lancet 2000;355:1048–52.

[64] Abernethy DR, Schwartz JB, Plachetka JR, Todd EL, Egan JM. Comparison in young and elderly patients of pharmacodynamics and disposition of labetalol in systemic hypertension. Am J Cardiol 1987;60:697–702.

[65] Lakatta EG. Cardiovascular aging research: The next horizons. J Am Geriatr Soc 1999;47:613–25.

[66] Maciel LMZ, Polikar R, Rohrer D, Popovich BK, Dillmann WH. Age-induced decreases in the messenger RNA coding for the sarcoplasmic reticulum Ca$^{2+}$-ATPase of the rat heart. Circ Res 1990;67:230–4.

[67] van Harten J, Burggraaf J, Ligthart GJ, van Brummelen P, Breimer DD. Single- and multiple-dose nisoldipine kinetics and effects in the young, the middle-aged, and the elderly. Clin Pharmacol Ther 1989;45:600–7.

[68] ACC/AHA Task Force Report. Guidelines for the evaluation and management of chronic heart failure in the adult. Circulation 2001;104:2996–3007.

[69] Tresch DD. The clinical diagnosis of heart failure in older patients. J Am Geriatr Soc 1997;45:1128–33.

[70] Bonow RO, Udelson JE. Left ventricular diastolic dysfunction as a cause of congestive heart failure: Mechanisms and management. Ann Intern Med 1992;117:502–10.

[71] van Kraaij DJW, Jansen RWMM, Bouwels LHR, Hoefnagels WHL. Furosemide withdrawal improves postprandial hypotension in elderly patients with heart failure and preserved left ventricular systolic function. Arch Intern Med 1999;159:1599–605.

[72] Cangiano JL, Martinez-Maldonado M. Isolated systolic hypertension in the elderly. In: Martinez-Maldonado M, editor. Hypertension and renal disease in the elderly. Oxford: Blackwell Scientific Publications; 1992. p. 79–94.

[73] Andrawis NS, Jones DS, Abernethy DR. Aging is associated with endothelial dysfunction in the human forearm vasculature. J Am Geriatr Soc 2000;48:193–8.

[74] Pan HYM, Hoffman BB, Porshe RA, Blaschke TF. Decline in beta-adrenergic receptor mediated vascular relaxation with aging in man. J Pharmacol Exp Ther 1986;239:802–7.

[75] Hosmane BS, Maurath CJ, Jordan DC, Laddu A. Effect of age and dose on the incidence of adverse events in the treatment of hypertension in patients receiving terazosin. J Clin Pharmacol 1992;32:434–43.

[76] Abernethy DR, Gutkowska J, Winterbottom LM. Effects of amlodipine, a long-acting dihydropyridine calcium antagonist in aging hypertension: Pharmacodynamics in relation to disposition. Clin Pharmacol Ther 1990;48:76–86.

[77] Abernethy DR, Schwartz JB, Todd EL, Luchi R, Snow E. Verapamil pharmacodynamics and disposition in young versus elderly hypertensive patients. Ann Intern Med 1986;105:329–36.

[78] Schwartz JB, Abernethy DR. Responses to intravenous and oral diltiazem in elderly versus younger patients with systemic hypertension. Am J Cardiol 1987;59:1111–7.

[79] Verza M, Cacciapuoti F, Spiezia R, D'Avino M, Arpino G, D'Errico S, et al. Effects of the angiotensin converting enzyme inhibitor enalapril compared with diuretic therapy in elderly hypertensive patients. J Hypertens 1988;6(Suppl. 1):S97–9.

[80] Crane MG, Harris JJ. Effect of aging on renin activity and aldosterone excretion. J Lab Clin Med 1976;87:947–59.

[81] Hall JE, Coleman TG, Guyton AC. The renin–angiotensin system: Normal physiology and changes in older hypertensives. J Am Geriatr Soc 1989;37:801–13.

[82] Agency for Health Care Policy and Research (AHCPR). Heart failure: Evaluation and treatment of patients with left ventricular systolic dysfunction. J Am Geriatr Soc 1998;46:525–9.

[83] Lindeman RD. Overview: Renal physiology and pathophysiology of aging. Am J Kidney Dis 1990;26:275–82.

[84] Miller M. Hyponatremia: Age-related risk factors and therapy decisions. Geriatrics 1998;53:32–48.

[85] Rowe JW, Minaker KL, Levi M. Pathophysiology and management of electrolyte disturbances in the elderly. In: Martinez-Maldonado M, editor. Hypertension and renal disease in the elderly. Boston, MA: Blackwell Scientific Publications; 1992. p. 170–84.

[86] Gurwitz JH, Avorn J, Ross-Degnan D, Lipsitz LA. Nonsteroidal anti-inflammatory drug associated azotemia in the very old. JAMA 1990;264:471–5.

[87] Field TS, Gurwitz JH, Glynn RJ, Salive ME, Gaziano JM, Taylor JO, Hennekens CH. The renal effects of nonsteroidal anti-inflammatory drugs in older people: Findings from the Established Populations for Epidemiologic Studies of the Elderly. J Am Geriatr Soc 1999;47:507–11.

[88] Whelton A, Schulman G, Wallemark C, Drower EJ, Isakson PC, Verburg KM, et al. Effects of celecoxib and naproxen on renal function in the elderly. Arch Intern Med 2000;160:1465–70.

[89] Swan SK, Rudy DW, Lasseter KC, Ryan CF, Buechel KL, Lambrecht LJ, et al. Effect of cyclooxygenase-2 inhibition on renal function in elderly persons receiving a low salt diet. Ann Intern Med 2000;133:1–9.

[90] Reardon LC, Macpherson DS. Hyperkalemia in outpatients using angiotensin-converting enzyme inhibitors. Arch Intern Med 1998;158:26–32.

[91] Sunderam SG, Mankikar GD. Hyponatremia in the elderly. Age Ageing 1983;12:77–80.

[92] Fichman M, Vorherr H, Kleeman G. Diuretic-induced hyponatremia. Ann Intern Med 1971;75:853–63.

[93] Ashraf N, Locksley R, Arieff A. Thiazide-induced hyponatremia associated with death or neurologic damage in outpatients. Am J Med 1981;70:1163–8.

[94] Dixon DO, Neilan B, Jones SE, Lipschitz DA, Miller TP, Grozea PN, et al. Effect of age on the therapeutic outcome in advanced diffuse histiocytic lymphoma: The Southwest Oncology Group experience. J Clin Oncol 1986;4:295–305.

[95] Tirelli U, Errante D, Van Glabbeke M, Teodorovic I, Kluin-Nelemans JC, Thomas J, et al. CHOP is the standard regimen in patients > or = 70 years of age with intermediate-grade and high-grade non-Hodgkin's lymphoma: Results of a randomized study of the European Organization for Research and Treatment of Cancer Lymphoma Cooperative Study Group. J Clin Oncol 1998;16:27–34.

[96] Ibrahim NK, Frye DK, Buzdar AU, Walters RS, Hortobagyi GN. Doxorubicin-based chemotherapy in elderly patients with metastatic breast cancer. Tolerance and outcome. Arch Intern Med 1996;156:882–8.

[97] Balducci L, Lyman GH. Patients aged ≥ 70 are at high risk for neutropenic infection and should receive hemopoietic growth

factors when treated with moderately toxic chemotherapy. J Clin Oncol 2001;19:1583–5.

[98] Balducci L, Yates J. General guidelines for the management of older patients with cancer. Oncology (Huntingt) 2000;14:221–7.

[99] Lyman GH, Kuderer NM, Djulbegovic B. Prophylatic granulocyte colony-stimulating factor in patients receiving dose-intensive cancer chemotherapy: A meta-analysis. Am J Med 2002;112:406–11.

[100] Lyman GH, Kuderer N, Agboola O, Balducci L. Evidence-based use of colony-stimulating factors in elderly cancer patients. Cancer Control 2003;10:487–99.

[101] Ania BJ, Suman VJ, Fairbanks VF, Rademacher DM, Melton III LJ. Incidence of anemia in older people: an epidemiologic study in a well defined population. J Am Geriatr Soc 1997;45:825–31.

[102] Schrijvers D, Highley M, De Bruyn E, Van Oosterom AT, Vermorken JB. Role of red blood cells in pharmacokinetics of chemotherapeutic agents. Anticancer Drugs 1999;10:147–53.

[103] Winn RJ, McClure J. The NCCN clinical practice guidelines in oncology: A primer for users. J Natl Compr Cancer Network 2003;1:5–13.

[104] Satariano WA, Ragland DR. The effect of comorbidity on 3-year survival of woman with primary breast cancer. Ann Intern Med 1994;120:104–10.

[105] Extermann M, Overcash J, Lyman GH, Parr J, Balducci L. Comorbidity and functional status are independent in older cancer patients. J Clin Oncl 1998;16:1582–7.

[106] Ferrucci L, Guralnik JM, Cavazzini C, Bandinelli S, Lauretani F, Bartali B, et al. The frailty syndrome: A critical issue in geriatric oncology. Crit Rev Oncol Hematol 2003;46:127–37.

[107] Eisenhauer EA, Vermorken JB, van Glabbeke M. Predictors of response to subsequent chemotherapy in platinum pretreated ovarian cancer: A multivariate analysis of 704 patients. Ann Oncol 1997;8:963–8.

[108] Wildiers H, Highley MS, de Bruijn EA, van Oosterom AT. Pharmacology of anticancer drugs in elderly population. Clin Pharmacokinet 2003;42:1213–42.

[109] Kintzel PE, Dorr RT. Anticancer drug renal toxicity and elimination: Dosing guidelines for altered renal function. Cancer Treat Rev 1995;21:33–64.

[110] Nakamura Y, Sekine I, Furuse K, Saijo N. Retrospective comparison of toxicity and efficacy in phase II trails of 3-h infusions of paclitaxel for patients 70 years of age or older and patients under 70 years of age. Cancer Chemother Pharmacol 2000;46:114–8.

[111] Miya T, Goya T, Fujii H, Ohtsu T, Itoh K, Igarashi T, et al. Factors affecting the pharmacokinetics of CPT-11: The body mass index, age and sex are independent predictors of pharmacokinetic parameters of CPT-11. Invest New Drugs 2001;19:61–7.

[112] O' Reilly S, Rowinsky EK, Slichenmyer W, Donehower RC, Forastiere AA, Ettinger DS, et al. Phase I and pharmacologic study of topotecan in patients with impaired renal function. J Clin Oncol 1996;14:3062–73.

[113] Gelman RS, Taylor SG. Cyclophosphamide, methotrexate, and 5-fluorouracil chemotherapy in women more than 65 years old with advanced breast cancer: The elimination of age trends in toxicity by using doses based on creatinine clearance. J Clin Oncol 1984;2:1404–13.

[114] Lichtman SM, Skirvin JA. Pharmacology of antineoplastic agents in older cancer patients. Oncology (Huntingt) 2000;14:1743–55.

[115] Miya T, Sasaki Y, Karato A, Saijo N. Pharmacokinetic study of mitomycin C with emphasis on the influence of aging. Jpn J Cancer Res 1992;83:1382–5.

[116] Looker AC, Johnston CC, Wahner HW, Dunn WL, Calvo MS, Harris TB, et al. Prevalence of low femoral bone density in older US women from NHANES III. J Bone Miner Res 1995;10:796–802.

[117] Colon-Emeric C, O'Connell MB, Haney E. Osteoporosis piece of the multi-morbidity puzzle in geriatric care. Mt Sinai J Med 2011;78:515–26.

[118] Moerman EJ, Teng K, Lipschitz DA, Lecka-Czernik B. Aging activates adipogenic and suppresses osteogenic programs in mesenchymal marrow stroma/stem cells: The role of PPAR-γ2 transcription factor and TGF-β/BMP signaling pathways. Aging Cell 2004;3:379–89.

[119] Lecka-Czernik B, Rosen CJ, Kawai M. Skeletal aging and the adipocyte program. Cell Cycle 2010;9:3648–54.

[120] Mundy GR, Elefteriou F. Boning up on ephrin signaling. Cell 2006;126:441–3.

[121] Teitelbaum SL, Ross FP. Genetic regulation of osteoclast development and function. Nature Rev Genetics 2003;4:638–49.

[122] Institute of Medicine. Dietary reference intakes for calcium and vitamin D. Report Brief. Washington DC: IOM (Internet at, www.iom.edu/~ /media/Files/Report%20Files/2010/Dietary-Reference-Intakes-for-Calcium-and-Vitamin-D/Vitamin%20D%20and%20Calcium%202010%20Report%20Brief.pdf; Revised March 2011).

[123] Holick MF. Vitamin D deficiency. N Engl J Med 2007;357:266–81.

[124] MacLean C, Newberry S, Maglione M, McMahon M, Ranganath V, Suttorp M, et al. Systematic review: Comparative effectiveness of treatments to prevent fractures in men and women with low bone density or osteoporosis. Ann Intern Med 2008;148:197–213.

[125] Gates BJ, Sonnett TE, DuVall CA, Dobbins EK. Review of osteoporosis pharmacotherapy for geriatric patients. Am J Geriatr Pharmacother 2009;7:293–323.

[126] Ettinger B, Black DM, Mitlak BH, Knickerbocker RK, Nickelsen T, Genant HK, et al. Reduction of vertebral fracture risk in postmenopausal women with osteoporosis treated with raloxifene: Results from a 3-year randomized clinical trial. JAMA 1999;282:637–45.

[127] Miyaura C, Kusano K, Masuzawa T, Chaki O, Onoe Y, Aoyagi M, Sasaki T, et al. Endogenous bone-resorbing factors in estrogen deficiency: Cooperative effects of IL-1 and IL-6. J Bone Mineral Res 1995;10:1365–73.

[128] Giuliani N, Sansoni P, Girasole G, Vescovini R, Passeri G, Passeri M, et al. Serum interleukin-6, soluble interleukin-6 receptor and soluble gp130 exhibit different patterns of age- and menopause-related changes. Exp Gerontol 2001;36:547–57.

[129] Cauley JA, Robbins J, Chen Z, Cummings SR, Jackson RD, LaCroix AZ, et al. Women's Health Initiative Investigators. Effects of estrogen plus progestin on risk of fracture and bone mineral density: The Women's Health Initiative Randomized Trial. JAMA 2003;290:1729–38.

[130] Nelson HD, Humphrey LL, Nygren P, Teutsch SM, Allan JD. Postmenopausal hormone replacement therapy: Scientific review. JAMA 2001;288:872–81.

[131] Chesnut CH, Silverman S, Andriano K, Genant H, Gimona A, Harris S, et al, for the PROOF Study Group. A randomized trial of nasal spray salmon calcitonin in postmenopausal women with established osteoporosis: The Prevent Recurrence of Osteoporotic Fractures Study. Am J Med 2000;109:267–76.

[132] Cummings SR, San Martin J, McClung MR, Siris ES, Eastell R, Reid IR, et al. Siddhanti S, Christiansen C. The FREEDOM Trial: Denosumab for prevention of fractures in postmenopausal women with osteoporosis. N Engl J Med 2009;361:756–65.

[133] Jilka RL. Molecular and cellular mechanisms of the anabolic effect of intermittent PTH. Bone 2007;40:1434–6.

[134] Canalis E, Giustina A, Bilezikian JP. Mechanisms of anabolic therapies for osteoporosis. N Engl J Med 2007;357:905–16.

[135] Shannon M, Lovejoy FH. The influence of age vs peak serum concentration on life-threatening events after chronic theophylline intoxication. Arch Intern Med 1990;150:2045–8.

[136] Schiff GD, Hegde HK, LaCloche L, Hryhoczuk DO. Inpatient theophylline toxicity: Preventable factors. Ann Intern Med 1991;114:748–53.

[137] Kopanoff DE, Snider Jr DE, Caras GJ. Isoniazid-related hepatitis: A US Public Health Service cooperative surveillance study. Am Rev Resp Dis 1979;117:992–1001.

[138] American Thoracic Society. Treatment of tuberculosis and tuberculosis infection in adults and children. Am J Respir Crit Care Med 1994;149:1359–74.

[139] Sorresso DJ, Mehta JB, Harvil LM, Bently S. Underutilization of isoniazid chemoprophylaxis in tuberculosis contacts 50 year of age and older. A prospective analysis. Chest 1995;108:706–11.

[140] American Thoracic Society. Targeted tuberculin testing and treatment of latent tuberculosis infection. MMWR 2000;49(No RR-6):1–51.

[141] Gabriel SE, Jaakkimainen L, Bombardier C. Risk for serious gastrointestinal complications related to use of nonsteroidal anti-inflammatory drugs. Ann Intern Med 1991;115:787–96.

[142] Cryer B, Lee E, Feldman M. Factors influencing gastroduodenal mucosal prostaglandin concentrations: Roles of smoking and aging. Ann Intern Med 1992;116:636–40.

[143] Shepherd AMM, Hewick DS, Moreland TA, Stevenson IH. Age as a determinant of sensitivity to warfarin. Br J Clin Pharmacol 1977;4:315–20.

[144] Fang MC, Chang Y, Hylek EM, Rosand J, Greenberg SM, Go AS, et al. Advanced age, anticoagulation intensity, and risk for intracranial hemorrhage among patients taking warfarin for atrial fibrillation. Ann Intern Med 2004;141:745–52.

[145] Palareti G, Hirsch J, Legnani C, Manotti C, D'Angelo A, Pengo V, et al. Oral anticoagulation treatment in the elderly: A nested, prospective, case–control study. Arch Intern Med 2000;160:470–8.

# Clinical Analysis of Adverse Drug Reactions

Michael Fotis and William Budris

*Drug Information Center, Department of Pharmacy, Northwestern Memorial Hospital, Chicago, IL 60611*

## INTRODUCTION

*Adverse drug reactions* (ADRs) are common, over-looked, expensive, serious, and under-reported. For the most part, our understanding of adverse reactions is based on anecdotal information that is reported on a voluntary basis, and these reports are commonly incomplete and even inaccurate [1–3]. However, Lazarou *et al.* [4] focused attention on the importance of ADRs in a careful meta-analysis of prospective ADR studies. These authors concluded that ADRs occurred in 10.9% of hospitalized patients, that serious ADRs accounted for 4.7% of hospital admissions, and that ADRs may rank somewhere between the fourth and sixth most common cause of death in the United States. Unfortunately, the frequency of ADRs remains unaffected by more than 10 years of process improvements such as use of order sets, care plans, computerized prescriber order entry, or other types of decision support systems [5].

There is general agreement that commonly used medications such as diuretics, anticoagulants, and antiplatelet and antidiabetic agents are implicated more often than high-risk agents [6–8]. Despite this, clinicians are left to make treatment decisions that usually are based on an imbalance of information about the benefit and harm of therapeutic options. Given the general lack of understanding of ADRs, clinicians may attribute a patient's symptoms to his or her underlying illness and not consider that these symptoms may be due to a potential ADR. By failing to consider an adverse drug reaction, even when faced with objective evidence to the contrary, clinicians may end up by adding a new agent to manage these symptoms instead of modifying the offending medication regimen [9]. This has the potential to initiate an entire cascade of adverse events [9, 10].

## DEFINITIONS AND CLASSIFICATION

The terminology used to describe ADRs is confusing and frequently used incorrectly [9, 11, 12]. The US Food and Drug Administration (FDA) defines an ADR as any undesirable experience associated with the use of a medical product in a patient [13]. Edwards and Aronson [12] define an ADR as "an appreciably harmful or unpleasant reaction, resulting from an intervention related to the use of a medicinal product, which predicts hazard from future administration and warrants prevention or specific treatment, or alteration of the dosage regimen or withdrawal of the product". When compared to an ADR, an *adverse event* (ADE) is a harmful outcome that presents during treatment with a medication and, as described in Chapter 28, includes some medication errors as well as ADRs. In an ADE there may not be enough information to even conclude that the event was caused by the medication [11, 12], Members of the Consolidated Standards of Reporting Trials (CONSORT) recommend use of the term *"Harms"* to refer to all possible adverse occurrences [11] (the sum of ADRs, ADEs, errors, plus other undesirable outcomes). Harms are the opposite of benefits [11].

*PRINCIPLES OF CLINICAL PHARMACOLOGY, THIRD EDITION*
DOI: http://dx.doi.org/10.1016/B978-0-12-385471-1.00027-1

## Classification by Severity

Classification of ADRs by severity allows comparisons to be made between medical teams or services, or, if standardized, to other medical centers, and a severity scale published by Hartwig *et al.* [14] is commonly used. A determination of severity is often necessary when setting priorities for actionable findings. The severity scale used by the authors of this chapter for clinical surveillance of adverse drug reactions is summarized in Table 27.1. This step-wise scale is graded by the expected consumption of resources in each level.

## Classification by Type

ADRs can be considered as dose related (Type A) or not dose related (Type B) [15]. Type B reactions can be further subdivided into immunologic and idiosyncratic. Additional categories include time related, withdrawal, and failure of therapy [12]. The classification scheme used by the chapter authors is summarized in Table 27.2.

### Pharmacologic ADRs

As pointed out over 40 years ago by Melmon [16], most pharmacologic ADRs are dose related and represent an exaggerated pharmacologic effect of the drug. This type of ADR can also be seen when reductions in renal clearance, due to renal insufficiency, or in non-renal clearance, due to

**TABLE 27.1  Definitions for the Determination of the Severity of an ADR**

*Minor*:

Prolongation of hospital stay is not required. Therapy might include stopping the medication, reducing the dose, and/or administering palliative therapy. Additional testing or increased hospitalization is not required.

*Moderate*:

Requires further testing or procedures, to evaluate patient, or increases hospitalization by at least 1 day, or results in admission.

*Serious*:

Results in persistent or significant disability (e.g., hemorrhage requiring transfusion or hospitalization but without symptoms of hemodynamic instability) or results in transfer to critical care.

*Serious life-threatening*:

ex. Hemorrhage associated with hypotension, hypoglycemic encephalopathy, profound hyponatremia, and acute renal failure requiring hospitalization.

*Serious lethal*:

Contributes to the death of the patient.

**TABLE 27.2  Surveillance Classification of ADRs by Type**

1. *Pharmacologic*: These adverse effects are dose related and represent an exaggerated pharmacologic effect of the drug — for example a hypoglycemic event following an excessive dose of insulin, or symptomatic hypotension following an excessive dose of an antihypertensive medication

2. *Intolerance*: Refers to exaggerated pharmacologic effects seen at low doses of medication — for example, drowsiness following a very low dose of morphine, or dizziness from a low dose of diphenhydramine

3. *Idiosyncratic*: Reactions that are not predictable, and not related to dose or pharmacology — for example, muscle pain associated with statins

4. *Allergic*: Medication allergies are most commonly seen with antibiotics and are immune mediated reactions, such as hives, rashes of other types, bronchospasm

hepatic disease or secondary to drug interactions, are not compensated for by reductions in the selected dose. Generally, these ADRs are predictable and reversible. They can be the result of a prescribing error, but are also seen during careful upward titration of doses to achieve a satisfactory therapeutic response.

### Idiosyncratic ADRs

Unlike pharmacologic ADRs, Type B ADRs, such as those described in Chapter 16, are not dose related and often are without an antidote. These ADRs include intolerance and allergic reactions as well as idiosyncratic drug reactions that cannot be explained by a known mechanism of drug action. Idiosyncratic ADRs are not seen at any dose in most patients, and thus are not classified as intolerance, but instead occur unpredictably and only in susceptible patients. It is important to be aware of idiosyncratic reactions because most severe and or life-threatening ADRs are idiosyncratic in nature and require discontinuation of treatment. As described in Chapter 16, these reactions result, in many cases, from patient differences in drug metabolism that result in accumulation of chemically reactive or otherwise toxic metabolites, or by variations in the human leukocyte antigen (HLA-B) complex. Severe dermatologic reactions to carbamazepine [17] and to allopurinol [18] are examples of HLA-B variation linked to ADRs. The Risk Evaluation and Mitigation Strategy (REMS), developed by the FDA and described later in this chapter, provides a systematic approach for improving medication safety, and tends to focus on these idiosyncratic reactions that are unpredictable yet severe.

*Allergic ADRs*

Medication allergies are considered as immune-mediated hypersensitivity and classified as one of the four types described by Gell and Coombs [19] and as expanded by Kay [20], or as an idiosyncratic drug hypersensitivity syndrome which generally involves fever, lymphadenopathy, rash, and internal organ involvement [21]. The Gell and Coombs Classification is summarized in Figure 27.1 [22].

## ADR Detection

Hospitals generally have protocol-based strategies for preventing and detecting ADRs. Prevention is frequently achieved by a combination of pharmacist review or involvement at the time of prescription. [23–25]. Detection is often accomplished by a clinician observing conditions, laboratory values, or other data points indicating an ADR. For example, elevated plasma drug concentrations or prescription of reversal agents, such as digoxin-specific antibody fragments, have been used to trigger identification of potential adverse reactions [26–31]. This mode of surveillance can be enhanced by combining triggers such as use of vitamin K in a patient with an elevated INR value. Combining search terms is an effective method for reducing the number of false alerts [32]. Systematic use of a trigger tool has been reported to result in a significant increase in the number of recognized adverse events [33, 34].

Surveillance has successfully identified a number of avoidable high-risk situations, as well as medications whose proper use is misunderstood. Digoxin, phenytoin, theophylline, and warfarin toxicities can be avoided by (1) reacting to predictable changes in drug clearance secondary to renal or hepatic insufficiency or due to drug–drug interactions, and (2) proper interpretation of non-steady-state or spurious serum concentration (e.g., due to improperly timed blood sampling) or other laboratory values such as the INR [28–30]. Careful assessment and documentation of medication allergy histories is necessary to prevent future allergic reactions, or to avoid use of unnecessary alternative medications when true allergy symptoms did not occur [35, 36].

Although ADRs have traditionally been identified by voluntary, retrospective reporting, several concurrent studies have found that adding a pharmacist to the medical team at the decision-making stage

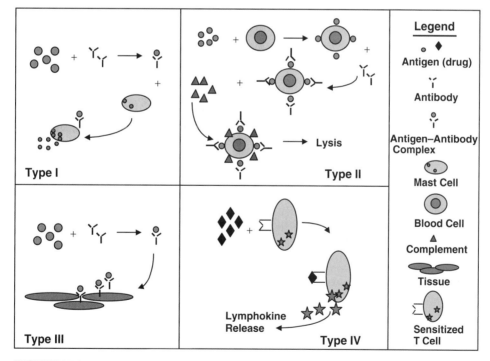

**FIGURE 27.1**   Mechanisms of hypersensitivity reactions. Type I: Antigens bind to antibodies on mast cells, causing degranulation and release of histamine and other mediators. Type II: Antibodies attach to cell-surface antigens, causing activation of complement or other effector cells (neutrophils, K lymphocytes, etc.) resulting in cell damage and cell death. Type III: Antigen–antibody complexes are deposited in tissue. Type IV: T cells are sensitized to a specific antigen, thereby causing lymphokine release. Reproduced with permission from Young LR, Wurtzbacher JD, Blankenship CS. Am J Manag Care 1997;3:1884–906 [22].

improves reporting and reduces the frequency of all adverse events [24, 27]. Decision support systems such as computerized physician order entry or pharmacy information systems are often used in a concurrent manner to identify at-risk scenarios [37]. Surveillance systems continue to add value to the medication-use process. Surveillance methods recently successfully identified bleeding risks associated with low molecular weight heparin dosing in patients with renal insufficiency [38], harms associated with epoetin alpha [39] and thiazolidinediones [40], and fatalities found with off-label use of dronedarone [41] and dabigatran [42]. An active retrospective approach, or even a prospective surveillance approach, is necessary, as many potential ADRs are unrecognized or are never reported, thus escaping detection and preventing flaws in the medication-use process from being corrected [26, 43].

## Determining Causality

It is difficult to determine if patients are experiencing an ADR to a medication or if the noted symptoms are caused by their underlying disorder or worsening of their condition, because the symptoms caused by ADRs are sometimes similar to disease symptoms (e.g., headache caused by excessive consumption of NSAIDs such as aspirin, or increases in patient temperature following administration of empiric broad-spectrum antibiotics) [44]. To overcome this problem, several rating scales have been developed to relate symptoms to medications [12, 45]. An ADR usually occurs shortly after the initiation of a treatment, and symptoms frequently begin to improve once treatment is stopped. It is clear that the event is an adverse drug reaction if administration of a specific antidote provides a dramatic improvement in symptoms. This is seen when naloxone is used to reverse excessive effects of an opioid. An ADR is often related to the mechanism of action of the medication, or is one of a series of known examples of intolerance or idiosyncratic reactions. Sometimes there is laboratory confirmation of the ADR (for example, elevated

**TABLE 27.3   Causality Checklist**

Is the reaction timely to medication initiation?

Is resolution timely to discontinuation?

Response to antidote or reversal agent?

Other plausible explanations and medications are ruled out?

Objective confirmation?

Reaction resumes if rechallenged?

blood concentrations of the medication), and at times the patient may describe a similar reaction to this medication in the past. This process of causality assessment is summarized in Table 27.3 and an example is provided in Table 27.4. Definitions are listed in Table 27.5, and the widely-used Naranjo scoring system is described in Table 27.6 [45]. Determining the proper diagnosis can prevent patient exposure to additional and unnecessary medications, and proper documentation of the diagnosis of an ADR can prevent future occurrences [9, 10].

## ASSESSING ADR RISK

The search for ADR information appropriately begins with the review of the approved labeling for the specific drug or drugs. Supplemental safety information also is provided by both the FDA and international regulatory agencies. In addition, ADR risk can be assessed from the published literature on ADRs, which is largely comprised of case reports and sometimes reviews. Tertiary drug resources, including books and databases, also can provide ADR information. Finally, one may consider contacting a drug's manufacturer for information beyond what appears in the approved labeling.

### Evaluating Drug Labels for ADR Risk

In addition to the Adverse Reactions section of the approved labeling, other sections of the label should

**TABLE 27.4   Clinical Example: Determining the Causality of an ADR**

Problem: Suspected corticosteroid induced hyperglycemia seen during rCHOP[a] regimen for non-Hodgkin's lymphoma.

Time frame: Hyperglycemia seen with scheduled lab work 1 week after first course. Resolved upon review of labs 2 weeks after first course. Repeats after rechallenge during second course of rCHOP. HA1C remains at baseline throughout six-course regimen.

Analysis: Reaction is timely to initiation, withdrawal and rechallenge with suspected agent. Confirmed by laboratory results. Patient does not have type 1 diabetes, and does not meet criteria for type 2 diabetes. Prednisone is the only component of rCHOP known to promote hyperglycemia.

*Conclusion:* Naranjo score of 8; probable hyperglycemic reaction to high-dose prednisone.

[a]rCHOP: rituximab, cyclophosphamide, hydroxydaunorubicin (doxorubicin), Oncovin®, (vincristine), prednisone.

**TABLE 27.5   Criteria for the Classification of Causality of Potential ADRs**

| Unlikely | • Untimely relationship to treatment or<br>• Reversible symptoms continue after stopping treatment |
| Possible | • Timely relationship to treatment and<br>• Therapy is continued or<br>• Reversible symptoms resolve upon discontinuation and negative response to rechallenge |
| Probable | • Timely relationship to treatment and<br>• Reversible symptoms resolve upon discontinuation<br>• No rechallenge |
| Definite | • Timely relationship to treatment and<br>• Reversible symptoms resolve upon discontinuation<br>• Positive response to rechallenge |

**TABLE 27.6   The Naranjo Adverse Drug Reaction Probability Scale**

| To assess the adverse drug reaction, please answer the following questionnaire and give the pertinent score | Yes | No | Do not know | Score |
|---|---|---|---|---|
| 1.  Are there previous *conclusive* reports on this reaction? | +1 | 0 | 0 | |
| 2.  Did the adverse event occur after the suspected drug was administered? | +2 | −1 | 0 | |
| 3.  Did the adverse reaction improve when the drug was discontinued or a *specific* antagonist was administered? | +1 | 0 | 0 | |
| 4.  Did the adverse reaction reappear when the drug was re-administered? | +2 | −1 | 0 | |
| 5.  Are there alternative causes (other than the drug) that could have on their own caused the reaction? | −1 | +2 | 0 | |
| 6.  Did the reaction reappear when a placebo was given? | −1 | +1 | 0 | |
| 7.  Was the medication detected in the blood (or other fluids) in concentrations known to be toxic? | +1 | 0 | 0 | |
| 8.  Was the reaction more severe when the dose was increased or less severe when the dose was decreased? | +1 | 0 | 0 | |
| 9.  Did the patient have a similar reaction to the same or similar drugs in *any* previous exposure? | +1 | 0 | 0 | |
| 10.  Was the adverse event confirmed by any objective evidence? | +1 | 0 | 0 | |
| The ADR is assigned to a probability category from the total score as follows: *definite* if the overall score is 9 or greater, *probable* for a score of 5–8, *possible* for 1–4, and *doubtful* if the score is 0 | | | Total | |

Reproduced with permission from Naranjo CA, Busto U, Sellers EM *et al*. Clin Pharmacol Ther. 1981; 30:239–45 [45].

be examined as these may contain important information along with important guidance. For example, the significant known ADRs also will usually be included in one or more of the sections for Contraindications, Precautions, or Warnings. Black Box Warnings are usually placed at the very beginning of the product information to give prominence to the most serious known risks. Because one study identified inconsistencies between drug information resources and the manufacturer's prescribing information, with some key elements of the official boxed warning missing in the drug information resources, the current label may be the most reliable source for the complete boxed warning for a given drug [46]. For this reason, clinicians are well advised to reach beyond the drug

resources they commonly use and to consult sources that provide the most up-to-date approved labeling, such as DailyMed or Drugs@FDA.

Drug labels use a number of methods to categorize ADRs, but the most common is to list ADRs by frequency of occurrence [47]. For example, the package insert for dronedarone (Multaq™) states that "Most common adverse reactions ($\geq 2\%$) are diarrhea, nausea, abdominal pain, vomiting and asthenia" (see Table 27.7) [48]. The frequency method provides an idea of what ADRs can be expected and of the frequency with which they can be anticipated. Unfortunately, since serious ADRs are rare for products that receive marketing approval, they are often missing from lists based on frequency. Also, this

**TABLE 27.7    Comparison of Frequency-Based ADR Reporting to a REMS**

Adverse effects: Dronedarone

Most common adverse reactions ($\geq$ 2%) are diarrhea, nausea, abdominal pain, vomiting and asthenia

(Official Prescribing Information Sanofi—Aventis, 2011, accessed May 17, 2011)

REMS: Dronedaron

There is a risk mitigation strategy in place for dronedarone

**Goals**:

- To **prevent** use in patients with NYHA Class IV heart failure or Class II—III heart failure with recent decompensation requiring hospitalization or referral to a specialized heart unit
- To inform healthcare professionals and patients about the serious risks including increased mortality in patients with severe unstable heart failure and signs and symptoms of liver injury

(FDA: Approved REMS accessed May 17, 2011)

Note the focus on prevention of serious adverse effects seen in the REMS

approach is a passive approach to understanding ADRs, and it would be more useful to include a risk-mitigation approach that specifies actions to prevent ADRs, such as shown in Table 27.7 for dronedarone.

The focus of drug labels does change to ADR prevention in the sections that specify contraindications, warnings, and precautions. Contraindications describe situations in which the drug should absolutely NOT be used. The warnings and precaution section provides a summary of clinically significant adverse reactions and how to avoid them [47]. All three of these sections should be considered when evaluating the potential for harm that is associated with each treatment option.

## Safety Alerts from FDA and International Regulators

FDA Safety Alerts are a valuable source of ADR risk information, and they can be easily accessed online at MedWatch Safety Alerts for Human Medical Products [49]. The following example illustrates the evolution of a drug safety issue. A May 21, 2007 FDA alert first described the differing rate of ischemic cardiovascular events (some fatal) associated with Avandia® (rosiglitazone) relative to other drugs used for the treatment of type 2 diabetes mellitus [50]. As additional data were analyzed, this led to the August 2007 notice of changes to the prescribing information for rosiglitazone that included a new boxed warning about the potential increased risk of myocardial ischemia [51]. Finally, in September 2010, the FDA announced its intent to significantly restrict the use of rosiglitazone and require that the manufacturer develop a restricted access program under a REMS [52].

The point of the above sequence is that one can be alerted to a safety issue at the very early stages of its recognition and can proactively adopt a more restrained and vigilant approach to the use of drugs with emerging safety concerns, particularly when safer therapeutic alternatives exist. Clinicians can obtain such emerging safety information by directly subscribing to the FDA's free e-mail subscription service and setting one of the preferences for MedWatch Safety Alerts (https://public.govdelivery.com/accounts/USFDA/subscriber/new). This will assure prompt delivery of new safety information for all human medical products, including prescription drugs, over-the-counter drugs, biologicals, and vaccines. The FDA also posts quarterly reports listing potential signals of the serious safety risks identified in FDA's Adverse Event Reporting System (AERS) database. These can be accessed at: www.fda.gov/Drugs/GuidanceComplianceRegulatoryInformation/Surveillance/AdverseDrugEffects/ucm082196.htm.

In addition, clinicians might find notice of medication issues that have not yet been raised by the FDA from international health regulators, such as Health Canada and EMEA. Health Canada's Advisories, Warnings, and Recalls for Health Professionals page can be accessed at www.hc-sc.gc.ca/dhp-mps/medeff/advisories-avis/prof/index-eng.php. An example is the advisory about the possible association of mycophenolate mofetil with red cell aplasia that was issued by Health Canada on June 3, 2009 [53]. This was later communicated by the FDA on August 14, 2009 [54]. Health Canada's website also offers a free e-mail subscription service to receive such notices. The European Medicines Agency (EMA) is responsible for the evaluation of medicines developed by pharmaceutical companies intended for use in the European Union. The EMA also provides notices of important patient safety information on their website at www.ema.europa.eu/ema/index.jsp?curl=pages/home/Home_Page.jsp&mid=.

## Evaluating Publications for ADR Risk

In theory, a published clinical trial provides the best opportunity for a clinician to obtain a systematic analysis of a particular medication's ADR risk. In practice, the reader should proceed cautiously and carefully to evaluate the provided safety information, as outlined in Table 27.8. The first step is to determine if ADRs are even reported in the publication, as a surprising percentage (20–30%) do not even report ADRs [55–59]. It should not be assumed that the absence of safety reporting is evidence of safety, and publications that exclusively report on favorable information should be discarded. Specialty publications and high-impact journals are equally implicated. When safety is reported, the methodology should be carefully assessed and the reader should note how adverse effects were identified by the investigators. Spontaneous reporting and other methods of passively collecting ADRs may overlook important information. The final step is to verify that the subjects in the study are similar to the patients you plan to treat. Age, severity of illness, other illnesses and medications are important exclusions to note.

A high-quality publication will follow a systematic approach to collect safety information and use an active adverse event surveillance system based upon a validated checklist. The publication should report results of prespecified objective safety endpoints, while accounting for all patient withdrawals because of ADRs. Unfortunately, only about 20% of publications report adverse effects using this systematic approach, and the usefulness of data from many clinical trials is compromised by the absence of ADR reporting and by weak methodology [11].

Although adverse reactions sections in a tertiary reference or drug database may be consulted (AHFS DI, Clinical Pharmacology, Micromedex, eFacts, etc.), it should be recognized that the ADR information found there is in great part taken from the clinical trials submitted to the FDA as part of a drug's approval process. As postmarket surveillance findings may emerge that supplement this initial information, these can result in important modifications of a drug's approved labeling by the FDA. However, retrieval of the primary literature is time consuming, so shortcuts to citations from tertiary resource references can help establish a starting point from which one can proceed to related articles. For example, when viewing such a citation in MEDLINE, one can examine the links to related citations or the Medical Subject Heading (MeSH) tags to further the search. Web of Science can similarly help map a given citation forward to subsequent articles that have referenced it.

## Risk Associated with Recently Approved Drugs

Clinicians should exercise caution before prescribing a recently approved medication, particularly when using it outside of the inclusion criteria used for the drug registration trial [10, 60, 61]. The design of the drug research studies that are conducted to obtain marketing approval limits their ability to detect rare yet serious ADRs. These studies are designed to see if the medication can show benefit under optimal circumstances, and a study with many fewer exclusion criteria would be needed in order to show benefit and safety under the usual conditions of clinical care [61]. Unfortunately, the cost and time necessary to conduct studies with this high level of external validity would be prohibitive, so most studies limit their enrollment to only the healthiest of eligible patients [62, 63]. These groups of included study patients often are not representative of the population that will receive the medication after marketing [62]. Jadad [64] reports that patients with multiple chronic diseases were excluded from 63% of published randomized controlled trials. Other limiting factors inherent in the design of these studies include the small numbers of patients receiving the study medication, and their short duration. Thus, the structure of drug development trials, including use of a controlled setting, documented patient compliance, short-term and intermediate outcomes, and low external validity, is very different from what is encountered in clinical practice, and ADR risk may be much higher in the clinical setting when compared to the research setting [10, 61]. For these reasons, prescribing decisions should be guided by giving first consideration to medications having an established track record of safety and efficacy, and clinicians should avoid succumbing to marketing-based claims, such as are often made for novel compounds with a unique mechanism of action [10].

**TABLE 27.8   Evaluating a Publication for ADRs**

Are adverse events actually reported?

Passive or active surveillance used to identify AE?

Is a validated checklist available?

Are pre-specified objective endpoints reported?

Are patient withdrawals because of adverse events reported?

Are AE reported in the abstract, methods, and results section?

Discussion includes a balanced discussion of harms and benefits?

Is there external validity?

Adapted from Ionnidis PA, Evans S, Gotzsche P *et al.* Ann Intern Med 2004;141:781–8 [11].

## Risk Associated with Off-Label Prescribing

The risk of an ADR is magnified when a drug is prescribed for an off-label indication or in a dose that exceeds that recommended in the package insert. Off-label prescribing is particularly likely to occur with new drugs. For example, an oral anticoagulant may be approved for thrombosis prevention, but not for treatment, and yet prescribers may try to use it for treatment. Both efficacy and safety evidence may be unavailable to support risk–benefit decisions for an unapproved use. Besides anticoagulants, many other drugs, due to their inherent high risk (antiarrhythmics, chemotherapeutics, hypoglycemics, opioids, skeletal muscle blockers, etc.), must be assumed to pose elevated risk with uncertain benefit when used off-label. Ultimate evidence may emerge that expected efficacy endpoints are not attained, yet patients are exposed to predictable adverse effects [65].

The enhanced risk of off-label prescribing can be evaluated by a *safety specification study* that compares the frequency of reported ADRs between patients receiving a medication for its labeled indications to the ADRs seen when the medication is used off-label. This information provides an early warning about types of patients or situations that are at a particularly high ADR risk [62]. Safety specification studies might also warn about drug–drug or drug–diet interactions and special risks for female patients, children, elderly, or other types of patients that are often excluded from registration trials. Both comparative effectiveness and safety specification studies offer new research opportunities for clinicians interested in identifying and preventing adverse drug reactions.

## MINIMIZING AND MANAGING ADRS

### Risk Evaluation and Mitigation Strategy (REMS)

In 2005, the FDA announced a plan to incorporate pharmacovigilance into its drug approval process. The plan was named *Risk Minimization Action Plans*, often referred to as RiskMAPs. A RiskMAP could be recommended for a particular medication because of the type or frequency of known risks when compared to expected benefits, such as for a drug that has a high risk of side effects but is the only option to treat a serious condition (e.g., an anticancer agent, particularly when failure to treat might be fatal). A RiskMAP might also be recommended for a high-risk medication used to treat elderly patients, children, or patients with renal failure for whom there is limited availability of alternative

treatments. Finally, a RiskMAP could be recommended for a high-risk drug when there is a remedy that can prevent or reverse the ADR (e.g., vitamin K used to reverse the effects of warfarin) [63].

In 2007, the Food and Drug Administration Amendments Act (FDAA) was signed into law and Title IX was enacted the following year to provide the FDA with the authority to place medication safety requirements on drug sponsors. As a result, the FDA developed Risk Evaluation and Mitigation Strategies (REMS) that evolved from and are very similar to RiskMAPs [63]. The FDA now has authority under REMS to include fines as an enforcement mechanism. Most products do not require a REMS or a RiskMAP, and it is not required as part of an FDA submission for marketing approval (although many applications do include a REMS). However, the availability of these risk-mitigation strategies is thought to be necessary to ensure that a drug's benefits outweigh its risks of serious ADRs, and a requirement for either can be identified after a medication is placed on the market [66, 67]. A REMS is unique to a medication, is a result of a negotiation between the FDA and the sponsor, and is based on the occurrence of ADRs either in clinical trials or subsequent to marketing.

Traditionally, contraindications are added to a drug's label for conditions or circumstances in which its risks are expected to outweigh its benefits. A Black Box Warning may subsequently be added to the label if prescribers do not adhere to these contraindications. Currently, there are more than 500 medications that have a Black Box Warning, often meaning that earlier contraindication warnings did not change prescribing in the face of known risk factors for adverse events. In fact, between 1995 and 2007 there were 174 biological products approved by the FDA and European regulatory agencies, and 19 Black Box Warnings were issued for 47 (23.6%) of these products [68]. However, under a REMS approach many potential contraindications can be spelled out initially under a REMS so that a new medication can be approved for marketing even before clear evidence has emerged that its benefits outweigh its risks. This has permitted faster approval of drugs for a broader range of indications and with warnings that are less restrictive than contraindications. A medication eligible for a REMS may have a unique REMS requirement since different drugs have different adverse effects, different mechanisms of action, and therefore different risks. Thus, a REMS for a cardiovascular medication may need to be very different from a REMS for an analgesic [69]. The goal of the REMS approach is to help clinicians avoid many serious ADRs by becoming aware of these warnings before they either prescribe or advise a prescriber to order a medication for a patient.

## Managing ADRs

Information on managing ADRs, other than discontinuation of suspected offending agents, can often be unsatisfactory, with little or no guidance to be found. Therefore, while information may well be acquired from an array of sources, answers remain lacking to many practical questions, such as if continued use will lead to progression or regression of an ADR, or how long after drug discontinuation will it take for ADRs to resolve. A practical approach to managing suspected ADRs is certainly needed. Whenever it is reasonably clear that a specific drug is causal, there should be a re-evaluation for its need and consideration of therapeutic alternatives with an unlikely association to the ADR. If the ADR is likely a dose-related one, a dose reduction may be all that is needed, rather than changing treatments. In a few cases, treatment with an antidote may be warranted (e.g., administration of vitamin K to a patient over-anticoagulated with warfarin). When a patient is taking multiple drugs that fall under ADR suspicion, eliminating those least essential to care one at a time is a reasonable approach to follow.

Actual clinical experience can provide useful insight into the types of ADRs that are commonly encountered. For example, a recent publication was based on a retrospective evaluation of queries related to ADRs received by the Drug Information Center (DIC) of a tertiary care teaching hospital over a period of three and a half years [70]. In that report, 600 (25.9%) of the 2312 DIC queries were related to ADRs. The organ system most commonly involved was the nervous system (14.7%), antibacterials were the most commonly drug class involved (18.6%), and phenytoin was the single drug that most frequently caused ADRs (35%).

The authors of this chapter have conducted a similar retrospective evaluation of 289 ADR-related inquiries that they received. The purpose of the ADR questions is summarized in Table 27.9, and was to obtain evidence for a particular suspected drug–ADR association or to request a review of a complete medication regimen in order to determine the likely drug or drugs that might be causing a specific ADR. Suspected neurologic ADRs were cited most frequently, in 14% of the questions, and the majority of those fell within the following types in descending order: hearing changes, neuromuscular issues, paresthesias, seizure-related, cognitive impairment, hallucinations, sedation, movement disorders, coma, and confusion. Allergy or hypersensitivity reactions were the next largest group of patient-specific ADR questions, and included questions about alternative therapy for patients who had experienced ADRs in the past.

Inquirers asked about specific drugs in 247 of the 289 patient-specific ADR questions. Psychiatric drugs were asked about most often (16%), followed by anti-infective drug questions (11%). The anti-infective drug

TABLE 27.9   Reasons for 289 Inquiries Concerning ADRs in Specific Patients

| Reason for inquiry | Patient currently suspected of having ADR occurrence | Patient had past ADR occurrence prompting screening to avoid recurrence with same or related drug | Screening for ADR issue in advance of planned initial drug exposure | Total |
|---|---|---|---|---|
| Locate evidence that a specific drug or drugs are associated with a specific ADR | 108 (37.4%) | | 7 (2.4%) | 115 (39.8%) |
| Help determine likely cause of a specific ADR (requiring review of regimen with > 1 medication) | 53 (18.3%) | | | 53 (18.3%) |
| Provide guidance on managing a specific ADR | 13 (4.5%) | | | 13 (4.5%) |
| Help determine suitable alternative to a medication that is causing or caused a specific ADR | 2 (0.7%) | 5 (1.7%) | 5 (1.7%) | 12 (4.2%) |
| Provide information to prevent or minimize a specific ADR of concern | 2 (0.7%) | 24 (8.3%) | 59 (20.4%) | 85 (29.4%) |
| Provide general information on a specific ADR or a range of ADRs | | | 11 (3.8%) | 11 (3.8%) |
| Total | 178 (61.6%) | 29 (10%) | 82 (28.4%) | 289 (100%) |

questions were primarily about renal effects or allergy/hypersensitivity reactions, but also included requests to locate evidence that a specific drug was associated with a particular ADR, or were requests for information to prevent or minimize a specific ADR of concern, such as prevention of an allergic or hypersensitivity reaction. The majority of the ADR inquiries came from physicians about specific patients who were suspected of having an ADR. These inquiries sought evidence about the strength of association of an ADR with a drug. Less frequently, the physician was attempting to screen for ADR issues in advance of starting therapy, in some cases prompted by a prior ADR occurrence.

# REFERENCES

[1] Bennett CL, Nebeker JR, Yarnold PR, Tigue CC, Dorr DA, McKoy JM. Evaluation of serious adverse drug reactions: A proactive pharmacovigilance program (RADAR) vs safety activities conducted by the Food and Drug Administration and pharmaceutical manufacturers. Arch Intern Med 2007;167:1041–9.

[2] Committee on Quality of HealthCare in America. To err is human: Building a safer health system. In: Kohn LT, Corrigan JM, Donaldson MS, editors. Washington, DC: National Academy Press; 1999.

[3] Moore N, Lecointre D, Noblet C, Mabille M. Frequency and cost of serious adverse drug reactions in a department of general medicine. Br J Clin Pharmacol 1998;45:301–8.

[4] Lazarou J, Pomeranz BH, Corey PN. Incidence of adverse drug reactions in hospitalized patients – A meta-analysis of prospective studies. JAMA 1998;279:1200–5.

[5] Landrigan CP, Parry GJ, Bones CB, Hackbarth AD, Goldmann DA, Share PJ. Temporal trends in rates of patient harm resulting from medical care. N Engl J Med 2010;363:2124–34.

[6] Davies EC, Green CF, Taylor S, Williamson PR, Mottram DR, Pirmohamed M. Adverse drug reactions in hospital inpatients: A prospective analysis of 3695 patient-episodes. PLoS One 2009;4:e4439.

[7] Davies EC, Green CF, Mottram DR, Pirmohamed M. Emergency re-admissions to hospital due to adverse drug reactions within 1 year of the index admission. Br J Clin Pharmacol 2010;70:749–55.

[8] Budnitz D, Lovegrove M, Shehab N, Richards C. Emergency hospitalizations for adverse drug events in older Americans. N Engl J Med 2011;365:2002–12.

[9] Nebeker JR, Barach P, Samore MH. Clarifying adverse drug events: A clinician's guide to terminology, documentation, and reporting. Ann Intern Med 2004;140:795–801.

[10] Schiff GD, Galanter WL, Duhig J, Lodolce AE, Koronkowski MJ, Lambert BL. Principles of conservative prescribing. Arch Intern Med 2011;171:1433–40.

[11] Ionnidis PA, Evans S, Gotzsche P, O'Neill R, Altman D, Schulz K, et al. Better reporting of harms in randomized trials: An extension of the CONSORT statement. Ann Intern Medicine 2004;141:781–8.

[12] Edwards IR, Aronson JK. Adverse drug reactions: Definitions, diagnosis, and management. Lancet 2000;356:1255–9.

[13] Postmarketing reporting of adverse drug experiences. In the US Code of Federal Regulations 21CFR314.80 (Internet at, www.accessdata.fda.gov/scripts/cdrh/cfdocs/cfCFR/CFRSearch.cfm?fr=314.80; April 1, 2011).

[14] Hartwig SC, Siegel J, Schneider PJ. Preventability and severity assessment in reporting adverse drug reactions. Am J Hosp Pharm 1992;49:2229–32.

[15] Rawlins MD, Thomas SHL. Mechanisms of adverse drug reactions. In: Davies DM, Ferner RE, de Glanville H, editors. Davies' textbook of adverse drug reactions. 5th ed. London: Chapman & Hill Medical; 1998. p. 40–64.

[16] Melmon KL. Preventable drug reactions – causes and cures. N Engl J Med 1971;284:1361–8.

[17] Bachot N, Roujeau JC. Differential diagnosis of severe cutaneous drug eruptions. Am J Clin Dermatol 2003;4:561–72.

[18] Shalom R, Rimbroth S, Rozenman D, Markel A. Allopurinol-induced recurrent DRESS syndrome: Pathophysiology and treatment. Ren Fail. 2008;30(3):327–9.

[19] Gell PGH, Coombs RRA. Classification of allergic reactions responsible for clinical hypersensitivity and disease. In: Gell PGH, Coombs RRA, Hachmann PG, editors. Clinical aspects of immunology. Oxford: Blackwell Scientific Publications; 1975. p. 161–81.

[20] Kay AB. Concepts of allergy and hypersensitivity in allergy and allergic diseases. In: Kay AB, editor. Allergy and allergic diseases, vol. 1. Oxford: Blackwell Science; 1997. p. 23–35.

[21] Knowles SR, Uetrecht J, Shear NH. Idiosyncratic drug reactions: The reactive metabolite syndromes. Lancet 2000;356:1587–91.

[22] Young LR, Wurtzbacher JD, Blankenship CS. Adverse drug reactions: A review for healthcare practitioners. Am J Manag Care 1997;3:1884–906.

[23] Folli HL, Poole RL, Benitz WE, Russo JC. Medication error prevention by clinical pharmacists in two children's hospitals. Pediatrics 1987;79:718–22.

[24] Leape LL, Cullen DJ, Clapp MD, Burdick E, Demonaco HJ, Erickson JI, et al. Pharmacist participation on physician rounds and adverse drug events in the intensive care unit. JAMA 1999;282:267–70.

[25] Bates DW, Leape LL, Cullen DJ, Laird N, Petersen LA, Teich JM. Effect of computerized physician order entry and a team intervention on prevention of serious medication errors. JAMA 1998;280:1311–6.

[26] Nilsen EV, Fotis MA. Developing a model to determine the effects of adverse drug events in hospital inpatients. Am J Health Syst Pharm 2007;64:521–5.

[27] Scarsi KK, Fotis MA, Noskin GA. Pharmacist participation in medical rounds reduces medication errors. Am J Health Syst Pharm 2002;59:2089–92.

[28] Piergies AA, Worwag EM, Atkinson AJ Jr. A concurrent audit of high digoxin plasma levels. Clin Pharmacol Ther 1994;55:353–8.

[29] Atkinson AJ Jr, Nadzam DM, Schaff RL. An indicator-based program for improving medication use in acute care hospitals. Clin Pharmacol Ther 1991;50:125–8.

[30] Greenberger PA, Cranberg JA, Ganz MA, Hubler GL. A prospective evaluation of elevated serum theophylline concentrations to determine if high concentrations are predictable. Am J Med 1991;91:67–73.

[31] Atkinson AJ Jr, Nordstrom K. The challenge of in-hospital medication use: An opportunity for clinical pharmacology. Clin Pharmacol Ther 1996;60:363–7.

[32] Szekendi MK, Sullivan C, Bobb A, Feinglass J, Rooney D, Barnard C, et al. Active surveillance using electronic triggers to detect adverse events in hospitalized patients. Qual Saf Health Care 2006;15:184–90.

[33] Classen DC, Resar R, Griffin F, Federico F, Frankel T, Kimmel N, et al. "Global trigger tool" shows that adverse events in hospitals may be ten times greater than previously measured. Health Aff (Millwood) 2011;30:581–9.

[34] Kaboli P, Hoth A, McClimon B, Schnipper J. Clinical pharmacists and inpatient medical care: A systematic review. Arch Intern Med 2006;166:955–64.

[35] Greenberger PA, Patterson R, Fotis MA. Penicillin allergy: Improving patient care and the medical record. Allergy Asthma Proc 2000;21:295–6.

[36] Lee CE, Zembower TR, Fotis MA, Postelnick MP, Greenberger PA, Peterson L, et al. The incidence of antimicrobial allergies in hospitalized patients: Implications regarding prescribing patterns and emerging bacterial resistance. Arch Intern Med 2000;160:2819–22.

[37] Raschke RA, Gollihare B, Wunderlich TA, Guidry JR, Leibowitz AI, Peirce JC, et al. A computer alert system to prevent injury from adverse drug events. JAMA 1998;280:1317–20.

[38] Enoxaparin Labeling Changes Approved By FDA Center for Drug Evaluation and Research (CDER) – July 2008. FDA US Food and Drug Administration. (Internet at, www.fda.gov/Safety/MedWatch/SafetyInformation/Safety-RelatedDrugLabelingChanges/ucm121933.htm).

[39] Epoetin Alpha. ASHP REMS Database (Internet at, www.ashp.org/Import/PRACTICEANDPOLICY/PracticeResourceCenters/REMSRDDS/quickguide.aspx#Epoetin_alfa. Accessed October 4, 2011).

[40] FDA Drug Safety Communication: Updated Risk Evaluation and Mitigation Strategy (REMS) to Restrict Access to Rosiglitazone-containing Medicines. FDA (Internet at, www.fda.gov/Drugs/DrugSafety/ucm255005.htm.; May 23, 2011).

[41] European Medicines Agency. Benefit Risk Review of Multaq (Internet at, www.ema.europa.eu; September 28, 2011).

[42] Pradaxa (dabigatran etexilate mesylate): Drug safety communication – safety review of post-market reports of serious bleeding events. FDA (Internet at, www.fda.gov/Safety/MedWatch/SafetyInformation/SafetyAlertsforHumanMedicalProducts/ucm282820.htm.; Dec. 7, 2011).

[43] Cullen DJ, Bates DW, Small SD, Cooper JB, Nemeskal AR, Leape LL. The incident reporting system does not detect adverse drug events: A problem for quality improvement. Jt Comm J Qual Improv 1995;21:549–52.

[44] Patel RA, Gallagher JC. Drug fever. Pharmacotherapy 2010;30:57–69.

[45] Naranjo CA, Busto U, Sellers EM, Sandor P, Ruiz I, Roberts EA. A method for estimating the probability of adverse drug reactions. Clin Pharmacol Ther 1981;30:239–45.

[46] Cheng CM, Fu C, Guglielmo BJ, Auerbach AD. Boxed warning inconsistencies between drug information resources and the prescribing information. Am J Health Syst Pharm 2011;68:1626–31.

[47] Kremzner M. An Introduction to the Improved FDA Prescription Drug Labeling. FDA (Internet at, http://www.fda.gov/Training/ForHealthProfessionals/ucm090801.htm; June 18, 2009).

[48] MULTAQ® (dronedarone) prescribing information. Sanofi-aventis US LLC. Bridgewater, NJ. (Internet at, www.multaq.com/docs/consumer_pdf/pi.aspx; 2011).

[49] MedWatch Safety Alerts for Human Medical Products. (Internet at, www.fda.gov/Safety/MedWatch/SafetyInformation/SafetyAlertsforHumanMedicalProducts/default.htm.)

[50] FDA. Safety alert for human medical products: Avandia (rosiglitazone) (Internet at, www.fda.gov/Safety/MedWatch/SafetyInformation/SafetyAlertsforHumanMedicalProducts/ucm150831.htm.; May 21, 2007).

[51] FDA. Safety alert for human medical products: Avandia (rosiglitazone maleate). Tablets. (Internet at, www.fda.gov/Safety/MedWatch/SafetyInformation/SafetyAlertsforHumanMedicalProducts/ucm150823.htm; August 14, 2007).

[52] FDA. Safety alert for human medical products: Avandia (rosiglitazone): REMS – Risk of cardiovascular events. Internet at,
www.fda.gov/Safety/MedWatch/SafetyInformation/SafetyAlertsforHumanMedicalProducts/ucm226994.htm; September 23, 2010).

[53] Reports of pure red cell aplasia in patients treated with CellCept® (mycophenolate mofetil) (Internet at, www.hc-sc.gc.ca/dhp-mps/medeff/advisories-avis/prof/_2009/cellcept_2_hpc-cps-eng.php).

[54] FDA. Safety alert for human medical products: CellCept (mycophenolate mofetil) (Internet at, www.fda.gov/Safety/MedWatch/SafetyInformation/SafetyAlertsforHumanMedicalProducts/ucm177397.htm).

[55] Loke YK, Derry S. Reporting of adverse drug reactions in randomised controlled trials – a systematic survey. BMC Clin Pharmacol 2001;1:3.

[56] de Vries TW, van Roon EN. Low quality of reporting adverse drug reactions in paediatric randomised controlled trials. Arch Dis Child 2009;95:1023–6.

[57] Gandhi S, TenBarge A, Caraher K, Winters-Williams L, Fotis M. Shining the light on drug safety. ASHP Connect (Internet at, http://connect.ashp.org/ASHP/Go.aspx?c=ViewDocument&DocumentKey=3e9737cd-f8a8-4f00-9ef5-fb793d7da9c8 November 2011).

[58] Nieto A, Mazon A, Pamies R, Linana JJ, Lanuza A, Jiménez FO. Adverse effects of inhaled corticosteroids in funded and non-funded studies. Arch Intern Med 2007;167:2047–53.

[59] Breau RH, Gaboury I, Scales Jr CD, Fesperman SF, Watterson JD, Dahm P. Reporting of harm in randomized controlled trials published in the urological literature. J Urol 2010 May;183:1693–7.

[60] Largent EA, Miller FG, Pearson SD. Going off-label without venturing off-course: Evidence and ethical off-label prescribing. Arch Intern Med 2009;169:1745–7.

[61] Schumock G. Comparative effectiveness research: Relevance and applications to pharmacy. Am J Health Syst Pharm 2009;66:1278–86.

[62] Goldman S, Hoffman J, Klein C, Dombrowski S. Discussion guide on risk evaluation and mitigation strategies (Internet at, www.remsupdates.org; 2011).

[63] US Food and Drug Administration. Managing the risks from medical product use: Creating a risk management framework: Report to the FDA Commissioner from the Task Force on Risk management. Rockville, MD, May 1999. (Internet at, www.fda.gov/Safety/SafetyofSpecificProducts/ucm180325.htm.)

[64] Jadad AR, To MJ, Emara M, Jones J. Consideration of multiple chronic diseases in randomized controlled trials. JAMA 2011;306:2670–2.

[65] Yank V, Tuohy CV, Logan AC, Bravata DM, Staudenmayer K, Eisenhut R, et al. Systematic review: Benefits and harms of in-hospital use of recombinant factor VIIa for off-label indications. Ann Intern Med 2011;154:529–40.

[66] Discussion guide on risk evaluation and mitigation strategies. (Internet at, www.remsupdates.org.)

[67] Approved REMS Strategies. FDA (Internet at, www.fda.gov/Drugs/DrugSafety/PostmarketDrugSafetyInformationforPatientsandProviders/ucm111350.htm; September 30, 2011).

[68] Giezen TJ, Mantel-Teeuwisse AK, Straus SM, Schellekens H, Leufkens HG, Egberts AC. Safety related regulatory actions for biologicals approved in the United States and the European Union. JAMA 2008;300:1887–96.

[69] Stubbings J, Joshi RA, Hoffman JM. Risk evaluation and mitigation strategies: Challenges and opportunities for health-system pharmacists. Am J Health Syst Pharm 2010;67:1547–54.

[70] Jimmy B, Jose J, Rao PG. Short communication: Pattern of adverse drug reaction related queries received by the drug information centre of a tertiary care teaching hospital. Pak J Pharm Sci. 2007;20:333–9.

# Quality Assessment of Drug Therapy

Charles E. Daniels

*Skaggs School of Pharmacy and Pharmaceutical Sciences, University of California–San Diego, La Jolla, CA 92093*

## INTRODUCTION

Dozens of new drugs, new combinations, and new dosage forms are approved each year in the USA and Europe. The availability of valuable new agents creates opportunities for improved therapeutic outcomes, but also creates increased opportunities for inappropriate medication use. The clinical pharmacologist must have generalized expertise in the use of medications that can be applied across the organization in clinical practice and in independent and collaborative research activities. Quality assessment and improvement of medication use constitute an important skill set.

The objective of this chapter will be to review medication-use quality issues in an institutional context and highlight their impact on patient care and clinical research. The focus is on three themes: understanding the medication-use system and organizational interests in medication use; understanding the application of drug-use monitoring as a tool to improve medication use; and understanding processes to identify and improve medication errors. Improvement in quality of medication use revolves around identifying and minimizing systematic risk of error, and improving outcomes through the use of relevant guidelines and benchmarking tools.

### Adverse Drug Events

In a 2001 publication, Ernst [1] projected that costs of $177 billion a year are attributable to medication misuse. Adverse drug events (ADEs) are instances when patient harm results from the use of medication. This includes both adverse drug reactions, which were discussed in Chapter 27, and medication errors, all of which are inherently preventable. A 1999 Institute of Medicine (IOM) report estimated that 98,000 Americans die each year due to medical error [2]. This includes diagnostic mistakes, wrong-site surgery, and other categories of error, including medication errors. A supplemental IOM report in 2007 estimated that hospitals experienced up to 450,000 preventable ADEs each year, and long-term care facilities experienced an estimated 800,000 per year. It further concluded that up to $3.5 billion is added to hospital costs due to preventable ADEs [3]. Approximately 20% of all medical errors are medication related [4, 5].

A medication error is any preventable event that may cause or lead to inappropriate medication use or patient harm while medication is in the control of a healthcare professional, patient, or consumer [6]. Not all medication errors reach the patient. These are sometimes referred to as "near misses". They are not usually considered to be ADEs only because no harm was done. Preventable ADEs are a subset of medication errors that cause harm to a patient [7]. Figure 28.1 depicts the relationship between ADEs, medication errors, and adverse drug reactions [8]. Because adverse drug reactions are generally unexpected, they are not presently considered to be a reflection of medication-use quality in a classic sense. However, as genetic variances become a more prominent consideration in drug selection and monitoring, it may be possible to predict and avoid some of the reactions that have been previously unexpected. This offers an opportunity to improve the quality of medication use.

*PRINCIPLES OF CLINICAL PHARMACOLOGY, THIRD EDITION*
DOI: http://dx.doi.org/10.1016/B978-0-12-385471-1.00028-3

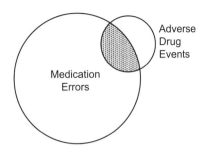

**FIGURE 28.1** Diagram showing the relationship between medication errors and adverse drug events. Because some adverse drug events are preventable, they are also considered to be medication errors (*shaded area*). Adapted from Bates DW, Boyle DL, Vander Vliet MB *et al*. J Gen Intern Med 1995;10:199–205 [8].

Medication errors are costly, and are a diversion from the intended therapeutic objective. Morbidity and mortality are possible outcomes of medication errors. A 1997 study by Bates *et al.* [9] found that 6.5 ADEs occurred for every 100 non-obstetric hospital admissions, and that 28% of them were preventable. It also was determined that 42% of life-threatening and serious ADEs were preventable. Preventable ADEs were responsible for an increased length of hospital stay of 4.6 days and $5857 per event. The cost for all ADEs was projected to be $5.6 million per year just for the institution in which the study was conducted. McDonnell [10] concluded from a separate dataset that ADE-related admissions resulted in a 6.1-day length of stay. Anderson *et al.* [11] conducted a simulation of the impact of an integrated medication-use system and projected $1.4 million in excess costs that might have been saved had the components of the system been effectively integrated. These findings imply that safer medication use, with fewer adverse medication events, is a cost-effective strategy.

## Medication-Use Process

Medications are prescribed, distributed, and consumed under the assumption that the therapeutic plan will work as intended to provide the expected outcome. It is clear from previous chapters that there are many biological system issues that will influence the success of the plan. Other organizational and societal system issues also influence the success of the therapeutic plan as profoundly as do those biological systems issues. A prescriber writes an order for a medication based on the best available information, the likely diagnosis, and the expected outcome. A pharmacist reviews the requested medication order (prescription), clarifies it based upon additional information about the patient or medication

(allergies, drug interactions, etc.), prepares the medication for use, counsels the patient about the drug, and gives it to the patient. The patient is responsible for understanding the therapeutic objective, knowing about the drug, creating a daily compliance plan (deciding when to take the drug), watching for good or bad results, and providing feedback to the prescriber or pharmacist regarding planned or unplanned outcomes. This process occurs over a variable period of time, in a system where the key participants of the process seldom speak with each other. Each action creates an opportunity for success or failure. Is there any wonder that the quality and integrity of the system are compromised on a regular basis?

The medication-use system in a hospital or long-term care setting offers even more complexity, with more chances for error. The five subsystems of the medication system in a hospital are selection and procurement of drugs, drug prescribing, preparation and dispensing, drug administration, and monitoring for medication or related effects [12]. Evaluation and improvement of medication-use quality require consideration of all of these subsystems.

Figure 28.2 is a flowchart of appropriate, safe, effective, and efficient use of medications in the hospital setting [13]. It incorporates the role of the prescriber, nurse, pharmacist, and patient in a typical inpatient environment. It also depicts the role of the organization's pharmacy and therapeutics committee and quality improvement functions, which will be discussed later in this chapter. The decision to treat a patient in a hospital or extended-care facility typically adds a nurse or other healthcare provider (respiratory therapist, etc.) to the trio described in the ambulatory care setting. Every time that individual has to read, interpret, decide, or act is yet another opportunity for a mistake to occur. Each of the steps in the medication-use process provides an opportunity for correct or incorrect interpretation and implementation of the tactics that support the therapeutic plan. With this many opportunities for medication misadventures to occur, it is easy to understand why tracking and improving quality are important aspects of medication use.

Phillips and colleagues [14] found a 236% increase in medication error-related deaths for hospitalized patients between 1983 and 1993. The same study showed an increase of over 800% for outpatient medication error deaths. The reported growth in medication error deaths may be partially attributed to more accurate reporting, but clearly represents a growth in the problem of medication errors from potent drugs. Phillips [15] has further proposed that

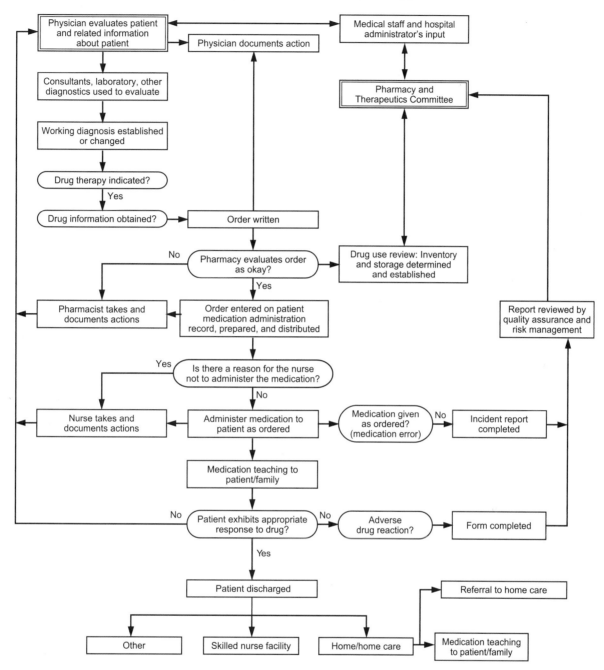

**FIGURE 28.2** Flow chart of the inpatient medication-use process showing the start and end points (*double-boxed rectangles*), intervening actions (*rectangles*) and decision-making steps (*ovals*) required for appropriate, safe, effective, and efficient medication use. Reproduced with permission from Atkinson AJ Jr, Nadzam DM, Schaff RL. Clin Pharmacol Ther 1991;50:125–8 [13].

impediments to reductions in medical error include perceptual, legal, and medical barriers. A 2002 poll commissioned by the American Society of Health-System Pharmacists concluded that the top two concerns of patients regarding hospitalization were related to drug–drug interactions and medication errors [16]. Winterstein [17] conducted a meta-analysis of 15 studies, and concluded that 4.3% of hospital admissions were drug related and that greater than 50% of them were preventable. A study by Bates *et al.* [18] determined that the 56% of medication errors in a hospital setting were associated with the ordering process, 6% with transcription of written orders, 4% with pharmacy dispensing, and 34% with administration of medications. Another study by Barker *et al.* [19] of medication administration in 36 healthcare settings identified a 19% total error rate during medication administration. Based on these findings, it is easily concluded that there is room for improvement in how medications are used in the inpatient and outpatient settings.

### Improving the Quality of Medication Use

There are multiple facets to the quality assessment of medication use. Among them are monitoring of adverse medication events and medication-use evaluation programs. To improve medication use, Berwick [20] has applied the industrial principles of continuous quality improvement to the healthcare setting. The critical elements of this approach are collection and use of data with a system focus. Deming [21] has championed the use of the Shewhart Cycle in continuous quality improvement. As shown in Figure 28.3, the Shewhart Cycle is an approach for implementing systematic change, based on data collection and evaluation, with each iteration of the cycle. Each time the work cycle is completed, the result is compared to the expected outcome or ideal target. Modifications that improve the result are permanently incorporated into the process. Changes with no impact or a negative result will be deleted in the next iteration. Deming's message is that ongoing process and system change, along with measurement of the result, provide the feedback loop to support continuous improvement of the product or service.

## ORGANIZATIONAL INFLUENCES ON MEDICATION-USE QUALITY

Several external organizations and internal elements of the healthcare system have an interest in optimizing medication use. These include the hospital or health system, the medical staff, the group purchasing organization with which the hospital participates for the contractual purchase of drugs, and external regulatory or accreditation organizations (e.g., Center for Medicare and Medicaid Services, Joint Commission on Accreditation of Healthcare Organizations, National Council on Quality Assurance, state and local public health agencies). There is interest in what drugs are used, when and how they are used, the economic impact of drug selection, and outcomes that result in safe and effective use of medications.

The Joint Commission (TJC) is the organization that accredits many hospitals, health systems, and home care agencies. A significant element of the overall JCAHO review of patient care involves medication-use quality and medication system safety. Accreditation standards for medication-related activities are applied across the organization. Organizations are expected to present evidence that ordering, dispensing, administering, and monitoring of medications are overseen by the medical staff. The organization must be able to demonstrate that policies for safe medication-use practices are in place. Quality-directed medication use is a key performance element for accreditation. Ongoing medication-use evaluation, adverse medication event investigation, medication-use performance improvement, and compliance with

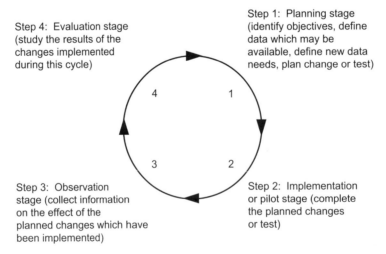

**FIGURE 28.3** The Shewhart Cycle. The cycle is repeated with desired improvements implemented with each iteration and the measured results used to guide the design of the next cycle. Reproduced with permission from Deming WE. Out of the crisis. Cambridge, MA: MIT Press; 2000. pp. 87–9 [21].

National Patient Safety Goals are required to meet the standards. The National Council on Quality Assurance accredits many managed care organizations. State professional boards (medicine, nursing, or pharmacy) provide oversight of specialized domains such as prescribing, dispensing, and administering medications. Most healthcare facilities are also regulated by state or local health departments that often have additional regulations on medication-related issues.

It is the shared responsibility of the medical staff and executive administration in a healthcare organization to oversee medication-use activities, ranging from product selection to long-term monitoring. This includes development of medication-use policies, selection of drug products that are appropriate to the needs of the patient population being served, and oversight of the quality of medication use. The pharmacy and therapeutics committee is frequently the focal point for medication-related activities within the organization. The pharmacy and therapeutics committee develops policies for managing drug use and administration, manages the formulary system, and evaluates the clinical use of drugs [22].

The structure of the pharmacy and therapeutics committee may vary to meet the unique needs and structure of the organization. It routinely reports to the medical staff executive committee or other leadership group within the medical staff organization. The committee is made up of representatives from the principal medication-using services (internal medicine, surgery, pediatrics, etc.) within the organization, plus representatives from the nursing services, pharmacy services, quality improvement program, and hospital administration. The chair of the committee is most frequently a clinician with experience in system-wide activities and, most important, an interest in quality use of medications. It is customary for the director of the pharmacy department to serve on the committee to assure a working link between pharmacy department and committee activities.

Pharmacy and therapeutics committees meet as frequently as needed to accomplish their mission, typically monthly. The schedule is dependent on the traditions of the organization and the amount of work included during the full committee meeting. The agenda should be prepared under the supervision of the committee chair and distributed well in advance of the meeting to allow all participants to read formulary drug monographs and drug-use reports before the meeting. Ongoing elements of many committees are special standing subcommittees or focused task-force workgroups. Typical standing subcommittees focus on drug formulary management, antimicrobial agents, and medication-use evaluation. Standing

subcommittees are appropriate for providing ongoing special expertise on matters that can be referred back to the full committee for action. A taskforce workgroup also may be used to address special limited-scope issues, such as *ad hoc* evaluations of agents within a given therapeutic drug class.

## Medication Policy Issues

The pharmacy and therapeutics committee is expected to oversee important policies and procedures associated with the use of medications. Medication policy includes a wide range of issues, from who may prescribe or administer drugs, to what prescribing direction and guidance are appropriate to assure safe and appropriate use of high-risk, high-volume, high-cost, or problem-prone drugs. Policies are often needed to identify who may prescribe or administer medications, to assure consistent supply or quality of drug products, or to allocate drugs in times of shortage. Responsibility for developing policies to address special circumstances or issues is often delegated to the pharmacy and therapeutics committee by the organization. Examples of this type of policy are special drug class restriction (e.g., antimicrobial agents), and use of agents for sedation during medical procedures.

## Formulary Management

The objective of an active formulary program is to direct medication use to preferred agents which offer a therapeutic or safety benefit or an economic advantage. This serves as a quality/benefit-driven opportunity when optimally implemented. A statement of principles of a Sound Drug Formulary System was developed in 2000 by a consortium composed of the US Pharmacopoeia, the Department of Veterans Affairs, the American Society of Health-System Pharmacists, the Academy of Managed Care Pharmacists, and the National Business Coalition on Health [23]. In this statement, a formulary is defined as "a continually updated list of medications and related information, representing the clinical judgment of physicians, pharmacists, and other experts in the diagnosis and or treatment of disease and promotion of health". A specific formulary is intended for use in a defined population. The defined population may consist of patients in a single hospital, patients seen within a group practice, a managed care patient population (local, regional, or national), or even an entire community.

Historically, formulary drug inclusion or exclusion has been used as an administrative barrier to discourage prescribers from using non-preferred drugs. The historical approach to formulary decision-making was based on a simple "on formulary" or "not-on formulary" approach. Formulary drugs were available immediately with no special requirements. Often a formulary drug was selected by the prescriber to avoid a prolonged waiting period for the non-formulary item to be ordered and made available for the patient. This approach was more effective when the array of effective drug choices was somewhat limited, and the principal cost and quality management need was to reduce the number of "me-too" products.

With the advent of many of the newest generation of products, including monoclonal antibodies and cytokine agents, it is not logical to simply deny the formulary availability of these novel agents. Accordingly, the standard for most institutions has been to include these novel drugs with committee-approved restrictions and guidelines for use. Continued expansion of prescriber order entry within an electronic medical record system offers growing opportunity for enhanced clinical decision support and evidence-based, diagnosis-specific formulary management. In the future, individual patient pharmacogenetic and pharmacogenomic characteristics that influence drug toxicity and effectiveness can be expected to play an important role in formulary drug management. As discussed in previous chapters, the ability to use this information to better customize patient-specific drug response will require an increasingly sophisticated approach in selecting the most appropriate drug.

### Drug Selection Process

Effective formulary development is based upon the scientific evaluation of drug safety, clinical effectiveness, and cost impact [23]. That information is used by the committee to determine the specific value and risk of the drug for the patient population to whom the drug will be administered. The committee evaluates a given drug relative to the disease states typically treated in this population. For instance, the presence or absence of certain tropical diseases may impact on the need to include some antimicrobial agents on the formulary. The evaluation of a drug should include discussion of what doses and duration of therapy might be most appropriate in order to establish guidelines for measuring prescribing quality. In some cases, it may be necessary to determine which healthcare professionals are appropriately trained or qualified to prescribe a particular drug. The committee may elect to restrict the use of a drug to certain specialists (e.g., board-trained cardiologists for high-risk anti-arrhythmic agents), or the drug may be restricted by the manufacturer or FDA to those prescribers who have received some drug-specific training and been approved by the supplier (e.g., thalidomide).

Economic evaluation of medications is a routine element of formulary development. The development of many effective but expensive drugs, which are likely to cost thousands of dollars for a single short course of therapy or tens of thousands for long-term therapy, has placed financial impact at center stage in product selection. The availability of these high-cost agents has created a new specialty discipline called pharmacoeconomics. A growing list of academic medical centers have established units that focus research and practice efforts on outcomes measurement of drug therapy. These programs often provide sophisticated evaluations of the economic or quality-of-life elements of drug use.

It is noteworthy that drug costs, and their impact, are perceived differently from different perspectives in the healthcare system. Each component of the healthcare system (hospital, home care, ambulatory provider) may have a different perspective on the cost of therapy. Hospitals are usually responsible for all drug-related costs (drug purchase, medication administration, laboratory monitoring, etc.) for the finite period of time that a patient is hospitalized. A stand-alone outpatient drug benefit manager might only worry about the drug cost for the non-hospitalized portion of the therapy. The overall health system may be at financial risk for all elements of outpatient and inpatient care. Because each element of the system may be responsible for a different component of the total cost of care, the cost impact of a given drug product selection may be different for each of them. The "societal perspective" often represents yet another view of drug costs in that it incorporates non-healthcare costs and the value of lost days of work and disability. Formulary inclusion is not routinely based on that level of evaluation, but public policy may be influenced by that information.

The cost-impact analysis of two hypothetical drug choices shown in Figure 28.4 demonstrates the role of cost perspective in the formulary selection process. Both regimens offer the same long-term clinical result and adverse reaction profile. This analysis shows that the decision as to which drug is the lower-cost option will vary with the perspective of the organization that is responsible for the different inpatient and outpatient components of care. This dilemma is a regular element of the formulary selection process in many institutions. The puzzle becomes more complex when trying

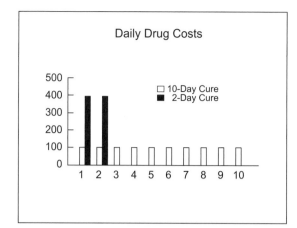

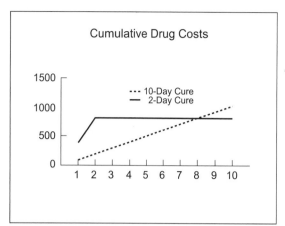

### Financial Responsibility at Discharge

|  | Daily Cost | 10-Day Total | Total at Hospital Discharge |
|---|---|---|---|
| 2-Day Cure | $400 | $800 | $800 |
| 10-Day Cure | $100 | $1000 | $300 |

### Perspective Based Financial Responsibility

|  | 2-Day Cure | 10-Day Cure |
|---|---|---|
| Hospital | $800 | $300 |
| Outpatient Payer | $0 | $700 |
| Total | $800 | $1000 |

**FIGURE 28.4**  Financial perspective in formulary decision-making. Comparison of two treatment options: 2-day cure at $400 day$^{-1}$ vs 10-day cure at $100 day$^{-1}$, with an anticipated hospital stay of 3 days.

to decide what elements of cost (e.g., laboratory tests or other monitoring activities) should be included. Despite of this lack of clarity, the cost impact of drug therapy on different stakeholders requires that this issue be considered in the decision process, and some hospitals have begun to use both expert guidelines and benchmarking data to guide formulary decision-making.

Most hospitals and healthcare organizations participate in a purchasing group to leverage volume-driven price advantages. The makeup and operations of these groups vary widely, but the price agreements and changing landscape of drug pricing add an additional dimension to the drug price factor. A specific drug may be the lowest price option for a given contract period, after which the choice may change. In another variation, a package of prices for bundled items may cause the price for a given item to change, depending on the use of yet another item. How this influences formulary decisions is a function of the drug and many other factors.

### Formulary Tactics

In addition to drug selection, the pharmacy and therapeutics committee is responsible for considering formulary tactics to support the overall goal of optimal medication use. Several of these tactics have been used successfully to direct drug use toward preferred agents. The most obvious tactic to direct use away from a given agent is to exclude it from the formulary. The use of non-formulary agents usually triggers some required override, or *post hoc* review of use, by the committee or designated individual. A second tactic involves a global management of medication use by therapeutic class. This tactic can be employed to minimize the use of drugs with a less clear profile of therapeutic efficacy or safety. A decision to limit the number of agents from a given drug class can also provide some advantages in price contracting, if formulary inclusion is effective in directing medication use to lower-cost agents.

Limiting prescribing rights for some specific drugs to a subset of prescribers who possess special expertise that qualifies them to use these drugs can improve the quality of their use. In many cases, drug restriction is managed by one or more gatekeepers whose approval is required prior to beginning therapy with the drug (e.g., infectious disease approval prior to start of a specified antibiotic). In some cases, direct financial incentives have been used to encourage use of a given drug or group of drugs. These formulary tactics have been used to influence decision-making by prescribers, pharmacists, and patients.

## Analysis and Prevention of Medication Errors

Reason [24] has described a model for looking at human error that portrays a battle between the sources of error and the system-based defenses against them. This model is often referred to as the "Swiss cheese model" because the defenses against error are displayed as thin layers with holes that are described as latent error in the system. Figure 28.5 demonstrates the model as applied to medication error. Each opportunity for error is defended by the prescriber, pharmacist, nurse, and patient. When a potential error is identified and corrected (e.g., dose error, route of administration error) the event becomes a "near miss" rather than an ADE. In those cases in which the holes in the Swiss cheese line up, a preventable medication error occurs. The Swiss cheese model provides an interesting framework for research in this field.

The latent errors in the medication-use system have been described in several studies. Major contributors to errors in medication use were found to be: knowledge gap related to drug therapy (30%); knowledge gap related to patient factors (30%); errors in dose calculations, placement of decimal points, and dosage units (18%); and nomenclature failures such as wrong drug name or misinterpreted abbreviation (13%) [25]. Cohen [26] describes six common causes of medication error based on his review of events reported to public

reporting databases. These causes of errors include failed communication practices (including verbal orders), poor drug distribution, dose miscalculations, drug- and device-related problems (such as name confusion, labeling, or poor design), and lack of patient education on the drugs that are prescribed for their use. Leape *et al.* [27] identified 13 proximal causes of medication errors in an academic medical center. They are detailed in Table 28.1.

### Medication Error Data

The rate and nature of medication errors has been studied by several authors. Nightingale *et al.* [28] found a medication error rate of 0.7% in a British National Health Service general hospital. Phillips *et al.* [29] evaluated all medication events reported to the FDA from 1993 through 1998 that were associated with a patient death, and found that 41% were associated with a wrong dose, 16% with the wrong drug, and 9.5% with the wrong route of administration. Rothschild *et al.* [30] found 36.2% preventable ADEs plus an additional 149.7 serious errors per 1000 patient days. Medication ordering or execution represented 61% of the serious errors. Slips and lapses rather than rule-based or knowledge errors were most common. Lesar *et al.* [31] describe the results of a review of 2103 clinically significant medication errors in an academic medical center. It was determined that 0.4% of medication orders were in error: 42% of the errors were overdosage, and 13% were the result of drug allergies that were not accounted for prior to prescribing. This work showed that medication errors result most frequently from failure to alter dose or drug after changes in renal or hepatic status, missed allergies, wrong drug name, wrong dosage form (e.g., IV for IM), use of abbreviations, or incorrect calculation of a drug dose. They concluded that an improved organizational focus on technological risk management

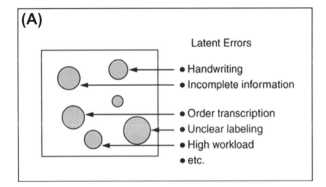
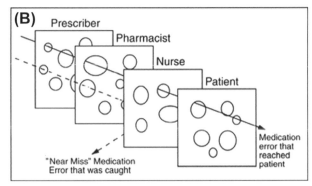

**FIGURE 28.5**   Latent medication system errors (A) and defensive layers against error (B) in the medication system.

**TABLE 28.1  Proximal Causes of Medication Errors**

| | |
|---|---|
| Lack of knowledge of the drug | Faulty dose-checking |
| Lack of information about the patient | Infusion pump and parenteral delivery problems |
| Violation of rules | Inadequate monitoring |
| Slips and memory lapses | Drug stocking and delivery problems |
| Transcription errors | Preparation errors |
| Faulty checking of identification | Lack of standardization |
| Faulty interaction with other services | |

Adapted from Leape LL, Bates DW, Cullen DJ *et al.* JAMA 1995;274:35–43 [27].

and training should reduce errors and patient risk of ADEs.

Given the latent errors associated with some elements of human performance, it seems likely that automation may reduce error. Several studies have demonstrated the value of computer assistance in the medication order entry process. Rules-based prescriber order entry systems have been shown to identify and reduce the chances of adverse medication events due to drug duplication, calculation errors, and drug–drug interactions [32–38]. Despite these demonstrated advantages to computer-assisted medication ordering, the process is still far from error free. MedMARx data from 2003 showed that nearly 20% of the medication errors reported to that national database were associated with problems in computerization and automation [39]. A large number of these were order entry errors associated with interruptions during order entry. Another study showed that an early-generation computerized prescriber order entry system facilitated some error types due to formatting and display limitations [40]. In still another study, Nebeker *et al.* [41] found that ADEs continued to occur following the implementation of a computerized prescriber order entry system. They concluded that effective decision support functions are required to prevent order entry-related medication errors associated with computerized prescribing systems.

Some therapeutic categories of medications might be predicted to be prone to error due to narrow therapeutic index, complexity of therapy, or other factors. Phillips *et al.* [14] found that analgesics, central nervous system agents, and non-tranquilizer psychotropic drugs were most frequently associated with deaths due to medication errors. Lesar *et al.* [42] found antimicrobials and cardiovascular drugs to be the most error-prone therapeutic categories in an academic medical center. Calabrese *et al.* [43] found vasoactive drugs and sedative/analgesics to be most problematic in the intensive care unit (ICU) setting. From the MedMARx reports, Hicks [44, 45] found

that opioid drugs were most frequently associated with reported errors causing patient harm, and that medication errors were fatal in geriatric patients at nearly twice the rate reported in the general population. Based on these non-converging findings, it might be concluded that the specific drugs of concern are unique to the institution or practice setting – a conclusion that is partially true. The JCAHO [46] has identified a list of drugs and drug practices that are associated with high risk for significant error based upon high report rates, and the Institute for Safe Medication Practices [47] also has identified drugs which should generate a high alert due to risk for medication errors. Lambert and colleagues [48, 49] have described a series of experiments that test the likelihood of drug name confusion based on fixed similarity patterns. This theoretical concept is providing the basis for selecting drug names that minimize the chance of sound-alike errors [50].

Research methods on medication error data are not standardized. Therefore, they are subject to some limitations in generalizability. Because widespread interest in developing scientific approaches for reducing medication error is relatively recent, there are few well-established methods for conducting research in this field. However, funding for research in safe medication use and error reduction is available from several public and private sources, including the Agency for Healthcare Research and Quality.

Medication error data collection and analysis for clinical use and quality improvement are also complex activities. Observational data, *post hoc* review of medical records, and self-reporting have all have been used with varying degrees of success for research and functional applications. Each offers strengths and weaknesses, and the appropriate method for data collection is in large part a function of its intended use and the resources available to collect it.

Most hospitals collect internal medication error data through a voluntary reporting mechanism. This

476

Daniels

system is used as the backbone of error reporting because it requires minimal resources for data collection and is supported by organizational risk-management programs. Voluntary reporting is presumed to under-report total errors. It is widely believed that most significant errors are reported when they are identified, but many mistakes are never recognized. Many other errors are determined to be insignificant and, therefore, are not formally reported. For these reasons, it is difficult to determine in the hospital setting if changes in a given series of numbers represent a real change or simply a different level of reporting.

Figure 28.6 illustrates a typical presentation of aggregated or high-level medication error data in an institutional setting. This presentation allows for general trends in total numbers to be plotted and tracked over time. Review of high-level data shows trends and provides a framework for the first level of error analysis. Major changes can be seen, which may trigger more intense analysis. However, this high-level data approach does not provide any detail to the analyst regarding the subcomponents of the composition of the reported errors. As a result, there are pitfalls in drawing conclusions from aggregated high-level data that can make these conclusions problematic. For instance, one might presume that administration of medication to the wrong patient is generally more serious than administration of a medication at the wrong time. However, an increase of five "wrong patient" errors and a decrease of five "wrong time" errors for a specific time period will register as a zero change for that period if only aggregated data

are used. If fact, it may represent a serious degradation in some element of the medication system that will not be seen through this level of error analysis.

Classification and analysis of medication error data by error type is recommended as a method to spot potentially important changes in system performance. The National Coordinating Council for Medication Error Reporting and Prevention system for classifying medication errors may be used [6]. Commercial systems for cataloging and analyzing medication errors are available. A potentially valuable element of some programs is the ability to share anonymous data with other hospitals for comparison with similar institutions [51]. Regardless of the system used to classify and analyze medication error data, clear and consistent classification must be made to avoid confounding conclusions regarding underlying problems.

*Reducing Medication Errors*

Collection and use of medication error data at the hospital level are challenging but important functions. A key organizational principle in quality improvement is to make reporting errors a non-punitive process. This usually increases the number of errors that will be reported, but not the number occurring. Making errors visible is an important step in the process of finding and fixing system-related problems [52]. The ongoing monitoring of ADE data (both medication errors and adverse drug reactions) is an important responsibility of the pharmacy and therapeutics committee. The committee is the organization's only convergence point for all medication-

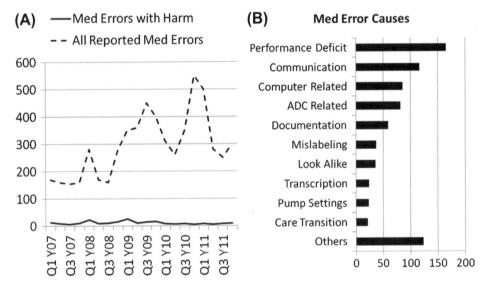

**FIGURE 28.6** Presentation of a typical approach to tracking medication error data. (A) Tracking data in aggregate form, separating errors that result in harm (*solid line*) from total reported errors (*broken line*). (B) Summary of medication errors categorized by error type.

related issues. This convergence allows for a full review of the medication-use process for system adjustments.

To identify opportunities for reducing medication errors, it is important that each error be carefully reviewed by a limited number of individuals to gain intimate knowledge of each reported incident. Collection and classification of error data must be followed by use of a careful epidemiological approach to problem-solving at the system level. Narrative data, which may not be seen by looking at the categorical data alone, can be used to provide important details about proximal causes and latent error that may have contributed to the event. Success in this type of error reduction requires the reviewers to read between the lines, look for common threads between reports, and link multiple errors which are the result of system weaknesses.

There is still work to be done in understanding errors in the medication-use process. However, available information provides suggestions on how to reduce medication errors. Bates's [53] ongoing studies of medication errors led to eight specific error-prevention strategies: (1) unit-dose medication dispensing; (2) targeted physician education on optimal medication use; (3) inclusion of the clinical pharmacist in decision-making patient activities; (4) computerized medication checking; (5) computerized order entry by the prescriber; (6) standardized processes and equipment; (7) automated medication dispensing systems; and (8) bar-coded medications for dispensing and administration. In addition, the IOM study on preventing medication errors [54] recommended a stronger role for consumers/patients in self-management, enhanced consumer information sources, complete patient information for providers, enhanced decision support, improved labeling, and standardization of technologies. They also encouraged further research in the field of medication-error prevention.

The more complex a patient's drug therapy regimen, the greater the likelihood that adverse medication events will occur. Cullen et al. [55] determined that the rate of preventable and potential adverse drug events was twice as high in ICUs, compared to non-intensive care units. This was attributed to the higher number of drugs used in the ICU. Lesar et al. [56] reviewed medication prescribing errors over a 9-year period, and concluded that the incidence of prescribing error increased as intensity of care increased and new drugs became available. Koechler et al. [57] reported that greater than 5 current medications, 12 or more doses day$^{-1}$, or medication regimen changes four or more times in a year were all

predictors for drug therapy problems in ambulatory patients. Transition between levels of care or components of the healthcare system put patients at risk for medication errors. Cornish [58] found that 53% of patients they studied had at least one medication unintentionally not ordered during the transition from home status to inpatient admission, but that dose errors were also a significant problem. Gray et al. [59] determined that the occurrence of an ADE was positively related to the number of new medications received at hospital discharge. The knowledge that some patients are at higher risk for ADEs suggests possible high-return intervention targets. When selecting improvement opportunities, it is wise to look for those areas most likely to yield results.

Examples of system improvements to reduce medication errors have been reported in several projects. Leape et al. [60] reduced medication errors in an ICU by including a pharmacist on the clinical rounding team. Flynn et al. [61] identified interruptions (telephone calls, conversations, etc.) during critical phases of pharmacist drug preparation activities as significant contributors to errors in medication preparation. Comprehensive efforts to prevent medication errors include the four-pronged medication error analysis program from the Institute for Safe Medication Practices [62]. This four-pronged approach includes evaluation of specific medication errors, evaluation of aggregated error data and near-miss data for the hospital, as well as evaluation of error reports from other hospitals. In addition, effective medication error prevention includes ongoing monitoring of drug therapy trends, changes in medication-use patterns, information from the hospital quality improvement or risk management program, and general hospital programmatic information.

Monitoring institutional trends in medication use can provide clues to possible high-risk or error-prone therapies. Increased use of drugs with a history of medication errors, such as patient-controlled analgesia, should alert organizations to develop safeguards to protect against errors before, rather than after, they become problems. Cohen and Kilo [47] describe a framework for improving the use of high-alert drugs, which is based on reducing or eliminating the possibility of error, making errors visible, and minimizing the consequences of errors. Table 28.2 presents change concepts for safeguarding against errors when using high-risk drugs.

Medication error prevention opportunities also may present themselves in unusual hospital programmatic information from sources not routinely applied to medication safety. For instance, reports of laboratory-related incidents or hospital information

**TABLE 28.2  Safeguarding Against Errors in High-Risk Drugs**

| Concept | Example |
| --- | --- |
| Build in System Redundancies | Independent calculation of pediatric doses by more than one person (e.g., prescriber and pharmacist) |
| Use Fail-Safes | IV pumps with clamps that automatically shut off flow during power outage |
| Reduce Options | Use of a single concentration of heparin for infusion (e.g., 25,000 units in 250 ml of saline) |
| Use Forcing Functions | Preprinted order forms for chemotherapy drugs which require patient height and weight information before preparation and dispensing |
| Externalize or Centralize Error-prone Processes | Prepare IV admixtures in the pharmacy instead of on nursing units |
| Use Differentialization | Supplemental labels for dosage forms which are not appropriate for intravenous use without dilution |
| Store Medications Appropriately | Store dopamine and dobutamine in separate locations |
| Screen New Products | Review new formulary requests for labeling, packaging and medication-use issues which may be error prone |
| Standardize and Simplify Order Communication | Avoid use of verbal orders |
| Limit Access | Restrict access to the pharmacy during "non-staffed" hours and follow-up on all medications removed from the pharmacy during this time |
| Use Constraints | Require approval before beginning therapy (e.g., attending signature on chemotherapy orders) |
| Use Reminders | Place special labels on products when they are dispensed by the pharmacy to remind of special procedures for use (e.g., double-check rate calculation of insulin infusions) |
| Standardize Dosing Procedures | Develop standardized dose and rate charts for products such as vasoactive drugs (e.g., infusion rate expressed as micrograms per kilogram per minute) |

Adapted from Cohen MR, Kilo CM. High-alert medications: Safeguarding against errors. In: Cohen MR, editor. Medication errors. Washington, DC: American Pharmaceutical Association; 1999. pp. 5.3–5.11 [47].

system problems may be indicators that medication-related problems can be expected. Thoughtful use of this information may prevent medication-related errors attributed to supplemental systems that are critical to safe and appropriate medication use. Reports of staff shortages within an institution (e.g., critical care nurses, nurse anesthetists) can be used to identify potential problem areas prior to medication error reports. Likewise, reports of planned construction or information system conversions may be an indicator that routines will be interrupted. Thus, use of hospital program information in a prospective way can be used to provide safe alternatives that avoid medication errors before they occur.

System improvements may improve the quality of prescribing by standardizing to an expert level. Morris [63] described the development, testing, and use of computerized protocols for managing intravenous fluid and hemodynamic factors in patients with acute respiratory distress syndrome. Evans *et al.* [64] used a computerized anti-infectives management program to improve the quality of medication use and reduce costs. In consideration of all that is currently known, Leape [65] provided a simple set of recommendations to reduce medical error: reduce reliance on memory, improve access to information, error-proof critical tasks, standardize processes, and instruct healthcare providers on possible errors in processes. These simple but thoughtful recommendations are an important concept that can help to reduce medication errors.

## Medication-Use Evaluation

Medication-use evaluation (also referred to as MUE or drug-use evaluation) is a required component of the medication-use quality improvement process. It is a performance improvement method with the goal of optimizing patient outcomes [66]. The first element of drug-use tracking is global monitoring of organizational drug use. This can be completed by routine evaluation of totals and changes in drug use within a therapeutic drug category. The American Hospital Formulary Service has created a comprehensive therapeutic classification system that is often used for drug-use monitoring [67], but other commercial medication databases are also available.

Figure 28.7 is an example of a global drug-use report that may be used to look for trends and variations in medication use. This report should be examined for changes that represent increases or decreases in comparison to previous reporting periods. A change in any specific category or group of drugs may be important and worthy of specific

| F | G | SPENT FY 06 | SPENT FY 07 | SPENT FY 08 | SPENT FY 09 | SPENT FY 10 | SPENT FY 11 |
|---|---|---|---|---|---|---|---|
| ANTIHISTAMINE | | $17,564 | $21,175 | $28,185 | $41,918 | $54,237 | $64,221 |
| ANTI-INFECTIVE AGENTS | | | | | | | |
| 80400 | AMEBICIDES | $0 | $1,522 | $332 | $884 | $1,321 | $746 |
| 80800 | ANTHELMINTICS | $2,510 | $996 | $2,623 | $1,231 | $1,834 | $2,702 |
| 81202 | AMINOGLYCOSIDES | $9,457 | $13,457 | $10,351 | $35,468 | $47,014 | $35,272 |
| 81204 | ANTIFUNGAL ANTIBIOTICS | $256,806 | $320,884 | $357,206 | $946,657 | $1,082,165 | $1,056,544 |
| 81206 | CEPHALOSPORINS | $221,196 | $197,231 | $162,850 | $180,186 | $188,435 | $146,069 |
| 81207 | B-LACTAMS | $59,322 | $77,722 | $77,703 | $90,073 | $112,235 | $81,442 |
| 81208 | CHLORAMPHENICOLS | $626 | $204 | $172 | $771 | $1,331 | $34 |
| 81212 | ERYTHROMYCINS | $52,106 | $69,377 | $89,793 | $112,984 | $109,499 | $92,816 |
| 81216 | PENICILLINS | $50,569 | $41,427 | $65,243 | $46,314 | $61,153 | $89,200 |
| 81224 | TETRACYLINES | $16,872 | $4,427 | $4,788 | $4,569 | $8,820 | $5,962 |
| 81228 | MISCELLANEOUS ANTIBIOTICS | $38,577 | $35,347 | $35,261 | $37,811 | $41,473 | $80,727 |
| 81600 | ANTITUBERCULOSIS AGENTS | $33,141 | $27,937 | $42,335 | $53,318 | $46,223 | $39,438 |
| 81800 | ANTIVIRALS | $658,157 | $1,399,246 | $2,472,982 | $3,251,543 | $3,417,004 | $3,775,675 |
| 82000 | ANTIMALARIAL AGENTS | $82,141 | $60,942 | $20,848 | $19,051 | $20,577 | $17,524 |
| 82200 | QUINOLONES | $82,319 | $113,064 | $94,705 | $117,380 | $116,301 | $119,356 |
| 82400 | SULFONAMIDES | $7,053 | $6,730 | $3,425 | $3,660 | $2,770 | $4,579 |
| 82600 | SULFONES | $5,207 | $4,839 | $4,651 | $4,972 | $5,366 | $3,735 |
| 83200 | ANTITRICHOMONAL AGENTS | $1,493 | $3,923 | $677 | $924 | $1,454 | $1,627 |
| 83600 | URINARY ANTI-INFECTIVES | $5,974 | $2,009 | $2,142 | $1,632 | $2,836 | $763 |
| 84000 | MISCELLANEOUS ANTI-INFECTIVES | $28,489 | $34,661 | $30,211 | $27,401 | $19,394 | $23,766 |
| | **TOTAL ANTI-INFECTIVE AGENTS** | $1,612,016 | $2,415,944 | $3,478,297 | $4,936,828 | $5,287,206 | $5,577,978 |
| **BLOOD DERIVATIVIES TOTAL** | | $212,109 | $188,350 | $204,843 | $236,087 | $348,825 | $11,095 |
| BLOOD FORMATION AND COAGULATION | | | | | | | |
| 200404 | IRON PREPARATIONS | $2,867 | $2,687 | $2,402 | $2,240 | $2,012 | $6,150 |
| 201204 | ANTICOAGULANTS | $41,207 | $66,851 | $75,294 | $114,764 | $179,357 | $146,496 |
| 201208 | ANTIHEPARIN AGENTS | $141 | $237 | $83 | $182 | $156 | $52,186 |
| 201216 | HEMOSTATICS | $56,030 | $21,246 | $27,266 | $48,408 | $75,817 | $65,886 |
| 201600 | HEMATOPOIETIC AGENTS | $1,228,251 | $1,526,711 | $1,471,910 | $1,515,326 | $2,027,767 | $1,406,002 |
| 202400 | HEMORRHEOLOGIC AGENTS | $3,179 | $2,717 | $2,046 | $3,014 | $6,683 | $1,109 |
| 204000 | THROMBOLYTIC AGENTS | $47,054 | $72,684 | $58,657 | $87,678 | $72,382 | $51,789 |
| | **TOTAL BLOOD FORMATION AND COAG.** | $1,378,728 | $1,693,133 | $1,637,657 | $1,771,613 | $2,142,912 | $1,729,616 |
| CARDIOVASCULAR DRUGS | | | | | | | |
| 240400 | CARDIAC DRUGS | $168,786 | $185,225 | $179,912 | $197,914 | $258,000 | $264,424 |
| 240600 | ANTILIPEMIC AGENTS | $237,143 | $237,827 | $298,091 | $269,520 | $298,957 | $333,476 |
| 240800 | HYPOTENSIVE AGENTS | $97,583 | $89,871 | $106,383 | $112,858 | $122,181 | $117,703 |
| 241200 | VASODILATING AGENTS | $20,063 | $21,023 | $28,385 | $39,040 | $26,947 | $25,841 |
| 241600 | SCLEROSING AGENTS | $0 | $0 | $0 | $0 | $0 | $220 |
| | **TOTAL CARDIOVASCULAR DRUGS** | $523,575 | $533,946 | $612,771 | $619,332 | $706,085 | $741,664 |

**FIGURE 28.7** Sample therapeutic category drug monitoring report based upon therapeutic classifications used by the American Hospital Formulary Service. (Internet at, www.ahfsdruginformation.com/class/index.aspx.)

follow-up. Smaller changes that support a trend over time can demonstrate ongoing changes in drug-use patterns. Changes seen in global-level monitoring may trigger a focused evaluation to further assess the appropriateness with which certain medications are used.

Medication-use evaluation has historically been categorized with regard to how and when data collection or intervention occurs (Table 28.3) [68–70]. Most medication-use evaluations are retrospective, as exemplified by an analysis of 8 years of emergency department prescribing data by Catarino *et al.* [68]. These authors found that, despite the availability of published lists of medications that are not generally appropriate for geriatric patients, one or more of those inappropriate medications were prescribed for 12.6% of elderly patients during their emergency department visits. Table 28.3 also describes concurrent and prospective reviews, classified based on the use and timing of intervention as part of the process that is used for screening and incorporating data.

### Focused Medication-Use Evaluation

Focused or targeted medication-use evaluation follows a reasonably well-established cycle: identification of a potential problem in the use of a specific drug or therapy, collection and comparison of data, determination of compliance with a pre-established guideline/expectation, and action as needed to improve discrepancies between expected and measured results. This type of medication-use evaluation provides an excellent opportunity to apply the Shewhart Cycle for continuous quality improvement (Figure 28.3). Focused medication-use projects are

**TABLE 28.3 Drug Use Review Categories**

| Review category | Data collection model(s) | Typical application | Comments |
|---|---|---|---|
| Retrospective | Data are collected for a fixed period, which may be archival or accumulation of new patients for a fixed period of time. | Data archive review of emergency department prescribing for geriatric patients [68]. | Supports large-scale epidemiologic approach. No active intervention to change medication-use patterns occurs due to the *post-hoc* data collection process. |
| Concurrent | Each new order generates an automatic review of previously approved criteria for use within a specified period of the initiation of therapy. | Review of naloxone to investigate possible nosocomial adverse medication event. | |
| | Laboratory or other monitoring criteria are reported for all patients on the drug. | Digoxin monitoring based upon daily review of digoxin serum levels [69]. | |
| | Abnormal laboratory or other monitoring criteria are reported for all patients on the drug on a regular basis. | Regular review of serum creatinine for patients on aminoglycosides. | |
| Prospective | Each new order for the drug is evaluated for compliance with previously approved criteria for use. Variance to the criteria requires intervention prior to initiation of therapy. | Medication-use guidelines (keterolac) [70]. Restricted antibiotics. | |

typically selected for a specific reason. Table 28.4 lists reasons to consider drugs for focused evaluation projects. A well-planned medication-use evaluation program includes a balance of high-volume, high-risk, high-cost, and problem-prone drugs.

### Concurrent or Prospective Focused Medication-Use Review

Concurrent or prospective focused medication-use review activities can be used to prevent medication-related adverse events and improve the quality of medication use. Focused concurrent review of potentially toxic digoxin concentration measurements has been used to monitor potential ADEs from this drug [70]. Information system support also has been used to warn of abnormalities in coagulation, or of predefined changes in renal function, blood glucose, and electrolytes, which are all potential indicators of medication-use problems in individual patients. When such laboratory test results are reported along with specific drugs, it is possible to respond to potential medication-related problems before serious negative outcomes occur. Kuperman *et al.* [71] concluded that incorporation of an automatic alerting system in the laboratory data system resulted in a 38% shorter response to appropriate treatment following alert to a critical value.

### Approaches for Improving Medication Use

Identification of best medication-use practices and benchmarking against best performers has become feasible over the last decade. Development and implementation of medication-use guidelines is one way for individual healthcare-provider organizations to apply evidence-based medicine to improve medication-use quality. This evidential approach to the use of medications is designed to rely on the best available clinical evidence to develop a treatment plan for a specific illness or use of a specific drug or drugs. Simple medication-use guidelines can be developed based on literature and the best judgment of in-house experts. Development of more formal clinical practice guidelines is a complex process that relies on well-defined methods to combine the results of multiple studies to draw statistically valid conclusions. These sophisticated products are often addressed by professional or governmental organizations. The National Guideline Clearinghouse, sponsored by the US Government Agency for Healthcare Research and Quality, hosts a website [72] with many evidence-based clinical practice guidelines. This guideline website supports searches by disease state, intervention type, and several other classifications. A representative clinical practice guideline contains systematically developed statements that include recommendations, strategies,

**TABLE 28.4    Selection of Targets for Focused Medication-Use Review**

- Medication is known or suspected to cause adverse reactions or drug interactions
- Medication-use process affects large number of patients or medication is frequently prescribed
- Medication is potentially toxic or causes discomfort at normal doses
- Medication is under consideration for formulary retention, addition, or deletion
- Medication use is expensive

- Medication is used in patients at high risk for adverse reactions
- Medication or process is a critical component of care for a specific disease, condition, or procedure
- Medication is most effective when used in a specific way
- Medication or process is one for which suboptimal use would have a negative effect on patient outcomes or system costs

Adapted from American Society of Health-System Pharmacists. Am J Health-Syst Pharm 1996;53:1953–5 [66]. (Also Internet at, www.ashp. org/DocLibrary/BestPractices/FormGdlMedUseEval.aspx.)

or information to assist physicians, other healthcare practitioners, and patients to make appropriate decisions about health care for specific clinical circumstances. These vetted guidelines are a valuable resource when considering plans for quality medication use.

The JCAHO Quality Check website [73] provides access to detailed information about an organization's performance on standardized performance measures, such as compliance with specific national patient safety goals. For instance, it is feasible to see how a particular organization is in compliance with standards for use of beta-blocker drugs for postmyocardial infarction patients. It is also possible to compare multiple organizations to look for best performers. Other organizations (e.g., Kaiser, VA Health System, University Healthsystem Consortium) have focused internal benchmarking systems to support improvements in medication use. Benchmarking use and outcome results and sharing of best medication-use practices provide among the strongest tools for quality improvement in medication use.

The use of "counter-detailing" by designated hospital staff [74] to offset the impact of pharmaceutical sales forces also has been an effective strategy for improving medication use. The objective of this category of quality improvement program is to educate prescribers regarding the organization's approved and preferred medication-use guidelines. This has been implemented by providing literature and prescriber contact from a pharmacist or other staff member to support the desired medication-use objective.

Several approaches have been described for improving medication use through the use of dosing service teams. Demonstrated enhancements in the quality of medication use have been reported for anticoagulants, antimicrobials, anticonvulsants, and other drugs. The common method of these programs is the use of expert oversight (physicians or pharmacists) to manage therapy with the targeted drug. Therapeutic management may rely on algorithms, pharmacokinetic models, or pre-approved collaborative plans [75–85].

Adoption of standardized medication order forms has been demonstrated to increase the quality of medication use and the effectiveness of medications that are prone to error [86, 87]. Chemotherapy, patient-controlled analgesia, and antimicrobial drug therapy are likely candidates for order standardization. Yet another approach to improved medication use is implementation of alert systems for sudden, unexpected actions, such as medication stop orders, or use of antidote-type drugs, such as diphenhydramine, hydrocortisone, or naloxone. A computerized application of this method was described by Classen et al. [88]. Another computerized system described by Paltiel et al. [89] improved outcomes by using a flashing alert on a computer monitor to highlight low potassium levels, thereby increasing the rate of therapeutic interventions and decreasing hypokalemia in patients at discharge.

## SUMMARY

The medication-use process is a complex system intended to optimize patient outcomes within organizational constraints. Quality medication use involves selection of the optimal drug, avoidance of adverse medication events, and completion of the therapeutic objective. Safe medication practices focus on the avoidance of medication errors. Medication-use review and ongoing medication monitoring activities focus on optimizing medication selection and use. These two approaches are important means of assessing and optimizing the quality of medication use.

## REFERENCES

[1] Ernst FR, Grizzle AJ. Drug-related morbidity and mortality: Updating the cost-of-illness model. J Am Pharm Assoc 2001;41:192–9.

[2] Committee on Quality of Health Care in America. To err is human: Building a safer health system. In: Kohn LT, Corrigan JM, Donaldson MS, editors. Washington, DC: National Academy Press; 1999. p. 223.

[3] Committee on Identifying and Preventing Medication Errors. Preventing medication errors. Washington, DC: National Academies Press; 2007.

[4] Leape LL, Brennan TA, Laird N, Lawthers AG, Localio AR, Barnes BA, et al. The nature of adverse events in hospitalized patients. Results of the Harvard Medical Practice Study II. N Engl J Med 1991;324:377–84.

[5] Thomas EJ, Brennan TA. Incidence and types of preventable adverse events in elderly patients: Population based review of medical records. BMJ 2000;320:741–4.

[6] National Coordinating Council for Medication Error Reporting and Prevention. Rockville, MD: U.S. Pharmacopoeia (Internet at, www.nccmerp.org/aboutMedErrors.html; 1999).

[7] American Society of Health-System Pharmacists. Suggested definitions and relationships among medication misadventures, medication errors, adverse drug events, and adverse drug reactions. Am J Health-Syst Pharm 1998;55:165–6.

[8] Bates DW, Boyle DL, Vander Vliet MB, Schneider J, Leape L. Relationship between medication errors and adverse drug events. J Gen Intern Med 1995;10:199–205.

[9] Bates DW, Spell N, Cullen DJ, Burdick E, Laird N, Petersen LA, et al. The costs of adverse drug events in hospitalized patients. JAMA 1997;277:307–11.

[10] McDonnell PJ, Jacobs MR. Hospital admissions resulting from preventable adverse drug reactions. Ann Pharmacother 2002;36:1331–6.

[11] Anderson JG, Jay SJ, Anderson M, Hunt TJ. Evaluating the capabilities of information technology to prevent adverse drug events: A computer simulation approach. J Am Med Inform Assoc 2002;9:479–90.

[12] Nadzam DM. A systems approach to medication use. In: Cousins DD, editor. Medication use: A systems approach to reducing errors. Oakbrook Terrace, IL: Joint Commission on Accreditation of Healthcare Organizations; 1998. p. 5–17.

[13] Atkinson AJ Jr, Nadzam DM, Schaff RL. An indicator-based program for improving medication use in acute care hospitals. Clin Pharmacol Ther 1991;50:125–8.

[14] Phillips DP, Christenfeld N, Glynn LM. Increase in US medication-error deaths between 1983 and 1993. Lancet 1998;351:643–4.

[15] Phillips P, Breder C. Morbidity and mortality from medical errors: An increasingly serious public health problem. Annu Rev Public Health 2002;23:135–50.

[16] Anon. Survey reveals patient concerns about medication-related issues. ASHP calls for increased patient access to pharmacists in hospitals and health systems. Bethesda, MD: American Society of Health System Pharmacists (Internet at, www.ashp.org/menu/AboutUs/ForPress/PressReleases/PressRelease.aspx?id=183; 2002).

[17] Winterstein AG, Sauer BC, Hepler CD, Poole C. Preventable drug-related hospital admissions. Ann Pharmacother 2002;36:1238–48.

[18] Bates DW, Cullen DJ, Laird N, Petersen LA, Small SD, Servi D, et al. Incidence of adverse drug events and potential adverse drug events. Implications for prevention. JAMA 1995;274:29–34.

[19] Barker KN, Flynn EA, Pepper GA, Bates DW, Mikeal RL. Medication errors observed in 36 health care facilities. Arch Intern Med 2002;162:1897–903.

[20] Berwick DM. Continuous improvement as an ideal in health care. N Engl J Med 1989;320:53–6.

[21] Deming WE. Out of the crisis. Cambridge, MA: MIT Press; 2000.

[22] American Society of Health-System Pharmacists. ASHP statement on the pharmacy and therapeutics committee and the formulary system. Am J Health-Syst Pharm 2008;65:2384–6. Also available through Internet at, www.ashp.org/DocLibrary/BestPractices/FormStPTCommFormSyst.pdf.

[23] Coalition Working Group. Principles of a sound formulary system. Rockville, MD: US Pharmacopoeia (Internet at, http://www.usp.org/pdf/EN/patientSafety/pSafetySndFormPrinc.pdf; 2000).

[24] Reason J. Human error. Cambridge, UK: Cambridge University Press; 1990.

[25] Lesar TS, Briceland L, Stein DS. Factors related to errors in medication prescribing. JAMA 1997;77:312–7.

[26] Cohen MR. Causes of medication errors. In: Cohen MR, editor. Medication errors. Washington, DC: American Pharmaceutical Association; 1999. p. 198–212.

[27] Leape LL, Bates DW, Cullen DJ, Cooper J, Demonaco HJ, Gallivan T, et al. Systems analysis of adverse drug events. JAMA 1995;274:35–43.

[28] Nightingale PG, Adu D, Richards NT, Peters M. Implementation of rules based computerised bedside prescribing and administration: Intervention study. BMJ 2000;320:750–3.

[29] Phillips J, Beam S, Brinker A, Holquist C, Honig P, Lee L, et al. Retrospective analysis of mortalities associated with medication errors. Am J Health-Sys Pharm 2001;58:1835–41.

[30] Rothschild JM, Landrigan CP, Cronin JW. The Critical Care Safety Study: The incidence and nature of adverse events and serious medical errors in intensive care. Crit Care Med 2005;33:1694–700.

[31] Lesar TS, Briceland L, Stein DS. Factors related to errors in medication prescribing. JAMA 1997;77:312–7.

[32] Bates DW, Leape LL, Cullen DJ, Laird N, Petersen NA, Teich JM, et al. Effect of computerized physician order entry and a team intervention on prevention of serious medication errors. JAMA 1998;280:1311–6.

[33] Bates DW, Teich JM, Lee J, Seger D, Kuperman GJ, Ma'Luf N, et al. The impact of computerized physician order entry on medication error prevention. J Am Med Inform Assoc 1999;6:313–21.

[34] Pestotnik SL, Classen DC, Evan RS, Burke JP. Implementing antibiotic practice guidelines through computer-assisted decision support: Clinical and financial outcomes. Ann Intern Med 1996;124:884–90.

[35] Raschke RA, Gollihare B, Wunderlich TA, Guidry JR, Leibowitz AI, Peirce JC, et al. A computer alert system to prevent injury from adverse drug events: Development and evaluation in a community teaching hospital. JAMA 1998;280:1317–20.

[36] Anderson JG, Jay SJ, Anderson M, Hunt TJ. Evaluating the capabilities of information technology to prevent adverse drug events: A computer simulation approach. J Am Med Inform Assoc 2002;9:479–90.

[37] Feldstein AC, Smith DH, Perrin N, Yang X, Simon SR, Krall M, et al. Reducing warfarin medication interactions: An interrupted time series analysis. Arch Int Med 2006;166:1009–15.

[38] Taylor JA, Loan LA, Kamara J, Blackburn S, Whitney D. Medication administration variances before and after implementation of computerized physician order entry in a neonatal intensive care unit. Pediatrics 2008;121:123–8.

[39] Zhan C, Hicks RW, Blanchette CM, Keyes MA, Cousins DD. Potential benefits and problems with computerized prescriber order entry: Analysis of a voluntary medication error-reporting database. Am J Health Syst Pharm 2006;63:353–8.

[40] Koppel R, Metlay JP, Cohen A, Abaluck B, Localio AR, Kimmel SE, et al. Role of computerized physician order entry systems in facilitating medication errors. JAMA 2005;293:1197–203.

[41] Nebeker JR, Hoffman JM, Weir R, Bennett CL, Hurdle JF. High rates of adverse drug events in a highly computerized hospital. Arch Intern Med 2005;165:1111–6.

[42] Lesar TS, Briceland L, Stein DS. Factors related to errors in medication prescribing. JAMA 1997;77:312–7.

[43] Calabrese AD, Erstad BL, Brandl K, Barletta JF, Kane SL, Sherman DS. Medication administration errors in adult patients in the ICU. Intensive Care Med 2001;27:1592–8.

[44] Hicks RW, Becker SC, Cousins DD. Harmful medication errors in children: A 5-year analysis of data from the USP MedMARx Program. J Ped Nursing 2007;21:290–8.

[45] Hicks RW, Cousins DD, Williams RL. Summary of information submitted to MedMARx in the year 2002: The quest for quality. Rockville, MD: USP Center for the Advancement of Patient Science (Internet at, www.usp.org/pdf/EN/patientSafety/capsLink2003–11–01.pdf; 2003).

[46] High-alert medications and patient safety. Sentinel Event Alert 11 (Internet at, www.jointcommission.org/sentinel_event_alert_issue_11_high-alert_medications_and_patient_safety November 19, 1999).

[47] Cohen MR, Kilo CM. High-alert medications: safeguarding against errors. In: Cohen MR, editor. Medication errors. Washington, DC: American Pharmaceutical Association; 1999. pp. 5.3 –5.11.

[48] Lambert BL. Predicting look-alike and sound-alike medication errors. Am J Health-Syst Pharm 1997;54:1161–71.

[49] Lambert BL, Lin SJ, Chang KY, Gandhi SK. Similarity as a risk factor in drug-name confusion errors: The look-alike (orthographic) and sound-alike (phonetic) model. Med Care 1999;37:1214–25.

[50] Lambert BL, Lin SJ, Tan H. Designing safe drug names. Drug Saf 2005;28:495–512.

[51] MedMaRx™. Milpitas, CA: Quantos, Inc (Internet at, www.medmarx.com/ 2009).

[52] Nolan TW. System changes to improve patient safety. BMJ 2000;320:771–3.

[53] Bates DW. Medication errors. How common are they and what can be done to prevent them? Drug Saf 1996;15:303–10.

[54] Committee on Identifying and Preventing Medication Errors. Preventing medication errors. Washington, DC: National Academies Press; 2007.

[55] Cullen DJ, Sweitzer BJ, Bates DW, Burdick E, Edmonson A, Leape LL. Preventable adverse drug events in hospitalized patients: A comparative study of intensive care and general care units. Crit Care Med 1997;25:1289–97.

[56] Lesar TS, Lomaestro BM, Pohl H. Medication-prescribing errors in a teaching hospital. A 9-year experience. Arch Intern Med 1997;157:1569–76.

[57] Koecheler JA, Abramowitz PW, Swim SE, Daniels CE. Indicators for the selection of ambulatory patients who warrant pharmacist monitoring. Am J Hosp Pharm 1989; 46:729–32.

[58] Cornish PL, Knowles SR, Marchesano R, Tam V, Shadowitz S, Juurlink DN, et al. Unintended medication discrepancies at the time of hospital admission. Arch Intern Med 2005; 165:424–9.

[59] Gray SL, Mahoney JE, Blough DK. Adverse drug events in elderly patients receiving home health services following hospital discharge. Ann Pharmacother 1999;33:1147–53.

[60] Leape LL, Cullen DJ, Clapp MD, Burdick E, Demonaco HJ, Erickson JI, et al. Pharmacist participation on physician rounds and adverse drug events in the intensive care unit. JAMA 1999;282:267–70.

[61] Flynn EA, Barker KN, Gibson JT, Pearson RE, Berger BA, Smith LA. Impact of interruptions and distractions on dispensing errors in an ambulatory care pharmacy. Am J Health Syst Pharm 1999;56:1319–25.

[62] Four-pronged medication error evaluation. ISMP Medication Safety Alert 1999;4(19):2. (Internet at, www.ismp.org/newsletters/acutecare/articles/19990922.asp.)

[63] Morris AH. Developing and implementing computerized protocols for standardization of clinical decisions. Ann Intern Med 2000;132:373–83.

[64] Evans RS, Pestotnik SL, Classen DC, Clemmer TP, Weaver LK, Orme JF, et al. A computer-assisted management program for antibiotics and other antiinfective agents. N Engl J Med 1998;338:232–8.

[65] Leape LL. Error in medicine. JAMA 1994;272:1851–7.

[66] American Society of Health-System Pharmacists. ASHP guidelines on medication-use evaluation. Am J Health Syst Pharm 1996;53:1953–5. (Internet at, www.ashp.org/DocLibrary/BestPractices/FormGdlMedUseEval.aspx.)

[67] AHFS Pharmacologic-Therapeutic Classification. Bethesda, MD: American Society of Health-System Pharmacists. (Internet at www.ahfsdruginformation.com/class/index.aspx.)

[68] Caterino JM, Emond JA, Camargo Jr CA. Inappropriate medication administration to the acutely ill elderly: A nationwide emergency department study, 1992–2000. J Am Geriatr Soc 2004;52:1847–55.

[69] Piergies AA, Worwag EM, Atkinson AJ Jr. A concurrent audit of high digoxin plasma levels. Clin Pharmacol Ther 1994;55:353–8.

[70] Krstenansky PM. Ketorolac injection use in a university hospital. Am J Hosp Pharm 1993;50:99–102.

[71] Kuperman GJ, Teich JM, Tanasijevic MJ, Ma'Luf N, Rittenberg E, Jha A, et al. Improving response to critical laboratory results with automation: Results of a randomized controlled trial. J Am Med Inform Assoc 1999;6:512–22.

[72] National Guideline Clearinghouse. Agency for Healthcare Research and Quality. (Internet at, www.guidelines.gov/.)

[73] Quality check and quality reports. The Joint Commission, 2012. (Internet at, www.qualitycheck.org/Consumer/SearchQCR.aspx.)

[74] Soumerai SB, Avorn J. Predictors of physician prescribing change in an educational experiment to improve medication use. Med Care 1987;25:210–21.

[75] Ellis RF, Stephens MA, Sharp GB. Evaluation of a pharmacy-managed warfarin-monitoring service to coordinate inpatient and outpatient therapy. Am J Hosp Pharm 1992;49:387–94.

[76] Dager WE, Branch JM, King JH, White RH, Quan RS, Musallam NA, et al. Optimization of inpatient warfarin therapy: Impact of daily consultation by a pharmacist-managed anticoagulation service. Ann Pharmacother 2000;34:567–72.

[77] Destache CJ, Meyer SK, Bittner MJ, Hermann KG. Impact of a clinical pharmacokinetic service on patients treated with aminoglycosides: A cost–benefit analysis. Ther Drug Monit 1990;12:419–26.

[78] Cimino MA, Rotstein CM, Moser JE. Assessment of cost-effective antibiotic therapy in the management of infections in cancer patients. Ann Pharmacother 1994;28:105–11.

[79] Okpara AU, Van Duyn OM, Cate TR, Cheung LK, Galley MA. Concurrent ceftazidime DUE with clinical pharmacy intervention. Hosp Formul 1994;29:392–4, 399, 402–4.

[80] Kershaw B, White RH, Mungall D, Van Houten J, Brettfeld S. Computer-assisted dosing of heparin. Management with a pharmacy-based anticoagulation service. Arch Intern Med 1994;154:1005–11.

[81] De Santis G, Harvey KJ, Howard D, Mashford ML, Moulds RF. Improving the quality of antibiotic prescription patterns in general practice. The role of educational intervention. Med J Aust 1994;160:502–5.

[82] Donahue T, Dotter J, Alexander G, Sadaj JM. Pharmacist-based i.v. theophylline therapy. Hosp Pharm 1989;24(440):442–8, 460.

[83] Ambrose PJ, Smith WE, Palarea ER. A decade of experience with a clinical pharmacokinetics service. Am J Hosp Pharm 1988;45:1879–86.

[84] Li SC, Ioannides-Demos LL, Spicer WJ, Spelman DW, Tong N, McLean AJ. Prospective audit of an aminoglycoside consultative service in a general hospital. Med J Aust 1992;157:308–11.

[85] McCall LJ, Dierks DR. Pharmacy-managed patient-controlled analgesia service. Am J Hosp Pharm 1990;47:2706–10.

[86] Lipsy RJ, Smith GH, Maloney ME. Design, implementation, and use of a new antimicrobial order form: A descriptive report. Ann Pharmacother 1993;27:856–61.

[87] Frighetto L, Marra CA, Stiver HG, Bryce EA, Jewesson PJ. Economic impact of standardized orders for antimicrobial prophylaxis program. Ann Pharmacother 2000;34:154–60.

[88] Classen DC, Pestotnik SL, Evans RS, Burke JP. Description of a computerized adverse drug event monitor using a hospital information system. Hosp Pharm 1992;27(774):776–9, 783.

[89] Paltiel O, Gordon L, Berg D, Israeli A. Effect of a computerized alert on the management of hypokalemia in hospitalized patients. Arch Intern Med 2003;163:200–4.

# DRUG DISCOVERY AND DEVELOPMENT

# Portfolio and Project Planning and Management in the Drug Discovery, Evaluation, Development, and Regulatory Review Process

Charles Grudzinskas[1] and Charles T. Gombar[2]

[1]*NDA Partners LLC, Annapolis, MD 21401*
[2]*Project Management, Development & Delivery, Endo Pharmaceuticals, Chadds Ford, PA 19317*

## INTRODUCTION

Drug discovery, evaluation, development and regulatory review are complex, lengthy, and costly processes that involve in excess of 10,000 interdependent activities. In order to be successful in biopharmaceutical new product development, one needs a set of general principles that provide guidance in (1) the construction of a *Research and Development (R&D) Portfolio*, (2) the construction of individual *Product Development Plans*, and (3) the subsequent updates required to keep the portfolio and product development plans current as learning occurs. The following five *Principles of Optimal Product Development* [1] form the basis for defining a decision-based operational model, identifying and quantifying the critical information required at each major decision-point, projecting the probabilities of various outcomes, and informing key stakeholders (management, board, and investors) with the clear and concise status information that is needed for effective product development governance. These five Principles are:

### Principle I: Market Advantage

The Product Development Program must produce data that clearly differentiate the new product from current therapies, products, or practices and demonstrate that the product will compete effectively in the market.

### Principle II: Product Readiness

Prior to commencing each phase of clinical studies, the appropriate *in vitro*, non-clinical, and clinical ADME, efficacy, pharmacokinetic, pharmacodynamic, toxicological, CMC, and clinical knowledge will be available, reviewed, verified, and integrated into a single coherent picture of the product's properties, with due emphasis on the types and magnitudes of key remaining uncertainties.

### Principle III: Value-Driven Program Execution

All studies (*in vitro*, non-clinical, clinical, and CMC) must be designed to produce knowledge that directly impacts expected product value, as specified in the Target Product Profile, and data to support the intended indications and claims.

### Principle IV: Learning and Confirming

Predictive knowledge of product properties essential to a decision theory-driven development program will be derived primarily from scientific learning studies which will form the knowledge needed to design the appropriate confirming studies, such as Proof of Concept. Use of study designs that allow "Learning while Confirming" should be maximized.

*PRINCIPLES OF CLINICAL PHARMACOLOGY, THIRD EDITION*
DOI: http://dx.doi.org/10.1016/B978-0-12-385471-1.00029-5

## Principle V: Regulatory Collaboration

Satisfaction of requirements and constraints from both US and non-US regulatory authorities must be addressed, coordinated and integrated into the program design and re-visited at every milestone and major decision-point.

These Principles are applicable to all medical product development programs regardless of technology, therapeutic area or indication, and can be applied to the development of devices and diagnostics as well. However, not all Principles are fully applicable to all product development programs, nor are they applied in precisely the same manner and to the same extent from program to program. Consequently, their use must be guided by adequate experience and judgment to adapt these principles to the specific needs of each program based on informed interpretation of study results in order to make mid-course corrections based upon accumulating knowledge. Each organization will need to develop corollaries for these principles that provide more specific guidance and help keep the product development effort focused on the critical success factors and key data and knowledge needed to support major decisions.

To operationalize these five principles and to manage and optimize the returns of this complex, lengthy and costly product development process, the biopharmaceutical industry has embraced the two disciplines of (1) portfolio design, planning, and management (PDPM), and (2) contemporary project planning and management (PPM). The obvious benefits of good portfolio and project planning and management are shown in Table 29.1. Achieving approval from global regulatory authorities to market a new biopharmaceutical product is no longer the only end-game for R&D organizations. Increasingly, the major hurdle to being able to deliver new medicines to patients is formulary access and/or reimbursement, be it by a government or private insurers. There are

**TABLE 29.1  Benefits of Good Portfolio and Project Planning and Management**

The organization is able to do more with less

The organization is able to optimize the value of a portfolio of projects

Better planning

Better decision-making

Projects meet expected outcomes

Projects finish on time

Projects finish within budget

more and more pressures to contain healthcare spending. For a new product to be successful it must address a true medical need, thereby bring true "value" to patients, healthcare providers, and payers. The expected market advance is often referred to as the "differentiation" of the new product, and the differentiation points are important goals that drive the design and construction of the product development plan. The differentiation points and value dimensions add even more complexity to an already complex process (for a discussion of Comparative Effectiveness, see Chapter 35). The level of complexity also demands a new level of collaboration between the R&D and the commercial groups such as marketing and manufacturing, as well as improved interaction between drug development organizations and payers. Understanding and accepting this new reality of complexity and collaboration increases the importance of portfolio planning and management and the role of project planning and management in ensuring effective, efficient, and timeline-driven development of new products.

## What Is R&D Portfolio Design, Planning and Management?

A *well-planned and managed* pharmaceutical R&D portfolio can be defined as: "The combination of *all* R&D projects, that based on past company, industry, and regulatory agency performance, *will predictably yield* valuable new products at the *rate needed* to support the planned growth of the organization." Portfolio design, planning, and management are the processes that the industry uses to ensure a well-balanced and value-optimized R&D pipeline. Balancing a portfolio now is far more challenging than in the past, and requires more diversification in the products being developed. This means not only diversification across therapeutic areas, but also a mix of traditional small molecule drugs, biological agents (large molecules such as proteins, peptides, monoclonal antibodies, and vaccines), and diagnostics, including companion diagnostics, devices, and services.

The lifespan of pharmaceutical products is limited by intellectual property duration and the competitive landscape. Loss of market exclusivity for products poses a major challenge to individual companies and to the industry as a whole. This limited product lifespan is being addressed by incorporating life-cycle management much earlier into product development programs. The variety of generic products now available across the therapeutic spectrum has led some to believe that pharmaceuticals are now a commodity market. We reject that view as there remain numerous unmet medical needs and the understanding of disease pathophysiology continues to expand at a staggering rate, creating new opportunities for developing improved therapeutic agents. The stakes for effective decision-making on *which products to develop* have never been higher – indeed, the survival of many companies will depend on how well they design and manage their respective portfolios. Therefore, better, more sophisticated portfolio design and management, along with highly efficient and rapid product development, is a requirement for sustainability.

Multiple pressures combine to constantly threaten the overall value for a product development program and the subsequent life-cycle management program, constituting what is termed "The AUC Value Problem". This is diagrammed in Figure 29.1, which depicts a typical revenue vs time forecast for a product under development, although the life-cycle management enhancement of additional indications and formulations are not represented. The figure illustrates that once a product receives regulatory approval, revenues are realized, and the revenues then increase as the new product gains market share. At a certain point sales will flatten and the revenues remain constant or might even decrease depending upon the competitive landscape. The sharp decline in revenues at the right side of the value curve is due to loss of patent protection, through either expiration or a successful patent challenge. This results in loss of market exclusivity, subsequent generic competition, and a sharp decline in revenues, termed the "generic cliff". Indeed, it has been reported that in some cases 90% of a product's annual sales are lost to generic competition within 6 months after patent protection is lost. The figure also shows the potential loss of market exclusivity and the revenue that might be associated with increased regulatory requirements or the inability of the company that is developing the product to achieve a "First-Cycle" marketing approval in major markets, as well as the combined potential loss in revenue and product value due to pressures from government and other third-party payers to force down the overall cost of biopharmaceuticals. It is the role of a Product Development Team (PDT) to identify and quantify these threats (see discussion of a *Risk Register* later in this chapter) and to develop proactive contingency plans that will ensure optimization of the product's value.

## What Is Project Planning and Management?

Project planning is an integral part of project management, which is defined in the Project Management Institute's *Guide to the Project Management Body of Knowledge* [2] as "the application of knowledge, skills, tools, and techniques to project activities in order to meet or exceed stakeholder needs and expectations from a project". As we will see later in this chapter, a project is defined by the specifications (i.e., a product label which drives product value), the required resources needed to achieve the desired specification, and the timelines, which are dependent on the combination of the specifications and resources.

For an excellent text on the application of project management principles and tools, the reader is referred to *Pharmaceutical Project Management* by Anthony Kennedy [3]. An excellent resource for those who would like to become actively involved in biopharmaceutical project management is the Drug Information Association's (DIA) Project Management Special Interest Advisory Committee (PM SIAC). Information on how to join the DIA PM SIAC can be found on the DIA website [4].

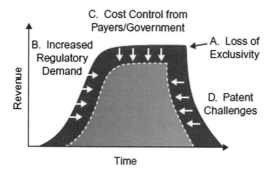

**FIGURE 29.1** "The AUC Value Problem" illustrates how the combined pressures of (A) Loss of Exclusivity, (B) Increased Regulatory Demand, (C) Cost Control from Payers/Government, and (D) Patent Challenges could affect the overall life-cycle value of a product.

## PORTFOLIO DESIGN, PLANNING, AND MANAGEMENT

*Portfolio management* is the term that is used to describe the overall process of program and franchise management. This process includes the three dimensions of portfolio design, portfolio planning, and portfolio management. Each of these three dimensions is described in this section. The five components needed for the successful use of PDPM are identified in Table 29.2. If any one (or more) of the five components is missing or not fully operational, then the likelihood of successful PDPM will be low.

**TABLE 29.2**   The Five Components of Successful Portfolio
Design, Planning, and Management

Portfolio Design

Portfolio Planning

Portfolio Management

Portfolio Management Teams (PMTs)

Portfolio Optimization using Sensitivity Analysis

**TABLE 29.3**   Discounted Cash Flows for a Hypothetical
Drug Development Project[a]

| | Year | 0 | 1 | 2 | 3 |
|---|---|---|---|---|---|
| Development | Expense | ($25) | ($75) | ($200) | ($200) |
| | Discounted expense | ($25) | ($71.4) | ($181.4) | ($172.8) |
| | Year | 4 | 5 | 6 | 7 |
| Marketing | Income | $50 | $100 | $200 | $300 |
| | Discounted income | $41.1 | $78.4 | $149.2 | $213.2 |

[a]Dollar amounts are in millions.

Most large organizations have now adopted the portfolio management team (PMT) concept. PMT membership consists of the senior management of the organization, and the mission of the PMT is to oversee the successful design, planning, and management of the organization's portfolio. The PMT usually has several working groups that focus on specific therapeutic areas. The ultimate responsibility of the PMT is to ensure that the portfolio has been optimized to maximize the potential expected value of the individual R&D projects and to meet the strategic growth goals of the organization.

## Maximizing Portfolio Value

*Portfolio value* is maximized by appropriately prioritizing the projects and the project value-drivers within the portfolio based on the future potential financial value of each project and project value-driver, multiplied by its probability of success (i.e., regulatory approval). The future value of each development project is based on a calculation of its net present value (NPV). In this calculation, the anticipated financial return from the project is compared with that of an alternative investment of an equivalent amount of capital [5]. The general equation for calculating NPV is:

$$\text{NPV} = I_0 + \frac{I_1}{1+r} + \frac{I_2}{(1+r)^2} \cdots + \frac{I_n}{(1+r)^n} \quad (29.1)$$

where the *I* values are given a negative sign for annual net cash outflow and a positive sign for projected net annual income. The subscripts and exponents correspond to the number of years of projected development and marketing time, and *r*, termed the *discount rate*, is the rate of return of an alternate investment, such as US Treasury Bills.

A NPV analysis using a 5% discount rate is summarized for a hypothetical drug in Table 29.3. It is assumed that the drug will be developed within 4 years at a total cost of $500 million. Because this investment is spread over 4-years, development funds budgeted for this project that are unexpended after year zero are assumed to be earning 5% interest until

spent, and are discounted accordingly. Marketing begins in Year 4 but income is similarly discounted as shown in Equation 29.1 and is assumed to be negligible when patent protection expires after Year 7. The NPV for the project is the sum of the discounted cash inflows and outflows over the life of the product, and in this case is $31.3 million. The NPV is far less than the $150 million difference between total income and expenditures for the project because this latter difference makes no allowance for potential alternative use of the money. The *internal rate of return* is another metric that may be helpful in evaluating different projects in a portfolio [5]. The internal rate of return is defined simply as the discount rate needed to yield an NPV of zero, and would be 6.78% for the hypothetical project shown in Table 29.3.

A note of caution is necessary in using NPV analyses because they are based on the *forecasted* value of products and the associated product value-drivers (i.e., differentiation points). For whatever reason, the forecasted values of pharmaceutical products are notoriously inaccurate. The sales of new products frequently are over- or underestimated, sometimes by orders of magnitude. So it is important to factor this into value calculations used for portfolio prioritization and to rely on no *single* metric to prioritize projects.

The probability of success is the second factor used to estimate portfolio value, and is calculated as the product of the probability of technical success, the probability of regulatory success, and the probability of commercial success. The criteria for these probabilities of success need to be clearly defined and characterized so that future PMTs can translate the impact of project progress and decisions, as well as the ever-changing regulatory and competitive landscapes, on the value of the projects in the portfolio (see section on Portfolio Optimization Using Sensitivity Analysis). Decision trees are a useful tool to estimate the probability of technical and regulatory success (see below).

It is easy to assess that projects for which application for marketing have been submitted to worldwide regulatory review bodies for review will most commonly have the highest probability of success. Therefore, they are likely to have the highest overall financial value in the portfolio (overall value equals possible future value times the probability of success), whereas projects that are in the discovery stage will have the lowest overall value in the portfolio (but are the life-blood of the organization 4–6 years in the future).

It is the role of the PMT to develop a "balanced portfolio" that supports the near-term, mid-term, and long-term needs of the organization. The R&D and commercial senior management teams need to ensure that organizational resources are properly allocated according to the agreed-upon project prioritization.

## Portfolio Design

It is not an overstatement to say that the near-term and long-term future of a biopharmaceutical company depends on the size and likelihood of success of its R&D pipeline. The pipeline is the totality of a company's portfolio, consisting of projects ranging from very early discovery to marketed products that are ending their current life-cycle and will need a line extension (new formulation or expanded indications) to remain competitive, or pharmacoecomic data to continue to support the product's value proposition. A pharmaceutical R&D portfolio begins with a vision of the intended growth rate of the organization. Based on the envisioned growth rate, a portfolio can be developed that is based on what the future pipeline will need to look like at each of the four phases of the drug development process described in Chapter 35,

and the factors associated with successful transition between these phases, termed *phase transition*. The size of the pipeline needed at each phase of drug development is estimated from both past industry and regulatory experiences and reported metrics.

The probability of a drug candidate maturing to an approved drug, as well as the average duration of development until approval, has been extensively studied by the Center for the Study of Drug Development (CSDD) at Tufts. In 2011 CSDD reported that on average only one compound reaches the market for every six (16% success rate) that enter the clinical development process [6]. In an earlier CSDD study of nearly 4000 drugs and biologics the odds of success for any one clinical candidate was found to depend on multiple factors, including (1) which therapeutic area was being studied, (2) whether the drug was self-originated or licensed-in, and (3) whether the drug being developed was a small or large molecule. As shown in Figure 29.2, the likelihood of overall clinical success rate (regulatory approval) for NCEs (new chemical entities) varies by therapeutic area, with the highest success rate observed for systemic antibiotics (23.9%) and the lowest success rate observed for CNS (central nervous system) (8.2%) [7]. In Figure 29.3 we see that the average development time until marketing approval for a new drug also depends on therapeutic area, and ranges from 6.1 to 10 years [6]. The probabilities for "phase transition" and the overall success rate for development candidates by *therapeutic class* are shown in Figure 29.4 [7]. In addition, the probabilities for "phase transition" and overall success rate for development candidates were found to be somewhat higher for licensed-in compared to self-originated compounds, and for large molecules compared to small molecules.

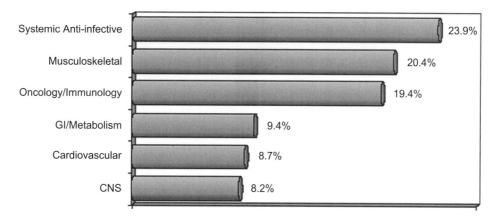

**FIGURE 29.2** Influence of the therapeutic class being studied upon the likely success rate from initiation of a first-in-human (FIH) study to regulatory approval for compounds with FIH studies between 1993 and 2004. Based on data from DiMasi JA, Feldman L, Seckler A, Wilson A. Clin Pharmacol Ther 2010;87:272–7 [7].

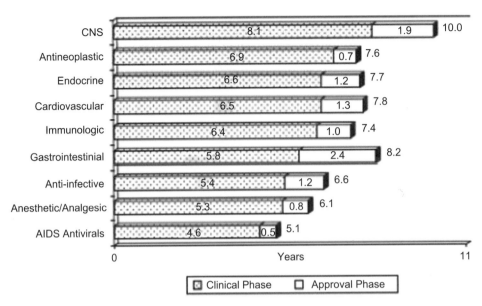

**FIGURE 29.3** Influence of the therapeutic class being studied on the likely timeline from FIH to regulatory approval for approved new molecular entities and significant biologicals during 2006–2009. Clinical phase times are given by the stippled bars and approval phase times by the empty bars. Note that the anti-infective group does not include AIDS and antivirals. (CNS, central nervous system.) Reproduced with permission from Kaitin KI, DiMasi JA. Clin Pharmacol Ther 2011;89:183–8 [6].

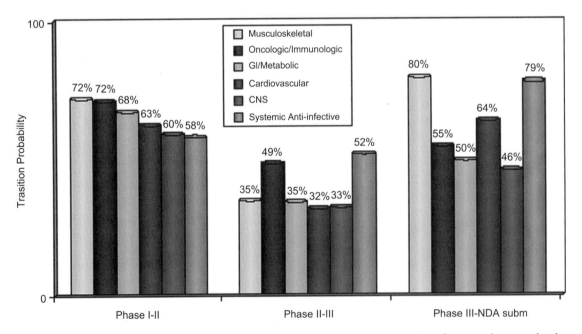

**FIGURE 29.4** Phase transition probabilities by therapeutic class based on the number of approved new molecular entities and significant biologicals for compounds with FIH studies between 1993 and 2004. Based on data from DiMasi JA, Feldman L, Seckler A, Wilson A. Clin Pharmacol Ther 2010;87:272–7 [7].

Therefore, as shown in the portfolio pyramid in Figure 29.5, a company that wants to produce one new approved product (NDA/BLA and MAA) each year would have to initiate on average a minimum of six new First-in-Human (FIH) clinical studies, and would need to adjust the size of the portfolio depending upon the likelihood for success of individual development projects, based on the compound type, therapeutic area, and whether self-originated or licensed-in. Naturally, if a company wanted to develop two or three new NDAs/BLAs and MAAs each year, it would have to have a pipeline portfolio that is, respectively, two or

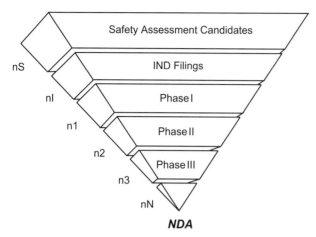

**FIGURE 29.5** Size of the drug development portfolio needed to support an NDA/BLA/MAA pipeline. ($nS$, number of compounds that will need to be screened each year; $nI$, number of INDs/CTCs that will need to be submitted each year for approval of a FIH clinical study; $n1$, number of Phase I projects that will need to be initiated each year; $n2$, number of Phase II projects that will need to be initiated each year; $n3$, number of Phase III projects that will need to be initiated each year; and $nN$, number of NDAs/BLAs/MAAs that will need to be submitted each year based on the portfolio of compounds screened, INDs/CTCs filed and Phase I–Phase III projects initiated each year.)

three times as large as is illustrated in Figure 29.5. However, this "shots-on-goal" approach has its limitations in that it must be supplemented by a robust assessment of the potential technical, regulatory, and commercial success of each product in the portfolio.

## Portfolio Planning

Once the portfolio vision and design have been defined, the organization can focus on how to build that portfolio. As projects mature from one stage to the next, or are terminated for lack of success, additional projects will need to be added to the various stages of the portfolio to ensure a portfolio of adequate size exists at each stage. To maintain an aggressive portfolio, companies have acknowledged that it is nearly impossible to fill the pipeline by being dependent solely on self-originated research. There are many sources for new products in addition to the organization's own discovery program. For example, companies can fill out their portfolios by entering into joint ventures and alliances with both established and startup organizations. Additional sources of new products include in-licensing early-stage research from the National Institutes of Health (NIH), universities, and foundations (e.g., the Juvenile Diabetes Foundation). Thus, the planning process includes both the identification and successful in-licensing of the candidates needed to populate the stages of the drug development process that we saw in Figure 29.5.

## Portfolio Management

Portfolio management is primarily focused on the prioritization of projects within an ever-changing portfolio, and the associated resource allocation decisions. Several consulting groups and software programs are available to aid in the management of a dynamic portfolio. These same tools can be used to evaluate "what-if" scenarios to determine how the addition or deletion of projects to the portfolio either increases or decreases the portfolio's overall value based on the trade-offs of project values, resource requirements and development timelines. As with most processes of this nature, the most important consideration is the quality of the information regarding the potential value and probability of success of each project. Precise evaluations of the commercial, regulatory, and technical probabilities need to come from those within the organization, as well as those outside of the organization, who have sufficient experience to be able to provide informed, realistic estimates of both expected values and probabilities of success.

As illustrated in Figure 29.6, organizations can graph the value that is expected to be gained vs the cost of the R&D needed to achieve the overall value that is calculated for each project. Organizations can then make decisions as to how to allocate resources based on the "steepness" of the slope of each project, which represents the ratio of added value per resource unit, keeping in mind that projects closest

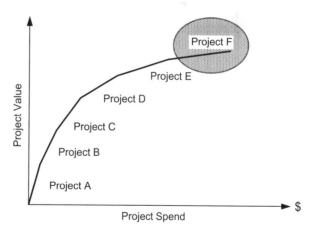

**FIGURE 29.6** Relationship between project value and R&D funds invested in their clinical development (project spend). The value of this hypothetical portfolio would be the cumulative value of its constituent projects. Project F clearly has the lowest expected value per "project spend". These low-value projects are usually considered as candidates for termination. In addition to termination as a possibility, effective companies evaluate the low-expected-value projects to identify the drivers that would lead to a significant increase in the project's expected value (see Figure 29.8 and discussion of Portfolio Optimization Using Sensitivity Analysis).

**TABLE 29.4    The Four Portfolio Quadrants**

| Quadrant I | A diamond mine |
| Quadrant II | Betting the ranch |
| Quadrant III | A sure bet |
| Quadrant IV | A turkey ranch |

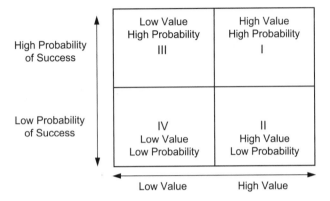

**FIGURE 29.7**    Four-quadrant table used for portfolio analysis in which projects are evaluated on the basis of their potential financial return (value) and probability of development success.

to the market (which have the highest probability of success) will likely have the steepest slope. In the next section, we examine how to avoid the pitfall of assuming that projects (such as the one identified in the oval in Figure 29.6) necessarily need to be terminated because they have less than acceptable expected value vs cost slopes. Indeed, we will describe how to increase the expected value of low-value projects.

Naturally, organizations will want to populate their portfolio with projects that balance potential value and probability of success, as illustrated in Figure 29.7 and described in Table 29.4. Clearly the most desirable projects are in Quadrant I (high value with a high probability of success). Projects in Quadrant IV, with low value and low probability of success, should either be examined for ways to increase the expected project value or probability of success, or be recommended for termination. Unfortunately, few projects fall into Quadrant I, so a typical portfolio is composed of projects mostly from Quadrants II and III (most organizations try to avoid Quadrant IV-type projects).

## Portfolio Optimization Using Sensitivity Analysis

Sensitivity analysis is used to identify and quantify project characteristics that are major factors in the expected commercial value of a project, and is one of the most powerful tools of modern portfolio management. Sensitivity analyses serve two goals. The first goal is to identify the project characteristics that were used to determine the project value – the so-called value drivers – and ensure that the project plan developed by the product development team solidly supports these value drivers. For example, a value driver for a potential sedative hypnotic might be that it has no potentiation or interaction with alcohol. Because much of the value of this project depends on this product characteristic, the product development team will design a development plan to assess this expected value driver as early as possible in the development cycle. Indeed, the absence of an interaction with alcohol could be adopted as a "Proof of Concept" milestone.

The second goal is to identify "differentiation" characteristics that, *if added* to the already existing project characteristics, would significantly increase the expected value of the project. This type of sensitivity analysis is important for all projects in the portfolio, but is critically important for those projects that are in danger of being terminated from the portfolio for lack of adequate value. The results of a sensitivity analysis are plotted with broad ranges of value for each criterion, and are called tornado charts because their shape resembles that of the meteorological phenomenon. As an example, Table 29.5 lists a set of "as planned" goals for a hypothetical antibiotic. We see from the tornado chart in Figure 29.8 that the portfolio analysis has determined that the "as planned" NPV for the project is $1 billion (represented by the dotted vertical axis on the chart). The stipulation of "as planned" underscores an important caveat, for the value determined was based on the project goals shown in Table 29.5.

What one can learn from this sensitivity analysis is that the scenario with the highest probability of occurring ("most likely") is the one that incorporates the following:

**TABLE 29.5    Example of "As Planned" Goals for a Hypothetical Oral Antibiotic**

| | |
| --- | --- |
| NDA submission | In 12 months |
| Dose regimen | Twice a day |
| Concomitant use | With some (but not all) drugs likely to be used by this population |
| Diagnostic kit | Available at launch |
| Cost of goods | ~$25,000/kg |
| IV formulation | Not available at launch |

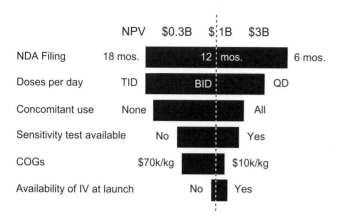

**FIGURE 29.8** "Tornado" chart illustrating a sensitivity analysis for the development of a hypothetical antibiotic. (NPV, net present value; COGs, cost of goods.)

- The NDA will be submitted in 12 months.
- Evidence supporting twice-a-day dosing will be established.
- The product can be administered concomitantly with many, but not all, of the drugs that might be expected to be used by this patient population.
- A diagnostic kit for antibiotic sensitivity will not be widely available at the time that product marketing is launched.
- The cost of goods will be in the range of $25,000/kg.
- It is unlikely that an intravenous form of the drug will be available at launch.

This "most likely" scenario values the oral antibiotic at $1 billion. The bars for each of the critical goals indicate that product value would be increased by $2 billion if the NDA could be submitted in 6 months. Likewise, the value would be reduced to $0.3 billion if the time required for NDA submission slips to 18 months. The sensitivity analysis also indicates that the product could have an increased value of $2.5 billion if a once-a-day formulation could be developed and made available at product launch. Although other changes would also increase the NPV of the product, the first two (a NDA submission within 6 months and a once-a-day formulation) provide the greatest increase in value. Clearly, the PMT and the senior management board would focus resources on these two high-value areas. If there were limited resources, then the project team would be asked which of the two increased value goals (6-month NDA submission or once-a-day formulation) would be the most likely to be achieved. Similar sensitivity assessment would be conducted for each of the development programs within the R&D portfolio, and a decision would be made as to which of the subprojects that would significantly increase the portfolio value should be funded.

## PROJECT PLANNING AND MANAGEMENT

Once the portfolio has been designed, planned, and managed for optimization, it is the job of the PDT to manage each development program. Project planning and management for the biopharmaceutical industry began in the early 1980s, and quickly became an integral part of the R&D organization by the mid-1980s. The paper entitled *Change - + Communication = Challenge − Management of New Drug Development* provides a review of the tools that are still used in biopharmaceutical project management [8]. Project planning and management have progressed to the point that there are now six dimensions of project planning and management that are routinely used to plan and manage biopharmaceutical projects (Table 29.6). An overview of each of these dimensions will be provided.

### Defining a Project

Biopharmaceutical projects, like all R&D projects, consist of three components, which must be planned and managed in an integrated manner. These three components are *project specifications*, *project resources*, and *project timelines*, and can be thought of as "the what?", "the how/where?", and "the when?" of a project, respectively. Recently, "project specification" has focused on the assessment of project value, which, as described earlier, is a requirement for commercial success. Once these three project components have been defined and agreed upon, they become known as the *baseline specifications*, the *baseline resource requirement*, and the *baseline timelines*.

### *Project Specifications (the What?)*
#### *Target Product Profile*

Project specifications include (1) the projected effectiveness, safety and especially the differentiation criteria (i.e., Market Advantage) of a project, (2) drug substance and formulation (e.g., oral, parenteral, transdermal, modified release), and (3) package styles

**TABLE 29.6  Project Management Dimensions in the Biopharmaceutical Industry**

Project Planning

Project Scheduling

Team Management

Resource Allocation

Decision-Making

Process Leadership and Benchmarking

(e.g., bottles, ampoules, blister packs). Drug development organizations typically use a *Target Product Profile* (TPP) to define and communicate the expectations of a particular development program. In some cases, TPPs are used as early as drug discovery to define the selection criteria for identifying "development leads" (e.g., orally active, does not inhibit CYP3A4, can be used in combination with drug X, etc.). The TPP frequently will include both the "optimal" criteria to drive the design of a development plan and "threshold" criteria for minimal acceptability. The threshold metric is identified as the criteria that if not achieved will prompt serious review of the project for possible termination.

*Target Package Insert and Target Summary of Product Characteristics*

A companion planning and decision-making tool to the TPP is the *Target Package Insert* (TPI) for US projects and the *Target Summary of Product Characteristics* (TSPC) for non-US projects. The TPI and TSPC reflect the target labeling that the organization hopes to achieve (see Figure 29.9). The TPP is used as a tool for planning the clinical and non-clinical activities needed to generate evidence of safety, efficacy, and quality, and to inventory the new knowledge that has been generated. This inventory of knowledge, along with the organization's level of confidence in the likelihood for product success, is used to assess whether adequate scientific evidence will exist to convince regulatory authorities that the product is deserving of market approval with the desired label. Thus,

the TPI/TSPC serves as a baseline for the desired labeling. A *Draft Package Insert* (DPI) and the corresponding *Draft Summary of Product Characteristics* (DSPC) begins to evolve as new knowledge is generated, and these drafts are constantly compared to the baseline TPI/TSPC to assess whether the drug candidate is still likely to achieve the prespecified value-level that was initially used to justify the selection of the drug candidate and the continued allocation of the organization's resources to the project.

In March 2007 the FDA issued a draft *Guidance for Industry and Review Staff Target Product Profile – A Strategic Development Process Tool* to encourage TPP-focused meetings with sponsors at the FDA [9]. The following is stated in the FDA TPP Guidance:

> An efficient dialogue between a sponsor and the FDA during the drug development process can minimize the risk of late-stage drug development failures, increase the probability that optimal safety and efficacy data are available in a timely manner, improve labeling content, and possibly decrease the total time involved with drug development.

### Project Timelines

Project timelines (the when?) consist of the timelines for both the overall project and for the subproject goals. In the context of drug development, time is a resource. However, time is the one resource that cannot be replaced. An organization can provide additional staff, funds, animals, clinical sites, and subjects, but the organization cannot recapture time

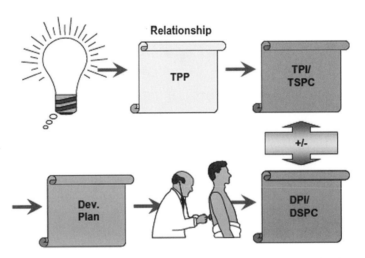

**FIGURE 29.9** The Target Product Profile (TPP) is a driver for the program development plan and is a tool for assessing whether the project is achieving the intended expectations and value (TPI, target package insert; TSPC, target summary of product characteristics; DPI, draft package insert; DSPC, draft summary of product characteristics.)

once it has been consumed. Project timelines can be established by three processes. The first process of establishing project timelines is by the forward planning process based on project specifications and available (usually limited) resources. The second process for establishing project timelines is by an impending deadline, which the organization uses to define the balance between (1) project specifications that can be accomplished within the specified project timeline and (2) the available project resources. The third process for establishing project timelines is to set a deadline, define what must be accomplished, and then resource accordingly to ensure the defined project can be completed by the deadline.

It needs to be noted that project planning and project scheduling are two separate, but interdependent, dimensions. The ideal way to craft a drug development program is to first define the goals of the project. This is often described as "label driven-question based" development planning, since the desired approved product label is used to define and drive the project goals. Once the project goals are defined, it is the role of a PDT to: (1) develop both a strategic plan and a tactical plan that define and support the major project objectives; (2) define the project Go/No-Go decisions with pre-specified decision-making criteria, as far as possible; (3) identify the individual activities, the supporting tasks, and the required resources (funding, people, and facilities) that will be needed to accomplish the project objectives; and (4) identify both the order (precedence) in which these tasks need to be carried out and any interdependencies between activities.

There are at least two approaches for defining the order of the activities. The first is the "plan for success" approach, in which as many activities as possible are conducted in parallel to provide the shortest timeline to the Go/No-Go decisions [proof of mechanism (PoM), proof of concept (PoC), confirmatory clinical studies, risk evaluation and mitigation studies (REMS)] and project completion (see Chapter 35 for a discussion of PoM and PoC). The second approach is used when there are very scarce resources or when there is a *low probability of project success*. This second approach defers resource-intensive activities until a PoC has been achieved for the project. Once the PoC has been achieved, then a plan-for-success style program for the project will be developed and implemented. One can also stage the development of lower prioritized projects in a portfolio, if resources are limited, or if the risk is still high and the project needs to be managed more conservatively by the organization.

### Project Resources (the How/Where?)

#### An Example of a Project Definition

An example of a project definition in the bio-pharmaceutical industry would be the development of a new chemical entity for the indication of treating mild to severe congestive heart failure (CHF), with both an oral and an intravenous formulation being developed, and with a projected development time of 3 years to NDA submission and a budget of $150 million. A subproject would be to complete a clinical PoC clinical study for the severe CHF indication for the intravenous formulation in 1 year with a budget of $9 million. It is important to note that product development teams have the responsibility to include in the inventory of desired product specifications not only those specifications that are required for regulatory approval and a successful product launch, but also product specifications that are required for clinical and postmarket studies conducted as part of REMS strategies (See Chapter 27 "Risk Evaluation and Mitigation Strategy (REMS)").

#### The Project Management Triangle

Project components can be represented as the three sides of a triangle, as illustrated in Figure 29.10. This representation is quite useful, since once the project components have been established, the length of each side (component) of the project management triangle is locked in and represents the baseline specifications. As usually happens with any project, changes constantly occur. If the project is changed by expanding the number of indications or formulations, then we realize from the geometric analogy that one or both of the other two components will need to change. Either

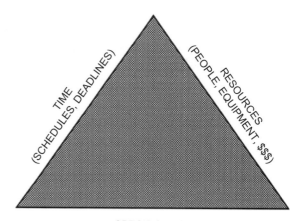

SPECIFICATIONS
(QUALITY AND QUANTITY)

**FIGURE 29.10** The project management triangle. A change in one side of the triangle necessitates changes in one or more of the other sides.

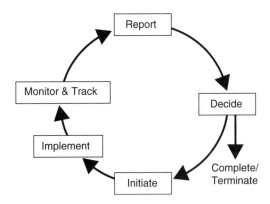

**FIGURE 29.11**   The project cycle. Adapted from Szakonyi R. How to successfully keep R & D projects on track. Mt Airy, MD: Lomond Publications, Inc.; 1988, p.103 [10].

the project resource component must be increased to adhere to the original timeline, or the project timeline component must be lengthened to maintain the project resource component as originally defined, or a balance needs to occur, involving a change in both the project timeline and project resource components. It is the role of a PDT to optimize these three project dimensions and present a proposal for any necessary project modification to their R&D governance team.

### The Project Cycle

As illustrated in Figure 29.11, the project cycle consists of six stages [10]. The first stage, the *initiation stage*, encompasses the design and planning of the project, including the definition of the three project components (specifications, resources, and timing) which, even in a preliminary fashion, are inventoried in the TPP. The project initiation stage also includes creation of a PDT composed of individuals representing the many disciplines needed to complete the project. This stage usually begins with a kickoff meeting in which the project goals, objectives, and components are presented, team members are introduced to each other, and agreement is reached regarding operating procedures for the project team. The second stage of the project cycle is called the *implementation stage*. During this stage, project planning, scheduling (timelines), and resource allocation actually start. For a drug development project, these first efforts will probably focus on the preparation of drug substance for formulation screening and animal safety studies, and the start of these studies (e.g., see Chapter 31). The third stage of the project cycle is called the *monitoring and tracking stage*. The critically important point to be made regarding monitoring and tracking is to focus and limit attention on what is tracked so that linkage is established to the major

milestones which will determine whether or not forward motion on the project is being made. The fourth stage of the project cycle is the *reporting stage*. The decision on what needs to be reported regarding project progress and variances, and to whom the information needs to be reported, should be based on what critical decisions will be made and by whom. Clearly, the level of detail reported to a PDT member is more than the level that senior management needs in order to make major decisions. Indeed, it is the role of the PDT to digest the current project information and to prepare Impact Reports and Actions Needed documents for those who make the resource allocation decisions necessary to keep the expected development program deliverables and timelines on track. The next stage is the *decision-making stage*. A key point to remember regarding the decision-making stage is that a useful definition of a decision is "an allocation of resources". When a decision is made, resources must be added to a project, or taken away from a project, or maintained for that project. The final stage is the *completion/termination stage*. This stage is reached for each project cycle, and the outcome is determined by whether or not the project goals and objectives of that particular project cycle have been achieved.

A full development program can be thought of as a series of projects and project cycles that each contain these stages. From that perspective, the last stage for a project in early-phase development will be "continue/ terminate" rather than "complete/terminate". For example, a critical Phase II dose–exposure–response clinical study must be planned carefully, with alignment and buy-in with key stakeholders in the organization, and then implemented, monitored, and reported. Based on the outcome of this Phase II study, a critical decision will be made as to whether or not to invest in a large, expensive, and lengthy Phase III confirmatory program.

## PROJECT PLANNING AND MANAGEMENT TOOLS

Several tools that are useful in the planning and management of biopharmaceutical projects are identified in Table 29.7. Definitions can be found in the PMI *A Guide to the Project Management Body of Knowledge* [2], and within the tutorial and help sections of Microsoft Project®. It is important to point out that these tools are useful only after the project objectives, goals, Go/No-Go decisions, decision criteria, and project critical operating assumptions have been established. Representative project planning and management tools are presented in Table 29.7 in the order in which they will

**TABLE 29.7   Project Planning and Management Tools**

Milestone charts

PERT charts

Gantt charts

Work breakdown structures (WBS)

Financial tracking

Risk register

Decision trees

be described. Each tool is intended for a specific purpose. Organizational context and culture are key considerations in selecting the tools to use and in deciding the level of rigor with which they will be applied. It is important *not* to force-fit the use of a tool into an organization that is not ready or willing to use it.

## Milestone Tables

Milestone tables consist of a tabulation of major drug development milestones. Whereas the Go/No-Go decisions discussed above are very project specific, development milestones are much more generic and can usually be applied to a wide variety of projects. Typical milestones for pharmaceutical development are shown in Table 29.8. It is important that each organization decides on the milestones that it wishes to use and that it defines them very clearly. Some companies distinguish between milestones (progress point to be noted) and stage gates (decision points for future resource investment). Typically, subsets of milestones are considered to be the stage gates.

**TABLE 29.8   Typical Project Milestones**

Potential therapeutic target identified

Chemical lead identified

Clinical candidate selected

Pre-IND meeting with FDA and scientific advice meeting with EMA

First in human (FIH) clinical study initiated

End of Phase IIa meeting with FDA

Effective dose and dose regimen characterized for safety and for effectiveness

End of Phase II meeting with FDA and meetings with EMEA

Phase III clinical studies initiated

Phase III clinical studies completed

Pre-NDA meeting with FDA

NDA/BLA/MAA submitted

Risk evaluation and mediation studies (REMS) agreed to by FDA

NDA/BLA/MAA approved

Product launched

Postmarket surveillance program initiated

## Work Breakdown Structures

A work breakdown structure (WBS) can be thought of as an organizational chart of tasks and activities needed in order to achieve the project objectives. The project WBS can be arranged either by deliverables (e.g., formulations, clinical trials) or by resource (e.g., formulation chemist, clinical study monitor). A common way of illustrating these different approaches is by analogy with the construction of a new house. One option for the construction WBS would include plumbing, and might be sorted either by house level or by room. A second option would be to sort the construction WBS by the activities needed to complete each room, with each room having as part of its WBS items such as framing, plumbing, wiring, flooring, drywall, painting, and so on.

The level of detail to track in plans and in WBSs varies greatly across organizations. Many companies have launched very elaborate, sophisticated tools to plan and track many detailed activities only to find that the resources required to maintain those plans exceeds the value that is gained from trying to monitor detailed activities. For this reason, the senior management of each organization needs to clearly define and articulate their philosophy with regard to the level of detail to be tracked and the allocation of resources needed for the creation, maintenance, and updating of detailed product development plans, schedules, and resource requirements.

## PERT/CPM Charts

PERT (Performance Evaluation, Review, and Tracking) and CPM (Critical Path Method) charts (flow charts) are based on the flow, connectivity, and interdependency of project tasks, activities, and goals. A PERT chart (Figure 29.12) depicts the activities in the order that they will need to be carried out, either in series or in parallel. These charts also identify which activities need to be completed (or initiated) before the next activity, which is dependent on it, can be initiated. It is important to point out that PERT and CPM charts are project planning and management tools that are used to ensure the integrity of the project design and planning process, but are rarely used as graphics to track and report on project progress. The Gantt chart is the main project graphic used to track project progress and decision points, and usually a PowerPoint® graphic of the key milestones and decision-points from the Gantt chart is prepared and used for PDT meetings and R&D management team updates.

CPM is the methodology used to identify the longest, or *critical*, path from project initiation to

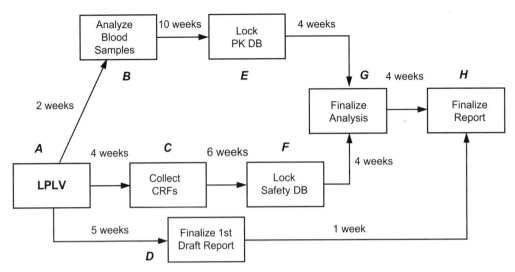

**FIGURE 29.12** A PERT chart showing three paths. Path 1 (A + D + H) will require 6 weeks. Path 2 (A + C + F + G + H) will require 18 weeks. Path 3 (A + B + E + G + H) is the longest, requiring 20 weeks, and is the critical path. (LPLV, last patient, last visit; CRF, case report forms; PK, pharmacokinetic; DB, database).

project completion. In Figure 29.12, the critical path is Path 3 (A + B + E + G + H) since this path is the longest path from "A" to "H". The significance of the critical path is two-fold. The first point is that if any activity on the critical path is delayed by 1 day, the whole project will be delayed by 1 day. The second point is that once the critical path activities have been identified, the PDT has four "critical path" jobs to focus on. The first job is to find a way to shorten the existing critical path. The second job is to track critical path activities very closely to ensure that there is no slippage. The third job is to track all of the activities that could possibly negatively impact the critical path to ensure that these "subcritical path" activities are initiated and completed as scheduled. The fourth job is to closely manage those activities that could create a new critical path if they were to be completed in a longer time frame than originally estimated.

## Gantt Charts

Gantt charts are horizontal bar charts (Figure 29.13) that are used to view (1) the timeline (duration) of each task, activity, and objective, (2) the temporal

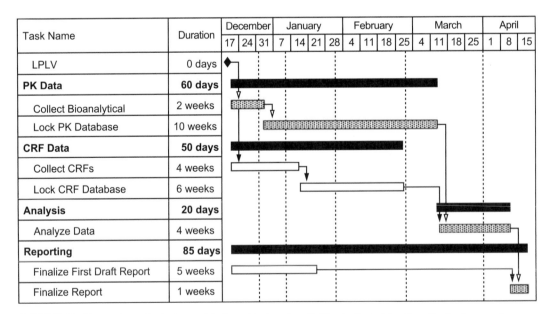

**FIGURE 29.13** A Gantt (bar) chart with the critical path activities indicated by the stipples bars and arrows (LPLV, last patient, last visit; PK, pharmacokinetic; CRF, case report form).

relationship and possible interdependencies between various activities, and (3) the actual progress made on each task, activity, and objective vs the original (baseline) project plan. A number of project-tracking software systems are available and provide the ability to view a chart of the whole project as well as just the high-level objectives (milestones and decision points).

Project progress is shown in a number of ways – for example, by shading a portion of the activity bar to indicate the proportion of the activity that has been completed (e.g., 75% shaded to represent that 75% of the subjects needed for a clinical study have been enrolled). A particularly effective way both to track project progress and to identify key activities that are lagging behind the agreed-upon schedule is to set up a comparison bar chart that includes the current bar chart schedule, the previous bar chart schedule, and the bar chart schedule that was originally planned. Project teams have found it very beneficial to view the project Gantt chart in a variety of presentations, such as a Gantt chart of all project activities that are scheduled to start within the next 90 days and a separate Gantt chart of all project activities that are scheduled to end within the next 90 days. To make the best use of PDT meeting time, it is advisable to have the project Gantt chart updated before each team meeting so that the team is fully informed of the current project timelines and any exceptions to the agreed-upon timelines. With a fully updated and informed project schedule, the project team can make the decisions and recommendations required to maintain the desired progress of the project.

As mentioned earlier, the project schedule is a consequence of the scope of the project objectives, availability of project resources, and timeline requirements. Projects can be scheduled to "complete no later than…", in which case objectives and resources have to be balanced appropriately. In other cases, the project objectives are established, the resources that are available for the project are allocated, and the product development team uses project management software to predict when the project is likely to be completed, given the limitations of the allocated resources. Clearly, allocation of more resources to a resource-limited project could accelerate the project significantly.

## Financial Tracking

The financial tracking of individual projects has become an increasingly important role for biopharmaceutical PDTs. In some organizations, a member of the R&D comptroller's office is a member of the team. In other cases, individuals from this office are available to support the team as requested. The

PDT is asked on an annual basis to estimate the funding and human resources needed for the project over the next 36 months in order for the project to meet the goals that have been approved by the organization. The team is also asked to help track the project costs on a real-time basis and to make regular (e.g., quarterly or monthly) projections as to the "spend rate" over the next 12 months. Although some organizations have developed financial tracking tools internally, a number of project-driven financial tracking tools are now commercially available (e.g., MS Project®, SAP).

## Risk Registers

Risk registers were formally introduced into biopharmaceutical project planning and management in the mid-2000s. A risk register is developed by a PDT as an inventory of critical activities, which if they were to have a negative outcome would significantly impede the project progress. By creating a project risk register, a product development team can use this valuable inventory of potential negative outcomes to proactively design well thought-out contingency project plans. Should adverse outcomes occur, these contingency plans could be rapidly deployed to maintain the forward motion of the project. This inventory of potentially negative impact outcomes also can be used proactively to modify the product development plan to minimize the risk posed by possible future negative outcomes. Thus, the risk register inventory is a valuable resource for driving PDT goals, objectives, plans, and project team-meeting agendas. Not all companies are ready to embrace risk registers. If the culture of a company can be characterized as "only good news is spoken here", then the company will likely not realize the value of a risk register.

## PROJECT TEAM MANAGEMENT AND DECISION-MAKING

### Industry Project Teams

In the pharmaceutical industry, the formal use of core product development teams (Core Team) to accelerate drug development began in the early 1980s. Rather than review the attributes and value of the team concept here, the reader is referred to an excellent text on the subject by Katzenbach and Smith [11]. The current standard for biopharmaceutical product development team structure is the matrix team, which is composed of core-team members from relevant functional organizations that are needed for the development of a new drug (i.e., discovery, toxicology, drug metabolism and pharmacokinetics, analytical, formulations, clinical, regulatory, manufacturing, and marketing), a PDT leader, and a project manager. Several alternatives for project leadership and project support are outlined in Table 29.9. Each alternative has its respective advantages and disadvantages, and each organization will need to choose the alternative that works best in its organizational culture.

It is the project manager's role to ensure that current project information has been incorporated into the various project planning and management tools that the organization is using. Using project management tools, the project manager develops various project scenarios for review at project decision-making meetings. Each core-team member represents the combined functions of his or her department and is supported by his or her own set of team members and project planners and managers in their department. Each core-team member is also a team leader of his or her respective functions that support the project, which may be called subteams (e.g., clinical subteam, regulatory subteam).

The term *matrix* refers to the fact that project team members have a dual reporting relationship and therefore are known as multiply supervised employees (MSEs). The traditional matrix team concept has performed adequately, but, as initially conceived, the performance evaluation of team members was conducted only by their departmental management, so that the focus of team members was usually centered on their functional department. However, this evaluation structure was modified in the early 1990s by having each team member's performance evaluated, at least in part, by his or her project team leader, and in some cases by other members of the project team. This change has greatly increased the effectiveness of the matrix team approach.

In the mid-1990s, Lilly introduced the concept of *heavyweight teams*. Heavyweight teams are formed at the end of Phase II, and members of these teams devote their entire time to the advancement of a single project to NDA/BLA/MAA submission, approval, and launch. Both matrix and heavyweight teams frequently adopt the concept of co-location or a "project village". Although the core-team members are formally part of a functional department, their "project team offices" are all within a few feet of each other. This project village concept has been particularly successful because it fosters rapid and frequent communication among the core-team members.

## FDA Project Teams

With the advent of the Prescription Drug User Fee Act (PDUFA) in 1992, which legislated timelines for NDA reviews, the FDA utilized the project team concept for both IND and NDA reviews. For INDs, an FDA project team is established upon IND submission, or earlier if there is a request for a pre-IND meeting. When an NDA/BLA is received, an important responsibility of the NDA/BLA review team is to determine whether the submission is adequate for review by the FDA. Within 45 days of submission, the review team will either accept the NDA/BLA for filing (review) or return the submission to the sponsor along with the reasons it was not acceptable for review (Refuse to File). The role of project manager has been created in both CDER and CBER. An FDA medical officer generally leads the technical review, and a regulatory project manager oversees the regulatory and logistical processes. Recently the FDA Office of

TABLE 29.9  Team Leadership and Project Support Alternatives

| Team leadership | Advantages | Disadvantages |
| --- | --- | --- |
| Dual leadership: Technical Process | Provides both strong technical AND process leadership | Two bosses, mixed signals |
| Technical (usually clinical) | Strong technical leadership | Limited management of process Usually a part-time role in a full-time job |
| Full-time team leader | Team leader is dedicated to one or more projects | Might not have strong technical knowledge of the project Might be leading multiple projects |
| *Team support* | *Advantages* | *Disadvantages* |
| Dedicated project manager | Provides both strong process and project planning & management support | None |
| None | None | Places excess burden on the project team leader to both lead and provide process and project planning & management support |

Safety and Epidemiology (OSE) has created the position of a safety project manager who participates on NDA/BLA review teams.

## Effective PDT Meetings

The ability to lead a meeting effectively is a skill that is most highly regarded in all types of organizations. Effective meetings rarely occur without good preparation and effective meeting management. A well-developed agenda is the most effective tool for holding a successful meeting. Indeed, in some organizations the mantra is becoming "no agenda, no attenda". Having the right people attend the meeting is as important as having an effective agenda. This means that the team leader, the project manager, and all of the team members have a special responsibility to ensure that those who are needed at the meeting do indeed attend and are appropriately informed regarding the status of their function's project activities and current results. With video-conferencing capabilities, many meetings can be very effective and productive even when not all the participants can be at the same physical site. It is important for one person to be responsible for ensuring that all of the remote-site participants receive meeting materials in advance of the meeting. It is not acceptable to delay a meeting while everyone is waiting for last minute e-mailing of critical documents to participants at another site. Most organizations have multimedia education tools in their libraries to help their staff develop effective meeting management skills.

## Resource Allocation

Resource allocation has become more important with the advent of prioritized portfolios. Once a portfolio is prioritized by the PMT, and the core project team has been informed of their project's priority, the core project team will allocate the resources made available for their project in a manner that will provide for the most rapid progress to be made over a given budget period – usually 12 months. For those who manage a department, resource allocation takes on an added dimension, for although a department head may have adequate resources for all of the approved projects for the next 12 months, the need for the resources might not be evenly spaced over that time period. For example, the portfolio of projects might need 75% of the department's annual resources in the first 6 months and the remaining 25% in the second 6 months. Ideally, project team leaders, project managers, and department project management staff will resolve

this mismatch by meeting and developing several alternative scenarios for senior management review and approval. For the decisions to be soundly based, management will ask each team to identify the impact of each alternative scenario on the project objectives, decisions, milestones, resources, and timelines.

## Effective Project Decision-Making

### Decision Trees

Decision trees began to be used in bio-pharmaceutical organizations during the mid-1990s as companies realized that a formalized decision-making process with pre-specified criteria for success at each decision-point could shorten the time needed for drug development program completion. Decision points for a specific biopharmaceutical project should focus on technical hurdles such as those in Table 29.10. An example of a high-level drug-development decision tree is provided in Figure 29.14 (certain elements from the decision tree are included in Table 29.10). The key features of this decision tree are: (1) the decision tree is driven by TPP criteria; (2) the decisions are "question-based"; (3) the early clinical program is designed to determine the dose–exposure–response relationship for both safety and efficacy; and (4) the decision tree follows the "learn and confirm" paradigm [12]. A decision tree that was developed by the FDA for the IND review process is shown in Figure 29.15. This example was obtained from the CDER Handbook website [13]. For each of the boxes shown in this figure, the website includes a narrative that can be accessed by clicking on the respective box. The website contains a similarly informative decision tree for the NDA

**TABLE 29.10   Examples of Project-Specific Go/No-Go Decisions[a]**

Serious toxicity observed in dogs is NOT observed in primates, and therefore **tolerability meets TTP criteria**

A stable IV formulation has now been identified

**PK & ADME profiles meet TPP criteria of adequate exposure**

**Dose–exposure–response (D–E–R) relationships for clinical safety and efficacy (S&E) established per TPP criteria**

A process to reduce the high cost of goods has been achieved

The human safety profile observed is as predicted

Clinical activity is observed at 1/20th the highest no adverse effect (NAE) human blood levels

Synergy is demonstrated with the new combination product

**Efficacy, safety and value meet TPP goals**

Highest survival ever observed is reported with this test medication

[a]Bold indicates go decision criteria from Figure 29.14.

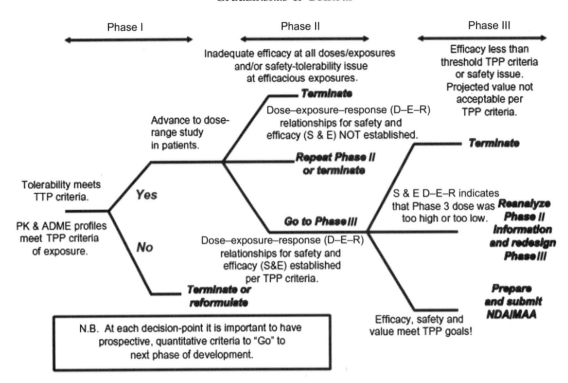

**FIGURE 29.14** Decision tree for a drug development project that illustrates that (1) decision trees are driven by TPP criteria, (2) decisions are question-based, (3) early clinical program should be designed to determine the dose–exposure–response (D–E–R) relationship for both safety and efficacy (S&E), and (4) decision trees should follow the "learn and confirm" paradigm. At each decision point it is important to have prospective, quantitative criteria to "Go" to the next phase of development.

review process. Similar decision trees are developed by project teams within the biopharmaceutical industry.

Project teams are now being asked not only to construct decision trees, but also to develop contingency plans based on multiple "what-if" scenarios far in advance of the next decision points. The goal is to ensure that the project will not lose forward motion in the event of a "No" decision that requires rework or another loop through the project cycle, or a management decision that resources for a particular project are more urgently needed for another project.

### Prespecified Decision Criteria

To facilitate the decision-making process, highly effective project teams should develop prespecified criteria for each decision point or contingency. These criteria provide the critical targets for the project and speed up the decision-making process. An example of clinical Go/No-Go decision criteria for a potential antihypertensive drug might be "lowers diastolic blood pressure by at least 10 mm Hg for at least 6 months in at least 80% of the subjects treated with the middle of three doses, with a side-effect profile lower by 25% than that observed for the active control". One can imagine the debate that will occur

if the blood-pressure lowering observed at 6 months is only 8 mm Hg. Finally, effective decision-making must include an assessment of resource allocation because, as previously emphasized, decision-making is in reality the selective allocation of resources.

### Process Leadership and Benchmarking

It is appropriate to conclude this chapter with some comments on process leadership and benchmarking. The ability to understand how all the complex pieces of drug development need to be integrated can only be learned through hands-on experience as a PDT team leader, project manager, or seasoned team member. Corporate management in the biopharmaceutical industry now counts on individuals with this experience to identify ways in which the drug development process can be improved to maximize the probability of commercial success and thereby add value to the organization.

Benchmarking has become an important tool that is being used to identify ways in which an organization can quantify, and then exceed, industry standards (best practices) for the time, cost, and quality of the R&D activities that are needed to discover, evaluate, develop,

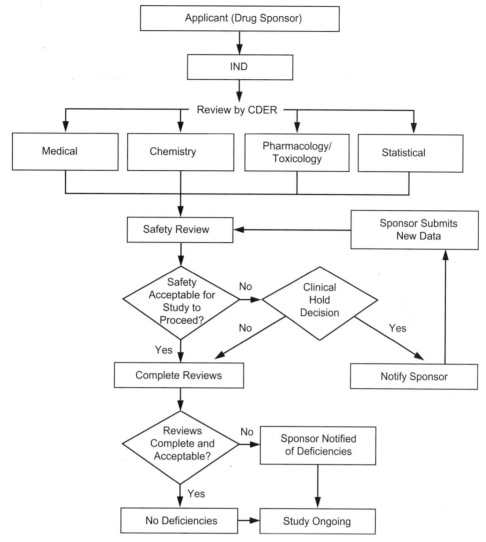

**FIGURE 29.15** Decision tree for the IND review process by the Center for Drug Evaluation and Research (CDER) that illustrates the importance of the safety assessment needed to allow the first clinical study for a new drug to begin in the US. Reproduced from the CDER handbook website at http://druganddevicelaw.net/CDER_handbook.pdf [13].

and bring a new drug to market. Benchmarks can be as broad as "How long should it take from the FIH study to NDA submission?" to "How long should it take to design an approvable clinical protocol and case report form for a one-site clinical study?" The Centre for Medicines Research (CMR International) has been formally conducting benchmarking studies for the industry, and additional information can be found on their website [14].

The emphasis on both process leadership and benchmarking in the project planning and management domain of biopharmaceutical R&D truly illustrates the level of maturity and sophistication that this discipline has achieved.

## REFERENCES

[1] NDA Partners LLC. Principles of Optimal Product Development (Internet at, www.ndapartners.com/principles/index.php).
[2] PMI Standards Committee. Guide to the project management body of knowledge (A PMBOK® Guide). Newtown Square, PA: Project Management Institute; 2000.
[3] Kennedy A, editor. Pharmaceutical project management. 2nd ed. New York, NY: Informa Healthcare; 2008.
[4] Drug Information Association (Internet at, www.diahome.org.)
[5] Baker SL. Perils of the internal rate of return (Internet at, http://sambaker.com/econ/invest/invest.html).
[6] Kaitin KI, DiMasi JA. Pharmaceutical innovation in the 21st century: New drug approvals in the first decade, 2000–2009. Clin Pharmacol Ther 2011;89:183–8.
[7] DiMasi JA, Feldman L, Seckler A, Wilson A. Trends in risks associated with new drug development: Success rates for investigational drugs. Clin Pharmacol Ther 2010;87:272–7.

[8]  Grudzinskas   C.   Change + Communication = Challenge –
     Management of new drug development. Clin Res Pract Drug
     Regu Affairs 1988;6:272–7.
[9]  CDER. Target product profile – A strategic development
     process tool. Draft guidance for industry. Rockville, MD:
     FDA   (Internet   at,   www.fda.gov/downloads/Drugs/
     GuidanceComplianceRegulatoryInformation/Guidances/
     ucm080593.pdf; 2007).
[10] Szakonyi R. How to successfully keep R & D projects on track.
     Mt Airy, MD: Lomond Publications Inc.; 1988.

[11] Katzenbach C, Smith D. The wisdom of teams: Creating the high–
     performance organization. New York, NY: HarperBusiness; 2003.
[12] Sheiner LB. Learning versus confirming in clinical drug devel-
     opment. Clin Pharmacol Ther 1997;61:275–91.
[13] CDER. The CDER handbook. Rockville, MD: FDA
     (Internet   at,   http://druganddevicelaw.net/CDER_
     handbook.pdf; 1998).
[14] CMR International. Reliable, authoritative performance
     metrics   and   trends   analysis   (Internet   at,   http://
     thomsonreuters.com/content/science/pdf/CMR-cfs-en.pdf).

# Drug Discovery

Edward A. Sausville

*Greenebaum Cancer Center, University of Maryland, Baltimore, MD 21201*

## INTRODUCTION

Drug discovery can be described as the process of identifying chemical entities that have the potential to become therapeutic agents. A key goal of drug discovery campaigns is the recognition of new molecular entities that may be of value in the treatment of diseases that qualify as presenting unmet medical needs. These diseases do not have definitively useful therapies, and are actually or potentially life-threatening. Marketed drugs at this point in time represent a relatively small number of drug target types. Drugs targeted against G-protein coupled receptors, nuclear (hormone) receptors, and ion channels represent slightly less than 50% of the marketed drugs. By far, drugs directed against enzymes represent the largest portion of marketed drugs [1]. Expansion into new types of drug targets may be necessary to fill certain therapeutic voids, but a matter of great intellectual challenge is how to choose a target likely to be of value, especially when venturing into less well-explored types of drug targets.

The traditional pharmaceutical research and development process suffers from a high attrition rate. For every new drug brought to the market, most estimates suggest that researchers will typically have employed over 100 screens looking for drug leads, winnowing down candidates from tens of thousands of compounds (Figure 30.1). Lead compound discovery research is also costly and time-consuming, taking by some estimates over 5 years and > $200 million, not including the even more substantial time and costs associated with drug development [2]. Even having an attractive lead compound in hand,

compounds then fail during the subsequent development phase for reasons that are unpredictable in the lead discovery phase. Reasons for failure may include unacceptable toxicity, lack of *in vivo* efficacy in models of the disease of interest, market-attractiveness reasons, and poor biopharmaceutical properties. Development can also slow down appreciably in the face of synthetic complexity, low potency, and ambiguous toxicologic findings [3]. Carefully thought-out and employed strategies for drug discovery are therefore needed, particularly when entering new drug target or disease arenas.

This chapter discusses four important considerations in drug discovery: definition of drug targets, generation of chemical diversity as sources of new molecular entities, definition of lead structures through screening strategies, and qualifying lead molecules for transition to early trials. Many of the examples will be drawn from the realm of cancer chemotherapy, but the principles are broadly applicable to a wide variety of disease types.

## DRUG DISCOVERY PHILOSOPHIES AND DEFINITION OF DRUG TARGETS

There are two historically contrasting philosophies underlying drug discovery. The first and more traditional is an "empirical" approach in which the initial drug lead is recognized by a functionally useful effect. Early drug discovery up through the 1960s largely utilized this approach and was exemplified by testing mixtures of natural products in bioassays, yielding drugs such as digitalis, rauwolfia, penicillins,

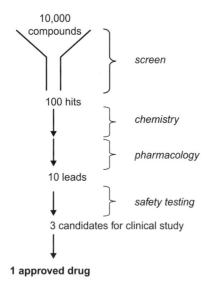

**FIGURE 30.1** The screening funnel. Loss of compounds is to be expected as candidates proceed through the preclinical process.

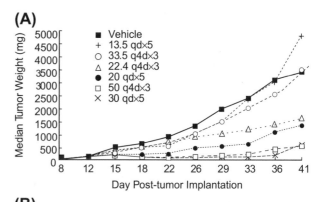

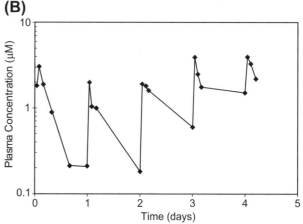

**FIGURE 30.2** Enthusiasm for an empirically active anticancer agent KRN5500. (A) Effect of drug on the rate of growth of COLO205 xenograft models in athymic mice (doses from 13.5 mg/kg to 50 mg/kg). (B) Mouse plasma concentrations at 20 mg/kg/d of KRN5500. Panel A reproduced with permission from Burger AM, Kaur G, Hollingshead M *et al.* Clin Cancer Res. 1997 Mar;3:455–63 [6]; Panel B Unpublished National Cancer Institute data provided by S. Stinson.

anthracyclines, vincas, paclitaxel, and camptothecins. Although natural product extracts are still screened for potential drug candidates, due to the complexities associated with identifying the active agent in the extract the screening efforts in most industrial sectors have moved in the direction of testing pure compounds. Having found a compound that produces a desired biological effect *in vitro*, one then goes on to optimize the molecule, its pharmacology, and the dosing schedule before proceeding to later-stage drug-development activities. This strategy has resulted in the discovery of drugs such as the sulfas, diuretics, hypoglycemics, and the newer antihypertensives.

As the technology became available, the use of bioassays evolved into the use of more focused enzymatic assays in which the targeted enzyme was known from physiological studies as being important in the pathogenesis of the intended disease. ACE inhibitors, cholesterol-lowering statins, and reverse transcriptase and protease inhibitors all emerged from this type of focused screening campaign. In a more recent evolution, investigators are also employing combinatorial methods to bring mixtures of compounds to bear against many targets, in some cases expressed in engineered organisms such as yeast or invertebrates [4].

## Empirical Drug Discovery

Empirical drug discovery, despite its successes, is not without intrinsic problems. The identification of a lead compound by bioassay is commonly divorced

from an understanding of its mechanism of action, making lead optimization difficult since there is no easily quantifiable way to ascertain whether an analog will have greater effect. Additionally, the value of an empirical screen depends on its predictive ability. In some cases, such as acid hyposecretion or $H_2$-receptor binding assays, a positive result in such an assay is now recognized to correlate highly with a prediction for a useful anti-ulcer therapy. On the other hand, an agent demonstrating activity in more than one-third of tested mouse models of anticancer activity still has at best a 50% chance of showing efficacy in a Phase II clinical trial [5].

As an example of the difficulties facing "empirical" discovery and development strategies, the spicamycin analog KRN5500 from Kirin Brewery was discovered through an empirical approach and had a broad spectrum of antitumor activity in *in vivo* anticancer models (Figure 30.2A) [6]. While efficacious

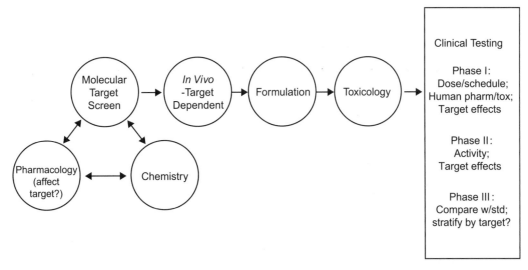

**FIGURE 30.3** The rational drug discovery paradigm directed at a molecular target.

concentrations of 2–5 µM were achievable in mice when administered daily for 5 consecutive days (Figure 30.2B), when the same schedule was used in the initial clinical trial the maximum tolerated dose produced concentrations of no more than 1 µM and a number of patients experienced unacceptable grade 4 toxicity, including interstitial pneumonitis not predicted in the animal models. In this case, then, the lack of a correspondence between tolerated rodent and human pharmacology allowed a compound to proceed all the way to human clinical trials only to produce unacceptable toxicity [7].

## Rational Drug Discovery

Rational drug discovery, by contrast, produces drug leads either by designing compounds to act against a particular biochemical target, or by screening compounds until candidates are identified that act against the target's function (Figure 30.3). In a rational approach, one returns at every step of development to the question of whether the drug candidate continues to act on the target. This hopefully allows one to identify failures at an earlier stage and continually adjust "organism"-related effects, such as distribution and pharmaceutic properties, while retaining core mechanistic features that allow activity. This approach was used very effectively in the identification of the initial HIV protease inhibitors, of metoprolol as an antihypertensive, and of methotrexate as an antifolate antitumor therapy.

The development of imatinib (Gleevec®), which has been extensively described [8–10], also serves as an excellent example of a rational approach to drug discovery. Briefly, the bcr–abl oncoprotein, with

increased tyrosine kinase activity, was identified as a potential target in certain leukemias due to its apparent pathogenicity in cells bearing translocations between chromosomes 9 and 22, which produces the "Philadelphia" chromosome present in chronic myelogenous leukemia (CML). It also occurs in certain cases of acute lymphocytic leukemia (ALL). Although the bcr–abl oncoprotein is able to modulate downstream signal transduction events, it is absent in normal tissues. Natural products such as erbstatin, lavendustin, and piceatannol were initially identified as bcr–abl directed agents. Alternative strategies to lead optimization which considered structural information available with respect to protein kinase ATP binding sites led in part to the compound now called imatinib [10]. Subsequent *in vivo* testing confirmed antitumor efficacy, but only on a schedule of administration that assured the continuous block of bcr–abl phosphorylating activity [9]. Clinical trials produced dramatic results in patients with chronic phase CML [8].

To proceed with a rational approach, however, begs the question of how to initially identify a suitable target around which rational discovery efforts might then be designed. The imatinib example could be said to exemplify a genetic or biological approach, proceeding from a cytogenetic observation through to identification of the target oncoprotein bcr–abl. Initiatives such as the Cancer Genome Anatomy Project (http://cgap.nci.nih.gov) allow other biological approaches to target definition, such as finding genes that are over- or underexpressed in cancer cells but not in normal cells. Such gene expression profiling allowed for the identification of distinct types of diffuse large B-cell lymphoma, and the stratification of patients into high- and low-risk groups [11]. The high-risk profiles can then indicate which expressed protein sets might be valuable as targets for new agents directed against aggressive lymphoma. In the non-cancer sphere, the recent availability of genomic sequencing methodologies has revealed the association of gene polymorphisms that are associated with the incidence or progression of a variety of diseases [12–14]. Genes with polymorphisms predisposing to the occurrence of these diseases could conceivably define targets that would modify their progression or severity, and therefore serve as targets for rational drug discovery. Likewise, the availability of genomic sequencing of pathogen genomes has led to novel target definition for infectious diseases [15].

A distinct approach to defining targets utilizes genetic manipulation of *in vitro* cell types or of entire organisms. A particular gene's expression in cell culture may be diminished ("knocked-down") by small interfering RNA (siRNA) technology to diminish gene expression, or by retroviral infection or transfection, to overexpress a particular gene. Isogenic cells are created that are identical except that the siRNA or transfected gene is absent. Ideally the under- or overexpression of the gene creates an assayable phenotype, and the manipulated cells can then be screened against compound sets to define those candidate drugs which modify the cells' behavior in the presence or absence of the gene product selected as the drug target [16, 17]. In the event that a desired target is unknown but one wishes to define a drug target that would enhance the activity of a known drug, siRNA technology can also be used to look for targets whose absence defines increased sensitivity to a particular drug ("synthetic lethals") [18]. Alternatively, one can define targets whose overexpression connotes altered sensitivity to an applied compound, and these would therefore reveal novel resistance targets in the case of antineoplastic or anti-infectious agents [19].

Occasionally a retroactive approach is possible, where one can start with a drug that was initially identified through more empirical means, and then identify its binding partners. Once identified, these targets can be screened to allow definition of additional candidates, particularly when the original candidate has failed at later stages of drug development for reasons such as unacceptable toxicity or formulation problems. The geldanamycins, members of the class of benzoquinoid ansamycin antibiotics, represent an example of such an approach. In the late 1980s, researchers saw that these compounds "reversed" the oncogene *src*-transformed phenotype of rat kidney cell and decreased steady-state phosphorylation levels without appearing to have any

direct effect on src kinases [20]. In an attempt to further explicate the mechanism of action of this class of compounds, a geldanamycin derivative was immobilized to a bead and affinity precipitated the molecular targets with which the drug interacted, thus teasing out heat shock protein 90 (HSP90) as the binding partner [21]. Consistent with these binding data, certain geldanamycins inhibited specifically the formation of a previously described src–HSP90 heteroprotein complex. HSP90 now is considered an active target for exploration for geldanamycin-like molecules as well as other classes of compounds [22].

In addition to biological and retroactive approaches to molecular target definition, one can also return to classical approaches of screening compounds against biochemical targets, and then explore their potential value in biologic assays. While these approaches do manipulate single targets, they can be inefficient. Chemical genetics approaches have recently been explored with libraries of molecules and precisely defined, genetically-modified organisms. These approaches have been, for example, valuable in defining modulators of DNA damage repair in yeast or cell strains bearing defined mutations in DNA-repair proteins [23, 24].

## GENERATING DIVERSITY

Not every drug lead will become a successful drug. Geldanamycin, for example, produced unacceptable hepatotoxicity. Ultimately, screening approaches defined new chemotypes with the capacity to modulate HSP90 function [22]. Having accepted HSP90 or any other molecular target as a viable lead for drug discovery, how does one find sufficient molecules to test in a target-directed assay, particularly if an initial lead looks like it may not pan out?

### Natural Products

Historically, natural products have been considered an excellent source of drug leads due to the amazing diversity found in microbes, plant and marine life. A single molecule found in an extract from these sources can contain lipophilic, hydrophilic, acidic, and basic elements, all of which can contribute to a molecule's value as a drug. Further, the diversity of available natural products has barely been scratched, even though, by some accounts, natural products and their derivatives comprise over a quarter of known drugs [25].

Natural products are not, however, without some issues to take into consideration. The collection of source materials can be problematic from several standpoints. Physical availability of the plant or organism can be a significant issue – for instance, in the case of a plant that can only be collected during its 2-week flowering interval in spring. Increasing attention has also been paid to the need to respect the rights of the source countries of the material. Further, on finding a "hit" in a natural product extract, the isolation and structural definition of the compound in the extract responsible for producing the activity is no trivial matter (Figure 30.4), even assuming that it is a single compound in the extract that is responsible.

## Chemical Compound Libraries

In addition to natural product sources, chemical compound libraries are used frequently in the drug discovery process. These libraries can range from small, focused libraries specifically synthesized with a particular target in mind, to massive, randomly generated libraries. While there is still the problem of deconvolution of an active library, synthetically generated libraries do have a few advantages over natural product extract mixtures. There are typically equal concentrations of the compounds. The chemical structures and synthetic pathway are known. Finally, some structure–activity relationships can be deduced by comparing active to inactive members of a library [26].

Many of the earliest combinatorial libraries were primarily composed of peptides, often without regard to the potential for success of these peptides as drugs. Lipinski's now commonly accepted "Rule of Five" provides guidelines for molecular characteristics likely to be associated with poor oral drug absorption (Table 30.1) [3]. Since the larger the peptide, the easier it is to create diversity, the initial peptide libraries were often composed of compounds with all of Lipinski's undesirable characteristics, such that even if a hit was identified in a screen it was unlikely to be viable for drug development. Further, by constructing libraries with hundreds to thousands of inactive compounds in a single well, along with only one or two active

**TABLE 30.1  Lipinski Rule of Five**

Compounds with two or more of the following characteristics are flagged as likely to have poor oral absorption:

- More than five hydrogen-bond donors
- Molecular weight > 500
- $c \log P$ (a measure of partitioning of compound between octanol and water) > 5
- Sum of Ns and Os ( a rough measure of hydrogen-bond acceptors) > 10

components, the potency of the mixture could be diluted to the point where the active compounds were undetectable. For this reason, many libraries now have fewer compounds per well. Later generations of libraries also have attempted to incorporate the Lipinski rules into their initial design by including more chemical functional groups in the scaffold and/or natural-product backbones. These newer libraries therefore are more readily amenable to a wide range of bioassays against soluble acceptors, membrane-bound receptors, microorganisms, and differentiation (stem cells), etc. [4].

## DEFINITION OF LEAD STRUCTURES

The next issue in the drug discovery process following definition of target and sources of diversity is the definition of a lead structure. Lead structures can arise from structure-based design or biochemical or cell-based screens against defined targets. Broach and Thorner [26] provide a more exhaustive description of screening strategies than is possible here.

### Structure-Based Drug Design

Current technology allows the molecular structures of even complex target proteins or protein fragments to be defined primarily through X-ray crystallography and nuclear magnetic resonance spectroscopic (NMR) techniques. The resulting three-dimensional

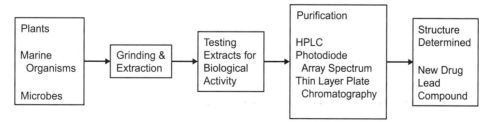

**FIGURE 30.4**  Steps in natural-product derived drug discovery.

information can provide a starting point for *a priori* drug design approaches for potential binding partners. The bcr–abl inhibitor imatinib was well understood in part through considerations of binding models of ATP to initial protein kinase substrates [10]. Other classes of agents whose definition was informed by structure-based design include HIV-related protease inhibitors, and DNA minor groove binding agents.

Alternatively, computer assisted drug design (CADD) approaches attempt to align protein structures with potential binding partners based on known sizes of potential small molecule ligands and algorithms that predict a basis for molecular interaction, such as bond distance along a small molecule scaffold, electronegativity at contact points, etc. [27]. The resulting structures identified as potentially binding to the larger molecule may then be tested for molecular interaction with the target, or one may proceed directly to biological assays in, for example, cellular assays that are dependent on target function. Examples of recently defined agent classes using CADD approaches include MAP kinase [28] and bcl6 [29] inhibitors.

A particularly powerful technique to utilize structural information consists of "Fragment Screening" by NMR techniques. In this approach, expressed target proteins are labeled with isotopes that can evoke an altered NMR signal after binding with a nearby small molecule. Upon interaction with candidate binding molecules, a change in the chemical shift of the target protein resonances is detected, and thus serves to define a molecular interactor [30]. Fragments may be selected so that they bind to nearby regions of the target molecule, and in this way it is possible to increase binding affinity by creating a larger drug lead that bears these fragments. This approach was used to successfully generate lead molecules directed at the bcl2 family of anti-apoptotic proteins, analogs of which have entered early clinical testing [31, 32].

## Biochemical Screens

Biochemical screens directed against purified enzymes or other protein targets in 96-well, 384-well, and even 1526-well formats are used quite commonly to identify drug leads. For example, phosphatases Cdc25A and B are overexpressed in many cultured cancer cell lines, and Cdc25A additionally suppresses apoptosis. Overexpression of CDC25A or B has been detected in human breast, head and neck, cervical, skin, lymph, lung, and gastric cancers. These phosphatases are therefore considered reasonable targets for eventual anticancer therapies. To quickly detect

potential Cdc25 phosphatase inhibitors, a high-throughput screen was developed in which fluorescein diphosphate is added to glutathione S-transferase (GST)-Cdc25 in assay buffer and the fluorescent output read as a measure of enzyme inhibition [33]. Both targeted array libraries and diverse chemical libraries were used, and a hit was identified. Validation of the potential hit from this assay was then done at the cellular, biochemical, and genetic levels, confirming that the hit from the initial screen binds tightly to the catalytic domain of Cdc25A and causes $G_2/M$ arrest.

## Cell-Based Screens

In an example from the cancer arena, a cell-based high-throughput screen was used in a study of small molecule inhibitors of hypoxia-inducible factor 1 (HIF-1), a transcription factor that plays key roles in the regulation of cell responses to hypoxia [34]. HIF-1 governs vascular endothelial growth factor (VEGF) and other angiogenic response genes. Overexpression of HIF-1 has been associated with tumor progression, treatment failure, and poor survival, leading to efforts to find pharmacologic modulators of HIF-1. One of the "hits" to emerge from this screening effort was topotecan, an S–phase-specific agent that causes cytotoxicity by a mechanism dependent on DNA replication-mediated DNA damage. In follow-up testing it was determined that topotecan inhibits HIF-1 accumulation independently of its effects on DNA [35]. Further, topotecan produced sustained inhibition of tumor growth in U251-hypoxia-responsive element (HRE) xenografts in a schedule-dependent fashion that was associated with a marked decrease of HIF-$1\alpha$ protein levels, angiogenesis, and the expression of HIF-1 target genes in tumor tissue.

While such cell-based screens can be used with molecularly defined reporter assays, in certain areas, such as cancer and early HIV-directed screens, cell-based screens also have been used in purely empirical screening efforts to detect agents with, for example, antiproliferative or antiviral activity. The National Cancer Institute's 60-cell line screen (NCI-60), which is described in Chapter 31 and elsewhere [36–39], consists of nine histologically-based panels of human tumor cell lines. In the typical screen, drugs are added to the cell lines at five different concentrations with a 48-hour drug exposure. The dose response of each individual cell line to the drug is then plotted, and the 50% growth inhibition ($GI_{50}$), total growth inhibition ($TGI$), and 50% lethal concentration ($LC_{50}$) indices are calculated. In an alternative method of viewing the data, the mean log $GI_{50}$, $TGI$ or $LC_{50}$ is placed as the center point of the so-called mean graph, and the individual values for a particular cell line are plotted as deflections from the mean. By means of a pattern recognition algorithm known as "COMPARE", which generates a Pearson correlation coefficient, it is then possible to compare the pattern of the tested drug with that of any other tested drug. The impetus to compare the patterns of activity of different drugs arose from the observation that drugs with similar mechanisms have similar patterns of activity. For instance, if a compound has a high correlation coefficient with the known tubulin binder paclitaxel, it is likely that the tested compound interacts with tubulin in some fashion. Confirmatory testing of the mechanism of action is, of course, necessary.

In addition to testing drugs in the 60-cell-line panel, numerous researchers have measured the levels of various molecular targets in each of the 60-cell lines. It is then possible to correlate the activity of a drug with the levels of a particular target. One of the first molecular targets measured in the 60-cell lines was the mRNA expression of the epidermal growth factor receptor (EGFR). A COMPARE analysis of this target profile with agents tested in the 60-cell-line screen produced positive correlations with agents known to inhibit EGFR or otherwise interact with this pathway. This type of COMPARE analysis can provide confirmation that the effect of a drug against a target seen in a biochemical assay translates to a cell-culture setting, thus helping to confirm the choice of a drug lead [40].

More recent cell-based screens have been developed to define the potential value of known compounds against new disease indications. For example, in a collection of several hundred lung cancer cell lines, crizotinib, a known *alk* oncogene protein kinase antagonist, was observed to be active against cell lines ultimately recognized as harboring the em4-*alk* fusion protein kinase [41]. This recognition promoted the rapid clinical development and FDA approval of crizotinib for this indication.

## QUALIFYING LEADS FOR TRANSITION TO EARLY TRIALS

The goal of the drug discovery process is ultimately to find molecules that could be suitable for eventual clinical testing. Following definition of an optimized lead structure, however, a substantial amount of drug development work remains to be done before the agent is ready to enter clinical testing. Once a drug lead is available, the dose, route, and schedule of administration of the drug should be optimized if possible in appropriate *in vivo* efficacy models. For molecules

designed under the "rational" philosophy, this optimization process should capitalize on target-directed effects. Initial pharmacokinetics determinations should provide verification that the concentration required to cause an effect *in vitro* is achievable *in vivo*. Development of an acceptable formulation is also important at this stage. It may even be necessary to consider additional analogs of the lead structure if any of the above testing indicates that the original lead is in any way untenable.

Following, or in conjunction with, these activities, preclinical pharmacology studies are typically conducted with the goals of developing sensitive analytical methods for drugs in biological fluids and tissues; determining *in vitro* stability and protein binding; determining pharmacokinetics in rodents and dogs; identifying and analyzing metabolites; defining an optimal dose schedule and blood sampling times; correlating peak plasma concentrations and/or AUC with efficacy, safety, and toxicity; and evaluating analogs if necessary to determine an optimal development candidate.

Safety testing is required by regulatory authorities before the drug lead is eligible for human testing. For an oncology therapeutic, the FDA currently requires that a drug be tested in two species, a rodent and non-rodent, in studies that follow the proposed clinical route and schedule. As discussed in Chapter 31, the objectives of these studies are to determine, in appropriate animal models, the maximum tolerated dose (MTD), dose-limiting toxicities (DLT), schedule-dependent toxicity, reversibility of adverse effects, and a safe clinical starting dose. Only after all these preclinical studies is it possible to proceed to clinical testing.

Among the drugs that have recently navigated all of these hurdles successfully is bortezomib (Velcade®, PS-341), a dipeptide boronic acid that inhibits the 20S proteasome. This molecule represents a paradigmatic illustration of an efficient cancer drug discovery and development program, as it proceeded from initial entry into preclinical studies to FDA approval in 7–8 years. The ubiquitin–proteasome pathway plays a critical role in the regulated degradation of proteins involved in cell-cycle control and tumor growth. The originating company selected PS-341 from a group of analogs because of its potent proteasome inhibitory activity, although there were other analogs that had slightly better efficacy in some *in vivo* models [42]. The company nevertheless demonstrated not only the ability of PS-341 to reduce the growth of a PC-3 prostate tumor in mice, but also that it did so concordant with its effect on the biochemical target. PS-341 did cause some toxicity in animals, so the question became whether the "safe" dose in animals was in the efficacy range for humans. During the course of the clinical trials, proteasome activity was measured *ex vivo* in human leukocytes and dose escalation proceeded to the point of proteasome inhibition, in contrast to standard clinical trials in which dose escalation proceeds to a maximum tolerated dose. Clinical activity was observed in patients with multiple myeloma, and botezomib was approved for this indication by the FDA in 2003.

## ACKNOWLEDGEMENT

Shannon Decker contributed to a prior version of this chapter in the second edition of this textbook, sections of which have been retained in this update.

## REFERENCES

[1] Verdine GL. The combinatorial chemistry of nature. Nature 1996;384(Suppl):11–3.

[2] Petsko GA. For medicinal purposes. Nature 1996;384(Suppl):7–9.

[3] Lipper RA. *E pluribus* product. Mod Drug Discov 1999;2:55–60.

[4] Houghten RA, Pinilla C, Giiulianotti MA, Appel JR, Dooley CT, Netzi A, et al. Strategies for the use of mixture-based synthetic combinatorial libraries: Scaffold ranking, direct testing *in vivo*, and enhanced deconvolution by computational methods. J. Comb Chem 2008;10:3–19.

[5] Johnson JI, Decker S, Zaharevitz D, Rubinstein LV, Venditti JM, Schepartz S, et al. Relationships between drug activity in NCI preclinical *in vitro* and *in vivo* models and early clinical trials. Br J Cancer 2001;84:1424–31.

[6] Burger AM, Kaur G, Hollingshead M, Fischer RT, Nagashima K, Malspeis L, et al. Antiproliferative activity *in vitro* and *in vivo* of the spicamycin analogue KRN5500 with altered glycoprotein expression *in vitro*. Clin Cancer Res 1997 Mar;3:455–63.

[7] Supko JG, Eder Jr JP, Ryan DP, Seiden MV, Lynch TJ, Amrein PC, et al. Phase I clinical trial and pharmacokinetic study of the spicamycin analog KRN5500 administered as a 1-hour intravenous infusion for five consecutive days to patients with refractory solid tumors. Clin Cancer Res 2003;9:5178–86.

[8] Druker BJ, Sawyers CL, Kantarjian H, Resta DJ, Reese SF, Ford JM, et al. Activity of a specific inhibitor of the BCR-ABL tyrosine kinase in the blast crisis of chronic myeloid leukemia and acute lymphoblastic leukemia with the Philadelphia chromosome. N Engl J Med 2001;344:1038–42.

[9] le Coutre P, Mologni L, Cleris L, Marchesi E, Buchdunger E, Giardini R, et al. Gambacorti-Passerini C. *In vivo* eradication of human BCR/ABL-positive leukemia cells with an ABL kinase inhibitor. J Natl Cancer Inst 1999;91:163–8.

[10] Capdeville R, Buchdunger E, Zimmermann J, Matter A. Glivec® (STI571, imatinib), a rationally developed, targeted anticancer drug. Nat Rev Drug Discov 2002;1:493–502.

[11] Alizadeh AA, Eisen MB, Davis RE, Ma C, Lossos IS, Rosenwald A, et al. Distinct types of diffuse large B-cell lymphoma identified by gene expression profiling. Nature 2000;403:503–11.

[12] Peters BJ, Pett H, Klungel OH, Stricker BH, Psaty BM, Glazer NL, et al. Genetic variability within the cholesterol lowering pathway and the effectiveness of statins in reducing the risk of MI. Atherosclerosis 2011;217:458–64.

[13] Farbstein D, Soloveichik YZ, Levy NS, Levy AP. Genetics of redox systems and their relationship with cardiovascular disease. Curr Atheroscler Rep 2011;13:215–24.

[14] Faberstein D, Levy AP. The genetics of vascular complications in diabetes mellitus. Cardiol Clin 2010;28:477–96.

[15] Cani PD, Delzenne NM. The gut microbiome as therapeutic target. Pharmacol Ther 2011;130:202–12.

[16] Iorns E, Lord CJ, Turner N, Ashworth A. Utilizing RNA interference to enhance drug discovery. Nat Rev Drug Discov 2007;6:556–68.

[17] Ngo VN, Davis RE, Lamy L, Yu X, Zhao H, Lenz G, et al. A loss-of function RNA interference screen for molecular targets in cancer. Nature 2006;441:106–10.

[18] Whitehurst AW, Bodemann BO, Cardenas J, Ferguson D, Girard L, Peyton M, et al. Synthetic lethal screen identification of chemosensitizer loci in cancer cells. Nature 2007;446:815–9.

[19] Koo Koo HM, Gray-Goodrich M, Kohlhagen G, McWilliams MJ, Jeffers M, Vaigro-Wolff A, et al. The ras oncogene-mediated sensitization of human cells to topoisomerase II inhibitor-induced apoptosis. J Natl Cancer Inst 1999;91:236–44.

[20] Uehara Y, Hori M, Takeuchi T, Umezawa H. Phenotypic change from transformed to normal induced by benzoquinonoid ansamycins accompanies inactivation of p60src in rat kidney cells infected with Rous sarcoma virus. Mol Cell Biol 1986;6:2198–206.

[21] Whitesell L, Mimnaugh EG, Costa BD, Myers CE, Neckers LM. Inhibition of heat shock protein HSP90-pp60$^{v-src}$ Heteroprotein complex formation by benzoquinone ansamycins: Essential role for stress proteins in oncogenic transformation. Proc Natl Acad Sci USA 1994;91:8324–8.

[22] van Montfort RLM, Workman P. Structure-based design of molecular cancer therapeutics. Trends Biotechnol 2009;27:315–44.

[23] Lord CJ, McDonald S, Swift S, Turner NC, Ashworth A. A high-throughput RNA interference screen for DNA repair determinants of PARP inhibitor sensitivity. DNA Repair (Amst) 2008;7:2010–9.

[24] Simon JA, Yen TJ. Novel approaches to screen for anticancer drugs using *Saccharomyces cerevisiae*. Methods Mol Biol 2003;223:555–76.

[25] Newman DJ, Cragg GM, Snader KM. Natural products as sources of new drugs over the period 1981–2002. J Nat Prod 2003;66:1022–37.

[26] Broach JR, Thorner J. High-throughput screening for drug discovery. Nature 1996;(Suppl):14–6.

[27] Dong X, Ebalunode JO, Yang SY, Zheng W. Receptor-based pharmacophore and pharmacophore key descriptors for virtual screening and QSAR modeling. Cur Comput Aided Drug Des 2011;7:181–9.

[28] Hancock CN, Macias AT, Mackerell Jr AD, Shapiro P. Mitogen activated protein (MAP) kinases: Development of ATP and non-ATP dependent inhibitors. Med Chem 2006;2:213–22.

[29] Cerchietti LC, Ghetu AF, Zhu X, Da Silva GF, Zhong S, Matthews M, et al. A small-molecule inhibitor of BCL6 kills DLBCL cells *in vitro* and *in vivo*. Cancer Cell 2010;17:400–11.

[30] Bruncko M, Oost TK, Belli BA, Ding H, Joseph MK, Kunzer A, et al. Studies leading to potent, dual inhibitors of Bcl-2 and Bcl-xL. J Med Chem 2007;50. 641–662.

[31] Hajduk PJ, Meadows RP, Fesik SW. NMR based screening in drug discovery. Q Rev Biophys 1999;32:211–40.

[32] Larsson A, Jansson A, Åberg A, Nordlund P. Efficiency of hit generation and structural characterization in fragment-based ligand discovery. Curr Opin Chem Biol 2011;15:482–8.

[33] Brisson M, Nguyen T, Vogt A, Yalowich J, Giorgianni A, Tobi D, et al. Discovery and characterization of novel small molecule inhibitors of human Cdc25B dual specificity phosphatase. Mol Pharmacol 2004;66:824–33.

[34] Rapisarda A, Uranchimeg B, Scudiero DA, Selby M, Sausville EA, Shoemaker RH, et al. Identification of small molecule inhibitors of hypoxia-inducible factor 1 transcriptional activation pathway. J Cancer Res 2002;62:4316–24.

[35] Rapisarda A, Zalek J, Hollingshead M, Braunschweig T, Uranchimeg B, Bonomi CA, et al. Schedule-dependent inhibition of hypoxia-inducible factor-1alpha protein accumulation, angiogenesis, and tumor growth by topotecan in U251-HRE glioblastoma xenografts. Cancer Res. 2004;64:6845–8.

[36] Alley MC, Scudiero DA, Monks PA, Hursey ML, Czerwinski MJ, Fine DL, et al. Feasibility of drug screening with panels of human tumor cell lines using a microculture tetrazolium assay. Cancer Res 1988;48:589–601.

[37] Boyd MR, Paull KD. Some practical considerations and applications of the national cancer institute *in vitro* anticancer drug discovery screen. Drug Dev Res 1995;34:91–109.

[38] Scherf U, Ross DT, Waltham M, Smith LH, Lee JK, Tanabe L, et al. A gene expression database for the molecular pharmacology of cancer. Nat Genet 2000;24:236–44.

[39] Weinstein JN, Myers TG, O'Connor PM, Friend SH, Fornace Jr AJ, Kohn KW, et al. An information-intensive approach to the molecular pharmacology of cancer. Science 1997;275:343–9.

[40] Wosikowski K, Schuurhuis D, Johnson K, Paull KD, Myers TG, Weinstein JN, et al. Identification of epidermal growth factor receptor and c-erbB2 pathway inhibitors by correlation with gene expression patterns. J Natl Cancer Inst 1997;89:1505–15.

[41] Gerber DE, Minna JD. ALK inhibition for non-small cell lung cancer: From discovery to therapy in record time. Cancer Cell 2010;18:548–51.

[42] Adams J, Palombella VJ, Sausville EA, Johnson J, Destree A, Lazarus DD, et al. Proteasome inhibitors: A novel class of potent and effective antitumor agents. Cancer Res 1999;59:2615–22.

# 31

# Non-Clinical Drug Development

**Chris H. Takimoto[1] and Michael J. Wick[2]**

[1]*Translational Medicine Early Development, Janssen Pharmaceutical Companies of Johnson & Johnson, Radnor, PA 19087*
[2]*Preclinical Research, South Texas Accelerated Research Therapeutics, San Antonio, TX 78229*

## INTRODUCTION

From the first time a promising molecule is identified in a drug discovery and screening program to the time it enters a first-in-human (FIH) clinical trial, an enormous amount of scientific work and evaluation must be performed. Non-clinical development, as defined in this chapter, encompasses all of the activities that must take place before a new chemical entity can be administered to humans, as well as the extensive toxicology testing that continues after clinical trial initiation. As such, it not only spans the gap between drug discovery and clinical testing, but also provides all the key non-human pharmacological and safety information that must be generated under tightly controlled experimental conditions in order to satisfy regulatory review requirements.

This chapter describes the general processes involved in the non-clinical development of a pharmaceutical agent, with specific examples taken from the field of oncology. From an industry perspective, the continuum of drug discovery and development can be subdivided into a series of interrelated steps outlined in Table 31.1. As described in Chapter 30, a typical small molecule drug discovery program begins this process by identifying and validating specific disease targets, followed by high-throughput screening of large chemical libraries containing a diversity of compounds. In the hit-to-lead stage, the most promising lead molecules or "hits" are identified, and during lead optimization these undergo chemical modification for further iterative testing. Ultimately, at the candidate selection or new molecular entity (NME)

declaration stage, drug discovery culminates with the selection of the agent with the most suitable pharmaceutical properties for future clinical testing. This candidate then undergoes a series of rigorous safety and toxicological tests that are required for filing an Investigation New Drug (IND) application with the US Food and Drug Administration (FDA), or with appropriate foreign regulatory organizations prior to initiating FIH studies. These specific IND-enabling tests are conducted during the preclinical stage of development. Biological therapeutics may share a similar series of targets, although the manufacturing and lead optimization processes differ substantially from the chemical modification of small molecules. Nonetheless, for both biological and small molecule therapeutics, the preclinical development period will encompass a similar diversity of safety and efficacy pharmacology studies, beginning roughly at the lead optimization stage and extending through to the initiation of clinical trials.

With the advent of the twenty-first century, advances in cancer biology and the complete sequencing of the human genome raised a public expectation that these seminal scientific achievements would be rapidly applied to the field of medicine, and this fostered the development of applied biomedical research necessary to move scientific investigation from the bench to the bedside … and back [1]. This area of applied biomedical science has been termed *translational research*, defined succinctly by Hait [1] as "the application of a discovery to the practice of medicine", and the growth of this field is dramatically impacting oncology discovery and development.

*PRINCIPLES OF CLINICAL PHARMACOLOGY, THIRD EDITION*
DOI: http://dx.doi.org/10.1016/B978-0-12-385471-1.00031-3

**TABLE 31.1  Stages of Drug Discovery and Non-Clinical Development**

1. Target Identification/Validation
2. High-Throughput Screening
3. Hit to Lead/Lead Identification
4. Lead Optimization
5. New Molecular Entity Declaration/Candidate Selection
6. Preclinical Development
7. Investigational New Drug Application

Under this new paradigm, tumors are viewed as complex biological systems comprised of malignant cells that co-opt host fibroblasts, stroma, and endothelial and inflammatory cells to collectively form the tumor microenvironment. Research into the nature of this microenvironment has led to an explosion in the number of molecular targets for therapeutic intervention. This has provided fertile ground for the discovery of molecularly targeted therapies that can be characterized by well-defined mechanisms of action and can be evaluated in clinical trials through the careful use of pharmacodynamic biomarkers [2]. Furthermore, the validation of predictive biomarkers that prospectively identify patient populations suitable for treatment underscores a more personalized approach to medical therapeutics. These advances have enabled well-designed pharmacology studies to be conducted during preclinical development, and have played an essential role in the formulation of rational translational research strategies.

## COMPONENTS OF NON-CLINICAL DRUG DEVELOPMENT

As outlined in the S9 FDA Guidance for non-clinical evaluation of anticancer pharmaceuticals, the goals of this testing are to (1) identify the pharmacological properties of a pharmaceutical, (2) establish a safe initial dose level for FIH exposure, and (3) understand the toxicological profile of a pharmaceutical [3]. Our current discussion will include these three key areas and touch upon their integration into the design of comprehensive translational scientific strategies for clinical development. Primary emphasis will be placed on those non-clinical studies referenced in the FDA guidance that include evaluation of safety and efficacy pharmacology, characterization of drug pharmacokinetics and pharmacodynamics, toxicology studies, and the selection of starting doses for clinical development. However, many additional components of non-clinical drug development are

required prior to clinical testing. For example, consistency in the chemical and physical properties of the active pharmaceutical ingredient (API) must be ensured from the earliest small-scale syntheses for pharmacological studies to bulk API manufacturing for large clinical trials. These processes, broadly referred to as chemistry, manufacturing, and controls (CMC), include the synthesis of the API under good manufacturing principles (GMP), bulk scale-up of the manufacturing process, and selection and formulation of the dosage format. It may also include impurity checks, solubility, and stability testing. These important CMC activities and related issues, such as packaging of clinical trial materials and analytical method development and validation, are beyond the scope of this chapter [4].

### *In Vitro* Assessment of Pharmacologic Efficacy

The earliest *in vitro* studies of a new pharmaceutical agent are often integral to the drug discovery and screening process. Historically, anticancer screening strategies used *in vitro* assays to identify agents with non-specific growth inhibitory or cytotoxic activities. Modern approaches now screen for specific pharmacological properties utilizing well-characterized high-throughput technologies. Thus, drug candidates are now selected on the basis of their pharmacological mechanism of action. In this process, molecular targets specific to cancer cells, but not present in normal tissues, are identified and used to screen drug libraries. As discussed in Chapter 30, these modern discovery programs are designed to identify molecularly targeted drug candidates with inherent pre-specified mechanisms of action.

In oncology, *in vitro* assessments of pharmacologic efficacy are used to evaluate mechanisms of action and resistance, measure potency, provide early indications of selectivity of action, and identify potential predictive biomarkers. The National Cancer Institute (NCI) has screened hundreds of thousands of compounds using an *in vitro* 60 human-tumor cell-line screen that incorporates a variety of cancer types, including colorectal, melanoma, lung, leukemia, renal, central nervous system, and ovarian malignancies [5]. Automated systems rapidly generate a unique pattern of relative sensitivity for each test compound by determining the drug concentration required to inhibit growth by 50% ($GI_{50}$) across the cell line panel. The COMPARE algorithm can rank in order these $GI_{50}$ sensitivity patterns and compare them to historical controls, thereby providing powerful insights into possible mechanisms of action [6, 7]. The relative sensitivity of cell lines derived from specific tumor types may suggest early directions for future clinical testing. Finally, the molecular characterization of the cell lines panel can identify potential predictive biomarkers associated with tumor sensitivity or resistance [8]. These *in vitro* efficacy studies are an important starting point for designing scientifically-sound translational research plans.

## *In Vivo* Assessment of Pharmacologic Efficacy

Research in cancer biology has identified many properties that distinguish malignant from normal cells, such as uncontrolled growth, metastasis, de-differentiation, genetic plasticity, and drug resistance. Of these, only uncontrolled growth has been extensively studied as a target for cancer chemotherapy. Several newer therapeutic strategies are now under investigation, and these include targets that interfere with the metastatic cascade, induce differentiation, interrupt autocrine or paracrine growth loops, block tumor angiogenesis, inhibit cell cycle and growth signaling cascades, enhance tumor immunogenicity, and reverse drug resistance. Non-clinical evaluation of these strategies using *in vitro* systems is routine; however, many of these approaches can only be adequately assessed using *in vivo* animal model systems.

Tumor initiation, progression, and metastasis rely on select aspects of the heterogeneous primary tumor [9, 10]. Therefore, successful evaluation of tumor biology and drug activity requires the appropriate selection of clinically relevant models. Mouse and rat models contain several advantages over other animals for investigating mammalian biology. The release of a draft sequence of the mouse genome in 2002 [11] and the ongoing efforts to sequence the rat genetic code have enabled the identification of important mutations involved in the pathogenesis of human diseases, such as cancer, diabetes, arterial atherosclerosis, and hypertension. In addition, numerous genetically well-defined rodent lines with distinct phenotypic characteristics are readily available. Short generation times and relatively modest maintenance costs make these non-clinical models extremely attractive for examining the targeted activity of potential therapeutic agents.

A number of animal model systems have been developed that mimic the tumor microenvironments found in clinical situations. However, there are no perfect animal models for drug development. The adequacy of any specific animal model depends on its validity, selectivity, predictability, and reproducibility [12]. In cancer chemotherapy, animal models are selected to simultaneously demonstrate antitumor

efficacy and acceptable systemic toxicity in an intact organism. Ideally, the tumor system under study should be genetically stable with homogeneous characteristics that mimic human tumor biology and do not vary over time. In oncology, a variety of diverse animal models for human tumors have been developed. These models can be broadly categorized into three groups: (1) spontaneous models, including those originating from natural or induced mutations; (2) genetically engineered models (GEMs), including transgenic and knockout animals; and (3) transplanted models, including implanted and orthotopic tumors.

### *Spontaneous* In Vivo *Models*

Models resembling human disease states may arise spontaneously in animals that reach a certain age or period of development, or they may be induced by invasive interventions such as treatments with drugs, chemical toxins, or radiation. Cardiovascular drug development routinely utilizes a number of these models for research on hypertension, hypertrophic cardiomyopathies, and heart failure. One well-defined cardiac animal model is the Spontaneously Hypertensive Rat (SHR), originating from a colony of hypertensive Wistar rats developed in Kyoto, Japan [13, 14]. Another example is the obese Zucker rat, an animal model of non-insulin-dependent type 2 diabetes [15, 16]. In the Zucker rat, a single defect in the gene coding the leptin receptor results in insulin resistance, hyperglycemia, and hypoinsulinemia.

In oncology, inbred or outbred animals with one or more naturally occurring genetic mutations comprise a majority of spontaneous animal tumor models. Examples include the spontaneous APC mutant Min mouse that develops adenomatous polyps which are precursors for invasive colon cancer [17], and the 7,12 diemethylbenz[α]anthracene (DMBA) or 1-methyl-1-nitrosourea (MNU) induced mammary carcinoma model for studying breast cancers [18]. Spontaneous models offer the advantages of orthotropic growth and clinically relevant metastatic spread via vascular and lymphatic vessels local to the primary tumor [19]. Although spontaneous tumors closely resemble the human clinical situation, a number of factors make these models poorly reproducible in controlled settings. For example, difficulties in experimental staging due to variability in the time and frequency of tumor induction can result in suboptimal animal numbers for comparative studies. Inconsistent tumor development due to local effects and extended experiment durations, ranging from several months to a year, also limit the utility of these specialized models [20].

### Genetically Engineered *In Vivo Models*

An exciting area of ongoing research is the increasing use of GEMs for preclinical drug testing. Transgenic and knockout mice are genetically altered to develop spontaneous endogenous tumors in a predictable fashion. Because of this, they can provide a versatile environment for testing novel experimental therapies. Advantages of these newer models include organ- or site-specific targeting, natural growth rates and patterns of growth, and the use of immunocompetent animals [21, 22]. Use of GEMs has also improved the understanding of the role that individual and cooperative gene mutations play in tumorigenesis. However, the cost of these specialized models can be prohibitive, and in some cases they may require a commercial license. Furthermore, the development of endogenous tumors often occurs later in the lifespan of these animals, which can delay experiment times. Finally, the diversity of available histological tumor types is low and the correlation between activity in GEM animal tumors and clinical anticancer activity has not been validated.

Transgenic mice provide a specialized tool and a model for a stepwise evolution of a particular disease state [23]. Transgenic mice arise from the introduction of a foreign gene into the pronucleus of a fertilized egg. This can be accomplished by microinjection [21, 22], retroviral infection [24], or embryonal stem cell transfer [25]. This latter technique involves the transfer of genetic material into embryonal stem cells that can then be transplanted into blastocysts to create a chimeric mouse. If the germ cells in the chimeric animal are derived from the embryonal stem cells, then the offspring of the animal will be transgenic and will express the inserted gene of interest. The capability of introducing and expressing a specific gene of interest in an intact organism provides a powerful means for manipulating the genetic milieu of an experimental animal.

Several transgenic models have been identified and characterized in recent years. One important example is the TG(mREN2)27 rat model, the genome of which contains the mouse renin transgene resulting in increased local angiotensin II concentrations and leading to hypertension and insulin resistance. Insertion of known oncogenes, such as *ras* [26] or *N-myc* [27], can generate transgenic animals that develop spontaneous tumors in a predictable fashion. For example, transgenic mice expressing a mutated *ras* gene frequently develop mammary tumors and can be used to screen for agents active in breast cancer [26].

This model is also useful for testing novel agents that specifically target abnormalities in the *ras* signaling pathway, such as farnesyl transferase inhibitors [28]. Use of organ-specific promoters can further enhance the power of these systems. For example, the association of the human *c-myc* oncogene with an immunoglobulin promoter can lead to the development of pre-B-cell lymphomas [29], while its association with a mouse mammary tumor virus promoter can result in mammary gland tumors [30]. Tumor resistance genes, such as the multiple drug resistance gene (*mdr*), have also been inserted and expressed in transgenic animals [31]. These animals are highly resistant to a variety of different natural product antitumor agents, are able to tolerate otherwise lethal doses of these drugs, and may be useful in screening for agents that can reverse the multidrug resistant phenotype. While these models are useful in answering specific questions, their utility in broader drug screening is limited due to the nature of the model [23]. Introduction of artificial promoters for gene expression can also influence the targeted cell type, thus extrapolation to human disease states should be done with caution [26].

Knockout mice are animals that have been genetically altered to remove both alleles of a specific gene [32]. This is accomplished by homologous recombination techniques that insert the defective gene into embryonic stem cells which are then isolated and injected into a blastocyst to generate heterozygous mice. Further inbreeding will generate homozygous "knockout" animals [32]. Knockout animals can be developed that are similar to transgenic animals in that they lack the function of a specific tumor suppressor gene, such as *p53*, and have a very high incidence of spontaneous tumor development [33]. If the tumor suppressor gene is required for viability of the animal during embryonic development, conditional knockout animals have been developed that selectively inactivate the gene of interest in specific tissues at defined periods in the animal's lifespan. Currently, these models are being extensively used in the study of carcinogenesis and chemoprevention, but their application in testing therapeutic agents is growing.

### Transplanted *In Vivo Models*

Transplanted animal or human tumor xenograft models are some of the most widely used tools for studying experimental therapeutics in cancer. Established transplantable murine tumors have been extensively characterized, and demonstrate excellent homogeneity and reproducibility [34]. However, many commonly used solid tumor models can be biased toward false positive results because their selection has been based on ease of implementation, rapidity of growth, published drug sensitivities, and other attributes that facilitate experimental study design rather than on clinical correlation. Examples of implanted syngeneic murine tumors commonly used in preclinical screening of antitumor agents include Lewis lung carcinoma, melanoma B16, sarcoma 180, L1210 leukemia, and P388 leukemia. A major advantage of these syngeneic murine models is that the host immune system remains intact. Although many of these tumor models have been successful in identifying active therapeutics against leukemia and some lymphomas, they may be inadequate for identifying therapeutics for solid tumors [35, 36]. For example, the L1210 leukemia model is insensitive to the widely used antitumor agent paclitaxel, most likely due to tumor physiology and differences in microenvironment compared with human tumors [37]. Variable pathophysiology and growth patterns of these models also limit their usefulness in developing agents for human cancers [38].

An important advance in preclinical models for anticancer agents was the development of immunosuppressed mouse strains that allowed for the reproducible implantation and growth of human tumor cells *in vivo*. The first xenograft of a human colon cancer cell line into immunocompromised "nude" mice was reported in 1969 by Rygaard and Povlsen [39]. These mouse strains contained an autosomal recessive mutation in the *nu* (for nude) gene on chromosome 11. Homozygous mutations in the *nu* gene resulted in the absence of hair, poor growth, decreased fertility, an absent thymus gland, and a shortened lifespan [39, 40]. These animals exhibit a severe T-cell immunologic defect that impair their ability to reject tissue transplants. Consequently, these animals tolerate the implantation and growth of human tumor cell xenografts because their suppressed immune system prevents the rejection of the human tumor cells. This discovery heralded a revolution in oncology experimental therapeutics [41]. Currently, xenograft tumors have been established for all common human solid tumors.

Severe combined immune deficiency (SCID) mice are another commonly employed immunosuppressed host for human tumor xenografts. These mice lack functional T and B cells and are more immunodeficient than nude mice. This may explain in part the increased ease of growth of some human tumor xenograft models in these animals [42]. The ability of SCID mice to support the growth of primary leukemia cell lines derived from patients with acute and chronic leukemia has led to the use of these animals as the

primary models for testing agents with antileukemic activity [43]. However, the greater sensitivity of SCID mice to toxic drug effects and their greater expense has made them less popular than their nude counterparts as a platform for screening agents for activity against solid tumors.

For studies designed to screen drug candidates *in vivo*, simplicity and ease of access make subcutaneous implantation the most common approach for growing human tumor xenografts in mice. After tumor cell suspensions are injected or tumor fragments implanted into the animal's flank, palpable subcutaneous tumors form over a period of days to weeks. Once a certain size is reached, screening studies are initiated and tumor growth and drug treatment effects are easily followed by monitoring the dimensions of these tumors. The reliability and reproducibility of these models allows for rapid, high-throughput screening of many test agents in multiple tissue types. While subcutaneous implantation is most common, human xenografts can also be implanted in other sites. Implantation in the renal subcapsule has the advantage of requiring a relatively short inoculation time prior to drug treatment, making it particularly useful for short-term *in vivo* assays. However, technical requirements and inability to follow tumor growth limit the utility of this assay in broader drug screening.

Orthotopic xenograft models involve injecting cancer lines or implanting tumor fragments into physiologic sites corresponding to the cancer tissue type. The premise is to create a tumor environment that reflects the clinical situation, thereby allowing for antitumor activity testing that is more predictive of clinical efficacy. These models also are more likely to produce tumor metastases than subcutaneous tumor models, which lack the microenvironment and well-defined vessel system of organ systems. Orthotopic xenograft models have been developed for a number of different tumors, including renal cell carcinoma [44], central nervous system tumors [45], and pancreatic, prostate, colon, and lung cancers [46]. However, because of technical challenges, orthotopic xenografts are not as widely used as subcutaneously implanted tumors.

The utility and predictive value of xenograft models is critically dependent on the source of the cells or tissue that is used. Models derived from cell lines continuously grown *in vitro* produce mostly undifferentiated tumors that rarely resemble the histological architecture of the original human disease. When injected subcutaneously, these models rapidly and reproducibly generate tumors for drug evaluation, but rarely metastasize or become invasive, and they lack the components of the tumor microenvironment that are necessary to mimic fully the clinical condition [47]. However, many of these models have well-characterized genotypes and phenotypes and are useful for the early characterization of targeted therapies. For example, cell-based xenograft models were used to identify drug leads targeting tumor cells with *BRAF* mutations, a useful target in melanoma [48].

Xenografts created from patient tumors directly implanted into mice and serially passaged in animals for a limited number of times (low-passage models) produce heterogeneous tumors that retain much of the histological architecture of the original sample. These models may better reflect the behavior of solid tumors in cancer patients. A recent review of low-passage models reported that they correctly predicted response in 90% (19 of 21 tumors) and resistance in 97% (57 of 59 tumors) of donor patients [49]. Additional studies have found strong clinical correlations between model sensitivity and patient response for a range of solid tumors [50, 51]. Interestingly, metastatic spread after subcutaneous implantation of these low passage models is much more common than for traditional xenografts, again suggesting that they may better recapitulate the clinical scenario. Further characterization and increased acceptance of low-passage models may lead to their more widespread preclinical use, thereby allowing for the prospective identification of those patient populations that are most likely to benefit from the test agent.

Despite their popularity, xenograft models still have limitations [52]. The required use of immuno-compromised animals limits their ability to screen for investigational therapies such as immunomodulators that require an intact immune response. Infections in these animals are common, requiring rigorous attention to maintaining a sterile laboratory environment. In addition, subcutaneous xenograft implants may have higher growth rates, better organized tumor vasculature, and less overall necrosis than their clinical counterparts [53]. Retrospective reviews of the power of these models to predict the results of subsequent Phase II clinical trials revealed various degrees of correlation based upon a number of factors, including tumor histology, drug class, and xenograft type. Breast tumor xenografts were generally not predictive of clinical activity; however, some lung adenocarcinoma xenografts did predict activity in human disease [49, 54–56]. In a retrospective study performed by the NCI of mostly cytotoxic chemotherapies, xenograft models predicted clinical activity about 33% of the time [49, 55]. Whether these models are as predictive for cytostatic and molecularly targeted therapies is unclear.

## Non-Clinical Pharmacokinetics

A fully integrated pharmacokinetic and pharmacodynamic strategy is the hallmark of a well-designed drug development program. Non-clinical pharmacokinetics can be evaluated using specialized *in vitro* assays predictive of drug absorption, distribution, metabolism, and elimination (ADME). For example, protein-binding studies can help interpret the kinetics of free and bound drug concentrations, and absorption and distribution can be predicted by assessing the transport properties of novel agents *in vitro* [57]. Specialized *in vitro* model systems can be used to assess the relevance of specific drug metabolism pathways and estimate the risk of future drug–drug interactions [58, 59]. Finally, *in vivo* non-clinical pharmacokinetic experiments can provide further guidance in designing future clinical trials.

The advent of the sensitive analytical methods described in Chapter 11 has made possible *in vitro* identification of potential drug metabolites using cell lines that express specific enzyme isoforms. Because the cytochrome P450 (CYP) enzyme system plays a prominent role in drug metabolism, CYP enzyme-mediated drug interactions of clinical significance are common. The risk of drug interactions due to metabolism by enzymes such as CYP3A4, 2D6, or 2C9 is now assessed *in vitro* using cell lines that express these specific enzyme isoforms [58, 59]. So it is now routine to conduct a battery of non-clinical *in vitro* tests of a drug candidate's potential to inhibit specific metabolic pathways, induce drug-metabolizing enzymes, or undergo metabolism by specific CYP isoforms. Finally, a drug that is metabolized by an enzyme with known pharmacogenetic polymorphisms may demonstrate predictable pharmacokinetic variability in certain patient populations [60].

In addition to *in vitro* metabolic assessments, there is a growing recognition of the importance of transporters in clinical pharmacokinetics and drug resistance. For example, oral bioavailability can be predicted by measuring drug transport across a monolayer of Caco-2 human colon carcinoma cells, as discussed in Chapter 4 [57]. Modified cell lines that differ from wild-type cells in their expression of specific drug resistance efflux transporters such as the P-glycoprotein-mediated multidrug-resistance (MDR) gene, or the multidrug-resistance protein (MRP), can be used to assess potential mechanisms of drug resistance [61]. Both MDR and MRP can confer drug resistance to a wide variety of natural-product anticancer agents. These tests can also provide early indications of the relative distribution of an agent, such as the likelihood of penetrating the blood–brain barrier.

Finally, non-clinical *in vivo* studies provide the first opportunity to perform detailed single-dose and multiple-dose studies in intact animals. Although the development plan has to be flexible and tailored for each individual agent, some broad generalizations can be made. The first step requires the development of a sensitive and reliable analytical assay for the test compound and any associated metabolites. The assay must be able to detect drug concentrations in the relatively small blood volumes obtained from animals such as rodents. Currently, the most commonly employed analytical methods utilize the liquid chromatography and mass spectrometry (LC/MS and LC/MS/MS) techniques as described in Chapter 11. These technologies have largely supplanted standard high-performance liquid chromatography (HPLC) methods because of their greater specificity and sensitivity.

After an appropriate assay is developed, formal pharmacokinetic studies can be designed in the animal species of interest. These early non-clinical pharmacokinetic and pharmacodynamic studies are typically conducted under non-GLP conditions [62]. In oncology, species selection should be based on the type of preclinical models employed for efficacy and toxicity testing. Ideally, the same formulation of drug planned for clinical use should be tested in these preclinical models. Defining the pharmacokinetics of a new agent in the same animal species used for efficacy and toxicity testing allows for pharmacodynamic data to be collected that relates systemic exposure to drug effects. Assessment of drug pharmacodynamics in xenograft studies is highly relevant because it allows drug effects to be evaluated directly in human tumors. This information is extremely valuable for the design of PK–PD studies. Finally, radiolabeled drug distribution/mass balance studies in animals provide early indications of the tissue distribution and the ADME profile of a new agent.

## Assessment of Pharmacologic Safety

Pharmacologic studies to assess drug safety are required to support the use of a new therapeutic in humans. The objectives of a safety pharmacology study are to identify undesirable pharmacodynamic effects of an agent that may have relevance to human safety, and to evaluate the pathophysiologic effects of a substance observed in previous *in vivo* studies. These studies evaluate the potential undesirable pharmacodynamic effects of a substance on

physiological process over a clinically relevant and even higher range of systemic drug exposures [63]. Safety endpoints can be included in ongoing non-clinical toxicology or pharmacokinetic studies, but dedicated safety pharmacology experiments may be required in some situations. However, extensive stand-alone safety pharmacology studies generally are not required for agents destined for use in late-stage cancer patients [63]. Experiments investigating the mechanisms of any adverse pharmacodynamic effects should only be designed after carefully considering all that is known about other agents in the same therapeutic class. *In vivo* and *in vitro* studies evaluating vital organ systems critical for life support, such as the cardiovascular, respiratory, and central nervous systems, form the safety pharmacology core battery and are given highest priority [63]. Additional follow-up and supplemental safety studies should be individualized for each drug after reviewing all available data. Formal safety pharmacology studies need to be conducted in compliance with GLP principles.

A common concern is the potential for a new agent to cause serious ventricular arrhythmias. Drug-induced prolongation of the QTc interval can increase the risk of ventricular arrhythmias, especially *torsade de pointes* [64]. The duration of the QT interval reflects the late repolarization phase of the cardiac action potential, which is mediated by the efflux of potassium ions through the delayed rectifier potassium channels in the cardiac ventricles. Agents that inhibit potassium ion efflux prolong the QTc interval and increase the risk of serious cardiac arrhythmias. The human ether-a-go-go related gene (*hERG*) encodes the alpha subunit of the human potassium ion channel protein responsible for ion efflux. Non-clinical tests in cell lines expressing this protein can estimate the risk of QTc prolongation [64]. The US FDA recommends preclinical hERG channel testing coupled with *in vivo* QT assessments in a non-rodent species. These data and all other relevant non-clinical information should be reviewed in a formal integrated risk-assessment process that also takes into consideration the compound's chemical and pharmacological class. The need for additional follow-up studies is determined on an individual basis. This assessment helps to define the necessary safeguards and precautions required for clinical testing, and will determine the need to perform a thorough QTc study.

## Non-Clinical Toxicology

After a drug's pharmacological properties have been characterized and deemed optimal, the next key decision point is the candidate selection or NME designation. This step identifies the specific compound for further clinical evaluation and it triggers a series of IND-enabling processes, the most extensive of which are the GLP toxicology studies. The IND-enabling toxicology studies should use the same drug formulation and route of administration that are planned for the clinical trial. The anticipated clinical schedule should also be approximated. For small molecules, toxicology testing usually includes a rodent and a non-rodent species, most often dogs. Biological agents often show large species-specific differences in activity, and may require specific toxicology studies performed in non-human primates. These experiments should be designed to assess both the severity of acute toxicities and the time to recovery. However, demonstration of complete resolution of any observed toxicities is not essential. Toxicokinetic evaluations are included in most formal toxicology studies [3].

For oncology agents, reproductive toxicology, including embryonic and fetal toxicology, studies may be deferred until the time of marketing application [3]. In rare cases these studies may not be needed at all, especially for known genotoxic agents that target rapidly dividing cells, or for known developmental toxins. Reproductive toxicology is typically performed in two different species, although biologicals may use only one relevant species when other options are not available. Fertility and early embryonic development studies are not required for use in patients with advanced cancer; likewise, pre- and postnatal toxicology studies are also not warranted for most oncology indications.

Genotoxicity experiments also are not essential for the initiation of FIH oncology trials, although they should be performed later to support an application for marketing approval [3]. Carcinogenicity trials are not needed for marketing approval in oncology patients, and immunotoxicity may be evaluated as a component of general toxicology studies. However, for known immunomodulators, more extensive studies may be required. Finally, the need for formal photosafety testing is based upon an initial phototoxic potential assessment conducted prior to clinical testing.

## Starting Dose Selection for FIH Studies in Oncology

An important goal of non-clinical development is to select a starting dose that is expected to have pharmacological effects yet is still reasonably safe. Allometric scaling, described in Chapter 32, is one approach that is commonly used for FIH dose selection. For most small molecules, body surface area is used to allometrically scale from animals to the equivalent human doses. However, biological therapeutics are typically scaled to body weight, AUC, or other exposure parameters [3]. In oncology, the highest anticipated dose in a clinical trial is *not* limited by the doses or exposures tested in nonclinical studies, but the planned dose escalation increments should reflect the steepness of the dose–toxicity curve. In Phase I trials in advanced-stage cancer patients, the duration of treatment may continue according to patient response and toleration of the experimental therapy and additional toxicology studies are not required for extended clinical use. Phase II studies may be supported by existing non-clinical data and the accumulated clinical Phase I experience. However, large Phase III studies may require additional non-clinical repeat-dose GLP toxicology studies of at least 3 months duration that can also be used to support the marketing application. New drug combination regimens do not require special toxicology studies; instead, *in vivo* efficacy pharmacology studies of the combination may suffice [3]. The recommended non-clinical toxicology treatment schedules required to support initiation of oncology clinical trials are shown in Table 31.2.

For small molecules, the FIH dose may be based upon 1/10 the dose that causes severe toxicity in 10% of animals ($STD_{10}$) in rodent studies. However, if non-rodents are the most appropriate species, then 1/6 the highest non-severely toxic dose (HNSTD) is used. The HNSTD is the highest dose level that does not produce evidence of life-threading toxicities or irreversible findings.

In Europe new recommendations for biologicals were established in 2007 after the Tegenero/Northwick Park incident, in which six volunteer subjects were severely injured in a Phase I trial [65, 66]. All were healthy volunteers participating in a FIH study of a super agonist anti-CD28 antibody that unexpectedly induced a cytokine storm after a single dose. The European Medicines Association now recommends that all biologicals consider an initial starting dose that is based on the minimal anticipated biological effect level, or MABEL [67]. The MABEL calculations should utilize all non-clinical information available, including (but not limited to) *in vitro* target binding and receptor occupancy, *in vivo* concentration–response curves, and dose–exposure and response data from relevant animal studies [68]. Whenever possible an integrated PK–PD modeling approach should be utilized, and the selection of the recommended starting dose should

**TABLE 31.2** Non-Clinical Toxicology Treatment Schedules of Anticancer Pharmaceuticals to Support Initial Clinical Trials

| Clinical schedule | Non-clinical treatment schedule[a] |
| --- | --- |
| Once every 3–4 weeks | Single dose |
| Daily for 5 days every 3 weeks | Daily for 5 days |
| Daily for 5–7 days, alternating weeks | Daily for 5–7 days, alternating weeks (two dose cycles) |
| Once a week for 3 weeks, 1 week off | Once a week for 3 weeks |
| Two or three times a week | Two or three times a week for 4 weeks |
| Daily | Daily for 4 weeks |
| Weekly | Once a week for 4–5 doses |

[a]The timing of the toxicity assessment(s) in the non-clinical studies should be scientifically justified based on the anticipated toxicity profile and the clinical schedule. For example, a sacrifice shortly after the dosing phase to examine early toxicity and a later sacrifice to examine late onset of toxicity should be considered. The treatment schedules described in the table do not specify recovery periods. The treatment schedules described in this table should be modified as appropriate for molecules with extended pharmacodynamic effects, long half-lives, or potential for anaphylactic reactions. In addition, the potential effects of immunogenicity should be considered.

Adapted from CDER, CBER. S9 Non-clinical evaluation for anticancer pharmaceuticals. Guidance for industry. Rockville, MD: FDA; 2010. (Internet at, www.fda.gov/downloads/ Drugs/Guidance ComplianceRegulatoryInformation/Guidances/UCM085389.pdf) [3].

incorporate a safety factor, such as 1/10 of the MABEL dose estimate [67].

## TRANSLATIONAL RESEARCH IN ONCOLOGY DRUG DEVELOPMENT

In the modern era of translational science-driven drug development, the clinical development plan is heavily influenced by the specific target and the pharmacological mechanism of action of the experimental therapeutic [1]. Inherent in this approach is the careful evaluation of the pharmacologic behavior of a new agent in early clinical trials. In this process, the flow of ideas from the laboratory bench to the patient bedside is not unidirectional because key clinical observations must also feed back to the laboratory, thereby generating new hypotheses for further clinical evaluation.

In oncology, translational research as applied to drug development can be organized around four basic principles. These are (1) molecularly targeted therapies, (2) biomarkers to guide clinical development, (3) PK–PD model-based drug development, and (4) Pharmacological Audit Trail evaluation in early clinical trials.

## Molecularly Targeted Therapies

The characterization of an increasing number of cancer-related molecular targets, coupled with high-throughput screening and sophisticated testing systems, has fundamentally altered the developmental paradigm for oncologic drugs. In the last century, anticancer agents were screened principally for cytotoxic effects against rapidly growing cells. Unsurprisingly, most of the chemotherapeutic agents that were developed lacked selectivity and caused substantial toxicity to normal tissues. However, our increased understanding of cancer biology has fundamentally changed this approach in the postgenomic era.

Modern discovery efforts start with the identification and validation of novel molecular targets present within cancer cells or in the tumor microenvironment. The characterization of these molecular targets is followed by an extensive screening and optimization effort to identify selective lead therapeutic agents. Thus, the resulting candidates for clinical testing have very specific molecular targets and well-characterized modes of action [69]. This understanding is reflected in an improved clinical development strategy in which target engagement and the proposed mechanism of action are evaluated in early clinical trials. In contrast, during the era of cytotoxic chemotherapy, drug mechanisms of action had little or no impact on clinical trial designs. Thus, clinical trials of molecularly targeted therapies are really translational research experiments that test scientific hypotheses and relate proposed drug mechanisms to the generation of clinical activity.

## Biomarker-Guided Drug Development

With a candidate molecule in hand, it is often advantageous to include biomarkers in the planning of early clinical trials. This discussion supplements the review of biomarkers presented in Chapter 18, and focuses on two biomarker types that are highly relevant for drug development: pharmacodynamic/mechanism of action (PD/MofA) biomarkers, and response-prediction biomarkers for optimizing patient selection. Ideally, these biomarkers will be identified during either non-clinical or early clinical development.

PD/MofA biomarkers are clinically applied assays that help define how a drug is impacting the target pathway in humans. These drug development tools inform about a drug's pharmacological properties and help determine drug effects within individual patients. As such, they are most useful in early clinical trials where demonstration of target engagement is an important milestone. Although target engagement does not guarantee clinical activity, it does increase the understanding of drug pharmacology and it can incrementally increase the likelihood of the development program's success. The PD/MofA biomarkers can also help with dose and schedule selection in Phase I studies, but they are generally not intended for use as companion diagnostics, and their clinical use diminishes as a molecule progresses into later stages of development where clinical activity and patient selection issues predominate.

In contrast, response-prediction biomarkers are used to select patients for treatment, and their importance increases as an agent advances in development. The identification of patient populations that can maximally benefit from a specific therapy can have a great impact on clinical development strategies. For example, in a recent Phase I trial of the cMET kinase inhibitor crizotinib, two patients with non-small cell lung (NSCL) cancer showed impressive tumor shrinkage while the majority of other patients, including those with lung cancer, did not [70]. Further investigation revealed that the tumors in the two responding patients uniquely harbored EML4/ALK translocations. This translocation results in the constitutive activation of ALK and is present in about 4% of NSCL cancers, where it appears to drive the malignant process. Although originally developed as an inhibitor of the cMET kinase, crizotinib is also a potent ALK inhibitor, which explains its activity in this setting. Crizotinib rapidly advanced into Phase III clinical trials in NSCLC using the EML4/ALK translocation as a predictive biomarker for patient selection. In cases such as this, the ultimate goal is to register the predictive biomarker as a companion diagnostic at the same time as the marketing application for the new therapeutic is filed. In oncology, essentially all drug development programs now include predictive biomarker/companion diagnostic strategies for identifying optimal treatment populations [71].

## Model-Based Drug Development and the Pharmacological Audit Trail

Biomarker tools are useful for the design of scientifically-sound early clinical trials, and the context for interpreting clinical biomarker data can be facilitated by a model-based drug development approach [72]. Because PD/MofA biomarker changes are no longer merely qualitative, this strategy uses modeling and simulation to provide a quantitative framework for the interpretation of these biomarkers in non-clinical and clinical studies, as shown in Figure 31.1. For example, preclinical trials of oncologic drugs in relevant animal models can relate systemic drug exposures to changes in PD/MofA biomarkers in target tumors. Changes in biomarker readouts can then be related to *in vivo* tumor growth inhibition, thereby providing a quantitative understanding of how biomarker perturbations correspond to a desired biological effect. PK–PD modeling of these non-clinical data can provide a valuable prospective framework for estimating clinical trial results, even before the first patient is dosed [73]. While PK–PD models based on *in vivo* animal models may not perfectly predict the clinical situation, they can be further refined as human data become available.

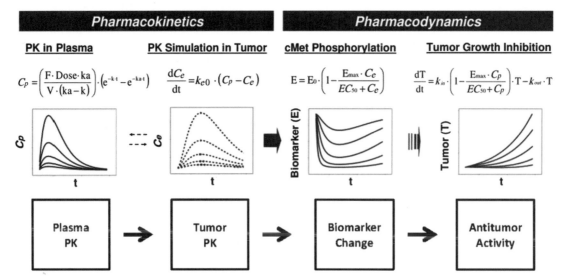

**FIGURE 31.1** Model-based drug development. Adapted with permission from Yamazaki S, Skaptason J, Romero D *et al*. Drug Metab Dispos 2008;36:1267–74 [73].

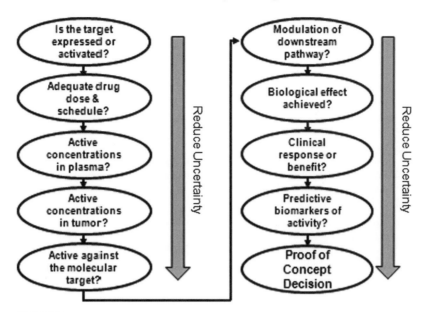

**FIGURE 31.2** Pharmacological Audit Trail. A color-coding system can be used to indicate the strength of clinical information supporting each audit point as a drug is evaluated in early clinical development. Reproduced with permission from Workman P. Mol Cancer Ther 2003;2:131–8 [74].

The clinical use of biomarkers in drug development can be further enhanced through the application of the Pharmacological Audit Trail (Figure 31.2). This concept, developed by Workman and colleagues [74], consists of a series of audit points tied to a drug's pharmacological behavior that can be evaluated during early clinical development. Key questions addressed in the audit trail include: Are sufficient drug concentrations achieved in blood or in tumor tissues? Is the target engaged? Is the downstream pathway modulated? Does this generate the expected biological effect? If these early milestones are met, additional questions are: Is there evidence of clinical activity? Are there biomarkers predictive of clinical benefit? Although each of these questions may not be fully answered for every agent in clinical development, the successful demonstration of each audit point advances the compound one step closer to the demonstration of proof of concept. Thus, the audit trail represents a valuable framework for organizing strategic thinking about biomarkers and translational research questions in early drug development.

## The Challenge: Molecularly Targeted Therapies and Translational Research in Drug Development

As translational scientists, clinical pharmacologists involved in the non-clinical and early clinical development of a new therapeutic are in an ideal position to span the interface between the laboratory and the clinic. Their greatest challenge is to develop safe and effective molecularly targeted therapies as expeditiously as possible. The non-clinical development processes described in this chapter form the basis of subsequent clinical development programs, and need to be carefully applied in order to design scientifically sound clinical development strategies that will provide the safety and efficacy information required for product registration. Although the optimal generation and use of this non-clinical information remains a daunting task, successfully meeting this challenge offers the best opportunity for efficiently developing improved treatments for human disease.

## REFERENCES

[1] Hait WN. Translating research into clinical practice: Deliberations from the American Association for Cancer Research. Clin Cancer Res 2005;11:4275–7.

[2] Hanahan D, Weinberg RA. Hallmarks of cancer: The next generation. Cell 144:646–74

[3] CDER, CBER. S9 Nonclinical evaluation for anticancer pharmaceuticals. Guidance for industry. Rockville, MD: FDA (Internet at, www.fda.gov/downloads/Drugs/Guidance ComplianceRegulatoryInformation/Guidances/UCM085389. pdf; 2010).

[4] Steinmetz KL, Spack EG. The basics of preclinical drug development for neurodegenerative disease indications. BMC Neurol 2009;9(Suppl. 1):S2.

[5] Monks A, Scudiero D, Skehan P, Shoemaker R, Paull K, Vistica D, et al. Feasibility of a high-flux anticancer drug screen

using a diverse panel of cultured human tumor cell lines. J Natl Cancer Inst 1991;83:757–66.

[6] Zaharevitz DW, Holbeck SL, Bowerman C, Svetlik PA. COMPARE: A web accessible tool for investigating mechanisms of cell growth inhibition. J Mol Graph Model 2002;20:297–303.

[7] Rixe O, Ortuzar W, Alvarez M, Parker R, Reed E, Paull K, et al. Oxaliplatin, tetraplatin, cisplatin, and carboplatin: Spectrum of activity in drug-resistant cell lines and in the cell lines of the National Cancer Institute's Anticancer Drug Screen panel. Biochem Pharmacol 1996;52:1855–65.

[8] Scherf U, Ross DT, Waltham M, Smith LH, Lee JK, Tanabe L, et al. A gene expression database for the molecular pharmacology of cancer. Nat Genet 2000;24:236–44.

[9] Talmadge JE, Fidler IJ. Cancer metastasis is selective or random depending on the parent tumour population. Nature 1982;297:593–4.

[10] Talmadge JE, Wolman SR, Fidler IJ. Evidence for the clonal origin of spontaneous metastases. Science 1982;217:361–3.

[11] Waterston RH, Lindblad-Toh K, Birney E, Rogers J, Abril JF, Agarwal P, et al. Initial sequencing and comparative analysis of the mouse genome. Nature 2002;420:520–62.

[12] Khleif SN, Curt GA. Animal models in drug development. In: Holland JF, Bast BR, Morton DL, Frei III E, Kufe DW, Weischelbaum RR, editors. Cancer medicine. Baltimore, MD: Williams & Wilkins; 1997. p. 855–68.

[13] Tsotetsi OJ, Woodiwiss AJ, Netjhardt M, Qubu D, Brooksbank R, Norton GR. Attenuation of cardiac failure, dilatation, damage, and detrimental interstitial remodeling without regression of hypertrophy in hypertensive rats. Hypertension 2001;38:846–51.

[14] Bing OH, Conrad CH, Boluyt MO, Robinson KG, Brooks WW. Studies of prevention, treatment and mechanisms of heart failure in the aging spontaneously hypertensive rat. Heart Fail Rev 2002;7:71–88.

[15] Kasiske BL, O'Donnell MP, Keane WF. The Zucker rat model of obesity, insulin resistance, hyperlipidemia, and renal injury. Hypertension 1992;19(Suppl. 1):I110–5.

[16] Van Zwieten PA, Kam KL, Pijl AJ, Hendriks MG, Beenen OH, Pfaffendorf M. Hypertensive diabetic rats in pharmacological studies. Pharmacol Res 1996;33:95–105.

[17] Thompson MB. The Min mouse: A genetic model for intestinal carcinogenesis. Toxicol Pathol 1997;25:329–32.

[18] Teicher BA. Molecular cancer therapeutics: Will the promise be fulfilled?. In: Prendergast GC, editor. Molecular cancer therapeutics: Strategies for drug discovery and development. Hoboken, NJ: John Wiley & Sons, Inc.; 2004. p. 8–40.

[19] Berger M. Is there a relevance of anticancer drug development? In: Fiebig H, Burger B, editors. Relevance of tumor models for anticancer drug development, vol. 54. Basel: Karger; 1999. p. 15–27.

[20] Talmadge JE, Lenz BF, Klabansky R, Simon R, Rigs C, Guo S. Therapy of autochthonous skin cancers in mice with intravenously injected liposomes containing muramyltripeptide. Cancer Res 1986;46:1160–3.

[21] Rosenberg MP, Bortner D. Why transgenic and knockout animal models should be used (for drug efficacy studies in cancer). Cancer Metastasis Rev 1998;17:295–9.

[22] Thomas H, Balkwill F. Assessing new anti-tumour agents and strategies in oncogene transgenic mice. Cancer Metastasis Rev 1995;14:91–5.

[23] Burger A, Fiebig H. Screening using animal systems. In: Baguley B, Kerr D, editors. Anticancer drug development. San Diego, CA: Academic Press; 2001. p. 285–97.

[24] Jaenisch R. Retroviruses and embryogenesis: Microinjection of Moloney leukemia virus into midgestation mouse embryos. Cell 1980;19:181–8.

[25] Hooper M, Hardy K, Handyside A, Hunter S, Monk M. HPRT-deficient (Lesch-Nyhan) mouse embryos derived from germline colonization by cultured cells. Nature 1987;326:292–5.

[26] Dexter DL, Diamond M, Creveling J, Chen SF. Chemotherapy of mammary carcinomas arising in ras transgenic mice. Invest New Drugs 1993;11:161–8.

[27] Sheppard RD, Samant SA, Rosenberg M, Silver LM, Cole MD. Transgenic N-myc mouse model for indolent B cell lymphoma: Tumor characterization and analysis of genetic alterations in spontaneous and retrovirally accelerated tumors. Oncogene 1998;17:2073–85.

[28] Mangues R, Corral T, Kohl NE, Symmans WF, Lu S, Malumbres M, et al. Antitumor effect of a farnesyl protein transferase inhibitor in mammary and lymphoid tumors overexpressing N-ras in transgenic mice. Cancer Res 1998;58:1253–9.

[29] Schmidt EV, Pattengale PK, Weir L, Leder P. Transgenic mice bearing the human c-myc gene activated by an immunoglobulin enhancer: A pre-B-cell lymphoma model. Proc Natl Acad Sci USA 1988;85:6047–51.

[30] Weaver ZA, McCormack SJ, Liyanage M, du Manoir S, Coleman A, Schröck E, et al. A recurring pattern of chromosomal aberrations in mammary gland tumors of MMTV-cmyc transgenic mice. Genes Chromosomes Cancer 1999;25:251–60.

[31] Dell'Acqua G, Polishchuck R, Fallon JT, Gordon JW. Cardiac resistance to adriamycin in transgenic mice expressing a rat alpha-cardiac myosin heavy chain/human multiple drug resistance 1 fusion gene. Hum Gene Ther 1999;10:1269–79.

[32] Majzoub JA, Muglia LJ. Knockout mice. N Engl J Med 1996;334:904–7.

[33] Donehower LA. The p53-deficient mouse: A model for basic and applied cancer studies. Semin Cancer Biol 1996;7:269–78.

[34] Rockwell S. In vivo–in vitro tumour cell lines: Characteristics and limitations as models for human cancer. Br J Cancer Suppl 1980;41(Suppl. 4):118–22.

[35] Schein PS, Scheffler B. Barriers to efficient development of cancer therapeutics. Clin Cancer Res 2006;12(11 Pt 1):3243–8.

[36] Schuh JC. Trials, tribulations, and trends in tumor modeling in mice. Toxicol Pathol 2004;32(Suppl. 1):53–66.

[37] Venditti JM, Wesley RA, Plowman J. Current NCI preclinical antitumor screening in vivo: Results of tumor panel screening, 1976–1982, and future directions. Adv Pharmacol Chemother 1984;20:1–20.

[38] Staquet MJ, Byar DP, Green SB, Rozencweig M. Clinical predictivity of transplantable tumor systems in the selection of new drugs for solid tumors: Rationale for a three-stage strategy. Cancer Treat Rep 1983;67:753–65.

[39] Rygaard J, Povlsen CO. Heterotransplantation of a human malignant tumour to "Nude" mice. Acta Pathol Microbiol Scand 1969;77:758–60.

[40] Flanagan SP. "Nude", a new hairless gene with pleiotropic effects in the mouse. Genet Res 1966;8:295–309.

[41] Neely JE, Ballard ET, Britt AL, Workman L. Characteristics of 85 pediatric tumors heterotransplanted into nude mice. Exp Cell Biol 1983;51:217–27.

[42] Liu M, Bishop WR, Wang Y, Kirschmeier P. Transgeneic versus xenograft mouse models of cancer: Utility and issues. In: Prendergast GC, editor. Molecular cancer therapeutics: Strategies for drug discovery and development. Hoboken, NJ: John Wiley & Sons, Inc.; 2004. p. 204–26.

[43] Uckun FM. Severe combined immunodeficient mouse models of human leukemia. Blood 1996;88:1135–46.

[44] Fidler IJ. Rationale and methods for the use of nude mice to study the biology and therapy of human cancer metastasis. Cancer Metastasis Rev 1986;5:29–49.

[45] Shapiro WR, Basler GA, Chernik NL, Posner JB. Human brain tumor transplantation into nude mice. J Natl Cancer Inst 1979;62:447–53.

[46] Hoffman RM. Fertile seed and rich soil: The development of clinically relevant models of human cancer by surgical orthotopic implantation of intact tissue. In: Teicher BA, editor. Anticancer drug development guide: Preclinical screening, clinical trials and approval. Totowa, NJ: Humana Press; 1997. p. 127–44.

[47] Solit DB, Garraway LA, Pratilas CA, Sawai A, Getz G, Basso A, et al. BRAF mutation predicts sensitivity to MEK inhibition. Nature 2006;439(7074):358–62.

[48] Gorelik B, Ziv I, Shohat R, Wick M, Hankins WD, Sidransky D, et al. Efficacy of weekly docetaxel and bevacizumab in mesenchymal chondrosarcoma: A new theranostic method combining xenografted biopsies with a mathematical model. Cancer Res 2008;68:9033–40.

[49] Voskoglou-Nomikos T, Pater JL, Seymour L. Clinical predictive value of the *in vitro* cell line, human xenograft, and mouse allograft preclinical cancer models. Clin Cancer Res 2003;9:4227–39.

[50] Hidalgo M, Bruckheimer E, Rajeshkumar NV, Garrido-Laguna I, De Oliveira E, Rubio-Viqueira B, et al. A pilot clinical study of treatment guided by personalized tumorgrafts in patients with advanced cancer. Mol Cancer Ther 2011;10:1311–6.

[51] Morelli P, Calvo E, Ordoñez E, Wick MJ, Viqueira BR, Lopez-Casas PP, et al. Prioritizing Phase I treatment options through preclinical testing in personalized tumorgrafts. J Clin Oncol 2012;30(4):e45–8.

[52] Gura T. Systems for identifying new drugs are often faulty. Science 1997;278:1041–2.

[53] Steel GG, Courtenay VD, Peckham MJ. The response to chemotherapy of a variety of human tumour xenografts. Br J Cancer 1983;47:1–13.

[54] Fiebig HH, Maier A, Burger AM. Clonogenic assay with established human tumour xenografts: Correlation of *in vitro* to *in vivo* activity as a basis for anticancer drug discovery. Eur J Cancer 2004;40:802–20.

[55] Johnson JI, Decker S, Zaharevitz D, Rubinstein LV, Venditti JM, Schepartz S, et al. Relationships between drug activity in NCI preclinical *in vitro* and *in vivo* models and early clinical trials. Br J Cancer 2001;84:1424–31.

[56] Peterson JK, Houghton PJ. Integrating pharmacology and *in vivo* cancer models in preclinical and clinical drug development. Eur J Cancer 2004;40:837–44.

[57] Wilson G. Cell culture techniques for the study of drug transport. Eur J Drug Meta Pharmacokinet 1990;15:159–63.

[58] Iwatsubo T, Hirota N, Ooie T, Suzuki H, Shimada N, Chiba K, et al. Prediction of *in vivo* drug metabolism in the human liver from *in vitro* metabolism data. Pharmacol Ther 1997;73:147–71.

[59] Thummel KE, Wilkinson GR. *In vitro* and *in vivo* drug interactions involving human CYP3A. Annu Rev Pharmacol Toxicol 1998;38:389–430.

[60] CDER, CBER. Drug metabolism/drug interaction studies in the drug development process: Studies *in vitro*. Guidance for industry. Rockville, MD: FDA (Internet at, www.fda.gov/downloads/Drugs/GuidanceComplianceRegulatoryInformation/Guidances/UCM072104.pdf; 1997).

[61] Jansen WJ, Hulscher TM, van Ark-Otte J, Giaccone G, Pinedo HM, Boven E. CPT-11 sensitivity in relation to the expression of P170-glycoprotein and multidrug resistance-associated protein. Br J Cancer 1998;77:359–65.

[62] Bjornsson TD, Callaghan JT, Einolf HJ, Fischer V, Gan L, Grimm S, et al. The conduct of *in vitro* and *in vivo* drug–drug interaction studies: A PhRMA perspective. J Clin Pharmacol 2003;43(5):443–69.

[63] ICH Expert Working Group. S7A Safety pharmacology studies for human pharmaceuticals. In: Guideline IHT, editor. International Conference on Harmonisation of Technical Requirements for Registration of Pharmaceuticals for Human Use; 2000. Vol. Step 4 Version.

[64] ICH Expert Working Group. S7B The non-clinical evaluation of the potential for delayed ventricular repolarization (QT interval prolongation) by human pharmaceuticals. In: Guideline IHT, editor. International Conference on Harmonisation of Technical Requirements for Registration of Pharmaceuticals for Human Use; 2005. Vol. Step 4 Version.

[65] Suntharalingam G, Perry MR, Ward S, Brett SJ, Castello-Cortes A, Brunner MD, et al. Cytokine storm in a Phase 1 trial of the anti-CD28 monoclonal antibody TGN1412. N Engl J Med 2006;355:1018–28.

[66] Walker M, Makropoulos D, Achuthanandam R, Bugelski PJ. Recent advances in the understanding of drug-mediated infusion reactions and cytokine release syndrome. Curr Opin Drug Discov Devel 2010;13:124–35.

[67] Committee for Medicinal Products for Human Use (CHMP). Guideline on strategies to identify and mitigate risks for first-in-human clinical trials with investigational medicinal products. London: European Medicines Agency; 2007.

[68] Muller PY, Milton M, Lloyd P, Sims J, Brennan FR. The minimum anticipated biological effect level (MABEL) for selection of first human dose in clinical trials with monoclonal antibodies. Curr Opin Biotechno 2009;20:722–9.

[69] Aggarwal S. Targeted cancer therapies. Nat Rev Drug Discov 9:427–8

[70] Kwak EL, Bang YJ, Camidge DR, Shaw AT, Solomon B, Maki RG, et al. Anaplastic lymphoma kinase inhibition in non-small-cell lung cancer. N Engl J Med 2010;363:1693–703.

[71] Yap TA, Sandhu SK, Workman P, de Bono JS. Envisioning the future of early anticancer drug development. Nat Rev Cancer 2010;10:514–23.

[72] Lalonde RL, Kowalski KG, Hutmacher MM, Ewy W, Nichols DJ, Milligan PA, et al. Model-based drug development. Clin Pharmacol Ther 2007;82:21–32.

[73] Yamazaki S, Skaptason J, Romero D, Lee JH, Zou HY, Christensen JG, et al. Pharmacokinetic–pharmacodynamic modeling of biomarker response and tumor growth inhibition to an orally available cMet kinase inhibitor in human tumor xenograft mouse models. Drug Metab Dispos 2008;36:1267–74.

[74] Workman P. Auditing the pharmacological accounts for Hsp90 molecular chaperone inhibitors: Unfolding the relationship between pharmacokinetics and pharmacodynamics. Mol Cancer Ther 2003;2:131–8.

# 32

# Preclinical Prediction of Human Pharmacokinetics

**Malcolm Rowland[1,2] and Robert L. Dedrick[3]**

[1]*Centre for Applied Pharmacokinetic Research, School of Pharmacy and Pharmaceutical Sciences, University of Manchester, Manchester M13 9PT, United Kingdom*
[2]*Department of Bioengineering and Therapeutic Sciences, Schools of Pharmacy and Medicine, University of California, San Francisco, CA 94117*
[3]*National Institute of Biomedical Imaging and Bioengineering, National Institutes of Health, Bethesda, MD 20892*

## INTRODUCTION

Pharmacokinetics is an important property of a drug. It determines the temporal profiles of drug and metabolites in blood and tissues, which in turn drive the magnitude and temporal pattern of response following drug administration. Poor pharmacokinetic properties of a drug limit its clinical utility. Too rapid elimination normally necessitates frequent administration and inconvenience for the patient; too slow elimination creates potential problems when trying to remove drug in the event of intoxication. Poor oral absorption may also limit the use of this common and convenient route of administration. For these and other reasons it is important to try to ensure that new drugs under development are likely to have desirable pharmacokinetic features at potential therapeutic doses, prior to actual administration to humans. In addition, accurate prediction of human pharmacokinetics from preclinical studies, often coupled with *in vitro* human receptor occupation data, helps to design Phase I studies and to calculate the appropriate drug doses that will be needed. This chapter contains a brief discussion of the three preclinical approaches to this prediction: allometry, microdosing, and physiologic modeling, incorporating *in vitro* and physiologic data. All three approaches involve scale-up of one form or another.

## ALLOMETRY

Allometry, which is the oldest of the approaches and still widely applied in biology, is concerned with the study of the relationship between the size and function of components of the body and growth or size of the whole body. Adolph [1] observed that many physiological processes and organ sizes show a relatively simple power–law relationship with body weight when these are compared among mammals. The allometric equation proposed by Adolph is:

$$P = a(BW)^m \qquad (32.1)$$

where $P$ = physiological property or anatomic size, $a$ = empirical coefficient, $BW$ = body weight and $m$ = allometric exponent. Note that $a$ is not dimensionless; its value depends on the units in which $P$ and $BW$ are measured, while the exponent, $m$, is dimensionless and independent of the system of units. Note further that if $m = 1$, then $P$ is directly proportional to $BW$, a common approximation when considering tissue or organ mass, such and heart weight (Figure 32.1A) and skeletal muscle mass. If $m < 1$, $P$ increases less rapidly than $BW$, or, expressed per unit of body weight, $P$ decreases as body weight increases. This is frequently found with physiologic functions, such as glomerular filtration rate (Figure 32.1B),

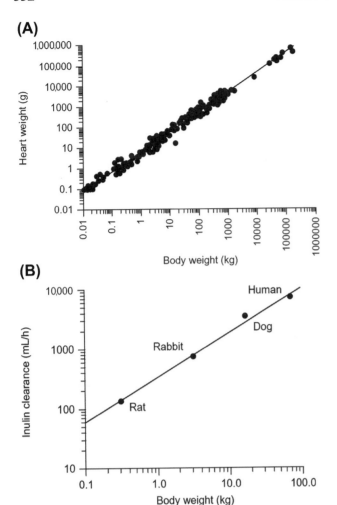

**(A)**

**(B)**

**FIGURE 32.1** Allometric relationships between body weight of mammals and: (A) heart weight, for 104 species spanning the weight range from mouse to blue whale; (B) inulin clearance, a measure of glomerular filtration rate. Note that the data are displayed as log–log plots, and that the slope of the line ($m$) is approximately 1 for heart weight and 0.75 for glomerular filtration rate. Data abstracted from Prothero J. Growth 1979;43:139–50 [2] (heart weight) and Adolf EF. Science 1949;109:579–85 [1] (inulin clearance).

cardiac output, tissue blood-flow rate, and daily heat production, with a value of $m$ centered on 0.75 in all these cases [1, 2]. Note also that the data in Figure 32.1 are displayed as log–log plots. This not only allows data for mammals of widely differing body weights, ranging between 20 g for a mouse to about 200,000 kg for a blue whale (Figure 32.1A), to be displayed on one graph, but also linearizes Equation 32.1:

$$\log P = \log a + m \log BW \qquad (32.2)$$

with the slope of the line providing the value of $m$.

While useful, general allometric correlations, such as $m = 1$ for organ weight, can obscure some interesting and important interspecies differences. Brain

size in humans and non-human primates, for example, is considerable larger than would be expected from scaling data of other mammals. Some implications of this have been discussed with reference to regional drug delivery to the brain [3].

## Use of Allometry to Predict Human Pharmacokinetic Parameters

Allometry has been widely used to make interspecies pharmacokinetic predictions [4, 5]. Given that body composition tends to vary relatively little among mammalian species, it is expected that, as with muscle mass, the volume of distribution of a drug should vary in direct proportion to body weight (i.e., $m = 1$). This reflects the fact that a drug's distribution volume is simply a function of the affinity tissues have for the drug and the size of the various tissues. On the other hand, the value of $m$ for drug clearance, being a measure of functional activity, like glomerular filtration rate, is expected to be about 0.75. As shown in Figure 32.2, the chemotherapeutic agent, cyclophosphamide is a drug that meets these expectations.

Although the difference in $m$ between 0.75 and 1 appears small, as shown in Figure 32.3 [6], the predicted value of a physiologic property varies substantially across this range of the exponential coefficient in moving from mouse to man, given the 3500-fold difference in body weight (20 g vs 70,000 g). In more concrete terms, if $m = 0.75$ for clearance of a particular drug, the clearance per unit body weight in a 20-g mouse [$20^{0.75-1}$ or $1/20^{0.25}$] would be expected to be [$(70,000)/(20)]^{0.25}$, or almost 8 times that in a 70-kg human. Furthermore, if the distribution volume is similar on a L/kg basis between the two species (e.g., cyclophosphamide) then, as a rough approximation, the elimination half life [$0.693(V/BW)/(CL/BW)$] would be 8 times shorter in the mouse than human. For example, 8 hours in a human would be pharmacokinetically equivalent on a timescale to 1 hour in a mouse. This chronologic difference should be kept in mind when undertaking safety assessment studies in small animals in which, for example, twice-daily dosing may appear to be frequent but could be associated with substantial "drug holiday" periods, during which the drug has been largely eliminated well before the end of each 12-h dosing interval.

Another property for which $m$ is approximately 0.75 is body surface area, which is the reason why physiologic functions are often said to vary in direct proportion to body surface area, both across and within species. For example, clinical dose calculations based on drug clearance are often expressed per 1.73 m$^2$, which is the average body surface area of

**(A)**

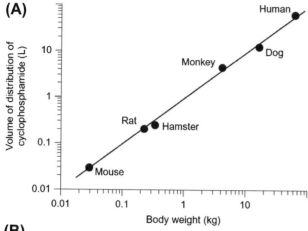

**(B)**

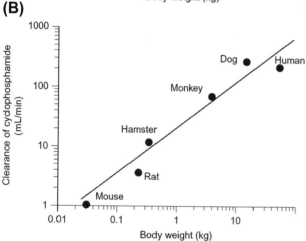

**FIGURE 32.2** Allometric relationship between (A) volume of distribution, and (B) clearance of cyclophosphamide and body weight among mammals. The exponents are 1.0 and 0.75, respectively. Note the differences in the scales of the y-axes of the two graphs. Redrawn from Boxenbaum H. J Pharmacokinet Pharmacodyn 1982;10:201–27 [4].

a 70-kg adult. Actually, the value of $m$ for surface area is closer to 0.67 ($^2/_3$) than 0.75 ($^3/_4$), but in practice the difference in prediction on scaling between 0.67 and 0.75 is acceptably small.

Dedrick *et al.* [7] used similar reasoning to demonstrate that methotrexate plasma concentration vs time data for several species were virtually superimposable, when plasma concentrations were normalized for dose/*BW* and chronological time was converted to an "equivalent time" by dividing it by species body weight raised to the 0.25 power (Figure 32.4). The form of the correlation should, in principle, be useful for interspecies plasma concentration data for other drugs. This is true for drugs that are primarily renally eliminated unchanged, because renal clearance is generally highly correlated with glomerular filtration rate [8]. However, it does not apply so well for many other drugs, especially those that are extensively metabolized.

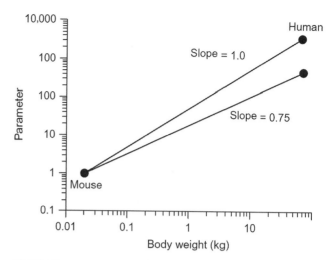

**FIGURE 32.3** Although exponents of 0.75 and 1 on relating a physiologic parameter to body weight do not appear to differ greatly, when applied across animal species that differ greatly in body weight, in this case from 0.02 kg (mouse) to 70 kg (human), the differences in the projected parameter values become large. The value of the parameter is arbitrarily set at 1 for mouse. Reproduced with permission from Rowland M, Tozer TN. Clinical Pharmacokinetics and Pharmacodynamics: Concepts and Application. Baltimore, MD: Lippincott Williams & Wilkins; 2010 [6].

## Deviation from Expectation

It is perhaps not surprising that allometric scaling frequently fails, given the simplistic assumptions set against the known complexity of biological systems. Various modifications of this scaling have been proposed to overcome discrepancies. One reason that predictions of human distribution volume fail is that there sometimes are large interspecies differences in plasma protein binding. Consequently, distribution volume predictions often are substantially improved when corrections for these differences are made, indicating that interspecies differences in overall tissue binding may be small.

Many proposals have been made for correcting clearance when the exponential coefficient $m$ deviates substantially from 0.75 [5]. However, these proposals have invariably been based on retrospective analysis of the body of combined animal *and* human data. Unfortunately, these proposals are of little value to those engaged in prospectively predicting human pharmacokinetics during preclinical drug development. Indeed, in a recent analysis of all the recommended correction strategies adopting the prospective approach, none systemically improved the allometric predictability over that with $m = 0.75$ and correcting for differences in plasma protein binding [9]. Failure to predict human clearance allometrically is particularly noticeable with relatively stable compounds – that is,

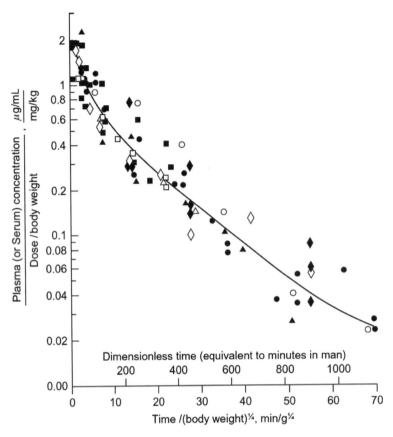

**FIGURE 32.4**   Plot of plasma concentrations of methotrexate after intravenous (IV) or intraperitoneal (IP) injection normalized for each species to dose per kg body weight vs time divided by kg body weight raised to the 0.25 power. Observations: mice, *diamonds* (IV 3 mg/kg; IP 4.5, 45, 450 mg/kg); rats, *circles* (IP 0.5, 6, 13.5, 25 mg/kg); rhesus monkey, *solid triangles* (IV 0.3 mg/kg); beagle dog, *open triangles* (IV 0.2 mg/kg); adult human patients, *squares* (IV 0.1, 1, 10 mg/ kg). Reproduced with permission from Dedrick RL, Bischof KB, Zaharko, DS. Cancer Chemother Rep 1970;54:95–101 [7].

ones with low clearance. This is because for such compounds clearance is heavily dependent on the activity of either metabolic enzymes or transporters, which often show large interspecies differences in both specificity and activity, whereas allometry assumes that the only variable is body weight. Today these are the more prevalent compounds emerging from early *in vitro* screens of stability (before *in vivo* studies), as these tend to have longer half-lives, facilitating once daily administration and lower doses to maintain therapeutic concentrations.

Beyond clearance, another common reason that allometric predictions fail is that most drugs are developed for oral administration, and gastrointestinal absorption is another major source of uncertainty. Unlike clearance and volume of distribution, the extent of oral absorption, bioavailability, is not dependent on body weight *per se*. In addition, the formulations of compounds used in preclinical

development are often very different from those given to humans. For example, it is not uncommon to administer to animals a suspension or a solution of the compound in a powerful water-miscible solvent, such as polyethylene glycol 400, whereas humans often receive capsules or tablets. This difference in formulation frequently becomes an important problem when dealing with sparingly soluble compounds, as formulation then has a profound effect on the absorption characteristics of the compound. Moreover, while the monkey might be thought to behave more similarly to humans than rats or dogs, this has not proved to be the case with respect to oral absorption, as the dog is the most reliable predictor among these species [9]. As a result of such discrepancies, considerable caution is warranted if only allometric scaling of pharmacokinetics is relied on to guide initial dose selection in Phase I clinical trials.

## MICRODOSING

Microdosing is a recent, novel, and essentially empirical approach to human pharmacokinetic prediction, which has been made possible by the development of the ultrasensitive analytical techniques discussed in Chapter 12 [10]. It involves administering to humans a minute, safe, sub-pharmacologic dose (a microdose) of the test compound (not greater than 0.1 mg) and proportionally scaling the observed pharmacokinetic profile, and hence dose, to the desired concentration–time profile intended to be evaluated in the Phase I study. Because microdosing is strictly neither a preclinical activity nor part of the normal Phase I program, it has been termed a Phase 0 study.

The microdose approach is based on two simple ideas: first, that there is no better pharmacokinetic predictor of humans than humans; and second, the assumption that the pharmacokinetics of the compound is dose proportional – that is, parameters, such as clearance, volume of distribution, and bioavailability, do not change with dose. Although essentially all processes within the body are eventually saturable if the dose is large enough, which clearly would violate the assumption of dose proportionality, it turns out that this assumption holds reasonably well for many compounds over the dose range of interest, as shown in Figure 32.5 for midazolam [11]. Exceptions to this assumption occasionally are encountered, and attempts are being made to improve predictions by coupling microdosing results with *in vitro* characterization of the saturable process. Another limitation of microdosing predictions is due to the fact that, at the minute doses administered, test compounds are invariably sufficiently soluble to dissolve in the dosing solution. As such, microdosing cannot be used to assess the performance of solid formulations, including tablets and capsules, a particular issue when dissolution of the drug critically determines its absorption. Nevertheless, early warning of a poor pharmacokinetic profile when a compound is given in solution is useful as it generally portends serious problems that are unlikely to be readily overcome by formulation efforts.

Neither microdosing nor allometry can predict pharmacokinetic events that may be encountered in studies beyond Phase I, such as the impact of genetics, disease, and age. This limitation does not apply in principle to the third approach, namely physiologically based prediction of human pharmacokinetics.

## PHYSIOLOGIC PHARMACOKINETICS

The absorption, distribution, and elimination of a drug result from a complex set of interactions that occur between drug and all tissues of the body which, together with recirculation, result in the observed concentration–time profile. In principle, it is possible to describe these events in mathematical terms and, if sufficient data are available, to predict the time course of drug and metabolite(s) in different species and at specific anatomic sites [12]. Such physiologic models have been developed to predict the pharmacokinetics of numerous compounds in humans, using a combination of anatomic, physiologic, and biochemical data, which are systems properties that are independent of the drug, coupled with drug-specific data comprising a mixture of physicochemical information, such as solubility, and *in vitro* metabolic and transporter experimental data gained using human tissue components, such as microsomes, hepatocytes, and enterocytes. Emphasis in the following section is on prediction of human pharmacokinetics, but much of the initial validation of the methods has been made in animals, and it is not uncommon to establish the appropriateness of a physiologic model for a particular drug in an animal, often the rat, prior to its application to predict events in humans.

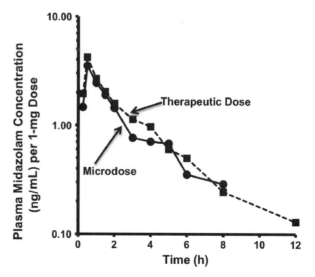

**FIGURE 32.5** An oral microdose (100 µg) (*circles*) successfully predicts the pharmacokinetics following a therapeutic oral dose of midazolam (7.5 mg) (*squares*), as evidenced by the virtual superposition of the plasma concentration–time profiles when normalized to a common 1-mg dose. Data are geometric means of observations in six subjects receiving the two 75-fold different doses on separate occasions. Redrawn from Lappin GKW, Kuhnz W, Jochemsen R *et al.* Clin Pharmacol Ther 2006;80:203–15 [11].

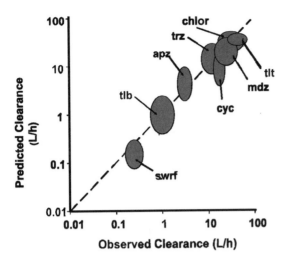

**FIGURE 32.6** Log–log plot showing a generally good accord between predicted and observed clearance in humans, including interindividual variability, for eight drugs predominantly eliminated by CYP enzymes. Prediction using a model of hepatic elimination is based on a combination of physiologic, biochemical, and demographic data together with drug-specific human data, including *in vitro* metabolic microsomal activity, and plasma and microsomal binding. The ellipses delineate the 90% confidence intervals for both predictions and observations; the dotted line is the line of identity. apz, alprazolam; chlor, chlorzoxazone; cyc, cyclosporine; mdz, midazolam; swarf, S-warfarin; tlb, tolbutamide; tlt, tolterodine; trz, triazolam. Abstracted from Howgate EM, Rowland Yeo K, Proctor NJ *et al.* Xenobiotica 2006;36:473–97 [14].

The use of *in vitro* methods to predict clearance is well established [13]. Figure 32.6 illustrates the application of the *in vitro* method to predict hepatic clearance, in this case using human hepatic expression systems containing minute amounts of the common CYP isoforms, which are primarily responsible for eliminating approximately 50% of all marketed drugs [14]. In this method, the *in vitro* metabolic activity data of the compound are scaled to the corresponding amount of enzyme in the liver and integrated in a mathematical model with other information, including binding of compound within blood, hepatic blood flow, and in some cases hepatocyte membrane permeability.

Tissue distribution estimates are an essential component of the model, but until recently their unavailability has been a major limitation in applying physiologic models due to the perceived need to obtain experimental human (or animal) drug tissue data. However, this limitation has been overcome for many compounds by the realization that tissue affinity is a function of the physicochemical properties of the compound, such as lipophilicity and degree of ionization in tissues, and the binding components within tissues, which are predominantly neutral lipids and phospholipids for neutral compounds and acidic

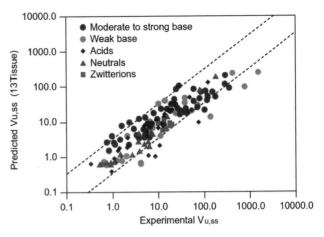

**FIGURE 32.7** Correlation between observed unbound volume of distribution at steady state ($V_{u,ss}$) and predicted values using a physiologic model of drug tissue distribution for a set of 140 diverse compounds in humans. The predicted values were based on a combination of the physicochemical properties of the compounds together with knowledge of the composition of the important binding constituents within tissues. The lines are three-fold on either side of the line of identity. Reproduced with permission from Rodgers T, Rowland M. Pharm Res 2007;24:918–33 [15].

phospholipids for bases, through ion pairing of the cation form of the base. The concentrations of these constituents vary among tissues, but are relatively fixed and known for a particular tissue. This knowledge has allowed the successful *in silico* prediction of tissue distribution in many cases, as shown in Figure 32.7 [15]. Exceptions are generally those in which the drug has a high affinity for a specific tissue-binding constituent that accounts for much of the drug in the body. Examples are some sulfonamide drugs, such as chlorthalidone, highly (and almost exclusively) bound to carbonic anhydrase, which resides predominantly within erythrocytes; doxorubicin, which extensively interacts with DNA; and digoxin, which binds to $Na^+$-$K^+$ ATPase.

Physiologic models of absorption, particularly oral absorption, are often more complex than those of elimination and tissue distribution, as can readily be seen in Figure 32.8 [16], where the gastrointestinal tract is divided into a series of sequentially connected compartments to accommodate the known heterogeneity of luminal dimension, content, structure, motility, and enzyme and transporter activity along the gastrointestinal tract. Again, much of this drug-independent information is now known. The net rate of absorption of a compound from the gastrointestinal tract is the sum of its rates of entry from each segment into the associated mesenteric blood, which then collectively drains into the hepatic portal vein and passes through the liver before entering the general

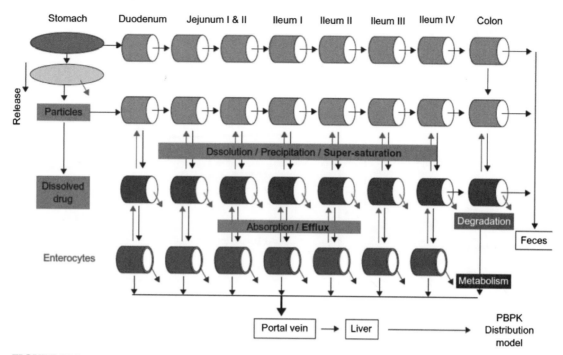

**FIGURE 32.8** An Advanced Dissolution Absorption and Metabolism (ADAM) model of events in the gastrointestinal tract. The intestine is divided into segments each comprising four compartments to account for luminal solid, particulate and dissolved drug, and drug passing through the enterocytes subject to metabolism and transport. Absorbed drug enters the physiologically based pharmacokinetic (PBPK) model characterizing systemic events via the hepatic portal vein. Modified from Jamei M, Turner D, Yang J et al. AAPS J. 2009;11:225–37 [16].

circulation. Hence, the overall systemic bioavailability of an oral dose is a function of three components operating in sequence: the fraction of the ingested dose that enters the apical membrane of the enterocyte (which is dependent on dissolution of the solid, stability in gut lumen, and permeation of the membrane); the fraction entering the enterocyte that avoids gut wall metabolism and intestinal efflux and enters the portal blood; and, finally, the fraction that escapes loss on single passage through the liver. Not surprisingly, developing drugs that are fully orally bioavailable is a challenge. Progress has also been profitably made towards development of physiologic models to accommodate other routes of drug administration, such as transdermal [17] and inhalation [18], and to represent events within specific target tissues such as brain [19] and solid tumors [20].

Physiologic pharmacokinetic models can be depicted with flow diagrams indicating the anatomic relationships among various organs and tissues, as shown in Figure 32.9. The degree of complexity of the model, in terms of the number of tissue compartments, varies with the application. In some cases, tissues such as those that are well perfused, which include the liver, kidneys, lungs and heart, and which have comparable kinetics of drug distribution, may be lumped together as a single compartment. Previously this was often done to reduce the complexity of the model to facilitate faster numerical integration of the rate equations, but with the computing power and speed now available this is less of a problem.

The accumulation of a drug within a compartment is described by an appropriate mass–balance equation, such as Equation 7.2, the equation for the well-stirred model of hepatic drug elimination that was derived in Chapter 7. As a further illustration, consider the accumulation with time of a drug in the kidney, which is assumed to eliminate the drug by a combination of glomerular filtration and saturable secretion. It is further assumed that the drug is unbound in plasma, that it is evenly distributed between plasma and blood cells, and that the concentration within the compartment is uniform and equal to that in the emergent venous blood.

$$V_K \frac{dC_{V,K}}{dt} = Q_K C_A - Q_K C_{V,K} - GFR \cdot C_A - \left[ \frac{T_{max,K} C_{V,K}}{K_{m,K} + C_{V,K}} \right]$$

(32.3)

where $V$ = volume of kidney compartment, $C$ = drug concentration, $t$ = time, $Q$ = blood flow rate, $T_{max}$ = maximum rate of secretion, $K_m$ = Michaelis-Menten

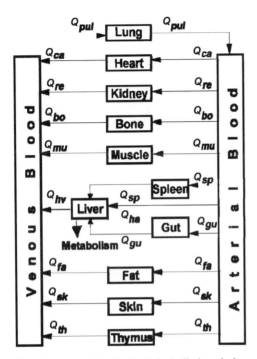

**FIGURE 32.9** A whole-body physiologically based pharmacokinetic model. $Q$ refers to blood flow. Input can be any site of the body. Elimination is depicted as occurring from only liver and kidneys, whereas it can occur also at other sites for some drugs. Some drugs can undergo enterohepatic cycling. The model can be extended to include a similar model for formed metabolites.

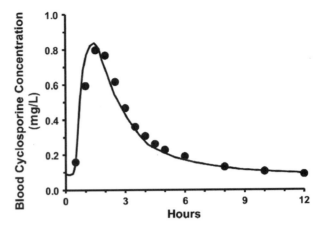

**FIGURE 32.10** Observed (●) and predicted (*solid line*) blood cyclosporine concentration–time profile within a dosing interval at steady state in renal transplant patients receiving 1.5 mg/kg orally twice daily. Measured data are the mean observations in 18 patients. The predictions were generated with the whole body physiologic model depicted in Figure 32.9, together with drug-specific information, including *in vitro* drug metabolism, intestinal permeability, binding within blood and dissolution data together with animal tissue distribution data. Redrawn from Kawai R, Mathew D, Tanaka C, Rowland M. J Pharmacol Exp Ther 1998;287:457–68 [21].

constant, $GFR$ = non-metabolic clearance, mL/min, and and the subscripts $K$, $A$ and $V$ refer to kidney, arterial and venous blood respectively.

Similar equations can be written for all relevant compartments. Once parameters are determined or chosen, the resulting set of non-linear ordinary differential equations can be solved numerically to yield predictions of the concentration of the drug in each of the compartments as a function of time. Of course, the simplifying assumptions above can be, and often are, refined to include much more detail concerning plasma and tissue binding, transport at the level of the blood capillary and cell membrane, and spatial non-uniformity, especially when dealing with gastrointestinal drug absorption. Similar equations can be written for metabolites.

Figure 32.10 compares a prediction of the expected blood concentration–time profile of cyclosporine with the observed concentrations measured in patients following oral administration of this immunosuppressive drug [21]. Cyclosporine is a neutral, lipophilic, sparingly soluble compound that is almost exclusively metabolized by CYP3A4. In this example, the prediction was based on a combination of tissue distribution information gained from animal studies, metabolism from

human hepatic tissue *in vitro*, and absorption from prior data for a micro-emulsion formulation of the drug. The compartment sizes and blood flow rates were taken from published data. In this case the prediction provides a good approximation to the observed data; however, had it been necessary or desired, the parameters of the model could have been updated to better fit the data, after first exploring the sensitivity of the blood profile to changes in each of the parameters.

Examination of Equation 32.3, or its counterpart for any eliminating organ, shows that blood flow and organ elimination interact. In general, clearance is taken to relate rate of elimination to systemic concentration. However, the driving force for elimination occurs within the cells of the eliminating organ, and the rate of the reaction related to the unbound concentration there is referred to as the *intrinsic clearance*, as it is independent of external factors such as blood flow and binding within blood. Because the organ cannot eliminate more drug than reaches it by blood flow, the absolute upper limit on the organ's contribution to rate of elimination is $QC_B$. This is known as a *blood flow or perfusion rate limitation*. This occurs when the drug is an excellent substrate for the elimination processes, in which case its intrinsic clearance is much greater than blood flow. Under these circumstances organ clearance approaches blood flow, and as organ blood flow scales well allometrically so too does the clearance of

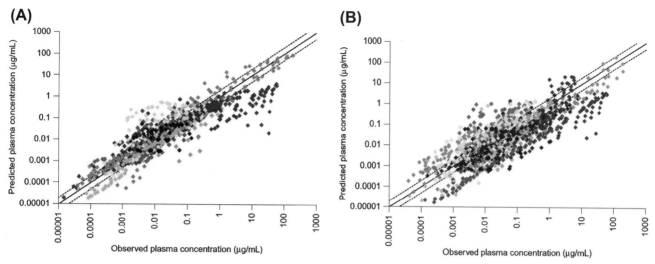

**FIGURE 32.11** Comparison of observed plasma concentrations at various times after administration of 19 compounds and those predicted by physiologically based modeling (A) and allometry (B). Each color represents the data set for a specific compound. Clinical data were available for these compounds at a range of doses after IV infusion or oral administration. The dashed lines are two-fold on either side of the line of identity. Individual concentration–time data summarized in Jones HM, Parrott N, Jorga K, Lavé T. Clin Pharmacokinet 2006;45:511–42 [22], obtained from Thierry Lavé (Roche).

such drugs. Also, for such drugs, because clearance is not limited by cellular eliminating activity, even if clearly seen *in vitro* the effects of enzyme induction or inhibition are expected to be attenuated *in vivo*. More often, however, the intrinsic clearances of drugs are relatively low, in which case the rate-controlling step is no longer blood flow but intrinsic clearance itself. Then, the impact of inhibitors and inducers should be readily apparent *in vivo*. In practice, these expectations are borne out experimentally.

As described in Chapter 3, the physiologic approach can be traced back to the 1930s but languished for many years, viewed by many in drug development as too complex and demanding, although it has been more widely employed in predicting human exposure to environmental chemicals, where often human data are lacking. However, recently the approach has gained substantial momentum and application in drug development with the availability of user-friendly commercially supported software platforms that provide not only the models but also a vast amount of relevant physiological, anatomic, and biochemical data [12]. The attractiveness of this physiological approach is several-fold. Being mechanistically based, it particularly lends itself to predict events with time for a whole array of situations, including the effects on pharmacokinetics of disease states and drug interactions. It is also both compound sparing and animal sparing, as there is often little need to study those compounds in animals that the

physiologic approach predicts would not have a pharmacokinetic profile that is relevant to humans. In addition, as Phase I and subsequent clinical data become available, the information gained can be incorporated to update and further inform the physiologic model and so improve its predictability.

Direct comparison between the physiologic model and allometry to predict first in human pharmacokinetics is limited. One such comparison, in which the physiologic approach is clearly seen to be superior to allometry, is shown in Figure 32.11 [22]. A more recent analysis of 107 orally administered compounds, representing typical drugs under current development, was more equivocal [23]. There were considerable failures with both allometry and the physiological approach, especially in the prediction of oral bioavailability, indicating that there is still need for improvement. However, further improvement is not possible with allometry, as it involves simple scaling, whereas it is with the physiologic approach. The performance of this latter method should improve as we learn more about the qualitative and quantitative factors controlling various physiological processes and continue to develop *in vitro* methods with improved *in vivo* predictability. Accordingly, because of their many advantages, physiologic models are likely to become the standard approach in the future for the preclinical prediction of human pharmacokinetics. In the meanwhile, all three methods, allometry, microdosing and physiologic pharmacokinetics, are needed.

# REFERENCES

[1] Adolph EF. Quantitative relations in the physiological constitutions of mammals. Science 1949;109:579–85.

[2] Prothero J. Heart weight as a function of body weight in mammals. Growth 1979;43:139–50.

[3] Dedrick RL, Oldfield EH, Collins JM. Arterial drug infusion with extracorporeal removal. I. Theoretic basis with particular reference to the brain. Cancer Treat Rep 1984;68:373–80.

[4] Boxenbaum H. Interspecies scaling, allometry, physiological time, and the ground plan of pharmacokinetics. J Pharmacokinet Pharmacodyn 1982;10:201–27.

[5] Mahmood I. Interspecies pharmacokinetic scaling: Principles and applications of allometric scaling. Rockville, MD: Pine House Publishers; 2005. 374pp.

[6] Rowland M, Tozer TN. Clinical pharmacokinetics and pharmacodynamics: Concepts and application. Baltimore, MD: Lippincott Williams & Wilkins; 2010.

[7] Dedrick R, Bischof KB, Zaharko DS. Interspecies correlation of plasma concentration history of methotrexate (NSC-740). Cancer Chemother Rep 1970;54:95–101.

[8] Mahmood I. Interspecies scaling of renally secreted drugs. Life Sci 1998;63:2365–71.

[9] Ring BJ, Chien JY, Adkison KK, Jones HM, Rowland M, Jones RDO, et al. PhRMA CPCDC Initiative on predictive models of human pharmacokinetics, Part 3: Comparative assessment of prediction methods of human clearance. J Pharm Sci 2011;100:4090–110.

[10] Lappin G. Microdosing: Current and the future. Bioanalysis 2010;2:509–17.

[11] Lappin GKW, Kuhnz W, Jochemsen R, Kneer J, Chaudhary A, Oosterhuis B, et al. Use of microdosing to predict pharmacokinetics at the therapeutic dose: Experience with 5 drugs. Clin Pharmacol Ther 2006;80:203–15.

[12] Rowland MP, Peck C, Tucker GT. Physiologically-based pharmacokinetics in drug development and regulatory science. Ann Rev Pharmacol Toxicol 2011;51:45–73.

[13] Ito KH, Houston JB. Comparison of the use of liver models for predicting drug clearance using *in vitro* kinetic data from hepatic microsomes and isolated hepatocytes. Pharm Res 2004;21:785–92.

[14] Howgate EM, Rowland Yeo K, Proctor NJ, Tucker GT, Rostami-Hodjegan A. Prediction of *in vivo* drug clearance from *in vitro* data. I: Impact of inter-individual variability. Xenobiotica 2006;36:473–97.

[15] Rodgers T, Rowland M. Mechanistic approaches to volume of distribution predictions: Understanding the processes. Pharm Res 2007;24:918–33.

[16] Jamei M, Turner D, Yang J, Neuhoff S, Polak S, Rostami-Hodjegan A, et al. Population-based mechanistic prediction of oral drug absorption. AAPS J 2009;11:225–37.

[17] McCarley KD, Bunge AL. Pharmacokinetic models of dermal absorption. J Pharm Sci 2001;90:1699–719.

[18] Avram MJ, Henthorn TK, Spyker DA, Krejcie TC, Lloyd PM, Casella JV, Rabinowitz JD. Recirculatory pharmacokinetic model of the uptake, distribution, and bioavailability of prochlorperazine administered as a thermally generated aerosol in a single breath to dogs. Drug Metab Dispos 2007;35:262–7.

[19] Liu X, Smith BJ, Chen C, Callegari E, Becker SL, Chen X, et al. Use of a physiologically based pharmacokinetic model to study the time to reach brain equilibrium: An experimental analysis of the role of blood–brain barrier permeability, plasma protein binding, and brain tissue binding. J Pharmacol Exp Ther 2005;313:1254–62.

[20] Modok S, Hyde P, Mellor HR, Roose T, Callaghan R. Diffusivity and distribution of vinblastine in three-dimensional tumour tissue: Experimental and mathematical modelling. Eur J Cancer 2006;42:2404–13.

[21] Kawai R, Mathew D, Tanaka C, Rowland M. Physiologically based pharmacokinetics of cyclosporine A: Extension to tissue distribution kinetics in rats and scale-up to human. J Pharmacol Exp Ther 1998;287:457–68.

[22] Jones HM, Parrott N, Jorga K, Lave T. A novel strategy for physiologically based predictions of human pharmacokinetics. Clin Pharmacokinet 2006;45:511–42.

[23] Poulin P, Jones RDO, Jones HM, Gibson CR, Rowland M, Chien JY, et al. PHRMA CPCDC initiative on predictive models of human pharmacokinetics, Part 5: Prediction of plasma concentration–time profiles in human by using the physiologically-based pharmacokinetic modeling approach. J Pharm Sci 2011;100:4127–57.

# 33

# Phase I Clinical Studies

**Jerry M. Collins**

*Developmental Therapeutics Program, Division of Cancer Treatment and Diagnosis, National Cancer Institute,*
*National Institutes of Health, Rockville, MD 20852*

## INTRODUCTION

In the drug development pipeline, Phase I clinical studies sit at the interface between the end of preclinical testing and the start of human exploration (Chapter 1, Figure 1.1). Somewhat surprisingly, this stage of drug development does not generally attract much attention. For clinical pharmacologists, as well as other practitioners of drug development, the entry of a novel molecular entity into human beings for the first time is unquestionably a very exciting event.

Some features of a Phase I study are invariant; others have changed considerably over time. On a periodic basis a set of new investigators enters the field, and almost everyone is inclined to reinvent the design features of Phase I studies. First-in-human studies are an extraordinary opportunity to integrate pharmacokinetic, pharmacodynamic, and toxicology information while launching the new molecule on a path for rational clinical development [1]. Above all, this is a major domain for application of the principles of clinical pharmacology.

The ongoing re-engineering of the entire drug development process places additional scrutiny on Phase I. Drug discovery and high-throughput screening have created a bulge in the pipeline as it heads towards the clinic. It is essential that truly useful medicines are not lost in the sheer numbers of compounds under evaluation, and it is just as essential that marginal candidates be eliminated as expeditiously as possible. Although the science generated via the discovery and development process can be dazzling, the "art" of Phase I trials requires continual focus on safety and probability of therapeutic effect [2].

The nomenclature for early clinical studies is not fully standardized. In addition to first-in-human evaluations, Phase I trials are appropriate throughout the drug development process as specific issues arise that require clinical pharmacologic investigation. Further, some exploratory first-in-human studies are currently being described as "Phase 0", in which the goals are somewhat different from classic Phase I trials.

## DISEASE-SPECIFIC CONSIDERATIONS

There is a large amount of conceptual similarity in the approach to Phase I trial design, regardless of the therapeutic area; however, there are some important differences. One major consideration is the selection of the population of human subjects for the Phase I study. For most therapeutic indications, healthy volunteers are the participants. They are compensated for the inconveniences of participating in the study, but they are not in a position to receive medical benefit. The use of healthy volunteers substantially limits the ability to observe the desired therapeutic goal. For example, if an agent is intended to correct metabolic deficiencies, or to lower elevated blood pressure, there may be no detectable changes in healthy subjects.

In several therapeutic areas, patients with the disease, rather than healthy volunteers, participate in Phase I studies,. This tradition is strongest in oncology, because many cytotoxic agents cause damage to DNA. For similar reasons, many anti-AIDS drugs are not tested initially in healthy persons. In neuropharmacology, some categories of drugs have an acclimatization or tolerance aspect, which makes them difficult to study in healthy persons [3]. On the other hand, as oncology drugs have shifted towards different targets and with milder side-effect profiles, more first-in-human trials are being conducted in healthy populations.

The primary goal of Phase I studies is always to evaluate safety in humans. When patients participate in a study, there is an additional element of therapeutic intent. In determining human safety, there has been an emphasis upon defining the maximum tolerated dose (MTD) as an endpoint of the study. Whereas determination of the MTD is important from the standpoint of clinical toxicology, the MTD has been selected in many cases as the dose for subsequent clinical trials, resulting in the registration and initial marketing of drug doses that are inappropriately high for some clinical conditions [4]. However, because the therapeutic index for anticancer drugs is so narrow, and because the disease is life-threatening, the concept of MTD has played a central role in Phase I studies of these drugs. A large portion of this author's experience with Phase I trials has been in the area of anticancer drugs; thus, the examples in this chapter will be taken from oncology.

## Starting Dose and Dose Escalation

Regardless of the details for Phase I trial design, the two essential elements are the starting dose and the dose escalation scheme. For a "first-in-human" study, selection of the starting dose is caught in a conflict between a desire for safety (leading to a cautious choice) vs an interest in efficiency. When patients take part in a Phase I trial, efficiency is also tied to a desire to provide therapeutic benefit, and can stimulate a more aggressive choice of starting dose.

The same conflicts exist for the escalation scheme. Once the current dose level has been demonstrated to be safe, the move to the next higher level is clouded by uncertainty about the steepness of the dose–toxic response curve. Recently, there has been an appreciation of the linkage between choices for starting dose and escalation rate. In particular, the combination of a cautious starting dose with a very conservative escalation rate can lead to trials that are so lengthy that they serve the interests of no one.

## Modified Fibonacci Escalation Scheme

Some version of the modified Fibonacci escalation scheme is probably the most frequently-used escalation scheme, particularly in oncologic Phase I studies. However, its pre-eminence is fading. The sequence of escalation steps for a typical scheme is shown in Figure 33.1. Implicit in the design of this scheme is an

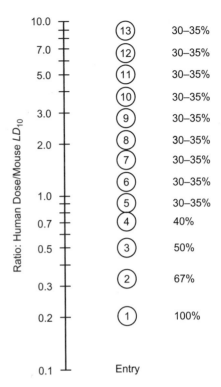

**FIGURE 33.1** Modified Fibonacci dose escalation procedure, expressed as a ratio of the human dose to a reference dose in mice [e.g., the 10% lethal dose ($LD_{10}$)]. Human studies typically start at one-tenth the murine dose, expressed on the basis of body surface area. If tolerated, the next dose is initially doubled, then the percentage change at each escalation step decreases. Reproduced from Collins JM, Zaharko DS, Dedrick RL, Chabner BA. Cancer Treat Rep 1986;70:73–80 [6].

attempt to balance caution and aggressiveness. Rapid increases in dose are prescribed at early stages of the trial (i.e., starting with a doubling of the dose), when the chance of administering a non-toxic dose is highest. The incremental changes in dose become more conservative at later stages (e.g., 30%) when the probability of encountering side effects has increased. When a modified Fibonacci design is submitted to the local review board and regulatory authorities for approval, the escalation rate is completely determined in advance and is adhered to throughout the trial, at least until toxicity intervenes.

Many variations of the Fibonacci scheme have arisen, driven by statistical and/or pharmacologic principles. In particular, accelerated titration designs have been replacing standard Fibonacci schemes in many oncologic studies [5]. From the perspective of clinical pharmacology, a particularly attractive goal is to integrate whatever is known about the properties of the drug into an adaptive design. One type of adaptive design modulates the rate of dose escalation based upon plasma concentrations of the drug, as described in the next section. The formal application of adaptive design has declined as empirical schemes have become more efficient, but the inclusion of specific pharmacokinetic, pharmacodynamic, and pharmaco-genetic tasks has risen steeply.

## Pharmacologically-Guided Dose Escalation

The pharmacologically-guided dose escalation (PGDE) design is based upon a straightforward pharmacokinetic–pharmacodynamic hypothesis: when comparing animal and human doses, expect equal toxicity for equal drug exposure [6, 7]. A fundamental principle of clinical pharmacology is that drug effects are caused by circulating concentrations of the unbound ("free") drug molecule, and are less tightly linked to the administered dose (see Chapter 2, Figure 2.1). The advantage of PGDE is that it mini-mizes the numbers of patients at risk, and pays more attention to the individual patient's risk of receiving too low a dose. A series of Phase I studies were found to be excessively lengthy because a starting dose was chosen that was too low, thus pushing the major portion of the trial into the conservative portion of the modified Fibonacci design.

As illustrated in Figure 33.2, for PGDE there is a continual evaluation of plasma concentrations as the trial is under way. Thus, unlike a modified Fibonacci design, the escalation rate is adapted throughout the procedure. Although the decisions are expressed in terms of pharmacokinetics (plasma concentrations of the drug), the design is named "pharmacologic" because it is intended to permit adjustments in the target plasma concentration, based upon pharmaco-dynamic information, such as species differences in the 90% inhibitory concentration ($IC_{90}$) for bone marrow or tumor cell proliferation.

A retrospective survey was conducted prior to embarking on "real-time" use of PGDE. The results shown in Figure 33.3 permit a comparison of limiting doses in humans vs mice. The doses used for this comparison were normalized for body surface area (e.g., $100 \, \text{mg/m}^2$) which is exceptional for any other therapeutic class. The use of body surface area in clinical dosing for oncology has faded substantially, but it remains an excellent metric for cross-species comparisons.

There are two major conclusions from an evaluation of the data in Figure 33.3:

1. There is enormous scatter in the ratio of human: murine tolerable doses. Thus, while murine doses may seem to give reasonable predictions for acceptable human doses on the average, there is no predictive consistency that could be relied upon for any specific drug about to enter Phase I study.
2. The drug exposure in terms of area under the plasma-level vs time curve ($AUC$) ratio at approxi-mately equitoxic doses has much less variability, indicating that pharmacokinetic differences account for almost all of the differences observed for toxic doses of this set of drugs between humans and mice.

What is the underlying cause for these interspecies differences? For equal doses, differences in plasma $AUC$ values simply indicate differences in total body clearance. Renal and metabolic elimination processes are the major contributors to total body clearance. When allometric scaling is used as described in Chapter 32, renal clearance tends to exhibit only small differ-ences across species, whereas there are many examples of interspecies differences in metabolism. Further, across many drug categories, metabolism is quantita-tively more important than renal elimination. There-fore, more emphasis on interspecies differences in drug metabolism could improve Phase I studies. The next two sections provide specific examples of the impact of monitoring metabolism during early human studies.

## Interspecies Differences in Drug Metabolism

The data in Table 33.1 for iododeoxydoxorubicin (I-Dox) were obtained during first-in-human studies conducted by Gianni *et al.* [8]. There was greater expo-sure to the parent drug in mice, and to the hydroxylated metabolite (I-Dox-ol) in humans. Overall, there was a 50-fold difference in the relative $AUC$ exposure ratios (metabolite : parent drug) for humans and mice. Because I-Dox and I-Dox-ol are approximately equi-effective and equitoxic, these exposure comparisons are also indicative of pharmacologic response. This extreme example of an interspecies difference in drug metabo-lism was comparable to studying one molecule (the

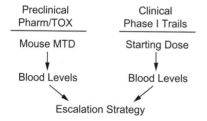

**FIGURE 33.2** Pharmacologically-guided dose escalation shown as an alternative to the fixed procedure for increasing doses (e.g., Figure 31.1). The size of each dose escalation step is based on current concentrations of drug in human blood, along with target concen-trations defined in preclinical studies. MTD, maximum tolerated dose.

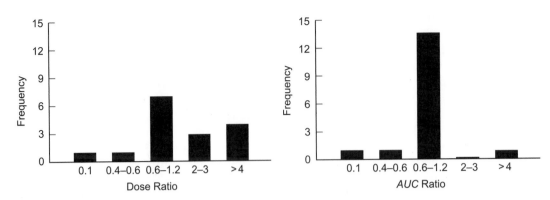

**FIGURE 33.3** Survey of acute toxicity of anticancer drugs in humans vs mice. Comparisons based upon dose (*left panel*) exhibit more scatter than do those based on drug exposure (*AUC*) (*right panel*).

**TABLE 33.1** *AUC* Values in Plasma for Iododeoxydoxorubicin (I-Dox) and Its Metabolite (I-Dox-ol) in Mouse and Human Equitoxic Doses

| Compound | Mouse (µM/h) | Human (µM/h) |
|----------|--------------|--------------|
| I-Dox    | 5.0          | 0.3          |
| I-Dox-ol | 1.2          | 4.0          |

Data from Gianni L, Vigano L, Surbone A *et al.* J Natl Cancer Inst 1990;82:469–77 [8].

parent) in mice, and then (unintentionally) studying a different molecule (the metabolite) in humans. The similarity in potency of the parent molecule and metabolite was fortuitous and not expected ordinarily, especially for both desirable and adverse effects.

Figure 33.4 illustrates an interspecies difference in paclitaxel metabolism [9]. The principal metabolite formed in humans was not produced by rat microsomes. This example illustrates the potential of *in vitro* studies to discover interspecies differences in metabolism. In most cases it is no longer necessary to wait for *in vivo* Phase I studies to discover such differences, and certainly not advisable. Regulatory authorities around the world have encouraged early consideration of interspecies metabolic comparisons.

## Active Metabolites

During first-in-human studies with the investigational anticancer drug penclomedine, it was discovered that exposure to parent drug concentrations was less than 1% of the exposure to its metabolite, demethylpenclomedine [10]. As shown in Figure 33.5, exposure to the parent drug was very brief, while the metabolite accumulated during the course of a 5-day treatment cycle. Because the toxicity of the parent molecule limits the amount of tolerable exposure to the metabolite, which provides the antitumor effect,

the penclomedine case clearly demonstrates the danger of not knowing which molecules are circulating in the body. If this type of information is determined early enough in drug development, the metabolite can be selected to replace the parent molecule as the lead development candidate.

There is stunning similarity of the penclomedine story to the history of terfenadine (Seldane™), a highly

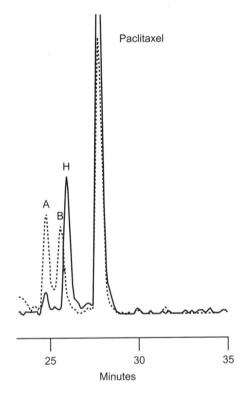

**FIGURE 33.4** High-performance liquid chromatograms comparing *in vitro* paclitaxel metabolism by hepatic microsomes from rats (*dotted line*) and humans (*solid line*). The major human metabolite, designated peak "H", was not formed by rats. Adapted from Jamis-Dow CA, Klecker RW, Katki AG, Collins JM. Cancer Chemother Pharmacol 1995;6:107–14 [9].

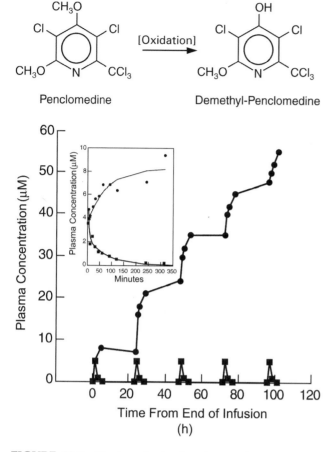

FIGURE 33.5  The investigational anticancer drug, penclomedine, was administered to patients once a day for 5 consecutive days. The parent drug disappeared rapidly from plasma, whereas the demethyl metabolite accumulated over the course of therapy. Adapted from Hartman NR, O'Reilly S, Rowinsky EK *et al.* Clin Cancer Res 1996;2:953–62 [10].

successful antihistamine product that was withdrawn from marketing. In early clinical studies, it was not appreciated that the major source of clinical benefit was its metabolite, fexofenadine (Allegra™; see structures in Chapter 1, Figure 1.2). It became obvious that the metabolite should have been the lead compound only after cardiotoxicity was subsequently discovered for the parent drug but not the metabolite.

## BEYOND TOXICITY

The study of toxicity without consideration of efficacy is inherently unsatisfying. Indeed, when patients participate in Phase I trials, there is always therapeutic intent. Realistically, there is only a low probability of success in many settings, but the obligation is to maximize that chance. As it becomes more common to seek "proof-of-concept" or mechanistic evaluations

during Phase I, an increased emphasis on demonstrating therapeutic activity – the usual domain for Phase II studies – looms on the horizon. By monitoring a target biomarker, both proof-of-concept and dose determination might be achieved simultaneously. Further, by enrolling in the trial patients that have favorable expression profiles of the target, an "enriched" population is obtained with a higher likelihood of response, if the therapeutic concept has merit.

For "accessible" targets such as blood pressure or heart rate, these concepts are not new. The techniques of external, non-invasive imaging described in Chapter 19 now permit real-time monitoring of targets such as *in situ* regions of the human brain that were previously considered inaccessible. Fowler *et al.* [11] reported a study of the inhibition of monoamine oxidase, type B (MAO-B) by lazabemide (Figure 33.6). A dose of 25 mg twice a day inhibited most MAO-B activity in subjects, and doubling the dose to 50 mg abolished all detectable activity. Also, brain activity for MAO-B had returned to baseline values within 36 hours of the last dose of lazabemide. This example of MAO-B inhibition demonstrates the successful investigation in early human studies of three areas of fundamental interest in developing drug therapy (Table 33.2): monitoring impact at the desired target, evaluating the dose–response relationship

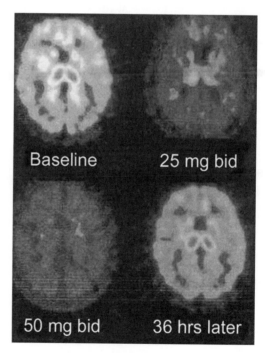

FIGURE 33.6  PET scans showing dose dependency and time dependency of lazabemide inhibition of monoamine oxidase, type B in human brain. Reproduced with permission from Fowler JS, Volkow ND, Wang G-J, Dewey SL. J Nucl Med 1999;40:1154–63 [11].

**TABLE 33.2 Therapeutic Issues for Drug Development**

- Does treatment impact the desired target?
- What is the minimum/maximum dose?
- What dose (therapeutic course) interval is appropriate?

(dose-ranging), and determining an appropriate dose interval from recovery of enzyme activity.

The expansion of Phase I studies to include goals formerly reserved for Phase II evaluation is only one direction of change. Simultaneously, the toxicity goals of Phase I studies are being decoupled from evaluations of drug absorption, distribution, metabolism, and excretion (ADME). As described in Chapter 32, both United States and European regulators now permit microdose studies that include both metabolism and excretion components as well as tracer doses for imaging [12, 13]. In both regulatory sectors, the preclinical requirements for first-in-human studies are substantially reduced for situations in which doses are kept low to minimize risk to study participants. This structural change facilitates the type of translational research that has been described as Phase 0 or Pre-Phase I.

Re-engineering of the entire drug development pipeline is stimulated by these opportunities to change the traditional goals of early drug development. However, this blurring of the traditional lines of demarcation between clinical phases of drug development has its pitfalls and disorienting aspects, and not all development organizations will adopt such changes. Indeed, there should always be a place for diversity in approaches to drug development. Nonetheless, the early harvesting of benefits from investments in biomarkers presents exciting new opportunities for clinical pharmacologists and other stakeholders in drug development.

# REFERENCES

[1] Peck CC, Barr WH, Benet LZ, Collins J, Desjardins RE, Furst DE, et al. Opportunities for integration of pharmacokinetics, pharmacodynamics, and toxicokinetics in rational drug development. Clin Pharmacol Ther 1992;51:465–73.

[2] Peck CC, Collins JM. First time in man studies: A regulatory perspective – art and science of Phase I trials. J Clin Pharmacol 1990;30:218–22.

[3] Cutler NR, Stramek JJ. Scientific and ethical concerns in clinical trials in Alzheimer's patients: The bridging study. Eur J Clin Pharmacol 1995;48:421–8.

[4] Rolan P. The contribution of clinical pharmacology surrogates and models to drug development – a critical appraisal. Br J Clin Pharmacol 1997;44:219–25.

[5] Simon R, Freidlin B, Rubinstein L, Arbuck SG, Collins J, Christian MC. Accelerated titration designs for Phase I clinical trials in oncology. J Natl Cancer Inst 1997;89:1138–47.

[6] Collins JM, Zaharko DS, Dedrick RL, Chabner BA. Potential roles for preclinical pharmacology in Phase I trials. Cancer Treat Rep 1986;70:73–80.

[7] Collins JM, Grieshaber CK, Chabner BA. Pharmacologically-guided Phase I trials based upon preclinical development. J Natl Cancer Inst 1990;82:1321–6.

[8] Gianni L, Vigano L, Surbone A, Ballinari D, Casali P, Tarella C, et al. Pharmacology and clinical toxicity of 4′-iodo-4′-deoxy-doxorubicin: An example of successful application of pharmacokinetics to dose escalation in Phase I trials. J Natl Cancer Inst 1990;82:469–77.

[9] Jamis-Dow CA, Klecker RW, Katki AG, Collins JM. Metabolism of taxol by human and rat liver *in vitro*: A screen for drug interactions and interspecies differences. Cancer Chemother Pharmacol 1995;6:107–14.

[10] Hartman NR, O'Reilly S, Rowinsky EK, Collins JM, Strong JM. Murine and human *in vivo* penclomedine metabolism. Clin Cancer Res 1996;2:953–62.

[11] Fowler JS, Volkow ND, Wang G-J, Dewey SL. PET and drug research and development. J Nucl Med 1999;40:1154–63.

[12] CDER Exploratory IND Studies. Draft guidance for industry, investigators, and reviewers. Rockville, MD: FDA (Internet at, www.fda.gov/downloads/Drugs/GuidanceCompliance RegulatoryInformation/Guidances/UCM078933.pdf.; 2006).

[13] CDER, CBER. M3(R2) Nonclinical safety studies for the conduct of human clinical trials and marketing authorization for pharmaceuticals. Guidance for industry. Silver Spring, MD: FDA. (Internet at, www.fda.gov/downloads/Drugs/GuidanceComplianceRegulatoryInformation/Guidances/UCM073246.pdf.; 2010).

# 34

# Pharmacokinetic and Pharmacodynamic Considerations in the Development of Biotechnology Products and Large Molecules

Pamela D. Garzone

*Clinical Research, Pfizer Inc., South San Francisco, CA 94080*

## INTRODUCTION

The original introduction of Chapter 32 started with the sentence "In 2004, the FDA approved 36 new medical entities and 5 new biologics". In 2011, this sentence can read: "In 2010, the FDA approved 15 new molecular entities and 6 new biologics" [1]. Biologics accounted for slightly more than 25% of the approved entities and this percentage is expected to increase. To support this notion, by the end of November 2011 the FDA had approved 34 new molecular entities and 13 biologics that included 3 monoclonal antibodies (mABs) [2]. For the purpose of this chapter, a macromolecule is defined as a large molecule, with a molecular mass in kilodaltons (kDa), such as a protein or glycoprotein, or a monoclonal antibody, either as an intact immunoglobulin or as its fragments.

Well-known macromolecules that have been approved and are currently marketed are listed in Table 34.1. This chapter presents information on proteins and mAbs currently marketed or under investigation and discusses methodology used to assay macromolecules, interspecies scaling of macromolecules, pharmacokinetic (PK) characteristics of macromolecules, and pharmacodynamics (PD) of macromolecules.

## MONOCLONAL ANTIBODIES

Monoclonal antibodies (mAbs) were initially considered "magic bullets" offering, for the first time, targeted therapy against specific tumor surface antigens. The development of mAbs as diagnostic aids and as therapy was made possible by advances in hybridoma technology [3]. The first murine monoclonal antibody trial was published in 1982 [4]. However, in the 1980s and early 1990s most of the murine mAbs failed in clinical trials. The major drawback was the inefficient interaction of the Fc component of the mouse antibody with human effector functions [5]. Also, the repeated administration of mouse antibodies to humans resulted in the production of a human antimouse antibody (HAMA) response that reduced the effectiveness of the murine antibody or resulted in allergic reactions in humans.

The first murine mAb was approved for marketing in 1986, when Orthoclone (CD3-specific antibody) or OKT3 was approved. Now, humanized and fully human antibodies, engineered so that HAMA response is neglible, have become mainstream therapy with such recent successes as Erbitux®, Avastin®, and Simponi® (Table 34.1). A successful antibody also needs to be potent and specific [6]. The following sections describe how engineered antibodies can be produced to meet these requirements.

### Antibody Structure and Production

The basic structure of an immunoglobulin (Ig) antibody, IgG, is shown in Figure 34.1 [7]. The IgG molecule consists of the Fc region and the Fab region allowing for multivalency, high avidity, and specificity.

**TABLE 34.1    Examples of Currently Marketed Macromolecules**

| Macromolecule | Abbreviation | Trade name |
|---|---|---|
| Adalimumab | | Humira |
| Alemtuzumab | | Campath |
| Belimumab | | Benlysta |
| Bevacizumab | | Avastin |
| Cetuximab | | Erbitux |
| Denosumab | | Prolia |
| Golimumab | | Simponi |
| Erythropoietin | Epo | Epogen |
| Factor VIII | | Advate |
| Factor IX | FIX | BeneFIX |
| Growth hormone | GH | Nutropin |
| Granulocyte colony-stimulating factor | G-CSF | Neupogen |
| Granulocyte-macrophage colony-stimulating factor | GM-CSF | Leukine |
| Interleukin-2 | IL-2 | Proleukin |
| Natalizumab | | Tysabri |

It should be noted that IgG sequences are conserved across species such that considerable homology between mouse and human variable regions exists [8]. Mouse antibodies can be further engineered by molecular cloning and expression of the variable region of IgG to be more human, or they can be fully human. Fully human mAbs, derived from transgenic mice or human antibody libraries, are the current state-of-the-art of mAb bioengineering.

Monoclonal antibodies, by definition, are produced by a single clone of hybridoma cells, i.e., a single species of antibody molecule (Figure 34.2) [9]. However, engineered monoclonal antibodies can be chimeras, in which the Fv region from mouse IgG is fused with the variable region of the human IgG. Monoclonal antibodies can be humanized so that only the complementary determining regions of the murine

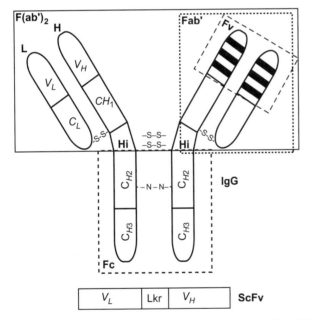

**FIGURE 34.1** Structure of prototypical IgG and single-chain FV (scFV) antibody molecules. The large solid-line box encloses the divalent Fab' molecules; the small dotted line box, the Fab' fragment; the large dashed-line box, the Fc components; and the small dashed-line box, the Fv components which are the antigen binding sites. The variable light-chain region is designated $V_L$ and variable heavy-chain region is designated $V_H$. Other definitions: constant region domains, $C_{H1}$, $C_{H2}$, $C_{H3}$; hinge, Hi; constant light region, $C_L$; linker region, Lkr. Conserved N-linked (–N–N–) carbohydrates are located in the Fc domain; cysteine bond (–S–S–) join heavy and light chains. Reproduced with permission from Colcher D, Goel A, Pavlinkova G et al. Q J Nucl Med. 1999;43:132–9 [7].

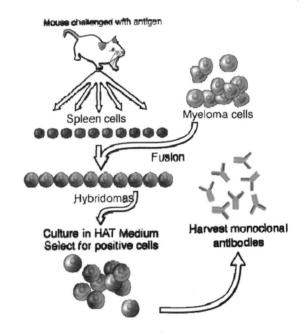

Abbreviations: **HAT** is a culture medium that contains hypoxanthine, aminopterin, and thymidine.
Ref: http://en.wikipedia.org/wiki/Monoclonal_antibodies

**FIGURE 34.2** Cartoon depicting monoclonal antibody production. A mouse is immunized by injection of an antigen to stimulate the production of antibodies targeted against it. The antibody-forming cells are isolated from the mouse's spleen. Monoclonal antibodies are produced by fusing single antibody-forming cells to tumor cells grown in culture. The resulting cell is called a *hybridoma*. Each hybridoma produces relatively large quantities of identical antibody molecules. By allowing the hybridoma to multiply in culture it is possible to produce a population of cells, each of which produces identical antibody molecules. These antibodies are called *monoclonal antibodies* because they are produced by the identical offspring of a single, cloned antibody-producing cell. Reproduced with permission from Access Excellence @ the National Health Museum;1999. (Internet at: http://www.accessexcellence.org/RC/VL/GG/monoclonal.html.) [9].

variable region are combined into the human variable region. In addition to being full length, mAbs can be single-chain IgG, the simplest fragment being the scFV (single-chain variable fragment). The scFV can be a monomer, dimer, or tetramer; this multivalency results in a significant increase in functional affinity [10]. Further, in addition to the diversity of engineered antibodies, other molecules can be attached to the antibody, such as enzymes, toxins, viruses, radionuclides, and biosensors for targeting, imaging or diagnosing. These are commonly referred to as antibody drug conjugates, or ADC.

The production of antibodies appears to be simple (Figure 34.2). However, their commercialization is challenging. The need for specificity makes the market small; thus, the costs of doing clinical trials for small markets are unattractive to most companies. Quality control of the production and manufacture of monoclonal antibodies is another issue, since a high degree of purification and low degree of contamination is necessary before approval. Finally, a major limitation is the stability of the mammalian cells expressing the immunoglobulin [7].

## Pharmacokinetic Properties of Monoclonal Antibodies

Many of the factors affecting the PK of mAbs are similar to those affecting other macromolecules, and these principles are explored in the following sections. However, the optimal mAb dose and schedule also are determined by several additional factors, such as the avidity of the antibody and the specific antibody–antigen system, the species being treated with the mAb, and the mAb itself. Dose selection influences mAb distribution into organs and tissues and liver uptake. At lower doses target-mediated clearance may be observed, particularly with mAbs directed at cell-surface targets. With increasing dose, saturation of binding sites, including non-specific binding, is expected to occur and results in decreased clearance and greater availability of the antibody to the target. The approved mAbs listed in Table 34.1 have diverse pharmacokinetic properties. For example, Avastin claims linear pharmacokinetics in a dose range of 1–10 mg/kg while Erbitux demonstrates non-linearity at doses greater than 200 mg/m$^2$.

The most characteristic features of mAbs are their low blood clearance and prolonged elimination half-life. It has been demonstrated for both intact mAbs and fragments that clearance is inversely related to molecular size (Table 34.2) [11, 12]. Detailed investigations have been undertaken to explore the specific IgG structures that may affect clearance and half-life.

**TABLE 34.2 Proposed Human Plasma Clearance of Different Antibody Molecules**

| Antibody molecule | Molecular weight (kD) | Relative plasma clearance (CL) |
|---|---|---|
| Native intact human IgG | 150 | ≈ 21 days |
| Fully human/humanized | 150 | |
| Chimeric human-mouse IgG | 150 | |
| Whole mouse IgG | 150 | |
| F(ab)$_2$ | 110 | |
| Fab' | 50 | |
| Single chain FV (scFV) | 25 | ≈ 1 day |

Adapted from Iznaga-Escobar N, Mishra Ak, Perez-Rodriguez R. Methods Find Exp Clin Pharmacol 2004; 26: 123–7 [12].

In particular, the Fc receptor, FcRn (neonatal MHC class I-related receptor), has been shown to play a central role in determining IgG half-life, and specific sequences in the $C_{H2}$ and $C_{H3}$ regions of IgG regulate clearance rate through their interaction with FcRn [13].

While the prolonged half-life of a mAb is usually advantageous, allowing for infrequent administration, it also has some disadvantages. For example, mAbs with the longest half-lives and lowest clearance rates diffuse poorly across tumor membranes. This feature can result in significant exposure to normal tissues and organs when effective antitumor doses are administered. In contrast, scFV fragments, one of the smallest functional amino acid sequences of antibodies, have more rapid clearance and better penetration of tumor mass than intact mAbs, yet retain high-affinity binding (Table 34.3) [13]. Also, tumor-to-blood concentration ratios appear to be higher and less heterogeneous with multivalent scFvs than with intact antibody. F(ab)$_2$ elimination clearance appears to be similar to intact IgG, but with a faster distribution to tissues from blood and a higher uptake in kidneys. Other fragments, such as Fab', sc(Fv)$_2$, (scFv)$_2$, and scFv have lower uptake in tissues due to their rapid elimination. For example, approximately 90% of scFvs are cleared from the body in 24 hours. Lastly, the charge of a mAb has been shown to affect PK and tissue distribution due to electrostatic and hydrophobic interactions between mammalian cell membrane lipid bilayers and negatively charged proteins [14]. Factors that may influence the effects of charge on mAb PK and tissue distribution include the magnitude of the change in isoelectric point (pI), the IgG isotype (i.e., IgG$_1$, IgG$_2$, IgG$_4$), the location of the charge (e.g., variable region vs the constant region of the IgG molecule), and the binding avidity. Cationization, the chemical conversion of surface carboxyl groups on aspartate or glutamate to primary amino groups, can raise the pI of

**TABLE 34.3** Tumor, Kidney and Blood Distribution, as Percentage of Dose per Gram of Iodinated Antibody Fragments of CC49

| Antibody fragment | Tissue | Time (h) | | | | |
|---|---|---|---|---|---|---|
| | | 0.5 | 4.0 | 24.0 | 48.0 | 72.0 |
| scFv | Tumor | 4.74 | 2.93 | 1.06 | 0.72 | 0.27 |
| | Blood | 4.66 | 1.32 | 0.06 | 0.04 | 0.05 |
| | Kidneys | 41.24 | 2.65 | 0.15 | 0.07 | 0.06 |
| (scFv)$_2$ | Tumor | 5.94 | 6.91 | 4.29 | 2.56 | 1.92 |
| | Blood | 19.27 | 2.56 | 0.10 | 0.07 | 0.07 |
| | Kidneys | 32.83 | 2.93 | 0.42 | 0.13 | 0.08 |
| Sc(Fv)$_2$ | Tumor | 6.12 | 6.78 | 4.29 | 2.62 | 1.94 |
| | Blood | 18.30 | 2.17 | 0.07 | 0.06 | 0.07 |
| | Kidneys | 27.85 | 2.32 | 0.36 | 0.12 | 0.07 |
| Fab′ | Tumor | 4.87 | 5.91 | 2.96 | 2.15 | ND[a] |
| | Blood | 9.63 | 2.38 | 0.1 | 0.06 | ND |
| | Kidneys | 138.34 | 21.50 | 0.37 | 0.16 | ND |
| F(ab′)$_2$ | Tumor | 14.63 | 25.82 | 28.06 | 19.42 | 13.11 |
| | Blood | 30.15 | 16.32 | 1.68 | 0.36 | 0.16 |
| | Kidneys | 11.48 | 9.78 | 2.10 | 0.52 | 0.25 |
| IgG | Tumor | 8.95 | 30.66 | 37.83 | 42.42 | ND |
| | Blood | 28.32 | 24.20 | 11.01 | 5.34 | ND |
| | Kidneys | 7.0 | 5.29 | 2.19 | 1.18 | ND |

[a]ND, not determined.
Adapted from Colcher D, Pavlinkova G, Beresford G *et al.* Ann NY Acad Sci 1999;880:263–80 [13].

macromolecules [15]. Raising the pI of mAbs has been shown to increase the rate of clearance of an IgG2a cationized mAb from the blood, resulting in higher tissue concentrations relative to a native IgG2a mAb in mice [15, 16]. In contrast, in mice given IgG4 antibodies with pIs ranging from 7.2 to 9.2, the elimination half-life increased with increasing pI [17].

As noted earlier, the earliest mAbs were derived entirely from mouse proteins and caused highly immunogenic reactions in patients. This reaction, the HAMA response, was against both the constant and the variable regions of the proteins. In addition to the signs and symptoms of the HAMA response that included the classic allergic hallmarks of urticaria, anaphylaxis, and fever, this response resulted in attenuated mAb activity due to the formation of neutralizing antibodies and rapid clearance of the resulting immune complex. Although the HAMA response has been mitigated by the development of humanized or fully human antibodies, these antibodies still can elicit anti-allotypic or anti-idiotypic antibody responses [12].

## ASSAY OF MACROMOLECULES

The most common types of assays employed to quantitate protein and mAb concentrations in biologic matrices are listed in Table 34.4. Radioimmunoassays

(RIA), radioreceptor assays (RRA), and immunoradiometric assays (IRMA) require radioactivity and have been largely replaced by enzyme-linked immunoabsorbent assays (ELISAs), which are based on antibody recognition of an antigenic epitope (i.e., a molecular region on the surface of a molecule capable of binding to the specific antibody). More recently, electrochemiluninescence (ECL) immunoassays have been developed and utilized in drug development because they provide a modest improvement in sensitivity and extended dynamic assay range.

The bioanalysis of biologics is far more complex than the assays of small molecules that are described in Chapter 12. Unlike small molecules, which can be extracted from matrices and subsequently analyzed, biologics are analyzed in a matrix containing other proteins that may cause interference, or soluble ligands that can be upregulated and prevent binding of the

**TABLE 34.4** Examples of Immunoassays Used to Quantitate Macromolecules

| Assay acronym | Assay description |
|---|---|
| ECL Immunoassay | Electrochemiluminescence immunoassay |
| ELISA | Enzyme-linked immunosorbent assay |
| RIA | Radioimmunoassay |
| IRMA | Immunoradiometric assay |
| RRA | Radioreceptor assay |

protein's or mAb's eptitope. An example of an interfering substance is rheumatoid factor (RF), a heterophilic antibody that is a normal secondary immune response to many antigens. RF interferes with many assays of IgG mAbs by binding to the Fc portion of IgG, but this interference can be circumvented by using anti-idiotype (anti-ID) antibodies in the assay construct. Anti-idiotype antibodies are antigenic determinants created by the combining site of an antibody, called *idiotypes*, and the antibodies elicited to the idiotypes, called anti-Id antibodies. Anti-idiotypic antibodies are those directed against the hypervariable regions of an antibody.

Macromolecules that have a particularly complex structure – such as trastuzumab-DMI, a humanized IgG1 specific for human EGF receptor that is conjugated to the cytotoxic maytansine derivative DM1which binds to microtubules – require orthogonal assay methods to fully characterize their PK/PD and to further our understanding of the biology of these molecules. Such orthogonal methods include multiple ELISAs, to measure total, bound, and free antibody; liquid chromatography; tandem mass spectrometry (LC-MS/MS) for free cytotoxin; bioactivity assays; and affinity capture–mass spectrometry (AC-MS). For further detail, the reader is referred to a review of the bioanalysis of macromolelcules [18] and to a report on the consensus of the AAPS Ligand-binding Assay Bioanalytical Focus Group on strategies for determing total and free concentrations of mAbs [19].

## INTERSPECIES SCALING OF MACROMOLECULES: PREDICTIONS IN HUMANS

As discussed in Chapter 32 and elsewhere [20], interspecies scaling is based upon allometry or physiology. Protein PK parameters such as volume of distribution ($V_d$), elimination half-life ($t_{1/2}$), and elimination clearance ($CL$) have been scaled across species using the standard allometric equation [21]:

$$Y = aW^b \tag{34.1}$$

In this equation, $Y$ is the parameter of interest, the coefficient $a$ is the value of the parameter at one unit of body weight, $W$ is body weight, and $b$ is the allometric exponent. For convenience, this equation is linearized to:

$$\log Y = \log a + b \log W \tag{34.2}$$

In this form, $\log a$ is the $y$-intercept and $b$ is the slope of the line. In Figure 34.3, representative linearized

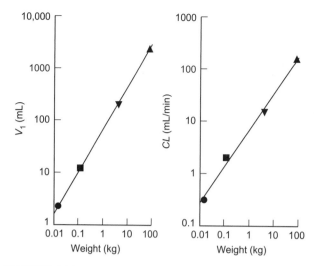

**FIGURE 34.3** Log–log plots of $V_1$ and $CL$ vs body weight for recombinant human growth hormone: mouse (●), rat (■), cynomolgous monkey (▼), human (▲). Reproduced with permission from Mordenti J, Chen SA, Moore JA *et al.* Pharm Res 1991;8:1351–9 [21].

plots of $CL$ and initial volume of distribution ($V_1$) are shown for recombinant growth hormone (GH) across four species.

Allometric equations for $V_1$ and $CL$ for some representative macromolecules are depicted in Table 34.5 [22–26]. The theoretical exponent approximations for $V_1$ (mL) and $CL$ (mL/min) are $aW^{0.8}$–$aW^{1.0}$ and $aW^{0.6}$–$aW^{0.8}$, respectively. Parameter estimates can be normalized for body weight simply by subtracting 1.0 from the exponent. In Table 34.6 the predicted parameter estimates derived from the allometric equations in Table 34.5 are compared with the corresponding parameter estimates reported in humans [27, 28]. The observed values of $V_1$ for the macromolecules listed fall within the expected range of observed results. However, the observed clearances of FIX and IL-12 were not predicted

**TABLE 34.5    Allometric Equations for Fepresentative Macromolecules**

| Macromolecule | Allometric equations | | Ref(s) |
| | $V_1$ (mL) | $CL$ (mL/h) | |
|---|---|---|---|
| Factor IX[a] | 87 W$^{1.26}$ | 14 W$^{0.68}$ | [22, 23] [b] |
| Factor VIII[a] | 44 W$^{1.04}$ | 10 W$^{0.69}$ | [24] |
| Interleukin-12[a] | 65 W$^{0.85}$ | 8 W$^{0.62}$ | [25, 26] [b] |
| Growth hormone[c] | 68 W$^{0.83}$ | 7 W$^{0.71}$ | [21] |
| Tissue plasminogen activator[c] | 91 W$^{0.93}$ | 17 W$^{0.84}$ | [21] |

[a]Based on parameter estimates in at least two species.

[b]Allometric equations determined from PK parameter estimates reported in published literature.

[c]Based on parameter estimates in at least four species.

TABLE 34.6    Prediction of Human Pharmacokinetic Parameters Based on Allometric Scaling

| Macromolecule | $V_1$ | | | $CL$ | | | Ref. |
|---|---|---|---|---|---|---|---|
| | Predicted (mL) | Observed (mL) | Expected range[a] (mL/kg) | Predicted (mL/h) | Observed (mL/h) | Expected range[a] (mL/h) | |
| Factor IX | 18,380 | 10,150[†] | 9190–27,570 | 248 | 434[b] | 124–372 | [27] |
| Factor VIII | 3617 | 3030 | 1809–5426 | 195 | 174 | 98–293 | [24] |
| Interleukin-12 | 2406 | 3360 | 1203–3609 | 113 | 406 | 57–170 | [28] |
| Growth hormone | 2243 | 2432 | 1122–3365 | 148 | 175 | 74–222 | [21] |
| Recombinant tissue plasminogen activator | 5814 | 4450 | 2907–8721 | 646 | 620 | 323–969 | [21] |

[a]For comparison with observed results, an expected range is chosen that is 0.5 to 1.5 times the predicted value.
[b]Calculated from Figure 1 of White G, Shapiro A, Ragni M *et al.* Semin Hematol 1998;35(Suppl 2):33–8 [27].

from allometry. Factors such as species specificity in the endothelial binding of FIX [29] or saturation of clearance mechanisms, may account for the inability to predict these parameters in humans.

Allometric scaling also has been applied to mAbs [30, 31]. Duconge and coworkers conducted PK studies in mice, rats, rabbits, and dogs after a single administration of 16 mg/kg, 8 mg/kg, 1.5 mg/kg, and 0.2 mg/kg, respectively, of a murine mAb ior EGF/r³ [32]. Three female patients with non-small cell lung cancer were also studied. They were participating in a Phase I trial and received a single IV infusion of 400 mg. EGF concentrations were analyzed either by a radioreceptor assay (mice and rats) or a sandwich ELISA method (rabbits, dogs, and humans). The allometric equations for $V_d$ and $CL$ were calculated according to the standard methods and with incorporation of a complex Dedrick plot, similar to that used in Figure 32.4. The results of the allometric analysis are shown in Table 34.7. A comparison between the predicted and calculated PK parameters in cancer patients is shown in Table 34.8. The actual clearance in patients with cancer was four-fold greater than the predicted value. The authors proposed that the observed variance suggests that patients with cancer possess additional clearance processes that are not present in healthy subjects or predictable from studies in normal animals. However, even with this disparate result the authors

used their 0.85 allometric scaling factor for $CL$ to assist in designing dose regimens for a clinical trial [32].

Mahmood *et al.* [31] further demonstrated that simple allometry using PK parameter estimates from at least three species, resulting in an exponent for $CL$ in the range of 0.5–0.9, predicted human clearance reasonably well. Recently, others have proposed that allometry based on single-species studies of macromolecules in monkeys, and using the theoretical exponent of 0.8 for $CL$, accurately predicts human $CL$ [33, 34]. In both cases, the authors determined PK parameters within a dosage range that was assumed to be linear. Recently, it has been shown that classifying mAbs based on whether or not the mAb antigen target was either soluble or membrane bound enables human $CL$ to be reasonably predicted with an exponent of either 0.85 for solid or 0.90 for membrane-bound targets [35]. Other factors to be considered in deciding whether or not interspecies scaling would be predictive of human PK parameter estimates include: (1) binding characteristics, (2) receptor density, (3) size and charge of molecule, (4) end-terminal carbohydrate characteristics, (5) degree of sialylation, and (6) saturation of elimination pathways. These factors are known to influence clearance and distribution volumes, as will be discussed in subsequent sections.

TABLE 34.7    Allometric Equations for EGF mAb PK Parameters

| Parameter (Y) | Coefficient (*a*) | Exponent (*b*) | *r* |
|---|---|---|---|
| $V_d$ (mL) | 219 | 0.84 | 0.92 |
| $CL$ (mL/h) | 4.07 | 0.85 | 0.94 |

Adapted from Duconge J, Fernandez-Sanchez E, Alvarez D. Biopharm Drug Dispos 2004;25:177–86 [30].

TABLE 34.8    Comparison of EGF PK Parameters Predicted from Allometric Equations and Estimated in Cancer Patients

| Parameter (Y) | Predicted PK parameter estimate[a] | Estimated PK parameter in cancer patients |
|---|---|---|
| $V_d$ (L/kg) | 0.01 | 0.04 |
| $CL$ (mL/h/kg) | 0.22 | 0.98 |

Calculated from the allometric equations in Table 7, Duconge J, Fernandez-Sanchez E, Alvarez D *et al.* Biopharm Drug Dispos 2004;25:177–86 [30].

For example, clearance may involve several mechanisms, including immune-mediated clearance that results in non-constant clearance rates. The interspecies predictability of clearance in this situation would be questionable.

In spite of the limitations, interspecies scaling can be used to relate dosages across species in toxicology studies, to predict human PK parameter estimates for macromolecules, and, as discussed in Chapters 32 and 33, to guide dose selection in Phase I clinical trials. However, an understanding of the characteristics of the macromolecule is important for the interpretation and application of these results.

## Safe Starting Doses of Monoclonal Antibodies in First-in-Human (FIH) Studies

In a 2006 Phase I study, TGN1412, an agonist mAb targeting CD-28, was administered to healthy volunteers and resulted in cytokine storm, an adverse event that is often fatal [36]. As this event had not been predicted by preclinical studies, the selection of safe starting doses for mAbs has subsequently received considerable attention and discussion in the pharmaceutical and regulatory communities. In response to this case, the Committee for Medicinal Product (CHMP) of the European Medicines Agency (EMEA) issued guidelines highlighting considerations that should be taken to mitigate safety risks, such as that seen with TGN1412 [37]. In particular, the guidelines emphasize application of the concept of "minimum anticipated biological effect", or MABEL. The steps for determining MABEL are outlined in Table 34.9. The integration of all information, including toxicology, mAb pharmacology, PK/PD modeling, and interspecies scaling, will result in improved decisions regarding safe starting doses and dose-escalation intervals in both healthy volunteers and subjects with disease [38].

An even more sophisticated mechanism-based PK/PD model has been proposed for FIH dose selection that incorporates factors such as receptor occupancy

and target cell (blood) depletion [39]. The purpose of the model is to predict a mAb's pharmacology at the proposed dosages in order to guide both initial and subsequent dose selection. The model incorporates *in vitro* measures of affinity binding of the mAb to blood cells and *in vivo* monkey PK and target cell depletion data. These data were fit to the PK/PD model and the resulting PK parameters were allometrically scaled to humans. The human model used the same structure as that for the monkey, but the mAb binding affinity was adjusted to that of humans in order to simulate PK, receptor occupancy, and target cell depletion profiles (Figure 34.4). Prior to building models of this type, it is important to establish that the humanized or fully human mAb being studied cross-reacts with monkey, in order to reliably extrapolate *in vivo* PK and PD, and that its binding affinity to the target cell is similar in the two species.

## PHARMACOKINETIC CHARACTERISTICS OF MACROMOLECULES

### Endogenous Concentrations

Unlike chemically synthesized molecules, many of the macromolecules currently marketed or under investigation are naturally occurring substances in the body. This presents some unique challenges for estimating PK parameters. Most commercially available ELISAs were developed to quantitate exogenously administered proteins, and do not distinguish between the native protein in the body and the exogenously administered protein. Clearly, concentrations of endogenous proteins, which can fluctuate because of stimulation or feedback control (such as insulin growth factor, IGF-1), can result in erroneous parameter estimates. There are several approaches to deal with the problem posed by detectable endogenous protein concentrations.

In a study by Cheung *et al.* [40], the investigators administered erythropoietin subcutaneously to 30 healthy volunteers. Blood sampling times included

TABLE 34.9   Steps in Determining MABEL

1. Assess relevant *in vitro* binding characteristics (e.g., via Biacore)
2. Determine receptor occupancy either by *in vitro* or *in vivo* methods, or by both (i.e, confirm *in vivo*, the *in vitro* findings)
3. Obtain concentration–effect data from *in vivo* studies
4. Establish the mechanism-based PK/PD model and integrate the pharmacology data
5. Account for species differences in binding affinity, potency, target expression and rate of turnover, target-mediated clearance, duration of effects
6. Use allometry to scale PK parameters to humans and refine PK/PD model to predict human dosages
7. Identify maximum recommended starting dose (MRSD)

Adapted from Muller PY, Milton M, Lloyd P *et al.* Curr Opin Biotech 2009; 20:722–9 [38].

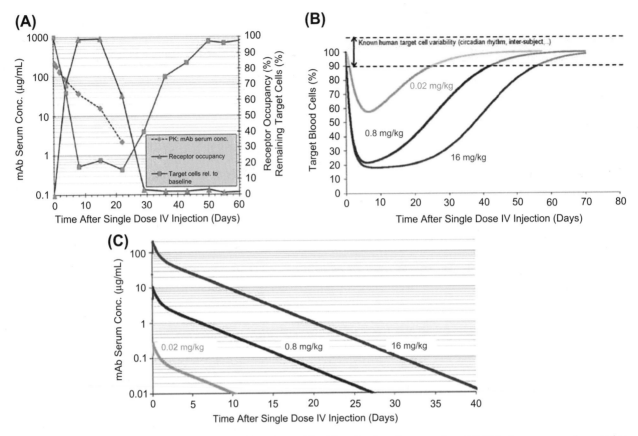

**FIGURE 34.4**   MABEL determination for a mAb binding to blood-based cell surface receptors. (A) Data from one monkey used to build the PK/PD monkey model. Depletion of target cells as percentage of remaining target cells in circulation, relative to baseline (on right axis) is modulated by receptor occupancy (RO), expressed as % occupied receptors from all available receptors at a specific time point. When mAb serum concentration (on left axis, logarithmic scale) falls below ≈ 10 μg/mL for this mAb, a decrease in RO is observed followed by recovery of target cell counts. (B) Simulation of human PK following three single IV doses with a half-life hypothesized to be ≈ 3.5 days. (C) Simulation of human target cell depletion dose–response for the three IV doses. On this figure, MABEL corresponds to a dose < 0.02 mg/kg, where suppression of target cells is minimal and transient. Reproduced with permission from Yu J, Karcher H, Feire AL, Lowe PJ. AAPS J 2011;13:169–78 [39].

a pre-dose sample and samples collected multiple times postadministration. In the pre-dose sample, erythropoietin was detected in all subjects at concentrations in the physiological range (< 7 to 30 IU/mL) with the exception of a subject whose baseline concentration of 48 IU/mL exceeded the normal physiologic range. Prior to estimating PK parameters, the investigators subtracted each pre-dose concentration from all concentrations detected postadministration. The underlying assumption for this approach was that the low endogenous concentrations remained relatively stable over the postadministration times. However, data were not presented to confirm or refute this assumption.

Another approach for dealing with this problem has been proposed for GH by Veldhuis and colleagues [41]. These investigators used a deconvolution method to minimize the influence of circulating endogenous

GH on PK parameter estimates derived from exogenously administered growth hormone. In this method, diurnal variation in the 24-hour secretory rate of GH is estimated by approximating endogenous plasma GH concentration data with cubic spline smoothing controlled by setting a maximum limit for the weighted residual square sum [42]. Patient-specific parameters can be estimated from individual endogenous hormone concentrations or from group means.

Another option is to estimate PK parameters from the sum of exogenous and endogenous protein concentrations detected after the exogenous administration of the protein. The basic assumption is that the PK parameter estimates are not significantly altered by the presence of endogenous protein concentrations. This generally is true in the very early part of the concentration vs time profile when the endogenous concentration may represent less than 10% of the total concentration. However, in the example depicted in Figure 34.5 endogenous concentrations are oscillating and pulsatile, reaching peaks during the sampling period that are greater than 100-fold the initial basal values [43]. This illustrates how changes in endogenous protein concentrations over the sampling period can influence model fitting and confound PK parameter estimation.

Finally, a cross-over study design can be employed such that subjects are randomized to placebo or treatment on one occasion and to the alternate regimen on a second occasion, assuring an adequate washout period between the two occasions. The endogenous concentrations determined in the same subjects after placebo administration can be subtracted from the matching sample collected after treatment administration. This design accommodates intrasubject variability and variations in endogenous concentrations due to pulsatile secretion, but assumes that the two separate study days are similar.

Thus, it is important to recognize that current analytical methods cannot distinguish endogenous protein concentrations from exogenous concentrations. Administering radiolabeled proteins would allow for exogenous and endogenous proteins to be distinguished, but there are experimental limitations to the use of radiolabeled proteins. Although the accuracy of PK parameter estimation may be impacted by the presence of endogenous concentrations, study designs and data analysis methods can be employed that take endogenous concentration into consideration.

## Absorption

The absolute bioavailability of representative macromolecules following extravascular administration is shown in Table 34.10 [44–51]. It is apparent that bioavailability is variable with different molecules and with different routes of administration, reflecting individual molecule characteristics. However, the bioavailability of mAbs generally has been found to be in the 50–60% range after subcutaneous (SC) administration [52, 53]. In one report, the bioavailability of interferon α after SC or intramuscular (IM) administration was actually greater than 100% relative to an intravenous (IV) bolus injection [47]. This implausible result may reflect the inability of the immunoradiometric assay to distinguish proteolytic fragments of interferon α from the intact molecule, the slow absorption phase of either the SC or IM routes, or a saturable elimination process. The authors did not elucidate which of these factors might have contributed to their observation.

### Flip-Flop Pharmacokinetics of Macromolecules

When the absorption rate constant ($k_a$) is greater than the elimination rate constant ($k_e$), elimination of the molecule from the body is the rate-limiting step and the terminal portion of the concentration–time curve is primarily determined by the elimination rate. However, as discussed in Chapter 4, if $k_a$ is less than $k_e$, absorption is rate limiting and the terminal of the curve reflects the absorption rate. This phenomenon is illustrated for several molecules in Table 34.11 [43, 47, 54–56].

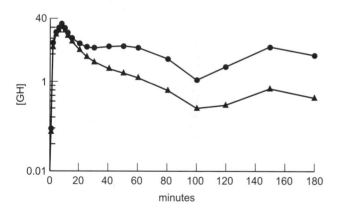

**FIGURE 34.5** Simulated effects of increasing basal growth hormone (GH) concentrations on measured total GH concentrations at various times during and after an 8-minute infusion of recombinant human growth hormone (rhGH) using basal concentrations 10 times (▲) and 100 times (●) the observed pre-infusion value of 0.042 ng/mL. Reproduced with permission from Bright GM, Veldhuis JD, Iranmanesh A *et al.* J Clin Endocrinol Metab 1999;84:3301–8 [43].

**TABLE 34.10 Bioavailability of Macromolecules after Extravascular Routes of Administration**

| Macromolecule | Route of administration | | | Ref(s) |
| --- | --- | --- | --- | --- |
| | SC[a] | IP[a] | Other | |
| Erythropoietin | 22.0% | 2.9% | — | [44] |
| Granulocyte-macrophage colony-stimulating factor | 83.0% | — | — | [45] |
| GH | 49.5% | — | 7.8–9.9%[b] | [46] |
| Interferon α₂ᵦ | >100% | 42.0% | >100 %[c] | [47, 48] |
| Interleukin-11 | 65% | — | — | [49] |
| Alemtuzumab[d] | 53% | — | — | [50] |
| Golimumab | 51% | — | — | [51] |

[a]SC, subcutaneous; IP, intraperitoneal.
[b]Nasal administration.
[c]Intramuscular administration.
[d]Calculated from *AUC* after IV administration (Summary Basis of Approval; Drugs@FDA), and after SC administration (Montagna M, Montillo M, Avanzini MA *et al.*, Haematologia 2011; 96:932–6 [50]).

**TABLE 34.11   Absorption and Apparent Elimination Rates of Macromolecules after SC and IV Administration**

| Macromolecule | Route of administration | $k_a$ (h$^{-1}$) | Apparent $k_e$ (h$^{-1}$) | Ref. |
|---|---|---|---|---|
| GH | SC | $0.23 \pm 0.04$ | $0.43 \pm 0.05$ | [54] |
|  | IV | — | 2.58 | [43] |
| IFN-$\alpha_{2b}$ | SC | 0.24 | 0.13 | [47] |
|  | IV | — | 0.42 |  |
| Erythropoietin | SC | $0.0403 \pm 0.002$ | $0.206 \pm 0.004$ | [55] |
|  | IV | — | 0.077 | [56] |

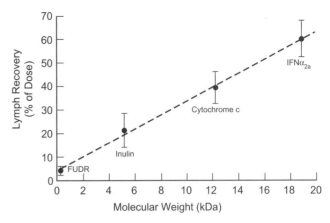

**FIGURE 34.6** Correlation between molecular weight (MW) and cumulative recovery of IFN-α-2a (MW 19,000), cytochrome c (MW 12,300), inulin (MW 5200) and 5-fluoro-2′-deoxyuridine (FUDR, MW 246.2) in the efferent lymph from the right popliteal lymph node following SC administration into the lower part of the right hind leg of sheep. Each point and bar show the mean and standard deviation of three experiments performed in three separate sheep. The line drawn represents a least-squares fit of the data ($r = 0.988$, $P < 0.01$). Reproduced with permission from Supersaxo A, Hein WR, Steffen H. Pharm Res 1990;7:167–9 [57].

In the absence of concentration–time profiles after IV administration, it is impossible to estimate the actual elimination rate constant, and the interpretation of absorption and elimination rates after SC administration of macromolecules must be performed cautiously. It is for this reason surprising that so few published pharmacokinetic studies include IV administration to assess whether or not the macromolecule follows flip-flop pharmacokinetics.

*Factors Affecting Absorption from Subcutaneous Sites*

Two very important principles on the absorption of macromolecules after SC administration were elucidated by Supersaxo *et al.* [57]. First, in the range of the molecular weight of the various molecules tested (246–19,000 Da), there was a linear relationship between molecular weight and absorption by the lymphatic system (Figure 34.6). Second, the authors concluded that molecules with a molecular weight greater than 16,000 Da are absorbed mainly by the lymphatic system that drains the SC injection site, whereas molecules with a molecular weight of less than 1000 Da are absorbed almost entirely by blood capillaries. The authors hypothesized that macromolecules are absorbed preferentially by lymphatic rather than blood capillaries because lymphatic capillaries lack the subendothelial basement membrane present in continuous blood capillaries, and also may have 20- to 100-nm gaps between adjacent endothelial cells.

Others have proposed that absorption from the lymphatics cannot be the only factor contributing to the observed bioavailabililty of macromolecules after SC administration, and that other factors such as an increase in blood flow, proteolysis at the site of injection, or the physical and electrostatic interaction of macromolecules with other components of the interstitum, such as the fibrous collagen network and glycosaminoglycans, also play a role [51, 58, 59]. In the case of mAbs, there is no evidence to suggest the

proteolysis occurs at the injection site since the binding of IgG isotypes to the FcRN may protect mAbs from degradation or contribute to transport across the interstitum to blood capillaries.

Although molecular weight is a key factor affecting the absorption of SC administered macromolecules, injection site may also influence the absorption. For example, the absorption half-life was significantly longer, 14.9 vs 12.3 hours, after injection of recombinant human erythropoeitin (RhEPO) into the thigh than after injection into the abdomen [60]. Also, the concentration vs time profile displayed a double peak after injection into the thigh that was more pronounced than after the abdominal injection (Figure 34.7). However, these differences are clinically irrelevant, and no statistically significant differences were observed in the area under the curve (*AUC* 5684 vs 6185 U·h/L), in the maximum concentration ($C_{max}$ 175 vs 212 U/L), or in the time of maximum concentration ($t_{max} = 10$ h) for thigh vs abdomen, respectively.

In another study, recombinant human GH was absorbed faster after SC injection into the abdomen compared with the absorption after SC injection into the thigh [61]. $C_{max}$ was higher ($29.7 \pm 4.8$ mU/L) and $t_{max}$ was faster ($4.3 \pm 0.5$ h) after injection into the abdomen than after injection into the thigh ($23.2 \pm 3.9$ mU/L and $5.9 \pm 0.4$ h, respectively). It is possible that these absorption differences may be dependent on lymphatic drainage at the two injection

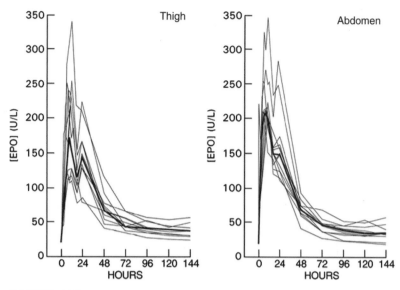

**FIGURE 34.7** Serum erythropoietin (EPO) concentrations as a function of time after SC injection of 100 U/kg of recombinant human erythropoietin into the thigh and abdomen of 11 healthy volunteers. The bold curve represents the median. Reproduced with permission from Jensen JD, Jensen LW, Madsen JK *et al.* Eur J Clin Pharmacol 1994;46:333–7 [60].

sites and may reflect differences in lymph flow. However, mean IGF-1 and insulin growth factor-binding protein 1 (IGFBP-1) concentrations, a PD marker of GH effect, were unaffected by the site of injection. Other effects independent of injection site were blood glucose, and serum insulin and glucagon levels. Thus, site of injection is clinically irrelevant for GH, as well as for recombinant erythropoeitin.

The influence of injection site on mAb absorption also has been studied [51]. In an open-label, random-ized, and parallel designed PK study, 100-mg doses of golimumab were administered either SC to the upper arm, abdomen, or thigh, or IV to healthy adult men. Similar to the results with protein macromolecules, the bioavailability of golimumab was not significantly different, suggesting that injection site had little effect on bioavailabililty. The mean absolute bioavailability of golimumab was 52% following SC injection in the upper arm, 47% following SC injection into the abdomen, and 54% following SC injection into the thigh, and no significant differences in $C_{max}$, $t_{max}$, or $AUC_{0-\infty}$ were observed. Further, the coefficient of variation (CV) in $AUC_{0-\infty}$ following SC injection was approximately 30% and was only slightly greater than that associated with IV administration (approximately 25% CV), suggesting the SC administration does not result in increased observed variability in estimates of these PK parameters.

In summary, there is no single factor that can account for the finding that macromolecules have reduced bioavailability after SC administration. However, molecular weight, injection site, proteolysis of proteins at injection site, or interactions of exoge-nously administered macromolecules with constitu-ents within the interstitium may affect their absorption characteristics, and should be considered both in designing clinical trials and in treating patients.

## Distribution

As discussed in Chapter 3, proteins and mAbs distribute initially into the plasma volume and then more slowly into the interstitial fluid space. It can be seen from Table 34.12 that the initial distribution volume of interleukin-2 (IL-2), IL-12, granulocyte colony-stimulating factor (G-CSF), and recombinant tissue plasminogen activator (rt-PA) approximates that of plasma volume. In contrast, the initial distri-bution volume of FIX is approximately twice that of plasma volume. On the other hand, the volume of distribution at steady state ($V_{d(ss)}$) for IL-12, G-CSF), and rt-PA are considerably smaller than the $V_{d(ss)}$ of inulin, a marker for extracellular fluid space (ECF) [22, 25, 62–67]. When distribution volume estimates are much less than expected values for ECF, they could reflect the slow transport of large molecules across membranes and the fact that either assay sensitivity or sampling time have been inadequate to characterize the true elimination phase of the compound.

TABLE 34.12    Distribution Volume of Representative Macromolecules

| Macromolecule | MW (kDa) | $V_1$ (mL/kg) | $V_{d(ss)}$ (mL/kg) | Ref(s) |
|---|---|---|---|---|
| Inulin[a] | 5.2 | 55 | 164 | [62] |
| Factor IX | 57 | 136[b] | 271[b] | [22] |
| Interleukin-2 | 15.5 | 60 | 112 | [63, 64] |
| Interleukin-12 | 53 | 52 | 59 | [25] |
| Granulocyte colony-stimulating factor | 20 | 44 | 60 | [65, 66] |
| Recombinant tissue plasminogen activator | 65 | 59 | 106 | [67] |

[a]Inulin values used as a reference for plasma volume ($V_1$) and extracellular fluid space ($V_{d(ss)}$).

[b]Calculated from Figure 1 of White G, Shapiro A, Ragni M. Semin Hematol 1998;35(Suppl 2):33–8 [27].

The issue of inadequate sampling time is exemplified by the PK results for mAbs that are shown in Table 34.13 [68]. The reported values of $V_1$ and $V_{ss}$ are not that different, and both are similar to intravascular space estimates that usually range from 2 to 3 L/m². These low $V_{ss}$ estimates for macromolecules suggest not only that equilibrium between the intravascular and extravascular compartments is slow but also that measured plasma concentrations at steady state may not be a good guide to the actual, active concentrations at the site of action. On the other hand, binding of macromolecules and mAbs to receptors or other binding sites could significantly increase apparent

TABLE 34.13    Pharmacokinetics of Marketed Monoclonal Antibodies

| mAbs | Molecular weight (kD) | $t_{1/2}$[a] (Days) | $V_1$[a] (L) | $V_{ss}$[a] |
|---|---|---|---|---|
| Avastin | 149 | 13–15 | 3 | 3.5–4.5 L |
| Erbitux | 152 | ND[b] | 2.7–3.4 | 2–3 L/m² |
| Raptiva | 150 | 6–7.5[c] | NR[d] | 9 L[e] |
| Humira | 148 | 12–18 | 3 | 5 L |
| Campath | 150 | 1–14[f] | NR[d] | 7–28 L |

[a]All values extracted from the Summary Basis for Approval review posted on www.accessdata.fda.gov/scripts/cder/drugsatfda/.

[b]Used clearance instead of $T_{1/2}$ since it has non-linear PK at dosages greater than 200 mg/m².

[c]Average $t_{1/2}$ based on non-compartmental methods and after subcutaneous administration (see [68]).

[d]NR, not reported.

[e]Calculated as $V/F$.

[f]Campath has non-linear PK in the range of 3–30 mg three times weekly.

distribution volumes that would otherwise be much smaller (e.g., Factor IX in Table 34.12) [69].

Finally, it is important to note that the PK studies submitted to support approval of a New Drug Application (NDA) for the most part are based on non-compartmental methods that assume linear, first-order kinetics, even though this clearly is not the case for the majority of the monoclonal antibodies currently marketed, such as cefuximab (Erbitux). Unfortunately, little attention has been paid to the fact that the use of non-compartmental methods to describe the PK of mAbs greatly oversimplifies their complex properties and, as pointed out in Chapter 8, is inappropriate.

### Binding to $\alpha_2$-Macroglobulin

$\alpha_2$-Macroglobulin, one of the major proteins in the serum, is highly conserved across species and can bind many molecules, such as cytokines, enzymes, lipopolysaccharide (LPS), and ions such as zinc and nickel [70]. $\alpha_2$-Macroglobulin is found in extravascular secretions, such as lymph. It exists in two forms: an electrophoretically slow native form, and a fast form, an $\alpha_2$-macroglobulin-protease complex that results in a conformational change that increases electrophoretic mobility. This conformational change results in exposure of a hydrophobic region that can bind to cell surface receptors such as those on hepatocytes.

There is evidence suggesting that $\alpha_2$-macroglobulin plays an important role in human immune function. Specifically, studies have shown that the fast form can inhibit antibody-dependent cellular toxicity and natural killer (NK) cell-mediated cytolysis [71], as well as superoxide production by activated macrophages [72].

As shown in Table 34.14, $\alpha_2$-macroglobulin can bind to a number of exogenously administered proteins. Three different mechanisms for this binding have been identified [73]. The binding can be non-covalent and reversible. An example of this type of binding is seen

TABLE 34.14    Binding of Macromolecules to Alpha$_2$-Macroglobulin

| Macromolecule | Physiological effect | Relevance of binding |
|---|---|---|
| Nerve growth factor | Stimulates nerve growth | Interferes with assay |
| Interleukin-1 | Regulates proliferation of thymocytes | Regulates cell activity |
| Interleukin-2 | Impairs proliferation of T cells | Inactivates cytokine |
| Tissue growth factor β | Stimulates growth of kidney fibroblasts | Functions as carrier; accelerates clearance |

with growth factors such as tissue growth factor-β (TGF-β). Second, the binding to α₂-macroglobulin can be covalent [74], and the third mechanism involves covalent linkages with proteinase reactions [75]. Subsequent to the binding, the PK and PD properties of the macromolecule may be altered. The binding of α₂-macroglobulin is associated with variable results: the α₂-macroglobulin–cytokine complex may interfere with bioassay results (e.g., nerve growth factor) [73], serve as a carrier (e.g., TGF-β) (73), prevent proteolytic degradation (e.g., IL-2) [76], or enhance removal of the protein from the circulation (e.g., tissue necrosis factor-α) [70].

### Binding to Other Proteins

Insulin-like growth factor-1 (IGF-1) is produced by many tissues in the body and has approximately 50% structural homology with insulin. In plasma, IGF-1 exists as "free" IGF-1 and "bound" IGF-1, and its physiology, as depicted in Figure 34.8, is very complex [77]. To date, eight binding proteins (designated IGFBP-1 through 8) have been identified, with IGFBP-3 being the most abundant. The binding proteins vary in

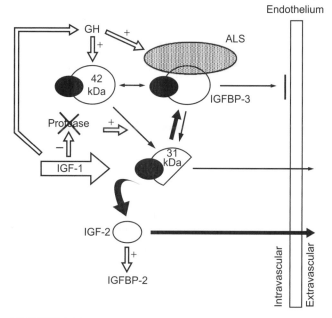

**FIGURE 34.8** Hypothetical model of the effects of insulin-like growth factor (IGF-1). Open arrows show regulating influences. Plasma IGF-1 consists of free and bound IGF-1. Insulin-like growth factor-binding protein-3 (IFGBP-3) exists in two forms, a 42-kDa complete form or a 31-kDa fragment. IGF-1 drives the reaction towards binding with the acid-labile subunit (ALS) to form a ternary complex, which is retained in the intravascular space. IFG-1 also suppresses growth hormone (GH) secretion, decreasing the synthesis of IGFBP-3. Reproduced with permission from Blum WF, Jensen LW, Madsen JK. Acta Paediatr Suppl 1993;82(Suppl 391):15–9 [77].

molecular weight, distribution, concentration in biological fluids, and binding affinity [78]. It is important to note that the interactions between the binding proteins and their physiologic role are poorly understood, but probably serve to modulate the clearance and/or biological effects of IGF-1.

### Metabolism

Table 34.15 summarizes the effects of various cytokines on the cytochrome P450 (CYP) mixed function oxidase system [79]. With the exception of IL-2, these cytokines depress the activity of CYP enzymes. Data on cytokine-mediated depression of drug-metabolizing ability has been obtained primarily in rodents under conditions of inflammation or infection [80]. The reduction in drug biotransformation capacity parallels a decrease in total CYP content and enzyme activity, and is due primarily to a downregulation of CYP gene transcription, but modulation of RNA and enzyme inhibition may also be involved [80, 81].

As shown in Table 34.15, the expression of CYP2C11 and CYP2D isoenzymes is frequently suppressed by cytokines. These two CYP gene families are constitutively expressed in male and female rats. In the rat, CYP2C is under developmental and pituitary hormone regulation. Although there is approximately 70% cDNA-deduced amino acid sequence homology with the human CYP2C, caution is needed in extrapolating these observations on CYP2C regulation from rats to humans [82]. In both rats and humans, there is polymorphic expression of the CYP2D and CYP2D1 isoenzymes which exhibit debrisoquine 4-hydroxylase activity. However, this gene family has evolved differently in rats than in humans. Specifically, the rat has four genes that are approximately 73–80% similar while the human has three genes that are 89–95% similar. Thus, results in rat studies may not be predictive of results in humans because of the

**TABLE 34.15  Effect of Various Macromolecules on P450 Isoenzymes**

| Macromolecule | Isoenzyme | Effects |
|---|---|---|
| Interferon-α | CYP2C11 | Decreased mRNA and enzyme levels |
| Interleukin-1 | CYP2C11 | Decreased mRNA and enzyme levels |
| | CYP2D | Decreased mRNA and enzyme levels |
| Interleukin-2 | CYP2D1 | Increased mRNA and enzyme levels |
| Interleukin-6 | CYP2C11 | Decreased mRNA and enzyme levels |
| Tumor necrosis factor | CYP2C11 | Decreased enzyme levels |

difference in number of genes, their regulation, and their complexity [83].

*In vitro* study results have been consistent with those obtained *in vivo*. For example, in primary rat hepatocyte cultures IL-1, tumor necrosis factor (TNF), and interleukin-6 (IL-6) concentrations ranging from 0.5 to 10.0 ng/mL suppressed the expression of CYP2C11 mRNA [82]. It is interesting to note that in rat liver microsomes, IL-2 increased both the amount of immunoreactive CYP2D protein and its mRNA [83]. In human primary hepatocytes, IL-1β, IL-6, and TNF-α caused a decrease in all mRNAs and CYP isoenzyme activities. Moreover, interferon γ (IFN-γ) was shown to decrease CYP1D2 and CYP2E1 mRNA, but had no effect on CYP2C or CYP3A mRNAs [79].

The *in vitro* effects of IL-6 on the CYP 450 isoenzymes were confirmed by Dickmann *et al.* [84], who found that IL-6 increased acute phase reactants (e.g., C-reactive protein), downregulated all CYP P450 isoform mRNA expression and, at concentrations greater than 500 pg/mL, suppressed induction of CYP1A2 by omeprazole and of CYP3A4 by rifampicin. In addition, in the presence of an anti-IL-6 mAb in the human primary hepatocyte culture, IL-6 suppression of CYP1A2 activity was completely abolished but the suppression of CYP3A4 was not, although there was a shift in the $EC_{50}$ to the right by approximately 19-fold and 13-fold, respectively, in two different donors.

The clinical significance of the aforementioned findings is unknown. A report by Khakoo *et al.* [85] did not demonstrate a PK interaction between IFN-$\alpha_{2b}$ and ribavirin, or an additive effect of the combination therapy on safety assessments. In another study, administration of IFN-α prior to cyclophosphamide administration significantly impaired the metabolism of cyclophosphamide and 4-hydroxycyclophosphamide. In contrast, the administration of IFN-α after cyclophosphamide resulted in higher 4-hydroxycyclophosphamide concentrations and produced a significant decrease in leukocyte count [86].

The interaction between IL-2 and doxorubicin was explored in patients with advanced solid tumors [87]. Doxorubicin was given alone, and 3 weeks later patients received the combination of rhIL-2 (18 mIU/m$^2$ given SC on days 1–5) and doxorubicin. Doxorubicin PK was assessed for 48 hours after each administration period. SC injections of rhIL-2 did not affect doxorubicin PK, but doxorubicin given before IL-2 prevented IL-2-induced lymphocyte rebounds, although it did not qualitatively alter non-major histocompatibility complex-restricted cytotoxicity.

Schmitt *et al.* [88] evaluated the effects of an anti-IL-6 antibody, tocilizumab, in patients with rheumatoid arthritis (RA), a disease characterized by elevated concentrations of IL-6. In this study of 12 patients with RA, the effects of tocilizumab on simvastatin, a CYP3A4 substrate, were used as an indirect measure of CYP3A4 activity. Simvastatin was administered on days 1, 13, and 43, and tocilizumab was given IV on Day 8. Tocilizumab reduced simvastatin *AUC* by one-half, corresponding to a doubling of simvastatin clearance over baseline values. In addition, C-reactive protein (CRP) levels that were markedly elevated at baseline were observed to be maximally reduced 1 week after tocilizumab administration, and this nadir occurred at the same time that the effects of tocilizumab on simvastatin were maximal. Taken together, these results constitute one of the first reports of a concurrent drug–disease and drug–drug interaction. Finally, since mAbs persist in the body for a long time, patients should be monitored for a prolonged period of time, even after stopping the mAb, since the effects on CYP activity may also persist.

Although these examples illustrate that various cytokines administered exogenously can affect CYP protein content, mRNA, and enzyme activities, and reports that evaluate the extent and clinical significance of corresponding PK or PD changes are emerging in the literature with increasing frequency [89], little is known regarding the catabolism of proteins that are either currently marketed or under investigation. The absence of suitable biological assays or other analytical methods for identifying and quantitating protein degradation products obviously limits evaluation of this catabolism. Similarly, the catabolism of mAbs, in particular the catabolism of the IgG molecule, is complex and not well understood [90]. Monoclonal antibody catabolism reflects the basal metabolic rate of the body as well as the function of phagocytic cells [monocytes, macrophages of the reticuloendothelial system (RES)]. There is also a relationship between IgG concentration and catabolism that is specific for each IgG molecule – the higher the IgG concentration, the shorter the survival time. To explain this characteristic of immunoglobulins, Brambell *et al.* [91] hypothesized, and Junghans and Anderson [92] have confirmed, that there is a specific, saturable receptor (FcRn) for each immunoglobulin that, when bound, protects the IgG from degradation. The IgG isotypes differ from one another in their amino acid sequence and Fc-fragment with survival half-lives of approximately 20 days for IgG$_1$, IgG$_2$ and IgG$_4$, but 7 days for IgG$_3$ [7]. The location and mechanism of IgG metabolism is not known but is believed to involve uptake by pinocytic vacuoles, release of proteolytic enzymes, and subsequent degradation of unbound IgG.

## Elimination

### Renal Excretion

The renal excretion of proteins is size dependent and glomerular filtration is rate limiting. It has been suggested that the renal clearance rate of macromolecules, relative to the glomerular filtration rate of inulin, decreases with increasing molecular radius [93]. The following general conclusions are based on studies using indirect methods to estimate glomerular sieving coefficients. Small proteins (< 25 kDa) cross the glomerular barrier, and filtration accounts for most of their plasma clearance; the degree of sieving is independent of biologic activity, and the filtered load of protein is directly related to plasma concentration. The effect of molecular charge is negligible for these small proteins, whereas charge retards glomerular filtration of anionic proteins as large as albumin (approximately 70 kDa). Subsequent to glomerular filtration, macromolecules may undergo hydrolysis and tubular reabsorption, mainly in endocytotic vesicles located in the apical regions of renal tubular cells [94].

### Hepatic Clearance

In addition to physical characteristics, the clearance of glycoproteins, structural components of macromolecules, is mediated by cell surface receptors for specific terminal carbohydrates and monosaccharides (Table 34.16). There are at least eight such receptors, the most well known of these being the Ashwell or asialoglycoprotein receptor [95]. Once the glycoprotein ligand binds to its receptor, it is internalized by endocytosis and degraded. The degrees of glycosylation, sialylation, or fucosylation are all factors that determine the clearance of these glycoproteins.

Clearance of rt-PA appears to mediated by the mannose/N-acetylglucosamine specific receptor on hepatic reticuloendothelial cells. To confirm that the mannose receptor is involved, Lucore et al. [96]

evaluated the clearance of rt-PA from the blood circulation of rabbits. Analysis of sequential blood samples by fibrin autography indicated that circulating free tissue plasminogen activator (t-PA) (approximately 55 kDa) was predominant, but that minimal amounts of high molecular weight complexes of approximately 110 and 170 kDa also were present. Competition experiments were conducted to determine the effect of glycosylation on rt-PA clearance. As shown in Figure 34.9, co-administration of rt-PA with p-aminophenyl-α-D-mannopyranoside-BSA (BSA-Man) prolonged both the α-phase and β-phase half-lives of rt-PA. The fact that BSA-Man inhibits the clearance of rt-PA suggests that the MAN-GlcNAc specific glycoprotein receptor contributes to its clearance. In contrast, co-administration of rt-PA with asialofetuin did not alter the α-phase and β-phase half-lives of rt-P, suggesting that the galactose receptor does not mediate clearance. This study demonstrates that the nature and extent of the glycosylation have a direct effect on the clearance of rt-PA and its interaction with the mannose receptors in the liver.

Production of recombinant proteins using Chinese hamster ovary (CHO) cells, or other mammalian cells, results in a glycosylation pattern that differs from that of recombinant proteins produced by bacteria such as Escherichia coli in that CHO-produced proteins are

**TABLE 34.16  Cell Surface Receptors for the Clearance of Carbohydrates and Monosaccharides**

| Specificity[a] | Cell type |
|---|---|
| Gal/Gal/NAc | Liver parencymal cells (asialoglycoprotein receptor) |
| Gal/GalNAc | Liver Kupfer and endothelial cells, peritoneal macrophages |
| Man/GlcNAc | Liver Kupfer and endothelial cells, peritoneal macrophages |
| Fuc | Liver Kupfer cells |

[a]Abbreviations: Gal, D-galactose; NAc, N-Acetylglucosamine; Glc, D-glucose; Man, D-mannose; Fuc, Fucose.

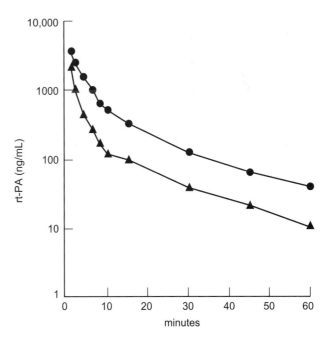

**FIGURE 34.9** Clearance of different forms of recombinant tissue plasmin activator (rt-PA) in rabbits after administration of rt-PA alone (▲) or in combination with p-aminophenyl-α-D-mannoside bovine serum albumin (●). Reproduced with permission from Lucore CL, Fry ETA, Nachowiak DA, Sobel BE et al. Circulation 1988;77:906–14 [96].

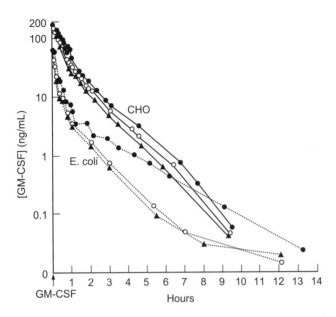

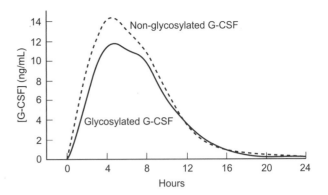

**FIGURE 34.11** Comparison of serum concentration vs time profiles in healthy subjects after SC administration of glycosylated G-CSF (—) and non-glycosylated G-CSF (- - -). Reproduced with permission from Watts MJ, Addison L, Long SG *et al.* Eur J Haematol 1997;98:474–9 [100].

**FIGURE 34.10** Granulocyte-macrophage colony-stimulating factor (GM-CSF) serum concentration vs time profiles for three patients after IV bolus injection of 8 µg/kg Chinese hamster ovary (CHO)-produced GM-CSF (*solid lines*), and for three patients who received E. *coli*-produced GM-CSF (*dotted lines*) (one patient received 5.5 µg/kg and two patients received 3 µg/kg). Reproduced with permission from Hovgaard D, Mortensen BT, Schifter S, Nissen NI. Eur J Haematol 1993;50:32–6 [97].

heavily glycosylated whereas those produced by bacteria are not glycosylated. Figure 34.10 depicts the results of an experiment comparing the plasma-concentration vs time profile of granulocyte-macrophage colony-stimulating factor (GM-CSF) produced by CHO cells with that produced by E. coli [97]. After IV administration, the E. *coli*-produced GM-CSF had a significantly shorter α-phase half-life than did CHO-produced GM-CSF, but there was no significant difference in the terminal half-life. The *AUC* of the glycosylated GM-CSF was approximately four to five times higher (6.3 µg·min/mL) than the *AUC* of the non-glycosylated product (1.27 µg·min/mL). However, since no difference in neutrophil counts was observed, the choice of one product over the other may only be a theoretical concern.

Similar to GM-CSF, granulocyte colony-stimulating factor (G-CSF) is available as either the glycosylated or non-glycosylated form of the protein. *In vitro* studies suggest that the glycosylated form is more stable and of a higher potency than the non-glycosylated form [98, 99]. The PK of these two forms of G-CSF were evaluated in 20 healthy volunteers [100]. As shown in Figure 34.11, the non-glycosylated form was more rapidly absorbed after SC administration and produced a higher $C_{max}$ (14.23 vs 11.85 pg/mL), but there was little difference in the elimination-phase

half-life (2.75 vs 2.95 h, respectively). The *AUC* for the non-glycosylated form was approximately 1.2 times higher than that of the glycosylated form. However, despite these PK differences, the progenitor cell count was significantly higher with the glycosylated product, confirming the *in vitro* potency results.

The results with G-CSF are dissimilar from those produced after IV administration of GM-CSF, where it was found that the $C_{max}$ was higher and the α-half life was longer for the glycosylated than for the non-glycosylated form. The reason for these differences is unknown, but it is apparent that the comparison and subsequent interpretation of study results is dependent on knowing the production source of the protein and the structural features that may influence the potency, PK, and/or PD of individual proteins.

Monoclonal antibody structural features, such as carbohydrate side chains, influence tissue uptake and clearance [12]. For example, Morell and colleagues [101] demonstrated that removal of sialic acid residue from the carbohydrate side chain of mouse $IgG_1$ increased its clearance and shortened its half-life. They also demonstrated increased clearance and liver uptake of asialo-$\alpha_2$ macroglobulin and asialohaptoglobin. Elimination of intact mAbs by the kidney is restricted so clearance is mainly due to catabolism, even though catabolytes may be renally eliminated.

Finally, clearance may change over time for macromolecules whose clearance is mediated by cell surface receptors and, in the case of mAbs, antigens. This is illustrated by an experiment in three patients with metastatic breast cancer who received a continuous infusion of G-CSF for 2 consecutive days [66]. Absolute neutrophil counts were obtained every morning, and there was a very strong positive

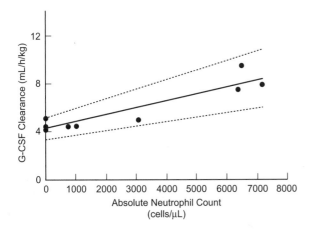

**FIGURE 34.12** Relationship between G-CSF clearance and absolute neutrophil count ($r = 0.85$, $P = 0.00025$). The dotted lines represent the 95% confidence intervals of the regression. Reproduced with permission from Ericson SG, Gao H, Gericke GH, Lewis LD. Exp Hematol 1997;25:1313–25 [66].

correlation between neutrophil count and G-CSF clearance (Figure 34.12). Clearance on day 2 was 4.6 mL/h/kg, increasing to 8.3 mL/h/kg on day 9. Thus, neutrophil production may mediate the clearance of G-CSF.

In summary, there are multiple characteristics of proteins that influence their PK; some of these are listed in Table 34.17.

## Application of Sparse Sampling and Population Kinetic Methods

There have been attempts to study the PK of macromolecules by applying the sparse sampling strategy and population kinetic methods described in Chapter 10 [55, 102, 103]. In one study, erythropoietin was administered SC to 48 healthy adult male Japanese volunteers [55]. The population mean values estimated for $k_a$, $k_e$, $V_d$, and the endogenous erythropoietin production rate were $0.043\,\text{h}^{-1}$, $0.206\,\text{h}^{-1}$,

**TABLE 34.17  Characteristics that Affect the Pharmacokinetics of Macromolecules**

| Physical characteristics | Size, structure, net charge |
| --- | --- |
| Post-translational modifications | Degree of glycosylation, sialylation, fucosylation |
| Protein binding | Plasma proteins, induced proteins |
| Route of administration | Transient peaks and trough, sustained concentrations |
| Duration of administration | Time-dependent changes in elimination clearance |
| Frequency of administration | Up- or downregulation of receptors |

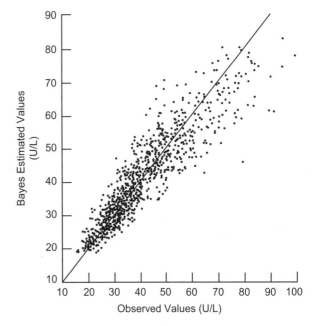

**FIGURE 34.13** Correlation between observed and predicted erythropoietin concentration values analyzing sparse sampling data with a population pharmacokinetic model (no $r$ value given). Reproduced with permission from Hayashi W, Kinoshita H, Yukawa E, Higuchi S. Br J Clin Pharmacol 1998;46:11–9 [55].

$3.14\,\text{L}$, and $15.7\,\text{IU}\,\text{h}^{-1}$, respectively. The good correlation between predicted and observed concentration values shown in Figure 34.13 supports the choice of model, as does the fact that the values for $k_e$ and $V_d$ determined by this analysis were similar to those reported for IV erythropoietin with the standard two-stage method of determining population PK parameters described in Chapter 10. However, given the flip-flop PK characteristics of erythropoietin (Table 34.10), the comparison to the IV parameter estimates may be misleading. In fact, the population PK estimates for $k_e$ are dissimilar to those obtained by other authors after SC administration of erythropoietin [40].

Population PK methods also were used to analyze the concentration vs time profiles of IFN-α in 27 patients with chronic hepatitis C virus infection who received an SC injection of this macromolecule [102]. The investigators reported that the absorption rate was best described by two processes: an initial zero-order process, accounting for 24% of net absorption, followed by a first-order process that had a rate constant of $0.18\,\text{h}^{-1}$. The authors noted that this value for $k_a$ is consistent with the $0.13\,\text{h}^{-1}$ reported by Radwanski et al. [47], and both results confirm that IFN-α is slowly absorbed after SC administration.

Population PK of sibrotuzumab, a humanized mAb directed against fibroblast activation protein (FAP), which is expressed in the stromal fibroblasts in > 90%

of malignant epithelial tumors, was analyzed in patients with advanced or metastatic carcinoma after multiple IV infusions of doses ranging from $5\,mg/m^2$ to a maximum of 100 mg [103]. The PK model consisted of two distribution compartments with parallel first-order and Michaelis–Menten elimination pathways from the central compartment. Body weight was significantly correlated with both central and peripheral distribution volumes, the first-order elimination clearance, and $V_{max}$ of the Michaelis–Menten pathway. Of interest was the observation that body surface area (BSA) was inferior to body weight as a covariate in explaining interpatient variability.

It is well known that for IV mAbs in general, and mAbs used in oncology in particular, dosing is based on weight or BSA. In recent years, the concept of BSA-based dosing for small molecules in oncology has been questioned [104]. The purpose of adjusting dosages based on BSA is the observation that clearance of many anticancer agents was related to glomerular filtration rate. However, the correlation of non-renal clearance with BSA has not been demonstrated and the clearance of many anticancer agents is a function of hepatic enzyme activity. So although the objective of adjusting dosages based on weight or BSA is to reduce the pharmacokinetic variability, this has been disputed by Baker et al. [105], who found that only 5 of 33 drugs evaluated demonstrated a reduction in interpatient variability with BSA-adjusted dosages. Currently, oncologic $IgG_1$ mAbs such as trastuzumab, bevacizumab, and rituximab are dosed based on body weight, but it has been proposed by several authors [106, 107] that fixed dosing of mAbs performs as well as weight-based dosing, and may offer advantages over weight-based dosing. This illustrates that it is important to assess during early development the contribution of differences in weight, BMI, or BSA to the observed intersubject variability in PK parameter estimates in order to make better decisions regarding the optimal basis for dose selection in late-stage clinical trials and in subsequent clinical practice.

## PHARMACODYNAMICS OF MACROMOLECULES

The relationship between circulating protein concentrations following exogenous administration and PD endpoints, either for efficacy or for safety, has been explored for a number of proteins, such as IGF-1, recombinant Factor IX and Factor VIII, interleukins (IL-2), and mAbs, such as rituximab, golimlumab, and omalizumab. Several conclusions emerge from the

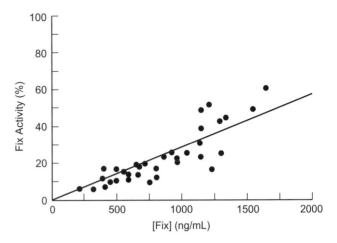

**FIGURE 34.14**   The relationship between Factor IX (FIX) activity (determined by a modified one-stage partial thromboplastin assay) and FIX concentration in hemophilia B dogs after an infusion of 50 μg/kg FIX over 10 minutes. Reproduced with permission from Schaub R, Garzone P, Bouchard P et al. Semin Hematol 1998;35(suppl 2):28–32 [22].

currently published data: these relationships are complex and not easily explained by a simple $E_{max}$ model, the endpoints are not clear cut (except for those macromolecules intended to substitute for endogenous proteins that are deficient), effects of disease on PD must be evaluated, and there is a high likelihood of regimen dependency.

## Models

The principles of receptor occupancy discussed in Chapter 20 and several of the PK/PD models described in Chapter 21 have been employed to explore the relationship between circulating protein or mAb concentrations and pharmacodynamic endpoints. For example, a dog model of hemophilia was used to study the activity of recombinant FIX [108]. Activity was determined in a bioassay, a modified one-stage partial thromboplastin time assay with pooled human plasma as the internal standard. As shown in Figure 34.14, the relationship between activity and recombinant FIX concentration was linear ($r^2 = 0.86$), suggesting that for every 34.5 ng/mL of FIX there is a corresponding 1% increase in FIX activity. In 11 males with hemophilia B, it was necessary to use a sigmoid $E_{max}$ model to describe the relationship between FIX activity and concentration (unpublished observations) and FIX serum concentrations of approximately 46 ng/mL were necessary to obtain a 1% increase in FIX activity. This translates into a 20% increase in the dosage of recombinant FIX necessary to achieve the same efficacy as plasma-derived FIX.

Model of rhGH Pharmacokinetics

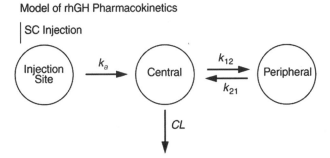

Indirect Response Model of IGF-1 Induction by rhGH

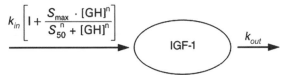

**FIGURE 34.15** Pharmacokinetic model for recombinant human growth hormone (rhGH) coupled with an indirect response model for IGF-1 induction by rhGH. The Hill equation was used to model IGF-1 induction by rhGH. Abbreviations: $k_a$, absorption rate of rhGH after SC injection; $CL$, elimination clearance of rhGH; $k_{12}$ and $k_{21}$, intercompartmental transfer rates of rhGH; IGF-1, total IGF concentration; and $k_{in}$, basal formation rate of IGF-1. Stimulation of IGF-1 production is modeled by the Hill function shown in brackets, where $S_{max}$ = maximum IGF stimulation of $k_{in}$ by rhGH, $S_{50}$ = rhGH concentration for 50% maximal stimulation of $k_{in}$, [GH] = rhGH concentration, $n$ = the Hill coefficient, and $k_{out}$ = elimination rate of IGF-1. Modified from Sun YN, Lee JH, Almon RR, Jusko WJ. J Pharmacol Exp Ther 1999;289:1523–32 [109].

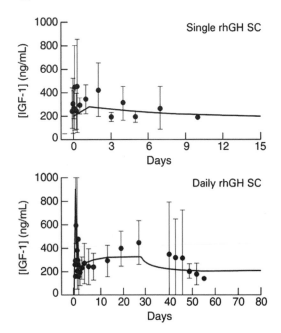

**FIGURE 34.16** Total IGF-1 concentrations resulting from single (*upper panel*) and daily (*lower panel*) SC injections of rhGH. Data points and bars represent the mean and standard deviation of results from four monkeys. Solid lines are the values that were simulated from the model shown in Figure 32.15. Reproduced with permission from Sun YN, Lee JH, Almon RR, Jusko WJ. J Pharmacol Exp Ther 1999;289:1523–32 [109].

paradigms that can be the basis for more sophisticated, complex models capable of describing complex dynamic interactions between administered macro-molecules, cells, and disease states.

### Regimen Dependency

Regimen dependency was first shown for the antitumor efficacy of IL-2. Mice given 12 injections of a 1500-unit dose of this cytokine showed greater tumor inhibition than those mice that received 2 doses of 9000 units [121]. Similar results were obtained in a Phase I clinical trial in which patients with renal cell carcinoma were given one of three schedules of IL-2 at an IV dosage of 1.0 or $3.0 \times 10^6 \, U/m^2/day$ given either as a 24-hour continuous infusion, as a single daily bolus injection, or as a combination of one-half of the dose by bolus injection and the remaining one-half by 24-hour infusion [122]. At least three patients received each schedule. Two of the 23 patients with renal cell carcinoma had a partial response and acceptable toxicity with the combined bolus and continuous infusion regimen. On the other hand, disease progressed in the patients that received the same dose as a daily bolus injection.

Other investigators have also described regimen dependency for IL-12 given IV [27, 123] and SC [124].

The indirect response model shown in Figure 34.15 was used to describe the relationship between the administration of GH and IGF-1 in non-human primates [109]. The realistic assumption was made that the production of IGF-1 varied over time and, as shown in Figure 34.16, the model provided a reasonable characterization of the induction of IGF-1 after both single and multiple GH doses. However, one limitation to this simple model is its inability to account for the role of the IGFBPs in the responses to both GH and IGF-1. Thus, others have proposed more complex models that account for the induction of IGFBPs [110–112] that can have an impact on IGF-1 and GH dosage regimens [111–113] and, more recently, for mAbs targeting the IGF-1 receptor [113].

Table 34.18 displays the PK/PD models used to predict dosage regimens for different mAbs with different IgG isotypes [114–120]. The models use population PK methods to describe the mAb concentration time course and include parameters describing receptor occupancy and binding, biomarker expression, downstream cell-signaling events, and disease severity indexes. These publications establish PK/PD

**TABLE 34.18  Pharmacokinetic and Pharmacodynamic Models Used to Predict Dosing Regimens of mAbs**

| mAb/IgG Isotype | Target | Disease | PD endpoint | PK/PD model | Ref. |
|---|---|---|---|---|---|
| Abciximab Fab fragment | GP 11b/111a (CD41) | Coronary artery disease (angioplasty) | *Ex-vivo* platelet aggregation | Mechanism-based model with target mediated disposition | [114] |
| Efalizumab[a] IgG$_1$ | CD11a | Psoriasis | CD11a | Mechanism based receptor mediated Pop PK | [115] |
| Golimumab IgG$_1$ | TNF-$\alpha$ | RA | ACRN | Inhibitory indirect response model Pop PK | [116] |
| Omalizumab IgG$_1$ | IgE | Asthma | Total and free IgE | Feedback model Pop PK | [117] |
| Otelixizumab IgG$_1$ (aglycosylated) | CD3 | Psoriasis Type 1 Diabetes | CD4$^+$ & CD8$^+$ T-cell counts CD3 T-cell receptors | Direct response PD Pop MM PK | [118] |
| Rituximab IgG$_1$ | CD20 | Follicular NHL | Progression-free survival | Drug–disease time to event model Pop PK TPP model | [119] |
| Volociximab IgG$_4$ | $\alpha_5\beta_1$ integrin | Cancer | Free $\alpha_5\beta_1$ (on monocytes) | Mechanism-based receptor binding Pop PK | [120] |

Abbreviations: Pop, population PK; RA, rheumatoid arthritis; MM, Michaelis-Menton; NHL, non-Hodgkin's lymphoma; TPP, time to progression.

[a]Withdrawn from the market in 2009.

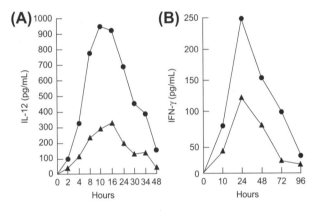

**FIGURE 34.17** Regimen dependency of IL-12 pharmacokinetics and IFN-$\gamma$ stimulating effects. (A) IL-12 serum concentrations are compared in patients who received an SC dose of 1.0 g/ml IL-12 on day 1 of their therapy (●) with levels obtained in other patients who received the same dose on day 15 of an escalating-dose scheme (▲). (B) the IFN-$\gamma$ responses of these two patient groups are compared. Reproduced with permission from Motzer RJ, Rakhit A, Schwartz LH, Olencki T *et al.* Clin Cancer Res 1998;4:1183–91 [124].

For example, Motzer and colleagues [124] treated patients with renal cell carcinoma with IL-12, administered on days 1, 8, and 15 either as a fixed dose of 1.0 µg/kg or as a series of escalating doses. As shown in Figure 34.17, IL-12 concentrations and IFN-$\gamma$ response were greater after patients received their initial 1.0-µg/kg dose on the fixed-dose regimen than after they received the same dose on day 15 as part of the dose-escalation scheme. However, more severe

toxicity was encountered with the single, fixed-dose regimen, and the maximum tolerated dose was lower (1.0 µg/kg) than that achievable with the escalation scheme (1.5 µg/kg). As a result, Phase II trials with this cytokine were begun with a regimen in which doses were escalated to 1.25 µg/kg.

## REFERENCES

[1] Internet at, http://pharmastrategyblog.com/2011/02/2010-fda-drug-approvals.html.

[2] Mullard A. 2010 FDA Drug approvals. Nat Rev Drug Discov 2011;10:83–5.

[3] Coté RJ, Morrissey DM, Houghtone AN, Beattie EJ, Oettgen HF, Old LJ. Generation of human monoclonal antibodies reactive with cellular antigens. Proc Natl Acad Sci USA 1983;80:2026–30.

[4] Sears HF, Atkinson B, Mattis J, Ernst C, Herlyn D, Steplewski A, et al. Phase-1 clinical trial of monoclonal antibody in treatment of gastrointestinal tumours. Lancet 1982;1:762–5.

[5] Mellstedt H. Monoclonal antibodies in human cancer. Drugs Today (Barc) 2003;39(Suppl. C):1–16.

[6] Hoet RM, Cohen EH, Kent RB, Rookey K, Schoonbroodt S, Hogan S, et al. Generation of high-affinity human antibodies by combining donor-derived and synthetic complementarity-determining-region diversity. Nat Biotechnol 2005;23:344–8.

[7] Colcher D, Goel A, Pavlinkova G, Beresford G, Booth B, Batra SK. Effects of genetic engineering on the pharmacokinetics of antibodies. QJ Nucl Med 1999;43:132–9.

[8] Clark M. Antibody humanisation for therapeutic applications. Cambridge UK: Cambridge University. Internet at, www.path.cam.ac.uk/~mrc7/ humanisation/index.html; 2000.

[9] Anon. Monoclonal antibody production. Washington DC: Access Excellence @ the National Health Museum. Internet at, www.accessexcellence.org/RC/VL/GG/monoclonal.html; 1999.

[10] Batra SK, Jain M, Wittel UA, Chauhan SC, Colcher D. Pharmacokinetics and biodistribution of genetically engineered antibodies. Curr Opin Biotechnol 2002;13:603–8.

[11] Miller K, Meng G, Liu J, Hurst A, Hsei V, Wong WL, et al. Design, construction, and in vitro analysis of multivalent antibodies. J Immunol 2003;170:4854–61.

[12] Iznaga-Escobar N, Mishra Ak, Perez-Rodriguez R. Factors affecting the pharmacokinetics of monoclonal antibodies: A review article. Methods Find Exp Clin Pharmacol 2004;26:123–7.

[13] Colcher D, Pavlinkova G, Beresford G, Booth BJ, Batra SK. Single-chain antibodies in pancreatic cancer. Ann NY Acad Sci 1999;880:263–80.

[14] Putnam WS, Prabhu S, Zheng Y, Subramanyam M, Wang YMC. Pharmacokinetic, pharmacodynamic and immunogenicity comparability assessment strategies for monoclonal antibodies. Trends Biotech 2010;28:509–16.

[15] Pardridge WM, Kang YS, Yang J, Buciak JL. Enhanced cellular uptake and in vivo biodistribution of a monoclonal antibody following cationization. J Pharm Sci 1995;84:943–8.

[16] Lee HJ, Pardridge WM. Monoclonal antibody radiopharmaceuticals: Cationization, pegylation, radiometal chelation, pharmacokinetics, and tumor imaging. Bioconj Chem 2003;14:546–53.

[17] Igawa T, Tsunoda H, Tachibana, Maeda A, Mimoto F, Moriyama C, et al. Reduced elimination of IgG antibodies by engineering the variable region. Protein Eng Des Sel 2010;23:385–92.

[18] Myler HA, Given A, Kolz K, Mora JR, Hristopoulos G. Biotherapeutic bioanalysis: A multi-indication case study review. Bioanalysis 2011;3:623–43.

[19] Lee JW, Kelley M, King LE, Yang J, Salimi-Moosavi H, Tang MT, et al. Bioanalytical approaches to quantify "total" and "free" therapeutic antibodies and their targets: Technical challenges and PK/PD applications over the course of drug development. AAPS J 2011;13:99–110.

[20] Chappell WR, Mordenti J. Extrapolation of toxicological and pharmacological data from animals to humans. Adv Drug Res 1991;20:1–116.

[21] Mordenti J, Chen SA, Moore JA, Ferraiolo BL, Green JD. Interspecies scaling of clearance and volume of distribution data for five therapeutic proteins. Pharm Res 1991;8:1351–9.

[22] Schaub R, Garzone P, Bouchard P, Rup B, Keith J, Brinkhous K, et al. Preclinical studies of recombinant factor IX. Semin Hematol 1998;35(Suppl. 2):28–32.

[23] Brinkhouse KM, Sigman JL, Read MS, Stewart PF, McCarthy KP, Timony GA, et al. Recombinant human Factor IX: Replacement therapy, prophylaxis, and pharmacokinetics in canine hemophilia B. Blood 1996;88:2603–10.

[24] Mordenti J, Osaka G, Garcia K, Thomsen K, Licko V, Meng G. Pharmacokinetics and interspecies scaling of recombinant human factor VIII. Toxicol Appl Pharmacol 1996;136:75–8.

[25] Nadeau RR, Ostrowski C, Ni-Wu G, Liberator DJ. Pharmacokinetics and pharmacodynamics of recombinant human interleukin-12 in male rhesus monkeys. J Pharmacol Exp Ther 1995;274:78–83.

[26] Rakhit A, Yeon MM, Ferrante J, Fettner S, Nadeau R, Motzer R, et al. Down-regulation of the pharmacokinetic–pharmacodynamic response to interleukin-12 during long-term administration to patients with renal cell carcinoma and evaluation of the mechanism of this "adaptive response" in mice. Clin Pharmacol Ther 1999;65:615–29.

[27] White G, Shapiro A, Ragni M, Garzone P, Goodfellow J, Tubridy K, et al. Clinical evaluation of recombinant factor IX. Semin Hematol 1998;35(Suppl. 2):33–8.

[28] Atkins MB, Robertson MJ, Gordon M, Lotze MT, DeCoste M, DuBois JS, et al. Phase 1 evaluation of intravenous recombinant human interleukin 12 (rhIL-12) in patients with advanced malignancies. Clin Cancer Res 1997;3:409–17.

[29] Wolberg AS, Stafford DW, Erie DA. Human factor IX binds to specific sites on the collagenous domain of collagen IV. J Biol Chem 1997;272:16717–20.

[30] Duconge J, Fernandez-Sanchez E, Alvarez D. Interspecies scaling of the monoclonal anti-EGF receptor ior EGF/r$^3$ antibody disposition using allometric paradigm: Is it really suitable? Biopharm Drug Dispos 2004;25:177–86.

[31] Mahmood I. Interspecies scaling of protein drugs: Prediction of clearance from animals to humans. J Pharm Sci 2004;93:177–85.

[32] Duconge J, Castillo R, Crombet T, Alvarez D, Matheu J, Vecino G, et al. Integrated pharmacokinetic–pharmacodynamic modeling and allometric scaling for optimizing the dosage regimen of the monoclonal ior EGF/r$^3$ antibody. Eur J Pharm Sci 2004;21:261–70.

[33] Wang W, Prueksaritanont T. Prediction of human clearance of therapeutic proteins: Simple allometric scaling method revisited. Drug Dispos 2010;31:253–63.

[34] Oitate M, Masubuchi N, Ito T, Yabe Y, Karibe T, Aoki T, et al. Prediction of human pharmacokinetics of therapeutic monoclonal antibodies from simple allometry of monkey data. Drug Metab Pharmacokinet 2011;26:423–30.

[35] Ling J, Zhou H, Jiao Q, Davis HM. Interspecies scaling of therapeutic monoclonal antibodies: Initial look. J Clin Pharmacol 2009;49:1382–402.

[36] Suntharalingam G, Perry MR, Ward S, Brett SJ, Castello-Cortes A, Brunner MD, et al. Cytokine Storm in a Phase 1 trial of the anti-CD28 monoclonal antibody TGN1412. New Engl J Med 2006;355:1018–28.

[37] Committee for Medicinal Products for Human Use. Guideline on strategies to identify and mitigate risks for first-in-human clinical trials with investigational medicinal products. London: EMEA/CHMP. Internet at, www.emea.europa.eu/docs/en_GB/document_library/Scientific_guideline/2009/09/WC500002988. pdf; July 19, 2007.

[38] Muller PY, Milton M, Lloyd P, Sims J, Brennan FR. The minimum anticipated biological effect level (MABEL) for selection of first human dose in clinical trials with monoclonal antibodies. Curr Opin Biotech 2009;20:722–9.

[39] Yu J, Karcher H, Feire AL, Lowe PJ. From target selection to minimum acceptable biological effect level for human study: Use of mechanism-based PK/PD modeling to design safe and efficacious biologics. AAPS J 2011;13:169–78.

[40] Cheung WK, Goon BL, Guilfoyle MC, Wacholtz MC. Pharmacokinetics and pharmacodynamics of recombinant human erythropoietin after single and multiple subcutaneous doses to healthy subjects. Clin Pharmacol Ther 1998;64:412–23.

[41] Veldhuis JD, Evans WS, Johnson ML. Complicating effects of highly correlated model variables on nonlinear least-squares estimates of unique parameter values and their statistical confidence intervals: Estimating basal secretion and neurohormone half-life by deconvolution analysis. Methods Neurosci 1995;28:130–8.

[42] Albertsson-Wikland K, Rosberg S, Libre E, Lundberg LO, Groth T. Growth hormone secretory rates in children as estimated by deconvolution analysis of 24-h plasma concentration profiles. Am J Physiol 1989;257:E809–14.

[43] Bright GM, Veldhuis JD, Iranmanesh A, Baumann G, Maheshwari H, Lima J. Appraisal of growth hormone (GH) secretion: Evaluation of a composite pharmacokinetic model that discriminates multiple components of GH input. J Clin Endocrinol Metab 1999;84:3301–8.

[44] Macdougall IC, Roberts DE, Neubert P, Dharmasena AD, Coles GA, Williams JD. Pharmacokinetics of intravenous, intraperitoneal, and subcutaneous recombinant erythropoietin in patients on CAPD. A rationale for treatment. Contrib Nephrol 1989;76:112–21.

[45] Cetron JS, Bury RW, Lieschke GJ, Morstyn G. The effects of dose and route of administration on the pharmacokinetics of granulocyte-macrophage colony stimulating factor. Eur J Cancer 1990;26:1064–9.

[46] Lauresen T, Grardjean B, Jørgensen JOL, Christiansen JS. Bioavailability and bioactivity of three different doses of nasal growth hormone (GH) administered to GH-deficient patients:

Comparison with intravenous and subcutaneous administration. Eur J Endocrinol 1996;135:309–15.

[47] Radwanski E, Perentisis G, Jacobs S, Oden E, Affrime M, Symchowicz S, et al. Pharmacokinetics of interferon alpha-2b in healthy volunteers. J Clin Pharmacol 1987;27:432–5.

[48] Schuller J, Czejka MJ, Schernthaner G, Wirth M, Bosse C, Jager W, et al. Pharmacokinetics of interferon-alfa-2b after intrahepatic or intraperitoneal administration. Semin Oncol 1992;19(Suppl. 3):98–104.

[49] Aoyama K, Uchida T, Takanuki F, Usui T, Watanabe T, Higuchi S, et al. Pharmacokinetics of recombinant human interleukin-11 (rhIL-11) in healthy male subjects. Br J Clin Pharmacol 1997;43:571–8.

[50] Montagna M, Montillo M, Avanzini MA, Tinelli C, Tedeschi A, Visai L, et al. Relationship between pharmacokinetic profile of subcutaneously administered alemtuzumab and clinical response in patients with chronic lymphocytic leukemia. Haematologia 2011;96:932–6.

[51] Xu Z, Wang Q, Zhuang Y, Frederick B, Yan H, Bouman-Thio E, et al. Subcutaneous bioavailability of golimumab at 3 different injection sites in healthy subjects. J Clin Pharmacol 2010;50:276–84.

[52] Plosker GL, Keam SJ. OmalizuMab: A review of its use in the treatment of allergic asthma. BioDrugs 2008;22:189–204.

[53] Smith DA, Minthorn EA, Beerahee M. Pharmacokinetics and pharmacodynamics of mepolizumab, an anti-interleukin-5 monoclonal antibody. Clin Pharmacokinet 2011;50:215–27.

[54] Kearns GL, Kemp SF, Frindik JP. Single and multiple dose pharmacokinetics of methionyl growth hormone in children with idiopathic growth hormone deficiency. J Clin Endocrin Metabol 1991;72:1148–56.

[55] Hayashi W, Kinoshita H, Yukawa E, Higuchi S. Pharmacokinetic analysis of subcutaneous erythropoietin administration with non-linear mixed effect model including endogenous production. Br J Clin Pharmacol 1998;46:11–9.

[56] Kindler J, Eckardt KU, Ehmer B, Jandeleit K, Kurtz A, Schreiber A, et al. Single-dose pharmacokinetics of recombinant human erythropoietin in patients with various degrees of renal failure. Nephrol Dial Transplant 1989;4:345–9.

[57] Supersaxo A, Hein WR, Steffen H. Effect of molecular weight on the lymphatic absorption of water-soluble compounds following subcutaneous administration. Pharm Res 1990;7:167–9.

[58] Kagan L, Turner MR, Balu-Iyer SV, Mager DE. Subcutaneous absorption of monoclonal antibodies: Role of dose, site of injection, and injection volume on rituximab pharmacokinetics in rats. Pharm Res 2012;29:490–9.

[59] Porter CJ, Charman SA. Lymphatic transport of proteins after subcutaneous administration. J Pharm Sci 2000;89:297–310.

[60] Jensen JD, Jensen LW, Madsen JK. The pharmacokinetics of recombinant human erythropoietin after subcutaneous injection at different sites. Eur J Clin Pharmacol 1994;46:333–7.

[61] Laursen T, Jørgensen JOL, Christiansen JS. Pharmacokinetics and metabolic effects of growth hormone injected subcutaneously in growth hormone deficient patients: Thigh versus abdomen. Clin Endocrinol 1994;40:373–8.

[62] Odeh YK, Wang Z, Ruo TI, Wang T, Frederiksen MC, Pospisil PA, et al. Simultaneous analysis of inulin and $^{15}N_2$-urea kinetics in humans. Clin Pharmacol Ther 1993;53:419–25.

[63] Sculier JP, Body JJ, Donnadieu N, Nejai S, Glibert F, Raymakers N, et al. Pharmacokinetics of repeated i.v. bolus administration of high doses of r-met-Hu interleukin-2 in advanced cancer patients. Cancer Chemother Pharmacol 1990;26:355–8.

[64] Konrad MW, Hemstreet G, Hersch EM, Mansell PW, Mertelsmann R, Kolitz JE, et al. Pharmacokinetics of recombinant interleukin 2 in humans. Cancer Res 1990;50:2009–17.

[65] Watari K, Ozawa K, Takahashi S, Tojo A, Tani K, Kamachi S, et al. Pharmacokinetic studies of intravenous glycosylated recombinant human granulocyte colony-stimulating factor in various hematological disorders: Inverse correlation

between the half-life and bone marrow myeloid cell pool. Int J Hematol 1997;66:57–67.

[66] Ericson SG, Gao H, Gericke GH, Lewis LD. The role of PMNs in clearance of granulocyte colony-stimulating factor (G-CSF) in vivo and in vitro. Exp Hematol 1997;25:1313–25.

[67] Tanswell P, Seifried E, Su PCAF, Feuerer W, Rijken DC. Pharmacokinetics and systemic effects of tissue-type plasminogen activator in normal subjects. Clin Pharmacol Ther 1989;46:155–62.

[68] Mortensen DL, Walicke PA, Wang X, Kwan P, Kuebler P, Gottlieb AB, et al. Pharmacokinetics and pharmacodynamics of multiple weekly subcutaneous efalizumab doses in patients with plaque psoriasis. J Clin Pharmacol 2005;45:286–8.

[69] Huang JD. What can the volume of distribution of macromolecular drugs indicate? Drug Metab Pharmacokinet 2010;25:510–20.

[70] James K. Interactions between cytokines and alpha-2 macroglobulin. Immunol Today 1990;11:163–6.

[71] Dickinson AM, Shenton BK, Alomran AH, Donnelly PK, Proctor SJ. Inhibition of natural killing and antibody-dependent cell-mediated cytotoxicity by the plasma protease inhibitor alpha 2-macroglobulin (alpha 2M) and alpha 2M protease complexes. Clin Immunol Immunopathol 1985;36:259–65.

[72] Hoffman M, Feldman SR, Pizzo SV. $\alpha_2$-macroglobulin "fast" forms inhibit superoxide production by activated macrophages. Biochim Biophys Acta 1983;760:421–3.

[73] Feige JJ, Negoescu A, Keramidas M, Souchelnitskiy S, Chambaz EM. Alpha 2-macroglobulin: A binding protein for transforming growth factor-beta and various cytokines. Horm Res 1996;45:227–32.

[74] Huang JS, Huang SS, Deuel TF. Specific covalent binding of platelet-derived growth factor to human plasma alpha 2-macroglobulin. Proc Natl Acad Sci USA 1984;81:342–6.

[75] LaMarre J, Wollenberg GK, Gonias SL, Hayes MA. Cytokine binding and clearance properties of proteinase-activated alpha 2-macroglobulin. Lab Invest 1991;65:3–14.

[76] Legrès LG, Pochon F, Barray M, Gay F, Chouaib S, Delain E. Evidence for the binding of a biologically active interleukin-2 to human alpha 2-macroglobulin. J Biol Chem 1995;83:81–4.

[77] Blum WF, Jensen LW, Madsen JK. Growth hormone insensitivity syndromes: A preliminary report on changes in insulin-like growth factors and their binding proteins during treatment with recombinant insulin-like growth factor I. Kabi Pharmacia Study Group on Insulin-like Growth Factor I Treatment in Growth Hormone Insensitivity Syndromes. Acta Paediatr Suppl 1993;82(Suppl. 391):15–9.

[78] Kostecka Y, Blahovec J. Insulin-like growth factor binding proteins and their functions. Endocr Regul 1999;33:90–4.

[79] Abdel-Razzak ZA, Loyer P, Fautrel A, Gautier JC, Corcos L, Turlin B, et al. Cytokines down-regulate expression of major cytochrome P-450 enzymes in adult human hepatocytes in primary culture. Mol Pharmacol 1993;44:707–15.

[80] Morgan ET. Regulation of cytochrome P450 during inflammation and infection. Drug Metab Rev 1997;9:1129–88.

[81] Chen JQ, Ström A, Gustafsson JA, Morgan ET. Suppression of the constitutive expression of cytochrome P-450 2C11 by cytokines and interferons in primary cultures of rat hepatocytes: Comparison with induction of acute-phase genes and demonstration that CYP2C11 promoter sequences are involved in the suppressive response to interleukins 1 and 6. Mol Pharmacol 1995;47:940–7.

[82] Gonzalez FJ. Molecular biology of cytochrome P450s. Pharmacol Rev 1989;40:243–87.

[83] Kurokohchi K, Matsuo Y, Yoneyama H, Nishioka M, Ichikawa Y. Interleukin-2 induction of cytochrome P450-linked monooxygenase systems of rat liver microsomes. Biochem Pharmacol 1993;45:585–92.

[84] Dickmann LJ, Patel SK, Dan RA, Wienkers LC, Slatter JG. Effects of interleukin-6 (IL-6) and an anti-IL-6 monoclonal

antibody on drug-metabolizing enzymes in human hepatocyte culture. Drug Metab Disp 2011;39:1415–22.

[85] Khakoo S, Glue P, Grellier L, Wells B, Bell A, Dash C, et al. Ribivarin and interferon alfa-2b in chronic hepatitis C: Assessment of possible pharmacokinetic and pharmacodynamic interactions. Br J Clin Pharmacol 1998;46:563–70.

[86] Hassan M, Nilsson C, Olsson H, Lundin J, Osterborg A. The influence of interferon-alpha on the pharmacokinetics of cyclophosphamide and its 4-hydroxy metabolite in patients with multiple myeloma. Eur J Haematol 1999;63:163–70.

[87] Le Cesne A, Vassal G, Farace F, Spielmann M, Le Chevalier T, Angevin E, et al. Combination interleukin-2 and doxorubicin in advanced adult solid tumors: Circumvention of doxorubicin resistance in soft-tissue sarcoma? J Immunother 1999;22:268–77.

[88] Schmitt C, Kuhn B, Zhang X, Kivitz AJ, Grange S. Disease–drug–drug interaction involving tocilizumab and simvastatin in patients with rheumatoid arthritis. Clin Pharmacol Ther 2011;89:735–40.

[89] Huang SM, Zhao H, Lee JI, Reynolds K, Zhang L, Temple R, et al. Therapeutic protein–drug interactions and implications for drug development. Clin Pharmacol Ther 2010;87:497–503.

[90] Morell A, Terry WD, Waldmann TA. Metabolic properties of IgG subclasses in man. J Clin Invest 1970;49:673–80.

[91] Brambell FWR, Hemmings WA, Morris LG. A theoretical model of γ-globulin catabolism. Nature 1964;203:1352–5.

[92] Junghans RP, Anderson CL. The protection receptor for IgG catabolism is the β2 microglobulin-containing neonatal intestinal transport receptor. Proc Natl Acad Sci USA 1996;93:5512–6.

[93] Venkatachalam MA, Rennke HG. The structural and molecular basis of glomerular filtration. Circ Res 1978;43:337–47.

[94] Maack T, Johnson V, Kau ST, Figueiredo J, Sigulem D. Renal filtration, transport, and metabolism of low-molecular-weight proteins: A review. Kidney Intl 1979;16:251–70.

[95] Ashwell G, Harford J. Carbohydrate-specific receptors of the liver. Annu Rev Biochem 1982;51:531–54.

[96] Lucore CL, Fry ETA, Nachowiak DA, Sobel BE. Biochemical determinants of clearance of tissue-type plasminogen activator from the circulation. Circulation 1988;77:906–14.

[97] Hovgaard D, Mortensen BT, Schifter S, Nissen NI. Comparative pharmacokinetics of single dose administration of mammalian and bacterially-derived recombinant human granulocyte-macrophage colony stimulating factor. Eur J Haematol 1993;50:32–6.

[98] Moonen P, Mermod JJ, Ernst JF, Hirschi M, DeLamarter JF. Increased biological activity of deglycosylated recombinant human granulocyte-macrophage colony stimulating factor produced by yeast or animal cells. Proc Natl Acad Sci USA 1987;84:4428–31.

[99] Kauskansky K. Role of carbohydrate in the function of human granulocyte-macrophage colony stimulating factor. Biochemistry 1987;26:4861–7.

[100] Watts MJ, Addison L, Long SG, Hartley S, Warrington S, Boyce M, et al. Crossover study of the haematological effects and pharmacokinetics of glycosylated and non-glycosylated G-CSF in healthy volunteers. Br J Haematol 1997;98:474–9.

[101] Morell AG, Gregoriadis G, Scheinberg HI, Hickman J, Ashwell G. The role of sialic acid in determining the survival of glycoproteins in the circulation. J Biol Chem 1971;246:1461–7.

[102] Chatelut E, Rostaing L, Grégoire N, Payen JL, Pujol A, Izopet J, et al. A pharmacokinetic model for alpha interferon administered subcutaneously. Br J Clin Pharmacol 1999;47:365–7.

[103] Kloft C, Graefe E-U, Tanswell P, Scott AM, Hofheinz R, Amelsberg A, et al. Population pharmacokinetics of sibrotuzumab, a novel therapeutic monoclonal antibody, in cancer patients. Invest New Drugs 2004;22:39–52.

[104] Felici A, Verweij J, Sparreboom A. Dosing strategies for anticancer drugs: The good, the bad and body-surface area. Eur J Cancer 2002;38:1677–84.

[105] Baker SD, Verweij J, Rowinsky EK, Donehower RC, Schellens JHM, Grochow LB, et al. Role of body surface area in dosing of investigational anticancer agents in adults 1991–2001. J Natl Cancer Inst 2002;94:1883–7.

[106] Ng CM, Lum BI, Gimenez V, Kelsey S, Allison D. Rationale for fixed dosing of pertuzumab in cancer patients based on population pharmacokinetic analysis. Pharmaceut Res 2006;23:1275–84.

[107] Wang DD, Zhang S, Zhao H, Men AY, Parivar K. Fixed dosing versus body size-based dosing of monoclonal antibodies in adult clinical trials. J Clin Pharmacol 2009;49:1012–24.

[108] Evans JP, Brinkhouse KM, Brayer GD, Reisner HM, High KA. Canine hemophilia B resulting from a point mutation with unusual consequences. Proc Natl Acad Sci USA 1989;86:10095–9.

[109] Sun YN, Lee JH, Almon RR, Jusko WJ. A pharmacokinetic/pharmacodynamic model for recombinant human growth hormone. Effects on induction of insulin-like growth factor 1 in monkeys. J Pharmacol Exp Ther 1999;89:1523–32.

[110] Baxter RC. Insulin-like growth factor (IGF) binding proteins: The role of serum IGFBPs in regulating IGF availability. Acta Paediatr Scand Suppl 1991;372:107–14.

[111] Carroll PV, Umpleby M, Alexander EL, Egel VA, Callison KV, Sonksen PH, et al. Recombinant human insulin-like growth factor-I (rhIGF-I) therapy in adults with type 1 diabetes mellitus: Effects on IGFs, IGF-binding proteins, glucose levels and insulin treatment. Clin Endocrinol 1998;49:739–46.

[112] Mandel SH, Moreland E, Rosenfeld RG, Gargosky SE. The effect of GH therapy on the immunoreactive forms and distribution of IGFBP-3, IGF-I, the acid-labile subunit, and growth rate in GH-deficient children. Endocrine 1997;7:351–60.

[113] Gualberto A. Figitumumab (CP-751,871) for cancer therapy. Expert Opin Biol Ther 2010;10:575–85.

[114] Mager DE, Mascelli MA, Kleiman NS, Fitzgerald JF. Simultaneous modeling of abciximab plasma concentration and ex vivo pharmacodynamics in patients undergoing coronary angioplasty. J Pharmacol Exp Ther 2003;307:969–76.

[115] Ng CM, Joshi A, Dedrick RL, Garovoy MR, Bauer RJ. Pharmacokinetic–pharmacodynamic–efficacy analysis of efalizumab in patients with moderate to severe psoriasis. Pharmaceut Res 2005;22:1088–100.

[116] Hu C, Xu A, Zhang Y, Rahman MU, Davis HM, Zhou H. Population approach for exposure–response modeling of golimumab in patients with rheumatoid arthritis. J Clin Pharmacol 2011;51:639–48.

[117] Lowe PJ, Renard D. Omalizumab decreases IgE production in patients with allergic (IgE-mediated) asthma; PK/PD analysis of a biomarker, total IgE. Br. J Clin Pharmacol 2011;72:306–20.

[118] Wiczling P, Rosenzweig M, Vaickus L, Jusko WJ. Pharmacokinetics and pharmacodynamics of a chimeric/humanized anti-CD3 monoclonal antibody, Otelixizumab (TRX4), in subjects with psoriasis and with type 1 diabetes mellitus. J Clin Pharmacol 2010;50:494–506.

[119] Ternant D, Hénin E, Cartron G, tod M, Paintaud G, Girard P. Development of a drug–disease simulation model for rituximab in follicular non-Hodgkin's lymphoma. Br J Clin Pharmacol 2009;68:561–73.

[120] Ng CM, Bai S, Takimoto CH, Tang MT, Tolcher AW. Mechanism-based receptor-binding model to describe the pharmacokinetic and pharmacodynamic of an anti-α5β1 integrin monoclonal antibody (volociximab) in cancer patients. Cancer Chemother Pharmacol 2010;65:207–17.

[121] Vaage J, Pauly JL, Harlos JP. Influence of the administration schedule on the therapeutic effect of interleukin-2. Intl J Cancer 1987;39:530–3.

[122] Sosman JA, Køhler PC, Hank J, Moore KH, Bechhofer R, Storer B, et al. Repetitive weekly cycles of recombinant human interleukin-2: Responses of renal carcinoma with acceptable toxicity. J Natl Cancer Inst 1988;80:60–3.

[123] Leonard JP, Sherman ML, Fisher GL, Buchanan LJ, Larsen G, Atkins MB, et al. Effects of single dose interleukin-12 exposure on interleukin-12-associated toxicity and interferon-gamma production. Blood 1997;90:2541–8.

[124] Motzer RJ, Rakhit A, Schwartz LH, Olencki T, Malone TM, Sandstrom K, et al. Phase 1 trial of subcutaneous human interleukin-12 in patients with advanced renal cell carcinoma. Clin Cancer Res 1998;4:1183–91.

# 35

# Design of Clinical Development Programs

Steven W. Ryder[1] and Ethan S. Weiner[2]

[1]*Astellas Pharma Global Development, Deerfield, IL 60015*
[2]*Latimer Brook Pharmaceutical Consultants, LLC, East Lyme, CT 06333*

## INTRODUCTION

Clinical development is the scientific process of exploring and confirming the product attributes and therapeutic role of potential new medical treatments. This chapter provides an overview of the clinical development of a pharmaceutical product for medical use, introducing and discussing the principles of clinical development and application of those principles on both a programmatic and a study level. While the development process is continuous, beginning during the discovery of an innovative potential pharmaceutical product and ending with the replacement of the innovative pharmaceutical by a more effective or safer alternative treatment, the process follows an orderly path of evidence-based, goal-directed development.

This chapter focuses on the clinical development and registration of an innovative pharmaceutical product in the treatment of patients or of an additional indication for an existing pharmaceutical product. The chapter covers clinical development spanning the traditional phases that are diagrammed in Figure 1.1 (Chapter 1). Coverage includes the conduct of proof of mechanism (PoM), proof of concept (PoC), and confirmatory clinical trials, registration and post-approval programs, including new indications and new formulations, risk-management plans, post-market studies and clinical trials conducted as part of risk evaluation and mitigation strategies authorized by the Food and Drug Administration Amendments Act (FDAAA) of 2007 [1]. The chapter also covers the development of both biological agents and small molecules, noting some areas that distinctly apply to each of these two therapeutic classes, but does not cover the development of non-pharmaceutical treatments, medical procedures, or medical devices, and does not discuss non-human development, although some development principles involving medical device and veterinary use products may be similar.

The clinical development process has allowed the introduction of many important new medical treatments that have improved public health and offered relief to countless patients. A recent example of the substantial public health impact of clinical development is the progress made in the treatment of patients with multiple sclerosis. Multiple sclerosis is the most common autoimmune disorder of the nervous system, has the potential to cause significant disability, and contributes significant public health morbidity [2]. Prior to the 1990s, therapy was non-specific and supportive. As noted in a 1951 medical textbook [3]:

> As yet there is no satisfactory treatment for the syndrome of multiple sclerosis, despite the large amount of published material concerning this subject.

Following a prescribed clinical development pathway, a number of agents have now been introduced to modify the course of multiple sclerosis [2]. While not able to repair already existing damage, the agents reduce the frequency and intensity of relapse. The first drug specifically approved for use in relapsing MS was interferon beta-1β[2,4,5], and the first oral drug specifically approved for use in relapsing MS was fingolomid

[6–8]. The medical introduction of both of these agents was the result of comprehensive and systematic clinical development programs [2, 8].

Importantly, the clinical development process is not stagnant. Rather, it is dynamic and evolves as science and medicine advance and as the information needs required by regulators, prescribers, patients, and payers continue to expand. It is the dynamic and improving capability of the clinical development process that assures its ability to continue to support significant medical and public health advancements.

# PRINCIPLES OF CLINICAL DEVELOPMENT

Clinical development is a scientific process that adheres to the principles of proper scientific conduct, to ethical principles applying to human research, to legal and regulatory requirements, and to the numerous technical guidances provided by governments and professional societies.

## Proper Scientific Conduct

Proper scientific conduct requires adherence to the principles of scientific excellence and integrity. All research should be soundly based on well-grounded prior evidence and, in accordance with this, clinical development requires a solid scientific foundation for the intervention being tested. The pathology and pathophysiology of the disorder under study should be examined and the actions of the studied intervention appropriately understood. Occasionally, empiric observations arise in clinical or preclinical studies that are unexpected and poorly understood on the basis of known pathophysiology and pharmacology. In these cases, attempts should be made to further understand the pharmacology and physiology underlying the observation. If this is not possible, or if studies fail to advance understanding, clinical development should proceed cautiously and with full consideration of the benefit/risk of the intervention.

Scientific misconduct, violation of integrity, and the occurrence of fraud have been reported in both preclinical and clinical investigations throughout the world. There is appropriate and particularly intense scrutiny of clinical development, since it involves human subjects and is closely linked with clinical therapeutics. This has caused an increasing emphasis on ensuring integrity through training, guidance, oversight, regulation, and law. It is the obligation of all scientists engaged in clinical development to assure that the highest standards of scientific conduct and integrity are always maintained.

## Ethical Principles

Ethical issues and concerns are prominent in the conduct of clinical development. Numerous agencies have issued reviews of the ethical principles of clinical research. These include ethical guidance issued by the US Department of Health, Education, and Welfare (now the Department of Health and Human Services) in the Belmont Report [9], by the World Medical Association in the Declaration of Helsinki [10], and by the Council for International Organizations of Medical Sciences in its International Ethical Guidelines for Biomedical Research Involving Human Subjects [11]. It is a fundamental requirement that clinical development respects the rights and well-being of all participating human subjects. External, objective review of the proposed clinical study by an independent review body (e.g., institutional review boards, regulatory agencies) is always required along with ongoing assessment of risks and benefits as substantial new information becomes available. This requires proper clinical study monitoring, data integration and review, and, for larger trials, may require an external, independent data safety monitoring board. A final rule on the Investigational New Drug Safety Reporting Requirements for Human Drug and Biological Products recently issued by the US Food and Drug Administration (FDA) [12] notes that, among other criteria, sponsors of clinical development must report an adverse event as a suspected adverse reaction if:

> an aggregate analysis of specific events observed in a clinical trial (such as known consequences of the underlying disease or condition under investigation or other events that commonly occur in the study population independent of drug therapy) indicates those events occur more frequently in the drug treatment group than in a concurrent or historical control group.

Adherence to this final rule requires diligent and regular study monitoring, data review, and analysis.

# LEGAL AND REGULATORY REQUIREMENTS

Clinical development occurs within a framework of increasing international, national, and local laws and regulation. The legal framework surrounding clinical development is substantially focused on pre-approval investigational activities, regulatory submission for approval, the approval process, and post-approval commitments and requirements. Although laws and regulations affecting these areas have been most notably increased in the EU, US, Japan, and affiliated regions such as Australia, New Zealand, and Canada, laws and regulations also are becoming increasingly stringent in emerging market areas such as China, India, Latin America, and Russia.

In the US, the FDA is the agency primarily charged with overseeing the regulation of clinical development activities, regulatory submissions, drug approval, and post-approval activities. The evolution of the legal framework impacting FDA-regulated clinical development in the US is discussed in Chapter 36 and has been summarized elsewhere [13]. A substantial recent addition to this legislation is the Food and Drug Administration Amendments Act (FDAAA) that in 2007 greatly increased the responsibilities of the FDA, provided it with new authorities, and reauthorized several FDA critical programs such as PDUFA, BPCA, and PREA. The Act [1]:

- Extensively expands the authority of the FDA to require sponsors to conduct and report on post-marketing studies and clinical trials. It defines a postmarketing requirement (PMR) as a study or trial that a sponsor is required by statute or regulation to conduct post-approval, and a post-marketing commitment (PMC) as a study or trial that a sponsor agrees to in writing, but is not required by law, to conduct post-approval;
- Introduces Risk Evaluation and Mitigation Strategies (REMS) as a tool to be used when "necessary to ensure that the benefits of the drug outweigh the risks of the drug";
- Requires the FDA to develop and maintain a website with comprehensive safety information about approved drug products. Among other things, the FDA must prepare a summary analysis of adverse reaction reports received for each drug 18 months after approval or after use of the drug by 10,000 individuals, whichever is later;
- Requires the FDA to conduct a regular bi-weekly screening of the Adverse Event Reporting System database and post a quarterly report on its website of "any new safety information or potential signal of a serious risk" identified within the last quarter;
- Requires the NIH (through the National Library of Medicine) to issue regulations that markedly expand the clinical trial registry and results databank;
- Establishes the Reagan-Udall Foundation to advance regulatory science and product safety; and

- Creates templates to immediately implement provisions regarding conflicts of interest waivers and disclosure of financial information for Advisory Committee members.

The body of Congressional Acts authorizes the FDA to issue regulations that have the strength of law and are codified in the Code of Federal Regulations (CFR) [14]. Particularly pertinent to clinical development are CFR Title 21, Part 50: Protection of Human Subjects; Part 56: Institutional Review Boards; Part 312: Investigational New Drug Application; Part 314: Applications for FDA Approval to Market a New Drug; and Part 316: Orphan Drugs.

In addition to these acts and amendments, the Patient Protection and Affordable Care Act (PPACA) [15] and the Health Care and Education Reconciliation Act of 2010 [16] include numerous health-related provisions to take effect over a 4-year period, including expanding Medicaid eligibility, subsidizing insurance premiums, providing incentives for businesses to provide health care benefits, prohibiting denial of coverage/claims based on pre-existing conditions, establishing health insurance exchanges, and support for medical research including a specific focus on comparative treatment clinical research. These substantive changes in US health care will have an impact on clinical development that is uncertain but will almost assuredly increase the emphasis on rigorously demonstrating the additional and comparative benefit of proposed new pharmaceutical treatments.

## Regulatory Guidance

In addition to regulation, the FDA issues guidance documents and other notes, representing the Agency's current thinking on a particular subject. Several guidances are issuances of the International Conference on Harmonization (ICH) approved guidelines. These documents cover both broad and focused areas. Guidances covering broad areas include the Content and Format of INDs, a number of ICH position papers, and a series of guidances describing Good Review Practices. Guidances are also regularly issued that focus on specific diseases (e.g., irritable bowel syndrome, lupus erythematosus), clinical trial design (e.g., adaptive design, establishment and operation of clinical trial data monitoring committees), or specific issues of efficacy (e.g., non-inferiority designs) or safety (e.g., assessment of abuse potential or suicidality). Guidances also outline the meetings between the FDA and sponsors that occur during the clinical development of a new pharmaceutical therapeutic. Typically, these meetings occur at the pre-IND, post-Phase I, end-of-Phase IIA, end-of-Phase II, and pre-NDA clinical development time points, and play a key role in effective clinical development. The FDA maintains a website with a comprehensive listing and current status of all guidance documents [17].

Directives, guidelines, and position papers pertinent to clinical development are also regularly issued by the European Medicines Agency (EMA), established by the European Union (EU) and beginning operations in 1995. The EMA guides, evaluates, and oversees pharmaceutical development, approval, and post-approval activities in EU member states. The directives, guidelines, and position papers of the EMA assume legal and regulatory status as they are approved by the EU Parliament and as they are adopted by EU member states. Although independent national regulatory agencies continue to exist, the EMA brings a comprehensive EU viewpoint on issues of clinical development and regulatory applications. The EMA also provides the opportunity for scientific advice meetings with clinical development sponsors. In addition, meetings with national regulatory agencies can also assist clinical development in the EU. The EMA website presents a complete listing of directives, guidelines, and position papers [18].

Since its establishment in April 2004, the Japanese Pharmaceuticals and Medical Devices Agency (PMDA) has become increasingly transparent and informative on the clinical development of new pharmaceutical products [19]. The PMDA is the Japanese regulatory agency which works together with the Japanese Ministry of Health, Labour and Welfare to protect the public health by assuring the safety, efficacy, and quality of pharmaceuticals and medical devices. The PMDA conducts scientific reviews of pharmaceutical and medical device regulatory applications and oversees and assists in their clinical development in Japan. Scheduled meetings between sponsors and the PMDA also are important in facilitating clinical development of pharmaceutical products in Japan.

For global clinical development programs, regulatory advice and guidance should routinely be obtained from the EU, US, and Japanese pharmaceutical regulatory authorities prior to the initiation of clinical development and periodically throughout the development process.

### International Conference on Harmonisation of Technical Requirements for Registration of Pharmaceuticals for Human Use (ICH)

In the early 1990s, the International Conference on Harmonisation of Technical Requirements for Registration of Pharmaceuticals for Human Use (ICH) was initiated to harmonize the drug development regulatory guidances in the EU, US, and Japan. ICH membership includes academic, regulatory, and pharmaceutical industry experts from the EU, the US, and Japan [20]. Six ICH conferences have been held since 1991 along with many meetings of the Steering Committee and Expert Working Groups. ICH guidelines have been issued on quality, safety, efficacy, and multidisciplinary topics, with the five-step process for implementation outlined by ICH for each of the three corresponding regions [21]. Formal implementation in the US occurs with the issuance of an approved FDA guidance such as Structure and Content of Clinical Study Reports (ICH E3), Good Clinical Practice: Consolidated Guideline (ICH E6), General Considerations for Clinical Trials (ICH E8), Statistical Principles for Clinical Trials (ICH E9), and Organization of the Common Technical Document (ICH M4).

### Good Clinical Practice

Clinical research is the core activity of clinical development, and it is essential that clinical development scientists adhere to the principles of good clinical research design, conduct, analysis, and reporting. The ICH Guideline for Good Clinical Practice (GCP) (ICH E6) [22] presents many of these principles and has been adopted by regulatory authorities in the EU, US, Japan and many other nations as the guideline for clinical research. Among the topics and functions covered in the guideline are the following:

- Institutional Review Board/Independent Ethics Committee (responsibilities, composition, functions, operations, procedures, and records);
- Investigator (qualifications, resources, compliance, handling of investigational product(s), informed consent of trial subjects, records, and reports);
- Sponsor (trial management, data handling, record keeping, quality control/assurance, financing, monitoring, handling of safety information, and reporting obligations);
- Clinical Trial Protocol (trial design and objective, selection and treatment of subjects, assessment of efficacy and safety, statistics, data handling, and clinical trial reporting);
- Investigator's Brochure (general considerations and contents for this document, which contains a summary of preclinical and clinical data known up to that point for use by investigators in clinical trials);

- Essential Documents (essential documents and their handling before, during, and after clinical trial conduct); and
- Standards for data quality and integrity.

GCP areas of particular focus for clinical development include:

- Ethics committee/IRB approval of protocols and updates during study conduct;
- Subject informed consent and privacy protection; protocol violations;
- Sponsor monitoring of investigative sites as required by standard procedures;
- Source data verification, including the verification of patients, matching of case report form data to source documents (e.g., medical records), record retention, and the audit trail for all case report form changes (i.e., who made them, why, and when);
- Timely reporting of serious adverse events to sponsors, ethics committees, and regulatory authorities; and
- The conduct of audits to assure GCP compliance by both sponsor and regulatory authorities.

## International (outside EU, US, Japan) and US State Regulation

The laws and regulations guiding and impacting clinical development are rapidly increasing as clinical research expands to more commonly involve areas outside of the EU, US, and Japan [23]. These laws and regulations should be reviewed and considered before planning a global clinical development program. In addition, state regulations may impact clinical development in the US, and most often address investigator financial disclosure [24] or agreements requiring health plans to pay for the routine medical care a patient receives while participating in a clinical trial [25].

## Business Regulation

For clinical development sponsors that are for-profit pharmaceutical firms, not-for-profit business organizations, or academic or governmental institutions, numerous laws and regulations addressing intellectual property, business conduct, or conflict of interest may also impact clinical development. Intellectual property concerns are increasingly important and are becoming increasingly complex with the global expansion of clinical research operations. They are important to consider as clinical development is planned, reviewed, and analyzed.

A number of laws and regulations govern the interactions of sponsors with investigators and with governmental officials. The US Federal Corrupt Practices Act specifically addresses relationships with foreign government officials. The US anti-trust regulations are particularly important because of the increasing importance of across-sponsor cooperation in the advancement of numerous pre-competitive scientific areas, such as the validation of biomarkers for use in clinical development. Several groups have directly addressed this issue through the creation of innovative, carefully defined structures. One example is the Biomarkers Consortium, a public–private partnership created to identify and qualify new biological markers. Members include the Foundation for the National Institutes of Health (FNIH), the National Institutes of Health (NIH), the FDA, the US Centers for Medicare & Medicaid Services (CMS), the Pharmaceutical Research and Manufacturers of America (PhRMA), the Biotechnology Industry Organization (BIO), and patient advocacy organizations [26, 27]. Projects sponsored by the consortium include adiponectin as a biomarker predictive of pharmaceutical glycemic efficacy [28, 29] and I-SPY 2 (Investigation of Serial Studies to Predict Your Therapeutic Response with Imaging and molecular Analysis 2), an adaptive Phase II clinical trial design in the neoadjuvant setting for women with locally advanced breast cancer that provides advice on the clinical development of paired anticancer pharmaceuticals and tumor biomarkers [30]. Continued support for broad-based, across-sponsor precompetitive collaboration is essential to advancing biomarkers, and proteomic and pharmacogenomic markers.

Sponsors of clinical development that are publicly held firms must also consider securities regulations that govern the release and sharing of information. Compliance with these regulations is mandatory and is determined by the materiality of the information. For a small biotechnology organization with few projects, the results of a single study or the occurrence of a single adverse reaction may be material, while the same information may not be material to a larger pharmaceutical organization with multiple projects.

## Data Privacy

Clinical development must also consider the impact of laws and regulations concerning data privacy, including the European Commission's Directive on Data Protection [31] and the US Privacy Rule enacted under the Health Insurance Portability and Accountability Act of 1996 (HIPAA) [32]. The increasingly multinational conduct of clinical development programs enhances the importance of adhering to privacy regulations. Clinical development design, conduct, analysis, and reporting must consider data privacy, while maintaining auditable data verification, allowing the composite pooling of appropriate data, and supporting the clinical trial data usage in all global areas. Informed consent is essential with full disclosure of the extent of necessary data collection, the need for verification, and the use of the data to support appropriate monitoring and regulatory requirements. Knowledge of and adherence to the scientific, ethical, legal, and regulatory principles of clinical development not only is essential, but also assures full support for the clinical research enterprise and allows for continuous improvements of the clinical development process within this framework.

## EVIDENCE-BASED, GOAL-DIRECTED CLINICAL DEVELOPMENT

Clinical development of a drug or biologic candidate is traditionally divided into four phases: Phase I, in which the pharmacokinetic, pharmacodynamic and early safety properties of the drug are determined, generally in healthy volunteers; Phase II, in which proof of efficacy along with safety and toleration are demonstrated in the targeted disease state and a dose response is determined; Phase III, in which selected doses are tested in larger numbers of subjects in order to confirm safety and efficacy; and post-approval Phase IV, in which new indications or use of the drug in special situations are examined. Over the years, it has been recognized that this paradigm is overly simplistic and gives the incorrect impression that these activities are chronologically separated and that drug development is a linear process. In fact, many "Phase I" studies, such as drug–drug interaction studies or bioequivalence studies, are often done later in development, and many Phase I studies, even first-in-human studies, are done in patients, not healthy volunteers.

Modern drug development programs therefore have come to be characterized as having different somewhat overlapping stages, focused first on "learning" and then on "confirming", as outlined below [33]:

- Nomination for development by discovery – after it has been demonstrated that the molecule in question has adequately characterized *in vitro* and *in vivo* pharmacology and has the appropriate pharmaceutic properties. This includes suitable potency and specificity for the desired target and effectiveness in animal models of the intended disease states to be treated, if such models exist. It also often includes demonstration of an acceptable genetic and short-term toxicology profile.

- Proof of mechanism (PoM) – demonstrating that the drug or biologic candidate in man gets to its target tissues at levels sufficient to have an effect on pharmacodynamic markers or biomarkers, showing that the agent exerts its intended mechanism (i.e., blocks or stimulates the appropriate receptors, inhibits the relevant enzymes or has an effect on a closely-related downstream activity). Typically, tens of study subjects are treated short term (days to weeks) to establish PoM.

- Proof of concept (PoC) – demonstrating that the candidate has a desirable effect on the appropriate endpoints in the relevant disease state(s) at a dose that is adequately tolerated with an acceptable level of serious adverse events. Generally, hundreds of study subjects are treated for weeks to months in order to establish PoC.

- Confirmatory clinical trials – demonstrating with a high degree of rigor, often with replicate studies, that the candidate has desirable effects on efficacy endpoints suitable for registration and has an acceptable safety profile, with risks that are out-weighed by the benefit conferred. Such programs typically involve thousands of study subjects, many of which may be treated for one to several years if chronic diseases are being targeted.

As emphasized in Chapter 18, the appropriate choice of biomarkers or clinical endpoints suitable for PoM, PoC, or confirmation trials is integral to the candidate development program. However, the demonstration of an "acceptable safety profile" or "tolerability" is also a critical factor in designing a development program.

Two major issues inform the design of all development programs: the resource requirements for each development phase, and candidate drug attrition.

### Exponential Growth of Resource Requirements as a Clinical Development Program Progresses

The cost of a complete development program adequate to meet regulatory requirements for registration costs was estimated to be $800 million in 2003, and is likely well over $1 billion for current candidates [34, 35]. Clinical trials account for the largest proportion of this cost, and this is a function of the number of study subjects enrolled, the duration of the trial, and the complexity of the endpoints being measured. The clinical activities required for PoC trials generally take 2–3 years and have direct costs in the range of $10–$50 million. Confirmatory clinical trials generally require 2 to > 5 years to complete, at a direct cost of $100–$500 million or more.

## High Attrition at All Phases of Clinical Development

Of every 100 molecules nominated for development, about 15 will become marketed pharmaceuticals. Failures occur in all phases of development, and candidate drug "survival" rate is roughly 50–65% in Phase I, 25–40% in Phase II, and 50–66% in Phase III. Furthermore, about 15–20% of candidates submitted for regulatory approval never become marketed. These percentages have not shown improvement over the past one to two decades, and if anything have recently become somewhat worse. Candidate survival rates vary somewhat by therapeutic area, and are somewhat higher for biologics (overall survival about 30%) vs small molecules (overall survival about 15%) [36, 37].

The primary reasons for attrition at the PoM phase are failure to achieve suitable tissue penetration or failure to affect desired pharmacodynamic endpoints or biomarkers, followed by adverse preclinical toxicology findings that emerge during long-term toxicology studies. Lack of tolerability or other safety issues are additional causes of early failure in early clinical trials. The predominant reasons for failure at the PoC phase are lack of effectiveness in the disease being tested followed by issues of clinical safety. Even in the confirmatory phase, failure to demonstrate benefit remains a primary cause for failure, as do safety issues which arise as larger populations are examined [Arrowsmith and Mooney, personal communication (Pfizer Global R&D, 2006)].

With all the advances over the past two decades in understanding the underlying basic science of disease pathways, one would have expected attrition rates to improve rather than to stagnate or worsen. The continuing high attrition rate is partly due to more stringent evidentiary requirements for evaluating drug candidates because of an intensified focus on the safety of drug candidates in development, and partly due to the fact that most candidates currently are developed for diseases for which treatments already exist. Hence market acceptance, if not regulatory acceptance, requires most new agents to have either a better safety profile or more pronounced efficacy than existing drugs. This presents an ever higher hurdle as our therapeutic armamentarium improves. The high failure rates are also partly due to the massive proliferation of previously unexplored targets that basic

science has produced over the past two decades as hundreds of new cytokine, kinase, and other enzymatic and signal transduction pathways have been elucidated. For example, agents to inhibit the effect of IL-1, TNF-α, and P-38 MAP kinase all showed good efficacy in preclinical models of rheumatoid arthritis. However, in clinical trials only anti-TNF-α showed a high degree of effectiveness and revolutionized therapy for the disease [38, 39], whereas anti-IL-1 showed modest efficacy [40], and P-38 MAP kinase inhibitors failed to have any lasting positive impact on the disease and are no longer being developed for rheumatoid arthritis [41, 42]. Unfortunately, ways to predict a priori which of these mechanisms will be successful, before undertaking clinical development, still lag behind the underlying science which identifies new targets. Similar problems plague pharmaceutical development in most therapeutic areas.

## Key Milestones: Proof of Mechanism, Proof of Concept, and Confirmation

Since failure is the norm and resource requirements rise exponentially as programs progress, clinical development programs are designed to fail as early as possible, but are also designed so that failure at each step yields critical information for follow-on programs. Programs that make it through stringent early hurdles are then run to succeed. Therefore, a well-designed program should focus on establishing or failing to establish PoM and PoC, and then on building the basis for success during confirmatory clinical trials. PoC is the inflection point after which a well-designed program which has not failed should be designed for success in the confirmatory phase. A well-designed program which does fail at the PoM or PoC stage also should provide key feedback for the drug-discovery scientists. In particular, it should provide answers as to whether the agent failed because it did not reach the target tissue in adequate levels or because of unanticipated toxicity, both of which can possibly be designed out of a follow-on candidate, or whether it failed to impact the disease in question because the pharmacologic rationale underlying target selection was flawed. With this information in hand, drug-discovery scientists can either produce new candidates that have the same mechanism of action but which correct the particular defect that caused the prior molecule to fail, or abandon the target and move on to new ones.

### Proof of Mechanism Trials

This approach informs the clinical trial designs for the studies which make up the development program.

Studies to assess PoM have designs and endpoints to answer the following questions:

- Does the candidate at a tolerated dose achieve suitable tissue levels at the target tissues, and does it bind to or inhibit its target?
- Does the agent have its desired pharmacologic activity at the site of action?
- Is there evidence that the mechanism targeted has a clinically relevant effect on the disease?
- Are safety and tolerability acceptable?

A well-designed trial should either confirm that the candidate meets all of the above requirements, or, if not, which hurdle failed and why. It should do so by exposing the fewest study subjects to the candidate for the shortest possible time, both to minimize human exposure to an unknown new agent and to minimize resource usage since at this stage failure is the likely outcome. As discussed in Chapter 18, endpoints for early trials are generally biomarkers but there generally is progression to more clinically established trial endpoints in later phases of development. Several examples of how endpoints evolve from pharmaco-dynamic markers or biomarkers to more established clinical endpoints as development progresses are shown in Table 35.1 [43–46].

### Proof of Concept Trials

Should the candidate achieve PoM, studies to assess PoC should focus on answering related questions:

- Is the pharmacologic activity of relevance to treating the symptoms of the disease, and for chronic diseases, is it likely to be of relevance to the natural history or progression of the disease?

- Is the drug adequately tolerated at a dose achieving the desired pharmacologic effects, taking into account the inherent limitations of relatively small trial size (hundreds of subjects) and short duration (weeks to months)?

Since these studies should be of the shortest possible duration to answer these questions, endpoints are focused on factors which can respond fairly quickly to an intervention, but which are also predictive of longer-term benefit. Sometimes these endpoints will be "hard clinical endpoints" that measure symptom improvement; sometimes they will be biomarkers or imaging tests that predict longer-term improvement. Examples for various chronic diseases are provided in Table 35.1, along with possible endpoints that would be examined in a PoC trial.

There are other considerations which also enter into deciding whether a drug candidate has achieved PoC, such as whether the agent is sufficiently well behaved from a pharmaceutic and pharmacokinetic perspective, whether it shows signs of differentiation from existing agents, and whether there is a clear set of endpoints and study designs accepted by regulatory authorities for the claims being sought [47].

Should the candidate fail in this phase, information again is passed back to drug discovery regarding whether this was a failure of the target to impact the disease, despite prior PoM showing that the pharmaceutical affected the target (as was the case with the P-38 MAP kinase inhibitors), or whether this was a failure due to a toxicity. If the latter, the data generated by a well-designed program should also be able to address whether the toxicity was related to the target itself or to the particular agent being used.

Should a candidate pass the PoC phase, subsequent trials enroll more subjects who are treated for

TABLE 35.1  Endpoint Selection in a Development Program[a]

| Disease to be treated | Possible PoM endpoints | Possible PoC endpoints | Regulatory approval endpoints |
|---|---|---|---|
| Rheumatoid arthritis | CRP, cytokine levels in blood or joint | DAS, ACR-20 | DAS, ACR-20, radiographic change, functional outcomes |
| Alzheimer's disease | Hippocampal imaging | ADAS-cog | ADAS-cog, clinician global change score |
| Multiple sclerosis | CNS and systemic markers of inflammation | MRI lesions | Number of relapses, neurological status |
| Osteoarthritis disease modification | Cartilage degradation products, anabolic markers (none yet validated) | Possibly signs and symptoms (e.g., WOMAC), possibly imaging modalities (e.g., MRI) | Radiographic change (joint space narrowing), functional status |

[a]Abbreviations: CRP, C-reactive protein; DAS, disease activity score for RA [43]; ACR-20, American College of Rheumatology 20% improvement score for an individual study subject which shows a 20% improvement over their baseline score in terms of the number of affected joints and other related factors [44]; ADAS-cog, Alzheimer's Disease Assessment Scale, Cognitive Subscale [45]; MRI, magnetic resonance imaging; WOMAC, Western Ontario and McMaster University osteoarthritis index [46].

longer durations. However, before moving to confirmatory Phase III trials, additional trials, sometimes called "Phase IIb" trials, are often conducted. The major purpose of such trials is to refine selection of the dose that optimally balances efficacy and safety, to "de-risk" the confirmation phase by conducting larger, longer-duration trials to ascertain whether beneficial effects observed in PoC trials can be replicated, and to acquire a larger safety database. Dose selection is sometimes folded into pre-PoC trials, especially if adaptive designs are used, as discussed below.

### Confirmatory Trials to Support Registration

Phase III confirmatory trials are often designed after consulting with regulatory authorities at an "end of Phase II meeting" with the appropriate review division at the US FDA, at a scientific advice session with the Committee on Human Medicinal Products of the EMA, or at meetings with national regulatory agencies in Europe and the Japanese PMDA. By this point, there should be sufficient knowledge of how the drug candidate behaves that agreement can be reached with regulatory authorities regarding the *a priori* specification of clinically relevant endpoints that will be included in designing the confirmatory trials. There must also be agreement on many of the study design aspects reviewed later in this chapter.

Examples of possible endpoints for confirmatory trials are included in Table 35.1. These endpoints are usually widely accepted scales of clinical benefit in a given disease state, such as the ACR-20 for rheumatoid arthritis [44] or the Alzheimer's Disease Assessment Scale cognitive subscale (ADAS-cog) for Alzheimer's disease [45]. Often it is required that the candidate shows benefit in more than one endpoint in order to establish claims, such as improvement in ADAS-cog plus improvement in the physician's global assessment for Alzheimer's disease [48]. Specific recommended endpoints for selected disease states are outlined in both FDA [17] and EMA [18] development guidances. Because confirmatory trials provide the vast majority of patient exposure to the pharmaceutical candidate, they also are instrumental in meeting registration requirements for an adequate safety database.

### Subsequent Clinical Trials

At the time the candidate is under review for marketing approval, and even after the drug is marketed, there are new questions which are raised:

- *Will very rare adverse effects occur that were not seen in the pre-registration database?* This question is often best answered by pharmacovigilance and epidemiologic surveillance, rather than by clinical trials, and such activities form an integral part of the risk management plan for the drug.
- *Will the agent be safe and effective in a more broadly defined population than was studied in the pre-registration development program?* For instance, can it be given to patients with concomitant morbidity, such as congestive heart failure? Clinical trials to address this question often make up part of what traditionally was called "Phase IV".
- *Will adverse events with an initially low background rate in the population being treated increase with prolonged drug treatment?* Such effects, for example a 30% increase in the incidence of stroke, MI, or cardiac death, are very hard to detect in a preregistration program. Large event-based outcomes trials often will be needed after registration to answer this question.
- *Will the agent be effective in conditions similar to those studied in the initial development program?* For example, will a drug developed for rheumatoid arthritis be useful in ankylosing spondylitis or psoriatic arthritis? Such separate development programs with both PoC and confirmatory phases often are conducted after an agent is initially marketed for a related condition. Because such programs take advantage of the vast knowledge developed in the initial dossier, such as safety data, dose response for the parent disease, and PK/PD data, these programs can be smaller and faster than the original program.

Clinical development of a drug candidate spans the gamut from the time the candidate is first introduced into man through its life cycle as a marketed agent. Throughout the process, the questions being asked by clinical trials, and the trial design and endpoints being measured, evolve with the specific needs of the program at that time. Initially the program is designed around likely failure, so early clinical trials seek to assess the relevance of the underlying pharmacology. During the next development phase, clinical trials are designed to learn the optimum dose and regimen for drug administration. Subsequently, the program seeks to establish efficacy, based on specific endpoints that have been agreed upon in meetings with regulatory authorities as representing effectiveness in the relevant disease state, while establishing an adequate safety database. Finally, the same process is used to conduct additional trials to look at related indications or broader populations and enhance knowledge of the agent's safety.

## SPECIFIC DESIGN ISSUES IN CLINICAL DEVELOPMENT PROGRAMS

Individual clinical trials are the building blocks of the development program, and, in addition to the above, there are many other design factors that must be considered for each clinical trial if it is to play its role effectively in the development program.

### Ethical Design Considerations

Ethical principles are embodied in the Declaration of Helsinki as well as in GCP guidelines, and designers of a clinical program must consider the ethical implications of study design as each clinical protocol is written. Every study is required to have a valid, testable hypothesis. For example, does treatment with the drug candidate have a specified impact on a given endpoint? Generally, studies testing therapeutic efficacy are done in patients with the disease who stand to benefit from the treatment. Often, however, early trials in humans to assess pharmacokinetic and pharmacodynamic parameters are done in healthy volunteers, since this provides a more standardized, more predictable population with less co-morbidity. However, if the drug candidate has high potential risks, ethical considerations dictate doing even these early trials in patients. In some areas, such as oncology, even first-in-human trials are designed to be of sufficient length to provide potential benefit to cancer patients.

There has been much controversy over the ethical use of placebos. The Declaration of Helsinki justifies the use of a placebo only if no other treatment exists, or if compelling scientific reasons dictate its use. In general, placebo-controlled trials are performed in non-progressive, non-life-threatening conditions, or if performed in progressive chronic disease, such trials are of short duration (often 12 weeks or less) and are usually followed by an extension phase in which every study subject receives an active treatment. Placebo-controlled trials are often necessary to provide a clear assessment of drug effect, and in many circumstances are required by regulatory agencies for proof of effectiveness. The alternative to a placebo-controlled trial is a non-inferiority trial, which compares an active drug with a known alternative. Such trials present both design and interpretation issues, as discussed later in this chapter. The ideal study design has been stated to be a design that includes both placebo and active control: the placebo arm to provide the reference for the population, and the active control to confirm that the trial is capable of demonstrating efficacy.

Temple and Ellenberg [49, 50] summarize the issues with the use of placebos and conclude that placebos generally remain necessary to establish the efficacy of a new pharmaceutical candidate, and that placebo use also generally remains ethically acceptable when used for a limited duration of time not associated with significant morbidity.

### Study Populations

Considerations in selecting a study population with a given disease include the choice of including either a patient population with little co-morbidity and limited complications of the disease, or a population with more co-morbidity or more disease complications. The former population oftentimes provides a clearer assessment of drug effect, since there are fewer confounders in the assessment of both safety and efficacy. However, it leaves open the question of whether the observed therapeutic benefits and safety profile can be generalized to more "real world" disease populations who often have complications and co-morbidities. Studying the latter population introduces more confounders but provides a more realistic assessment. In general, early-phase development programs focus on a restricted population (i.e., before PoC), but during the confirmatory phase include a broader population, so that by the time of dossier submission a population has been treated that is more representative of the patients who will use the agent in medical practice. In addition, there are regulatory expectations that the elderly, the young, and other special populations will be included in adequate numbers by the time a development program is completed.

### Study Design Paradigms

There are several fundamental trial designs that are reviewed from a regulatory and statistical perspective in the ICH E9 guidelines [51]. Each trial design has its advantages and disadvantages. However, in general trials are randomized, so that subjects are assigned to different treatment regimens by an algorithm rather than by the investigator's choice, and double-blind, so that neither the investigator treating the study subjects nor the subjects themselves know which treatment regimen they are allocated to.

#### Cross-Over Studies

Early development-phase studies frequently use a cross-over design in which subjects receive each of several different treatments for several days, often with a several-day washout period between treatments, and then are assigned to another of the treatment regimens. The different arms of the study to which subjects are randomized receive the treatments in different order. Such studies allow each subject to serve as his or her own control, eliminating confounding patient selection factors due to imbalances in age, gender, genetic makeup, disease duration and severity, and other individual factors. However, interpretation of cross-over studies can be confounded because key measurements may change over the time of the study or the effects of the prior treatment may linger beyond the washout period. As a result, cross-over designs are generally feasible only for small numbers of study subjects and are mainly used in early-phase development.

## Cohort Studies

Another design predominantly used in early development is the cohort study, in which small groups of subjects (often 10–12) are randomized either to the active agent or to placebo, often with more subjects receiving drug than placebo. Subsequent cohorts often are treated with higher doses of the study drug or different combinations of study drug and other agents. These studies afford the assessment of safety and PK in one cohort before the next cohort is treated, and lend themselves to early evaluation of agents about which little safety data exist. By incorporating different dosing regimens, cohort studies allow rapid ascertainment of the maximum tolerated dose and rapidly add key PK and PD insights. It also is common to pool the placebo groups from the various cohorts and compare that entire placebo group to the various cohorts receiving the candidate drug. As with cross-over designs, these studies are generally limited to short treatment durations and small numbers of subjects, and can be confounded by temporal shifts between cohorts. In addition, a large amount of variability is introduced if the different cohorts are evaluated by different investigators at different study sites, often making results difficult or impossible to interpret. Hence, as with cross-over studies, cohort studies best lend themselves to early development and are best suited to single-investigator settings.

## Parallel Group Studies

Most safety and efficacy data in a development program are acquired by means of parallel group studies in which subjects are randomly allocated to two or more treatment arms. Patients in each arm usually receive one treatment regimen for the duration

of the study, but there are variations in which the regimens are modified for each treatment arm at a prespecified study time-point. Parallel group studies are amenable to any treatment duration and can be scaled up over multiple sites, since any confounding introduced by time or by study-site differences will be more or less equally applied to each arm of the study. Since regulatory agencies often require studies of 1 year or longer to show evidence of durable efficacy and acceptable toxicity in many chronic diseases, such studies, almost by definition, must be parallel group studies. The major drawback of these studies is that the treatment arms can be imbalanced by factors that can affect the outcome, such as significant co-morbidity that can affect safety assessments or the fact that patients with the most severe disease at baseline tend to show the greatest improvement during the study as they "regress to the mean". Enrolling larger numbers of study subjects and stratifying them by prognostic factors known to affect the study outcome (i.e., putting equal numbers from each stratification factor into each treatment group) are two common ways to mitigate these confounders.

## Adaptive Study Designs

Increasing use is being made of adaptive study designs in which the study data are sampled and the study modified under controlled circumstances that are specified in the study protocol. Examples include early termination of a study for futility (statistical demonstration based on partial results that there is a very low probability of showing a drug effect), modification of study size based on observed variability in results (more variability than planned will require a larger study size, less variability a smaller study size), or reallocation of study subjects to various treatment arms or cohorts based on prior results in order to maximize the number of patients allocated to treatment-dose groups or regimens with the highest therapeutic index [52]. These techniques can be very powerful in increasing the efficiency of clinical development. At the same time they can become quite challenging from an operational perspective, as the repeated interim analyses called for by some of the more complex adaptive designs require extraordinary steps to protect data integrity while data are being rapidly acquired and analyzed [53]. Some adaptive design features, such as futility analysis and modification of study size based on a blinded assessment of variability, are well accepted by regulatory authorities even in pivotal confirmatory trials. However, other adaptive designs, especially those that seek to combine the learning (pre-PoC) and confirming phases into one study, are generally still considered only suitable for exploratory trials both by the FDA [54] and by regulators elsewhere [55]. Despite these caveats, elements of adaptive design, while rarely used just a decade ago, are now finding their way into most clinical development programs because of the increased efficiency that they can add to these programs.

## Statistical Considerations Underlying the Number of Study Subjects

As noted previously, every clinical trial should have a hypothesis to be tested. Generally, such a hypothesis for a superiority study is that the active treatment will have a specified difference, or *effect size*, compared to placebo or the comparator drug. For example, for a rheumatoid arthritis study it could be postulated that the active agent in the trial will produce an ACR-20 response (see Table 35.1) in at least 25% more of the study subjects given the experimental therapy than those receiving placebo [44]. Generally, the study is designed to validate the hypothesis that the observed difference has a 95% chance of being more than 25 units if any similar population is studied, and that the likelihood of the observed difference in the study being due to chance or confounders alone is less than 5% ($\alpha = 0.05$), the level most commonly required to conclude that a result is "statistically significant". The larger the number of study subjects enrolled, the more

likely the findings will achieve this level of certainty, because increasing the number of subjects reduces the impact of variability due to random "noise". Likewise, the larger the effect size is for a given number of study subjects, the more likely the effect will achieve this degree of certainty because the "signal to noise ratio" is larger. The likelihood that a study will achieve the desired goal based on a given effect size is termed the study *power*. The number of study subjects per treatment arm required to achieve a given power is a function of the inherent variability of the study population, the study endpoint, and the effect size. Generally, studies are powered to 80–90%, meaning that the designers expect 80–90% certainty that if the agent they are testing truly has the desired effect size designed into the study, it will manifest itself with statistical significance when the study is completed.

These concepts are illustrated in Figure 35.1. While it is impossible to generalize over the vast array of study designs, diseases, endpoints, and pharmaceuticals, generally tens to hundreds of subjects per arm are required. If one intends to impact an infrequent outcome, the number of study patients can be in the thousands or tens of thousands. Small increases in variability, small decreases in anticipated effect size, or small changes in desired power (e.g., going from 80% to 90%) have very large impacts on the number of patients required for each treatment group – often many-fold the size of the change in the input parameter.

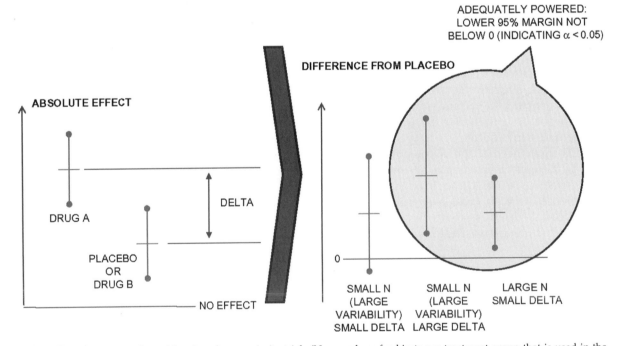

**FIGURE 35.1**  Statistical considerations for superiority trials (N = number of subjects per treatment group that is used in the power calculations, Delta = expected effect size).

Non-inferiority studies, in which one active agent is compared to another to show that their effect is similar, add additional complexities. The approach is outlined in Figure 35.2. These studies are powered to demonstrate that the lower 95% confidence bound of the difference between the experimental agent and the established agent is no worse than a specified amount. For instance, if two antibiotics are being compared for community acquired pneumonia, the study might be powered to show that the lower 95% confidence bound of the cure rate for the experimental agent stays above the −5% non-inferiority margin. That way we can say with 95% confidence that the experimental agent at worst cures 5% fewer pneumonias than the established antibiotic. At best, it may cure the same amount or more, but it is the worst-case scenario that the study must be powered for. How much worse the experimental agent can be and still be considered "non-inferior" can become a major issue, involving clinical judgment, health policy, and statistics. A large non-inferiority margin is of little use because it allows for the experimental agent to be sufficiently worse than the established agent that the clinical relevance of the findings is called into question. Conversely, very small non-inferiority margins, requiring very tight confidence bounds, require inordinately large numbers of patients per treatment arm. The right balance is often difficult to ascertain, and sometimes may not exist. The FDA, for instance, in its influenza

guidance does not consider non-inferiority studies to be valid evidence of effectiveness partly because there is no consensus on what a meaningful non-inferiority margin might be [56]. In other areas, such as community-acquired pneumonia [57], where sufficient data on effectiveness of active agents exist and placebo studies would be unethical, regulatory agencies accept non-inferiority studies, but in this and other conditions caution the sponsor that extensive justification of the non-inferiority margin used is required [58]. Despite the issues associated with these trials, many recent new drug applications, particularly for antibacterial agents, have relied on non-inferiority designs in the key pivotal trials that support the registration dossier [59]. These study designs will also be heavily relied upon in any comparative effectiveness program.

## The Impact of Safety Assessment on Development Programs

Whereas efficacy is measured with specific endpoints and prespecified differences between treatments that are incorporated into the hypothesis testing of a clinical trial, safety is holistic, oftentimes unpredictable, and its evaluation must be comprehensive. While many unsafe potential drug candidates are weeded out in preclinical assessment, this does not assure safety in the clinic and many types of adverse events are difficult to predict from *in vitro* or *in vivo*

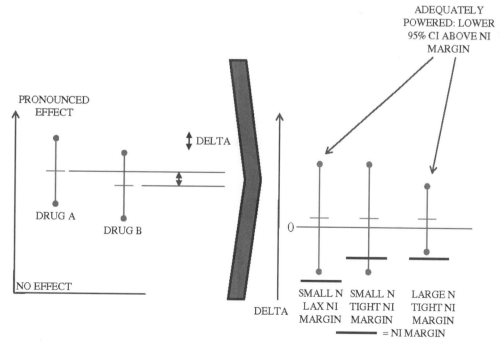

**FIGURE 35.2** Statistical considerations for non-inferiority trials (delta = between treatment difference in effect, CI = confidence interval, NI = non-inferiority).

preclinical data. While studies can be designed to test specific safety-related hypotheses using a formal statistical powering method (e.g., there will be x% fewer cases of renal failure on an experimental transplant drug vs standard of care), most preregistration knowledge of candidate drug safety is accrued by treating as many patients as possible for as long as possible. Modern drug development programs typically vastly exceed the minimum requirements set by ICH for the amount of required patient exposure to an experimental agent by the time the dossier is filed for approval, as shown in Table 35.2 [60], which compares a typical recent development program for a chronic disease to the ICH guidelines [61].

Large databases are required not only to characterize more common adverse events, but also to detect rare but severe events such as agranulocytosis, toxic epidermal necrolysis, or fulminant hepatic necrosis. These life-threatening conditions often occur at rates of 1 in 10,000 to 1 in 100,000 for drugs known to cause them. For instance, a database with 6,000 patients exposed to an experimental agent would have about a 50% chance of detecting an adverse event that occurs at a rate of 1 in 10,000, and a single event could be dismissed as chance alone. The likelihood of such a database containing two such events, which would begin to raise serious concerns about the candidate, is only about 12%. Therefore, drug development programs must be constructed to be of adequate size to characterize safety with a reasonable degree of certainty.

Power calculations based on efficacy hypotheses generally dictate the size of the component studies in a drug development program. Often the aggregate drug exposure provided by these studies is inadequate

either in number of subjects treated or duration of treatment, or in both, to fully characterize safety to a degree suitable for registration. Hence, the development program must incorporate other types of studies to accrue adequate exposure data. For example, additional efficacy studies can be performed that test alternate hypotheses while adding to the size of the safety database. Such studies also have the advantage of providing exposure to placebo and/or additional comparative agents, helping to place safety data observed with the experimental candidate in a broader context. Alternatively, it is common practice to allow subjects completing double-blind studies to enter extension studies. Such studies provide long-term exposure and offer study subjects the opportunity to remain on treatment should they have a good response. This not only enhances patient recruitment into the studies but also places the entire program on a solid ethical foundation.

Many development programs must be designed to meet an even more difficult safety challenge than detecting very rare events by demonstrating that a drug candidate does not increase the amount of low-level background morbid events. Certain drug classes such as oral antidiabetic agents or cyclooxygenase inhibitors have the potential to increase the rate of major adverse cardiovascular events (MACE) (i.e., strokes, non-fatal myocardial infarctions, and cardiac deaths). These events occur at a background rate of several occurrences per 100 patient-years in many of the populations being treated for chronic diseases such as arthritis or diabetes. For example, design of an outcome trial to demonstrate that a drug candidate does not cause an increase in the rate of MACE events can take an approach similar to that of a non-inferiority study by being powered to show that the occurrence of MACE events in a population treated with the new agent (often for 1–2 years) at worst (upper confidence bound) does not exceed by more than a given percentage the rate observed with a comparator treatment. Thus, if the outcomes trial were powered for 20% and the background rate of MACE events was 5% per year, the trial would need to show with 95% confidence that MACE events for the experimental treatment were less than 6% (i.e., 20% more than 5%). These safety studies are major undertakings, and their size grows exponentially as the background rate of events of interest falls or the non-inferiority margin is reduced. As seen in Table 35.3, if the rate of MACE events is 4% per year for both the experimental drug and background therapy, it would take 743 study subjects per arm to show that the experimental drug did not increase MACE events by more than 80% with a 95% confidence level, and

TABLE 35.2 Size of a Preregistration Safety Database

| Study subjects' exposure to investigational drug | ICH guideline (# of subjects) | Size of a contemporary chronic use drug database (# of subjects)[a] |
|---|---|---|
| Total exposure to new drug | 1500 | 2498 |
| Duration > 3 months | | 2237 |
| Duration > 6 months | | 1979 |
| Duration > 1 year | 100 | 1698 |
| Duration > 2 years | | 821 |
| Duration > 3 years | | 153 |

[a]Data from Pfizer, Inc. Advisory Committee Briefing Document EXUBERA – Endocrinologic and Metabolic Drugs Advisory Committee 2005. Internet at, www.fda.gov/ohrms/dockets/ac/05/briefing/2005-4169B1_01_01-Pfizer-Exubera.pdf [60].

**TABLE 35.3  Size of Event-Based Outcomes Trials**

| Percent of subjects with event | Upper 95% CI = 1.1 | Upper 95% CI = 1.3 | Upper 95% CI = 1.8 | Upper 95% CI = 2.0 |
|---|---|---|---|---|
| 1% | 173,354 | 19,339 | 2747 | 1765 |
| 4% | 44,961 | 5076 | 743 | 483 |
| 10% | 19,414 | 2244 | 347 | 231 |
| 15% | 13,840 | 1630 | 264 | 178 |

Assumptions:
- Two arms – 1 : 1 randomization to treatments A or drug B
- Treatments A and B have equal risk – i.e., a true odds ratio of 1.0 is assumed
- Need to show that drug A is no worse (95% upper bound) than drug B to level of 1.1, 1.3, 1.8 or 2.0 with 90% power
- Study will be run until requisite number of events achieved
- Size of treatment arms not adjusted upwards to correct for potential early withdrawals from the study.

5076 subjects per arm to show that the same agent with a true rate identical to background therapy did not increase the rate of MACE events by more than 30%.

Current FDA guidelines for antidiabetic drug development require at the time of registration that the safety database is large enough, or that an outcomes trial exists, to demonstrate a no more than 80% increase in MACE events over background or comparator treatments, and that a post-approval commitment be made to study sufficient subjects to establish this at the 30% level [62]. As concerns for the cardiovascular safety of commonly used drugs increase, such requirements are likely to become more common features of other clinical development programs. This methodology can also be applied to address concerns that a pharmaceutical agent could potentially increase other major health events, such as infection or cancer, over an existing background rate. Finally, as in the above example of antidiabetic drugs, the clinical development program for drug safety does not end at the time of dossier submission but post-approval clinical trials, coupled with epidemiology and pharmacovigilance, continue as long as the agent remains in medical use.

## CONDUCT OF CLINICAL DEVELOPMENT

### Number and Location of Study Sites for Global Clinical Development Programs

Small trials conducted early in development are often conducted at one or only a few study sites. As programs progress into large parallel group trials, tens or hundreds of study sites become the norm. Modern large multicenter trials are often global in scope. Advantages of global trials include access to large numbers of qualified study subjects that would be difficult to recruit solely in North America or Western Europe. This also expands the diversity of the study population, making it more representative of the ultimate users of the drug. It may also enhance the validity of the development program to foreign regulatory authorities, provided that sufficient numbers of study subjects from their respective country or region are enrolled to give them confidence that the study results can be generalized to their jurisdiction [63].

Historically, data quality was suspect from trials conducted in regions outside of North America and Western Europe. However, with the adoption of electronic data capture and global standards such as GCP this is no longer a significant issue. Likewise, statistical methodologies have been developed for dealing with regional variability [64]. Despite these advances, cultural, regulatory, and operational barriers continue to impede the conduct of global trials [65]. However, large global trials that are coordinated with global development programs and use the same pivotal studies for simultaneous filing in major regions of the world are rapidly becoming the norm in clinical development programs.

### Data Flow and Data Quality

The flow of data in a clinical trial is schematized in Figure 35.3. A significant part of GCP is concerned with data quality and integrity. Sponsors of clinical trials must assure themselves and regulatory authorities through comprehensive and consistent monitoring of activities at every study site that GCP standards were maintained and that the data were collected as specified by the study protocol. These monitoring activities must also assure that every study subject's data is valid and can be verified by examination of source documents such as medical records and office notes. Data, whether entered on paper case report forms or electronically, must have an audit trail indicating when the data were entered, why and when any changes were made, and the persons who entered and changed the data. Before study data can be analyzed, the data must have been verified, inconsistencies checked with the study site and resolved, and the database "locked" for analysis.

The advent of electronic data capture has streamlined this process by enabling study sites to enter data directly through an internet portal into the study database, and has been one of the key enablers of global clinical trials. Data entry software has even provided automated recognition of some data

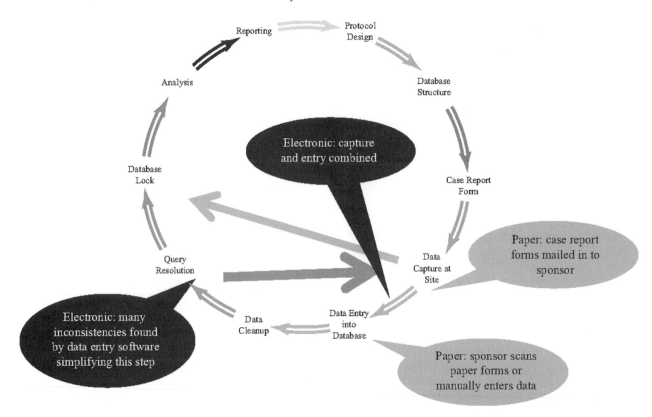

**FIGURE 35.3**   Clinical trial data flow.

inconsistencies (Figure 35.3). It also has facilitated the adoption of adaptive designs for which electronic data capture provides the rapid data turnaround that is required to make the protocol-specified changes in study design that are based on the acquired data.

## Use of Independent Data Monitoring Committees (IDMCs) and Adjudication Committees

For the past several decades, large clinical trials with outcomes related to survival, mortality, or major events such as myocardial infarction have used IDMCs to monitor unblinded data as these were acquired during a study and, under appropriate circumstances, advise the sponsor to modify or terminate the study. Although generally not required under regulatory law, IDMCs have become more widespread and are now used in the majority of large confirmatory trials, and even smaller PoC trials for some indications. Generally, an IDMC should be used for any trial in which a clinically important difference in significant morbidity is possible between treatment arms. An IDMC is equally appropriate to safeguard against the risk of increased adverse events or mortality in the experimental treatment arm or against

worse outcomes, such as more disease progression, in the non-experimental or placebo arms of a study.

The composition of IDMCs includes clinicians, preferably with experience in drug safety and expertise in the disease under study, and statisticians who operate independently of the sponsor. Their roles and responsibilities are defined by a charter that generally specifies committee membership and rules of operation, the milestones at which the board will review data, the specific data that the board will review, and what the board is allowed to communicate back to the sponsor without compromising the integrity of the study. It is critical that communication back to the sponsor be limited to what is absolutely necessary in order to avoid revealing information about how the respective study arms are performing, which could influence further conduct of the study outside of the specific IDMC remit and thus unblind the study. Often the board is restricted to simply recommending that the sponsor continue the study unchanged, eliminate one or more arms in the study, modify the dose of one of the treatments in the study, or terminate the study entirely. Occasionally boards are provided with specific "stopping rules", so that the board will recommend termination or modification of the study if a prespecified difference is observed between treatment groups. The FDA [66] and EMA [67] each have guidance documents for IDMCs that elaborate the benefits (independent oversight of study conduct, protection of patient safety) and risks (particularly the potential of interim analyses to bias future study conduct) and provide practical guidance regarding the composition, operation, and remit of these committees.

Somewhat related in function to IDMCs are adjudication committees, which are groups of independent experts who review study data, often in a blinded fashion unlike the case with IDMCs, in order to assess whether specific criteria are met for important study events. Most cardiovascular outcomes trials, for instance, have a committee to adjudicate data acquired about every suspected MACE event and use prespecified criteria to determine whether the incident under review truly represents a MACE event, to be counted as an endpoint for the trial, or some other type of adverse event. Similarly, a blinded adjudication committee might be used in an oncology study to provide an unbiased assessment of tumor progression.

## SPECIAL TOPICS

### Personalized Medicine

The optimal therapy of individual patients has been a long-standing goal of clinical pharmacologists and has been enhanced by the incorporation of therapeutic drug monitoring and pharmacokinetics into clinical care. Recent advances in pharmacogenetics and pharmacogenomics represent an extension of this effort to "personalize" medicine. As discussed in previous chapters, genomic and biological markers have played key roles in the clinical development of a number of drugs, and the evolving process and evidentiary standards of diagnostic validation and "fit-for-purpose" utilization are important considerations for clinical development scientists [68]. Recent examples include the HER2 assay for trastuzumab in the treatment of breast and gastric cancer, the KRAS mutation assay for cetuximab and pantitumumab in the treatment of colon cancer, the EGFR mutational assay for erlotinib in the treatment of lung cancer, the HIV CCR5 tropism assay for maraviroc in the treatment of HIV, and the HLA-B 5701 assay for abacavir in the treatment of HIV.

Incorporation of a genomic or biomarker diagnostic should be considered during exploratory development (pre-PoC) along with the development of a diagnostic assay that is validated, standardized, practical, scalable, and affordable at the time of regulatory registration. The pace and clinical development relevance of personalized medicine is anticipated to increase, so clinical development scientists must be aware of personalized medicine advances in the therapeutic and pharmacologic areas relevant to their research.

### Elderly and Pediatric Populations

Clinical development programs should gather sufficient information to assess benefit and risk and provide adequate treatment guidance for the population of patients likely to receive the new treatment following approval. Since most disease states occur more frequently in elderly patients, there has been special emphasis on assuring adequate participation of elderly subjects in clinical development programs. Advanced age alone should generally not exclude clinical trial participation, especially in confirmatory clinical trials. Rather, exclusion criteria should be medically appropriate and based on the pharmacology of the new treatment and the characteristics of the disease under study. The clinical development program should recognize that age-related physiological changes, as described in Chapter 26, may impact the pharmacokinetics or the pharmacodynamic response to a new treatment. In addition, elderly clinical trial participants generally use more concomitant medication and have more concurrent medical illness. For these reasons, clinical development programs should: (1) in early development, specifically investigate the comparative pharmacokinetics of a new pharmaceutical treatment in elderly and young patients; (2) include adequate numbers of elderly participants in clinical trials; and (3) specifically review the aggregate efficacy and safety results in elderly and young clinical trial participants. There is specific ICH guidance on the inclusion of elderly subjects in clinical development programs [69, 70].

It is important that infants and children have access to new pharmaceutical treatments and that adequate information be available on their use in the pediatric population. There is increasing focus on assuring these goals and on the pediatric clinical development of new pharmaceutical products. In the US, the Pediatric Research Equity Act (PREA) of 2003 requires the FDA and sponsor to agree on the conduct and timing of the pediatric studies, with their possible deferral pending the acquisition of appropriate preliminary information. If the new pharmaceutical treatment is not anticipated to have pediatric application, a specific FDA waiver of pediatric development must be obtained [71]. In addition, the Best Pharmaceutical for Children Act (BPCA) of 2002 incentivizes pediatric clinical development by providing an additional 6 months of marketing exclusivity for products that have a pediatric data package which is accepted by the FDA [72]. In the EU, regulatory approval applications must include the results of pediatric studies conducted in compliance with a Pediatric Investigation Plan (PIP), unless a deferral has been granted, or unless pediatric development is inappropriate or not necessary [73]. The PIP is binding, and must be agreed to in advance by the sponsor and the Pediatric Committee of the EMA. If changes are required during clinical development of the new pharmaceutical product, modification of the plan must be requested from the Pediatric Committee. Compliance with the PIP is checked at the time of application for marketing authorization but also provides the pharmaceutical product with eligibility for a 6-month extension of market exclusivity in the EU.

There are a number of ethical concerns particular to the conduct of pediatric clinical development. These include the process of obtaining informed consent, which raises issues of even subtle coercion or influence. In general, written informed consent must be obtained from both parents or a legal guardian, as well as assent from children able to understand, and consent from older children and adolescents. In each instance a full disclosure of risks and benefits

must be made using appropriate and understandable language [74, 75].

## Orphan Drugs

Specific legislative and regulatory actions have been taken in the EU, US, and Japan to support the development of new pharmaceutical treatments for patients with rare diseases [76–79]. These actions are intended to address and incentivize the clinical development of designated "orphan drug" candidates. Table 35.4 shows the specific orphan drug definitions, actions, and incentives for each of the three regions. In addition to the disease prevalence restriction, legislation enabling orphan product development in the US requires that applications for orphan product designation demonstrate that the candidate drug has "promise" for efficacy in treating the rare disease. As reported by the FDA, the Orphan Drug Act has been successful in promoting the development of more than 300 new pharmaceutical treatments for rare diseases since 1983, compared to fewer than 10 such treatments in the prior decade [80]. In the single area of rare neurological diseases, over 27 new treatments have been introduced in the US between 1983 and 2009, covering the areas of movement disorders (14 treatments), seizures (7 treatments), sleep (3 treatments),

**TABLE 35.4**  Orphan Drug Definitions, Regulatory Actions, and Incentives in the EU, US, and Japan

| Legislation (year) | Definition | Regulatory actions | Incentives |
|---|---|---|---|
| EU Orphan Medicinal Product Regulation (2000) | Disorder that affects < 5/10,000 people in the EU, or the treatment is intended for a life-threatening, seriously debilitating, or serious and chronic condition in the EU, and that without incentives it is unlikely that the marketing of the medicinal product would generate sufficient return to justify the necessary investment | • EMA Scientific Advice and protocol assistance<br>• Reduction of fees or fee waivers will be considered for all types of pre- and post-authorization activities | • 10-year period of market exclusivity for the orphan drug indication<br>• Tax incentives<br>• Incentives made available by EU and Member States |
| US Orphan Drug Act (1982) | Disorder that affects < 200,000 people in the US, or that affects > 200,000 persons but is not expected to recover the costs of developing and marketing the treatment drug | • Creation of Office of Orphan Products Development (OOPD)<br>• FDA written recommendations concerning required clinical studies<br>• Possible fast-track regulatory review of marketing application | • 7-year period of market exclusivity for the orphan drug indication<br>• Tax incentives<br>• Orphan Drug Product Grants Program |
| Japan Orphan Drug Pharmaceutical Affairs Law Revisions (1993) | Disorder that affects < 50,000 people in Japan (corresponding to < 4/10,000 people) and is incurable and without alternative treatment, or the efficacy and expected safety of the drug must be excellent in comparison with other available drugs | • Fast-track Marketing Authorization procedure<br>• Regulatory consultation<br>• Specific mention of global clinical trial acceptability | • Up to a 10-year period of market exclusivity for the orphan drug indication<br>• Tax incentives<br>• Possible financial support for development costs |

pain (2 treatments), and spinal cord spasticity (1 treatment) [81].

Clinical development programs for orphan drug indications should adhere to the same principles, guidance, and good practice that apply to all clinical development. In order to address the rarity of the diseases under study, combined and collaborative efforts are being proposed to accelerate biomarker validation, improve patient access, and accelerate research and development in rare diseases [82]. Clinical development scientists involved with orphan drug development should consider these and other available resources.

## Comparative Effectiveness

Increasing importance is being placed on comparing the efficacy and safety profiles of new pharmaceutical products with those of existing treatments, and there is particular emphasis on the need for direct comparative studies. In these studies, the active comparator serves as the reference for the proposed new pharmaceutical candidate, oftentimes instead of placebo. The importance of comparative effectiveness has been highlighted in the evaluations of many regulatory and reimbursement agencies, including the UK National Institute for Health and Clinical Excellence (NICE) [83] and the US Department of Health and Human Services Agency for Healthcare Research and Quality (AHRQ) [84]. Both NICE and AHRQ sponsor reviews in which the efficacy and safety data of newly approved treatments are compared to already existing therapies. The importance of comparative effectiveness is further emphasized by the fact that specific funding has been allocated by the US government for comparative effectiveness research in both the Patient Protection and Affordable Care Act (PPACA) of 2009 [15] and the American Recovery and Reinvestment Act of 2009, which includes the establishment of a US Federal Coordinating Council for Comparative Effectiveness Research [85].

There are significant challenges in the acquisition of the comparative effectiveness data that should be considered when planning a clinical development program. These include:

- Selection of the most appropriate comparator agent, which may depend on the medical practice environment in which the trials take place;
- Dose and administration regimen of the comparator and experimental agents;
- Specific endpoints for comparison;
- Specific population to be studied (e.g., allowed concurrent illness and concomitant medications, disease severity at baseline, demographic entry criteria); and

- Specific conditions under which the study is conducted. This is particularly important since the relatively strict conditions required for randomized, controlled clinical trials oftentimes cannot replicate the less controlled environment of medical practice. The most relevant comparative effectiveness data obviously are those data collected in an environment that most closely reflects medical practice.

In addition, there are a number of substantial issues in designing trials that are intended to show non-inferiority or therapeutic equivalence rather than superiority. One particular concern is in selecting a non-inferiority margin that is clinically meaningful and is supported by prior clinical investigation, yet also allows for feasible clinical trial design. Because of these substantial challenges, while most drug development programs include comparative data, they also continue to depend on the use of placebo to establish the effectiveness of the pharmaceutical candidate and to provide a reference point for determining the treatment-emergent safety and toleration profile. For many indications in the US, this is a required evidentiary standard for efficacy.

## Combination Treatments

It is becoming apparent that there often is value in using two or more pharmaceutical agents together to treat numerous diseases, including hypertension, diabetes, infectious disease, and cancer. While we will only discuss the combined use of two or more pharmaceutical agents administered as a single entity, there are other examples in which two different regulated entities are combined, such as a drug and device (e.g., a drug-eluting coronary stent) or a drug and diagnostic (e.g., the use of trastuzumab and the HER-2 diagnostic). As stated by the US FDA Office of Combination Products [86]:

Combination products have the potential to provide enhanced therapeutic advantages compared to single entity devices, drugs, and biologics. More and more combination products are incorporating cutting-edge, novel technologies that hold great promise for advancing patient care. Combination products may include drug-delivery systems, gene therapy systems, personalized medicine drug–device combinations, biological–device combinations, nanotechnology, and other innovative products for diagnostic and therapeutic treatments of cardiovascular, metabolic, oncologic, and other disorders.

Traditionally, combination pharmaceuticals were single entities that contained an investigational new drug and an already approved drug that was commonly used in the population for which the combination was targeted. The combination product generally would have the following characteristics:

- The constituents act on the same disease or symptom via different mechanisms and in doing so may act to produce a greater therapeutic effect than either one could individually, or may produce similar efficacy with improved safety/toleration than either one could individually (e.g., combined angiotensin-converting enzyme or angiotensin receptor blocker and calcium channel blocker agents);
- The constituents act on distinct diseases or symptoms that commonly occur together where the combination product may offer improved convenience and compliance (e.g., combined hypolipidemic and antihypertensive agents);
- One constituent is used to markedly improve the pharmacokinetic or pharmacodynamic profile of the investigational new drug. Examples include:
  - Ritonavir/lopinavir where lopinavir is an inhibitor of the HIV-1 protease and ritonavir inhibits the CYP3A-mediated metabolism of lopinavir, thereby providing increased plasma levels of lopinavir; and
  - Amoxicillin/clavulanate potassium which is an oral antibacterial combination consisting of the semisynthetic antibiotic, amoxicillin and the β-lactamase inhibitor, clavulanate potassium.

Initiation of combination product global development should begin after regulatory consultation with EU [87], US [55], and Japanese regulatory agencies, and generally occurs after the efficacy, safety, and toleration of the investigational drug has been established as a single agent for treating the disease or symptom under study. This would usually require completion of a PoC trial and substantial confirmatory trial experience. The efficacy, safety, and toleration data of the already approved drug component would be summarized and available for review in the approval authorization submission. After completing some preclinical animal safety studies with the combination product, clinical development traditionally began with a study of the PK/PD response of the investigational and approved drugs given alone and in combination. Based on these results, a broad, dose-ranging clinical study then would be conducted to examine the efficacy, safety, and toleration of the investigational and approved agents given alone and in combination. One example is a broad dose-ranging study that was conducted to examine the combined

use of the calcium channel blocker amlodipine and the angiotensin receptor blocker valsartan [88]. Using a two-study paradigm, the dose-ranging covered a four-fold range of amlodipine doses (2.5 to 10 mg once daily) and an eight-fold range of valsartan doses (40 to 320 mg once daily) administered alone and in combination. Depending on the required efficacy, safety, and toleration database, and the required combination product labeling, further confirmatory trials might need to be conducted based on the results of the broad dose-ranging studies.

It is now increasingly recognized that new pharmaceutical treatments for certain diseases or conditions require combination use in order to show meaningful efficacy that cannot be obtained when either agent is used alone. For example, combination therapy may be needed because an infectious agent develops resistance to single-agent therapy or because redundant pathophysiological mechanisms reduce the effectiveness of single-agent antihypertensive therapy. To respond to this need, the FDA has issued draft guidance for the combined development of two or more investigational pharmaceutical agents [89]. The guidance notes that this approach generally should be used: (1) for agents to treat a serious disease; (2) where there is a strong pathophysiological rationale; (3) where there are favorable preclinical data supporting the combination use; and (4) where there are data supporting the inappropriateness of single-agent use. Xavier and Sander [90] note that while combination drug therapy may be more effective, it may also be antagonistic or suppressive, and emphasize that the thorough understanding of the pathophysiology of the disease to be treated and the selection of drugs with appropriate mechanisms of action form the foundation for the clinical development of rational combination therapy.

## Transparency

There is increasing emphasis on the transparency of clinical development, including clinical trial conduct, clinical trial reporting, and regulatory review and oversight. There not only is general support for more timely reporting of all clinical trial results but greater transparency is also advocated to address concerns regarding key issues such as the selective reporting of clinical trial results and patient access to clinical development programs. As a result of the 1997 FDA Modernization Act, the National Institutes of Health (NIH), through its National Library of Medicine (NLM), collaborated with the FDA to develop a clinical trials registry (www.ClinicalTrials.gov). The basic registry contains information about a trial's purpose, participant entry criteria, investigative site location, and contact information for obtaining more details. The 2008 FDA Amendments Act [91] required the NLM to markedly expand the clinical trial registry and results databank, which now presents information on the following:

- Clinical studies of all diseases and studies of devices (previously, only trials of drugs and biologics for serious or life-threatening diseases or conditions were required to be registered);
- An increased amount of clinical trial information and summary data tables including the following:

  - Baseline participant characteristics taken at the beginning of a trial that may include demographic and physiologic characteristics,
  - Participant flow to indicate the number of participants at each stage of the trial,
  - Outcomes data, including prespecified primary and secondary outcomes and relevant statistical analyses,
  - Tables for reporting serious adverse events and other frequent adverse events observed during the trial.

Trial results posting now is required for Phase II through IV interventional studies involving drugs, biological products, and medical devices approved by the FDA that have at least one trial site in the US or are conducted under a US IND [92].

In addition to the NLM website and publication, additional clinical trial result registries include web sites sponsored by the US National Cancer Institute (www.cancer.gov/clinicaltrials) as well as a number of individual pharmaceutical organizations. In the EU, EudraCT (https://eudract.ema.europa.eu/index. html) is a database of all clinical trials in the European Community that was established in accordance with Directive 2001/20/EC.

## REFERENCES

[1] US Food and Drug Administration. Food and Drug Administration Amendments Act (FDAAA) of 2007. Internet at, www.fda.gov/RegulatoryInformation/ Legislation/Federal FoodDrugandCosmeticActFDCAct/SignificantAmendmentsto theFDCAct/FoodandDrugAdministrationAmendmentsActof 2007/default.htm.

[2] Greenberg BM, Ratchford JN, Calebresi PA. Multiple sclerosis. In: Waldman S, Terzic A, editors. Pharmacology and therapeutics: Principles to practice. Philadelphia, PA: Saunders, Elsevier; 2009. p. 685–702.

[3] Schumacher G. Multiple sclerosis. In: Cecil RL, Loeb RF, editors. Textbook of medicine. 8th ed. Philadelphia, PA: WB Saunders; 1951. p. 1431–5.

[4] The IFNB. Multiple Sclerosis Study Group. Interferon beta-1b is effective in relapsing remitting multiple sclerosis. I. Clinical results of a multicenter, randomized, double-blind, placebo-controlled trial. Neurology 1993;43:655–61.

[5] Paolicelli D, Direnzo V, Trojano M. Review of interferon beta-1b in the treatment of early and relapsing multiple sclerosis. Biologics 2009;3:369–76.

[6] Kappos L, Radue E-W, O'Connor P, Polman C, Hohlfeld R, Calabresi P, et al. A placebo-controlled trial of oral fingolimod in relapsing multiple sclerosis. N Engl J Med 2010; 362:387–401.

[7] US Food and Drug Administration. FDA News Release: FDA approves first oral drug to reduce MS relapses (September 22, 2010) (Internet at, www.fda.gov /NewsEvents/Newsroom/ PressAnnouncements/ucm226755.htm.)

[8] Francis G, Collins W, Burtin P. Fingolimod (NDA 22–527) Briefing Document (Prepared by Novartis Pharmaceuticals for the Peripheral and Central Nervous System Drugs Advisory Committee Meeting 10 June 2010) (Internet at, /www. fda.gov/downloads/AdvisoryCommittees/Committees MeetingMaterials/Drugs/PeripheralandCentralNervous SystemDrugsAdvisoryCommittee/UCM214675.pdf.)

[9] US Department of Health, Education, and Welfare. The Belmont report, (Internet at, www.ohsr.od.nih.gov/guidelines/ belmont.html.)

[10] World Medical Association. Declaration of Helsinki (Internet at, www.wma.net/en/30publications/10policies/b3/index.html).

[11] Council for International Organizations of Medical Sciences (CIOMS). International ethical guidelines for biomedical research involving human subjects (Internet at, www.cioms. ch/publications/layout_guide2002.pdf.)

[12] Investigational new drug safety reporting requirements for human drug and biological products and safety reporting requirements for bioavailability and bioequivalence studies in humans. In: Federal Register Vol. 75, No. 188, Wednesday, September 29, 2010/Rules and Regulations 59935 21 CFR Parts 312 and 320. (Internet at, http//edocket.access.gpo.gov/2010/ pdf/2010-24296.pdf.)

[13] US Food and Drug Administration. Legislation (Internet at, www.fda.gov/RegulatoryInformation/Legislation/default. htm.)

[14] Code of Federal Regulations. Title 21 Food and Drugs (Internet at, www.access.gpo.gov/cgi-bin/cfrassemble.cgi?title=200621.)

[15] Public Law 111–148 – Patient Protection and Affordable Care Act. (Internet at, www.gpo.gov/fdsys/pkg/PLAW-111publ148/ content-detail.html.)

[16] Public Law 111–152 – Health Care and Education Reconciliation Act of 2010 (Internet at, www.gpo.gov/fdsys/pkg/ PLAW-111publ152/content-detail.html.)

[17] US Food and Drug Administration. Guidance, compliance and regulatory information (Internet at, www.fda.gov/Drugs/ GuidanceComplianceRegulatoryInformation /default.htm.)

[18] European Medicines Agency. Regulatory and procedural guidance index (Internet at, www.ema.europa.eu/ema/index.jsp? curl=pages/regulation/general/general_content_000316.jsp&; murl=menus/regulations/regulations. jsp&mid=WC0b01ac05800a4902.)

[19] Pharmaceutical and Medical Devices Agency. Japan. Home website (Internet at, www.pmda.go.jp/english/index.html.)

[20] International Conference on Harmonisation of Technical Requirements for Registration of Pharmaceuticals for Human Use. Home website (Internet at, www.ich.org.)

[21] International Conference on Harmonisation of Technical Requirements for Registration of Pharmaceuticals for Human Use. ICH guidelines (Internet at, www.ich.org/products/ guidelines.html.)

[22] International Conference on Harmonisation of Technical Requirements for Registration of Pharmaceuticals for Human

Use. Guidelines for good clinical practice – E6(R1). Internet at, www.ich.org/fileadmin/Public_Web_Site/ICH_Products/Guidelines/Efficacy/E6_R1_Guideline.pdf.

[23] McAuslane N, Cone M, Collins J, Walker S. Emerging markets and emerging agencies: A comparative study of how key regulatory agencies in Asia, Latin America, the Middle East and Africa are developing regulatory processes and review models for new medicinal products. Drug Inf J 2009;3:349–59.

[24] National Conference of State Legislatures. State legislation relating to transparency and disclosure of health and hospital charges. Internet at, www.ncsl.org/default.aspx?tabid=14512.

[25] National Conference of State Legislatures. Clinical trials: what are states doing? (Internet at, wwwncsl.org/default.aspx?tabid=14331.)

[26] Zerhouni E, Sanders C, Von Eschenbach A. The biomarkers consortium: Public and private sectors working in partnership to improve the public health. Oncologist 2007;12:250–2.

[27] Altar C. The biomarkers consortium: On the critical path of drug discovery Clin Pharmacol Ther 2009;83:361–4.

[28] Wagner J, Wright E, Ennis M, Prince M, Kochan J, Nunez DJR, et al. Utility of adiponectin as a biomarker predictive of glycemic efficacy is demonstrated by collaborative pooling of data from clinical trials conducted by multiple sponsors. Clin Pharmacol Ther 2009;86:619–25.

[29] Wagner J, Prince M, Kelloff C, Ennis MM, Kochan J, Nunez DJ, et al. The biomarkers consortium: Practice and pitfalls of open-source precompetitive collaboration. Clin Pharmacol Ther 2010;87:539–42.

[30] Barker AD, Sigman CC, Kelloff C, Hylton NM, Berry DA, Esserman LJ. I-SPY 2: An adaptive breast cancer trial design in the setting of neoadjuvant chemotherapy. Clin Pharmacol Ther 2009;86:97–100.

[31] European Commission. Data protection homepage. Internet at, http://ec.europa.eu/justice/policies/privacy/index_en.htm.

[32] US Department of Health & Human Services. The Health Insurance Portability and Accountability Act of 1996 (HIPAA) privacy and security rules. Internet at, www.hhs.gov/ocr/privacy/.

[33] Sheiner LB. Learning versus confirming in clinical drug development. Clin Pharmacol Ther 1997;61:275–9.

[34] DiMasi JA, Hansen RW, Grabowski HG. The price of innovation: New estimates of drug development costs. J Health Econ 2003;22:151–85.

[35] Adams CP, Brantner V. Estimating the cost of new drug development: Is it really $802 million? Health Aff 2006;25:420–8.

[36] Global R&D performance metrics programme: Industry success rates report. CMR International May 2005:p.7.

[37] DiMasi JA, Feldman L, Seckler A, Wilson A. Trends in risks associated with new drug development: Success rates for investigational drugs. Clin Pharmacol Ther 2010;87:272–7.

[38] Smolen JS, Landewe R, Breedveld FC, Dougados M, Emery P, Gaujoux-Viala C, et al. EULAR recommendations for the management of rheumatoid arthritis with synthetic and biological disease-modifying antirheumatic drugs. Ann Rheum Dis 2010;69:964–75.

[39] Saag KG, Teng GG, Patkar NM, Anuntiyo J, Finney C, Curtis JR, et al. American College of Rheumatology 2008 recommendations for the use of nonbiologic and biologic disease-modifying antirheumatic drugs in rheumatoid arthritis. Arthritis Rheum 2008;59:762–84.

[40] Gartlehner G, Hansen RA, Jonas BL, Thieda P, Lohr KN. The comparative efficacy and safety of biologics for the treatment of rheumatoid arthritis: A systematic review and meta-analysis. J Rheumatol 2006;33:2398–408.

[41] Damjanov N, Kauffman RS, Spencer-Green GT. Efficacy, pharmacodynamics, and safety of VX-702, a novel p38 MAPK inhibitor, in rheumatoid arthritis: Results of two randomized, double-blind, placebo-controlled clinical studies. Arthritis Rheum 2009;60:1232–41.

[42] Cohen AB, Cheng T, Chindalore V, Damjanov N, Burgos-Vargas R, Delora P, et al. Evaluation of the efficacy and safety of pamapimod, a p38 MAP kinase inhibitor, in a double-blind methotrexate-controlled study of patients with active rheumatoid arthritis. Arthritis Rheum 2009;60:335–44.

[43] Fransen J, van Riel PL. The disease activity score and the EULAR response criteria. Rheum Dis Clin North Am 2009;35:745–57.

[44] Felson DT, Anderson JJ, Boers M, Bombardier C, Furst D, Goldsmith C, et al. American College of Rheumatology preliminary definition of improvement in rheumatoid arthritis. Arthritis Rheum 1995;38:1–9.

[45] Rosen WG, Mohs RC, Davis KL. A new rating scale for Alzheimer's disease. Am J Psychiatry 1984;141:1356–64.

[46] New Bellamy N, Buchanan WW, Goldsmith CH, Campbell J, Stitt L. Validation study of WOMAC: A health status instrument for measuring clinically important patient relevant outcomes to antirheumatic drug therapy in patients with osteoarthritis of the hip or knee. J Rheumatol 1988;15:1833–40.

[47] Cartwright ME, Cohen S, Fleishaker JC, Madani S, McLeod JF, Musser B, et al. Proof of concept: A PhRMA position paper with recommendations for best practice. Clin Pharmacol Ther 2010;87:278–84.

[48] Reisberg B, Schneider L, Doody R, Anand R, Feldman H, Haraguchi H, et al. Clinical global measures of dementia. Position paper from the International Working Group on Harmonization of Dementia Drug Guidelines. Alzheimer Dis Assoc Disord 1997;11(Suppl. 3):8–18.

[49] Temple R, Ellenberg S. Placebo-controlled trials and active-controlled trials in the evaluation of new treatments, Part 1: Ethical and scientific issues. Ann Intern Med 2000;133:455–63.

[50] Ellenberg S, Temple R. Placebo-controlled trials and active-controlled trials in the evaluation of new treatments, Part 2: Practical issues and specific cases. Ann Intern Med 2000;133:464–70.

[51] International Conference on Harmonisation of Technical Requirements for Registration of Pharmaceuticals for Human Use. Statistical principles for clinical trials – E9. Internet at, www.ich.org/fileadmin/Public_Web_Site/ICH_Products?Guidelines/Efficacy?E9/Step4/E0_Guideline.pdf.

[52] Dragalin V. An introduction to adaptive designs and adaptation in CNS trials. Eur Neuropsychopharmacol 2010;21:153–8.

[53] Wang S-J, Hung HMS, O'Neill R. Adaptive design clinical trials and trial logistics models in CNS drug development. Eur Neuropsychopharmacol 2010;21:159–66.

[54] CDER, CBER. Adaptive design clinical trials for drugs and biologics. Guidance for industry. Silver Spring and Rockville, MD: FDA. Internet at, www.fda.gov/downloads/Drugs/GuidanceComplianceRegulatoryInformation/Guidances/UCM201790.pdf.; 2010.

[55] Ando Y, Hirakawa A, Uyama Y. Adaptive clinical trials for new drug applications in Japan. Eur Neuropsychopharmacol 2010;21:175–9.

[56] CDER. Influenza: Developing drugs for treatment and/or prophylaxis. Guidance for industry. Rockville, MD: FDA. Internet at, www.fda.gov/downloads/Drugs/GuidanceComplianceRegulatoryInformation/Guidances/ucm091219.pdf.; 2010.

[57] CDER. Community acquired pneumonia. Guidance for industry. Silver Spring, MD: FDA. Internet at, www.fda.gov/downloads/Drugs/GuidanceComplianceRegulatoryInformation/Guidances/ucm123638.pdf.; 2009.

[58] CDER. Antibacterial drug products: Use of noninferiority trials to support approval. Guidance for industry. Silver Spring, MD: FDA. Internet at, www.fda.gov/downloads/Drugs/GuidanceComplianceRegulatoryInformation/Guidances/UCM070951.pdf.; 2009.

[59] New Drug Approval: FDA's consideration of evidence from certain clinical trials. United States Government Accountability Office: 2010; Report 10–798.

[60] Pfizer, Inc. Advisory Committee Briefing Document EXUBERA – Endocrinologic and Metabolic Drugs Advisory Committee. Internet at, www.fda.gov/ohrms/dockets/ac/05/briefing/2005-4169B1_01_01-Pfizer-Exubera.pdf.

[61] International Conference on Harmonisation of Technical Requirements for Registration of Pharmaceuticals for Human Use. The extent of population exposure to assess clinical safety for drugs intended for long-term treatment of non-life-threatening conditions – E1. Internet at, www.ich.org/fileadmin/Public_Web_Site/ICH_Products/Guidelines/Efficacy/E1/Step4/E1_Guideline.pdf.

[62] CDER. Diabetes mellitus – evaluating cardiovascular risk in new antidiabetic therapies to treat type 2 diabetes. Guidance for industry. Rockville, MD: FDA. Internet at, www.fda.gov/downloads/Drugs/GuidanceComplianceRegulatoryInformation/Guidances/ucm071627.pdf.; 2008.

[63] Uyama Y, Shibata T, Nagai N, Hanaoka H, Toyoshima S, Mori K. Successful bridging strategy based on ICH E5 guideline for drugs approved in Japan. Clin Pharmacol Ther 2005;78:102–13.

[64] Quan H, Li M, Chen J, Gallo PP, Binkowitz B, Ibia EO, et al. Assessment of consistency of treatment effects in multiregional clinical trials. Drug Inf J 2010;44:617–32.

[65] Saillot JL, Paxton M. Industry efforts on simultaneous global development. Drug Inf J 2009;43:339–48.

[66] CDER, CBER, CDRH. Establishment and operation of clinical trial data monitoring committees. Guidance for industry. Rockville, MD: FDA. Internet at, www.fda.gov/RegulatoryInformation/Guidances/ucm127069.htm.; 2006.

[67] Committee for Medicinal Products for Human Use. Guideline on data monitoring committees. London: EMA. Internet at, www.ema.europa.eu/docs/en_GB/document_library/Scientific_guideline/2009/09/WC500003635.pdf.; 2006.

[68] Woodcock J. Assessing the clinical utility of diagnostics used in drug therapy. Clin Pharmacol Ther 2010;88:765–73.

[69] International Conference on Harmonisation of Technical Requirements for Registration of Pharmaceuticals for Human Use. Studies in support of special populations: geriatrics – E7. Internet at, www.ich.org/fileadmin/Public_Web_Site/ICH_Products/Guidelines/Efficacy/E7/Step4/E7_Guideline.pdf.

[70] International Conference on Harmonisation of Technical Requirements for Registration of Pharmaceuticals for Human Use. Studies in support of special populations: geriatrics – Questions & answers – E7 (Current version dated July 6, 2010). Internet at, www.ema.europa.eu/docs/en_GB/document_library/Scientific_guideline/2009/10/WC500005218.pdf.

[71] CDER, CBER. How to comply with the pediatric research equity act. Guidance for industry. Rockville, MD: FDA. Internet at, www.fda.gov/downloads/Drugs/GuidanceComplianceRegulatoryInformation/Guidances/ucm079756.pdf.; 2005.

[72] CDER, CBER. Qualifying for pediatric exclusivity under section 505A of the Federal Food, Drug, and Cosmetic Act. Guidance for industry. Rockville, MD: FDA. Internet at, www.fda.gov/downloads/Drugs/GuidanceComplianceRegulatoryInformation/Guidances/UCM080558.pdf.; 1999.

[73] European Medicines Agency. Medicines for Children home page. Internet at, www. ema.europa.eu/ema/index.jsp?curl=pages/special_topics/general/general_content_000302.jsp&murl=menus/special_topics/special_topics.jsp&mid=WC0b01ac058002d4ea.

[74] International Conference on Harmonisation of Technical Requirements for Registration of Pharmaceuticals for Human Use. Clinical investigation of medicinal products in the pediatric population – E11. Internet at, http://private.ich.org/LOB/media/ MEDIA487.pdf.

[75] Gill D, Kurz R. Practical and ethical issues in pediatric clinical trials. Appl Clin Trials 2003;12:41–4.

[76] US Food and Drug Administration. Regulatory information: Orphan Drug Act. Internet at, www.fda.gov/RegulatoryInformation/Legislation/FederalFoodDrugandCosmeticActFDCAct/SignificantAmendmentstotheFDCAct/OrphanDrugAct/default.htm.

[77] European Medicines Agency. Orphan designation. Internet at, www.ema.europa.eu/ema/index.jsp?curl=pages/regulation/general/general_content_000029.jsp&;murl=menus/regulations/regulations.jsp&mid=WC0b01ac05800240ce&jsenabled=true.

[78] Shah RR. Regulatory framework for the treatment of orphan diseases. In: Mehta A, Beck M, Sunder-Plassmann G, editors. Fabry disease: Perspectives from 5 years of FOS (Fabry Outcome Survey). Oxford: Oxford PharmaGenesis. Chapter 11. (Internet at, www.ncbi.nlm.nih.gov/books/NBK11586/.; 2006.

[79] Shiragami M, Kiyohito N. Analysis of orphan drug development in Japan. Jpn J Clin Pharmacol Ther 1999;30:681–8.

[80] US Food and Drug Administration. Office of Orphan Product Development. Home page. Internet at, www.fda.gov/AboutFDA/CentersOffices/OC/OfficeofScienceandHealthCoordination/OfficeofOrphanProductDevelopment/default.htm.

[81] Burke K, Freeman S, Imoisili M, Cote T. The impact of the orphan drug act on the development and advancement of neurological products for rare diseases: A descriptive review. Clin Pharmacol Ther 2010;88:449–53.

[82] Institute of Medicine. Rare diseases and orphan products: Accelerating research and development. Washington DC: National Academies Press; 2010.

[83] National Institute for Health and Clinical Excellence. Home page. Internet at, www.nice.org.uk/.

[84] Agency for Healthcare Research and Quality. Home page. Internet at, www.ahrq.gov/.

[85] American Recovery and Reinvestment Act of 2009. (Internet at, http://frwebgate.access.gpo.gov/cgi-bin/getdoc.cgi?dbname=111_cong_bills&docid =f:h1enr.pdf.)

[86] US Food and Drug Administration. Combination products. Home page. Internet at, www.fda.gov/CombinationProducts/default.htm.

[87] Committee for Medicinal Products for Human Use. Guideline on fixed combination medicinal products (draft). Guideline. London: EMA. Internet at, www.ema.europa.eu/docs/en_GB/document_library/Scientific_guideline/2009/09/WC500003689.pdf.; 2008.

[88] Philipp T, Smith TR, Glazer R, Wernsing M, Yen J, Jin J, et al. Two multicenter, 8-week, randomized, double-blind, placebo-controlled, parallel-group studies evaluating the efficacy and tolerability of amlodipine and valsartan in combination and as monotherapy in adult patients with mild to moderate essential hypertension. Clin Ther 2007;29:563–80.

[89] CDER. Codevelopment of two or more unmarketed investigational drugs for use in combination (draft). Silver Spring, FDA: Guidance for Industry. Internet at, www.fda.gov/downloads/Drugs/GuidanceComplianceRegulatoryInformation/Guidances/UCM236669.pdf.; 2010.

[90] Xavier JB, Sander C. Principle of system balance for drug interactions. N Engl J Med 2010;362:1339–40.

[91] National Library of Medicine. ClinicalTrials.gov. Home page. Internet at, www.clinicaltrials.gov.

[92] Tse T, Williams RJ, Zarin DA. Reporting '"basic results"' in clinical trials. Chest 2009;136:295–303.

# 36

# The Role of the FDA in Guiding Drug Development

**Chandrahas G. Sahajwalla[1], Lawrence J. Lesko[2] and Shiew-Mei Huang[1]**

[1]*Office of Clinical Pharmacology, Office of Translational Sciences, Center for Drug Evaluation and Research, Food and Drug Administration, Silver Spring, MD 20993*
[2]*Center for Pharmacometrics and Systems Pharmacology, College of Pharmacy, University of Florida, Lake Nona in Orlando, FL 32832*

The drug development process is defined here as one that includes the preclinical and clinical phases of drug development following the selection of a lead molecule by the sponsor and includes the regulatory review phase that is intended to lead to marketing authorization. As discussed in Chapter 29, this process is complex, time-consuming, and costly. A typical new molecular entity (NME), if approved for marketing, has gone through extensive preclinical pharmacology/toxicology evaluation followed by a clinical evaluation stage that lasts, on average, 5–7 years. With an average of 6–10 months required for regulatory review, the entire process, from preclinical evaluation to market approval, may take up to 15 years, with a cost that may exceed $990 million dollars in direct and lost-opportunity costs [1–3]. Given the current high attrition rate of drugs that enter into clinical testing (~50% in Phase 3), the need for more predictive and informative drug development is obvious.

One of the goals of the drug development process is to provide effective drugs to patients as quickly as possible, and to manage the risks associated with these drugs in the best way possible. That is, the benefit/risk ratio should be appropriate for the indication. Another goal is to make sure that ineffective drugs, unsafe drugs, drugs with inappropriate benefit/risk ratios, or drugs for which risk management after marketing authorization is too difficult, do not get to the marketplace. In addition, it is critical to obtain data during drug development to achieve individualization of dose and dosing regimen for specific patient populations (e.g., pediatric or elderly patients), especially those not studied in the pivotal registration trials. To achieve these goals, there needs to be a transparent and accountable review process. The Food and Drug Administration (FDA) not only reviews the designs and results of studies submitted by the sponsor in a submitted New Drug Application (NDA) or Biologics License Application (BLA) but also plays a critical role in guiding drug development decisions by providing sponsors with advice, insights, and scientific knowledge regarding drug development, all gleaned from past experience.

Effective communication and mutual trust between the FDA and sponsors is essential to achieving the goals of the drug development process in an efficient, successful, and informative manner. Well-constructed meetings held face-to-face between sponsor representatives and FDA staff are a key part of direct communication. However, less direct but critical communications can also occur through domestic and international guidances, telephone conferences, FDA presentations at public professional meetings and advisory committee meetings, FDA-authored, peer-reviewed publications, and information posted on the FDA website. These sources of information combine to provide transparency and accountability that should facilitate drug development and help to reduce uncertainty about the regulatory review process by enabling sponsors to learn about the FDA's thinking.

This chapter reviews the various ways that the FDA gets involved in guiding drug development and communicating with sponsors. This chapter is written from the perspective of the submitted NDAs and BLAs that are the responsibility of the Center for Drug Evaluation and Research (CDER) in FDA.

## WHY DOES THE FDA GET INVOLVED IN DRUG DEVELOPMENT?

In the United States, the development and marketing of drug products for human use are regulated by legislation enacted by the US Congress. The FDA is responsible for interpreting and enforcing this legislation. To facilitate that process, the FDA implements rules and regulations which are published in the Federal Register and coded in the US Code of Federal Regulations (CFR). According to 21 USC 393, the FDA has a dual mission of promoting the public health by promptly and efficiently reviewing clinical research, and by taking appropriate and timely action on the marketing of regulated products.

The 2004 FDA Critical Path White Paper ("Innovation/Stagnation: Challenge and Opportunity on the Critical Path to New Medical Products") [4] addressed the recent slowdown in innovative medical therapies submitted to the FDA for approval. The report describes the urgent need to modernize the medical product development process, the "critical path", to make product development more predictable and less costly. In this regard, the FDA and the pharmaceutical industry have basically the same goals – namely, to promote public health by getting safe and effective drugs to patients as quickly as possible and to protect public health by assuring that drugs with inadequate benefit/risk attributes do not get into the marketplace. In addition, both the FDA and the industry maintain pharmacovigilance programs to monitor adverse drug reactions after a new drug is marketed, and risk-management strategies have been a part of the FDA's 5-year plan that is outlined in the 2002 Prescription Drug User Fee Act III (PDUFA III) and subsequent PDUFAs that undergo a renewal process every 5 years. PDUFA IV (FDAAA) defined "twenty-first century review" and outlined a process for efficient and timely review of applications. The most recent PDUFA V draft addresses issues related to increased communications (e.g., with sponsors for NME NDAs and original BLAs at pre-submission meetings, mid-cycle meetings, and late-cycle meetings), and includes recommendations to promote innovation and advance the science of drug development to meet emerging scientific and technologic challenges in various areas (e.g., by advancing greater use of biomarkers and pharmacogenomics, and by promoting the development of drugs for rare diseases) [5].

The chronology of legislation regulating drug development is summarized in Table 36.1. Beginning in 1906 with the Food and Drugs Act [6] that prohibited interstate commerce in misbranded and adulterated foods, drinks, and drugs, the FDA has had an important role in protecting public health. Over the years, a number of public health safety disasters have contributed to the evolution of the drug regulations that currently impact drug development. For example, the sulfanilamide elixir disaster in 1937, in which sulfanilamide was dissolved in the poisonous solvent diethylene glycol, killed 107 persons and highlighted the need to establish drug safety before marketing. The Federal Food, Drug and Cosmetic Act of 1938, which contained provisions to require sponsors to demonstrate that new drugs are safe before marketing, ushered in a new system of drug regulation. The thalidomide tragedy of 1962, in which birth defects occurred in thousands of babies whose mothers took thalidomide during pregnancy, aroused public support for stronger drug regulations. As a result, the Kefauver-Harris Drug Amendments were passed to ensure drug efficacy and greater drug safety. The bioavailability problems with digoxin reported by Lindenbaum *et al.* [7] in 1971, which included substantial variability in rate and extent of absorption between different manufacturers and between different lots produced by the same manufacturer, led to a greater awareness of the need for better regulatory standards in manufacturing to ensure high-quality drug products for the American public. Dissolution-rate testing requirements for digoxin tablets were initiated by the FDA in 1974 and effectively improved the uniformity of performance of digoxin tablets from various manufacturers. More recently, drug regulations have focused on the individualization of drug therapy in patient subsets defined by age, sex, and race. With the pharmacogenomic advances in molecular biology, the next stage in the evolution of drug regulations may well focus on individualization of drug therapy based on knowledge of both disease genetics and drug-response pharmacogenetics. With the various cardiovascular safety issues associated with the postmarketing use of Vioxx® and Avandia® [8, 9], there have been new calls to strengthen premarketing safety assessments and postmarketing surveillance, including the establishment of various systems (e.g., Mini-Sentinel) to leverage public and private healthcare databases to quickly evaluate drug safety issues [10]. In addition, various public–private partnerships have been formed to collectively address

TABLE 36.1  Chronology and Key Components of Selected Pharmaceutical Legislation

| Date | Legislation | Key components |
|---|---|---|
| 1906 | Food and Drug Acts | Drugs meet standards of strength and purity |
| 1938 | Food, Drug and Cosmetic Act (FD&C Act) | Manufacturers need to show safety of a drug before marketing |
| 1962 | Kefauner-Harris Amendments | Drugs need to be safe and effective |
| 1983 | Orphan Drug Act | Incentives (tax deduction and market exclusivity) for developing drugs for rare diseases |
| 1992 | Prescription Drug User Fee Act (PDUFA) | Provides FDA resources and defines review timelines |
| 1997 | FDA Modernization Act (FDAMA) | Significant amendments to the FD&C Act[a] |
| 2007 | FDA Amendments Act (FDAAA) | Reauthorization of PDUFA, MDUFA/MA, FDAMA, BPCA, PREA and amendments related to FDA to assess/manage drug risks and to create a foundation (Reagan-Udall)[b] |
| 2009 | Biologics Price Competition and Innovation (BPCI) Act | Establishes an abbreviated approval pathway for "biosimilars" |
| 2012 | PDUFA V | Reauthorization of PDUFA |

[a]Details of the amendments can be found in the following website: www.fda.gov/RegulatoryInformation/Legislation/FederalFoodDrugand CosmeticActFDCAct/SignificantAmendmentstotheFDCAct/FDAMA/default.htm.

[b]MDUFA/MA, Medical device User Fee and Modernization Act; BPCA, Best Pharmaceuticals for Children Act; PREA: Pediatric Research Equity Act.

risk factors (e.g., those related to genomics) in specific patient groups that have a high propensity to experience rare and serious adverse events, such as Steven-Johnson syndrome [11, 12].

## WHEN DOES THE FDA GET INVOLVED IN DRUG DEVELOPMENT?

For over 30 years, the FDA has had a formal process for holding meetings with sponsors to discuss scientific and clinical issues related to drug development. These formal meetings are consistent with the FDA's goal of facilitating drug development by providing advice and assuring a transparent review process. Although these meetings are voluntary, they are quite common and generally helpful. The meetings are referred to by the time frame in which they occur during the drug development process, and meetings at different times have different purposes and goals. Examples are meetings held before the submission of an Investigational New Drug Application (IND), at the end of Phase 1 (EOP1), the end of Phase 2A (EOP2A) and the end of Phase 2 (EOP2), and pre-NDA submission.

Each of these meetings can have a major impact on decisions made during the drug development process, including those related to regulatory review of an IND or an NDA. The questions that are raised and discussed at each of these meetings need to be appropriate for the drug's stage of development. For example, pre-IND meetings that are held early in the drug development process are extremely valuable to both the FDA and the sponsor because they routinely focus on critical issues (e.g., drug safety) in the drug development program, before the sponsor has expended substantial resources in the conduct of clinical trials. These meetings may help sponsors minimize the risk of a *clinical hold*, which the FDA may impose on a study or study site during any phase of clinical development if it finds that human subjects are or would be exposed to unreasonable and significant risk of illness or injury.

Because of great interest on the part of sponsors to obtain early advice and the FDA's goal of facilitating drug development, EOP2A meetings were recently introduced [13]. These meetings are held at the request of the sponsor when the sponsor is seeking advice or non-binding consultations at a time when there is uncertainty related to the limited data that are available during that point in drug development. For the FDA, the primary objectives of these meetings are to help optimize the drug development process by reducing the potential for Phase 2 and Phase 3 clinical trial failures, for example by improving dose selection for these pivotal trials. At this meeting, the sponsor's plans for Phase 2 and/or 3 trials are reviewed and recommendations are made based on available preclinical, clinical, and literature data, and on the experience that FDA staff may have with the same class of compounds. Often, the FDA, in conjunction with sponsors, develops disease-state models that can be used to simulate different clinical trial designs. These models allow the probability of a favorable outcome to be estimated for different study designs and can be constructed to evaluate the impact of tradeoffs in terms of number of doses or number of patients studied. Strategies for conducting additional clinical studies in specific populations are also discussed at this meeting, which could provide the basis for dose recommendations in package inserts. EOP2A meetings are usually focused more on clinical pharmacology issues related to modeling and simulation approaches for dose selection, and/or other clinical pharmacology issues that need to be addressed prior to initiating Phase 2B or Phase 3 clinical trials. At any of the meetings held during this phase of drug development the sponsor could seek advice on the utility or acceptability of emerging scientific tools, such as pharmacogenetics and pharmacogenomics, advice on designing an enrichment trial to demonstrate efficacy, or a study to evaluate biomarkers predictive of specific adverse effects (e.g., electrocardiographic QT intervals).

During subsequent clinical development, the EOP2 meeting is critical to discuss any remaining product development issues, including safety risks and the efficiency and appropriateness of the study design, especially with respect to the endpoints to be assessed in the pivotal Phase 3 efficacy studies. Acceptable statistical analysis approaches to provide evidence of efficacy that should be specified in advance are also discussed. These meetings also play an important role in resolving any outstanding manufacturing issues, or questions regarding dose, dose regimen selection, or major modifications to the drug development plan that are contemplated to support anticipated label claims. Pre-NDA meetings are intended to focus on the content and format of the sponsor's marketing application, and to familiarize the reviewers from various disciplines with the NDA that will be submitted. Any issues that remain to be resolved [e.g., problems or questions related to CMC (chemistry, manufacturing, and control)] may also be discussed at this meeting. Pre-NDA meetings serve as a means to identify any other pending issues which may result in a *refuse-to-file* (RTF) action when an NDA is submitted to the Agency for review.

Important interactions between a pharmaceutical company and the FDA also occur at the end of the marketing application review process, when meetings and discussions take place to sort out the content and language of the label or package insert. Risk Evaluation and Mitigation Strategies (REMS) and the need for postmarketing commitments or requirements (PMC or PMR) are further discussed prior to approval. Following market authorization, the FDA continues to be involved with the development and approval of new uses or new dosage forms for an approved product and maintains the MedWatch postmarketing surveillance program of adverse drug reactions [14]. In addition, through the Office of Surveillance and Epidemiology (OSE), the FDA performs ongoing pharmacovigilance activities.

## HOW DOES THE FDA GUIDE DRUG DEVELOPMENT?

As previously indicated, the FDA guides drug development in many different ways, such as by interpreting laws, rules, and regulations; by disseminating policy statements that may otherwise be vague or unclear; by providing advice and sharing experiences and expertise in face-to-face meetings, and via written agreements and letters; by issuing domestic and international guidances; and by planned telephone conferences and/or scheduled videoconferences [15]. Policies and procedures for requesting, scheduling, and conducting formal meetings between CDER and a sponsor are described in the FDA Guidance for Industry entitled "Formal Meetings Between the FDA and Sponsors or Applicants" [16]. CDER now holds more than 2000 formal meetings a year with sponsors [17]. Depending on the type of meeting, these meetings occur within 30–75 days following a meeting request and the FDA prepares official minutes for these meetings within 4 weeks after the meeting. According to the formal meeting guidance, sponsors have the option to contact the appropriate FDA project manager to arrange for discussion of any differences of opinion expressed in the minutes of the meeting. There is also a formal pathway described in the guidance for dispute resolution if this is necessary.

One or more formal meetings with the FDA generally occur for every development plan for a new chemical entity. Given the relatively short time available for meetings (1–2 hours), the agenda, topics, and quality of these meetings are important determinants of their impact on the drug development process. Both the sponsor and the FDA review division that is involved in the meeting share the responsibility for planning and conducting these meetings in an optimally productive way. To ensure a high-quality meeting with substantive agreements or understanding about issues, the meetings should be focused on the most important questions or issues, designed with a specific purpose in mind, and have the necessary background data available that are appropriate for the agenda. Proper timing of the meeting is important if the meeting involves a discussion of drug development plans. For example, in planning a meeting to discuss a clinical trial protocol, the sponsor should allow sufficient time so that the meeting is held before the clinical study has begun, otherwise the sponsor's and the FDA's resources may be wasted. The EOPIIA meetings, for example, are extremely resource-intensive for the FDA and the sponsor. The FDA may conduct extensive data analysis, including modeling and simulation, in order to provide recommendations on options for the drug development plan. Sponsors are often joined by their consultants or investigators at meetings that are expected to have a significant impact on drug development or approval, and they should request attendance by discipline-specific reviewers from the FDA review divisions that are appropriate for the agenda.

In the past 20 years, the FDA has implemented regulatory initiatives that have impacted the drug development process. These include fast-track drug development programs, accelerated approval (21 CFR 314.500–560), and priority reviews. The Subpart E (21 CFR 312.80–88) and fast-track regulations (21 CFR 356), respectively, have expedited the drug development process and market access for new drugs for severely debilitating and serious conditions or life-threatening diseases without approved alternative treatments. An additional requirement for fast-track status is that there is an unmet medical need. In these instances, multiple meetings between sponsors and the FDA early in the development process are recommended to gain agreement on the development plan. The accelerated approval regulations were developed as a complementary program to the Subpart E initiative, and encourage the use of surrogate endpoints as a basis for accelerated approval. Applications designated for fast-track approvals can be submitted as continuous marketing applications (CMA) whereby the FDA will accept and review individual sections (e.g., preclinical, chemistry, clinical pharmacology) of the NDA prior to submission of the full application. The newer meetings, such as the EOPIIA and the voluntary genomic submission meetings, require much more forward planning and are limited in number by available FDA resources. However, the PDUFA of 1992 [18] has allowed CDER to increase the number of reviewers as the meeting workload has increased, and CDER has made a commitment to schedule the planned meetings that sponsors request in a reasonable time, so that the drug development process can be advanced expeditiously.

The FDA also guides drug development by holding closed or open advisory committee meetings. These meetings facilitate the regulatory review and FDA approval process by bringing together external experts to assess data, to recommend need for new studies, and to address specific questions formulated by the FDA to help resolve scientific or clinical issues related to the drug development process or a specific product approval. Slides and handouts presented at public meetings and publications are generally available to anyone who requests them, and are placed on an FDA website such as the FDA genomics website [19] and the drug interaction website [20].

## WHAT ARE FDA GUIDANCES?

Perhaps the most widespread, effective, and important way that the FDA communicates with sponsors and guides drug development is through guidances issued either by the FDA or by the International Conference on Harmonization (ICH). Guidances represent a wealth of knowledge, consensus, and experience, generally drawn collectively from academia, industry, and FDA. The FDA published the first guidance to industry in 1949, and this guidance was related to procedures for appraising the toxicity of chemicals in food.

The development of guidances proceeds by a process known as Good Guidance Practices, which is intended to ensure that there is the appropriate level of meaningful public participation in the guidance development process [21, 22]. Recent guidance development was motivated, in part, by the Food and Drug Administration Modernization Act of 1997 (FDAMA) that reauthorized the PDUFA of 1992 and mandated the most wide-ranging reforms in FDA practices since 1938 [23]. Since 1997, significant numbers of final or draft guidances have been published, and information on over 400 guidance documents can be found on the FDA website [24]. For example, under FDAMA, Section 111, guidance has been developed that deals with the important application of "bridging studies" for pediatric drug approval, in which a pharmacokinetic study can serve to bridge to children the efficacy and safety database that has been established in adults under circumstances described in the guidance. Another key provision of FDAMA, Section 115, deals with clinical investigations in which data from *one* adequate and well-controlled clinical investigation, and *confirmatory evidence*, are sufficient to establish effectiveness.

The FDA recognizes the value to sponsors of transparency, consistency, and predictability in regulatory decision-making, and guidances for industry are developed as good-faith efforts to share with sponsors the current thinking on a given scientific topic. Guidances are intended to provide sponsors with assurances that FDA staff will interpret statutes and regulations in a consistent manner across its various clinical divisions. However, if inconsistent interpretations of guidances occur among CDER's therapeutic review divisions, the sponsors should communicate with the FDA about the inconsistencies and try to understand or resolve them. Additional factors, such as the number of regulatory filings, FDA division workload, and sponsor submission quality, have impacted drug sponsors' regulatory review experience [25]. However, the FDA has implemented various measures, including good review management practices [26], twenty-first century performance standards [27], and organizational changes [28], to improve the review process.

Guidances cover a wide range of topics that focus on standards of quality, such as CMC, preclinical animal toxicology requirements, ethical standards for the conduct of clinical trials, and documentary requirements for INDs, Abbreviated New Drug Applications (ANDAs), and NDAs [15]. Other guidances focus on the clinical phase of drug development, including biopharmaceutics, clinical pharmacology, and clinical trial design. Many of the newer clinical pharmacology guidances issued by the FDA are based on the principles of risk management.

One of the most important guidances, issued by the FDA in 1998, is entitled "Providing Clinical Evidence of Effectiveness for Human Drug and Biological Products" [24]. This guidance puts forth advice and experience in drawing evidence of effectiveness from all clinical phases of drug development. In particular, it provides examples to demonstrate how exposure–response relationships may be used to provide the primary evidence of efficacy in drug development. Among these examples are recommendations regarding requests for approval of new formulations and new doses or dosing regimens of approved drug products. Other noteworthy guidances include those relating to exposure–response, which can be found on the FDA website [15]. The clinical pharmacology guidance page includes specific guidances that address the need to consider whether dose adjustments are needed for specific clinical settings or patient groups (e.g., patients taking concomitant medications or with certain genetic make-ups) and the related study-design issues and labeling consequences [29].

Through its guidances, the FDA also facilitates and encourages the use of emerging scientific technology and knowledge. For example, to enable scientific progress in the field of pharmacogenomics and to facilitate the use of pharmacogenomic data in informing regulatory decisions, FDA has issued a guidance on when pharmacogenomic data are to be submitted, the format of the data, and how the data will be used [30]. In addition, a draft guidance has been published that encourages the sponsors to collect DNA samples during early drug development [31].

In the area of biopharmaceutics, two guidances are noteworthy because they are the culmination of a decade of public discussion of scientific principles related to the documentation of product quality. The General Bioavailability (BA) and Bioequivalence (BE) Guidance [32] provides guidance on the design, analysis, and utility of BA and BE studies in new and generic drug development, including the use of replicate design studies. Another guidance on the biopharmaceutical classification system (BCS) offers advice on when BA and BE studies may be waived on sound principles of drug absorption science as it relates to the solubility and permeability characteristics of drug substances, and the dissolution of drug products (see Chapter 4) [33]. Together, these guidances, along with the Scale-Up and Post Approval Changes (SUPAC), provide a framework for the biopharmaceutical development of new and generic drug dosage forms.

The recently enacted Biologics Price Competition and Innovation (BPCI) Act [34] authorizes the FDA to oversee an "abbreviated pathway" for approval of biologics that are "biosimilar" to marketed US reference products. The FDA has published a "totality of evidence" approach to evaluating biosimilars [35], and a public hearing concerning implementation of this Act has been held to understand specific issues raised by sponsors, investigators, patient groups, specific disease foundations, and professional societies [36]. Specific guidance documents relating to the development and review of biosimilar products have been published [15].

## THE ROLE OF THE FDA OFFICE OF CLINICAL PHARMACOLOGY

The role of clinical pharmacology at the FDA has expanded over the past 20 years. The Division of Biopharmaceutics, which reviewed basic PK and BA/BE studies, has evolved to the Office of Clinical Pharmacology, which is focused on ensuring that the right dose is given to the right patient. To this end, the Office of Clinical Pharmacology has prepared various guidance documents based on advances in understanding the clinical importance of BA/BE, drug metabolism, drug transporters, and biomarkers, and scientific progress in the areas of genomics and modeling and simulation that enable drug and biologics dosing to be individualized for patients with varying intrinsic (e.g., renal impairment, hepatic impairment) and extrinsic (e.g., taking concomitant medications, dietary supplements) complicating factors.

In addition to preparing guidance documents that address these clinical pharmacology issues, the Office of Clinical Pharmacology initiated "Clinical Pharmacology Advisory Committee" meetings that have been held at least annually since 2002 to discuss contemporary regulatory science issues. For example, the 2010 meeting discussed recommendations for conducting PK studies to evaluate the effects of renal impairment and drug–drug interactions on drug dosing, and the use of systems biology in interpreting and predicting adverse drug reactions [37]. In 2011, the meeting focused on the utility and applications of various clinical pharmacology tools to the regulatory review of orphan drug products for rare diseases [38, 39].

## Future Development of Regulatory Science at the FDA

Because of its regulatory vantage point, the FDA is uniquely positioned to work with companies, patient groups, academic researchers, and other stakeholders to coordinate, develop, and/or disseminate solutions to scientific hurdles that are impairing the industry-wide efficiency of product development. The FDA commissioner, Dr Hamburg, recently indicated that "our nation is at an important crossroads, where the science before us presents unprecedented opportunities to create new and better medical products and promote better health for the public" [40]. To achieve this goal, the FDA has undertaken an initiative to modernize the tools and methods that it uses to evaluate whether the products it regulates are effective and safe [41, 42]. This initiative emphasizes the critical need for regulatory scientists to be equipped with innovative approaches to make science-based regulatory decisions and expedite drug development. In addition, a new regulatory paradigm, "adaptive licensing", has been proposed to address the root cause of the overall high cost of drug development and to encourage innovative drug development strategies [43]. In fact, some measures of staged approval are already in place in the US that balance regulatory requirements for developing evidence of both efficacy and safety with patient's need for early access [44]. However, drug regulatory paradigms incorporating novel regulatory science will need to continue to evolve if they are to reduce the uncertainties currently inherent in evaluating drug response. The key to the future successful development of regulatory science will be an understanding of the drivers and challenges underlying drug development, and this will require intense collaboration among all stakeholders [45]. The ultimate value of these efforts will be reflected in the quality of the data and of the NDA, BLA, and ANDA submissions provided by sponsors.

## DISCLAIMER

The views expressed in this chapter do not necessarily represent the FDA's official view.

## REFERENCES

[1] PhRMA 2005. An industrial revolution in R&D. London: Pricewaterhouse Coopers; 1998.
[2] Vernon JA, Golec JH, DiMasi JA. Drug development costs when financial risk is measured using the FAMA-French three-factor model. Health Econ 2010;19:1002–5.
[3] Lesko LJ, Sahajwalla C. Introduction to drug development and regulatory-decision making. In: Sahajwalla CG, editor. New drug development, regulatory paradigms for clinical pharmacology and biopharmaceutics. New York, NY: Marcel Dekker; 2004. p. 1–12.
[4] US Food and Drug Administration The critical path initiative: Report on key achievements in 2009. FDA Report (Internet at, www.fda.gov/downloads/ScienceResearch/SpecialTopics/CriticalPathInitiative/UCM221651.pdf).
[5] PDUFA V. Internet at, www.fda.gov/NewsEvents/Testimony/ucm261396.htm and www.thepinksheet.com/nr/FDC/SupportingDocs/Pink/2011/PDUFA_V_draft_commitment_letter.pdf.
[6] US Food and Drug Administration. Overview on FDA history. Silver Spring, MD: FDA; (Internet at, www.fda.gov/AboutFDA/WhatWeDo/History/Overviews/default.htm).
[7] Lindenbaum J, Mellow MH, Blackstone MO, Butler Jr VP. Variation in biologic availability of digoxin from four preparations. N Engl J Med 1971;285:1344–7.
[8] US Food and Drug Administration. COX-2 selective (includes Bextra, Celebrex, and Vioxx) and non-selective non-steroidal anti-inflammatory drugs (NSAIDS). Postmarket drug safety information for patients and providers. Silver Spring, MD: FDA. (Internet at, www.fda.gov/drugs/drugsafety/postmarketdrugsafetyinformationforpatientsandproviders/ucm103420.htm; April 7, 2005).
[9] US Food and Drug Administration. Updated risk evaluation and mitigation strategy (REMS) to restrict access to rosiglitazone-containing medicines including Avandia, Avandamet, and Avandaryl. FDA Drug Safety Communication. Silver Spring, MD: FDA. (Internet at, www.fda.gov/Drugs/DrugSafety/ucm255005.htm; May 18, 2011).
[10] Staffa JA, Dal Pan GJ. Regulatory innovation in postmarketing risk assessment and management. Clin Pharmacol Ther 2012;91:555–7.
[11] Buckman S, Huang S-M, Murphy S. Medical product development and regulatory science for the 21st century: The critical path vision and its impact on health care. Clin Pharmacol Ther 2007;81:141–4.
[12] Barratt RA, Bowens SL, McCune SK, Johannessen JN, Buckman SY. The critical path initiative: Leveraging collaborations to enhance regulatory science. Clin Pharmacol Ther 2012;91:380–3.
[13] CDER. End-of-phase 2A meetings. Guidance for industry. Silver Spring, MD: FDA. (Internet at, www.fda.gov/downloads/Drugs/GuidanceComplianceRegulatoryInformation/Guidances/UCM079690.pdf; September 2009).
[14] MedWatch. The FDA medical products reporting program. Rockville, MD: FDA (Internet at, www.fda.gov/medwatch; 2005).
[15] FDA Drug Guidance Page, www.fda.gov/Drugs/GuidanceComplianceRegulatoryInformation/Guidances/default.htm.

[16] CDER, CBER. Formal meetings between the FDA and sponsors or applicants. Guidance for industry. Rockville, MD: FDA (Internet at, www.fda.gov/downloads/Drugs/GuidanceComplianceRegulatoryInformation/Guidances/UCM153222.pdf; May 2009).

[17] US Food and Drug Administration. FY. performance report to the president and congress for the prescription drug user fee act. FDA report. Rockville, MD: FDA (Internet at, www.fda.gov/downloads/AboutFDA/ReportsManualsForms/Reports/UserFeeReports/PerformanceReports/PDUFA/UCM243358.pdf; 2010).

[18] Prescription Drug User Fee Act of 1992. Public Law 102–571. In the US Code of Federal Regulations 21 CFR 379.106 Stat 4491; Oct 29, 1992.

[19] Genomics at the FDA website. (Internet at, www.fda.gov/drugs/scienceresearch/researchareas/pharmacogenetics/default.htm)

[20] Drug interaction website. (Internet at, www.fda.gov/Drugs/DevelopmentApprovalProcess/DevelopmentResources/DrugInteractionsLabeling/ucm080499.htm)

[21] Good guidance practices (Notice): The FDA's development, issuance, and use of guidance documents. Federal Register 62 FR 8961; February 17, 1977.

[22] Good guidance practices (Final Rule). Federal Register 65FR182; September 29, 2000.

[23] Food and Drug Cost of Administration Modernization Act of 1997. Public Law 105–115. In the US Code of Federal Regulations 21 CFR 355a.111 Stat 2296 (Internet at, www.fda.gov/dber/fdama.htm; Nov 21, 1997).

[24] FDA guidance page (Internet at, www.fda.gov/Drugs/GuidanceComplianceRegulatoryInformation/Guidances/default.htm).

[25] Milne CP, Kaitin KI. FDA review divisions: Performance levels, and the impact on drug sponsors. Clin Pharmacol Ther 2012;91:393–404.

[26] CDER, CBER. Good review management: Principles and practices for PDUFA products. Guidance for Review Staff and Industry. Rockville, MD: FDA (Internet at, www.fda.gov/downloads/Drugs/GuidanceComplianceRegulatoryInformation/Guidances/UCM079748.pdf; April 2005).

[27] CDER. Using the 21st century review process desk reference guide. Manual of policies and procedures. Silver Spring, MD: FDA. (Internet at, www.fda.gov/downloads/AboutFDA/CentersOffices/OfficeofMedicalProductsandTobacco/CDER/ManualofPoliciesProcedures/UCM233003.pdf; November 8, 2010).

[28] US Food and Drug Administration. FDA announces changes in Drug Center's oncology office. News Release. Silver Spring, MD: FDA. (Internet at, www.prnewswire.com/news-releases/fda-announces-changes-in-drug-centers-oncology-office-129654298.html; September 12, 2011).

[29] FDA Clinical Pharmacology Guidance Page. Internet at, www.fda.gov/Drugs/GuidanceComplianceRegulatoryInformation/Guidances/ucm064982.htm.

[30] CDER, CBER. CDRH, Pharmacogenomic data submissions. Guidance for Industry. Rockvillle, MD: FDA. (Internet at, www.fda.gov/cder/guidance/6400fnl.htm; March 2005).

[31] CDER, CBER CDRH. Clinical pharmacogenomics: Premarket evaluations in early phase clinical studies. Draft Guidance for Industry. Silver Spring, MD: FDA (Internet at, www.fda.gov/downloads/Drugs/GuidanceComplianceRegulatoryInformation/Guidances/UCM243702.pdf; February 2011).

[32] CDER. Guidance for industry. Bioavailability and bioequivalence studies for orally administered drug products – general considerations. Rockville, MD: FDA (Internet at, www.fda.gov/downloads/Drugs/GuidanceComplianceRegulatoryInformation/Guidances/UCM070124.pdf; March 2003).

[33] CDER. Guidance for industry. Waiver of *in vivo* bioavailability and bioequivalence studies for immediate-release solid oral dosage forms based on a biopharmaceutics classification system. Rockville, MD: FDA (Internet at, www.fda.gov/downloads/Drugs/GuidanceComplianceRegulatoryInformation/Guidances/UCM070246.pdf; 2000).

[34] The Biologics Price Competition and Innovation Act. (Internet at, http://dpc.senate.gov/healthreformbill/healthbill70.pdf.)

[35] Kozlowski S, Woodcock J, Midthun K, Sherman RB. Developing the nation's biosimilar program. N Engl J Med 2011;365:385–8.

[36] Public hearing on biosimilars. Minutes at, www.regulations.gov/ November 2–3, 2010.

[37] US Food and Drug Administration. March 17, 2010. FDA CDER Clinical Pharmacology Advisory Committee meeting. 2010 Meeting Materials, Pharmaceutical Science and Clinical Pharmacology Advisory Committee (Internet at, http://www.fda.gov/AdvisoryCommittees/CommitteesMeetingMaterials/Drugs/AdvisoryCommittforPharmaceuticalScienceandClinicalPharmacology/ucm201700.htm).

[38] US Food and Drug Administration. March 2, 2011. FDA CDER Clinical Pharmacology Advisory Committee meeting. 2011 Meeting Materials, Pharmaceutical Science and Clinical Pharmacology Advisory Committee (Internet at, www.fda.gov/AdvisoryCommittees/CommitteesMeetingMaterials/Drugs/AdvisoryCommitteeforPharmaceuticalScienceandClinicalPharmacology/ucm240583.htm).

[39] Bashaw ED, Huang S-M, Coté TR, Pariser AR, Garnett CE, Burckart G, et al. Clinical pharmacology as a cornerstone of orphan drug development. Nat Rev Drug Discov 2011;10:795–6.

[40] US Food and Drug Administration. Driving biomedical innovation: Initiatives to improve products for patients. FDA report. Rockville, MD: FDA (Internet at, www.fda.gov/AboutFDA/ReportsManualsForms/Reports/ucm274333.htm; October 2011).

[41] US Food and Drug Administration. Strategic priorities 2011–2015: Responding to the public health challenges of the 21st century. FDA report. Rockville, MD: FDA (Internet at, www.fda.gov/AboutFDA/ReportsManualsForms/Reports/ucm227527.htm updated; April 20, 2011).

[42] US Food and Drug Administration. Advancing regulatory science at FDA. Rockville, MD: FDA (Internet at, www.fda.gov/downloads/ScienceResearch/SpecialTopics/RegulatoryScience/UCM268225.pdf; August 2011).

[43] Eichler H-G, Oye K, Baird LG, Abadie E, Brown J, Drum CL, et al. Adaptive licensing: Taking the next step in the evolution of drug approval. Clin Pharmacol Ther 2012;91:426–37.

[44] Woodcock J. Evidence vs access: Can twenty-first century drug regulation refine the tradeoffs? Clin Pharmacol Ther 2012;91:378–80.

[45] Honig PK, Huang S-M. Regulatory science and the role of the regulator in biomedical innovation. Clin Pharmacol Ther 2012;91:347–52.

# I

# Abbreviated Tables of Laplace Transforms

**TABLE I.1  Table of Operations ($\mathscr{L}$)**

| Time domain | Laplace domain |
|---|---|
| $F(t)$ | $f(s) = \int_0^\infty F(t)e^{-st}dt$ |
| 1 | $1/s$ |
| $A$ | $A/s$ |
| $F'(t)$ | $sf(s) - F(0)$ |
| $F''(t)$ | $s^2f(s) - sF(0) - F'(0)$ |

**TABLE I.2  Table of Inverse Operations ($\mathscr{L}^{-1}$)**

| Laplace domain | | Time domain |
|---|---|---|
| $\dfrac{1}{s}$ | | 1 |
| $\dfrac{1}{s-a}$ | | $e^{at}$ |
| $\dfrac{1}{(s-a)^2}$ | | $te^{at}$ |
| $\dfrac{1}{s(s-a)}$ | | $\dfrac{1}{a}(e^{at} - 1)$ |
| $\dfrac{1}{(s-a)(s-b)}$ | $a \neq b$ | $\dfrac{1}{a-b}(e^{at} - e^{bt})$ |

# II

# Answers to Study Problems

**Arthur J. Atkinson, Jr.**

*Department of Molecular Pharmacology & Biochemistry, Feinberg School of Medicine,*
*Northwestern University, Chicago, IL 60611*

## ANSWERS TO STUDY PROBLEMS – CHAPTER 2

Note how dimensional analysis has been performed by including units in the calculations.

### Problem 1: Answer – E

$$V_d = \frac{\text{Dose}}{C_0} = \frac{80 \text{ mg}}{4 \text{ mg/L}} = 20 \text{ L}$$

### Problem 2: Answer – A

$$V_d = 2.0 \text{ L/kg} \cdot 80 \text{ kg} = 160 \text{ L}; \quad t_{1/2} = 3 \text{ h}$$

Therefore,

$$CL_E = \frac{\ln 2 \cdot V_d}{t_{1/2}} = \frac{\ln 2 \cdot 160 \text{ L}}{3 \text{ h}} = 37 \text{ L/h}$$

and the infusion rate should be

$$I = C_{ss} \cdot CL = 4 \text{ mg/L} \cdot 37 \text{ L/h} = 148 \text{ mg/h}$$
$$= 2.5 \text{ mg/min}$$

### Problem 3: Answer – C

The gentamicin plasma level fell to half of its previous value in the 5-hour interval between blood draws. Therefore, $t_{1/2} = 5 \text{ h}$ and $k = \ln 2/t_{1/2} = 0.139 \text{ h}^{-1}$

$$CF = \frac{1}{(1 - e^{-k\tau})}$$

Since $\tau = 8 \text{ h}$,

$$CF = \frac{1}{(1 - e^{-1.11})} = \frac{1}{0.67} = 1.49$$

Therefore, the expected steady state peak level is: $1.49 \cdot 10 \text{ μg/mL} = 15 \text{ μg/mL}$.

### Problem 4: Answer – C

The target level of $12 \text{ μg/mL}$ is one-half the toxic level of $24 \text{ μg/mL}$. Therefore, one should wait one half-life before restarting the aminophylline infusion.

$$t_{1/2} = \frac{0.693 \, V_d}{CL} \quad V_d = 60 \text{ kg} \cdot 0.45 \text{ L/kg} = 27 \text{ L}$$

$$CL = \frac{I}{C_{ss}} = \frac{(0.5 \text{ mg/kg} \cdot \text{h}) \cdot (60 \text{ kg})}{24 \text{ mg/L}} = 1.25 \text{ L/h}$$

Therefore,

$$t_{1/2} = \frac{0.693 \cdot 27 \text{ L}}{1.25 \text{ L/h}} = 15 \text{ h}$$

### Problem 5: Answer – D

Given that once-daily doses are administered, it requires 3.3 half-lives to reach 90% of the eventual steady-state level:

$$3.3 \cdot 7 \text{ days} = 23 \text{ days}$$

### Problem 6: Answer – B

On admission the digoxin plasma level was $3.2 \text{ ng/mL}$ and it fell to $2.7 \text{ ng/mL}$ 24 hours later.

Hence, the daily excretion fraction is $0.5/3.2 = 0.156$ (the excretion fraction with normal renal function $= 1/3$). Therefore, levels can be expected to fall by 0.156 every 24 hours as follows:

| Hospital day: | 0 | 1 | 2 | 3 | 4 |
|---|---|---|---|---|---|
| Digoxin level: | 3.2 ng/ mL | 2.7 ng/ mL | 2.28 ng/ mL | 1.92 ng/ mL | 1.62 ng/ mL |
| "More days": | — | — | 1 | 2 | 3 |

We can see that levels can be expected to reach the 1.6 ng/mL target on the fourth hospital day, or *3 more days after the level of 2.7 ng/mL was measured.*

## Problem 7: Answer – E

Three half-lives are needed for plasma levels to fall from 8 µg/mL to 1 µg/mL:

| Level: | 8 µg/mL | → | 4 µg/mL | → | 2 µg/mL | → | 1 µg/mL |
|---|---|---|---|---|---|---|---|
| Half-lives: | 0 | | 1 | | 2 | | 3 |

Since the elimination-phase half-life is given as 2 hours, three half-lives would require 6 hours. However, the question asks for a dosing interval that would allow peak levels *to exceed 8 µg/mL and fall below 1 µg/mL.* The only dosing interval offered that is longer than 6 hours is 8 hours. Currently, most patients would be treated with gentamicin by administering this drug in larger doses at a 24-hour interval (see Chapter 3).

## Problem 8: Answer – D

Since phenytoin is eliminated by Michaelis-Menten kinetics, Equation 2.6 applies:

$$Dose / \tau = \frac{V_{max}}{K_m + \overline{C}_{ss}} \cdot \overline{C}_{ss} \qquad (II.1)$$

Rearranging:

$$(Dose/\tau)K_m + (Dose/\tau)\overline{C}_{ss} = V_{max} \overline{C}_{ss}$$

Two simultaneous equations can be set up, one for the concentration measured at each previously administered dose.

$$300 \text{ mg/day} \cdot K_m + 300 \text{ mg/day} \cdot 5 \text{ µg/mL}$$
$$= 5 \text{ µg/mL} \cdot V_{max} \qquad (II.2)$$

$$600 \text{ mg/day} \cdot K_m + 600 \text{ mg/day} \cdot 30\text{µg/mL}$$
$$= 30\text{µg/mL} \cdot V_{max} \qquad (II.3)$$

These can be simplified to:

$$300 \text{ mg/day} \cdot K_m + 1500 \text{ mg}^2/ \text{L} \cdot \text{day}$$
$$= 5 \text{ mg/L} \cdot V_{max} \qquad (II.4)$$

$$600 \text{ mg/day} \cdot K_m + 18,000 \text{ mg}^2/ \text{L} \cdot \text{day}$$
$$= 30 \text{ mg/L} \cdot V_{max} \qquad (II.5)$$

By multiplying Equation II.4 by 2 and subtracting it from Equation II.5 we obtain:

$$15,000 \text{ mg}^2/ \text{L} \cdot \text{day} = 20 \text{ mg/L} \cdot V_{max}$$

Therefore,

$$V_{max} = 750 \text{ mg/day}$$

Substituting this value for $V_{max}$ into Equation II.4 yields:

$$300 \text{ mg/day} \cdot K_m + 1500 \text{ mg}^2/ \text{L} \cdot \text{day}$$
$$= 5 \text{ mg/L} \cdot 750 \text{ mg/day}$$

$$300 \text{ mg/day} \cdot K_m = 2250 \text{ mg}^2/ \text{L} \cdot \text{day}$$

$$K_m = 7.5 \text{ mg/ L}$$

We can now substitute these parameters into Equation II.1 to estimate the dose that will provide a phenytoin level of 15 µg/mL.

$$Dose/\tau = \frac{750 \text{ mg/day}}{7.5 \text{ mg/L} + 15.0 \text{ mg/L}} \cdot 15 \text{ mg/L}$$

$$Dose/\tau = 500 \text{ mg/day}$$

## ANSWERS TO STUDY PROBLEMS – CHAPTER 3

### Problem 1

We are given that $CF_{obs} = 1.29$ and $\tau = 12$ h. Since

$$k_{eff} = \frac{1}{\tau} \ln \left[ \frac{CF_{obs}}{CF_{obs} - 1} \right]$$

$$k_{eff} = \frac{1}{12} \ln \left[ \frac{1.29}{0.29} \right] = 0.124$$

Therefore,

$$t_{1/2\,\text{eff}} = \frac{\ln 2}{0.124} = 5.6\,\text{h}$$

## Problem 2

### Part a

Although a number of software packages are available to facilitate analysis of this type of data, most of them require the kineticist to provide initial estimates of the parameter values. The technique of "curve peeling" is widely used for this purpose, and also provides an initial evaluation of data quality.

The first step is to graph the experimental data (●) in a semilogarithmic plot of drug-concentration vs time as shown in Figure II.1. Then draw a line (beta line) through the terminal exponential phase and back-extrapolate it to the $y$-axis. Read the $y$-intercept ($B'$) and half-life of this line ($\beta_{t_{1/2}}$) from the graph. Next, as shown in Table II.1, obtain the difference (alpha values in the table) between the experimental data points lying above the back-extrapolated line and the corresponding values on the back-extrapolated beta line (beta values in the table) at each data time point.

The alpha values (○) are then plotted on the graph (Figure II.1) and are used to draw a second line (alpha line) from which the $y$-intercept ($A'$) and $\alpha_{t_{1/2}}$ are

**TABLE II.1    Results of Curve Peel**

| Time (h) | [Plasma] (μg/mL) | Beta value (μg/mL) | Alpha value (μg/mL) |
|---|---|---|---|
| 0.10 | 6.3 | 1.7 | 4.6 |
| 0.25 | 5.4 | 1.7 | 3.7 |
| 0.50 | 4.3 | 1.6 | 2.7 |
| 0.75 | 3.5 | 1.6 | 1.9 |
| 1.0 | 2.9 | 1.5 | 1.4 |
| 1.5 | 2.1 | 1.43 | 0.67 |
| 2.0 | 1.7 | 1.34 | 0.36 |
| 2.5 | 1.4 | 1.25 | 0.15 |

obtained. Criteria that can be used to assess data quality at this point are: (1) the number of points that lie on each of the exponential lines, and (2) the scatter of the points about the alpha and beta lines.

The values for $\alpha$ and $\beta$ are obtained from their half-life estimates as follows:

$$\alpha = \frac{\ln 2}{\alpha_{t_{1/2}}} = \frac{\ln 2}{0.5\,\text{h}} = 1.39\,\text{h}^{-1}$$

$$\beta = \frac{\ln 2}{\beta_{t_{1/2}}} = \frac{\ln 2}{5.3\,\text{h}} = 0.131\,\text{h}^{-1}$$

*Please Note:* Although it might seem easier to calculate $\alpha$ and $\beta$ directly from the graph as slopes, this is complicated by the fact that most semilogarithmic graph paper uses a $\log_{10}$ scale rather than a natural log scale on the $y$-axis. The best way to circumvent this difficulty is to calculate the values of $\alpha$ and $\beta$ from their respective half-lives.

The intercept values of $A' = 5.50\,\mu\text{g/mL}$ and $B' = 1.74\,\mu\text{g/mL}$ are normalized as follows:

$$A = \frac{A'}{A' + B'} = \frac{5.50}{5.50 + 1.74} = 0.76$$

$$B = \frac{B'}{A' + B'} = \frac{1.74}{5.50 + 1.74} = 0.24$$

As shown here, normalization is a technique for converting the sum of $A$ and $B$ to 1 and is required because we have stipulated that the administered dose is 1 in our derivation of the equations for calculating the model parameters.

### Part b

The parameters of the two-compartment model shown in Figure II.2 can be calculated as follows.

From Equation 3.11:

$$k_{01} = \frac{1}{A/\alpha + B/\beta} = \frac{1}{\dfrac{0.76}{1.39} + \dfrac{0.24}{0.131}} = 0.42\,\text{h}^{-1}$$

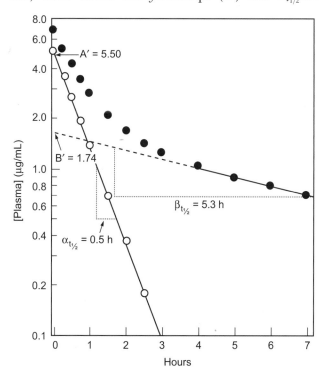

**FIGURE II.1**  Curve peel of the data (●) that are plotted on semilogarithmic coordinates. The points for the $\alpha$ curve (○) are obtained by subtracting back-extrapolated $\beta$ curve values from the experimental data, as shown in Table II.1.

The y-axis label reads [Plasma] (μg/mL) and x-axis label reads Hours. Annotations on the figure: A' = 5.50, B' = 1.74, $\beta_{t_{1/2}}$ = 5.3 h, $\alpha_{t_{1/2}}$ = 0.5 h.

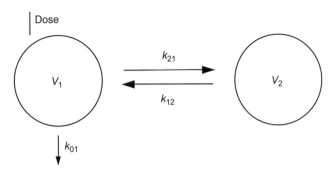

**FIGURE II.2** Diagram of the two-compartment model used to analyze the experimental data.

From Equation 3.14:

$$k_{12} = \beta A + \alpha \beta = (0.131)(0.76) + (1.39)(0.24)$$
$$= 0.43 \, h^{-1}$$

From Equation 3.15:

$$k_{21} = \frac{AB(\alpha - \beta)^2}{k_{12}} = \frac{(0.76)(0.24)(1.39 - 0.13)^2}{0.43}$$
$$= 0.67 \, h^{-1}$$

**Part c**

$$V_1 = \frac{Dose}{A' + B'} = \frac{100 \, mg}{(5.50 + 1.74) mg/L} = 13.8 \, L$$

The elimination clearance is:

$$CL_E = k_{01} \cdot V_1 = (0.42 \, h^{-1})(13.8 \, L) = 5.8 \, L/h$$

Similarly,

$$CL_I = k_{21} \cdot V_1 = (0.67 \, h^{-1})(13.8 \, L) = 9.25 \, L/h$$

**Part d**

$$V_2 = \frac{CL_I}{k_{12}} = \frac{9.25 \, L/h}{0.43 \, h^{-1}} = 21.5 \, L$$

$$V_{d(ss)} = V_1 + V_2 = 13.8 \, L + 21.5 \, L = 35.3 \, L$$

Compare this value with

$$V_{d(area)} = \frac{CL_E \cdot t_{1/2\beta}}{\ln 2} = \frac{5.8 \, L/h \cdot 5.3 \, h}{\ln 2} = 44 \, L$$

and

$$V_{d(extrap)} = \frac{Dose}{B'} = \frac{100 \, mg}{1.74 \, mg/L} = 57.5 \, L$$

The reason that $V_{d(ss)}$ is smaller than either of these two estimates is that neither the half-life equation used to calculate $V_{d(area)}$ nor the single compartment model implied in calculating $V_{d(extrap)}$ makes any provision for the contribution of intercompartmental clearance to the prolongation of the elimination-phase half-life. Therefore, these estimates must compensate for this by increasing the estimate of distribution volume, which in these approaches is the only way that half-life can be prolonged without affecting elimination clearance.

## ANSWERS TO STUDY PROBLEMS – CHAPTER 4

### Problem 1

**AUC after a single intravenous drug dose**

We have shown that after a single drug dose,

$$F \cdot D = CL \cdot AUC$$

When the dose is administered intravenously it is completely absorbed, so $F = 1$, and

$$AUC_{IV} = \frac{D_{IV}}{CL}$$

**$AUC_{0 \to \tau}$ after an oral dose at steady state**

The mean steady state concentration ($\overline{C}_{ss}$) with oral dosing is $\overline{C}_{ss} = \dfrac{F \cdot D_{oral}/\tau}{CL}$ where the dose ($D_{oral}$) divided by the dosing interval ($\tau$) is the dosing rate. As shown in Figure II.3, the area under the plasma-level vs time curve during a steady-state dosing interval is equivalent to the area of a rectangle whose height equals $\overline{C}_{ss}$ and whose base equals $\tau$. In other words,

$$AUC_{0 \to \tau \, (oral)} = \overline{C}_{ss} \cdot \tau$$

Substituting for $\overline{C}_{ss}$,

$$AUC_{0 \to \tau \, (oral)} = \frac{F \cdot D_{oral}/\tau}{CL} \cdot \tau = \frac{F \cdot D_{oral}}{CL}$$

Therefore, it can be seen by inspection that

$$\frac{AUC_{0 \to \tau \, (oral)}}{D_{oral}} = F \cdot \frac{AUC_{IV}}{D_{IV}}$$

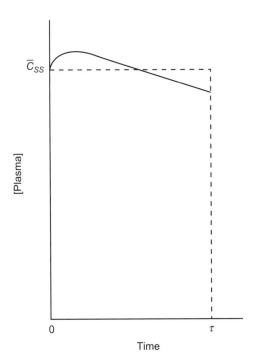

**FIGURE II.3** Diagram of a plasma-level vs time curve during a dosing interval at steady state. $\overline{C}_{ss}$ is the average plasma concentration during the dosing interval $\tau$. $AUC_{0-\tau}$ is equal to the area given by the product $\overline{C}_{ss} \cdot \tau$.

and that the extent of absorption of the oral dose formulation is

$$\% \text{ Absorption} = \frac{D_{IV} \cdot AUC_{0 \to \tau \, (oral)}}{D_{oral} \cdot AUC_{IV}} \times 100$$

## Problem 2

We are asked to obtain $X(t)$ from the convolution of $G(t)$ and the disposition function $H(t)$, where the input function $G(t)$ is a constant intravenous drug infusion:

$$X(t) = G(t) * H(t)$$

Since the operation of convolution in the time domain corresponds to multiplication in the domain of the subsidiary algebraic equation given by Laplace transformation, we can write the subsidiary equation as

$$x(s) = g(s) \cdot h(s)$$

The intravenous infusion provides a constant rate of drug appearance in plasma ($I$), so

$$G(t) = I$$

Since $\mathscr{L} \, 1 = 1/s$,

$$g(s) = \frac{I}{s}$$

We have shown previously (see derivation of Equation 4.3) that the Laplace transform of the disposition function is

$$h(s) = \frac{1}{s + k}$$

Therefore, the subsidiary equation for the output function is

$$x(s) = \frac{I}{s} \cdot \frac{1}{s + k}$$

and $\mathscr{L}^{-1} \, x(s)$ is

$$X(t) = \frac{I}{k} \, (1 - e^{-kt})$$

## Problem 3

### Part a

From the equation derived above for $X(t)$, we see that steady state is only reached when $t = \infty$. At infinite time

$$X_\infty = \frac{I}{k}$$

Since $C_{ss} = X_\infty / V_d$ and $k = CL_E / V_d$,

$$C_{ss} = \frac{I}{CL_E}$$

Note that this is Equation 2.2 that we presented in Chapter 2. In the problem that we are given, $I = 2 \, \text{mg/min}$, and $V_{d(area)} = 1.9 \, \text{L/kg} \cdot 70 \, \text{kg} = 133 \, \text{L}$. Therefore,

$$CL_E = \frac{\ln 2 \cdot V_{d(area)}}{t_{1/2}} = \frac{0.693 \cdot 133 \, \text{L}}{90 \, \text{min}} = 1.02 \, \text{L/min}$$

and

$$C_{ss} = \frac{2 \, \text{mg/min}}{1.02 \, \text{L/min}} = 2.0 \, \mu\text{g/mL}$$

*Note:* Many nurses who work in cardiac intensive care units know that the expected steady state lidocaine level in μg/mL simply equals the infusion rate in mg/min (usual therapeutic range: 2–5 μg/mL). Somewhat higher levels occur in patients with congestive heart failure or severe hepatic dysfunction.

### Part b

Since

$$X(t) = \frac{I}{k} \, (1 - e^{-kt})$$

When $t = \infty$,

$$X_\infty = \frac{I}{k}$$

Therefore, for any fraction of the eventual steady state,

$$X(t)/X_\infty = (1 - e^{-kt})$$

When 90% of the eventual steady state level is reached,

$$0.90 = (1 - e^{-kt_{0.90}})$$

$$e^{-kt_{0.90}} = 0.10$$

$$kt_{0.90} = \ln 10 = 2.30$$

Since

$$k = \frac{\ln 2}{90 \text{ min}} = 0.0077 \text{ min}^{-1}$$

it follows that

$$t_{0.90} = \frac{2.30}{0.0077 \text{ min}^{-1}} = 299 \text{ min}$$

*Note:* Because it takes so long for an infusion to provide stable therapeutic drug concentrations, lidocaine therapy of life-threatening cardiac arrhythmias is usually begun by administering an intravenous loading dose together with an infusion.

### Part c

Since $t_{1/2} = 90$ min, this corresponds to 3.3 half-lives. Note: This result for a continuous intravenous infusion was previously presented in Chapter 2.

## ANSWER TO STUDY PROBLEM – CHAPTER 5

### Part a

$t_{1/2} = 6.2$; $CL_E = 233$ mL/min $= 14.0$ L/hr;

% Renal excretion $= 85.5\%$.

$$CL_R = 0.855\, CL_E = 12.0 \text{ L/h}$$

$$CL_{NR} = 0.145\, CL_E = 2.03 \text{ L/h}$$

$$V_{d(area)} = \frac{CL_E \cdot t_{1/2}}{\ln 2} = \frac{(14.0 \text{ L/h})(6.2 \text{ h})}{\ln 2} = 125 \text{ L}$$

Therefore, if $CL_{NR}$ for $N$-acetylprocainamide (NAPA) is unchanged in functionally anephric patients, the expected elimination-phase half-life would be

$$t_{1/2} = \frac{(\ln 2)V_{d(area)}}{CL_{NR}} = \frac{(\ln 2)(125 \text{ L})}{2.03 \text{ L/h}} = 42.7 \text{ h}$$

*Note:* The mean NAPA elimination half life measured in six functionally anephric patients was 41.9 hours (Stec GP, Atkinson AJ Jr, Nevin MJ, Thenot J-P, Ruo TI, Gibson TP, Ivanovich P, del Greco F. $N$-Acetylprocainamide pharmacokinetics in functionally anephric patients before and after perturbation by hemodialysis. Clin Pharmacol Ther 1979;26:618–28).

### Part b

*From Figure II.4:*
when $CL_{CR} = 50$ mL/min, expected $CL_E = 8.0$ L/h

*By direct calculation:*
when $CL_{CR} = 50$ mL/min, $CL_R = (50/100)(12 \text{ L/h}) = 6.0$ L/h
since $CL_{NR} = 2.0$ L/h: $CL_E = CL_R + CL_{NR} = 8.0$ L/h

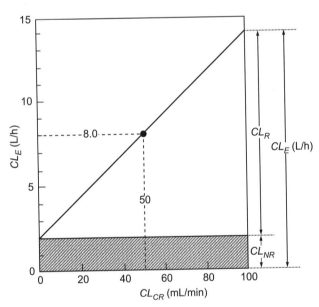

**FIGURE II.4** Nomogram for estimating $N$-acetylprocainamide (NAPA) elimination clearance in patients with impaired renal function. The hypothetical patient described in Part b of the problem has a creatinine clearance of 50 mL/min and would be expected to have a NAPA elimination clearance of 8.0 L/h.

### Part c

The 8-hour dosing interval is maintained.

Adjusted dose $= (8/14)(1\text{g}) = 0.57$ g

This would reduce fluctuation between peak and trough levels, but would be awkward if only 0.5-g tablets were available.

### Part d

The 1-g dose is maintained and the interval is adjusted. The usual 8-hour interval corresponds to: $8\,h/6.2\,h = 1.3$ half-lives when renal function is normal.

Expected half-life when $CL_{CR} = 50\,mL/min$:

$$t_{1/2} = \frac{(\ln 2)\,V_{d(area)}}{CL_E} = \frac{(\ln 2)(125\,L)}{8.0\,L/hr} = 10.8\,h$$

Adjusted dose interval $= (1.3)(10.8\,h) = 14\,h$.

In practice, a 12-hour dose interval would be selected to increase patient convenience.

# Subject Index